A
MODERN HERBAL

A
MODERN HERBAL

THE MEDICINAL, CULINARY, COSMETIC AND ECONOMIC
PROPERTIES, CULTIVATION AND FOLKLORE
OF HERBS, GRASSES, FUNGI, SHRUBS
AND TREES WITH ALL THEIR
MODERN SCIENTIFIC USES

By

MRS M. GRIEVE
F.R.H.S.

Edited and introduced by

MRS C. F. LEYEL

JONATHAN CAPE
THIRTY BEDFORD SQUARE LONDON

FIRST PUBLISHED 1931
REPRINTED 1974, 1975

JONATHAN CAPE LTD
30 BEDFORD SQUARE, LONDON WCI

ISBN O 224 00998 2

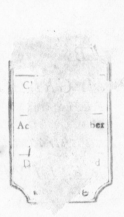

PRINTED IN GREAT BRITAIN BY
LOWE AND BRYDONE (PRINTERS) LTD
THETFORD, NORFOLK

LIST OF PLATES

Aconite (*Aconitum Napellus*), PLATE I — *Facing page* 6
Aloe (*Aloe Vulgaris*), PLATE II — 7
Almond (*Amygdalus Communis*), PLATE III — 40
Anise (*Pimpinella Anisum*), PLATE III — 40
Angelica (*Angelica Archangelica*), PLATE IV — 41
Apple, Bitter (Colocynth) (*Citrullus Colocynthis*), PLATE IV — 41
Angostura, True (*Cusparia Febrifuga*), PLATE V — 50
Arnica (*Arnica Montana*), PLATE V — 50
Arrach, Stinking (*Chenopodium Olidum*), PLATE VI — 51
Asafetida, Persian (*Ferula Persica*), PLATE VI — 51
Asarabacca (*Asarum Europæum*), PLATE VII — 78
Avens (*Geum Urbanum*), PLATE VII — 78
Balsam of Gilead (*Commiphora Opobalsamum*), PLATE VIII — 79
Balsam of Peru (*Myroxylon Pereiræ*), PLATE VIII — 79
Benzoin (*Styrax Benzoin*), PLATE IX — 102
Bindweed, Syrian (Scammony) (*Convolvulus Scammonia*), PLATE IX — 102
Bindweed, Greater (Convolvulus) (*Convolvulus Sepium*), PLATE X — 103
Bindweed, Jalap (*Convolvulus Jalapa*), PLATE X — 103
Bladderwrack (*Fucus Vesiculosis*), PLATE XI — 112
Bistort (*Polygonum Bistorta*), PLATE XII — 113
Bogbean (*Menyanthes Trifoliata*), PLATE XII — 113
Broom (*Cytisus Scoparius*), PLATE XIII — 134
Bryony, European White (*Bryonia Alba*), PLATE XIII — 134
Buchu (*Barosma Betulina*), PLATE XIV — 135
Buckthorn, Alder (*Rhamnus Frangula*), PLATE XIV — 135
Cajuput (*Melaleuca Leucadendron*), PLATE XV — 152
Calumba (*Jateorhiza Calumba*), PLATE XVI — 153
Cabbage Tree (*Andira Inermis*), PLATE XVII — 156
Camphor (*Cinnamonum Camphora*), PLATE XVII — 156
Cardamom (*Elettaria Cardamomum*), PLATE XVIII — 157
Caraway (*Carum Carvi*), PLATE XIX — 162
Carrot (*Daucus Carota*), PLATE XIX — 162
Cascarilla (*Croton Eleuteria*), PLATE XX — 163
Castor Oil Plant (*Ricinus Communis*), PLATE XX — 163
Catechu, Black (*Acacia Catechu*), PLATE XXI — 178
Cayenne (*Capsicum Minimum*), PLATE XXI — 178

Celandine, Greater (*Chelidonium Majus*), PLATE XXII   *Facing page* 179

Centaury (*Erythræa Centaurium*), PLATE XXII   179

Chamomile, Common (*Anthemis Nobilis*), PLATE XXIII   192

Chestnut, Horse (*Æsculus Hippocastanum*), PLATE XXIII   192

Cinnamon (*Cinnamonum Zeylanicum*), PLATE XXIV   193

Cinnamon, White (Canella) (*Canella Alba*), PLATE XXIV   193

Cloves (*Eugenia Caryophyllata*), PLATE XXV   208

Coffee (*Coffea Arabica*), PLATE XXV   208

Coltsfoot (*Tussilago Farfara*), PLATE XXVI   209

Contrayerva (*Dorstenia Contrayerva*), PLATE XXVII   218

Copaiba (*Copaifera Langsdorffii*), PLATE XXVII   218

Coriander (*Coriandrum Sativum*), PLATE XXVIII   219

Cowhage (*Mucuna Pruriens*), PLATE XXIX   234

Croton Tree (*Croton Tiglium*), PLATE XXIX   234

Crowfoot, Upright Meadow, and Lesser Spearwort (*Ranunculus Acris* and *Ranunculus Flammula*), PLATE XXX   235

Cubebs (*Piper Cubeba*), PLATE XXXI   238

Cuckoo-Pint (*Arum Maculatum*), PLATE XXXII   239

Cucumber, Squirting (*Echallium Elaterium*), PLATE XXXIII   256

Dandelion (*Taraxacum Officinale*), PLATE XXXIV   257

Dill (*Peucedanum Graveolens*), PLATE XXXIV   257

Dropwort, Hemlock Water (*Œnanthe Crocata*), PLATE XXXV   264

Dropwort, Water (*Œnanthe Phellandrium*), PLATE XXXV   264

Elder (*Sambucus Nigra*), PLATE XXXVI   265

Elecampane (*Inula Helenium*), PLATE XXXVII   278

Flax – Linseed and Mountain Flax (*Linum Usitatissimum* and *Linum Catharticum*), PLATE XXXVIII   279

Foxglove (*Digitalis Purpurea*), PLATE XXXIX   326

Frankincense (*Boswellia Thurifera*), PLATE XXXIX   326

Fungi (*Agaricus Bulbosus*), PLATE XL   327

Fungi (*Agaricus Semiglobatus*), PLATE XL   327

Fungi (*Amanita Muscaria, Var.*), PLATE XLI   334

Fungi (Fly Agaric) (*Amanita Muscaria*), PLATE XLI   334

Fungi – Ergot of Rye (*Claviceps Purpurea*), PLATE XLII   335

Gamboge (*Garcinia Hanburyii*), PLATE XLIII   342

Garlic (*Allium Sativum*), PLATE XLIII   342

Gentian (*Gentiana Lutea*), PLATE XLIV   343

Ginger (*Zingiber Officinale*), PLATE XLV   362

Grass, Darnel (*Lolium Temulentum*), PLATE XLVI   363

Golden Rod (*Solidago Virgaurea*), PLATE XLVI   363

Guaiacum (*Guaiacum Officinale*), PLATE XLVII   380

Hellebore, Black (*Helleborus Niger*), PLATE XLVIII   *Facing page* 381

Hellebore, White (*Veratrum Album*), PLATE XLVIII   381

Hellebore, (Black) Stinking (English Bearsfoot) (*Helleborus Fœtidus*), PLATE XLIX   390

Hellebore, (White) Oriental (*Helleborus Orientalis*), PLATE XLIX   390

Hemlock (*Conium Maculatum*), PLATE L   391

Hemlock, Water (Cowbane) (*Cicuta Virosa*), PLATE L   391

Henbane (*Hyoscyamus Niger*), PLATE LI   406

Holly, Sea (*Eryngium Campestre*), PLATE LI   406

Horehound, White (*Marrubium Vulgare*), PLATE LII   407

Horseradish (*Cochlearia Armoracia*), PLATE LII   407

Hyssop, Hedge (*Gratiola Officinalis*), PLATE LIII   436

Ipecacuanha (*Psychotria Ipecacuanha*), PLATE LIII   436

Iris, Florentine (*Iris Florentina*), PLATE LIV   437

Ivy, Poison (*Rhus Toxicodendron*), PLATE LIV   437

Juniper (*Juniperus Communis*), PLATE LV   464

Kino, African (*Pterocarpus Marsupium*), PLATE LV   464

Laurel, Cherry (*Prunus Laurocerasus*), PLATE LVI   465

Laurel (*Laurus Nobilis*), PLATE LVI   465

Lavender, Spike (*Lavandula Spica*), PLATE LVII   474

Lemon (*Citrus Limonum*), PLATE LVII   474

Lettuce, Wild (*Lactuca Virosa*), PLATE LVIII   475

Liquorice (*Glycyrrhiza Glabra*), PLATE LVIII   475

Loosestrife, Purple (*Lythrum Salicaria*), PLATE LIX   522

Mallow, Marsh (*Althæa Officinalis*), PLATE LIX   522

Marjoram, Wild (*Origanum Vulgare*), PLATE LX   523

Mastic (*Pistacia Lentiscus*), PLATE LX   523

Mercury, Dog's (*Mercurialis Perennis*), PLATE LXI   530

Mezereon (*Daphne Mezereum*), PLATE LXI   530

Mints (*Mentha Viridis, Mentha Pulegium, Mentha Piperita*), PLATE LXII   531

Moss, Iceland (*Cetraria Islandica*), PLATE LXIII   552

Mustards, Black and White (*Brassica Nigra* and *Brassica Alba*), PLATE LXIII   552

Nightshade, Deadly (Belladonna) (*Atropa Belladonna*), PLATE LXIV   553

Nightshade, Woody (Bittersweet) (*Solanum Dulcamara*), PLATE LXIV   553

Nutmeg (*Myristica Fragans*), PLATE LXV   592

Nux Vomica (*Strychnos Nux-Vomica*), PLATE LXVI   593

Oak Galls (*Quercus Infectoria*), PLATE LXVI   593

Olive (*Olea Europœa*), PLATE LXVII   598

Orange, Sweet (*Citrus Aurantium*), PLATE LXVII   598

Opoponax (*Opoponax Chironium*), PLATE LXVIII   *Facing page* 599
Parsley, Fools' (*Æthusa Cynapium*), PLATE LXVIII   599
Paris, Herb (*Paris Quadrifolia*), PLATE LXIX   628
Pepper, Black (*Piper Nigrum*), PLATE LXIX   628
Paradise, Grains of (Hungarian Pepper) (*Amomum Melegueta*), PLATE
    LXX   629
Peruvian Bark (*Cinchona Succirubra*), PLATE LXX   629
Pellitory (*Anacyclus Pyrethrum*), PLATE LXXI   636
Pimpernel, Scarlet (*Anagallis Arvensis*), PLATE LXXI   636
Pine, Larch (*Pinus Larix*), PLATE LXXII   637
Pine, Wild (*Pinus Sylvestris*), PLATE LXXII   637
Pink Root (*Spigelia Marilandica*), PLATE LXXIII   652
Pomegranate (*Punica Granatum*), PLATE LXXIII   652
Poppy, White (*Papaver Somniferum*), PLATE LXXIV   653
Quassia (*Picræna Excelsa*), PLATE LXXV   662
Rhatany, Peruvian (*Krameria Triandra*), PLATE LXXVI   663
Rhododendron, Yellow (*Rhododendron Chrysanthum*), PLATE LXXVII   676
Rhubarb, East Indian (*Rheum Palmatum*), PLATE LXXVII   676
Rhubarb, French (*Rheum Undulatum*), PLATE LXXVIII   677
Rosemary (*Rosmarinus Officinalis*), PLATE LXXIX   698
Rue (*Ruta Graveolens*), PLATE LXXIX   698
Saffron (*Crocus Sativus*), PLATE LXXX   699
Saffron, Meadow (*Colchicum Autumnale*), PLATE LXXX   699
Sarsaparilla, Jamaica (*Smilax Ornata*), PLATE LXXXI   714
Sassafras (*Sassafras Officinale*), PLATE LXXXI   714
Sedge, Sweet (*Acorus Calamus*), PLATE LXXXII   715
Senna (*Cassia Acutifolia*), PLATE LXXXIII   734
Senega (*Polygala Senega*), PLATE LXXXIV   735
Simaruba (*Simaruba Amara*), PLATE LXXXIV   735
Snakeroot (*Aristolochia Serpentaria*), PLATE LXXXV   766
Spurge (Euphorbium) (*Euphorbia Resinifera*), PLATE LXXXVI   767
Squill (*Urginea Scilla*), PLATE LXXXVI   767
Stavesacre (*Delphinium Staphisagria*), PLATE LXXXVII   776
Storax (*Liquidambar Orientalis*), PLATE LXXXVII   776
Tamarind (*Tamarindus Indica*), PLATE LXXXVIII   777
Tansy (*Tanacetum Vulgare*), PLATE LXXXVIII   777
Thistle, Holy (*Carbenia Benedicta*), PLATE LXXXIX   796
Thornapple (*Datura Stramonium*), PLATE XC   797
Tobacco (*Nicotiana Tabacum*), PLATE XC   797
Tormentil (*Potentilla Tormentilla*), PLATE XCI   818
Wood Sorrel (*Oxalis Acetosella*), PLATE XCI   818

Tragacanth (*Astragalus Gummifer*), PLATE XCII   *Facing page* 819

Bearberry (Uva-Ursi) (*Arbutus Uva-Ursi*), PLATE XCII   819

Valerian, Common (*Valeriana Officinalis*), PLATE XCIII   850

Willow (*Salix Russeliana*), PLATE XCIII   850

Wintergreen (*Chimophila Umbellata*), PLATE XCIV   851

Winter's Bark (*Drimys Winteri*), PLATE XCIV   851

Wormseed, Levant, and Levant Wormwood (*Artemisia Cina* and *Artemisia Absinthium*), PLATE XCV   858

Zedoary (*Curcuma Zedoaria*), PLATE XCVI   859

BIBLIOGRAPHICAL NOTE

I T is impossible to give a complete list of the works consulted for reference in the compiling of this HERBAL.

Mrs. Grieve has of course drawn her knowledge from books as well as from plants.

As Editor I have confirmed her facts with those in Bentley and Trimen's *Medicinal Plants* in four volumes, Clarke's *Dictionary of Materia Medica* in three volumes, and Potter's *Cyclopædia of Botanical Drugs and Preparations*.

I have also consulted Anne Pratt's *Flowering Plants of Great Britain* in four volumes, Stephenson and Churchill's *Medical Botany* in three volumes, Dr. Fernie's *Herbal Simples*, Rhind's *History of the Vegetable Kingdom*, and the English and French official Pharmacopœias.

HILDA LEYEL

EDITOR'S INTRODUCTION

Botany and medicine came down the ages hand in hand until the seventeenth century; then both arts became scientific, their ways parted, and no new herbals were compiled. The botanical books ignored the medicinal properties of plants and the medical books contained no plant lore.

The essence of a herbal was the combination of traditional plant lore, the medicinal properties of the herbs, and their botanical classification. From the time of Dioscorides down to Parkinson in 1629 this herbal tradition was unbroken. Culpeper's popular herbal was discredited with scientific people because it was astrological.

The death of the herbal was one of the reasons why, with a few exceptions, the only plants which have retained their place in the Allopaths' pharmacopœias are poisonous ones like Aconite, Belladonna, Henbane and the Opium Poppy.

Dandelion, Gentian and Valerian for some reason have survived and the Homeopaths use many more, but such useful plants as Agrimony, Slippery Elm, Horehound, Bistort, Poplar, Bur Marigold, Wood Betony, Wood Sanicle, Wild Carrot, Raspberry leaves, and the Sarsaparillas are now only used by Herbalists.

All serious Herbalists have long realized that a new Herbal is badly needed – a herbal which must include the traditional lore and properties of plants, and the modern use of properly standardized extracts and tinctures which were unknown in the days of Gerard and Parkinson, and even in the days of Culpeper, and which have been made possible by the development of modern chemistry.

The interest for the amateur can only be an historical one, because the herbal tinctures and extracts are too potent to be prescribed or experimented with by the unskilled or the inexperienced; in fact, it is as dangerous for amateurs to doctor themselves indiscriminately with herbs, as it would be for them to administer drugs in their alkaloid form.

A knowledge of herbs is as necessary as a knowledge of Pathology, if herbal treatment for all but the simplest ailments is to be successful.

Each herb has its own indications for use, and successful prescribing depends upon the correspondence between these indications and the patient's symptoms. Then, and only then, will the result be altogether successful.

Most of the modern scientific work on the right use of herbs we owe to Hahnemann and his successors.

★

That famous head master, Edward Thring, first taught me botany when I was a baby, in the School House garden and Uppingham fields. I still remember the pride I felt when he strapped the black japanned tin lined with green to my tiny back, and though at the time I was only four and much too young to enjoy searching in the heat for rare plants like Ladies' Tresses and Green Hellebore, the names of the plants, like the dates of the English kings, were impressed upon my mind so vividly that it has been impossible for me ever to forget them.

After Edward Thring's death, his daughter Sarah carried on my lessons, and I have never lost touch with the subject.

At one time there was an idea of my entering the medical profession, but I was put off by my first lesson in dissection.

I have always experimented in the innocent alchemy of scent blending and cooking, but it was not until I had written my first book on herbs that the idea came to me to found the Society of Herbalists, and since 1926 I have done nothing else but research work in herbal medicine.

Just before I opened Culpeper House, a list of Mrs. Grieve's monographs on herbs came to me through the post. I made her acquaintance, and after examining the pamphlets, thought they might be the nucleus of the much-needed modern herbal.

I took the monographs and the suggestion to Mr. Cape, who agreed to publish them if I would collate and edit them and see that the American herbs were also included.

Mrs. Grieve's original pamphlets only included the English herbs, many of which she grew in her Buckinghamshire garden.

During the War, when there was a shortage of medicinal plants because they could no longer be imported from abroad, Mrs. Grieve made practical use of her knowledge and trained pupils in the work of drying and preparing herbs for the chemists' market.

She did a great deal to revive the herb industry in England.

The arrangement and the editing of the vast quantity of material which Mrs. Grieve had accumulated has been a task of some difficulty. I have arranged the plants alphabetically under their most familiar names, hoping to interest flower-lovers as well as doctors, and in this way they are as easily found as the words in a dictionary. The country names are in the index.

This is not the orthodox arrangement either from the Herbalist's, or the Homeopath's, or the Allopath's, point of view.

Herbalists talk about Jalap and Black Haw, but to the uninitiated Bindweed and Guelder Rose are far more familiar, and it is under these names that they will be found in this herbal.

In homeopathy the Anemone and the Forget-me-not are known as Pulsatilla and Myosotis, and chemists accustomed to the Latin names may be shocked to find Taraxacum under Dandelion, Podophyllum under Mandrake, and Calendula under Marigold.

The very names of the plants are so interesting; the names are often derived from their original use in medicine, and the traditional use has been derived from some peculiarity of the plant based on the doctrine of signatures, its shape, growth, colour, scent or taste, or habitat.

For instance, the flower of the Scullcap, one of the best cures for insomnia, has a strong resemblance to the shape of the human skull. The Yellow Cedar has a curious sinister appearance and is used to cure fungoid growths. The little blue flower of the Eyebright with its yellow centre suggests the human eye, and is so useful for tired eyes that the French have called it 'casse lunettes.'

The flowers of many of the herbs which purify the blood are red in colour, e.g. the Scarlet Pimpernel, the Burdock, the Red Clover.

The medicinal value of Nettles is indicated by their sting; they are used internally to stimulate the circulation.

When a plant has a particularly unpleasant smell like the stinking Arrach, it usually points to a particular use – the stinking Arrach is used for foul ulcers.

The bark of the Willow cures rheumatism brought on by damp, and the tree grows in wet places.

Most of the flowers used for jaundice are yellow, like the Dandelion, Agrimony, Celandine, Hawkweed and Marigold.

Viper's Buglass is considered an antidote to snake-bite, and its seed is not unlike the reptile's head.

Lungwort, because of its spotted leaves, was used for diseased lungs.

The classical names often embody the tradition which goes

back to legendary times. For instance, Bellis Perennis chronicles the wound-healing properties of the Daisy. Tussilago Farfara is the botanical name for the Coltsfoot, which is used to cure coughs and colds, and Valerian is derived from the Latin word *Valere*.

Surely it makes a garden more romantic and wonderful to know that Wallflowers, Irises, Lupins, Delphiniums, Columbines, Dahlias and Chrysanthemums, every flower in the garden from the first Snowdrop to the Christmas Rose, are not only there for man's pleasure but have their compassionate use in his pain.

HILDA LEYEL

A
MODERN HERBAL

VOLUME I

ABSCESS ROOT

Polemonium reptans (LINN.)
N.O. Polemoniaceæ

Synonyms. American Greek Valerian. Blue Bells. False Jacob's Ladder. Sweatroot
Part Used. Root
Habitat. United States

¶ *Description.* This plant grows from New York to Wisconsin, in woods, damp grounds, and along shady river-banks. It has creeping roots, by which it multiplies very quickly. The stems are 9 to 10 inches high, much branched, bearing pinnate leaves with six or seven pairs of leaflets. The nodding, blue flowers are in loose, terminal bunches.

The slender rootstock, when dried and used as the drug, is 1 to 2 inches long and $\frac{1}{8}$ inch in diameter, with the bases of numerous stems on the upper surface, and tufts of pale, slender, smooth, wiry, brittle roots on the underside. The rootstock has a slightly bitter and acrid taste.

¶ *Medicinal Action and Uses.* Astringent, alterative, diaphoretic, expectorant. The drug has been recommended for use in febrile and inflammatory cases, all scrofulous diseases, in bowel complaints requiring an astringent, for the bites of venomous snakes and insects, for bronchitis and laryngitis, and whenever an alterative is required. It is reported to have cured consumption; an infusion of the root in wineglassful doses is useful in coughs, colds and all lung complaints, producing copious perspiration.

The tincture of the root is made of whisky.

¶ *Dosage.* 1 to 2 fluid ounces, two or three times a day.

ACACIAS

N.O. Leguminosæ

Acacias (nat. order, Leguminosæ) are composed of handsome trees and shrubby bushes scattered over the warmer regions of the globe. The flowers are arranged in rounded or elongated clusters, the leaves generally compoundly pinnate, i.e. divided into leaflets up to the mid-rib and each leaflet similarly cut into narrow segments.

In several of the Australian species the leaflets are suppressed and the leaf stalks, vertically flattened, serve the purpose of leaves. Some species afford valuable timber: the black wood of Australia, which is used for furniture because it takes such a high polish, is the wood of the *A. melanoxylon.* The bark of another Australian species, known as Wattles, is rich in tannin and forms a valuable article of export. The pods of other species are employed in Egypt and Nubia for their tannin. The pods of the *A. Concuine* are used by Indian women in the same way as the soapnut for washing the head; and the leaves of the same tree are employed in cookery for their acidity.

Certain tribes on the Amazon use the seeds of another species, the *Acacia Niopo,* for snuff combined with lime and cocculus. Various species of acacia yield gum; but the best gum arabic used in medicine is an exudation from the *A. Senegal.* This species grows abundantly in East and West tropical Africa, forming forests in Senegambia north of the River Senegal. Most of the gum acacia collected in Upper Egypt and the Sudan is produced by the *A. verek,* and is known locally as Hachah.

ACACIA BARK

Acacia decurrens
Acacia arabica
N.O. Leguminosæ

Synonym. Wattle Bark

Acacia Bark, known as Wattle Bark, is obtained from the chief of the Australian Wattles, *A. decurrens* (Willd.), the Black Wattle, and, more recently, *A. arabica* has been similarly used in East Africa for its astringency.

The bark is collected from wild or cultivated trees, seven years old or more, and must be allowed to mature for a year before being used medicinally.

¶ *Description.* The bark of *A. decurrens* is usually in curved pieces, externally greyish brown, darkening with age, often with irregular longitudinal ridges and sometimes transverse cracks. Inner surface longitudinally striated, fracture irregular and coarsely fibrous. It has a slight tan-like odour and astringent taste.

The bark of *A. arabica* is hard and woody, rusty brown and tending to divide into several layers. The outer surface of older pieces is covered with thick blackish periderm, rugged and fissured. The inner surface is red, longitudinally striated and fibrous. Taste, astringent and mucilaginous.

¶ *Constituents*. Acacia Bark contains from 24 to 42 per cent. of tannin and also gallic acid. Its powerful astringency causes it to be extensively employed in tanning.

¶ *Medicinal Action and Uses*. Medicinally it is employed as a substitute for Oak Bark. It has special use in diarrhœa, mainly in the form of a decoction, the British Pharmacopœia preparation being 6 parts in 100, administered in doses of $\frac{1}{2}$ to 2 fluid ounces.

ACACIA CATECHU. See CATECHU

ACACIA (FALSE)

Synonym. Locust Tree

In common language, the term Acacia is often applied to species of the genus *Robinia*, which also belongs to the family *Leguminosæ*, though to a different section.

R. pseudacacia, the False Acacia or Locust Tree, one of the most valuable timber trees of the American forest, where it grows to a very large size, was one of the first trees introduced into England from America, and is cultivated as an ornamental tree in the milder parts of Britain, forming a large tree, with beautiful pea-like blossoms.

The timber is supposed to unite the qualities of strength and durability to a degree unknown in any other kind of tree, being very hard and close-grained. It has been extensively used for ship-building, being superior for the purpose to American Oak, and is largely used in the construction of the wooden pins called *trenails*, used to fasten the planks to the ribs or timber of ships. Instead of decaying, it acquires an extraordinary degree of hardness with time. It is also suitable for posts and fencing and other purposes where durability in contact with the ground is essential, and is used for axle-trees and other mechanical purposes, though not for general purposes of construction.

The roots and inner bark have a sweetish,

ACACIA (GUM)

Part Used. Gummy Exudation from stem

ACACIA NILOTICA (LINN.)

All the gum-yielding Acacias exhibit the same habit and general appearance, differing only in technical characters. They are spiny shrubs or small trees, preferring sandy or sterile regions, with the climate dry during the greater part of the year.

The gum harvest from the various species lasts about five weeks. About the middle of November, after the rainy season, it exudes spontaneously from the trunk and principal

The decoction also is used as an astringent gargle, lotion, or injection.

A liquid extract is prepared from the bark of *A. arabica*, administered in India for its astringent properties in doses of $\frac{1}{2}$ to 1 fluid drachm, but the use of both gum and bark for industrial purposes is much larger than their use in medicine. The bark, under the name of *Babul*, is used in Scinde for tanning, and also for dyeing various shades of brown.

Robinia pseudacacia
N.O. Leguminosæ

but somewhat offensive and nauseating taste, and have been found poisonous to foraging animals.

¶ *Medicinal Action and Uses*. The inner bark contains a poisonous proteid substance, *Robin*, which possesses strong emetic and purgative properties. It is capable of coagulating the casein of milk and of clotting the red corpuscles of certain animals.

Tonic, emetic and purgative properties have been ascribed to the root and bark, but the locust tree is rarely, if ever, prescribed as a therapeutic agent.

Occasional cases of poisoning are on record in which boys have chewed the bark and swallowed the juice: the principal symptoms being dryness of the throat, burning pain in the abdomen, dilatation of the pupils, vertigo and muscular twitches; excessive quantities causing also weak and irregular heart action. Though the leaves of *Robinia* have also been stated to produce poisonous effects, careful examination has failed to detect the presence of any soluble proteid or of alkaloids, and by some the leaves have been recorded as even affording wholesome food for cattle.

The flowers contain a glucoside, *Robinin*, which, on being boiled with acids, is resolved into sugar and quercetin.

Acacia Senegal (WILLD.)
Acacia nilotica (LINN.)
N.O. Leguminosæ

branches, but the flow is generally stimulated by incisions in the bark, a thin strip, 2 to 3 feet in length and 1 to 3 inches wide being torn off. In about fifteen days it thickens in the furrow down which it runs, hardening on exposure to the air, usually in the form of round or oval tears, about the size of a pigeon's egg, but sometimes in vermicular forms, white or red, according to whether the species is a white or red gum tree.

About the middle of December, the Moors

commence the harvesting. The masses of gum are collected, either while adhering to the bark, or after it falls to the ground, the entire product, often of various species, thus collected, is packed in baskets and very large sacks of tanned leather and brought on camels and bullocks to the centres of accumulation and then to the points of export, chiefly Suakin, Alexandria, or – in Senegambia – St. Louis. It is then known as 'Acacia sorts,' the term being equivalent to 'unassorted Acacia.' The unsorted gums show the widest variation as to size of fragments, whiteness, clearness, freedom from adhering matter, etc. It is next sorted or 'picked' in accordance with these differences.

There are many kinds of Acacia Gum in commerce:

KORDOFAN GUM, collected in Upper Egypt and the Sudan, in Kordofan, Dafur and Arabia, and exported from Alexandria, is considered the best and is the kind generally used in pharmacy. It consists of small, irregular pieces, commonly whitish, or slightly tinged with yellow, and is freer from impurities than most other commercial varieties. But those known in commerce as 'Turkey sorts' and 'Trieste picked,' which are brought from the Sudan by way of Suakin, are equally suitable for medicinal use.

SENEGAL GUM, of two varieties, produced by two different trees, one yielding a white, the other a red gum, is usually in roundish or oval unbroken pieces of various sizes, larger than those of Turkey Gum, less brittle and pulverizable, less fissured and often occurs in long, cylindrical or curved pieces.

The term 'Gum Senegal' is not, strictly speaking, synonymous with Gum Acacia, though it is commonly so used. Gum Acacia is the name originally pertaining to Sudan, Kordofan or Egyptian (hashabi) Gum, which possesses properties rendering it superior and always preferred to any other known to commerce. During the political and military disturbances in Egypt between 1880 and 1890, this gum became so nearly unobtainable that occasional packages only were seen in the market. Among the many substitutes then offered, the best was Gum Senegal, which was adopted as the official equivalent of Gum Acacia. In this way, it came about that the names were regarded as synonymous. In 1890, the original Acacia again came into the market and eventually became as abundant as ever, but it is no longer possible to entirely separate the two names. Most of the characteristically distinct grades of Acacia Gum are now referred to particular species of the genus Acacia. Most works state that both the Kordofan and Senegal Gums are products of

A. Senegal (Willd.), the range of which is thus given as Senegambia in West Africa, the Upper Nile region in Eastern Africa, with more or less of the intervening central region.

A. glaucophylla (Staud.) and *A. Abyssinica* (Hochst.) are said to yield an equally good gum, but little of it is believed to reach the market.

Mogadore Gum, from *A. gummifera* (Willd), a tall tree found in Morocco and in the Isle of Bourbon, occurs in rather large pieces, closely resembling Kordofan Gum in appearance.

Indian Gum, the product of *A. arabica*, the Gum Arabic tree of India. The gum of this and other Indian species of Acacia is there used as a substitute for the official Gum Acacia, to which it is, however, inferior. Indian Gum is sweeter in taste than that of the other varieties, and usually contains portions of a different kind of gum.

Cape Gum is also imported. It is of a pale yellow colour and is considered of inferior quality.

Australian Gum, imported from South Australia, is in elongated or globular pieces, rough and even wrinkled on the surface and of a violet tint, which distinguishes it from other varieties. It is not entirely soluble in water, to which it imparts less viscidity than ordinary Gum Acacia. It frequently contains tannin.

Gum Acacia for *medicinal* purposes should be in roundish 'tears' of various sizes, colourless or pale yellow, or broken into angular fragments with a glass-like, sometimes iridescent fracture, often opaque from numerous fissures, but transparent and nearly colourless in thin pieces; taste insipid, mucilaginous; nearly inodorous. It should be almost entirely soluble in water, forming a viscid, neutral solution, or mucilage, which, when evaporated, yields the gum unchanged. It is insoluble in alcohol and ether, but soluble in diluted alcohol in proportion to the amount of water present. It should be slowly but completely soluble in two parts of water: this solution shows an acid reaction with litmus-paper. The powdered gum is not coloured blue (indicating absence of starch) or red (indicating absence of dextrin) by the iodine test solution. It should not yield more than 4 per cent. of ash.

¶ *Adulteration.* Adulteration in the crude state is confined almost wholly to the addition of similar and inferior gums, the detection of which requires only familiarity with the genuine article.

In the ground condition, it is adulterated oftenest with starch and dextrins, tests for which are given in the official description.

Tannin is present in inferior gums and can be detected by the bluish-black coloration produced on adding ferric chloride. Gums of a yellow or brown colour usually contain tannin, and these, together with such as are incompletely soluble in water and which yield ropy or glairy solutions, should not be used for medicinal purposes.

¶ *Chemical Constituents.* Gum Acacia consists principally of *Arabin*, a compound of Arabic acid with calcium, varying amounts of the magnesium and potassium salts of the same acid being present. It is believed, also, that small amounts of other salts of these bases occur. (Arabic acid can be obtained by precipitating with alcohol from a solution of Acacia acidulated with hydrochloric acid.) The gum also contains 12 to 17 per cent. of moisture and a trace of sugar, and yields 2·7 to 4 per cent. of ash, consisting almost entirely of calcium, magnesium and potassium carbonates.

¶ *Medicinal Action and Uses.* Gum Acacia is a demulcent and serves by the viscidity of ·its solution to cover and sheathe inflamed surfaces.

It is usually administered in the form of a mucilage – *Mucilago Acaciæ*, British Pharmacopœia and United States Pharmacopœia – made from small pieces of Gum Acacia dissolved in water and strained (1 in 8·75).

¶ *Dose* in syrup, 1 to 4 drachms of the gum. Mucilage of Acacia is a nearly transparent, colourless or scarcely yellowish, viscid liquid, having a faint, rather agreeable odour and an insipid taste. It is employed as a soothing agent in inflammatory conditions of the respiratory, digestive and urinary tract, and is useful in diarrhœa and dysentery. It exerts a soothing influence upon all the surfaces with which it comes in contact. It may be diluted and flavoured to suit the taste. In low stages of typhoid fever, this mucilage, sweetened, is greatly recommended. The ordinary dose of the mucilage is from 1 to 4 fluid drachms.

In dispensing, Mucilage of Acacia is used for suspending insoluble powders in mixtures, for emulsifying oils and other liquids which are not miscible with water, and as an ingredient of many cough linctures. The British Pharmacopœia directs it to be used as an excipient in the preparation of troches. Compound Mucilage of Acacia – Pill-coating Acacia – is made from Gum Acacia, 1 in 10, with tragacanth, chloroform and water, and is used for moistening pills previous to coating.

Gum Acacia is an ingredient of the official *Pilula Ferri, Pulvis Amygdalæ compositus, Pulvis Tragacanthæ compositus,* all the official *Trochisci,* and various syrups, pastes and pastilles or jujubes.

Acacia Mixture, *Mistura Acaciæ* of the British Pharmacopœia Codex, is made from Gum Acacia (6 in 100) with syrup and diluted orange-flower water, employed as a demulcent in cough syrups and linctures.

¶ *Dose,* 1 to 4 fluid drachms.

Syrup of Acacia, British Pharmacopœia Codex, used chiefly as a demulcent in cough mixtures, is freshly prepared as required, from 1 part of Gum Acacia Mucilage and 3 of syrup; the dose, 1 to 4 fluid drachms.

The United States Pharmacopœia Syrup of Acacia, though regarded as a useful demulcent, is chiefly employed as an agent for suspending powders in mixtures.

The French Pharmacopœia has a Syrup of Acacia and a *potion gommeuse* made from powdered Acacia, syrup and orange-flower water.

As a dry excipient, powdered Acacia is employed, mixed in small proportion with powdered Marsh Mallow root, or powdered Liquorice root. A variation of this is a mixture of Acacia, 50 parts; Liquorice root, 34 parts; Sugar, 16 parts, all in fine powder. Another compound Acacia Powder, used sparingly as an absorbent pill excipient, is made of equal parts of Gum Acacia and Tragacanth.

Gum Acacia is highly nutritious. During the time of the gum harvest, the Moors of the desert are said to live almost entirely on it, and it has been proved that 6 oz. is sufficient to support an adult for twenty-four hours. It is related that the Bushman Hottentots have been known in times of scarcity to support themselves on it for days together. In many cases of disease, it is considered that a solution of Gum Arabic may for a time constitute the exclusive drink and food of the patient.

ACONITE (POISON)

Aconitum Napellus (LINN.)
N.O. Ranunculaciæ

Synonyms. Monkshood. Blue Rocket. Friar's Cap. Auld Wife's Huid
Part Used. The whole plant
Habitat. Lower mountain slopes of North portion of Eastern Hemisphere. From Himalayas through Europe to Great Britain

Aconite is now found wild in a few parts of England, mainly in the western counties and also in South Wales, but can hardly be considered truly indigenous. It was very early introduced into England, being mentioned in all the English vocabularies of plants from the tenth century downwards, and in Early English medical recipes.

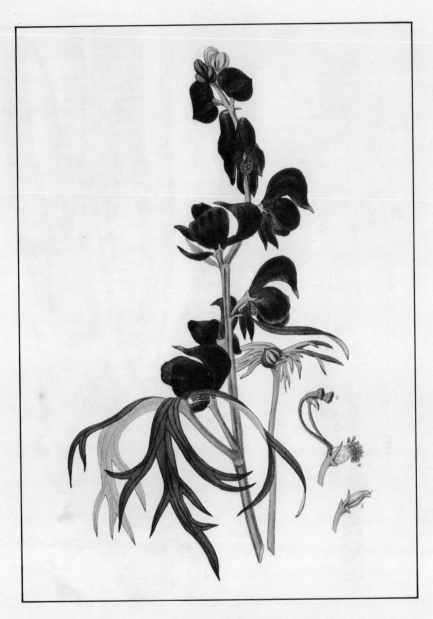

ACONITE
Aconitum Napellus

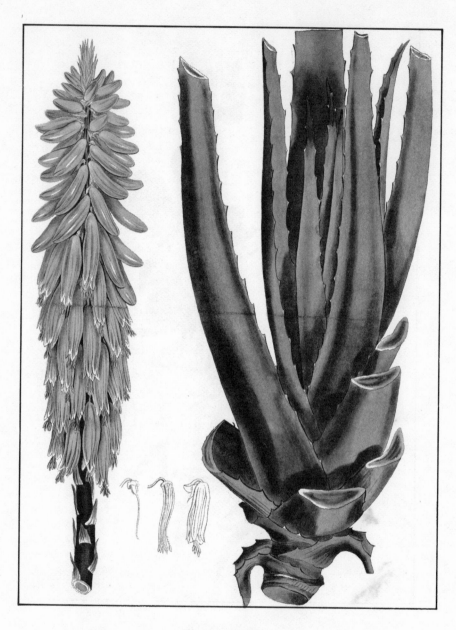

ALOE
Aloe Vulgaris

¶ *Description*. The plant is a hardy perennial, with a fleshy, spindle-shaped root, pale-coloured when young, but subsequently acquiring a dark brown skin. The stem is about 3 feet high, with dark green, glossy leaves, deeply divided in palmate manner and flowers in erect clusters of a dark blue colour. The shape of the flower is specially designed to attract and utilize bee visitors, especially the humble bee. The sepals are purple – purple being specially attractive to bees – and are fancifully shaped, one of them being in the form of a hood. The petals are only represented by the two very curious nectaries within the hood, somewhat in the form of a hammer; the stamens are numerous and lie depressed in a bunch at the mouth of the flower. They are pendulous at first, but rise in succession and place their anthers forward in such a way that a bee visiting the flower for nectar is dusted with the pollen, which he then carries to the next flower he visits and thereby fertilizes the undeveloped fruits, which are in a tuft in the centre of the stamens, each carpel containing a single seed.

In the Anglo-Saxon vocabularies it is called *thung*, which seems to have been a general name for any very poisonous plant. It was then called Aconite (the English form of its Greek and Latin name), later Wolf's Bane, the direct translation of the Greek *lycotonum*, derived from the idea that arrows tipped with the juice, or baits anointed with it, would kill wolves – the species mentioned by Dioscorides seems to have been *Aconitum lycotonum*. In the Middle Ages it became Monkshood and Helmet-flower, from the curious shape of the upper sepal overtopping the rest of the flower. This was the ordinary name in Shakespeare's days.

The generic name is said to have been derived from *akontion*, a dart, because it was used by barbarous races to poison their arrows, or from *akone*, cliffy or rocky, because the species grow in rocky glens. Theophrastus, like Pliny, derived the name from *Aconæ*, the supposed place of its origin. The specific name, *Napellus*, signifies a little turnip, in allusion to the shape of the roots.

¶ *Cultivation*. The chief collecting centres for foreign Aconite root have been the Swiss Alps, Salzburg, North Tyrol and Vorarlberg. Much was also formerly collected in Germany. Supplies from Spain and Japan are imported, so that the demand for English Aconite is somewhat restricted. The official Aconite is directed by the British Pharmacopœia to be derived only from plants cultivated in England, and a certain amount of home-grown Aconite has been regularly produced by the principal drug-farms,

though good crops are grown with some difficulty in England, and cultivation of Aconite has not paid very well in recent years.

Aconite prefers a soil slightly retentive of moisture, such as a moist loam, and flourishes best in shade. It would probably grow luxuriantly in a moist, open wood, and would yield returns with little further trouble than weeding, digging up and drying.

In preparing beds for growing Aconite, the soil should be well dug and pulverized by early winter frosts – the digging in of rotten leaves or stable manure is advantageous.

It can be raised from seed, sown $\frac{1}{2}$ inch deep in a cold frame in March, or in a warm position outside in April, but great care must be exercised that the right kind is obtained, as there are many varieties of Aconite – about twenty-four have been distinguished – and they have not all the same active medicinal properties. It takes two or three years to flower from seed.

Propagation is usually by division of roots in the autumn. The underground portion of the plants are dug up after the stem has died down, and the smaller of the 'daughter' roots that have developed at the side of the old roots are selected for replanting in December or January to form new stock, the young roots being planted about a foot apart each way. The young shoots appear above ground in February. Although the *plants* are perennial, each distinct root lasts only one year, the plant being continued by 'daughter' roots.

This official Aconite is also the species generally cultivated in gardens, though nearly all the species are worth growing as ornamental garden flowers, the best perhaps being *A. Napellus*, both white and blue, *A. paniculatum*, *A. Japonicum* and *A. autumnale*. All grow well in shade and under trees. Gerard grew four species in his garden: *A. lycotonum*, *A. variegatum*, *A. Napellus* and *A. Pyrenaicum*.

¶ *Part Used. – Collection and Drying*. The leaves, stem, flowering tops and root: the leaves and tops fresh, the root dried. The leaves and flowering tops are of less importance; they are employed for preparing Extract of Aconitum, and for this purpose are cut when the flowers are just breaking into blossom and the leaves are in their best condition, which is in June.

The roots should be collected in the autumn, after the stem dies down, but before the bud that is to produce the next year's stem has begun to develop. As this bud grows and forms a flowering stem, in the spring, some of the lateral buds develop into short shoots, each of which produces a long, slender, descending root, crowned with a bud. These roots rapidly thicken, filled with reserve material produced by the parent plant, the root of which dies as the 'daughter' roots increase in size. Towards the autumn, the parent plant dies down and the daughter roots which have then reached their maximum development are now full of starch. If allowed to remain in the soil, the buds that crown the daughter roots begin to grow, in the late winter, and this growth exhausts the strength of the root, and the proportion of both starch and alkaloid it contains is lessened.

On account of the extremely poisonous properties of the root, it is considered desirable that the root should be grown and collected under the same conditions, so that uniformity in the drug is maintained. The British Pharmacopœia specifies, therefore, that the roots should be collected in the autumn from plants cultivated in Britain and should consist of the dried, full-grown 'daughter' roots: much of the Aconite root that used to come in large quantities from Germany was the exhausted parent root of the wild-flowering plants.

When the roots are dug up, they are sorted over, the smallest laid aside for replanting and the plumper ones reserved for drying. They are first well washed in cold water and trimmed of all rootlets, and then dried, either entire, or longitudinally sliced to hasten drying.

Drying may at first be done in the open air, spread thinly, the roots not touching. Or they may be spread on clean floors or on shelves in a warm place for about ten days, turning frequently. When somewhat shrunken, they must be finished more quickly by artificial heat in a drying room or shed, near a stove or gas fire, care being taken that the heated air can escape at the top of the room. Drying in an even temperature will probably take about a fortnight or more. It is not complete till the roots are dry to the core and brittle, snapping when bent.

Dried Aconite root at its upper extremity, when crowned with an undeveloped bud, enclosed by scaly leaves, is about ¾ inch in diameter, tapering quickly downwards. It is dark brown in colour and marked with the scars of rootlets. The surface is usually longitudinally wrinkled, especially if it has been dried entire. The root breaks with a short fracture and should be whitish and starchy within. A transverse section shows a thick bark, separated from the inner portion by a well-marked darker line, which often assumes a stellate appearance. Aconite root as found in commerce is, however, often yellowish or brownish internally with the stellate mark-

ings not clearly shown, probably from having been collected too early. It should be lifted in the autumn of the second year.

Aconite root is liable to attack by insects, and after being well dried should be kept in securely closed vessels.

¶ *Chemical Constituents.* Aconite root contains from 0·3 to 1 per cent. alkaloidal matter, consisting of Aconitine – crystalline, acrid and highly toxic – with the alkaloids Benzaconine (Picraconitine) and Aconine.

Aconitine, the only crystallizable alkaloid, is present to the extent of not more than 0·2 per cent., but to it is due the characteristic activity of the root. Aconite acid, starch, etc., are also present. On incineration, the root yields about 3 per cent. ash.

The Aconitines are a group of highly toxic alkaloids derived from various species of Aconite, and whilst possessing many properties in common are chemically distinguishable according to the source from which they are obtained. The Aconitines are divided into two groups: (1) the Aconitines proper, including Aconitine, Japaconitine and Indaconitine, and (2) the Pseudaconitines – Pseudaconitine and Bikhaconitine.

This disparity between Aconites is a very important matter for investigation, though perhaps not so serious from a pharmaceutical point of view as might at first appear, since in the roots of several different species the alkaloid is found to possess similar physiological action; but this action varies in degree and the amount of alkaloid may be found to vary considerably. It is considered that the only reliable method of standardizing the potency of any of the Aconite preparations is by a physiological method: the lethal dose for the guinea-pig being considered to be the most convenient and satisfactory standard. Tinctures vary enormously as to strength, some proving seven times as powerful as others.

The Aconite which contains the best alkaloid, *A. Napellus*, is the old-fashioned, familiar garden variety, which may be easily recognized by its very much cut-up leaves, which are wide in the shoulder of the leaf – that part nearest the stem – and also by the purplish-blue flowers, which have the 'helmet' closely fitting over the rest of the flower, not standing up as a tall hood. All varieties of Aconite are useful, but this kind with the close set in helmet to the flower is the most valuable.

The Aconite derived from *German* root of *A. Napellus* appears to possess somewhat different properties to that prepared from English roots. The German roots may be recognized by the remains of the stem which crown the root. They are also generally less starchy, darker externally and more shrivelled than the English root and considered to be less active, probably because they are generally the exhausted parent roots.

¶ *Medicinal Action and Uses.* Anodyne, diuretic and diaphoretic. The value of Aconite as a medicine has been more fully realized in modern times, and it now ranks as one of our most useful drugs. It is much used in homœopathy. On account of its very poisonous nature, all medicines obtained from it come, however, under Table I of the poison schedule: Aconite is a deadly poison.

Both tincture and liniment of Aconite are in general use, and Aconite is also used in ointment and sometimes given as hypodermic injection. Preparations of Aconite are employed for outward application locally to the skin to diminish the pain of neuralgia, lumbago and rheumatism.

The official tincture taken internally diminishes the rate and force of the pulse in the early stages of fevers and slight local inflammations, such as feverish cold, larnyngitis, first stages of pneumonia and erysipelas; it relieves the pain of neuralgia, pleurisy and aneurism. In cardiac failure or to prevent same it has been used with success, in acute tonsilitis children have been well treated by a dose of 1 to 2 minims for a child 5 to 10 years old; the dose for adults is 2 to 5 minims, three times a day.

¶ *Note.* The tincture of Aconite of the British Pharmacopœia 1914 is nearly double the strength of that in the old Pharmacopœia of 1898.

Externally the linament as such or mixed with chloroform or belladonna liniment is useful in neuralgia or rheumatism.

¶ *Poisoning from, and Antidotes.* The symptons of poisoning are tingling and numbness of tongue and mouth and a sensation of ants crawling over the body, nausea and vomiting with epigastric pain, laboured breathing, pulse irregular and weak, skin cold and clammy, features bloodless, giddiness, staggering, mind remains clear. A stomach tube or emetic should be used at once, 20 minims of Tincture of Digitalis given if available, stimulants should be given, and if not retained diluted brandy injected per rectum, artificial respiration and friction, patient to be kept lying down.

All the species contain an active poison, Aconitine, one of the most formidable poisons which have yet been discovered: it exists in all parts of the plant, but especially in the root. The smallest portion of either root or leaves, when first put into the mouth, occasions burning and tingling, and a sense of numbness immediately follows its continuance. One-fiftieth grain of Aconitine will kill a sparrow in a few seconds; one-tenth grain a rabbit in five minutes. It is more powerful than prussic acid and acts with tremendous rapidity. One hundredth grain will act locally, so as to produce a well-marked sensation in any part of the body for a whole day. So acrid is the poison, that the juice applied to a wounded finger affects the whole system, not only causing pains in the limbs, but a sense of suffocation and syncope.

Some species of Aconite were well known to the ancients as deadly poisons. It was said to be the invention of Hecate from the foam of Cerberus, and it was a species of Aconite that entered into the poison which the old men of the island of Ceos were condemned to drink when they became infirm and no longer of use to the State. Aconite is also supposed to have been the poison that formed the cup which Medea prepared for Theseus.[1]

Various species of Aconite possess the same narcotic properties as *A. Napellus*, but none of them equal in energy the *A. ferox* of the East Indies, the root of which is used there as an energetic poison under the name of Bikh or Nabee. Aconite poisoning of wells by *A. ferox* has been carried out by native Indians to stop the progress of an army. They also use it for poisoning spears, darts and arrows, and for destroying tigers.

All children should be warned against Aconite in gardens. It is wiser not to grow Aconite among kitchen herbs of any sort. The root has occasionally been mistaken for horse-radish, with fatal results – it is, however, shorter, darker and more fibrous – and the leaves have produced similar fatal results. In Ireland a poor woman once sprinkled powdered Aconite root over a dish of greens, and one man was killed and another seriously affected by it.

In 1524 and 1526 it is recorded that two criminals, to whom the root was given as an experiment, quickly died.

The older herbalists described it as venomous and deadly. Gerard says: 'There hath beene little heretofore set down concerning the virtues of the Aconite, but much might be saide of the hurts that have come thereby.' It was supposed to be an antidote against other poisons. Gerard tells us that its power was 'So forcible that the herb only thrown

---

[1] Aconite and Belladonna were said to be the ingredients in the witches' 'Flying ointments.' Aconite causes irregular action of the heart, and Belladonna produces delirium. These combined symptoms might give a sensation of 'flying.'—EDITOR.

before the scorpion or any other venomous beast, causeth them to be without force or strength to hurt, insomuch that they cannot moove or stirre untill the herbe be taken away.' Ben Jonson, in his tragedy *Sejanus*, says:

'I have heard that Aconite
Being timely taken hath a healing might
Against the scorpion's stroke.'

Linnæus reports Aconite to be fatal to cattle and goats when they eat it fresh, but when dried it does no harm to horses, a peculiarity in common with the buttercups, to which the Aconites are related. Field-mice are well aware of its evil nature, and in hard times, when they will attack almost any plant that offers them food, they leave this severely alone.

¶ *Other Varieties. Japanese Aconite* – syn. *Aconitum Chinense* – is regularly imported in considerable quantities. It used formerly to be ascribed to *A. Fischeri* (Reichb.), but is now considered to be derived from *A. uncinatum*, var. *Japonicum* (Regel.) and possibly also from *A. volubile* (Pallas). It has conical or top-shaped, gradually tapering tuberous roots, 1 to 2 inches long, $\frac{1}{3}$ to 1 inch in thickness at the top, externally covered with a brown, closely adhering skin, internally white. Dried roots do not contain much alkaloid, if steeped when fresh in a mixture of common salt, vinegar and water. The poisonous alkaloid present is called Japaconitine, to distinguish it from the official Aconitine and the Pseudaconitine of *A. laciniatum*. Japaconitine is similar in constituents and properties with the Aconitine of *A. Napellus*.

Indian Aconite root or Nepal Aconite consists of the root of *A. laciniatum* (Staph.). It is also called Bikh or Bish, and is collected in Nepal. It is much larger than the English variety, being a conical, not suddenly tapering root, 2 to 4 inches long and an inch or more at the top, of a lighter brown than the official variety, the rootlet scars much fewer than the official root. Internally it is hard and almost resinous, the taste intensely acrid and is much shrivelled longitudinally. This root yields a very active alkaloid, *Pseudoaconitine*, which is allied to Aconitine and resembles it in many of its properties; it is about twice as active as Aconitine. Indian Aconite root was formerly attributed to *A. ferox* (Wall). Their large size and less tapering character sufficiently distinguish these from the official drug.

Other varieties of Aconite are *A. chasmanthum* (Staph.), known in India as Mohri, which contains Indaconitine, and *A. spica-*

tum, another Indian species containing Bikhaconitine, resembling Pseudaconitine.

Russian Aconite, A. orientale, grows abundantly in the Crimea and Bessarabia. It has a small, compact, greyish-black root with a transverse section similar to that of *A. Napellus*. Its taste is hot and acrid. When treated by a process which gave 0·0526 per cent. of crystalline Aconitine from a sample of powdered root of *A. Napellus*, the dried root of *A. orientale* yielded 2·207 per cent. of total alkaloids, which were, however, amorphous. The total alkaloid has not yet been investigated further.

A. heterophyllum (Wall), Atis root, is a plant growing in the Western temperate Himalayas. This species does not contain Aconitine and is said to be non-poisonous. Its chief constituent is an intensely bitter alkaloid – *Atisine* – possessing tonic and antiperiodic principles. *A. palmatum*, of Indian origin, yields a similar alkaloid, Palmatisine.

The province of Szechwen in West China grows large quantities of medicinal plants, among them *A. Wilsoni*, which is worth about 4*s.* per cwt., of which 55,000 lb. a year can be produced in this province; *A. Fischeri*, about four times the price, of which rather less are yearly available, and *A. Hemsleyan*, about the same price as the latter, of which about 27,000 lb. are available in an average year.

¶ *Other Species.* The Anthora, or Wholesome Aconite described by Culpepper, is a small plant about a foot high, with pale, divided green leaves, and yellow flowers – a native of the Alps. Its stem is erect, firm, angular and hairy; the leaves alternate and much cut into. The flowers are large, hooded, with fragrant scent, growing on top of the branches in spikes of a pale yellow colour, smaller than the ordinary Monkshood and succeeded by five horn-like, pointed pods, or achenes, containing five angular seeds. It flowers in July and the seeds ripen at the end of August. The root is tuberous.

Culpepper tells us that the herb was used in his time, but not often. It was reputed to be very serviceable against vegetable poisons, and 'a decoction of the root is a good lotion to wash the parts bitten by venomous creatures.' . . . 'The leaves, if rubbed on the skin will irritate and cause soreness and the pollen is also dangerous if blown in the eyes.'

As a matter of fact, this species of Aconite by no means deserves its reputation of harmlessness, for it is only poisonous in a less degree than the rest of the same genus, and the theory that it is a remedy against poison, particularly that of the other Aconites, is now an exploded one.

Parkinson, speaking of the Yellow Monkshood, calls it:

'The "counter-poison monkeshood" – the roots of which are effectual, not only against the poison of the poisonful Helmet Flower and all others of that kind, but also against the poison of all venomous beasts, the plague or pestilence and other infectious diseases, which raise spots, pockes, or markes in the outward skin, by expelling the poison from within and defending the heart as a most sovereign cordial.'

The so-called Winter Aconite, *Æranthis hyemalis*, is not a true Aconite, though closely allied, being also a member of the Buttercup family, whose blossoms it more nearly resembles.

Also see DELPHINIUM, FIELD LARKSPUR, STARVEACRE.

ADDER'S TONGUE (AMERICAN)

Erythronium Americanum (KER-GAWL)
N.O. Liliaceæ

Synonyms. Serpent's Tongue. Dog's Tooth Violet. Yellow Snowdrop
Parts Used. Leaves, bulbs
Habitat. Eastern United States of America, from New Brunswick to Florida, and westwards to Ontario and Arkansas

The American Dog's Tooth Violet or Adder's Tongue, *Erythronium Americanum* (Ker Gawl), is a very beautiful early spring flower of the Eastern United States of America, belonging to the Lily family. It grows in damp, open woodlands from New Brunswick to Florida and westwards to Ontario and Arkansas.

¶ *Description.* The plant, which is quite smooth, grows from a small, slender, ovoid, fawn-coloured corm, ¼ to 1 inch long, which is quite deeply buried in the soil and is of solid, firm consistence and white and starchy internally.

The stem is slender, a few inches high, and bears near the ground, on footstalks 2 to 3 inches long, a pair of oblong, dark-green, purplish-blotched leaves, the blades about 2½ inches long and 1 inch wide, minutely wrinkled, with parallel, longitudinal veins. The stem terminates in a handsome, large, pendulous, lily-like flower, an inch across, with the perianth divisions strongly recurved, bright yellow in colour, often tinged with purple and finely dotted within at the base, and with six stamens. It flowers in the latter part of April and early in May.

¶ *Medicinal Action and Uses.* The constituents of the plant have not yet been analysed. The fresh leaves and corm, and to a lesser degree the rest of the plant, are emetic.

The fresh leaves having emollient and anti-scrofulous properties are mostly used in the form of a stimulating poultice, applied to swellings, tumours and scrofulous ulcers.

The infusion is taken internally in wineglassful doses. It is reputed of use in dropsy, hiccough and vomiting.

The recent bulbs have been used as a substitute for colchicum. They are emetic in doses of 25 to 30 grains.

ADDER'S TONGUE (ENGLISH). *See under* FERNS

ADONIS. *See* HELLEBORE (FALSE)

ADRUE

Cyperus articulatus (LINN.)
N.O. Cyperaceæ

Part Used. The drug Adrue is the tuberous rhizome of the Guinea Rush (*Cyperus articulatus* Linn.), a tall sedge, common in Jamaica, and on the banks of the Nile.

¶ *Description.* The blackish-red, somewhat top-shaped tubers are ¾ to 1 inch long, ½ to ¾ inch in diameter, sometimes in a series of two or three, connected by an underground stem ⅛ inch in diameter and 1 to 2 inches long. Internally, the tubers are pale in colour, a transverse section showing a central column with darker points indicating vascular bundles. The dried tubers often bear the bristly remains of former leaves on their upper ends. The drug has a bitterish, aromatic taste, recalling that of Lavender. The odour of the fresh tubers has been likened to that of the Sweet Sedge, *Calamus aromaticus.*

¶ *Medicinal Action and Uses.* Carminative, sedative, very useful in vomiting of pregnancy.

The aromatic properties of the drug cause a feeling of warmth to be diffused throughout the whole system and it acts as a sedative in dyspeptic disorders.

¶ *Preparations.* A fluid extract is made from the tubers. Dose, 10 to 30 minims.

AGAR-AGAR

Gelidium Amansii (KUTZ)
N.O. Algæ

Synonyms. Japanese Isinglass
Part Used. The mucilage dri ed, after boiling the seaweed
Habitat. Japan, best variety; Ceylon and Macassar

¶ *Description*. A seaweed gathered on the East Indian coast and sent to China, it is derived from the various species of *Sphærococcus Euchema* and *Gelidium*. It is brownish-white in colour with thorny projections on its branches; the best variety, known as Japanese Isinglass, contains large quantities of mucilage. The seaweed after collection is spread out on the shore until bleached, and then dried; it is afterwards boiled in water and the mucilaginous solution strained, the filtrate being allowed to harden, and then it is dried in the sun. The time for collection of the Algæ is summer and autumn when the bleaching and drying can take place, but the final preparation of Agar-Agar is carried out in winter from November to February. The Japanese variety is derived from several kinds of Algæ and comes into European commerce in two forms: (1) In transparent pieces 2 feet long, the thickness of a straw, prepared in Singapore by treating it in hot water. (2) In yellowish white masses about 1 inch wide and 1 foot long. The latter is the form considered the more suitable for the culture of bacteria.

¶ *Constituents*. Agar-Agar contains glose, which is a powerful gelatinizing agent. It is precipitated from solution by alcohol. Glose is a carbohydrate. Acetic, hydrochloric and oxalic acids prevent gelatinization of Agar-Agar.

¶ *Medicinal Action and Uses*. Agar-Agar is widely used as a treatment for constipation, but is usually employed with Cascara when atony of the intestinal muscles is present. It does not increase peristaltic action. Its therapeutic value depends on the ability of the dry Agar to absorb and retain moisture. Its action is mechanical and analogous to that of the cellulose of vegetable foods, aiding the regularity of the bowel movements. It is sometimes used as an adulterant of jams and jellies.

¶ *Dosage and Preparations*. It is usually administered in small shreds mixed with fruit, milk or any convenient vehicle. It is not wise to give it in powder, as this gives rise to irritation in some cases. ½ to 1 ounce may be taken at a time. 1 ounce to a pint of boiling water makes a suitable jelly for invalids and may be flavoured with lemon.

¶ *Other Species*. Ceylon Agar-Agar, or Agal Agal, which is the native name of *Gracillaria lichenoides*, is largely used in the East for making soups and jellies. *Gigartina speciosa*, a variety found on the Swan River, was erroneously supposed to have formed the edible swallow's nest, but it has been ascertained that this delicacy comes from a peculiar secretion in the birds themselves. Macassar Agar-Agar comes from the straits between Borneo and Celebes and consists of impure *Euchema Spinolum* incrusted with salt.

AGARIC. *See* FUNGI. **LARCH AGARIC.** *See* FUNGI.

AGAVE. *See* ALOES

AGRIMONY

Agrimonia Eupatoria (LINN.)
N.O. Rosaceæ

Synonyms. Common Agrimony. Church Steeples. Cockeburr. Sticklewort. Philanthropos
Part Used. The herb
Habitat. The plant is found abundantly throughout England, on hedge-banks and the sides of fields, in dry thickets and on all waste places. In Scotland it is much more local and does not penetrate very far northward

Agrimony has an old reputation as a popular, domestic medicinal herb, being a simple well known to all country-folk. It belongs to the Rose order of plants, and its slender spikes of yellow flowers, which are in bloom from June to early September, and the singularly beautiful form of its much-cut-into leaves, make it one of the most graceful of our smaller herbs.

¶ *Description*. From the long, black and somewhat woody perennial root, the erect, cylindrical and slightly rough stem rises 1 or 2 feet, sometimes more, mostly unbranched, or very slightly branched in large specimens. The leaves are numerous and very rich in outline, those near the ground are often 7 or 8 inches long, while the upper ones are generally only about 3 inches in length. They are pinnate in form, i.e. divided up to the mid-rib into pairs of leaflets. The graduation in the size and richness of the leaves is noticeable: all are very similar in general character, but the upper leaves have far fewer leaflets than the lower, and such leaflets as there are, are less cut into segments and have altogether a simpler outline. The leaflets vary very considerably in size, as besides the six or eight large lateral leaflets and the terminal one, the mid-rib is fringed with several others that are very much smaller than these and ranged in the intervals between them. The main leaflets increase in size towards the apex of the leaf, where they are 1 to 1½ inches long. They are oblong-oval in shape, toothed, downy above and more densely so beneath.

The flowers, though small, are numerous, arranged closely on slender, terminal spikes, which lengthen much when the blossoms have withered and the seed-vessels are maturing. At the base of each flower, which is placed stalkless on the long spike, is a small bract, cleft into three acute segments. The flowers, about ⅜ inch across, have five conspicuous and spreading petals, which are egg-shaped in form and somewhat narrow in proportion to their length, slightly notched at the end and of a bright yellow colour. The stamens are five to twelve in number. The flowers face boldly outwards and upwards towards the light, but after they have withered, the calyx points downwards. It becomes rather woody, thickly covered at the end with a mass of small bristly hairs, that spread and develop into a burr-like form. Its sides are furrowed and nearly straight, about ¼ inch long, and the mouth, about as wide, is surmounted by an enlarged ring armed with spines, of which the outer ones are shorter and spreading, and the inner ones longer and erect.

The whole plant is deep green and covered with soft hairs, and has a slightly aromatic scent; even the small root is sweet scented, especially in spring. The spikes of flowers emit a most refreshing and spicy odour like that of apricots. The leaves when dry retain most of their fragrant odour, as well as the flowers, and Agrimony was once much sought after as a substitute or addition to tea, adding a peculiar delicacy and aroma to its flavour. Agrimony is one of the plants from the dried leaves of which in some country districts is brewed what is called 'a spring drink,' or 'diet drink,' a compound made by the infusion of several herbs and drunk in spring time as a purifier of the blood. In France, where herbal teas or *tisanes* are more employed than here, it is stated that Agrimony tea, for its fragrancy, as well as for its virtues, is often drunk as a beverage at table.

The plant is subject to a considerable amount of variation, some specimens being far larger than others, much more clothed with hairs and with other minor differences. It has, therefore, by some botanists, been divided into two species, but the division is now scarcely maintained. The larger variety, having also a greater fragrance, was named *Agrimonia odorata*.

The long flower-spikes of Agrimony have caused the name of 'Church Steeples' to be given the plant in some parts of the country. It also bears the title of 'Cockeburr,' 'Sticklewort' or 'Stickwort,' because its seed-vessels cling by the hooked ends of their stiff hairs to any person or animal coming into contact with the plant. It was, Gerard informs us, at one time called Philanthropos, according to some old writers, on account of its beneficent and valuable properties, others saying that the name arose from the circumstance of the seeds clinging to the garments of passers-by, as if desirous of accompanying them, and Gerard inclines to this latter interpretation of the name.

The whole plant yields a yellow dye: when gathered in September, the colour given is pale, much like that called nankeen; later in the year, the dye is of a darker hue and will dye wool of a deep yellow. As it gives a good dye at all times and is a common plant, easily cultivated, it seems to deserve the notice of dyers.

Sheep and goats will eat this plant, but cattle, horses and swine leave it untouched.

¶ *History.* The name Agrimony is from *Argemone*, a word given by the Greeks to plants which were healing to the eyes, the name *Eupatoria* refers to Mithridates Eupator, a king who was a renowned concoctor of herbal remedies. The magic power of Agrimony is mentioned in an old English medical manuscript:

'If it be leyd under mann's heed,
He shal sleepyn as he were deed;
He shal never drede ne wakyn
Till fro under his heed it be takyn.'

Agrimony was one of the most famous vulnerary herbs. The Anglo-Saxons, who called it Garclive, taught that it would heal wounds, snake bites, warts, etc. In the time of Chaucer, when we find its name appearing in the form of Egrimoyne, it was used with Mugwort and vinegar for 'a bad back' and 'alle woundes': and one of these old writers recommends it to be taken with a mixture of pounded frogs and human blood, as a remedy for all internal hæmorrhages. It formed an ingredient of the famous arquebusade water as prepared against wounds inflicted by an arquebus, or hand-gun, and was mentioned by Philip de Comines, in his account of the battle of Morat in 1476. In France, the *eau de arquebusade* is still applied for sprains and bruises, being carefully made from many aromatic herbs. It was at one time included in the London Materia Medica as a vulnerary herb, but modern official medicine does not recognize its virtues, though it is still fully appreciated in herbal practice as a mild astringent and tonic, useful in coughs, diarrhœa and relaxed bowels. By pouring a pint of boiling water on a handful of the dried herb – stem, leaves and flowers – an excellent gargle may be made for a relaxed throat, and a teacupful of the same infusion is recommended, taken cold three or four times in the day for looseness in the bowels, also for passive losses of blood. It may be given either in infusion or decoction.

¶ *Constituents*. Agrimony contains a particular volatile oil, which may be obtained from the plant by distillation and also a bitter principle. It yields in addition 5 per cent. of tannin, so that its use in cottage medicine for gargles and as an astringent applicant to indolent ulcers and wounds is well justified. Owing to this presence of tannin, its use has been recommended in dressing leather.

¶ *Medicinal Action and Uses*. Astringent, tonic, diuretic. Agrimony has had a great reputation for curing jaundice and other liver complaints. Gerard believed in its efficacy. He says: 'A decoction of the leaves is good for them that have naughty livers': and he tells us also that Pliny called it a 'herb of princely authoritie.' Dioscorides stated that it was not only 'a remedy for them that have bad livers,' but also 'for such as are bitten with serpents.' Dr. Hill, who from 1751 to 1771 published several works on Herbal medicine, recommends 'an infusion of 6 oz. of the crown of the root in a quart of boiling water, sweetened with honey and half a pint drank three times a day,' as an effectual remedy for jaundice. It gives tone to the system and promotes assimilation of food.

Agrimony is also considered a very useful agent in skin eruptions and diseases of the blood, pimples, blotches, etc. A strong decoction of the root and leaves, sweetened with honey or sugar, has been taken successfully to cure scrofulous sores, being administered two or three times a day, in doses of a wineglassful, persistently for several months. The same decoction is also often employed in rural districts as an application to ulcers.

¶ *Preparation*. Fluid extract dose, 10 to 60 drops.

In North America, it is said to be used in fevers with great success, by the Indians and Canadians.

In former days, it was sometimes given as a vermifuge, though that use of it is obsolete.

In the Middle Ages, it was said to have magic powers, if laid under a man's head inducing heavy sleep till removed, but no narcotic properties are ascribed to it.

Green (*Universal Herbal*, 1832) tells us that 'its root appears to possess the properties of Peruvian bark in a very considerable degree, without manifesting any of its inconvenient qualities, and if taken in pretty large doses, either in decoction or powder, seldom fails to cure the ague.'

Culpepper (1652) recommends it, in addition to the uses already enumerated, for gout, 'either used outwardly in an oil or ointment, or inwardly, in an electuary or syrup, or concreted juice.' He praises its use externally, stating how sores may be cured 'by bathing and fomenting them with a decoction of this plant,' and that it heals 'all inward wounds, bruises, hurts and other distempers.' He continues: 'The decoction of the herb, made with wine and drunk, is good against the biting and stinging of serpents . . . it also helpeth the colic, cleanseth the breath and relieves the cough. A draught of the decoction taken warm before the fit, first relieves and in time removes the tertian and quartian ague.' It 'draweth forth thorns, splinters of wood, or any such thing in the flesh. It helpeth to strengthen members that are out of joint.'

There are several other plants, not actually related botanically to the Common Agrimony, that were given the same name by the older herbalists because of their similar properties. These are the COMMON HEMP AGRIMONY, *Eupatorium Cannabinum* (Linn.), called by Gerard the Common Dutch Agrimony, and by Salmon, in his *English Herbal* (1710), *Eupatorium Aquaticum mas*, the Water Agrimony; also the plant now called the Trifid Bur-Marigold, *Bidens tripartita* (Linn.), but by older herbalists named the Water Hemp, Bastard Hemp and Bastard Agrimony. The name Bastard Agrimony has also been given to a species of true Agrimony, *Agrimonium Agrimonoides*, a native of Italy, growing in moist woods and among bushes.

AGRIMONY (HEMP)

Eupatorium Cannabinum (LINN.)
N.O. Compositæ

Synonyms. Holy Rope. St. John's Herb
Part Used. Herb

The Hemp Agrimony, *Eupatorium Cannabinum*, belongs to the great Composite order of plants. It is a very handsome, tall-growing perennial, common on the banks of rivers, sides of ditches, at the base of cliffs on the seashore, and in other damp places in most parts of Britain, and throughout Europe.

¶ *Description.* The root-stock is woody and from it rises the erect, round stems, growing from 2 to 5 feet high, with short branches springing from the axils of the leaves, which are placed on it in pairs. The stems are reddish in colour, covered with downy hair and are woody below. They have a pleasant aromatic smell when cut.

The root-leaves are on long stalks, but the stem-leaves have only very short foot-stalks. They are divided to their base into three, more rarely five, lance-shaped toothed lobes, the middle lobe much larger than the others, the general form of the leaf being similar to that of the Hemp (hence both the English name and the Latin specific name, deriven from *cannabis*, hemp). In small plants the leaves are sometimes undivided. They have a bitter taste, and their pungent smell is reminiscent of an umbelliferous rather than of a composite plant. All the leaves bear distinct, short hairs, and are sparingly sprinkled with small inconspicuous, resinous dots.

The plant blooms in late summer and autumn, the flower heads being arranged in crowded masses of a dull lilac colour at the top of the stem or branches. Each little composite head consists of about five or six florets. The corolla has five short teeth; though generally light purple or reddish lilac, it sometimes may be nearly white; it is covered with scattered resinous points. The anthers of the stamens are brown, and the very long style is white. The crown of hairs, or pappus, on the angled fruit is of a dirty white colour.

We sometimes find the plant called 'St. John's Herb,' and on account of the hempen-shaped leaves, it was also formerly called, in some districts, 'Holy Rope,' being thus named after the rope with which the Saviour was bound.

¶ *Constituents.* The leaves contain a volatile oil, which acts on the kidneys, and likewise some tannin and a bitter chemical principle which will cut short the chill of intermittent fever.

¶ *Medicinal Action and Uses.* Alternative and febrifuge. Though now little used medicinally, herbalists recognize its cathartic, diuretic and anti-scorbutic properties, and consider it a good remedy for purifying the blood, either used by itself, or in combination with other herbs. A homœopathic tincture is prepared, given in frequent small well-diluted doses with water, for influenza, or for a similar feverish chill, and a tea made with boiling water poured on the dry leaves will give prompt relief if taken hot at the onset of a bilious catarrh or of influenza.

In Holland it was used by the peasants for jaundice with swollen feet, and given as an alternative or purifier of the blood in the spring and against scurvy. The leaves have been used in infusion as a tonic, and in the fen districts where it prevails, such medicines are very necessary. Country people used to lay the leaves on bread, considering that they thus prevented it from becoming mouldy

¶ *Preparation.* Fluid extract, 10 to 60 drops.

According to Withering, an infusion of a handful of the fresh herb acts as a strong purgative and emetic. Boerhaave, the famous Dutch physician (1668–1738), recommends an infusion of the plant for fomenting ulcers and putrid sores, and Tournefort (*Materia Medica*, 1708) affirmed that the fresh-gathered root, boiled in ale, purges briskly, but without producing any bad effects, and stated that there were many instances of its having cured dropsy.

It had also the reputation of being a good wound herb, whether bruised or made into an ointment with lard.

Goats are said to be the only animals that will eat this plant.

See BONESET, EUPATORIUM, GRAVEL ROOT.

AGRIMONY (WATER)

Bidens tripartita (LINN.)
N.O. Compositæ.

Synonym. Bur Marigold
Part Used. Whole plant

The Water Agrimony, now called the Bur Marigold, is an annual, flowering in late summer and autumn, abounding in wet places, such as the margins of ponds and ditches, and common in England, but rather less so in Scotland.

¶ *Description.* The root is tapering, with many fibres attached to it. The erect stem grows about 2 feet high, sometimes more, and is wiry and nearly smooth, angular, solid and marked with small brown spots, so as to almost give it the dark purple appearance described by Culpepper. It is very leafy and the upper portion branches freely from the axils of the leaves, which are placed opposite one another and are of a dark green colour, 2 to 3 inches in length. All except the uppermost are narrowed into winged foot-stalks at the bases, which are united together across the stem. They are smooth and sharp-pointed, with coarsely toothed margins, and are divided into three segments (hence the specific name of the plant), occasionally into five, the centre lobe much larger and also often deeply three-cleft. The uppermost leaves are sometimes found undivided.

The composite flowers are in terminal heads, brownish-yellow in colour and somewhat drooping, usually without ray florets, the disk florets being perfectly regular. The heads are surrounded by a leafy involucre, the outer leaflets of which, about eight in number, pointed and spreading, extend much behind the flower-head. The fruits have four ribs, which terminate in long, spiky projections, or awns, two of which, as well as the ribs, are armed with reflexed prickles, causing them to cling to any rough substance they touch, such as the coat of an animal, thus helping in the dissemination of the seeds. From these burr-like fruits, the plant has been given the name it now universally bears. These burrs, when the plant has been growing on the borders of a fish-pond, have been known to destroy gold fish by adhering to their gills. The flower-heads smell rather like rosin or cedar when burnt.

¶ *Medicinal Action and Uses.* This plant was formerly valued for its diuretic and astringent properties, and was employed in fevers, gravel, stone and bladder and kidney troubles generally, and was considered also a good

stypic and an excellent remedy for ruptured blood-vessels and bleeding of every description, of benefit to consumptive patients.

Culpepper tells us that it was called *Hepatorium* 'because it strengthens the liver':

'it healeth and drieth, cutteth and cleanseth thick and tough humours of the breast, and for this I hold it inferior to few herbs that grow . . . it helpeth the dropsy and yellow jaundice; it opens the obstruction of the liver, mollifies the hardness of the spleen, being applied outwardly. . . it is an excellent remedy for the third day ague; . . . it kills worms and cleanseth the body of sharp humours which are the cause of itch and scab; the herb being burnt, the smoke thereof drives away flies, wasps, etc. It strengthens the lungs exceedingly. Country people give it to their cattle when they are troubled with cough or are broken-winded.'

It has sometimes been employed on the Continent as a yellow dye, but the colour yielded is very indifferent. The yarn or thread must be first steeped in alum water, then dried and steeped in a decoction of the plant and afterwards boiled in the decoction.

A nearly-allied species, *Bidens bipinnata* (Linn.), popularly called Spanish Needles, is a native of North America, where the roots and seeds have been used as emmenagogues and in laryngeal and bronchial diseases.

MARIGOLD (NODDING). Another species of *Bidens*, called *B. cernua*, popularly known as the Nodding Marigold. The flowers are somewhat larger than *B. tripartita*, and have a much more decided droop, hence the name 'Nodding.' The leaves are not made up of three leaflets but are of lanceolate form, deeply serrated. It is found by streams and ditches, and flowers during the later summer and autumn.

ALDER, BLACK AMERICAN

Prinos Verticillatus (LINN.)
N.O. Aquiloliaceæ

Synonyms. Ilex Verticillata. Black Alder Winterberry. Deciduous Winterberry. Virginian Winterberry. P. Gronovii. P. Confertus. Fever Bush. Apalachine a feuilles de Prunier

Parts Used. The fresh bark and fruit

Habitat. The United States, from western Florida northwards

¶ *Description.* This shrub is the most ornamental of the American deciduous hollies. It grows from 6 to 10 feet in height, with thin, oval or lanceolate leaves, white flowers, and bright scarlet berries the size of a large pea, causing it to be very conspicuous in the autumn, when the surrounding vegetation is leafless.

The bark is found in thin fragments, the outer surface brownish, with whitish patches and black dots and lines, the cork layer easily separating from the pale-greenish or yellowish white inner tissue. The fracture is short, the odour almost imperceptible, and the taste bitter and slightly astringent.

It was widely used by the aborigines of

North America for its astringent properties.
¶ *Constituents*. The bark contains about 4·8 per cent. tannin, two resins, the one soluble and the other insoluble in alcohol, albumen, gum, sugar, and a bitter principle and a yellow colouring matter not yet isolated. There is no berberine.

The fresh bark and fruit are gathered before the first autumnal frost.
¶ *Medicinal Action and Uses*. Cathartic, antiseptic, tonic, and astringent bitter. The decoction of the bark is prepared by boiling 2 ounces of bark in 3 pints of water down to 2 pints, this being given internally in diarrhœa and malarial disorders, and externally in indolent sores and chronic skin disease. The berries should not be used as a substitute for the bark. In intermittent fever it can be used like Peruvian Bark, and is valuable in jaundice, gangrenous affections, dropsy, and when the body is devitalized by discharges. The bark is well known as an ingredient in several alternative syrups.

The berries are cathartic, and with Cedar-apples form a mild anthelmintic for children.

An observed case, after eating twenty-five berries, had a sensation of nausea, not interfering with appetite, vomiting of bile without retching, painless and profuse evacuation of the bowels, followed by a second evacuation in half an hour, and as a result, a feeling of great lightness and well-being, with appetite and digestion better than usual.

For dyspepsia, 2 drachms of the powdered bark, and 1 drachm of powdered Golden Seal infused in a pint of boiling water, taken, when cold, in the course of one day in wine-glassful doses, will be found very helpful.
¶ *Dosage*. Of the decoction, 2 to 3 fluid ounces. Of the powdered bark, ½ to 1 drachm.

ALDER, COMMON

Alnus Glutinosa (GAERTN.)
N.O. Betulaceæ

Synonym. Betula Alnus
Parts Used. The bark and the leaves
Habitat. Europe south of the Arctic Circle, including Britain, Western Asia, North Africa

¶ *History*. The English Alder is a moderately-sized tree or large shrub of dark colour, usually growing in moist woods or pastures or by streams. The leaves are broadly ovate, stalked, and usually smooth. The catkins are formed in the autumn, the fruiting ones having scales rather like a tiny-fir-cone; the flowers appear in early spring, before the leaves are fully out. The woody, nearly globular female catkins are the so-called 'berries.' The trees are often grown in coppices, which afford winter shade for stock on mountain grazings without appearing to injure the grass beneath, and can be cut down for poles every nine or ten years.

The wood is much used. When young it is brittle and very easily worked. When more mature it is tinted and veined; in the Highlands of Scotland it is used for making handsome chairs, and is known as Scottish mahogany. It has the quality of long endurance under water, and so is valuable for pumps, troughs, sluices, and particularly for piles, for which purpose it is said to have been used in sixteenth-century Venice and widely in France and Holland. The roots and knots furnish good material for cabinet-makers, and for the clogs of Lancashire mill-towns and the south of Scotland the demand exceeds the supply, and birch has to be used instead. It is also used for cart and spinning wheels, bowls, spoons, wooden heels, her-ring-barrel staves, etc. On the Continent it is largely used for cigar-boxes, for which its reddish, cedar-like wood is well adapted. After lying in bogs the wood has the colour but not the hardness of ebony. The branches make good charcoal, which is valuable for making gunpowder.

The bark is used by dyers, tanners, leather dressers, and for fishermen's nets.
¶ *Dyeing*. The *bark* is used as a foundation for blacks, with the addition of copperas. Alone, it dyes woollens a reddish colour (Aldine Red). The Laplanders chew it, and dye leathern garments with their saliva. An ounce dried and powdered, boiled in three-quarters of a pint of water with an equal amount of logwood, with solution of copper, tin, and bismuth, 6 grains of each, and 2 drops of iron vitriol, will dye a deep *boue de Paris*.

Both *bark* and *young shoots* dye yellow, and with a little copper as a yellowish-grey, useful in the half-tints and shadows of flesh in tapestry. The shoots cut in March will dye cinnamon, and if dried and powdered a tawny shade. The *fresh wood* yields a pinkish-fawn dye, and the *catkins* a green.

The *leaves* have been used in tanning leather. They are clammy, and if spread in a room are said to catch fleas on their glutinous surface.
¶ *Constituents*. The bark and young shoots contain from 16 to 20 per cent. of tannic

acid, but so much colouring matter that they are not very useful for tanning. This tannin differs from that of galls and oak-bark, and does not yield glucose when acted upon by sulphuric acid, which, it is stated, resolves it into almine red and sugar.

¶ *Medicinal Action and Uses.* Tonic and astringent. A decoction of the bark is useful to bathe swellings and inflammations, especi-

ally of the throat, and has been known to cure ague.

Peasants on the Alps are reported to be frequently cured of rheumatism by being covered with bags full of the heated leaves.

Horses, cows, sheep and goats are said to eat it, but swine refuse it. Some state that it is bad for horses, as it turns their tongues black.

ALDER BUCKTHORN. *See* BUCKTHORN

ALDER, TAG

Alnus serrulata (WILLD.)
N.O. Betulaceæ

Synonyms. Alnus rubra (obsolete). Smooth Alder. Red Alder
Parts Used. Bark. Cones
Habitat. United States and Europe

¶ *Description.* A well-known shrub, growing in clumps and forming thickets on the borders of ponds or rivers, or in swamps. It bears flowers of a reddish-green colour in March and April. The bark is blackish grey, with small, corky warts, the inner surface being orange-brown, striated. The taste is astringent and somewhat bitter. It is almost odourless.

The name *Alnus rubra* should no longer be applied to *Alnus serrulata*, though some authorities retain it. That is the correct name of the Oregon Alder.

¶ *Medicinal Action and Uses.* Alterative, tonic, astringent, emetic. A decoction or extract is useful in scrofula, secondary syphilis and several forms of cutaneous disease. The inner bark of the root is emetic, and a decoction of the cones is said to be astringent, and useful in hæmaturia and other hæmorrhages.

When diarrhœa, indigestion and dyspepsia are caused by debility of the stomach, it will be found helpful, and also in intermittent fevers.

It is said that an excellent ophthalmic powder can be made as follows: bore a hole from ½ to 1 inch in diameter, lengthwise, through a stout piece of limb of Tag Alder. Fill the opening with finely-powdered salt, and close it at each end. Put into hot ashes, and allow it to remain until the Tag is almost charred (three to four days), then split it open, take out the salt, powder, and keep it in a vial. To use it, blow some of the powder upon the eye, through a quill.

¶ *Dosage.* Of fluid extract, ½ to 1 drachm. Infusion of 1 oz. of bark in 1 pint of boiling water – in wineglassful doses. Almim, 4 to 10 grains.

ALECOST. *See* TANSY

ALEXANDERS. *See* (BLACK) LOVAGE

ALKANETS

Alkanna tinctoria (TAUSCH.)
Lithosfermum tinctorium (VAH L.)
N.O. Boraginaceæ

Synonyms. Anchusa. Dyer's Bugloss. Spanish Bugloss. Orchanet
Part Used. Root

The name *Anchusa* is derived from the Greek *anchousa*=paint, from the use of the root as a dye.

The species are hispid or pubescent herbs, with oblong, entire leaves, and bracteated racemes, rolled up before the flowers expand. The corolla is rather small, between funnel and salver-shaped; usually purplish-blue, but in some species yellow or whitish; the calyx enlarges in fruit. The root, which is often very large in proportion to the size of the

plant, yields in many of the species a *red dye* from the rind.

Alkanet (*A. tinctoria*) is cultivated in Central and Southern Europe for its dye, which is readily extracted by oils and spirit of wine. It is employed in *pharmacy* to give a red colour to salves, etc., and in staining wood in imitation of rosewood, or mahogany. This is done by rubbing it with oil in which the Alkanet root has been soaked. About 8 to 10 tons were annually imported from France

18

and Germany. The plant is sometimes also cultivated in Britain, but by far the greater portion of the Alkanet used here is imported either from the Levant or from the neighbourhood of Montpellier, in France.

Though Alkanet imparts a fine deep red colour to oily substances and to spirit of wine, it tinges *water* with a dull brownish hue. Wax tinged with Alkanet, and applied to the surface of warm marble, stains it flesh-colour and sinks deep into the stone. It is also used in colouring spurious 'port-wine,' for which purpose it is perfectly harmless.

Our British species, the Common Alkanet (*A. officinalis*), is a soft, hairy plant with an angular stem; narrow, lanceolate leaves; and forked, one-sided cymes of violet flowers; calyx longer than the funnel-shaped corolla. It is an occasional escape from gardens. It is a biennial, and flowers from June to July.

The Evergreen Alkanet (*A. sempervireus*) is also found in Great Britain. This is a stout bristly plant, with deep green, ovate leaves, and long-stalked axillary, crowded clusters of rather large flowers, which are of an intense azure blue and have a short tube to the corolla. It is not generally considered a native, but it is not an uncommon hedgeplant in Devonshire. It is a perennial and flowers from May to August.

Parkinson says that the French ladies of his day coloured their faces with an ointment containing *anchusa* and the colour did not last long.

¶ *Medicinal Action and Uses.* Culpepper says:

'It is an herb under the dominion of Venus, and indeed one of her darlings, though somewhat hard to come by. It helps old ulcers, hot inflammations, burnings by common fire and St. Anthony's fire . . . for these uses your best way is to make it into an ointment; also if you make a vinegar of it, as you make a vinegar of roses, it helps the morphy and leprosy . . . it helps the yellow jaundice, spleen, and gravel in the kidneys. Dioscorides saith, it helps such as are bitten by venomous beasts, whether it be taken inwardly or applied to the wound; nay, he saith further, if any that hath newly eaten it do but spit into the mouth of a serpent, the serpent instantly dies. . . . It also kills worms. Its decoction made in wine and drank, strengthens the back, and easeth the pains thereof. It helps bruises and falls, and is as gallant a remedy to drive out the smallpox and measles as any is; an ointment made of it is excellent for green wounds, pricks or thrusts.'

ALLSPICE

Pimento officinalis (LINDL.)
N.O. Myrtaceæ

Synonyms. Pimento. Jamaica Pepper
Part Used. Fruit, particularly the shell
Habitat. Pimento, or Jamaica Pepper, familiarly called Allspice, because it tastes like a combination of cloves, juniper berries, cinnamon and pepper, is the dried full-grown, but immature fruit of *Pimento officinalis* (Lindl.), or *Eugenia Pimenta*, an evergreen tree about 30 feet high, a member of the natural order *Myrtaceæ*, indigenous to the West Indian Islands and South America, and extensively grown in Jamaica, where it flourishes best on limestone hills near the sea. In this country, it only grows as a stove plant

It is also cultivated in Central America and surrounding states, but more than half the supply of the spice found in commerce comes from Jamaica, where the tree is so abundant as to form in the mountainous districts whole forests, which require little attention beyond clearing out undergrowth

¶ *Description.* The tree begins to fruit when three years old and is in full bearing after four years. The flowers appear in June, July and August and are quickly succeeded by the berries.

The special qualities of the fruit reside in the rind of the berries. It loses its aroma on ripening, owing to loss of volatile oil, and the berries are therefore collected as soon as they have attained their full size, in July and August, but while unripe and green.

Gathering is performed by breaking off the small twigs bearing the bunches; these are then spread out and exposed to the sun and air for some days, after which the stalks are

removed and the berries are ready for packing into bags and casks for exportation.

The spice is sometimes dried in ovens (Kiln-dried Allspice), but the method by evaporation from sun-heat produces the best article, though it is tedious and somewhat hazardous, requiring about twelve days, during which the fruit must be carefully guarded against moisture, being housed at night and during rainy and damp weather.

The green colour of the fresh fruit changes on drying to reddish brown. If the fruit is allowed to ripen, it loses almost the whole of its aromatic properties, becoming fleshy, sweet and of a purple-black colour. Such

Pimento, to render it more attractive, is then often artificially coloured with bole or brown ochre, a sophistication which may be detected by boiling for a few seconds with diluted hydrochloric acid, filtering and testing with potassium ferrocyanide; the liquid should assume at most a bluish-green colour.

The fruits as found in commerce are small, nearly globular berries, about $\frac{3}{16}$ inch in diameter, somewhat like black pepper in appearance, with a rough and brittle surface and crowned by the remains of the calyx teeth, surrounding the short style. The fruit is two-celled, each cell containing a single, kidney-shaped seed. The remains of the calyx crowning the fruit and the presence of two single-seeded cells are features that distinguish Pimento from Cubebs, the fruit of which is one-celled, one-seeded and grey, and from Black Peppercorns, which are also one-celled and one-seeded.

The spice derives its name from the Portuguese *pimenta*, Spanish *pimienta*=pepper, which was given it from its resemblance to peppercorns.

¶ *Constituents.* The chief constituent of Pimento is from 3 to 4·5 per cent. of a volatile oil, contained in glands in the pericarp of the seeds and obtained by distillation from the fruit.

It occurs as a yellow or yellowish-red liquid, becoming gradually darker on keeping and having a pleasant aromatic odour, somewhat similar to that of oil of cloves, and a pungent, spicy taste. It has a slightly acid reaction. It is soluble in all proportions of alcohol. The specific gravity is 1·030 to 1·050. Its chief constituent is the phenol Eugenol, which is present to the extent of 60 to 75 per cent., and a sesquiterpene, the exact nature of which has not yet been ascertained. The specific gravity to some extent indicates the amount present; if lower than 1·030, it may be assumed that some eugenol has been removed, or that the oil has been adulterated with substitutes having a lower specific gravity than that of eugenol. The eugenol can be determined by shaking the oil with a solution of potassium hydroxide and measuring the residual oily layer. The United States Pharmacopœia specifies that at least 65 per cent. by volume of eugenol should be present. On shaking the oil with an equal volume of strong solution of ammonia, it should be converted into a semi-solid mass of eugenol-ammonium.

The clove-like odour of the oil is doubtless due to the eugenol, but the characteristic odour is due to some other substance or substances as yet unknown. A certain amount of resin is also present, but the oil has not yet been fully investigated.

Bonastre obtained from the fruit, a volatile oil, a green fixed oil, a fatty substance in yellowish flakes, tannin, gum, resin, uncrystallizable sugar, colouring matter, malic and gallic acids, saline matter and lignin. The green fixed oil has a burning, aromatic taste of Pimento and is supposed to be the acrid principle. Upon this, together with the volatile oil, the medicinal properties of the berries depend, and as these two principles exist most in the shell, this part is the most efficient. According to Bonastre, the shell contains 10 per cent. of the volatile and 8 per cent. of the fixed oil; the seeds only 5 per cent. of the former and 2·5 of the latter. Berzelius considered the green fixed oil of Bonastre to be a mixture of the volatile oil, resin, fixed oil and perhaps a little chlorophyll.

On incineration, the fruits yield from 2·5 to 5 per cent. of ash.

They impart their flavour to water and all their virtues to alcohol. The infusion is of a brown colour and reddens litmus paper.

The leaves and bark abound in inflammable particles.

¶ *Medicinal Action and Uses.* The chief use of Pimento is as a spice and condiment: the berries are added to curry powder and also to mulled wine. It is popular as a warming cordial, of a sweet odour and grateful aromatic taste.

The oil inaction resembles that of cloves, and is occasionally used in medicine and is also employed in perfuming soaps.

It was formerly official in both the British and United States Pharmacopœias. Both Pimento Oil and Pimento Water were official in the British Pharmacopœia of 1898, but Oil of Pimento was deleted from the British Pharmacopœia of 1914, though the Water still has a place in the British Pharmacopœia Codex.

Pimento has also been dropped from the United States Pharmacopœia, but admitted to the National Formulary IV. Pimento is one of the ingredients in the Compound Tincture of Guaic of the National Formulary IV.

Pimento is an aromatic stimulant and carminative to the gastro-intestinal tract, resembling cloves in its action. It is employed chiefly as an addition to tonics and purgatives and as a flavouring agent.

The Essential Oil, as well as the Spirit and the distilled Water of Pimento are useful for flatulent indigestion and for hysterical paroxysms. Two or three drops of the oil on sugar are given to correct flatulence. The oil is also given on sugar and in pills to correct the griping tendencies of purgatives: it was formerly added to Syrup of Buckthorn to prevent griping.

Pimento Water (*Aqua Pimentæ*) is used as a vehicle for stomachic and purgative medicines. It is made by taking 5 parts of bruised Pimento to 200 parts of water and distilling down to 100, the dose being 1 to 2 fluid ounces.

¶ *Concentrated Pimento Water of the British Pharmacopœia Codex.*

Oil of Pimento	1 fl. oz.
Alcohol	12 fl. oz.
Purified Talc	1 oz.
Distilled Water	up to 20 fl. oz.

Dissolve the oil in the alcohol, contained in a suitable bottle, add the water gradually, shaking after each addition; add the talc, shake, allow to stand for a few hours, occasionally shaking, and filter.

One part of this solution corresponds to about 40 parts of Pimento Water.

¶ *Other Preparations.* The powdered fruit: dose, 10 to 30 grains. Fluid extract: dose, ½ to 1 drachm. Oil: dose, 2 to 5 drops.

Pimento is one of the ingredients of Spice Plaster. An extract made from the crushed berries by boiling them down to a thick liquor is, when spread on linen, a capital stimulating plaster for neuralgic or rheumatic pains.

The fruits of four other species of the genus *Pimento*, found in Venezuela, Guiana and the West Indies, are employed in their native countries as spices.

The 'Bay Rum,' used as a toilet article, is a tincture scented with the oil of the leaves of an allied species, *P. acris*, commonly known as the Bayberry tree.

¶ *Adulterations.* Although ground Pimento is sometimes used to adulterate powdered cloves, it is itself little subject to adulteration in the entire condition, though the ground article for household consumption as a spice is subject to the same adulteration as other similar substances, it is sometimes adulterated with the larger and less aromatic berries of the Mexican *Myrtus Tobasco*, Mocino, called Pimienta de Tabasco.

At one time the fruit of the common American Spice Bush, 'Benzoin,' was used for this purpose. The powdered berries of this American plant, a member of the natural order *Lauraceæ, Lindera Benzoin*, occurring in damp woods throughout the Eastern and Central States, were used during the War of Independence by the Americans as a substitute for Allspice and its leaves as a substitute for tea, hence the plant was often called 'Wild Allspice.' All parts of the shrub have a spicy, agreeable flavour, which is strongest in the bark and berries. The leaves and berries are also used in decoction in domestic practice as a febrifuge and are considered to have tonic and also anthelmintic properties. A tincture prepared from the fresh young twigs before the buds have burst in the spring, is still used in homœopathy, but no preparation is employed officially.

The 'Carolina Allspice,' or Sweet Bush (*Calycanthis floridus*, Lindl.), is a shrub 6 to 8 feet high, which inhabits the low, shady woods along the mountains of Georgia and North Carolina and in Tennessee. The whole plant is aromatic, having the odour of strawberries when crushed.

It is asserted that the shrub is important as a source of poisoning to cattle and sheep. The alkaloid it contains exercises a powerfully depressant action upon the heart.

It has been used as an antiperiodic, in fluid extract.

ALMONDS

N.O. Rosaceæ

1. SWEET ALMOND	Amygdalus communis (LINN.) var. dulcis
2. BITTER ALMOND	Amygdalus communis (LINN.) var. amara

Habitat. The Almond tree is a native of the warmer parts of western Asia and of North Africa, but it has been extensively distributed over the warm temperate region of the Old World, and is cultivated in all the countries bordering on the Mediterranean. It was very early introduced into England, probably by the Romans, and occurs in the Anglo-Saxon lists of plants, but was not cultivated in England before 1562, and then chiefly for its blossom

¶ *History.* The tree has always been a favourite, and in Shakespeare's time, as Gerard tells us, Almond trees were 'in our London gardens and orchards in great plenty.' There are many references to it in our early poetry. Spenser alludes to it in the *Fairy Queen*:

'Like to an Almond tree ymounted hye,
On top of greene Selinis all alone,
With blossoms brave bedecked daintly;
Whose tender locks do tremble every one
At everie little breath that under Heaven is blowne.'

Shakespeare mentions it only once, very casually, in *Troilus and Cressida*: – 'The parrot will not do more for an Almond' – 'An Almond for a parrot' being an old simile in his days for the height of temptation.

The early English name seems to have been Almande: it thus appears in the *Romaunt of the Rose*. Both this old name and its more modern form came through the French *amande*, derived from the late Latin *amandela*, in turn a form of the Greek *amygdalus*, the meaning of which is obscure.

The tree grows freely in Syria and Palestine: it is mentioned in Scripture as one of the best fruit trees of the land of Canaan, and there are many other biblical references to it. The Hebrew name, *shakad*, is very expressive: it signifies 'hasty awakening,' or 'to watch for,' hence 'to make haste,' a fitting name for a tree, whose beautiful flowers appearing in Palestine in January, herald the wakening up of Creation. The rod of Aaron was an Almond twig, and the fruit of the Almond was one of the subjects selected for the decoration of the golden candlestick employed in the tabernacle. The Jews still carry rods of Almond blossom to the synagogues on great festivals.

As Almonds were reckoned among 'the best fruits of the land' in the time of Jacob, we may infer they were not then cultivated in Egypt. Pliny, however, mentions the Almond among Egyptian fruit-trees; and it is not improbable that it was introduced between the days of Jacob and the period of the Exodus.

Almonds, as well as the oil pressed from them, were well known in Greece and Italy long before the Christian era. A beautiful fable in Greek mythology is associated with the tree. Servius relates that Phyllis was changed by the gods into an Almond tree, as an eternal compensation for her desertion by her lover Demophoon, which caused her death by grief. When too late, Demophoon returned, and when the leafless, flowerless and forlorn tree was shown him, as the memorial of Phyllis, he clasped it in his arms, whereupon it burst forth into bloom – an emblem of true love inextinguishable by death.

During the Middle Ages, Almonds became an important article of commerce in Central Europe. Their consumption in mediæval cookery was enormous. An inventory, made in 1372, of the effects of Jeanne d'Evreux, Queen of France, enumerates only 20 lb. of sugar, but 500 lb. of Almonds.

The ancients attributed many wonderful virtues to the Almond, but it was chiefly valued for its supposed virtue in preventing intoxication. Plutarch mentions a great drinker of wine, who by the use of Bitter Almonds escaped being intoxicated, and Gerard says: 'Five or six, being taken fasting, do keepe a man from being drunke.' This theory was probably the origin of the custom of eating salted Almonds through a dinner.

¶ *Description.* The Almond belongs to the same group of plants as the rose, plum, cherry and peach, being a member of the tribe *Prunæ* of the natural order *Rosaceæ*. The genus *Amygdalus* to which it is assigned, is very closely allied to *Prunus* (Plum) in which it has sometimes been merged; the distinction lies in the fruit, the succulent pulp attached to the stone in the plum (known botanically as the mesocarp) being replaced by a leathery separable coat in the almond, which is hard and juiceless, of a dingy green tinged with dull red, so that when growing it looks not unlike an unripe apricot. When fully ripe, this green covering dries and splits, and the Almond, enclosed in its rough shell (termed the endocarp) drops out. The shell of the Almond is a yellowish buff colour and flattened-ovoid in shape, the outer surface being usually pitted with small holes; frequently it has a more or less fibrous nature. Sometimes it is thin and friable (soft-shelled Almond), sometimes extremely hard and woody (hard-shelled Almond). The seed itself is rounded at one end and pointed at the other, and covered with a thin, brown, scurfy coat. The different sorts of Almonds vary in form and size, as well as in the firmness of the shell. The fruit is produced chiefly on the young wood of the previous year, and in part on small spurs of two and three years growth.

The tree is of moderate size, usually from 20 to 30 feet high, with spreading branches, the leaves lance-shaped, finely toothed (or serrated) at the edges. The flowers are produced before the leaves – in this country early in March – and in great profusion. There are two principal forms of the Almond, the one with entirely pink flowers, *Amygdalus communis*, var. *dulcis*, producing Sweet Almonds; the other, *A. communis*, var. *amara*, with flowers slightly larger, and the petals almost white towards the tips, deepening into rose at the base, producing Bitter Almonds. Botanically, they are considered merely variations of the one type, and the difference in variety has been supposed originally to be mainly owing to climate, the Bitter Almond being a native of Barbary. The Sweet Almond is the earliest to flower, and is cultivated more largely than the Bitter Almond. It is valuable as a food and for confectionery purposes, as well as in medicine, being rich in a bland oil, and sustaining as a nutriment:

the staying power conferred by a meal of Almonds and raisins is well known. It is only the Bitter Almond in the use of which caution is necessary, especially with regard to children, as it possesses dangerous poisonous properties.

¶ *Cultivation*. The early, delicate flowers of the Almond give it a unique position among ornamental trees, and it should have a place in every shrubbery, for it will flourish in any ordinary, well-drained soil, both in open and somewhat sheltered situations, and does well in town gardens.

There are several varieties, differing in colour and size of the flowers: one dwarf variety, *A. nana*, a native of the Lower Danube, is especially decorative, and is often planted in the forefront of shrubberies. All the species are deciduous.

Sicily and 'Southern Italy are the chief Almond-producing countries; Spain, Portugal, the South of France, the Balearic Islands and Morocco also export considerable quantities.

In the southern counties of England it is not uncommon for the tree to produce a fair crop of fruit, though it is mostly very inferior to that which is imported, but in less favoured districts in this country the production of fruit is rare.

The tree is liable to destruction by frosts in many parts of Central Europe. In France and Belgium, when grown in gardens for its fruit, the tender-shelled varieties are preferred, and the cultivation is the same as for the peach.

SWEET ALMOND. There are numerous varieties of the Sweet Almond in commerce, the chief being: (1) the Jordan Almonds, the finest and best of the Sweet variety. These, notwithstanding their Oriental name (derived really from the French *jardin*), we receive from Malaga, imported without their shells. They are distinguished from all other Almonds by their large size, narrow, elongated shape and thin skin; (2) Valentia Almonds, which are broader and shorter than the Jordan variety, with a thicker dusty brown, scurfy skin, usually imported in their shell, and sometimes called in consequence, 'Shell Almonds'; (3) and (4) Sicilian and Barbary Almonds, which closely resemble the Valentia Almonds, but are rather smaller and of an inferior quality. They occasionally contain an admixture of Bitter Almonds.

The annual import of Sweet Almonds into this country is normally over 500 tons.

Sweet Almonds have a bland taste, and the white emulsion formed when they are bruised with water is characterized by no marked odour, the seeds being thus distinguished from Bitter Almonds.

¶ *Medicinal Action and Uses*. Fresh Sweet Almonds possess demulcent and nutrient properties, but as the outer brown skin sometimes causes irritation of the alimentary canal, they are blanched by removal of this skin when used for food. Though pleasant to the taste, their nutritive value is diminished unless well masticated, as they are difficult of digestion, and may in some cases induce nettlerash and feverishness. They have a special dietetic value, for besides containing about 20 per cent. of proteids, they contain practically no starch, and are therefore often made into flour for cakes and biscuits for patients suffering from diabetes.

Sweet Almonds are used medicinally, the official preparations of the British Pharmacopœia being Mistura Amygdalæ, Pulvis Amygdalæ Compositus and Almond Oil.

On expression they yield nearly half their weight in a bland fixed oil, which is employed medicinally for allaying acrid juices, softening and relaxing solids, and in bronchial diseases, in tickling coughs, hoarseness, costiveness, nephritic pains, etc.

When Almonds are pounded in water, the oil unites with the fluid, forming a milky juice – Almond Milk – a cooling, pleasant drink, which is prescribed as a diluent in acute diseases, and as a substitute for animal milk: an ounce of Almonds is sufficient for a quart of water, to which gum arabic is in most cases a useful addition. The pure oil mixed with a thick mucilage of gum arabic, forms a more permanent emulsion; one part of gum with an equal quantity of water being enough for four parts of oil. Almond emulsions possess in a certain degree the emollient qualities of the oil, and have this advantage over the pure oil, that they may be given in acute or inflammatory disorders without danger of the ill effects which the oil might sometimes produce by turning rancid. Sweet Almonds alone are employed in making emulsions, as the Bitter Almond imparts its peculiar taste when treated in this way.

Blanched and beaten into an emulsion with barley-water, Sweet Almonds are of great use in the stone, gravel, strangury and other disorders of the kidneys, bladder and biliary ducts.

By their oily character, Sweet Almonds sometimes give immediate relief in heartburn. For this, it is recommended to peel and eat six or eight Almonds.

Almonds are also useful in medicine for uniting substances with water. Castor oil is rendered palatable when rubbed up with pounded Almonds and some aromatic distilled water.

The fixed *Oil of Almonds* is extracted from

both Bitter and Sweet Almonds. If intended for external use, it must, however, be prepared only from Sweet Almonds.

The seeds are ground in a mill after removing the reddish-brown powder adhering to them and then subjected to hydraulic pressure, the expressed oil being afterwards filtered and bleached, preferably by exposure to light.

¶ *Constituents.* Almond oil is a clear, pale yellow, odourless liquid, with a bland, nutty taste. It consists chiefly of Olein, with a small proportion of the Glyceride of Linolic Acid and other Glycerides, but contains no Stearin. It is thus very similar in composition to Olive Oil (for which it may be used as a pleasant substitute), but it is devoid of Chlorophyll, and usually contains a somewhat larger proportion of Olein than Olive Oil.

It is used in trade, as well as medicinally, being most valuable as a lubricant for the delicate works of watches, and is much employed as an ingredient in toilet soap, for its softening action on the skin. It forms a good remedy for chapped hands.

Gerard says:

'The oil newly pressed out of Sweet Almonds is a mitigator of pain and all manner of aches, therefore it is good in pleurisy and colic. The oil of Almonds makes smooth the hands and face of delicate persons, and cleanseth the skin from all spots and pimples.'

And Culpepper writes:

'The oil of both (Bitter and Sweet) cleanses the skin, it easeth pains of the chest, the temples being annointed therewith, and the oil with honey, powder of liquorice, oil of roses and white wax, makes a good ointment for dimness of sight.'

Culpepper also tells us of Almond butter, saying:

'This kind of butter is made of Almonds with sugar and rose-water, which being eaten with violets is very wholesome and commodious for students, for it rejoiceth the heart and comforteth the brain, and qualifieth the heat of the liver.'

BITTER ALMOND. There are several varieties of the Bitter Almond, the best being imported from the south of France, and others from Sicily and Northern Africa (Barbary), where it forms a staple article of trade. The annual imports of Bitter Almonds to this country amount normally to about 300 tons.

The seeds are used chiefly as a source of Almond Oil, but also yield a volatile oil, which is largely employed as a flavouring agent.

Bitter Almonds are usually shorter, proportionately broader and smaller, and less regular than the Sweet Almonds. They contain about 50 per cent. of the same fixed oil which occurs in the Sweet Almond, and are also free from starch. The bitter taste is characteristic.

¶ *Constituents.* The Bitter Almond differs from the Sweet Almond in containing a colourless, crystalline glucoside, Amygdalin, of which the Sweet are entirely destitute. This substance is left in the cake obtained after the oil has been expressed, and can be extracted from it by digestion with alcohol. Many other Rosaceous plants contain Amygdalin, such as the peach, apricot, plum, etc., not only in the seed, but also in the young shoots and flower-buds.

The Bitter Almond seed also contains a ferment Emulsin, which in presence of water acts on the soluble glucoside Amygdalin, yielding glucose, prussic acid and the essential oil of Bitter Almonds, or Benzaldehyde, which is not used in medicine. Bitter Almonds yield from 6 to 8 per cent. of Prussic Acid. About 5 lb. of the seeds yield on the average half an ounce of the essential oil.

The term 'prussic acid' owes its origin to the fact of its having been first obtained from Prussian blue. This acid is contained in small quantities in the leaves and seeds of some of our commonest fruits, especially in apple-pips. While it is a valuable remedy for some diseases, it is also a deadly poison and its action is extremely rapid.

The leaves of the Cherry-laurel (*Prunus lauro-cerasus*) owe their activity to the prussic acid they contain. The laurel water made by distillation is a dangerous poison, and is so variable in strength, that it is unsuited for administration as a medicinal agent. Several fatal cases have occurred from its injudicious use.

The once famous 'Macassor Oil' consisted chiefly of Oil of Almonds, coloured red with Alkanet root, and scented with Oil of Cassia.

This essential volatile oil of Bitter Almonds, under the name of 'Almond flavouring' and 'Spirit of Almonds,' is used in confectionery and as a culinary flavouring, but on account of its poisonous nature, great care ought to be exercised in its use, and for the same reason, Bitter Almonds and ratifia biscuits and Marchpane (made largely of Bitter Almonds) should be eaten sparingly.

Bitter Almonds and their poisonous properties were well known to the ancients, who used them in intermittent fevers and as a vermifuge, and they were also employed by them, and in the Middle Ages as an aperient and diuretic, and as a cure for hydrophobia, but from the uncertainty of their operation and the risk attending it, we seldom see them administered now. Taken freely in substance they occasion sickness and vomiting, and to dogs, birds and some other animals, they are poisonous. A simple water, strongly impregnated by distillation with the volatile oil, will cause giddiness, headache and dimness of sight, and has been found also poisonous to animals, and there are instances of cordial spirits flavoured by them being poisonous to man.

Of the several varieties under which they exist, none in size and form resembles the long, sweet Jordan Almond, and it is to avoid Bitter Almonds being used instead of Sweet, that the British Pharmacopœia directs that Jordan Almonds alone shall be employed when Sweet Almonds are used medicinally.

Culpepper says that Bitter Almonds

'do make thin and open, they remove stoppings out of the liver and spleen, therefore they be good against pain in the sides. . . . The same doth likewise kill tetters in the outward parts of the body (as Dioscorides addeth) if it be dissolved in vinegar.'

He also tells us that mixed with honey, these Almonds 'are good for bitings of a mad dog.'

¶ *Adulterations and Substitutes.* The adulteration of Bitter Almonds with Sweet Almonds is a frequent source of loss and annoyance to the pressers of Almond Oil, whose profit largely depends on the amount of volatile oil they are able to extract from the residual cake.

Apricot and peach kernels contain constituents similar to those of the Bitter Almonds. They are imported in large quantities from Syria and California, and are often used by confectioners in the place of Bitter Almonds.[1]

The fixed oil expressed from them is known as Peach Kernel Oil (*Ol. Amygdæ Pers.*). From the cake, an essential oil is distilled (*Ol. Amygdæ Essent. Pers.*), as from Bitter Almond cake.

True Oil of Almonds is frequently distinguished from these by being described as 'English,' since the bulk of it has hitherto been pressed in this country. The kernels of the peach and apricot are with difficulty distinguished from those of the Almond, and the oils obtained from them closely resemble the so-called English, and much more expensive oil.

To make Almond Cake (Seventeenth Century)

'Take one pound of Jordan almonds, Blanch ym into cold water, and dry ym in a clean cloth: pick out these that are nought and rotten: then beat ym very fine in a stone mortar, puting in now and then a little rose water to keep ym from oyling: then put it out into a platter, and half a pound of loaf sugar beaten fine and mixt with ye almonds, ye back of a spoon, and set it on a chafing dish of coals, and let it stand till it be hott: and when it is cold then have ready six whites of eggs beaten with too spoonfuls of flower to a froth, and mix it well with ye almonds: bake ym on catt paper first done over with a feather dipt in sallet oyle.'

Almond Butter (Seventeenth Century)

'Seeth a little French Barly with a whole mace and some anniseeds to sweeten but not to give any sensible tast: then blanch and beat the almonds with some of the clearest of the liquor to make the milke the thicker, and strain them, getting forth by often beating what milk you can: seeth the milke till it thicken and bee ready to rise, and turne it with the juice of a lemon or salt dissolved in rose water: spread the curd on a linnen cloath that the whey may run out, and let it hang till it leave dropping: then season the butter that is left with rose water, and sugar to your liking.'

This is a seventeenth-century recipe for *Almond Milk*:

To make Almond Milk

'Take 3 pints of running water, a handfull of Raisins of the Sun stoned, halfe a handfull of Sorrell, as much violet and strawberry leaves, halfe a handfull of the topps and flowers of burrage (borage), as much of Buglass, halfe a handfull of Endive, as much Succory, some Pauncys (Pansies), a little broad time and Orgamen (Marjoram), and a branch or two of Rosemary; lett all these boyle well together; then take a good handfull of French Barley, boyling it in three waters, put it to the rest, and lett them boyle till you think they are enough; then pour the liquor into a basin, and stampe the barley and reasons, straining them thereto; then take a quarter of a pound of Sweet Almonds, blanch them and pound them thrice, straining them to the other liquor; then season it with damask rosewater to your liking.'

[1] A very large proportion of the so-called ground Almonds sold are prepared from peach kernels, and this is the reason why in good cookery the whole Almonds are used, though the pounding is a long and tedious business.–EDITOR

A seventeenth-century recipe:

A Paste for ye Hands

'Take a pound of sun raysens, stone and take a pound of bitter Almonds, blanch ym and beat ym in stone morter, with a glass of sack take ye peel of one Lemond, boyle it tender; take a quart of milk, and a pint of Ale, and make therewith a Possett; take all ye Curd and putt it to ye Almonds: yn putt in ye Rayson: Beat all these till they come to a fine Past, and putt in a pott, and keep it for ye use.'

ALOES

Aloe Perryi (J. G. BAKER)
Aloe vera (LINN).
N.O. Liliaceæ

Part Used. Leaves

Habitat. Aloes are indigenous to East and South Africa, but have been introduced into the West Indies (where they are extensively cultivated) and into tropical countries, and will even flourish in the countries bordering on the Mediterranean

The drug *Aloes* consists of the liquid exuded from the transversely-cut bases of the leaves of various species of Aloes, evaporated to dryness.

¶ *Description*. They are succulent plants, belonging to the Lily family, with perennial, strong and fibrous roots and numerous, persistent, fleshy leaves, proceeding from the upper part of the root, narrow, tapering, thick and fleshy, usually beset at the edges with spiney teeth. Many of the species are woody and branching. In the remote districts of S.W. Africa and in Natal, Aloes have been discovered 30 to 60 feet in height, with stems as much as 10 feet in circumference.

The flowers are produced in erect, terminal spikes. There is no calyx, the corolla is tubular, divided into six narrow segments at the mouth and of a red, yellow or purplish colour. The capsules contain numerous angular seeds.

The true Aloe is in flower during the greater part of the year and is not to be confounded with another plant, the *Agave* or American Aloe (*Agave Americana*), which is remarkable for the long interval between its periods of flowering. This is a succulent plant, without stem, the leaves being radical, spiney, and toothed. There is a variety with variegated foliage. The flower-stalk rises to many feet in height, bearing a number of large and handsome flowers. In cold climates there is usually a very long interval between the times of its flowering, though it is a popular error to suppose that it happens only once in a hundred years, for when it obtains sufficient heat and receives a culture similar to that of the pineapple, it is found to flower much more frequently. Various species of Agave, all of which closely resemble each other, have been largely grown as ornamental plants since the first half of the sixteenth century in the south of Europe, and are completely acclimatized in Spain, Portugal and Southern Italy, but though often popularly called Aloes, all of them are plants of the New World, whereas the true Aloes are natives of the Old World. From a chemical point of view there is also no analogy at all between Aloes and Agaves.

Although the Agave is not employed medicinally, the leaves have been used in Jamaica as a substitute for soap, the expressed juice (a gallon of the juice yields about 1 lb. of the soft extract), dried in the sun, being made into balls with wood ash. This soap lathers with salt water as well as fresh. The leaves have also been used for scouring pewter and kitchen utensils. The inner spongy substance of the leaves in a decayed state has been employed as tinder and the fibres may be spun into a strong, useful thread.

The fleshy leaves of the true *Aloe* contain near the epidermis or outer skin, a row of fibrovascular bundles, the cells of which are much enlarged and filled with a yellow juice which exudes when the leaf is cut. When it is desired to collect the juice, the leaves are cut off close to the stem and so placed that the juice is drained off into tubs. This juice thus collected is concentrated either by spontaneous evaporation, or more generally by boiling until it becomes of the consistency of thick honey. On cooling, it is then poured into gourds, boxes, or other convenient receptacles, and solidifies.

Aloes require two or three years' standing before they yield their juice. In the West Indian Aloe plantations they are set out in rows like cabbages and cutting takes place in March or April, but in Africa the drug is collected from the wild plants.

¶ *Constituents*. The most important constituents of Aloes are the two Aloins, Barbaloin and Isobarbaloin, which constitute the so-called 'crystalline' Aloin, present in the drug at from 10 to 30 per cent. Other constituents are amorphous Aloin, resin and Aloe-emodin. The proportion in which the Aloins are present in the respective Aloes is not accurately known.

The manner in which the evaporation is conducted has a marked effect on the appearance of the Aloes, slow and moderate concentration tending to induce crystallization of the Aloin, thus causing the drug to appear opaque. Such Aloes is termed 'livery' or hepatic, and splinters of it exhibit minute crystals of Aloin when examined under the microscope. If, on the other hand, the evaporation is carried as far as possible, the Aloin does not crystallize and small fragments of the drug appear transparent; it is then termed 'glassy,' 'vitreous,' or 'lucid' Aloes and exhibits no crystals of Aloin under the microscope.

¶ *Varieties*. The chief varieties of Aloes are Curacao or Barbados, Socotrine (including Zanzibar) and Cape. Other varieties of Aloes, such as black 'Mocha' Aloes, occasionally find their way to the London market. *Jafferabad* Aloes, supposed to be the same as 'Mocha' Aloes, is of a black, pitch-like colour and a glassy, somewhat porous fracture; it is the product of *Aloe Abyssinica* and is imported to Bombay from Arabia. It does not enter into English commerce. *Musambra* Aloes is made in India from *A. vulgaris*. *Uganda* Aloes, imported from Mossel Bay, not from Uganda, is a variety of Cape Aloes produced by careful evaporation. *Natal* Aloes, another South African variety, is no longer a commercial article in this country. The *A. Purificata* of the United States Pharmacopœia is prepared by adding Alcohol to melted Aloes, stirring thoroughly, straining and evaporating the strained liquid. The product occurs in irregular, brittle, dull-brown or reddish pieces and is almost entirely soluble in Alcohol.

Curacoa Aloes is obtained from *A. chinensis* (Staud.) *A. vera* (Linn.) and probably other species. It was formerly produced on the island of Barbados, where it was largely cultivated, having been introduced at the beginning of the sixteenth century, and is still frequently, but improperly called *Barbados Aloes*. It is now almost entirely made on the Dutch islands of Curacoa, Aruba and Bonaire by boiling the Aloe juice down and pouring the viscid residue into empty spirit cases, in which it is allowed to solidify. Formerly gourds of various sizes were used (usually containing from 60 to 70 lb.) but Aloes in gourds is now seldom seen. It is usually opaque and varies in colour from bright yellowish or rich reddish brown to black. Sometimes it is vitreous and small fragments are then of a deep garnet-red colour and transparent. It is then known as 'Capey Barbados' and is less valuable, but may become opaque and more valuable by keeping. Curacoa Aloes possesses the nauseous and bitter taste that is characteristic of all Aloes and a disagreeable, penetrating odour. It is almost entirely soluble in 60 per cent. alcohol and contains not more than 30 per cent. of substances insoluble in water and 12 per cent. of moisture. It should not yield more than 3 per cent. of ash.

Commercial Aloin is obtained usually from Curacoa Aloes.

Solutions of Curacoa and other Aloes gradually undergo change, and may after a month no longer react normally, and may also lose the bitterness natural to Aloes.

Socotrine Aloes is prepared to a certain extent on the island of Socotra, but probably more largely on the African and possibly also on the Arabian mainland, from the leaves of *A. Perryi* (Baker). It is usually imported in kegs in a pasty condition and subsequent drying is necessary. It may be distinguished principally from Curacoa Aloes by its different odour. Much of the dry drug is characterized by the presence of small cavities in the fractured surface, but the variety of Socotrine Aloes distinguished as *Zanzibar Aloes* often very closely resembles Curacoa in appearance and is usually imported in liver-brown masses which break with a dull, waxy fracture, differing from that of Socotrine Aloes in being nearly smooth and even. When it is prepared, it is commonly poured into goat skins, which are then packed into cases.

¶ *Constituents*. The name 'Socotrine' Aloes is officially applied to both Socotrine and Zanzibar Aloes. Its chief constituents are Barbaloin (formerly called Socaloin and Zanaloin) and B. Barbaloin, no Isobarbaloin being present in this variety of Aloes. Resin, water-soluble substances other than Aloin and Aloe-emodin are also present.

Socotrine Aloes should be of a dark, reddish-brown colour, and almost entirely soluble in alcohol. Not more than 50 per cent. should be insoluble in water and it should yield not more than 3 per cent. of ash. Garnet-coloured, translucent Socotrine Aloes is not now found in commerce, though fine qualities of Zanzibar Aloes are sometimes slightly translucent. Samples of the drug which are nearly black are unfit for pharmaceutical purposes. The odour of Zanzibar Aloes is strong and characteristic, and its taste nauseous and bitter.

Cape Aloes is prepared in Cape Colony from *A. ferou* (Linn.), *A. spicata* (Thumb.) *A. Africana*, *A. platylepia* and other species of Aloe. It possesses more powerfully purgative properties than any other variety of the drug and is preferred to other varieties on the Continent, but is chiefly employed in this country for veterinary purposes only, though for this purpose the Curacoa Aloes is as a rule preferred. Another form of the drug used for veterinary purposes, called *Caballine* or *Horse Aloes*, usually consists of the residue from the purification of the more valuable sorts.

Cape Aloes almost invariably occurs in the vitreous modification; it forms dark coloured masses which break with a clean, glassy fracture and exhibit in their splinters a yellowish, reddish-brown or greenish tinge. Its translucent, glossy appearance and very characteristic, red-currant like odour sufficiently distinguish it from all other varieties of Aloes.

Uganda Aloes is also obtained from *A. ferox*. It occurs in bricks or fragments of hepatic, yellowish-brown colour, with a bronze gold fracture and its odour resembles that of Cape Aloes.

Cape Aloes contains 9 per cent. or more of Barbaloin (formerly known as Capaloin) and *B*. Barbaloin. Only traces of Capalores not annol combined with paracumaric acid. Cape Aloes should not contain more than 12 per cent. of water; it should yield at least 45 per cent. of aquoeus extract but not more than 2 per cent. of ash. Uganda Aloes yields about 6 per cent. of Aloin, part of which is *B*. Barbaloin. The leaves of the plants from which Cape Aloes is obtained are cut off near the stem and arranged around a hole in the ground, in which a sheepskin is spread, with smooth side upwards. When a sufficient quantity of juice has drained from the leaves it is concentrated by heat in iron cauldrons and subsequently poured into boxes or skins in which it solidifies on cooling. Large quantities of the drug are exported from Cape Town and Mossel Bay.

Natal Aloes. The source of this variety, which is seldom imported, is not yet definitely ascertained, but it is probably prepared from one or more species of Aloe, probably including *A. ferox*. Natal Aloes is prepared with greater care than Cape Aloes, the leaves being cut obliquely into slices and the juice allowed to exude in the hot sunshine, after which it is boiled down in iron pots, the liquid being stirred until it becomes thick and then poured into wooden cases to solidify. Natal Aloes is much weaker than any other variety, having little purgative action on human beings, apparently because it contains no Emodin. It is no longer of commercial importance. It resembles Cape Aloes in odour and occurs in irregular pieces, which are almost always opaque and have a characteristic, dull greenish-black or brown colour. It is much less soluble than Cape Aloes. It has not a glassy fracture like that of Cape Aloes and when powdered is of a greenish colour.

Good Aloes should yield 40 per cent. of soluble matter to cold water.

Both Curacoa and Cape Aloes in powder give a crimson colour with nitric acid; Socratine Aloes powder touched with nitric acid does *not* give a crimson colour.

¶ *History.* The Mahometans, especially those in Egypt, regard the Aloe as a religious symbol, and the Mussulman who has made a pilgrimage to the shrine of the Prophet is entitled to hang the Aloe over his doorway. The Mahometans also believe that this holy symbol protects a householder from any malign influence.

In Cairo, the Jews also adopt the practice of hanging up the Aloe.

In the neighbourhood of Mecca, at the extremity of every grave, on a spot facing the epitaph, Burckhardt found planted a low shrubby species of Aloe whose Arabic name, *saber*, signifies *patience*. This plant is evergreen and requires very little water. Its name refers to the waiting-time between the burial and the resurrection morning.

All kinds of Aloes are admirably provided by their succulent leaves and stems against the drought of the countries where they flourish. The cuticle which covers every part of the plant is, in those which contain a great quantity of pulpy material, formed so as to imbibe moisture very easily and to evaporate it very slowly. If the leaf of an Aloe be separated from the parent plant, it may be laid in the sun for several weeks without becoming entirely shrivelled; and even when considerably dried by long exposure to heat, it will, if plunged into water, become in a few hours plump and fresh.

¶ *Medicinal Action and Uses.* The drug Aloes is one of the safest and best warm and stimulating purgatives to persons of sedentary habits and phlegmatic constitutions. An ordinary small dose takes from 15 to 18 hours to produce an effect. Its action is exerted mainly on the large intestine, for which reason, also it is useful as a vermifuge. Its use, however, is said to induce Piles.

From the *Chemist and Druggist* (July 22, 1922):

'*Aloes*, strychnine and belladonna in pill form was criticized by Dr. Bernard Fautus in a paper read before the Chicago branch of the American Pharmaceutical Society. He pointed out that when given at the same time they cannot possibly act together because of the different speed and duration of the three agents. *Aloin is slow in action*, requiring from 10 to 12 hours. Strychnine and Atropine, on the other hand, are rapidly absorbed, and have but a brief duration of action.'

Preparations of Aloes are rarely prescribed alone; they require the addition of carminatives to moderate the tendency to griping. The compound preparations of Aloes in use generally contain such correctives, but powdered Aloes and the extracts of Aloes represent the crude drug.

Aloes in one form or another is the commonest domestic medicine and is the basis of most proprietary or so-called 'patent' pills.

There is little to choose medicinally between the Curacoa and Socotrine varieties, but the former is somewhat more powerful, 2 grains of Curacoa Aloes being equal to 3 grains of Socotrine Aloes in purgative action. The latter is more expensive, but varies much in quality.

Aloes is the purgative in general uses for horses; it is also used in veterinary practice as a bitter tonic in small doses, and externally as a stimulant and desiccant.

Aloes was employed by the ancients and was known to the Greeks as a production of the island of Socotra as early as the fourth century B.C. The drug was used by Dioscorides, Celsus and Pliny, as well as by the later Greek and Arabian physicians, though it is not mentioned either by Hippocrates or Theophrastus.

From notices of it in the Anglo-Saxon leech-books and a reference to it as one of the drugs recommended to Alfred the Great by the Patriarch of Jerusalem, we may infer that its use was not unknown in Britain as early as the tenth century. At this period the drug was imported into Europe by way of the Red Sea and Alexandria. In the early part of the seventeenth century, there was a direct trade in Aloes between England and Socotra, and in the records of the East Indian Company there are notices of the drug being bought of the King of Socotra, the produce being a monopoly of the Sultan of the island.

The word Aloes, in Latin *Lignum Aloes*, is used in the Bible and in many ancient writings to designate a substance totally distinct from the modern Aloes, namely the resinous wood of *Aquilaria agallocha*, a large tree growing in the Malayan Peninsula. Its wood constituted a drug which was, down to the beginning of the present century, generally valued for use as incense, but now is esteemed only in the East.

A beautiful violet colour is afforded by the leaves of the Socotrine Aloe, and it does not require a mordant to fix it.

¶ *Preparations.* Fluid extract: dose, 5 to 30 drops. Powdered extract: dose, 1 to 5 grains. Comp decoc., B.P.: dose, ½ to 2 oz. Tincture B.P.: dose, ¼ to 2 drachms. Tincture aloes myrrh, U.S.P.: dose, 30 drops.

ALSTONIA

Alstonia scholaris (R. BR.)
N.O. Apocynaceæ

Synonyms. Echites scholaris (Linn.). Dita Bark. Bitter Bark. Devil Tree. Pale Mara
Part Used. The bark
Habitat. India and the Philippines

¶ *Description.* The tree grows from 50 to 80 feet high, has a furrowed trunk, oblong stalked leaves up to 6 inches long and 4 inches wide, dispersed in four to six whorls round the stem, their upper side glossy, under side white, nerves running at right angles to the mid-rib. The bark is almost odourless and very bitter, in commerce it is found in irregular fragments ⅛ to ½ inch thick, texture spongy, fracture coarse and short, outside layer rough uneven fissured brownish grey and sometimes blackish spots; inside layer bright buff, transverse section shows a number of small medullary rays in inner layer.

¶ *Constituents.* It contains three alkaloids, Ditamine, Echitamine or Ditaine, and Echitenines, and several fatty and resinous substances; the second is the strongest base and resembles ammonia in chemical characters.

¶ *Medicinal Action and Uses.* The bark is used in homœopathy for its tonic bitter and astringent properties; it is particularly useful for chronic diarrhœa and dysentry.

¶ *Preparations and Dosages.* Infusion of Alstonia, 5 parts to 100 parts water. Dose, 1 fluid ounce. Powdered bark, 2 to 4 grains.

In India the natives use the bark for bowel complaints. In Ceylon its light wood is used for coffins. In Borneo the wood close to the root of the same species is very light and of white colour and is used for net floats, household utensils, trenchers, corks, etc.

¶ *Other Species.* A bark called Poele is obtained from *Alstonia spectabilis*, habitat Java; it contains the same alkaloids as dita and an additional crystalline, Alstonamine.

ALSTONIA BARK
Alstonia constricta (F. MUELL.)
N.O. Apocynaceæ

Synonyms. Fever Bark. Australian Quinine
Part Used. The dried bark
Habitat. New South Wales and Australia

¶ *Description*. The name is derived from Alston, a professor of botany in Edinburgh. In commerce the bark is usually in curved pieces or quills 2½ inches wide and ½ inch thick. Periderm $\frac{1}{10}$ to ¼ of an inch; rusty brown, rugose, deeply fissured recticulations; internally the bark is cinnamon brown with strong coarse longitudinal stripes. Transverse section shows dark brown periderm covering the inner orange-brown tissues. Fracture short granular in outer layers and fibrous inner ones, slight aromatic odour, very bitter taste.

¶ *Constituents*. Contains three alkaloids, Alstonine, Porphrine and Astonidine, and traces of others.

¶ *Medicinal Action and Uses*. Used for chronic diarrhœa, dysentery and in intermittent fever; also as an anthelmintic. Scientific investigation has failed to show why it is of such service in malaria, but herbalists consider it superior to quinine and of great use in convalescence, also much used by homœopaths.

¶ *Preparations and Dosages*. Powdered bark, 2 to 8 grains. Fluid extract, 4 to 40 minims.

AMARANTHS
Amaranthus hypochondriacus (LINN.)
N.O. Amaranthaceæ

Synonyms. Love-Lies-Bleeding. Red Cockscomb. Velvet Flower
Habitat. The Amaranths are met with most abundantly in the tropics, especially in tropical America, but are not plentiful in cold countries.

Many species are widely distributed as pernicious weeds. Their economic importance is slight, their properties chiefly proteid nutrient. Many abound in mucilage and sugar and many species are used as pot-herbs, resembling those of *Chenopodiaceæ*. Many, also, are excellent fodder-plants, though not cultivated.

¶ *Constituents*. Their constituents are indefinite; none are poisonous; none possess very distinct medicinal properties, though many have use in native practice as alteratives, and as antidotes to snake-bite, etc.

¶ *Medical Action and Uses*. Some species have slightly astringent properties, others are diaphoretics and diuretics, and a few are tonics and stimulants.

In ancient Greece, the Amaranth was sacred to Ephesian Artemis: it was supposed to have special healing properties and as a symbol of immortality was used to decorate images of the gods and tombs. The name, from the Greek signifying *unwithering*, was applied to certain plants which from their lasting for ever, typified immortality.

Some of the species are old favourites as garden flowers, viz., *Amaranthus hypochondriacus*, known as Prince's Feather, an Indian annual – with deeply-veined, lance-shaped leaves, purple on the under side with deep crimson flowers, densely packed on erect spikes, and *A. caudatus* (Jacq.) (Love-lies-bleeding), a native of Africa and Java, a vigorous hardy annual with dark purplish flowers crowded in handsome drooping spikes. It is considered astringent and a decoction of the flowers has been administered in spitting of blood and various hæmorrhages and has been said to be so energetic that it may be used in cases of menorrhagia. With several other species belonging to the closely allied genus *Ærva*, natives of India, it has also been used as an anthelmintic.

A. spinosa (Linn.), *A. campestris* (Willd.) and many others are used in India as diuretics. *A. oleraceus* (Linn.) is used in India in diarrhœa and menstrual disorders and the young leaves and shoots are also eaten as a vegetable, similarly to spinach. *A. polygonoides*, a common garden weed in India, is also used as a pot-herb and considered so wholesome that convalescents are ordered it in preference to all other kinds.

AMARANTH, WILD
Amaranthum blitum (LINN.)
N.O. Amaranthaceæ

Synonym. Strawberry Blite

Amaranthum blitum (Linn.), the wild Amaranth admitted to the list of British plants, is an inconspicuous weed, often mistaken for an Orache or Goosefoot, sometimes found on rubbish-heaps near towns and probably a remnant of ancient cultivation as a pot-herb.

It is an annual, with trailing stems a foot or two in length and more or less oval leaves with long stalks. The numerous green flowers are clustered in the angles between leaf and stem and are unisexual, without petals, both male and female flowers occurring on the same plant.

The female flower develops into a juicy, crimson capsule containing a single seed. The clusters of these fruits have in some localities suggested the name of Strawberry Blite for the plant.

It flowers in August.

In France, its leaves are still eaten in the same way as spinach.

Culpepper, speaking of the garden Amaranths and especially of the Love-lies-bleeding, which he calls Flower Gentle, Flower Velure, Floramor and Velvet flower, says:

'The flowers dried and beaten into powder stops the terms in women, and so do almost all other red things. And by the icon or image of every herb, the ancients at first found out their virtues. Modern writers laugh at them for it; but I wonder how the virtues of herbs came at first to be known, if not by their signatures; the moderns have them from the writings of the ancients; the ancients had no writings to have them from. – The flowers stop all fluxes of blood, whether in man or woman, bleeding either at the nose or wound.'

¶ *Medicinal Uses*. In modern herbal medicine, a fluid extract is employed, the dose being $\frac{1}{2}$ to 1 drachm, and also a decoction, taken in wineglassful doses, which is used externally as an application in ulcerated conditions of the throat and mouth and as an injection in leucorrhœa, and as a wash for ulcers, sores, etc. For its astringency it is much recommended in diarrhœa, dysentery and hæmorrhages from the bowels.

AMMONIACUM   Dorema ammoniacum (D. DON.)
                                      N.O. Umbelliferæ

Synonyms. Gum Ammoniac
Part Used. The gum resin exuding from the flowering and fruiting stem of *Dorema ammoniacum* and probably other species
Habitat. Persia, extending into Southern Siberia

¶ *Description*. The plant grows to height of about 7 feet and in spring and early summer contains a milky juice. It is visited by numbers of beetles which puncture the stem and thus cause an exudation, part of which dries on the stem, the rest falling to the ground where it becomes mixed with stones and other impurities found in the gum collected by the natives. The gum resin is found in special cavities in the tissues of the stem, root and petioles of the leaves. The name of the drug is said to be derived from the Temple of Jupiter Ammon in the Libyan Desert where it was collected by the ancients. The gum resin occurs in commerce in two forms, tear ammoniacum and lump or block ammoniacum. The former alone is official in England and consists of pale yellow nodular masses varying in size from a pea to a walnut, brittle when cold but softens on warming, fractured surface, milky white or pale brown in colour. The lump ammoniacum, which is that collected from the ground, is used sometimes but is not official in medicine. The odour of the drug is slight, taste acrid and persistent.

¶ *Constituents*. The drug contains volatile oil, resin and gum. The resin consists of an indifferent resene associated with ammoresinotannol combined with salicylic acid.

¶ *Medicinal Action and Uses*. Taken internally, it acts by facilitating expectoration and is of value in chronic bronchitis, especially in the aged when the secretion is tough and viscid. The resin has a mild diuretic action. It is antispasmodic and stimulant and is given sometimes as a diaphoretic and emmenagogue, used as a plaster for white swellings of the joints and for indolent tumours. Its use is of great antiquity and is mentioned by Hippocrates.

¶ *Preparations and Dosages*. Ammoniacum mixture, B.P.4 to 8 drachms. Ammoniacum in powder, 1 part; syrup of balsam of tolu, 2 parts; distilled water, 30 parts. Dose, $\frac{1}{2}$ to 1 fluid ounce. Dose of the powdered gum, 5 to 15 grains, B.P.C. Dose of the powdered gum, 10 to 30 grains, U.S.P.

¶ *Other Species*. African Ammoniacum or 'feshook,' from *Ferula Communis* is not a commercial article. The Mahommedans use if for incense; this variety grows well in the author's garden at Chalfont St. Peter.

ANCHUSA. *See* ALKANET

ANEMONES

N.O. Ranunculaceæ

The Anemones are represented in our native British flora by only two species, the dainty little Wood Anemone (*Anemone nemorosa*) and the Pasque Flower (*A. pulsatilla*), both possessing medicinal properties, though the former is little used now.

There are, however, about seventy species in the genus *Anemone*, including the subgenus *Hepatica*, now also reckoned as Anemones, though formerly ranking as a separate genus, the chief representative of which, *A. hepatica*, is of some considerable medicinal value. *A. pratensis*, a continental species, is employed medicinally for the same purposes as *A. pulsatilla*, and the number of species familiar to us as garden flowers is very great, the most popular among these being, perhaps, the Poppy or Garden Anemone, *A. coronavria* a native of the Levant and Southern Europe, introduced here in 1596, and the Star Anemone, *A. hortensis*, a native of Italy, brought to England from Holland about the same time. *A. apennina* and *A. blanda* are also particularly charming, the latter with large flowers of various shades of blue being the earliest to open.

¶ *Description*. The distinguishing characteristics of the genus Anemone are the presence of three entire leaflets arranged in a whorl just under the flowers, forming an involucre, and the fact that the flowers themselves have no real petals, but a calyx of six to eight petal-like sepals. All species share the acrid and bitter nature of almost all plants of the Ranunculus order to which they belong, and the leaves and flowers should not be eaten. The toxic principle has been extracted from three species: the two British species and one foreign one, though no actually fatal results have been recorded. A yellow-flowered foreign species, *A. ranunculoides*, found in almost all parts of the Continent, has been used for poisoning arrows, and in France, swelling and blistering of the hands has resulted from using the juice as a stimulant to ulceration.

¶ *Cultivation*. Anemones flourish best in a rich, sandy loam, but will thrive in any garden soil which is well-drained and tolerably light; it should also be enriched with decayed manure. Sea sand, or a little salt mixed with the soil is a good preventive of mildew.

Propagation is by division of the rootstocks and cuttings of the root in autumn and early spring – from October to the end of March – and also from seed, which should be sown within a month of ripening, as it deteriorates with keeping. Sow thinly in lines on the surface and merely rake the seeds in with a very light hand. Germination is slow. Thin the plants to 6 inches apart. Thinnings will bear transplanting if carefully handled and helped with water afterwards. The first flowers are generally produced the first spring after sowing, but soil and situation have always a great effect on them.

Some persons take up Anemone tubers as soon as the leaf has died down, and replant in the early part of the year, but this is not necessary: those that have been two or three years in the ground attain a large size – they are solid, flattened masses, not unlike ginger. When planting, cover with soil to the depth of 3 inches.

Most garden Anemones can be treated in this way. The best time for transplanting *A. pulsatilla* is considered. to be directly after it has flowered, or at any rate during the summer, while it is in growth; autumn is a bad time and early spring not much better.

ANEMONE PULSATILLA

Anemone pulsatilla (LINN.)
N.O. Ranunculaceæ

Synonyms. Pasque Flower. Wind Flower. Meadow Anemone. Passe Flower. Easter Flower

Part Used. Whole herb

Habitat. *Anemone pulsatilla* is found not in woods, but in open situations. It grows wild in the dry soils of almost every Central and Northern country of Europe, but in England is rather a local plant, abounding on high chalk downs and limestone pastures, mostly in Yorkshire, Berkshire, Oxford and Suffolk, but seldom found in other situations and other districts in this country

¶ *Description*. It has a thick and somewhat woody root-stock, from which arises a rosette of finely-divided, stalked leaves, covered with silky hairs, especially when young, the foot-stalk often being purplish.

The flowers, which are about 1½ inches across, are borne singly on stalks 5 to 8 inches in height, with an involucre of three sessile (i.e. stalkless) deeply-cut leaflets or bracts. The sepals are of a dull violet-purple colour,

32

very silky on the under surfaces. The seed-vessels are small, brown hairy achenes, with long, feathery tails, like those of the Travel-ler's Joy or Wild Clematis.

The whole plant, especially the bases of the foot-stalks, is covered with silky hairs. It is odourless, but possesses at first a very acrid taste, which is less conspicuous in the dried herb and gradually diminishes on keeping. The majority of the leaves devel-op after the flowers; they are two to three times deeply three-parted or pinnately cleft to the base, in long, linear, acute segments.

The juice of the purple sepals gives a green stain to paper and linen, but it is not per-manent. It has been used to colour the Paschal eggs in some countries, whence it has been supposed the English name of the plant is derived. Gerard, however, expressly in-forms us that he himself was 'moved to name' this the Pasque Flower, or Easter Flower, because of the time of its appearance, it being in bloom from April to June. The specific name, *pulsatilla*, from *pulse*, I beat, is given in allusion to its downy seeds being beaten about by the wind.

Varieties of *pulsatilla* when cultivated in this country like a well-drained, light, but deep soil, and will flourish in a peat or leaf soil, with the addition of lime rubble.

¶ *Part used Medicinally*. The drug Pulsa-tilla, which is of highly valuable modern curative use as a herbal simple, is obtained not only from the whole herb of *A. pulsatilla*, but also from *A. pratensis*, the Meadow Anemone, which is closely allied to the Pasque Flower, differing chiefly in having smaller flowers with deeper purple sepals, inflexed at the top. It grows in Denmark, Germany and Italy, but not in England. It is recommended for certain diseases of the eye, like Pulsatilla, and is used in homœo-pathy, but has been considered somewhat dangerous. The whole plant has a strong acrid taste, but is eaten by both sheep and goats, though cows and horses will not touch it. The leaves when bruised and applied to the skin raise blisters. *A. patens*, var. *Nutalliana* is also used for the same purpose as *A. pulsatilla*.

In each case, the whole herb is collected, soon after flowering, and should be carefully preserved when dried; it deteriorates if kept longer than one year.

¶ *Constituents*. The fresh plant yields by distillation with water an acrid, oily prin-ciple, with a burning, peppery taste, Oil of Anemone. A similar oil is obtained from *Ranunculus bulbosus*, *R. flammula* and *R. sceleratus*, which belong to the same order of plants. Its therapeutic value is not con-sidered great. When kept for some time, this oily substance becomes decomposed into Anemonic acid and Anemonin. Anemonin is crystalline, tasteless and odourless when pure and melts at 152°. The action of Pulsatilla is virtually that of this crystalline substance, Anemonin, which is a powerful irritant, like cantharides, in overdoses causing violent gastro-enteritis. It is volatile in water vapour and is then irritative to the eyes and mouth. The Oil acts as a vesicant when applied to the skin. Anemonic acid appears to be inert. Ane-monin sometimes causes local inflammation and gangrene when subcutaneously injected, vomiting and purging when given internally. It is, however, uncertain whether these symptoms are due to Anemonin itself or to some impurity in it. The chief action of pure Anemonin is a depressant one on the circulation, respiration and spinal cord, to a certain extent resembling that of Aconite. The symptoms are slow and feeble pulse, slow respiration, coldness, paralysis and death without convulsions. In poisoning by extract of Pulsatilla, convulsions are always present. Their absence in poisoning by pure Anemonin appears to be due to its paralysing action on motor centres in the brain.

¶ *Medicinal Action and Uses*. Nervine, anti-spasmodic, alterative and diaphoretic. The tincture of Pulsatilla is beneficial in disorders of the mucous membrane, of the respiratory and of the digestive passages. Doses of 2 to 3 drops in a spoonful of water will allay the spasmodic cough of asthma, whooping-cough and bronchitis.

For catarrhal affection of the eyes, as well as for catarrhal diarrhœa, the tincture is serviceable. It is also valuable as an em-menagogue, in the relief of headaches and neuralgia, and as a remedy for nerve exhaus-tion in women.

It is specially recommended for fair, blue-eyed women.

It has been employed in the form of extract in some cutaneous diseases with much success; it is included in the British Pharma-copœia and was formerly included in the United States Pharmacopœia.

In homœopathy it is considered very efficacious and even a specific in measles. It is prescribed as a good remedy for nettlerash and also for neuralgic toothache and earache, and is administered in indigestion and bilious attacks.

¶ *Preparation*. Fluid extract, 5 to 10 drops.

Parkinson says of this species: 'There are five different kinds of Pulsatilla, which flower in April: they are sometimes used for tertian ague and to help obstructions.'

See LIVERWORT, HELLEBORE (FALSE).

Other Species

PULSATILLA NUTTALIANE   N.O. Ranunculaceæ

> *Synonym*. American Pulsatilla
> *Parts Used*. Whole plant
> *Habitat*. The bed of the Mississippi

¶ *Description*. Flowers pale purple; odour of flowers camphoraceous; taste sweetish; of leaves, sweetish and astringent.

¶ *Constituents*. Grape sugar, gum resin, an alkaloid and anemonic acid, sulphate of potash, carbonate of potash, chlorate of potassium, carbonate of lime, magnesia and 'proto salt of iron.'

¶ *Medicinal Action and Uses*. Amenorrhœa; has also proved successful in warding off colds, and in rheumatism of the knees.

ANEMONE (WOOD)

Anemone nemorosa (LINN.)
N.O. Ranunculaceæ

> *Synonyms*. Crowfoot. Windflower. Smell Fox
> *Parts Used*. Root, leaves, juice

The Wood Anemone is one of the earliest spring flowers.

¶ *Description*. It has a long, tough, creeping root-stock, running just below the surface; it is the quick growth of this root-stock that causes the plant to spread so rapidly, forming large colonies in the moist soil of wood and thicket. The deeply-cut leaves and star-like flowers rise directly from it on separate unbranched stems. Some distance below the flower are the three leaflets, often so deeply divided as to appear more than three in number and very similar to the true leaves. They wrap round and protect the flower-bud before it unfolds, but as it opens, its stalk lengthens and it is carried far above them.

The flower has no honey and little scent, and apparently relies little on the visits of insects for the fertilization of its one-celled seed-vessels, which are in form like those of the butter-cup, arranged in a mass in the centre of the many stamens, and are termed achenes. As in all the Anemones, there are no true petals, what seem so are really the sepals, which have assumed the colouring and characteristics of petals. They are six in number, pure white on the upper surfaces and pale rose-coloured beneath.

In sunshine, the flower is expanded wide, but at the approach of night, it closes and droops its graceful head so that the dew may not settle on it and injure it. If rain threatens in the daytime, it does the same, receiving the drops upon its back, whence they trickle of harmlessly from the sepal tips. The way the sepals then fold over the mass of stamens and undeveloped seed-vessels in their centre has been likened to a tent, in which, as used fancifully to be said by country-folk, the fairies nestled for protection, having first pulled the curtains round them.

The plant is very liable to attack from certain fungi: at times, a species of *Puccinia* settles on it, the result being that the stalks of infected leaves grow rapidly, high above the others, though the leaves themselves dwindle and lose their divisions. A species of *Sclerotinia* attacks the swollen tubers of the root, doing still more harm, for in the spring there arise not the delicate white flowers, but the ugly fructifications of the fungus.

Though so innocent in appearance, the Wood Anemone possesses all the acrid nature of its tribe and is bitter to the tongue and poisonous. Cattle have been poisoned, Linnæus tells us, by eating it in the fresh state after having been underfed and kept on dry food during the winter, so that they were ready to browse on the first leaves they saw. A vinegar made from the leaves retains all the more acrid properties of the plant, and is put in France to many domestic purposes: its rubifacient effects have caused it to be used externally in the same way as mustard.

The Egyptians held the Anemone as the emblem of sickness, perhaps from the flush of colour upon the backs of the white sepals. The Chinese call it the 'Flower of Death.' In some European countries it is looked on by the peasants as a flower of ill-omen, though the reason of the superstition is obscure. The Romans plucked the first Anemones as a charm against fever, and in some remote districts this practice long survived, it being considered a certain cure to gather an Anemone saying, 'I gather this against all diseases,' and to tie it round the invalid's neck.

Greek legends say that Anemos, the Wind, sends his namesakes the Anemones, in the earliest spring days as the heralds of his coming. Pliny affirmed that they only open when the wind blows, hence their name of Windflower, and the unfolding of the blossoms in the rough, windy days of March has been the theme of many poets:

'Coy anemone that ne'er uncloses
Her lips until they're blown on by the wind.'

Culpepper also uses the word 'windflower.' In Greek mythology it sprang from the tears of Venus, as she wandered through the woodlands weeping for the death of Adonis –

'Where streams his blood there blushing springs a rose
And where a tear has dropped, a windflower blows.'

The old herbalists called the Wood Anemone the Wood Crowfoot, because its leaves resemble in shape those of some species of Crowfoot. We also find it called Smell Fox. The specific name of *nemorosa* refers to its woodland habits.

[*'Anemone nemorosa*, Varieties in,' by E. J. Salisbury (*Ann. Bot.*, October 1916, Vol. xxx, No. cxx: figs.) – Two varieties distinct from the common form are mentioned as being fairly numerous in some of the Hertfordshire woodlands, and for which the author has proposed the names *A. nemorosa*, var. *robusta* and *A. nemorosa*, var. *apetala*. The former differs from the normal type in the lighter green colour and larger size of the vegetative organs and in the perianth segments, which are broadest above the middle and rounded towards the apex. The latter bears inconspicuous flowers, which are small purplish-green structures, and it is noted that these plants are usually associated with the more deeply shaded situations, but as this character is maintained when the coppice in which the variety grows is felled, it is not considered a mere effect of inadequate illumination. – G.D.L.]

¶ *Medicinal Action and Uses*. Though this species of Anemone has practically fallen out of use, the older herbalists recommended application of various parts of the plant for headaches, tertian agues and rheumatic gout. Culpepper practically copies verbatim the some half-dozen uses of the Anemone that Gerard gives, saying:

'The body being bathed with the decoction of the leaves cures the leprosy: the leaves being stamped and the juice snuffed up the nose purgeth the head mightily; so doth the root, being chewed in the mouth, for it procureth much spitting and bringeth away many watery and phlegmatic humours, and is therefore excellent for the lethargy. . . . Being made into an ointment and the eyelids annointed with it, it helps inflammation of the eyes. The same ointment is excellent good to cleanse malignant and corroding ulcers.'

Culpepper also advises the roots to be chewed because it 'purgeth the head mightily'; he adds, 'And when all is done, let physicians prate what they please, all the pills in the dispensary purge not the head like to hot things held in the mouth.'

Parkinson writes:

'there is little use of these (the Anemones) in physic in our days, either for inward or outward diseases; only the leaves are used in the ointment called Marciatum, which is composed of many other hot herbs. . . . The root by reason of the sharpness is apt to draw down rheum if it be tasted or chewed in the mouth.'

Modern authorities would, however, hesitate to recommend the chewing of the root, on account of the acrid, irritant poison known to be present in it.

Linnæus noticed that in Sweden the Wood Anemone flowered at the same time as the return of the swallow, and that the Marsh Marigold was contemporaneous with the cuckoo. A British naturalist in this country has also remarked this. Another naturalist, who took an annual account of the days on which various flowers came into bloom in spring, found that the Wood Anemone never blossomed earlier than March 16, and never later than April 22. His observations were made each spring during thirty years.

The English name is derived from its Greek signification (wind) and is due to the fact that so many of its species grow on elevated places exposed to high winds; other writers attribute the name to the trembling of the flower before the blasts of spring.

ANGELICA

Angelica Archangelica (LINN.)
N.O. Umbelliferæ

Synonyms. Garden Angelica. Archangelica officinalis
Parts Used. Root, leaves, seeds
Habitat. By some botanists, this species of Angelica is believed to be a native of Syria, from whence it has spread to many cool European climates, where it has become naturalized. It is occasionally found native in cold and moist places in Scotland, but is more abundant in countries further north, as in Lapland and Iceland. It is supposed to have come to this country from northern latitudes about 1568. There are about thirty varieties of Angelica, but this one is the only one officially employed in medicine

Parkinson, in his *Paradise in Sole*, 1629, puts Angelica in the forefront of all medicinal plants, and it holds almost as high a place among village herbalists to-day, though it is not the native species of Angelica that is of such value medicinally and commercially, but an allied form, found wild in most places in the northern parts of Europe. This large variety, *Angelica Archangelica* (Linn.), also known as *Archangelica officinalis*, is grown abundantly near London in moist fields, for the use of its candied stems. It is largely cultivated for medicinal purposes in Thuringia, and the roots are also imported from Spain.

¶ *History.* Its virtues are praised by old writers, and the name itself, as well as the folk-lore of all North European countries and nations, testify to the great antiquity of a belief in its merits as a protection against contagion, for purifying the blood, and for curing every conceivable malady: it was held a sovereign remedy for poisons, agues and all infectious maladies. In Courland, Livonia and the low lakelands of Pomerania and East Prussia, wild-growing Angelica abounds; there, in early summer-time, it has been the custom among the peasants to march into the towns carrying the Angelica flower-stems and to offer them for sale, chanting some ancient ditty in Lettish words, so antiquated as to be unintelligible even to the singers themselves. The chanted words and the tune are learnt in childhood, and may be attributed to a survival of some Pagan festival with which the plant was originally associated. After the introduction of Christianity, the plant became linked in the popular mind with some archangelic patronage, and associated with the spring-time festival of the Annunciation. According to one legend, Angelica was revealed in a dream by an angel to cure the plague. Another explanation of the name of this plant is that it blooms on the day of Michael the Archangel (May 8, old style), and is on that account a preservative against evil spirits and witchcraft: all parts of the plant were believed efficacious against spells and enchantment. It was held in such esteem that it was called 'The Root of the Holy Ghost.'

Angelica may be termed a perennial herbaceous plant. It is biennial only in the *botanical* sense of that term, that is to say, it is neither annual, nor naturally perennial: the seedlings make but little advance towards maturity within twelve months, whilst old plants die off after seeding once, which event may be at a much more remote period than in the second year of growth. Only very advanced seedlings flower in their second year, and the third year of growth commonly completes the full period of life. There is another species, *Angelica heterocarpa*, a native of Spain, which is credited as truly perennial; it flowers a few weeks later than the biennial species, and is not so ornamental in its foliage.

¶ *Description.* The roots of the Common Angelica are long and spindle-shaped, thick and fleshy – large specimens weighing sometimes as much as three pounds – and are beset with many long, descending rootlets. The stems are stout, fluted, 4 to 6 feet high and hollow. The foliage is bold and pleasing, the leaves are on long, stout, hollow footstalks, often 3 feet in length, reddish purple at the much dilated, clasping bases; the blades, of a bright green colour, are much cut into, being composed of numerous small leaflets, divided into three principal groups, each of which is again subdivided into three lesser groups. The edges of the leaflets are finely toothed or serrated. The flowers, small and numerous, yellowish or greenish in colour, are grouped into large, globular umbels. They blossom in July and are succeeded by pale yellow, oblong fruits, $\frac{1}{6}$ to a $\frac{1}{4}$ inch in length when ripe, with membraneous edges, flattened on one side and convex on the other, which bears three prominent ribs. Both the odour and taste of the fruits are pleasantly aromatic.

Our native form, *A. sylvestris* (Linn.), is hairy in stalk and stem to a degree which makes a well-marked difference. Its flowers differ, also, in being white, tinged with purple. The stem is purple and furrowed. This species is said to yield a good, yellow dye.

Angelica is unique amongst the *Umbelliferæ* for its pervading aromatic odour, a pleasant perfume, entirely differing from Fennel, Parsley, Anise, Caraway or Chervil. One old writer compares it to Musk, others liken it to Juniper. Even the roots are fragrant, and form one of the principal aromatics of European growth; the other parts of the plant have the same flavour, but their active principles are considered more perishable.

In several London squares and parks, Angelica has continued to grow, self-sown, for several generations as a garden escape; in some cases it is appreciated as a useful foliage plant; in others, it is treated rather as an intruding weed. Before the building of the London Law Courts and the clearing of much slum property between Holywell Street and Seven Dials, the foreign population of that district fully appreciated its value, and were always anxious to get it from Lincoln's Inn Fields, where it abounded and where it still grows. Until very recent years, it was exceedingly common on the slopes bordering the Tower of London on the north and west sides; there, also, the inhabitants held the plant in high repute, both for its culinary and medicinal use.

¶ *Cultivation.* Cultivate in ordinary deep, moist loam, in a shady position, as the plant

36

thrives best in a damp soil and loves to grow near running water. Although the natural habitat is in damp soil and in open quarters, yet it can withstand adverse environment wonderfully well, and even endure severe winter frost without harm. Seedlings will even successfully develop and flower under trees, whose shelter creates an area of summer dryness in the surface soil, but, of course, though such conditions may be allowable when Angelica is grown merely as an ornamental plant, it must be given the best treatment as regards suitable soil and situation when grown for its use commercially. Insects and garden pests do not attack the plant with much avidity: its worst enemy is a small two-winged fly, of which the maggots are leaf-miners, resembling those of the celery plant and of the spinach leaf.

¶ *Propagation* should not be attempted otherwise than by the sowing of ripe, fresh seed, though division of old roots is sometimes recommended, and also propagation by off-shoots, which are thrown out by a two-year-old plant when cut down in June for the sake of the stems, and which transplanted to 2 feet or more apart, will provide a quick method of propagation, considered inferior, however, to that of raising by seed. Since the germinating capacity of the seeds rapidly deteriorates, they should be sown as soon as ripe in August or early September. If kept till March, especially if stored in paper packets, their vitality is likely to be seriously impaired. In the autumn, the seeds may be sown where the plants are to remain, or preferably in a nursery bed, which as a rule will not need protection during the winter. A very slight covering of earth is best. Young seedlings, but not the old plants, are amenable to transplantation. The seedlings should be transplanted when still small, for their first summer's growth, to a distance of about 18 inches apart. In the autumn they can be removed to permanent quarters, the plants being then set 3 feet apart.

¶ *Parts Used.* The *roots* and *leaves* for medicinal purposes, also the *seeds*.

The *stems* and *seeds* for use in confectionery and flavouring and the preparation of liqueurs.

The dried leaves, on account of their aromatic qualities, are used in the preparation of hop bitters.

The whole plant is aromatic, but the root only is official in the Swiss, Austrian and German Pharmacopœias.

Angelica roots should be dried rapidly and placed in air-tight receptacles. They will then retain their medicinal virtues for many years.

The *root* should be dug up in the autumn of the first year, as it is then least liable to become mouldy and worm-eaten: it is very apt to be attacked by insects. Where very thick, the roots should be sliced longitudinally to quicken the drying process.

The fresh root has a yellowish-grey epidermis, and yields when bruised a honey-coloured juice, having all the aromatic properties of the plant. If an incision is made in the bark of the stems and the crown of the root at the commencement of spring, this resinous gum will exude. It has a special aromatic flavour of musk benzoin, for either of which it can be substituted.

The dried root, as it appears in commerce, is greyish brown and much wrinkled externally, whitish and spongy within and breaks with a starchy fracture, exhibiting shining, resinous spots. The odour is strong and fragrant, and the taste at first sweetish, afterwards warm, aromatic, bitterish and somewhat musky. These properties are extracted by alcohol and less perfectly by water.

If the plants are well grown, the *leaves* may be cut for use the summer after transplanting. Ordinarily, it is the third or fourth year that the plant develops its tall flowering stem, of which the gathering for culinary or confectionery use prolongs the lifetime of the plant for many seasons. Unless it is desired to collect seed, the tops should be cut at or before flowering time. After producing seed, the plants generally die, but by cutting down the tops when the flower-heads first appear and thus preventing the formation of seed, the plants may continue for several years longer, by cutting down the stems right at their base, the plants practically become perennial, by the development of side shoots around the stool head.

The whole herb, if for medicinal use, should be collected in June and cut shortly above the root.

If the stems are already too thick, the leaves may be stripped off separately and dried on wire or netting trays.

The *stem*, which is in great demand when trimmed and candied, should be cut about June or early July.

If the *seeds* are required, they should be gathered when ripe and dried. The seed-heads should be harvested on a fine day, after the sun has dried off the dew, and spread thinly on sailcloth in a warm spot or open shed, where the air circulates freely. In a few days the tops will have become dry enough to be beaten out with a light flail or rod, care being taken not to injure the seed. After threshing, the seeds (or fruits) should be sieved to remove portions of the stalks and

37

allowed to remain for several days longer, spread out in a very thin layer in the sun, or in a warm and sunny room, being turned every day to remove the last vestige of moisture. In a week to ten days they will be dry. Small quantities of the fruits can be shaken out of the heads when they have been cut a few days and finished ripening, so that the fruits divide naturally into the half-fruits or mericarps which shake off readily when quite ripe, especially if rubbed out of the heads between the palms of the hands. It is imperative that the seeds be dry before being put into storage packages or tins.

¶ *Constituents.* The chief constituents of Angelica are about 1 per cent. of volatile oil, valeric acid, angelic acid, sugar, a bitter principle, and a peculiar resin called Angelicin, which is stimulating to the lungs and to the skin. The essential oil of the roots contains terebangelene and other terpenes; the oil of the 'seeds' contains in addition methyl-ethylacetic acid and hydroxymyristic acid.

Angelica balsam is obtained by extracting the roots with alcohol, evaporating and extracting the residue with ether. It is of a dark brown colour and contains Angelica oil, Angelica wax and Angelicin.

¶ *Uses.* Angelica is largely used in the grocery trade, as well as for medicine, and is a popular flavouring for confectionery and liqueurs. The appreciation of its unique flavour was established in ancient times when saccharin matter was extremely rare. The use of the sweetmeat may probably have originated from the belief that the plant possessed the power of averting or expelling pestilence.

The preparation of Angelica is a small but important industry in the south of France, its cultivation being centralized in Clermont-Ferrand. Fairly large quantities are purchased by confectioners and high prices are easily obtainable. The flavour of Angelica suggests that of Juniper berries, and it is largely used in combination with Juniper berries, or in partial substitution for them by gin distillers. The stem is largely used in the preparation of preserved fruits and 'confitures' generally, and is also used as an aromatic garnish by confectioners. The seeds especially, which are aromatic and bitterish in taste, are employed also in alcoholic distillates, especially in the preparation of Vermouth and similar preparations, as well as in other liqueurs, notably Chartreuse. From ancient times, Angelica has been one of the chief flavouring ingredients of beverages and liqueurs, but it is not a matter of general knowledge that the Muscatel grape-like flavour of some wines, made on both sides of the Rhine, is (or is suspected to be) due to the secret use of Angelica. An Oil of Angelica, which is very expensive, was prepared in Germany some years ago: it is obtained from the seeds by distillation with steam, the vapour being condensed and the oil separated by gravity. One hundred kilograms of Angelica seeds yield one kilolitre of oil, and the fresh leaves a little less, the roots yielding only 0·15 to 0·3 kilograms. Like the seeds themselves, the oil is used for flavouring. Besides being employed as a flavouring for beverages and medicinally, Angelica seeds are also used to a limited extent in perfumery.

¶ *Medicinal Action and Uses.* The root, stalks, leaves and fruit possess carminative, stimulant, diaphoretic, stomachic, tonic and expectorant properties, which are strongest in the fruit, though the whole plant has the same virtues.

Angelica is a good remedy for colds, coughs, pleurisy, wind, colic, rheumatism and diseases of the urinary organs, though it should not be given to patients who have a tendency towards diabetes, as it causes an increase of sugar in the urine.

It is generally used as a stimulating expectorant, combined with other expectorants, the action of which is facilitated, and to a large extent diffused, through the whole of the pulmonary region.

It is a useful agent for feverish conditions, acting as a diaphoretic.

An infusion may be made by pouring a pint of boiling water on an ounce of the bruised *root*, and two tablespoonsful of this should be given three or four times a day, or the powdered root administered in doses of 10 to 30 grains. The infusion will relieve flatulence, and is also of use as a stimulating bronchial tonic, and as an emmenagogue. It is used much on the Continent for indigestion, general debility and chronic bronchitis. For external use, the fresh leaves of the plant are crushed and applied as poultices in lung and chest diseases.

The following is extracted from an old family book of herbal remedies:

'Boil down gently for three hours a handful of Angelica root in a quart of water; then strain it off and add liquid Narbonne honey or best virgin honey sufficient to make it into a balsam or syrup and take two tablespoonsful every night and morning, as well as several times in the day. If there be hoarseness or sore throat, add a few nitre drops.'

A somewhat similar drink, much in use on the Continent in the treatment of typhus fever, is thus prepared:

'Pour a quart of boiling water upon 6 oz. of Angelica root cut up in thin slices, 4 oz. of honey, the juice of 2 lemons and ½ gill of brandy. Infuse for half an hour.'

Formerly a preparation of the roots was much used as a specific for typhoid.

Angelica *stems* are also grateful to a feeble stomach, and will relieve flatulence promptly when chewed. An infusion of Angelica *leaves* is a very healthful, strengthening tonic and aromatic stimulant, the beneficial effect of which is felt after a few days' use.

The yellow juice yielded by the stem and root becomes, when dry, a valuable medicine in chronic rheumatism and gout.

Taken in medicinal form, Angelica is said to cause a disgust for spirituous liquors.

It is a good vehicle for nauseous medicines and forms one of the ingredients in compound spirit of Aniseed.

Gerard, among its many virtues that he extols, says 'it cureth the bitings of mad dogs and all other venomous beasts.'

¶ *Preparations.* Fluid extract, herb: dose, 1 drachm. Fluid extract, root: dose, ¼ to 1 drachm.

RECIPES

¶ *To Preserve Angelica.* Cut in pieces 4 inches long. Steep for 12 hours in salt and water. Put a layer of cabbage or cauliflower leaves in a clean brass pan, then a layer of Angelica, then another layer of leaves and so on, finishing with a layer of leaves on the top. Cover with water and vinegar. Boil slowly till the Angelica becomes quite green, then strain and weigh the stems. Allow 1 lb. loaf sugar to each pound of stems. Put the sugar in a clean pan with water to cover; boil 10 minutes and pour this syrup over the Angelica. Stand for 12 hours. Pour off the syrup, boil it up for 5 minutes and pour it again over the Angelica. Repeat the process, and after the Angelica has stood in the syrup 12 hours, put all on the fire in the brass pan and boil till tender. Then take out the pieces of Angelica, put them in a jar and pour the syrup over them, or dry them on a sieve and sprinkle them with sugar: they then form candy.

Another recipe (from *Francatelli's Cook's Guide*):

'Cut the tubes or stalks of Angelica into six-inch lengths; wash them, then put them into a copper preserving-pan with hot syrup; cover the surface with vine-leaves, and set the whole to stand in the larder till next day. The Angelica must then be drained on a sieve, the vine-leaves thrown away, half a pint of water added to the syrup, in which, after it

has been boiled, skimmed, and strained into another pan, and the copper-pan has been scoured clean, both the Angelica and the boiling syrup are to be replaced and the surface covered with fresh vine-leaves, and again left to stand in this state till the next day; this process must be repeated 3 or 4 days running: at the end of which time the Angelica will be sufficiently green and done through, and should be put in jars without breaking the tubes. After the syrup has been boiled and skimmed, fill up the jars, and when they are become cold, cover them over with bladder and paper, and let them be kept in a very cool temperature.'

Another way of preserving Angelica: Choose young stems, cut them into suitable lengths, then boil until tender. When this stage is reached, remove from the water, and strip off the outer skin, then return to the water and simmer slowly until the whole has become very green. Dry the stems and weigh them, allowing one pound of white sugar to every pound of Angelica. The boiled stalks should be laid in an earthenware pan and the sugar sprinkled over them, allowing the whole to stand for a couple of days; then boil all together. When well boiling, remove from the fire and turn into a colander to drain off the superfluous syrup. Take a little more sugar and boil to a syrup again, then throw in the Angelica, and allow it to remain for a few minutes, and finally spread on plates in a cool oven to dry.

If a small quantity of the leaf-stalks of Angelica be cooked with 'sticks' of rhubarb, the flavour of the compound will be acceptable to many who do not relish plain rhubarb. The quantity of Angelica used may be according to circumstances, conditions and individual taste. If the stems are young and juicy, they may be treated like rhubarb and cut up small, the quantity used being in any proportion between 5 and 25 per cent. If the stalks are more or less fully developed, or even rather old and tough, they can be excellently used in economically small quantities for flavouring large quantities of stewed rhubarb, or of rhubarb jam, being added in long lengths before cooking and removed before sending to table. The confectioner's candied Angelica may be similarly utilized, but is expensive and not so good, whilst the home-garden growth in spring-time of fresh Angelica, with thick, stout leaf-stalks, and of still stouter flowering stems, is very easy to use and cheap. If this flowering stem be cut whilst very tender, early in May, later leaf-stalks will be plentifully available for use with the latter part of the rhubarb crop.

A well-known jam maker and confectioner, the late Mr. Robertson, of Chelsea, won considerable reputation by reason of his judicious blending of Angelica in jam-making and its combination in other confections, including temperance beverages. A pleasant form of Hop Bitters is made by taking 1 oz. of dried Angelica herb, combined with 1 oz. of Holy Thistle, and ½ oz. of hops, infused with 3 pints of boiling water and strained off when cold, a wineglassful being taken several times a day before meals, forming a good appetiser.

A delicious liqueur which is also a digestive, preserving all the virtues of the plant, is made in this way: 1 oz. of the freshly gathered stem of Angelica is chopped up and steeped in 2 pints of good brandy during five days, 1 oz. of skinned bitter almonds reduced to a pulp being added. The liquid is then strained through fine muslin and a pint of liquid sugar added to it.

Angelica is used in the preparation of Vermouth and Chartreuse.

Though the tender leaflets of the blades of the leaves have sometimes been recommended as a substitute for spinach, they are too bitter for the general taste, but the blanched mid-ribs of the leaf, boiled and used as celery, are delicious, and Icelanders eat both the stem and the roots raw, with butter. The taste of the juicy raw stems is at first sweetish and slightly bitter in the mouth, and then gives a feeling of glowing warmth. In Lapland, the inhabitants regard the stalks of Angelica as a great delicacy. These are gathered before flowering, the leaves being stripped off and the peel removed, the remainder is eaten with much relish. The Finns eat the young stems baked in hot ashes, and an infusion of the dried herb is drunk either hot or cold: the flavour of the decoction is rather bitter, the colour is a pale-greenish grey and the odour greatly resembles China Tea. It was formerly a practice in this country to put a portion of the fresh herb into the pot in which fish is boiled.

The Norwegians make bread of the roots.

Angelica may be made much use of in the garden by cutting the hollow stalks into convenient lengths and placing them amongst shrubs as traps for earwigs.

A drink much in use on the Continent for typhus fever: Pour a quart of boiling water on 6 oz. of Angelica root sliced thin; infuse for half an hour, strain and add juice of 2 lemons, 4 oz. of honey and ½ gill of brandy.

Other Angelicas.

AMERICAN ANGELICA or Masterwort (*A. atropurpurea*, Linn.), also used in herbal medicine in North America, grows throughout the eastern United States. The root has a strong odour and a warm aromatic taste. The juice of the fresh root is acrid and said to be poisonous, but the acridity is dissipated by drying.

The root, though lighter and less branched, is similar in appearance to that of *A. Archangelica*, with nearly allied constituents and properties, and the medicinal virtues of the whole plant are similar, so that it has been employed as a substitute, but it is inferior to the European Angelica, being less aromatic.

WILD ANGELICA (*A. sylvestris*, Linn.), yields a yellow dye.

The Angelica Tree of America (*Xanthoxylum Americanum*, Mill), the Prickly Ash, as it is more generally named, is not allied to the umbelliferous Angelicas. Its berries and bark are employed to prepare a tonic, and it is used in the treatment of rheumatism and skin diseases.

See ASH (PRICKLY), CHERVIL (SWEET), LOVAGE

ANGELICA TREE

Aralia spinosa
N.O. Araliaceæ

Synonyms. Hercules Club. Toothache Tree. Prickly Elder. Prickly Ash, though not to be confused with the better-known Prickly Ash
Parts Used. Bark, root and berries
Habitat. Virginia and Japan

¶ *Description*. Grows from 8 to 12 feet high, stem and leaves prickly, leaves doubly and triply pinnate, ovate, serrated leaflets, panicles much branched, downy, numerous umbels of white flowers, blooming in August and September, berries juicy and blackish.

The bark is used officially (is thin and ash-coloured), but other parts of the plant possess medical properties; odour fragrant and peculiar, slightly bitter taste.

¶ *Constituents*. *Aralia spinosa* contains a glucoside Araliin.

¶ *Medicinal Action and Uses*. Fresh bark causes vomiting and purging, but dried is a stimulating alterative. A tincture made from the bark is used for rheumatism, skin diseases and syphilis. The berries in tincture form, lull pain in decayed teeth and in other parts of the body, violent colic and rheumatism, useful in cholera when a cathartic is required in the following compound: 1 drachm compound powdered Jalap, 1 drachm *Aralia spinosa*, 2 drachms compound rhubarb powder or infused in ½ pint boiling water and

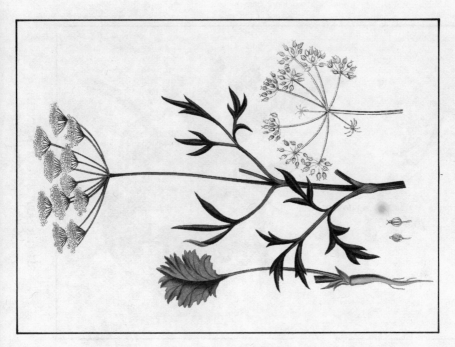

ANISE
Pimpinella Anisum

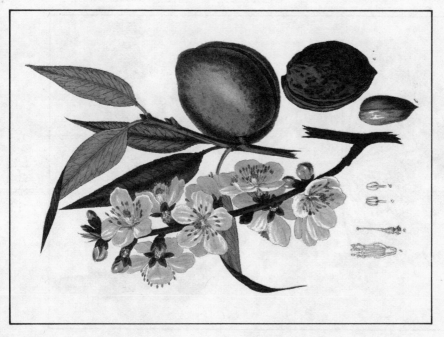

ALMOND
Amygdalus Communis

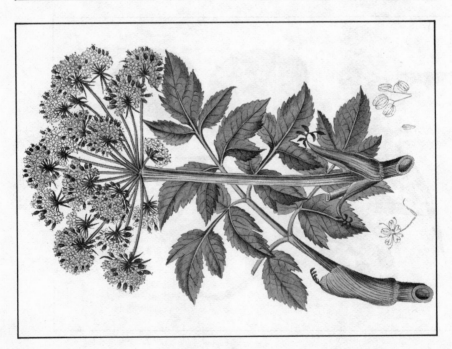

BITTER APPLE (COLOCYNTH)
Citrullus Colocynthis

ANGELICA
Angelica Archangelica

when cold taken in tablespoonful doses every half-hour. This does not produce choleric discharges. Also a powerful sialogogue and valuable in diseases where mouth and throat get dry, and for sore throat; will relieve difficult breathing and produce moisture if given in very small doses of the powder. The bark, root, and berries can all be utilized.

See also BAMBOO BRIER, AMERICAN DWARF ELDER, SPIKENARD (AMERICAN AND CALIFORNIAN), SARSAPARILLA.

ANGOSTURA (TRUE)

Cusparia febrifuga (D. C.)
N.O. Rutaceæ

Synonyms. Cusparia Bark. Galipea officinalis
Part Used. The dried bark
Habitat. Tropical South America

¶ *Description.* A small tree with straight stem irregularly branched, covered with a smooth grey bark, leaves alternate, petiolate and composed of three leaflets oblong and pointed, smooth, glossy and vivid green, sometimes with small white spots on them and in their first state having a tobacco-like aroma, this odour is one of the characteristics distinguishing the true Angostura from the false which is odourless. The flowers also have a peculiar nauseous smell; salver-shaped corollas and arranged in axillary, terminal, peduncled racemes. Fruit has five two-valved capsules, two or three of which are often abortive; two seeds in each capsule, round and black, one only is generally fertile. The tree was given the name of *Galipea officinalis* to denote the true variety of Angostura and thus distinguish it from the very dangerous substitute and adulterant. The characteristics of the true commercial bark are flattened curved pieces or quills 4 to 5 inches long, 1 inch wide and $\frac{1}{12}$ of an inch thick. The outer layer of bark is a yellowish-grey cork which is easily removed, often being soft, the inner surface is lighter brown and sometimes laminated, fracture short and resinous white, points being visible on broken surface; the transverse section shows numerous cells filled with circular crystals of Calcium Oxalate, small oil glands, small groups of bast fibres with a musty smell and bitter taste.

¶ *Constituents.* The chief bitter principle of Angostura bark is Angosturin, a colourless crystalline substance readily soluble in water, alcohol or ether. The bark also contains about 2·4 per cent. of the bitter crystalline alkaloids Galipine, Cusparine, Galipidine Cusparidine and Cuspareine, about 1·5 per cent. of volatile oil and a glucoside which yields a fluorescent substance when hydrolysed by heating with dilute sulphuric acid.

¶ *Medicinal Action and Uses.* The bark has long been known and used by the natives of South America and West Indies as a stimulant tonic. In large doses it causes diarrhœa and is often used as a purgative. Most useful in bilious diarrhœa, dysentery, and diseases which require a tonic. Commercially it is an ingredient of bitter liqueurs. The natives also employ it to stupefy fish in the same manner as Cinchona is used by the Peruvians. Some doctors prefer Angostura Bark to Cinchona for use in fever cases; it is also used in dropsy.

¶ *Dosages and Preparations.* Infusion Cuspariæ, B.P.: Angostura Bark in powder, 5 parts; distilled water, boiling, 100 parts; infuse for 15 minutes in a covered vessel and strain. Dose, 1 to 2 fluid ounces. This infusion is the most satisfactory way of taking the bark, but to obviate nausea it should be combined with aromatics. It may be given in powder, tincture or fluid extract. Dose of the powder, 5 to 15 grains. Fluid extract, 5 to 30 minims.

¶ *Other Species.* Dangerous substitutions are: The bark of the Nux Vomica Tree; this is known as False Angostura Bark; it is much more twisted and bent than the true, has no unpleasant smell, is not so heavy, and is more easily broken.

Copalchi Bark from Mexico, composition similar to *Cascarilla Esenbeckia febrifuga* (N.O. Rutaceæ), contains Ovodine.

ANISE

Pimpinella anisum (LINN.)
N.O. Umbelliferæ

Part Used. Seeds
Habitat. It is a native of Egypt, Greece, Crete and Asia Minor and was cultivated by the ancient Egyptians. It was well known to the Greeks, being mentioned by Dioscorides and Pliny and was cultivated in Tuscany in Roman times. In the Middle Ages its cultivation spread to Central Europe

¶ *Description.* Anise is a dainty, white-flowered umbelliferous annual, about 18 inches high, with secondary feather-like leaflets of bright green, hence its name (of mediæval origin), Pimpinella, from *dipinella*, or twice-pinnate, in allusion to the form of the leaves.

¶ *History*. In this country Anise has been in use since the fourteenth century, and has been cultivated in English gardens from the middle of the sixteenth century, but it ripens its seeds here only in very warm summers, and it is chiefly in warmer districts that it is grown on a commercial scale, Southern Russia, Bulgaria, Germany, Malta, Spain, Italy, North Africa and Greece producing large quantities. It has also been introduced into India and South America. The cultivated plant attains a considerably larger size than the wild one.

In the East, Anise was formerly used with other spices in part payment of taxes. 'Ye pay tithe of Mint, Anise and Cummin,' we read in the 23rd chapter of St. Matthew, but some authorities state that Anise is an incorrect rendering and should have been translated 'Dill.'

In Virgil's time, Anise was used as a spice. Mustacæ, a spiced cake of the Romans, introduced at the end of a rich meal, to prevent indigestion, consisted of meal, with Anise, Cummin and other aromatics. Such a cake was sometimes brought in at the end of a marriage feast, and is, perhaps, the origin of our spiced wedding cake.

On the Continent, especially in Germany, many cakes have an aniseed flavouring, and Anise is also used as a flavouring for soups. It is largely employed in France, Spain, Italy and South America in the preparation of cordial liqueurs. The liqueur Anisette, added to cold water on a hot summer's day, makes a most refreshing drink.

Anise is one of the herbs that was supposed to avert the Evil Eye.

The oil extracted from the seed is said to prove a capital bait for mice, if smeared on traps. It is poisonous to pigeons.

Turner's *Herbal*, 1551, says that 'Anyse maketh the breth sweter and swageth payne.' 'The seeds,' says Delamer, *Kitchen Garden*, 1861, 'are much used by distillers to give flavour to cordial liqueurs.' Anisette is a liqueur flavoured with aniseed. Langham, *Garden Health*, 1683, says: 'For the dropsie, fill an old cock with Polipody and Aniseeds, and seethe him well, and drink the broth.' The leaves are useful for seasoning some dishes. The essential oil of Anise is a good preventive of mould in paste. The ground seeds form an ingredient of sachet powders.

¶ *Cultivation*. Sow the seed in dry, light soil, on a warm, sunny border, early in April, where the plants are to remain. When they come up, thin them and keep them clean from weeds. Allow about a foot each way. The seeds may also be sown in pots in heat and removed to a warm site in May.

The seeds will ripen in England in good seasons if planted in a warm and favourable situation, though they are not successful everywhere, and can hardly be looked upon as a remunerative crop. The plant flowers in July, and if the season prove warm, will ripen in autumn, when the plants are cut down and the seeds threshed out.

¶ *Part Used*. The fruit, or so-called seeds. When threshed out, the seeds may be easily dried in trays, in a current of air in half-shade, out-of-doors, or by moderate heat. When dry, they are greyish brown, ovate, hairy, about one-fifth of an inch long, with ten crenate ribs and often have the stalk attached. They should be free from earthy matter. The taste is sweet and spicy, and the odour aromatic and agreeable.

The commercial varieties differ considerably in size, but the larger varieties alone are official. The Spanish Anise, sold as Alicante Anise, are the largest and the best adapted for pharmaceutical use, yielding about 3 per cent. of oil. Russian and German fruits are smaller and darker, and are the variety generally used for distillation of the volatile oil. Italian Anise is frequently adulterated with Hemlock fruit.

¶ *Constituents*. Anise fruit yields on distillation from 2·5 to 3·5 per cent. of a fragrant, syrupy, volatile oil, of which *anethol*, present to about 90 per cent., is the principal aromatic constituent. It has a strong Anise odour and separates in the form of shining white crystalline scales on cooling the oil. Other constituents of the fruit are a fixed oil, choline, sugar and mucilage.

Oil of Anise, distilled in Europe from the fruits of *Pimpinella anisum*, Anise, and in China from the fruits of *Illicium anisatum*, Star Anise, a small tree indigenous to China, is colourless, or very pale yellow, with taste and odour like the fruit. The oils obtainable from these two fruits are identical in composition, and nearly the same in most of their characters, but that from Star Anise fruit congeals at a lower temperature. The powdered drug from Star Anise is administered in India as a substitute for the official fruit, and the oil is employed for its aromatic, carminative and stimulant properties. The bulk of the oil in commerce is obtained from the Star Anise fruit in China. The fruits are also often imported into France and the oil extracted there. Chinese Anise oil is harsh in taste.

¶ *Medicinal Action and Uses*. Carminative and pectoral. Anise enjoys considerable reputation as a medicine in coughs and pectoral affections. In hard, dry coughs where expectoration is difficult, it is of much value.

It is greatly used in the form of lozenges and the seeds have also been used for smoking, to promote expectoration.

The volatile oil, mixed with spirits of wine forms the liqueur Anisette, which has a beneficial action on the bronchial tubes, and for bronchitis and spasmodic asthma, Anisette, if administered in hot water, is an immediate palliative.

For infantile catarrh, Aniseed tea is very helpful. It is made by pouring half a pint of boiling water on 2 teaspoonsful of bruised seed. This, sweetened, is given cold in doses of 1 to 3 teaspoonsful frequently.

Gerard said:

'Aniseed helpeth the yeoxing or hicket (hiccough) and should be given to young children to eat, which are like to have the falling sickness (epilepsy), or to such as have it by patrimony or succession.'

The stimulant and carminative properties of Anise make it useful in flatulency and colic.

It is used as an ingredient of cathartic and aperient pills, to relieve flatulence and diminish the griping of purgative medicines, and may be given with perfect safety in convulsions. For colic, the dose is 10 to 30 grains of bruised or powdered seeds infused in distilled water, taken in wineglassful doses, or 4 to 20 drops of the essential oil on sugar. For the restlessness of languid digestion, a dose of essence of aniseed in hot water at bedtime is much commended.

In the Paregoric Elixir (Compound Tincture of Camphor), prescribed as a sedative cordial by doctors, oil of Anise is also included – 30 drops in a pint of the tincture.

Anise oil is a good antiseptic and is used, mixed with oil of Peppermint or Gaultheria (Wintergreen) to flavour aromatic liquid dentrifrices.

Oil of Anise is used also against insects, especially when mixed with oil of Sassafras and Carbolic oil.

ANISE (STAR)

Illicuim verum (HOOK, F.)
N.O. Magnoliaceæ

Synonyms. Chinese Anise. Aniseed Stars. Badiana
Parts Used. Seeds, oil

Star Anise is so named from the stellate form of its fruit. It is often chewed in small quantities after each meal to promote digestion and sweeten the breath.

¶ *Medicinal Action and Uses.* Carminative, stimulant, diuretic.

The fruit is used in the East as a remedy

for colic and rheumatism, and in China for seasoning dishes, especially sweets.

The Japanese plant the tree in their temples and on tombs; and use the pounded bark as incense.

The homœopaths prepare a tincture from the seeds.

ANNATTO

Bixa orellana (LINN.)
N.O. Bixaceæ

Synonyms. Annotta Orellana Orleana
Part Used. The dried pulp of the fruit
Habitat. Tropical America, East and West Indies. Widely cultivated in Asia and Africa

ANTIRRHINUM. *See* SNAPDRAGON.

APPLE

Pyrus malus
N.O. Pomaceæ

Synonyms. Wild Apple. Malus communis
Parts Used. The fruit and the bark
Habitat. Temperate regions of the Northern Hemisphere

¶ *History.* The Apple is a fruit of the temperate zones and only reaches perfection in their cooler regions. It is a fruit of long descent and in the Swiss lake-dwellings small apples have been found, completely charred, but still showing the seed-valves and the grain of the flesh. It exists in its wild state in most countries of Europe and also in the region of the Caucasus: in Norway, it is found in the lowlands as far north as Drontheim.

The Crab-tree or Wild Apple (*Pyrus malus*), is native to Britain and is the wild ancestor of all the cultivated varieties of apple trees. It was the stock on which were grafted choice varieties when brought from Europe, mostly from France. Apples of some sort were abundant before the Norman Conquest and were probably introduced into Britain by the Romans. Twenty-two varieties were mentioned by Pliny: there are now about 2,000 kinds cultivated. In the Old

Saxon manuscripts there are numerous mentions of apples and cider. Bartholomeus Anglicus, whose *Encyclopedia* was one of the earliest printed books containing botanical information (being printed at Cologne about 1470), gives a chapter on the Apple. He says:

'Malus the Appyll tree is a tree yt bereth apples and is a grete tree in itself. . . it is more short than other trees of the wood wyth knottes and rinelyd Rynde. And makyth shadowe wythe thicke bowes and branches: and fayr with dyurs blossomes, and floures of swetnesse and lykynge: with goode fruyte and noble. And is gracious in syght and in taste and vertuous in medecyne . . . some beryth sourysh fruyte and harde, and some ryght soure and some ryght swete, with a good savoure and mery.'

¶ *Description.* The Crab-tree is a small tree of general distribution in Britain south of Perthshire. In most respects it closely resembles the cultivated Apple of the orchard, differing chiefly only in the size and flavour of the fruit. Well-grown specimens are not often met with, as in woods and copses it is cramped by other trees and seldom attains any considerable height, 30-foot specimens being rare and many being mere bushes. Those found in hedgerows have often sprung from the seeds of orchard apples that have reverted to ancestral type. The branches of the Crab-tree become pendant, with long shoots which bear the leaves and flowers. The leaves are dark green and glossy and the flowers, in small clusters on dwarf shoots, are produced in April and May. The buds are deeply tinged with pink on the outside, the expanded flowers an inch and a half across, and when the trees are in full bloom, they are a beautiful sight.

The blossoms, by their delightful fragrance and store of nectar, attract myriads of bees, and as a result of the fertilization effected by these visitors in their search for the buried nectar, the fruit develops and becomes in autumn the beautiful little Crab Apple, which when ripe is yellow or red in colour and measures about an inch across. It has a very austere and acid juice, in consequence of which it cannot be eaten in the raw condition, but a delicious jelly is made from it, which is always welcome on the table, and the fruit can also be used for jam-making, with blackberries, pears or quinces. In Ireland, it is sometimes added to cider, to impart a roughness. The fruit in some varieties is less acid than in others: in the variety in which the fruit hangs *down* from the shoots, the little apples are exceedingly acid, but in another kind, they stand more or less erect on their stalks and these are so much less acid as to give almost a suggestion of sweetness. The fruit of the Siberian Crab, or Cherry-apple, grown as an ornamental tree, makes also a fine preserve.

Cider Apples may be considered as a step in development from the Wild Apple to the Dessert Apple. Formerly every farmhouse made its cider. The apples every autumn were tipped in heaps on the straw-strewn floor of the pound house, a building of cob, covered with thatch, in which stood the pounder and the press and vats and all hands were busy for days preparing the golden beverage. This was the yearly process – still carried out on many farms of the west of England, though cider-making is becoming more and more a product of the factories. One of the men turned the handle of the pounder, while a boy tipped in the apples at the top. A pounder is a machine which crushes the apples between two rollers with teeth in them. The pulp and juice are then taken to the press in large shovels which have high sides and are scored bright by the acid. The press is a huge square tray with a lip in the centre of the front side and its floor slopes towards this opening. On either side are huge oaken supports on which rests a square baulk of the same wood. Through this works a large screw. Under the timber is the presser. Directly the pulp is ready, the farmer starts to prepare the 'cheese.' First of all goes a layer of straw, then a layer of apples, and so on until the 'cheese' is a yard high, and sometimes more. Then the ends of straw which project are turned up to the top of the heap. Now the presser is wound down and compresses the mound until the clear juice runs freely. Under the lip in the front of the cider press is put a vat. The juice is dipped from this into casks. In four months' time the cider will be ready to drink.

The demand for cider has increased rapidly of late years, chiefly on account of the dry varieties being so popular with sufferers from rheumatism and gout. As very good prices have been paid in recent seasons for the best cider apples, and as eight tons per acre is quite an average crop from a properly-managed orchard in full bearing, it is obvious to all progressive and up-to-date farmers and apple-growers that this branch of agriculture is well worthy of attention. In the last few years, with the object of encouraging this special Apple-growing industry, silver cups have been awarded to the owners of cider-apple orchards in Devon who make the greatest improvement in the cultivation of their orchards during the year, and it is hoped this will still further stimulate the planting of new orchards and the renovation of the old ones.

The peculiar winy odour is stimulating to many. Pliny, and later, Sir John Mandeville, tell of a race of little men in 'Farther India' who 'eat naught and live by the smell of apples.' Burton wrote that apples are good against melancholy and Dr. John Caius, physician to Queen Elizabeth, in his *Boke of Counseille against the Sweatynge Sicknesse* advises the patient to 'smele to an old swete apple to recover his strengthe.' An apple stuck full of cloves was the prototype of the pomander, and pomatum (now used only in a general sense) took its name from being first made of the pulp of apples, lard and rosewater.

In Shakespeare's time, apples when served at dessert were usually accompanied by caraway, as we may read in *Henry IV*, where Shallow invites Falstaff to 'a pippin and a dish of caraway,' In a still earlier *Booke of Nurture*, it is directed 'After mete pepyns, caraway in comfyts.' The custom of serving roast apples with a little saucerful of Carraways is still kept up at Trinity College, Cambridge, and at some of the old-fashioned London Livery dinners, just as in Shakespeare's days.

The taste for apples is one of the earliest and most natural of inclinations; all children love apples, cooked or uncooked. Apple pies, apple puddings, apple dumplings are fare acceptable in all ages and all conditions.

Apple cookery is very early English: Piers Ploughman mentions 'all the povere peple' who 'baken apples broghte in his lappes' and the ever popular apple pie was no less esteemed in Tudor times than it is to-day, only our ancestors had some predilections in the matter of seasonings that might not now appeal to all of us, for they put cinnamon and ginger in their pies and gave them a lavish colouring of saffron.

Apple Moyse is an old English confection, no two recipes for which seem to agree. One Black Letter volume tells us to take a dozen apples, roast or boil them, pass them through a sieve with the yolks of three or four eggs, and as they are strained temper them with three or four spoonfuls of damask (rose) water; season them with sugar and half a dish of sweet butter, and boil them in a chafing dish and cast biscuits or cinnamon and ginger upon them.

Halliwell says, upon one authority, that apple moyse was made from apples after they had been pressed for cider, and seasoned with spices.

Probably the American confection, *Apple Butter*, is an evolution of the old English dish? Apple butter is a kind of jam made of tart apples, boiled in cider until reduced to a very thick smooth paste, to which is added a flavouring of allspice, while cooking. It is then placed in jars and covered tightly.

The once-popular custom of 'wassailing the orchard-trees' on Christmas Eve, or the Eve of the Epiphany, is not quite extinct even yet in a few remote places in Devonshire. More than three centuries ago Herrick mentioned it among his 'Ceremonies of Christmas Eve':

'Wassaile the trees, that they may beare
You many a Plum and many a Peare:
For more or lesse fruits they will bring,
As you do give them Wassailing.'

The ceremony consisted in the farmer, with his family and labourers, going out into the orchard after supper, bearing with them a jug of cider and hot cakes. The latter were placed in the boughs of the oldest or best bearing trees in the orchard, while the cider was flung over the trees after the farmer had drunk their health in some such fashion as the following:

'Here's to thee, old apple-tree!
Whence thou may'st bud, and whence thou may'st blow,
Hats full! Caps full!
Bushel – bushel-bags full!
And my pockets full too! Huzza!'

The toast was repeated thrice, the men and boys often firing off guns and pistols, and the women and children shouting loudly.

Roasted apples were usually placed in the pitcher of cider, and were thrown at the trees with the liquid. Trees that were bad bearers were not honoured with wassailing, but it was thought that the more productive ones would cease to bear if the rite were omitted. It is said to have been a relic of the heathen sacrifices to Pomona. The custom also prevailed in Somersetshire and Dorsetshire.

Roast apples, or crabs, formed an indispensable part of the old-fashioned 'wassail-bowl,' or 'good brown bowl," of our ancestors.

'And sometime lurk I in a gossip's bowl
In very likeness of a roasted Crab'

Puck relates in *Midsummer's Night's Dream*.

The mixture of hot spiced ale, wine or cider, with apples and bits of toast floating in it was often called 'Lamb's wool,' some say from its softness, but the word is really derived from the Irish '*la mas nbhal*,' 'the feast of the apple-gathering' (All Hallow Eve), which being pronounced somewhat like 'Lammas-ool,' was corrupted into 'lamb's wool.' It was usual for each person who partook of the spicy beverage to take out an apple and eat it, wishing good luck to the company.

¶ *Constituents.* Various analyses show that the Apple contains from 80 to 85 per cent. of water, about 5 per cent. of proteid or nitrogenous material, from 10 to 15 per cent. of carbonaceous matter, including starch and sugar, from 1 to 1·5 per cent. of acids and salts. The sugar content of a fresh apple varies from 6 to 10 per cent., according to the variety. In spite of the large proportion of water, the fresh Apple is rich in vitamins, and is classed among the most valuable of the anti-scorbutic fruits for relieving scurvy. All apples contain a varying amount of the organic acids, malic acid and gallic acid, and an abundance of salts of both potash and soda, as well as salts of lime, magnesium, and iron.

It has been calculated that in 100 grams of dried apples, there are contained 1·7 milligrams of iron in sweet varieties and 2·1 milligrams in sour varieties. It has also been proved by analysis that the Apple contains a larger quantity of phosphates than any other vegetable or fruit.

The valuable acids and salt of the Apple exist to a special degree in and just below the skin, so that, to get the full value of an apple, it should be eaten unpeeled.

The bark of the Apple-tree which is bitter, especially the root-bark, contains a principle called Phloridzin, and a yellow colouring matter, Quercetin, both extracted by boiling water. The seeds give Amygdaline and an edible oil.

Apple oil is Amyl Valerate or Amyl-valeric Ester. An alcoholic solution has been used as a flavouring liquid, called Apple Essence.

Fresh apple-juice is employed for the N.F. Ferrated Extract of Apples.

¶ *Medicinal Uses.* The chief dietetic value of apples lies in the malic and tartaric acids. These acids are of signal benefit to persons of sedentary habits, who are liable to liver derangements, and they neutralize the acid products of gout and indigestion. 'An apple a day keeps the doctor away' is a respectable old rhyme that has some reason in it.

The acids of the Apple not only make the fruit itself digestible, but even make it helpful in digesting other foods. Popular instinct long ago led to the association of apple sauce

with such rich foods as pork and goose, and the old English fancy for eating apple pie with cheese, an obsolete taste, nowadays, is another example of instinctive inclination, which science has approved.

The sugar of a sweet apple, like most fruit sugars, is practically a predigested food, and is soon ready to pass into the blood to provide energy and warmth for the body.

A ripe raw apple is one of the easiest vegetable substances for the stomach to deal with, the whole process of its digestion being completed in eighty-five minutes.

The juice of apples, without sugar, will often reduce acidity of the stomach; it becomes changed into alkaline carbonates, and thus corrects sour fermentation.

It is stated on medical authority that in countries where unsweetened cider is used as a common beverage, stone or calculus is unknown, and a series of inquiries made of doctors in Normandy, where cider is the principal drink, brought to light the fact that not a single case of stone had been met with during forty years.

Ripe, juicy apples eaten at bedtime every night will cure some of the worst forms of constipation. Sour apples are the best for this purpose. Some cases of sleeplessness have been cured in this manner. People much inclined to biliousness will find this practice very valuable. In some cases stewed apples will agree perfectly well, while raw ones prove disagreeable. There is a very old saying:

'To eat an apple going to bed
Will make the doctor beg his bread.'

The Apple will also act as an excellent dentifrice, being a food that is not only cleansing to the teeth on account of its juices, but just hard enough to mechanically push back the gums so that the borders are cleared of deposits.

Rotten apples used as a poultice is an old Lincolnshire remedy for sore eyes, that is still in use in some villages.

It is no exaggeration to say that the habitual use of apples will do much to prolong life and to ameliorate its conditions. In the Edda, the old Scandinavian saga, Iduna kept in a box, apples that she gave to the gods to eat, thereby to renew their youth.

A French physician has found that the bacillus of typhoid fever cannot live long in apple juice, and therefore recommends doubtful drinking water to be mixed with cider.

A glucoside in small crystals is obtainable from the bark and root of the apple, peach and plum, which is said to induce artificial diabetes in animals, and thus can be used in curing it in human beings.

The original *pomatum* seems to date from Gerard's days, when an ointment for roughness of the skin was made from apple pulp, swine's grease, and rosewater.

The astringent verjuice, rich in tannin, of the Crab, is helpful in chronic diarrhœa.

The bark may be used in decoction for intermittent and bilious fevers.

Cider in which horse-radish has been steeped has been found helpful in dropsy.

Cooked apples make a good local application for sore throat in fevers, inflammation of the eyes, erysipelas, etc.

Stewed apples are laxative; raw ones not invariably so.

¶ *Dosages.* Of infusion of the bark, 1 to 4 fluid ounces. Of phloridzin, 5 to 20 grains.

¶ *Other Species.* APPLE OF SODOM (*Solanum sosomeum*). This is a prickly species found near the Dead Sea, full of dust when ripe, the result of insects' eggs deposited in the young fruit. Some regard the name as referring to *Colocynth*, and others again to *Calatropis procera*.

ADAM'S APPLE is a variety of the Lime (*Citrus limetta*). Superstition relates that a piece of the forbidden apple stuck in Adam's throat, and his descendants ever after had the lump in the front of the neck which is so named.

MAY APPLE. American Mandrake, Racoonberry, Hog-apple, Devil's Apple, Indian Apple, or Wild Lemon, a purgative used in liver complaints.

THORN-APPLE. *Datura stramonium*, Jamestown Weed, Stinkweed, or Apple of Peru, has narcotic, anodyne leaves and seeds.

CUSTARD APPLES, or Annonas, grow in hotter countries than common apples. Several species are edible, especially *Annona tripetela*, *A. squamosa* and *A. glabra*. *A. palustris* of Jamaica, also called Shining-leaved Custard Apple or Alligator Apple, is said to be a strong narcotic. The wood is so soft that it is used for corks.

PINE APPLE is the fruit of *Bromelia ananas*, deriving its name from its pine-cone shape.

LOVE APPLE, or Tomato Plant, is the fruit of *Solanum lycopersicum* or *Lycopersicum esculentum*.

MAD, or JEW'S APPLE is the fruit of *S. esculentum*.

RED ASTRACHAN APPLE is var. *Astracanica* of *P. malus*. Var. *Paradisiaca* and var. *Pendula* are also well-known.

Varieties of Crabs are Dartmouth or Hyslop, Fairy, John Downie, Orange, Transcendent and Transparent.

MALAY APPLE is the fruit of *Eugenia malaccensis*.

ROSE APPLE, or Jamrosade, is the fruit of *E. jambos*. The bark and seeds are employed in diarrhœa and diabetes. Dose, of fluid extract, 10 minims or more, in hot water.

THE STAR APPLE (*Chrysophyllum cainito*) of the West Indies has an astringent, milky juice.

APPLE OF ACAJOU is a name of *Anacardium occidentale*, which yields a caustic oil used like croton oil. It is used in marking-ink. It also supplies a gum like gum-arabic.

CEDAR APPLES are excrescences on the trunk of *Juniperus virginiana*, used as an anthelmintic in the dose of from 10 to 20 grains three times a day.

ELEPHANT APPLE is the fruit of *Feronia elephantum*.

KANGAROO APPLE is the fruit of *S. laciniatum*.

KAU, or KEL APPLE is the South African name for the fruit of *Abaria Kaffra*.

MAMMEE APPLE is the fruit of *Mammea americana*.

MANDRAKE APPLE is the fruit of *Mandragora officinalis*.

MONKEY APPLE is the West Indian name for *Clusia flava*.

OAK-APPLES are spongy excrescences on the branches of oak-trees.

OATAHETTE APPLE is the fruit of *Spondias dulcis*.

PERSIAN APPLE is the name by which the peach was first known in Europe.

PRAIRIE APPLE is *Psoralea esculenta*.

WILD BALSAM APPLE is *Echinocystis lobata*.

RECIPES

Plain *Apple Marmalade*, unspiced, is made by peeling, and coring and cutting up 12 lb. of apples and cooking very gently with 6 lb. of sugar and 1 quart of cider till the fruit is very soft. Then pour through a sieve and place in glass jars. This is delicious with cream as a sweet.

It is also possible to make a very delicious preserve called *Apple Honey,* by boiling apples slowly for a very long time without any addition of sugar. The people of Denmark make this in hayboxes, thus saving fuel. When cooked long enough it is thick and brown, and very sweet, and will keep any length of time.

Spiced Apples

Peel some nice-shaped firm apples, and for every 3 lb. allow 1 quart of vinegar, 4 lb. of sugar, 1 oz. of stick cinnamon, and ½ oz. of cloves. Boil sugar, vinegar, and spices together, then put in the apples, and let them cook until tender. Put them into a jar; boil down the syrup quite thick, and pour it over. Cover and keep for a few months in a cool place.

Apple Ginger

4 lb. apples.	3 pt. water.
4 lb. sugar.	2 oz. essence of ginger.

Boil sugar and water until they form a syrup. Add ginger. Pare, core and quarter apples, boil them in the syrup until transparent. Place in warm, clean, dry jars. Tie down at once.

Another recipe. 3 lb. of apples, ¼ lb. of preserved ginger. Pare apples and cut up in small pieces. Put in a basin of water till required; then put skins and cores into preserving pan, cover with water and boil till tender; strain and measure juice. To 3 pints of juice allow 2 lb. of sugar. Take next the cut apples and weigh them. To every 3 lb. allow 2 lb. of sugar. Put apples, juice, sugar and ginger all together into pan, and boil till ready.

Apple Jelly

6 lb. apples (any kind).
1 lemon.

Wipe and cut apples in four, remove bad parts. Place in preserving pan with lemon, well cover with water. Boil to a pulp. Place in a bag, allow to drip into a clean basin all night. Return to pan, adding 1 lb. sugar to each pint of juice. Boil for ¾ hour or until jelly will set. Pour into clean, dry, warm jar. Tie down at once.

Crab-apple Jelly

Cook the Crab-apples with 6 cloves and an inch of ginger until the fruit is soft. Strain, boil again and add ¾ lb. of sugar to a pint of liquid. Let boil until it jells. To make a successful jelly, the fruit should not be cooked too long, and the sugar should be added just before the strained liquid boils.

Apples Stewed Whole

Take 6 large red apples, wash carefully, and put in a fruit kettle, with just enough boiling water to cover. Cover the kettle, and cook slowly until the apples are soft, with the skins broken and the juice a rich red colour. After removing the apples, boil the juice to a syrup, sweeten, and pour over the apples. A better plan is to make a syrup with sugar and water in which apples are stewed whole or sliced. Some add a clove, others the rind of lemon to improve the flavour.

Apples with Raisins

Pare, core, and quarter a dozen or more medium-sized apples. Clean thoroughly one fourth the weight of apples in raisins, and pour over them a quart of boiling water. Let them steep until well swollen, then add the apples, and cook until tender. Sugar to sweeten may be added if desired, although little will be needed unless the apples are very tart. Dried apples soaked overnight may be made much more palatable by stewing with raisins or English currants in the same way for about 40 minutes.

Apple Sandwiches

Cut apples into very thin slices, and lay between slices of bread and butter.

Apple and Egg Cream

Stew and strain 1 large tart apple; when cold add the well-beaten white of an egg. Serve with cream.

Apple Water

The following is an excellent recipe for a suitable drink for all fevers and feverish conditions:

Slice thinly 3 or 4 apples without peeling. Boil in a saucepan with a quart of water and a little sugar until the slices become soft. The apple water must then be strained and taken cold.

Mutton Baked with Apples and Onions

2 lb. of mutton cutlets from neck, salt, 1 onion, 4 medium-sized apples. Prepare the meat by removing the bone and superfluous fat. Season with salt and lay in a baking dish. Cover the meat with finely-sliced sour apples and finely-chopped onions. Bake in a moderate oven until the meat is tender, which will be about 1 hour.

There is an old recipe for *Apple Bread*, wherein to the sponge was added one-third as much grated apple, which is perhaps worth reviving.

In some years, especially in a drought, the number of *windfalls* in the orchard is unusually large. They should never be allowed to lie on the ground, as most of them contain grubs which will hatch out into insect pests that ruin the fruit trees. But not a single windfall need be wasted. Those which are big enough to peel can be used for puddings or tarts. The small fruit can be used for making jelly, by cutting each in half so as to remove any grub that may be present, and then proceeding in the usual manner, as given above. The jelly will be a brilliant red colour, equal to Crab-apple Jelly in taste and appearance.

Excellent chutneys, syrups, and jams can also be made from windfalls, which curiously enough so many housewives use only for stewing and baking, neglecting less hum-drum methods, of which there are quite a number, of using the fruit. We give a few recipes:

Apple Fool

2 lb. of windfall apples, 4 oz. of brown sugar, 1 gill of water, a strip of lemon peel or 2 or 3 cloves or an inch of stick cinnamon, ½ pint of custard or cream.

Wash and wipe the fruit, remove any damaged portions, and cut into quarters, without peeling or coring. Put it into a pan with the sugar, water, and flavouring, bring to the boil, and simmer until the fruit is soft. If too dry add a little more water. Rub through a sieve, and mix the puree with custard or cream.

Pears (windfall) or plums of any kind may be used in the same way, or apples and pears mixed.

Apple, Pear and Plum Jam

8 lb. of each fruit, ½ pint of cider, ¼ oz. of powdered cloves (no sugar is required).

Cut the windfall apples and pears in quarters (do not peel or core), put into a preserving pan with the plums, and add enough water to cover the bottom of the pan. Bring to the boil, then simmer until soft. Press out all the juice by pouring the fruit on to a fine hair sieve. Strain the juice through muslin, and boil it quickly in an uncovered pan until thick like a syrup. Put the syrup into bottles and cork well. Tie bladder or run sealing wax over the corks, and store in a dry, cool place.

Apple Chutney

About 30 windfall apples, 2 oz. of salt, ¾ lb. of brown sugar, 4 oz. of onions, 1 clove of garlic, 3 oz. of powdered ginger, ½ oz. of dried chillies, 1 oz. of mustard seeds, 4 oz. of raisins, 1 quart of vinegar.

Peel, core and slice the apples, put them into a pan with the sugar and vinegar and simmer until the apples are soft. Wash the mustard seed with vinegar and dry in a cool oven. Stone and chop the raisins. Peel and slice the garlic and onions, slice the chillies and pound them all in a mortar with the ginger and mustard seeds. When the apples are soft add the rest of the ingredients and let the mixture become cold. Mix well and put into bottles. Cork and cover like jam.

Note.—Some prefer not to pound the chillies, but to add them just before putting the chutney into the bottles.

(*POISON*)
APPLE (BALSAM)

Momordica balsamina
N.O. Cucurbitaceæ

Synonyms. Balsamina
Part Used. The fruit deprived of the seeds
Habitat. East India

¶ *Description.* A climbing annual plant cultivated in gardens for the sake of its ornamental fruit, which is of a rich orange red colour, ovate attenuated towards each extremity, angular, warty, not unlike a cucumber. The name is derived from Mordio, to bite, so called from the bitten appearance.
¶ *Constituents.* Has not been examined qualitatively.
¶ *Medicinal Action and Uses.* A liniment is made by adding the pulped fruit (without the seeds) to almond oil. This is useful for piles, burns, chapped hands, etc. The pulp is also used as a poultice. The fluid extract is used for dropsy.

Caution is required in administering—large doses resulting in death.
¶ *Dosage and Preparation.* Dose, 6 to 15 grains.
¶ *Poisons and Antidotes.* As for Bitter Apple.

¶ *Other Species.*
Momordica charantia and East Indian species with bright orange yellow oblong fruits. *Momordica mixta* has fruit shaped like a bullock's heart, bright red in colour.

(*POISON*)
APPLE (BITTER)

Citrullus colocynthis (SCHRAD.)
N.O. Cucurbilaceæ

Synonyms. Colocynth Pulp. Bitter Cucumber
Part Used. The dried pulp
Habitat. Native of Turkey abounding in the Archipelago; also found in Africa (Nubia especially), Asia, Smyrna and Trieste

¶ *Description.* The Colocynth collected from the Maritime Plain between the mountains of Palestine and the Mediterranean, is mainly shipped from Jaffa and known as Turkish Colocynth. This is the best variety. It is an annual plant resembling the common watermelon. The stems are herbaceous and beset with rough hairs; the leaves stand alternately on long petioles. They are triangular, many-cleft, variously sinuated, obtuse, hairy, a fine green on upper surface, rough and pale under. Flowers yellow, appearing singly at axils of leaves; fruit globular, size of an orange, yellow and smooth, when ripe contains within a hard coriaceous rind, a white spongy pulp enclosing numerous ovate compressed white or brownish seeds.

¶ *Constituents.* The pulp contains Colocynthin, extractive, a fixed oil, a resinous substance insoluble in ether, gum, pectic acid or pectin, calcium and magnesium phosphates, lignin and water.

¶ *Medicinal Action and Uses.* It is a powerful drastic hydragogue cathartic producing, when given in large doses, violent griping with, sometimes, bloody discharges and dangerous inflammation of the bowels.

Death has resulted from a dose of $1\frac{1}{2}$ teaspoonsful of the powder. It is seldom prescribed alone. It is of such irritant nature that severe pain is caused if the powdered drug be applied to the nostrils; it has a nauseous, bitter taste and is usually given in mixture form with the tinctures of podophylum and belladonna. Colocynth fruits broken small are useful for keeping moth away from furs, woollens, etc.

¶ *Dosage and Preparation.* Dose of the powder, 2 to 5 grains.

It is an important ingredient in Extractum Colocynthidis Compositum, Pilula Colocynthidis Composita, and Pilula Colocynthidis et Hyosiyami.

¶ *Poison and Antidotes.* In case of poisoning by Colocynth the stomach should be emptied, opium given by mouth or rectum followed by stimulants and demulcent drinks.

APPLE, CUSTARD. *See* PAPAW

APLOPPAS. *See* (FALSE) DAMIANA

¶ *Description.* Bixa orillana is a small tree 20 to 30 feet high, leaves broad, heart-shape, pointed, flowers in bunches, rose-coloured fruit, heart-shaped, $1\frac{1}{4}$ inches long, reddish brown, covered with stiff prickles. Annatto is obtained by pulping the seeds, allowing the pulp to dry spontaneously and pressing it into cakes, or the seeds are soaked in water, allowed to ferment, and when the colouring matter subsides are collected and formed into cakes. There are two forms of Annatto used in commerce, the Spanish, made in Brazil, which is hard, brittle, odourless, and is usually sent over in rolls; and the French, or flag, Annatto which comes from Cayenne, and is bright yellow in colour, firm, soft, and evil-smelling, owing to the fermentive process used in which urine is utilized. The French is superior as a dye. Annatto has a dull fracture, a sweetish odour and a very disagreeable saline bitterish taste. It is inflammable, but does not melt with

heat; insoluble in water, though it colours it yellow.

¶ *Constituents.* The chief constituent is a red resinous substance named Bixin.

¶ *Medicinal Action and Uses.* In the past it was used internally as medicine, but is now only employed as a colouring agent for ointments and plasters, and sometimes as a substitute for saffron. In South America it is largely used by the Caribs and other Indian tribes to paint their bodies. South American Indians are said to produce directly from the seeds, without fermentation, a brilliant carmine-like colour.

In this country it is used for colouring cheese, inferior chocolate, etc., and by the Dutch as a butter colouring. It is also used as a dye for fabrics and in the manufacture of varnishes and lacquers.

¶ *Adulterants.* Annatto is adulterated with ochre, sand gypsum, and a farinaceous matter.

APOCYRUM. *See* (CANADIAN) HEMP

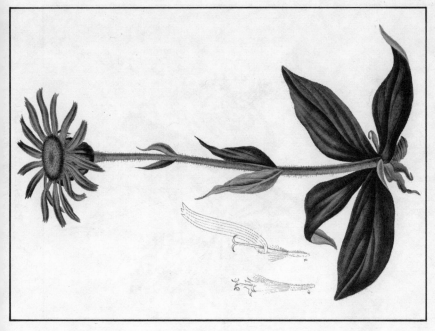

ARNICA
Arnica Montana

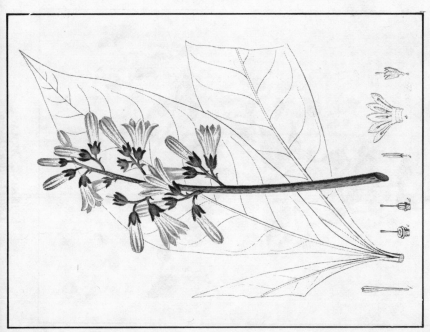

TRUE ANGOSTURA
Cusparia Febrifuga

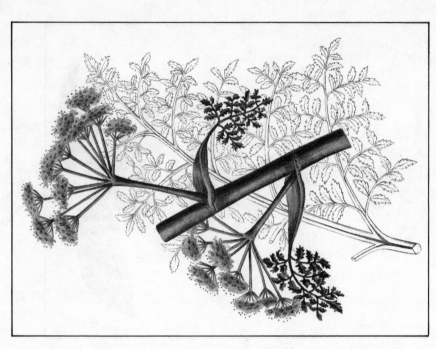

PERSIAN ASAFETIDA
Ferula Persica

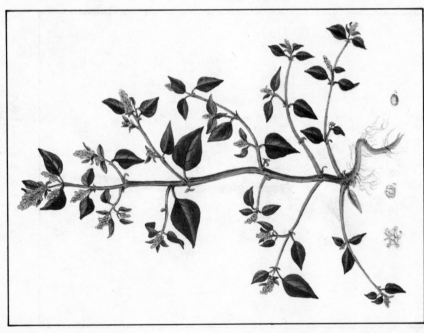

STINKING ARRACH
Chenopodium Olidum

APRICOT
Prunus Armeniaca (LINN.)
N.O. Rosaceæ

Synonyms. Apricock. *Armeniaca vulgaris*
Parts Used. Kernels, oil
Habitat. Although formerly supposed to come from Armenia, where it was long culti-vated, hence the name *Armeniaca*, there is now little doubt that its original habitat is northern China, the Himalaya region and other parts of temperate Asia. It is culti-vated generally throughout temperate regions. Introduced into England, from Italy, in Henry VIII's reign

¶ *Description.* A hardy tree, bearing stone fruit, closely related to the peach. The leaves are broad and roundish, with pointed apex; smooth; margin, finely serrated; petiole $\frac{1}{2}$ inch to an inch long, generally tinged with red. The flowers are sessile, white, tinged with the same dusky red that appears on the petiole, with five regular sepals and petals and many stamens, and open very early in the spring. The fruit, which ripens end of July to mid-August, according to variety, is a drupe, like the plum, with a thin outer, downy skin enclosing the yellow flesh (meso-carp), the inner layers becoming woody and forming the large, smooth, compressed stone, the ovule ripening into the kernel, or seed. As a rule in Britain, the fruit rarely ripens unless the tree is trained against a wall; when growing naturally, it is a medium-sized tree. It is propagated by budding on the mussel-plum stock. A great number of varieties are distinguished by cultivators. Large quanti-ties of the fruit are imported from France. The kernels of several varieties are edible and in Egypt, those of the Musch-musch variety form a considerable article of commerce. Like those of the peach, apricot kernels con-tain constituents similar to those of the bitter almond: they are imported in large quanti-ties from Syria and California and are often used by confectioners in the place of bitter almonds, which they so closely resemble as to be with difficulty distinguished.

The French liqueur *Eau de Noyaux* is pre-pared from bitter apricot kernels.

¶ *Constituents.* Apricot kernels yield by ex-pression 40 to 50 per cent. of a fixed oil, similar to that which occurs in the sweet almond and in the peach kernel, consisting chiefly of Olein, with a small proportion of the Glyceride of Linolic acid, and commonly sold as Peach Kernel oil (*Ol. Amygdæ Pers.*). From the cake is distilled, by digestion with alcohol, an essential oil (*Ol. Amygdæ Essent. Pers.*) which contains a colourless, crystalline glucoside, Amygdalin, and is chemically identical with that of the bitter almond. The essential oil is used in confectionery and as a culinary flavouring.

¶ *Medicinal Action and Uses.* Apricot oil is used as a substitute for Oil of Almonds, which it very closely resembles. It is far less expensive and finds considerable employ-ment in cosmetics, for its softening action on the skin. It is often fraudulently added to genuine Almond oil and used in the manu-facture of soaps, cold creams and other pre-parations of the perfumery trade.

ARALIAS. *See* ANGELICA TREE, BAMBOO BRIAR (AMERICAN), DWARF ELDER, SARSAPARILLAS (AMERICAN), SPIKENARD

ARAROBA
Andira araroba (AGUIAR.)
N.O. Leguminosæ

Synonyms. Goa Powder. Crude Chrysarobin. Bahia Powder. Brazil Powder. Ring-worm Powder. Chrysatobine. Goa. Araroba Powder. Voucapoua Araroba
Parts Used. The medullary matter of the stem and branches, dried and powdered
Habitat. Brazil

¶ *Description.* The powder is named Goa, after the Malabar port, and it was not real-ized until 1875 that the drug was Brazilian Araroba, and reached the East Indies through Portugal and her colonies. The tree from which it is obtained, *Andira Araroba*, is large, smooth, and quite commonly found in Bahia, Brazil. The yellowish wood has longitudinal canals and interspaces in which the powder is deposited in increasing quantity as the tree ages. It is probably due to a pathological condition. It is scraped out with an axe, after felling, sawing, and splitting the trunk, and is thus inevitably mixed with splinters and debris, so that it needs sifting, and is sometimes ground, dried, boiled, and filtered.

It irritates the eyes and face of the wood-men.

As it darkens quickly, the crude chrysa-robin is changed from primrose yellow to shades of dark brown before it is met with in commerce, when it often contains a large percentage of water, added to prevent the dust from rising.

An amber skin-varnish is made with 20 parts of amber to 1 of chrysarobin in turpentine.

¶ *Constituents.* The powder is insoluble in water, but yields up to 80 per cent. of its weight to solutions of caustic alkalies and to benzene. It contains 80 to 84 per cent. of chrysarobin (easily convertible into chrysophanic acid), resin, woody fibre, and bitter extractive. Goa Powder is usually regarded as crude chrysarobin, while the purified chrysarobin, or Araroba, is a mixture extracted by hot benzene, which melts when heated, and leaves not more than 1 per cent. of ash when it finally burns.

Chrysarobin is a reduced quinone, and chrysophanic acid (also found in rhubarb, yellow lichen, Buckthorn Berries, *Rumox Eckolianus*, a South African dock, etc., etc.), is a dioxymethylanthraquinone.

Chrysarobin contains at least five substances, and owes its power to one of these, chrysophanol-anthranol.

Lenirobin, a tetracetate,, and eurobin, a triacetate, are recommended as substitutes for chrysarobin, as they do not stain linen indelibly. (Benzin helps to remove the stains of chrysarobin.)

The action of chrysarobin on the skin is not due to germicidal properties, but to its chemical affinity for the keratin elements of the skin. The oxygen for its oxidation is abstracted from the epithelium by the drug.

Oxidized chrysarobin, obtained by boiling chrysarobin in water with sodium peroxide, can be used as an ointment for forms of eczema which chrysarobin would irritate too much.

¶ *Medicinal Action and Uses.* The internal dose in pill or powder is a gastro-intestinal irritant, producing large, watery stools and vomiting. It is used in eczema, psoriasis, acne, and other skin diseases.

In India and South America it has been esteemed for many years for ringworm, psoriasis, dhobi's itch, etc., as ointment, or simply moistened with vinegar or saliva. The application causes the eruption to become whitish, while the skin around it is stained dark.

In the crude form it should never be applied to the head, as it may cause erythema and œdema of the face. The 2 per cent. ointment is good in eczema (after exudation has ceased), fissured nipples, and tylosis of the palms and soles after the skin has been removed by salicylic acid plaster, etc.

A drachm of chrysarobin may be dissolved in a fluid ounce of official flexible collodion, painted over the parts with a camel's-hair brush, and the part coated with plain collodion to avoid staining the clothing; or chrysarobin may be dissolved in chloroform and the solution painted on the skin. For hæmorrhoids, an ointment mixed with iodoform, belladonna, and petrolatum is recommended.

It is said to have been used as a tænifuge.

¶ *Dosage.* One-half grain.

¶ *Other Species.*

A. Inermis, or Cabbage Tree of South America and Senegambia, has a narcotic, anthelmintic bark, known as Bastard Cabbage Bark or Worm Bark. The powder, in doses of 3 to 4 grains, purges like jalap. The decoction is usually preferred.

The symptoms of an overdose are feverish delirium and vomiting, which should be counteracted with lime-juice or castor oil.

It is no longer officially used in England. *See* CABBAGE TREE.

ARBUTUS (STRAWBERRY TREE)

Arbutus unede
N.O. Ericaceæ

Habitat. In the woods at Killarney and Bantry is found growing wild the beautiful evergreen shrub, known as the Arbutus, or Strawberry Tree (*Arbutus unede*), which for its attractiveness should gain a place in every well-planted garden. It would, indeed, be hard to find any other ornamental shrub or tree that has such a cheerful appearance throughout the autumn and early winter, when its dense mass of greenery is mingled with a profusion of flower clusters and ruddy, round fruit resembling small strawberries. The creamy-white, bell-shaped flowers, often tinged with pink, are intermixed with the orange-scarlet rough fruit, which owing to the length of time it takes to ripen, remains on the tree for twelve months, not maturing until the autumn succeeding that in which the flower is produced.

Although a native of South Europe, and only growing wild here in the South of Ireland on the rocks at Killarney, the Arbutus will thrive almost anywhere in this country, especially in warm and coast regions, where it will grow 20 feet high, making huge, globular masses of green, though ordinarily its height is only from 8 to 10 feet. In inland districts it is liable to be cut down during exceptionally severe winters, but this rarely happens, and if large bushes are apparently killed by cold, they almost invariably send up strong shoots again. When young, it requires in order to get it established, a slight protection during winter. It grows quickly in sheltered places, but dislikes shade, and seems to be most at home in a deep, light soil, flourishing best in a sandy loam.

When eaten in quantities this fruit is said to be narcotic, and the wine made from it in Spain has the same property.

The tree is common in the Mediterranean region, and the fruit was known to the ancients, but according to Pliny (who gave the tree the name of Arbutus) was not held in much esteem, as the name implies (*un ede*=one I eat), the fruits being considered so unpalatable, that no one tasting them for the first time would be tempted to repeat the experiment. Nevertheless, there is some evidence that at one time the fruit was an article of diet with the ancients. Horace praises the tree for its shade and Ovid for its loads of 'blushing fruit.' Virgil recommends the young shoots as winter food for goats and for basket-work.

Gerard speaks of it in his time as growing in 'some few gardens,' and says, 'the fruit being ripe is of a gallant red colour, in taste somewhat harsh, and in a manner without any relish, of which thrushes and blackbirds do feed in winter.'

In Spain, a sugar and spirit have been extracted from the fruit and a wine made from it in Corsica.

In the neighbourhood of Algiers it forms hedges, and in Greece and Spain the bark has been used for tanning. The wood of the tree makes good charcoal.

ARBUTUS, TRAILING

Epigæa repens (LINN.)
N.O. Ericaceæ

Synonyms. Mountain Pink. May Flower. Gravel Plant. Ground Laurel. Winter Pink

Part Used. The leaves, used dried to make an infusion, and fresh to make a tincture

Habitat. The Trailing Arbutus (*Epigæa repens*, Linn.) is a small evergreen creeping shrub, found in sandy soil in many parts of North America, in the shade of pines. Its natural home is under trees, and it will thrive in this country only in moist, sandy peat in shady places. It has long been known in cultivation here as an ornamental plant, having been introduced into Great Britain in 1736. Like the common Arbutus, or the Strawberry Tree and the Bearberry, it belongs to the order *Ericaceæ*, the family of the heaths

❡ *Description.* It grows but a few inches high, with a trailing, shrubby stalk, which puts out roots at the joints, and when in a proper soil and situation multiplies very fast. The evergreen leaves are stalked, broadly ovate, 1 to 1½ inches long, rough and leathery, with entire, wavy margins and a short point at the apex. Branches, leaf-stalks and nerves of the leaves are very hairy. The flowers are produced at the end of the branches in dense clusters. They are white, with a reddish tinge and very fragrant, divided at the top into five acute segments, which spread open in the form of a star. The plant flowers in April and May, but rarely produces fruit in England. It is stated to be injurious to cattle when eaten by them.

The name of the genus, *Epigæa*, derived from Greek words signifying 'upon the ground,' expresses the mode of growth and trailing habit of the species.

❡ *Cultivation.* The Trailing Arbutus generally does not do well when attempts are made to take it from its natural surroundings and place it under garden conditions. It needs partial shade and very free soil, composed mainly of decayed leaves, and perfect shelter from cold winds. In short grass, just within the shelter of oak trees, the overhanging boughs of which give a certain amount of shade, it will do well and is usually found at its best in sandy loam, on a gravelly, well-drained subsoil.

In removing it from its native haunts, dense tufts of low-growing and apparently young plants should be selected. These should be lifted intact, and to such a depth, that the roots are not disturbed, and placed in conditions in the home garden exactly similar to those from which they are taken. To plant in an ordinary herbaceous border means failure. They must not be choked out with long grass or coarse weeds. In dry weather water the plants occasionally, and in winter give a little mulching of leaves.

It may be increased by seeds, but they are slow in sprouting. By carefully dividing the well-established tufts in autumn, or by layering the branches, good plants are sometimes obtained. The trailing stalks, which put out roots at the joints, may be cut off from the old plant and placed in a shady situation and a moist soil. If done in autumn, the plants may be well rooted before the spring. Cuttings of previous year's wood are more successful inserted in sandy soil, under a glass in gentle heat in spring. As soon as rooted, plants should be grown on in pots until well established, and then transferred in early autumn, or spring, to their permanent positions outside, but they will never grow so well in the open (where they will always be more or less stunted specimens), as they will under conditions which closely imitate those which the plant enjoys in the woods of New England.

¶ *Medicinal Action and Uses.* Astringent and diuretic. Used in the same way as Buchu and *Uva ursi* for bladder and urinary troubles: of special value when the urine contains blood or pus, and when there is irritation.

The infusion of 1 oz. of the leaves to a pint of boiling water may be taken freely.

See BEARBERRY, UVA URSI.

ARCHANGEL. *See* NETTLES

ARECA NUT

Areca catechu (LINN.)
N.O. Palmacea

Synonyms. Betel Nut. Pinang
Part Used. The seed
Habitat. East Indies, cultivated in India and Ceylon

¶ *Description.* A handsome tree cultivated in all the warmer parts of Asia for its yellowish-red fruits the size of a hen's egg, containing the seed about the size of an acorn, conical shape with flattened base and brownish in colour externally; internally mottled like a nutmeg. The seeds are cut into narrow pieces and rolled inside Betel Pepper leaf, rubbed over with lime and chewed by the natives. They stain the lips and teeth red and also the excrement, they are hot and acrid when chewed.

¶ *Constituents.* Areca Nut contains a large quantity of tannin, also gallic acid, a fixed oil gum, a little volatile oil, lignin, and various saline substances. Four alkaloids have been found in Areca Nut – Arecoline, Arecain, Guracine, and a fourth existing in very small quantity. Arecoline resembles Pilocarpine in its effects on the system. Arecaine is the active principle of the Areca Nut.

¶ *Medicinal Actions and Uses.* Areca Nut is aromatic and astringent and is said to intoxicate when first taken. The natives chew these nuts all day. Whole shiploads are exported annually from Sumatra, Malacca, Siam and Cochin China. In this country Areca Nut is made into a dentrifrice on account of its astringent properties. Catechu is often made by boiling down the seeds of the plant to the consistency of an extract, but the proper Catechu used in Britain is produced from the *Acacia catechu.* The flowers are very sweet-scented and in Borneo are used in medicines as charms for the healing of the sick. In India the nut has long been used as a tænifuge for tapeworm. The action of Arecain resembles that of Muscarine and Pilocarpine externally, internally used it contracts the pupils.

Arecoline Hydrobromide, a commercial salt, is a stronger stimulant to the salivary glands than Pilocarpine and a more energetic laxative than Eserine. It is used for colic in horses.

¶ *Dosages and Preparations.* Of the powdered nut for tapeworm 1 to 2 teaspoonsful. Of the Fluid Extract of Areca Nut, 1 drachm. Of the Arecoline Hydrobromide, for colic in horses, 1 to 1½ grains. Of the Arecoline Hydrobromide, for human use, $\frac{1}{15}$ to $\frac{1}{10}$ grains.

¶ *Other Species.* In Malabar *Areca Dicksoni* is found growing wild and is used by the poor as a substitute for the true Betel Nut (*A. aleraceæ*). The Cabbage Palm, which grows profusely in the West Indies, derives its name from the bud topping the tall stem; this consists of leaves wrapped round each other as in the cabbage, the heart of which is white inside. It has a delicate taste and is cut and cooked as a vegetable, many of these beautiful palms being destroyed in this way. It is said that in the empty cavity a beetle lays its eggs. These turn into maggots which are eaten with great relish by the negroes of Guiana.

ARENARIA RUBRA. *See* SPERGULARIA

ARNICA

Arnica montana (LINN.)
N.O. Compositæ

Synonyms. Mountain Tobacco. Leopard's Bane
Parts Used. Root, flowers
Habitat. *Arnica montana* or Leopard's Bane is a perennial herb, indigenous to Central Europe, in woods and mountain pastures. It has been found in England and Southern Scotland, but is probably an escape

¶ *Description.* The leaves form a flat rosette, from the centre of which rises a flower stalk, 1 to 2 feet high, bearing orange-yellow flowers. The rhizome is dark brown, cylindrical, usually curved, and bears brittle wiry rootlets on the under surface.

¶ *Cultivation.* Arnica thrives in a mixture of loam, peat, and sand. It may be propagated by root division or from seed. Divide in spring. Sow in early spring in a cold frame, and plant out in May.

The flowers are collected entire and dried, but the receptacles are sometimes removed as they are liable to be attacked by insects.

The root is collected in autumn after the leaves have died down.

¶ *Constituents.* A bitter yellow crystalline principle, Arnicin, and a volatile oil. Tannin and phulin are also present. The flowers are said to contain more Arnicin than the rhizome, but no tannin.

¶ *Medicinal Action and Uses.* In countries where Arnica is indigenous, it has long been a popular remedy. In the North American colonies the flowers are used in preference to the rhizome. They have a discutient property. The tincture is used for external application to sprains, bruises, and wounds, and as a paint for chilblains when the skin is unbroken. Repeated applications may produce severe inflammation. It is seldom used internally, because of its irritant effect on the stomach. Its action is stimulant and diuretic, and it is chiefly used in low fevers and paralytic affections.

Arnica flowers are sometimes adulterated with other composite flowers, especially *Calendula officinalis*, *Inula brittanica*, *Kragapogon pratensis*, and *Scorzonera humilis*.

A homœopathic tincture, X6, has been used successfully in the treatment of epilepsy; also for seasickness, 3 X before sailing, and every hour on board till comfortable.

For tender feet a foot-bath of hot water containing ½ oz. of the tincture has brought great relief. Applied to the scalp it will make the hair grow.

Great care must be exercised though, as some people are particularly sensitive to the plant and many severe cases of poisoning have resulted from its use, especially if taken internally.

British Pharmacopœia Tincture, root, 10 to 30 drops. United States Pharmacopœia Tincture, flowers, 10 to 30 drops.

ARRACHS OR ORACHES

Chenopodium olidum (LINN.)
Chenopodium vulvaria (S. WATS.)
N.O. Chenopodiaceæ

Synonyms. Stinking Motherwort. Wild Arrach. Stinking Arrach. Stinking Goosefoot. Netchweed. Goat's Arrach
Part Used. Herb
Habitat. The Wild Arrach, or Netchweed (*Chenopodium olidum*, Linn.), (syn. *C. vulvaria*, S. Wats.), one of the common Goosefoots, is an annual herb, found on roadsides and dry waste ground near houses, from Edinburgh southward

¶ *Description.* Its stem is not erect, but partly lying, branched from the base, the opposite branches spreading widely, a foot or more in length.

The stalked leaves are oval, wedge-shaped at the base, about ½ inch long, the margins entire.

The small, insignificant green flowers are borne in spikes from the axils of the leaves and consist of five sepals, five stamens and a pistil with two styles. There are no petals and the flowers are wind-fertilized. They are in bloom from August to October.

The whole plant is covered with a white, greasy mealiness, giving it a grey-green appearance, which, when touched, gives out a very objectionable and enduring odour, like that of stale salt fish, and accounts for its common popular name: Stinking Goosefoot.

¶ *Medicinal Action and Uses.* The name of 'Stinking Motherwort' refers to the use of its leaves in hysteria and nervous troubles connected with women's ailments: it has emmenagogue and anti-spasmodic properties. In former days, it was supposed even to cure barrenness and in certain cases, the mere smelling of its fœtid odour was held to afford relief.

An infusion of 1 oz. of the dried herb in a

pint of boiling water is taken three or four times daily in wineglassful doses as a remedy for menstrual obstructions. It is also sometimes used as a fomentation and injection, but is falling out of use, no doubt on account of its unpleasant odour and taste.

The infusion has been employed in nervous debility and also for colic.

A fluid extract is prepared, the dose being ½ to 1 drachm.

The leaves have also been made into a conserve with sugar. Dr. Fuller's famous *Electuarium hystericum* was compounded by adding 48 drops of oil of Amber (*Oleum Succini*) to 4 oz. of the conserve of this *Chenopodium*. A piece of the size of a chestnut was prescribed to be taken when needed and repeated as often as required.

¶ *Constituents*. Chemical analysis has proved Trimethylamine to be a constituent, together with Osmazome and Nitrate of Potash. The plant gives off free Ammonia.

Culpepper speaks of two kinds of 'Arrach.' One he calls Garden Arrach, 'called also Orach, and Arage,' giving its Latin name as *Atriplex hortensis*. The other kind he calls 'Wild and Stinking Arrach' (*A. olida*), 'called also Vulvaria, Dog's Arrach, Goat's Arrach and Stinking Motherwort.' He is emphatic in his commendation of this 'Stinking Arrach' for every kind of women's diseases and troubles, though he describes its odour in his usual unvarnished language, saying: 'It smells like rotten fish, or something worse.'

The names 'Dog's Arrach,' 'Goat's Arrach' and 'Dog's Orache' point to a contemptuous scorn of its unfitness as a pot-herb compared with the true Orache (*Atriplex*), closely allied to it.

ARRACH (GARDEN)
Atriplex hortensis

Synonyms. Mountain Spinach. Garden Orache

The Garden Orache, or Mountain Spinach (*Atriplex hortensis*), is a tall, erect-growing hardy annual, a native of Tartary, introduced into this country in 1548. It is not much cultivated here now, but is grown a good deal in France, under the name of *Arroche*, for its large and succulent leaves, as a substitute for Spinach and to correct the acidity of Sorrel.

The quality of the spinach yielded by Orache is, however, far inferior to that of Common Spinach, or even of the New Zealand Spinach.

There are several varieties of Orache, of various colourings. The White and the Green are the most desirable kinds.

The plants should be grown quickly, in rich soil. They may be sown in rows, 2 feet apart, and thinned out to the same distance apart in the rows, sowings being in May, and for succession, again in June. If dry, water must be freely given so as to maintain a rapid growth.

'Orache is cooling,' says Evelyn, 'and allays the pituit humours.' Being set over the fire, neither this nor the lettuce needs any other water than their own moisture to boil them in.

The name Orache, given to this Goosefoot and others of the same tribe, is a corruption of *aurum*, gold, because their seeds, mixed with wine, were supposed to cure the ailment known popularly as the 'yellow jaundice.' They excite vomiting.

¶ *Uses*. Heated with vinegar, honey and salt and applied, the Orache was considered efficacious to cure an attack of gout.

ARRACH (HALBERD-LEAVED)
Atriplex hastata

The Halberd-leaved Wild Orache (*Atriplex hastata*) closely resembles the Spreading Orache and is often regarded merely as a sub-species, but is, however, of a more erect character and the lower leaves are broadly triangular, the lobes widely spread.

It is a troublesome weed in gardens and cultivated ground.

The leaves have been frequently eaten instead of spinach, but Culpepper says its chief virtues lie in the seed, employed in the same manner as that of the Garden Orache.

ARRACH (WILD)
Atriplex patula

Synonym. Spreading Orache

The Wild Orache (*Atriplex patula*) is a common native weed on clays and heavy ground. It has spreading stems, 2 to 3 feet long, sometimes prostrate, only occasionally erect (hence often called the Spreading Orache).

The leaves are triangular in outline, rather narrow, the lower ones in opposite pairs.

The very small, green flowers are in dense clusters.

The whole plant is more or less covered with a powdery meal, often tinged red. It is distinguished from the Goosefoot genus, *Chenopodium*, by the solitary seeds being enclosed between two triangular leaf-like valves.

56

'These are to be gathered when just ripe; for if suffered to stand longer, they lose part of their virtue. A pound of these bruised, and put into three quarts of spirit, of moderate strength, after standing six weeks, afford a light and not unpleasant tincture; a tablespoonful of which, taken in a cup of water-gruel, has the same effect as a dose of ipecacuanha, only that its operation is milder and does not bind the bowels afterwards. . . . It cures headaches, wandering pains, and the first attacks of rheumatism.'

See CHENOPODIUM, GOOD KING HENRY.

ARROWHEAD

Sagittaria sagittifolia (LINN.)
N.O. Alismaceæ

Synonyms. Wapatoo. Is'-ze-kn

The *Alismaceæ* group of plants in general contain acrid juices, on account of which, a number of species, besides the Water Plantain, have been used as diuretics and antiscorbutic.

Several species of *Sagittaria*, natives of Brazil, are astringent and their expressed juice has been used in making ink.

The rhizome of *Sagittaria sagittifolia* (Linn.), the Arrowhead, Wapatoo, and *S. Chinensis* (Is'-ze-kn) are used respectively by the North American Indians and the Chinese as starchy foods, as are some other species.

The Arrowhead is a water plant widely distributed in Europe and Northern Asia, as well as North America, and abundant in many parts of England, though only naturalized in Scotland.

The stem is swollen at the base and throws out creeping stolons or runners, which produce globose winter tubers, ½ inch in diameter, composed almost entirely of starch.

The leaves are borne on triangular stalks that vary in length with the depth of the water in which the plant is growing. They do not lie on the water, like those of the Water Lily, but stand boldly above it. They are large and arrow-shaped and very glossy.

The early, submerged leaves are ribbon-like.

The flower-stem rises directly from the root and bears several rings of buds and blossoms, three in each ring or whorl, and each flower composed of three outer sepals and three large, pure white petals, with a purple blotch at their base. The upper flowers are stamen-bearing, the lower ones generally contain the seed vessels only.

The root tubers are about the size of a small walnut. They grow just below the surface of the mud. The Chinese and Japanese cultivate the plant for the sake of these tubercles, which are eaten as an article of wholesome food. Bryant, in *Flora Dietetica*, writes of them:

'I cured some of the bulbs of this plant in the same manner that saloop is cured, when they acquired a sort of pellucidness, and on boiling afterwards, they broke into a gelatinous meal and tasted like old peas boiled.'

The tubers, it has been stated, may also be eaten in the raw state.

¶ *Medicinal Action and Uses.* Diuretic and antiscorbutic.

See PLANTAIN (WATER).

ARROWROOT

Maranta arundinaceæ (LINN.)
N.O. Marantaceæ

Synonyms. Indian Arrowroot. Maranta Indica. Maranta ramosissima. Maranta Starch or Arrowroot. East or West Indian Arrowroot. Araruta. Bermuda Arrowroot
Part Used. The fecula or starch of the rhizome
Habitat. Indigenous in the West Indian Islands and possibly Central America. Grows in Bengal, Java, Philippines, Mauritius, Natal, West Africa

¶ *Description.* The name of the genus was bestowed by Plumier in memory of Bartommeo Maranto (*d.* 1559, Naples), a physician of Venosa in Basilicata. The popular name is a corruption of the Aru-root of the Aruac Indians of South America, or is derived from the fact that the plant is said to be an antidote to arrow-poison.

The product is usually distinguished by the name of the place from which it is imported. Bermuda Arrowroot was formerly the finest, but it is now rarely produced, and the name is applied to others of high standard.

It was introduced into England about 1732, though it will only grow as a stove plant, with tanners' bark. The plant is an herbaceous perennial, with a creeping rhizome with upward-curving, fleshy, cylindrical tubers covered with large, thin scales that leave rings of scars. The flowering stem reaches a height of 6 feet, and bears creamy flowers at the ends of the slender branches that terminate the long peduncles. They grow in pairs. The numerous, ovate, glabrous leaves are from 2 to 10 inches in length, with long sheaths often enveloping the stem.

The starch is extracted from rhizomes not more than a year old. They are washed, pulped in wooden mortars, stirred in clean water, the fibres wrung out by hand, and the milky liquor sieved, allowed to settle, and then drained. Clean water is again added, mixed, and drained, after which the starch is dried on sheets in the sun, dust and insects being carefully excluded. The starch yield is about one-fifth of the original weight of the rhizomes. It should be odourless and free from unpleasant taste, and when it becomes mouldy, should be rejected. It keeps well if quite dry. The powder creaks slightly when rubbed, and feels firm. Microscopical examination of the starch granules is necessary for certainty of purity. Potato starch, which corresponds in chemical and nutritive qualities, is sometimes substituted, but it has a somewhat unpleasant taste, and a test with hydrochloric acid brings out an odour like French beans. Sago, rice, and tapioca starches are also found occasionally as substitutes.

The jelly is more tenacious than that of any other starch excepting *Tous-les-mois*.

Arrowroot is often used simply in the form of pudding or blanc-mange. The roots could be candied like Eryngo.

¶ *Constituents.* An 1887 analysis of the root of the St. Vincent Arrowroot gave starch 27·17 per cent., fibre, fat, albumen, sugar, gum, ash, and 62·96 per cent. water.

Of the starch was given: starch 83·70 per cent., fibre, fat, sugar, gum, ash and sand, and water 15·87 per cent.

The official granules, according to Pereira, are 'rarely oblong, somewhat ovate-oblong, or irregularly convex, from 10 to 70 microns in diameter, with very fine lamellæ, a circular hilium which is fissured in a linear or stellate manner.'

¶ *Medicinal Action and Uses.* Arrowroot is chiefly valuable as an easily digested, nourishing diet for convalescents, especially in bowel complaints, as it has demulcent properties. In the proportion of a tablespoonful to a pint of water or milk, it should be prepared by being first made into a smooth paste with a little cold milk or water, and then carefully stirred while the boiling milk is added. Lemon-juice, sugar, wine, or aromatics may be added. If thick, it will cool into a jelly that usually suits weaning infants better than other farinaceous foods.

It is said that the mashed rhizomes are used for application to wounds from poisoned arrows, scorpion and black spider bites, and to arrest gangrene.

The freshly-expressed juice, mixed with water, is said to be a good antidote, taken internally, for vegetable poisons, such as Savanna.

¶ *Other Species.*

Maranta ramosissima is the *M. arundinaceæ* of the East Indies.

M. allouya and *M. nobilis* are also West Indian species. The term arrowroot is applied to other starches.

BRAZILIAN ARROWROOT, or Tapioca Meal, is obtained from *Manihot utilissima* (bitter) and *M. palmata* (sweet). It is also called Bahia, Rio, or Para-Arrowroot. *See* MANDIOCA.

TAHITI ARROWROOT is from *Tacca oceanica* (*pinnatifida*). It is a favourite article of diet in the tropics, being found in the Sandwich and South Sea Islands, and is said to be the best arrowroot for dysentery.

EAST INDIAN ARROWROOT is from *Curcuma augustifolia*, or *longa*.

TOUS-LES-MOIS is from *Canna edulis* and *C. achiras*, of the West Indies, called Indian Shot, from their hard, black seeds, used as beads, and Balisier, from the use of their leaves for packing, in Brazil.

OSWEGO ARROWROOT, used in America, is from *Zea Mays*, Indian Corn.

MEXICAN ARROWROOT is from the seeds of *Dion edule*.

CHINESE ARROWROOT is said to be from the tubers of *Nelumbium speciosum*.

PORTLAND ARROWROOT was formerly obtained from *Arum maculatum*, but it was acrid and not very satisfactory.

M. dichotoma has stems used, when split, for making shade mats in India.

M. Malaccensis has poisonous roots used as an ingredient in a Borneo arrow-poison.

ARTICHOKE, JERUSALEM

Helianthus tuberosus
N.O. Compositæ

Synonym. Sunflower Artichoke

Habitat. The Jerusalem Artichoke (*Helianthus tuberosus*, Linn.), now commonly cultivated in England for its edible tubers, another of the numerous Sunflowers, is a native of the North American plains, being indigenous in the lake regions of Canada, as far west as Saskatchewan, and from thence southward to Arkansas and the middle parts of Georgia.

Though it rarely blossoms in England, it flowers profusely in its native country (blooming also freely in South Africa), the flowers, however, being small and inconspicuous, produced just above the last leaves. Its name, Jerusalem Artichoke, does not, as it seems, imply that it grows in Palestine, but is a corruption of the Italian *Girasola articiocco*, the Sunflower Artichoke, *Girasola* meaning 'turning to the sun,' an allusion to the habit it is supposed to have in common with many of the Sunflower tribe. The North Italian word *articiocco* – modern *carciofo* – comes through the Spanish, from the Arabic *Al-Kharshuf*. False etymology has corrupted the word in many languages: it has been derived (though wrongly) in English from 'choke' and 'heart,' or the Latin *hortus*, a garden; and in French, the form *artichaut* has been connected with *chaud*, hot, and *chou*, a cabbage.

¶ *History.* It appears to have been cultivated as an article of food by the Indians of North America before the settlement in that country of Europeans, and very soon attracted the attention of travellers. Sir J. D. Hooker, in the *Botanical Magazine*, July, 1897, gives the following account of its introduction:

'In the year 1617, Mr. John Goodyer, of Mapledurham, Hampshire, received two small roots of it from Mr. Franqueville, of London, which, being planted, enabled him before 1621 "to store Hampshire." In October of the same year, Mr. Goodyer wrote an account of it for T. Johnson, who printed it in his edition of Gerard's "Herball," which appeared in 1636, where it is called *Jerusalem Artichoke*. Previous to which, in 1629, it had been figured and described under that name by Parkinson in his "Paradisus," and he also mentions it in his "Theatrum" in 1640. From the last-given date to the present time, the Jerusalem Artichoke has been extensively cultivated in Europe, but rather as a garden vegetable than a field crop, and has extended into India, where it is making its way amongst the natives under Hindoo, Bengali, and other native names.'

Parkinson speaks of it as 'a dainty for a queen.' When first introduced, the mode of preparation of the tubers was to boil them till tender, and after peeling, they were eaten sliced and stewed with butter, wine and spices. They were also baked in pies, with marrow, dates, ginger, raisins, sack, etc. Parkinson called them 'Potatoes of Canada,' because the French brought them first from Canada. Their flavour is somewhat sooty when cooked and not agreeable to everyone, but they are very nutritious, and boiled in milk form an excellent accompaniment to roast beef.

The tuber, instead of containing starch like the potato, has the allied substance Inulin. The chief ingredients are water, 80 per cent.; albuminoids, 2 per cent.; gum, known as Lævulin, 9·1 per cent.; sugar, 4·2 per cent.; inulin, 1·1 per cent.

¶ *Cultivation.* In any odd bit of ground, shaded or open, that is unsuitable for other vegetables, a crop of the tubers of Jerusalem Artichoke will always be obtained, though like other things, it pays for a good position and generous culture and the largest tubers will be produced in a light, rich soil.

The ground should be well dug over and if at all heavy, or poor, should be lightened by incorporating some sand with it enriched with well-rotted manure.

For planting, which may be done in February, but not later than March, small tubers should be chosen and indeed reserved for this purpose when the crop is taken up, but almost any part of a tuber will grow and form a plant. The sets should be planted in rows, 3 feet apart and at a distance of 18 inches from each other in the rows; they should be set at least 6 inches deep. As a rule, a great number of plants is produced from one tuber.

The ground should be kept clean by hoeing and as the plants grow in height, a little earth should be drawn up around the stem.

Cut the plants down when the leaves are decayed, but not before, otherwise the tubers will cease to grow. The tubers may be left in the ground till wanted for use. If taken up towards the end of November, they may be stored in sand or earth, but they must be covered, so that the light and air may be effectually excluded, otherwise they will be of a dark colour when cooked.

The white-skinned variety, 'New White Mammoth,' is to be recommended. The tubers have a clean, white skin, instead of the purplish-red tint of the old variety. They are also rounder in shape and not so irregular in form as the tubers of the red sort. This variety is equally hardy, being in no way liable to injury from frost.

Jerusalem Artichokes afford a useful screen for a wooden fence, when planted along the foot of it, but the more open the spot, the more likely they are to prosper. When once planted, the difficulty is to get the ground clear of them again, for the smallest tuber will grow. It is desirable to change the ground allotted to their culture about once in three years, for when they are permitted to remain too long on the same spot, the tubers deteriorate in size and quality.

ARTICHOKE, GLOBE

Cynara Scolymus
N.O. Compositæ

The Globe Artichoke (*Cynara Scolymus*, Linn.) also has a tuberous root, but it is the large flower-buds that form the edible portion of the plant, and it is from a similarity in the flavour of the tuber of the Jerusalem Artichoke to that of the fleshy base of this flower that the Jerusalem Artichoke has obtained its name.

The expanded flower has much resemblance to a large thistle; the corollas are of a rich blue colour.

It is one of the world's oldest cultivated vegetables, grown by the Greeks and the Romans in the heyday of their power. It was introduced into this country in the early sixteenth century both as a vegetable and an ornamental plant in monastery gardens.

Gerard (1597) gives a good figure of the Artichoke. Parkinson (1640) alludes to a statement of Theophrastus (fourth century B.C.) that 'the head of Scolymus is most pleasant, being boyled or eaten raw, but chiefly when it is in flower, as also the inner substance of the heads is eaten.' Though this 'inner substance' – botanically the 'receptacle' – has a delicate flavour, it contains little nutritive matter.

Tournefort (1730) says:

'The Artichoke is well known at the table. What we call the bottom is the *thalamus* on which the *embryos* of the seeds are placed. The leaves are the scales of the empalement. The Choak is the florets, with a chaffy substance intermixt (the pappus). The French and Germans boil the heads as we do, but the Italians generally eat them raw with salt, oil and pepper.'

In Italy the receptacles, dried, are also largely used in soups.

The whole plant has a peculiar smell and a strong bitter taste. It was reputed to be aperient.

¶ *Cultivation.* It is grown either from *seed*, sown in March, in a deep, moist, rich soil, which may be greatly aided by wood-ashes and seaweed (for it is partial to saline manures, its home being the sandy shores of Northern Africa); or by planting *suckers* in April; the latter is preferable for a permanent plantation. Strong plants may be ensured by inserting them 4 feet each way, but market growers usually put out suckers in rows 4½ feet apart, and 2 feet distant in the rows. Suckers should be planted when about 9 inches high; put in rather deep in soil and planted firmly and covered with rough mulch. If the weather be dry, they will need watering, and during hot weather water and liquid manure should be given freely to ensure a good supply of large heads.

Seedlings that are started well in a suitable bed do better than plants from suckers, especially in a dry season.

Vigorous seedlings send down their roots to a great depth. To get large heads, all lateral heads should be removed when they are about the size of a large egg. After the heads are used, the plant should be cut down.

The Artichoke is hardy on dry soils in winters of only average severity. But on moist soils – so favourable to fine heads – a severe winter will kill the plantations unless they have some kind of protection. This is usually ensured by cutting down the stems and large leaves without touching the smaller central leaves, and when severe frost threatens, to partially earth up the rows with soil taken from between, also adding dry, light litter loosely thrown over; the latter is removed in the spring and the earth dug back, and a liberal supply of manure dug in. At the end of five years a plantation is worn out; the best method being to sow a bed annually and allow it to stand for two years.

The flower-stems grow erect and attain the height of 4 to 6 feet. They are each terminated by a large globular head of imbricated oval spiny scales of a purplish-green colour. These envelop a mass of flowers in the centre. These flowerheads in an immature state contain the parts that are eatable, which comprise the fleshy receptacle usually called the 'bottom,' freed from the bristles and seed-down, commonly called the 'choke,' and the thick lower part of the imbricated scales or leaves of the involucre.

Although Artichokes are a common vegetable, they are not so much in request with us as on the Continent.

In France, the bottoms are often fried in paste, and enter largely into râgouts. They are occasionally used for pickling, but for this purpose the smaller heads which are formed on the lateral shoots that spring in succession from the main stem, are generally preferred when about the size of a large egg.

The chard of Artichokes, or the tender central leaf-stalks, blanched, is by some considered to be equal to the Cardoon.

The flowers are very handsome, and are said to possess the property of coagulating milk.

ARTICHOKE, CHINESE

Stachys Sieboldii

The Chinese Artichoke (*Stachys Sieboldii*), is a comparatively new variety of vegetable of which the edible portion is the tuber.

This plant has nothing to do with either of the well-known Artichokes, both of which belong to the *Compositæ* family, whereas this belongs to the Mint family, *Labiatæ*, and to the same genus that is represented here by the Woundworts and Wood Betony. This species occurs wild in Northern China, where it is also cultivated, its native name being *Tsanyungtzu*, while in Japan it is called *Chorogi*. It was introduced as a culinary vegetable by the late Dr. M. T. Masters, F.R.S., in 1888. The tubers are eaten more in France than in this country.

The dietetic value resides especially in a carbonaceous substance, which reaches 16·6 per cent.; the nitrogenous ingredients amount to 3·2 per cent.; water forming 78·3 per cent. of the bulk.

¶ *Cultivation*. It is perfectly hardy and may be left in the ground until required for use. Planting should take place in the spring and the tubers dug through the winter as required. The plants are perfectly easily grown and extraordinarily productive.

ARTICHOKE, CARDOON

Scolymus Cardunculus (LINN.)
N.O. Compositæ

The Cardoon (*Scolymus Cardunculus*, Linn.) is by some botanists regarded as merely a variety of this plant, but by others as a distinct species. The blanched inner leafstalks and the top of the stalk, the receptacle, are the only parts eaten, used in soups, stews and salads. It is more cultivated on the Continent than here. Dioscorides refers to its cultivation on a large scale near Great Carthage, and Pliny speaks of its medicinal virtues. Dodoens, in his *History of Plants* (1559), describes it as much more spinescent than the *Articoca* of Italy and less used as food.

¶ *Cultivation*. It requires so much room that it is little grown in small gardens, and as a crop can hardly pay for the enormous extent of ground that it claims.

Its culture is very similar to that of celery, only on a rather larger scale, the trenches being made wider and slightly deeper than those for the latter, and the plants being placed about 18 inches to 2 feet apart in the rows and 6 feet between the rows. The trenches are prepared in just the same way as those for celery.

Sow three or four seeds in a 'large sixty' pot, in April, placing the pots in a gentle warmth, or in a cold frame, when the seed will soon germinate. Mice are very fond of the seed, consequently the frame must be kept close enough to prevent their entry, or the whole will be destroyed.

When the little plants appear, select the strongest plant in each pot and pull out all the others. In due course the plants are hardened off and planted out, usually in July, before they become potbound, in the previously prepared trenches, which have been well manured, about 18 inches or more apart, keeping them well supplied with water. Occasionally forking or hoeing between the plants to encourage growth and destroy weeds will be all that is required besides watering, until September or October, when they will be ready to earth up in order to blanch them.

Before doing this, it is usual to arrange the stalks upright and wind a hay-band round them closely, to within about a foot of the tops. This soil must then be earthed up nearly as high as the hay-bands. It is important that this operation should be performed on a dry day, when the hearts are free from water, or they will probably decay. No earth, also, must be allowed to fall between the leaves. When the plants have grown still further, the earthing up should be increased.

The plants will be fit for use in about a month after earthing up and may be taken up as required. Should Cardoons be in great demand, an earlier or later sowing may be made for successional crops; for spring crop, sow at midsummer. If the plants have to be kept for any length of time during winter, they must be protected from rain and frost by means of a covering of litter, or may be dug up and stored in a cool, dry place, the hay-bands being allowed to remain.

When taking up, remove the earth carefully and take up the plants by the roots, which must be cut off. The points of the leaves are also cut off to where they are solid and blanched. These latter are washed, the parts of the leaf-stalks remaining on the stem are tied to it, and they are ready for cooking.

The SPANISH CARDOON, with large solid ribs and spineless leaves, is the one most generally grown. It is not so liable to run to seed as the common variety.

In France, the TOURS CARDOON is much cultivated, but, on account of the long, sharp spines on the leaves, great care has to be exercised in working amongst them.

¶ *Uses.* Cardoons are said to yield a good yellow dye, and in some parts of Spain they substitute the down of this plant for rennet in making cheese; a strong infusion is made overnight and the next morning, when the milk is warm from the cow, they put nearly half a pint of the infusion to about 14 gallons of milk.

RECIPES
Artichoke Bottoms

If dried, they must be soaked, then stewed in weak gravy, and served with or without forcemeat in each. Or they may be boiled in milk, and served with cream sauce; or added to râgouts, French pies, etc.

To Dress Artichokes

Trim a few of the outside leaves off, and cut the stalk even. If young, half an hour will boil them. They are better for being gathered two or three days, first. Serve them with melted butter, in as many small cups as there are Artichokes, to help with each.

To keep Artichokes for the Winter

Artichoke bottoms, slowly dried, should be kept in paper bags.

Artichokes à la Barigoule

Trim some small Artichokes, and with the handle of an iron tablespoon scoop out all the fibrous part inside. Put about a pound of clean hog's-lard into a frying-pan on the fire, and when quite hot, fry the bottom of the Artichokes in it for about 3 minutes; then turn them upside down, and fry the tips of the leaves also; drain them upon a cloth to absorb all the grease, and fill them with a similar preparation to that directed for tomatoes à la Provençale; tie them up with a string, and place them in a large stewpan or *fricaudeaupan*; moisten with a little good stock; put the lid on; place them in the oven to simmer for about an hour; remove the strings; fill the centre of each Artichoke with some Italian sauce; dish them up with some of the sauce, and serve.

Artichokes à la Lyonnaise

Pull off the lower leaves without damaging the bottoms of the Artichokes, which must be turned smooth with a sharp knife; cut the Artichokes into quarters, remove the fibrous parts, trim them neatly, and parboil them in water with a little salt. Then put them in a saucepan on a slow fire to simmer very gently for about three-quarters of an hour, taking care that they do not burn; when done they should be of a deep yellow colour and nicely glazed. Dish them up in the form of a dome, showing the bottom of the Artichokes only; remove any leaves that may have broken off in the *sautapan*; add a spoonful of brown gravy or sauce, 2 pats of butter and some lemon-juice; simmer this over the fire, stirring it meanwhile with a spoon; and when the butter has been mixed in with the sauce, pour it over the Artichokes, and serve.

ARUM. *See* CUCKOO-PINT, (AMERICAN) WAKE-ROBIN

ASAFETIDA
Ferula fœtida (REGEL.)
N.O. Umbelliferæ

Synonyms. Food of the Gods. Devil's Dung
Part Used. An oleogum-resin obtained by incision of root
Habitat. Afghanistan and Eastern Persia

¶ *Description.* A coarse umbelliferous plant growing up to 7 feet high, large fleshy root covered with bristly fibres, has been for some time successfully cultivated in Edinburgh Botanical Gardens; stem 6 to 10 feet, numerous stem leaves with wide sheathing petioles; flowers pale greeny yellow; fruit oval, flat, thin, foliaceous, reddish brown with pronounced vittæ, it has a milky juice and a strong fœtid odour; was first found in the sandy desert of Aral in 1844, but has been known since the twelfth century. Several species of *Ferula* yield Asafetida. The bulk of the drug comes from the official plant, which is indigenous to Afghanistan and grows from two to four thousand feet above sea-level. These high plains are arid in winter but are thickly covered in summer with a luxuriant growth of these plants. The great cabbage-like folded heads are eaten raw by the natives. June is the month the juice is collected from plants about four years old. The roots of plants which have not flowered are exposed and slashed, then shaded from the sun for five or six weeks and left for the gummy oleoresin to leak out and harden. It is then scraped off in reddish lumps and put into leather bags and sent to Herat, where it is adulterated before being placed on the market. The fruit is sent to India for medicinal use. A very fine variety of Asafetida is obtained from the leaf bud in the centre of the root, but this does not come into European commerce, and is only used in India, where it is known in the Bazaars as Kandaharre Hing. It appears in reddish-yellow flakes and when squeezed gives out an oil.

¶ *Constituents.* Its chief constituent is about 62 per cent. of resin, 25 per cent. of gum and 7 per cent. oil. The drug also contains free ferulic acid, water, and small quantities of various impurities.

¶ *Medicinal Action and Uses.* The odour of Asafetida is stronger and more tenacious than that of the onion, the taste is bitter and acrid; the odour of the gum resin depends on the volatile oil. It is much used in India and Persia in spite of its offensive odour as a condiment and is thought to exercise a stimulant action on the brain. It is a local stimulant to the mucous membrane, especially to the alimentary tract, and therefore is a remedy of great value as a carminative in flatulent coliç and a useful addition to laxative medicine. There is evidence that the volatile oil is eliminated through the lungs, therefore it is excellent for asthma, bronchitis, whooping-cough, etc. Owing to its vile taste it is usually taken in pill form, but is often given to infants per rectum in the form of an emulsion. The powdered gum resin is not advocated as a medicine, the volatile oil being quickly dissipated.

ASARABACCA

Synonyms. Hazelwort. Wild Nard
Parts Used. Root and Herb

Asarabacca is the only British species of the Birthwort family (and perhaps not indigenous). It is a curious plant consisting of a very short fleshy stem, bearing two large, dark-green, kidney-shaped evergreen leaves, and a solitary purplish-green drooping flower.

Found in woods and very rare. Flowering in May – Perennial.

The herbs belonging to this order are chiefly plants or shrubs of a tropical habitat, very abundant in South America; but rare elsewhere.

¶ *Medicinal Action and Uses.* Tonic and stimulant, sometimes acrid or aromatic. The dried and powdered leaves of Asarabacca (*Asarum Europæum*) are used in the preparation of cephalic snuffs, exciting sneezing and giving relief to headache and weak eyes.

Mixed with Ribwort, this herb is used to remove mucous from the respiratory passages.

Virginian Snake-root (*Aristolochia serpentaria*) and other allied species are used as antidotes to the bite of venomous snakes.

The juice extracted from a South American species is said to have the power of stupefying serpents if placed in their mouths; and

¶ *Dosages and Preparations.* Emulsion, Asafetida 4 parts, water 100 parts. Tincture, ½ to 1 fluid drachm. In pills, 3 grains of the oleogum-resin to a pill.

¶ *Adulterants.* Asafetida is admittedly the most adulterated drug on the market. Besides being largely admixed with inferior qualities of Asafetida, it has often red clay, sand, stones and gypsum added to it to increase the weight.

¶ *Other Species.* The Thibetan Asafetida (*Narthex Asafetida*) is closely allied to the *Ferulas.* The umbels have no involucre, the limb of the calyx is suppressed, the stylopods depressed and cup-shaped, styles recurved, fruit compressed at back, dilated at margin. This variety produces some of the Asafetida used in commerce.

Scorodosma fœtida, another gigantic umbelliferous plant found on the sandy steppes of the Caspian, also supplies the market. The Persian *Sagapenum,* or *Serapinum,* a species of *Ferula* which was formerly imported from Bombay, is in appearance very similar to Asafetida, but does not go pink when freshly fractured, and in smell is less disagreeable than Asafetida. This species is an ingredient of Confection Rutea, British Pharmacopœia Codex.

Asarum Europæum (LINN.)
N.O. Aristolochiaceæ

African species are used by Egyptian jugglers for this purpose.

The British variety is said to be found wild in Westmorland and other places in the north of England.

Culpepper says of the European species:

'This herb, being drunk, not only provoketh vomiting but purgeth downward . . . both choler and phlegm. If you add to it some spikenard, with the whey of goat's milk, or honeyed water, it is made more strong; but it purgeth phlegm more manifestly than choler, and therefore doth much help pains in the hips and other parts; being boiled in whey they wonderfully help the obstructions of the liver and spleen, and are therefore profitable for the dropsy and jaundice: being steeped in wine and drank it helps those continual agues that come by the plenty of stubborn tumours; an oil made thereof by setting in the sun, with some laudanum added to it, provoketh sweating (the ridge of the back anointed therewith) and thereby driveth away the shaking fits of the ague. It will not abide any long boiling, for it loseth its chief strength thereby; nor much beating, for the finer powder doth provoke vomit and urine, and the coarser purgeth downwards. The common use hereof is to take the juice of five or seven leaves in a little drink to cause vomiting; the roots have also the same virtue, though they do not operate forcibly, they are very effectual against the biting of serpents, and therefore are put in as an ingredient both into Mithridate and Venice treacle. The leaves and root being boiled in lye, and the head often washed therewith while it is warm, comforteth the head and brain that is ill affected by taking cold, and helpeth the memory.

'I shall desire ignorant people to forbear the use of the leaves; the roots purge more gently, and may prove beneficial to such as have cancers, or old putrefied ulcers, or fistulas upon their bodies, to take a dram of them in powder in a quarter of a pint of white wine in the morning. The truth is, I fancy purging and vomiting medicines as little as any man breathing doth, for they weaken nature, nor shall ever advise them to be used unless upon urgent necessity. If a physician be nature's servant, it is his duty to strengthen his mistress as much as he can, and weaken her as little as may be.'

¶ *Constituents*. The root and leaves are acrid, and contain a volatile oil, a bitter matter, and a substance like camphor. Asarabacca was formerly used as a purgative and emetic, also to promote sneezing – but it is now rarely used, having been supplanted by safer and more certain remedies.

See (WILD) GINGER, (VIRGINIAN) SNAKE-ROOT.

ASCLEPIAS

This genus consists of herbaceous plants with a milky juice, which are for the most part natives of America. Several species are cultivated for the sake of their showy flowers. All of them are more or less poisonous. *Asclepias curassavica* is employed in the West Indies as an emetic, and goes by the name of Ipecacuanha: the drug known in medicine by that name is derived from quite a different plant and must not be confused with it. *A. tuberosa*, the Butterfly-weed, has mild purgative properties, and promotes perspiration and expectoration. *A. syriaca*, a plant misnamed, as it is a native of America and Canada, is frequently to be met with in gardens; its dull red flowers are very fragrant, and the young shoots are eaten as asparagus in Canada, where a sort of sugar is also prepared from the flowers, while the silk-like down of the seeds is employed to stuff pillows. Some of the species furnish excellent fibre, which is woven into muslins, and in certain parts of India is made into paper.

In Hindu mythology, Soma – the Indian Bacchus – and one of the most important of the Vedic gods, is a personification of the Soma plant, *A. acida*, from which an intoxicating milky juice is squeezed. All the 114 hymns of the ninth book of the Rig Veda are in his praise. The preparation of the Soma juice was a very sacred ceremony and the worship of the god is very old. The true home of the plant was fabled to be in heaven, Soma being drunk by gods as well as men, and it is under its influence that Indra is related to have created the universe and fixed the earth and sky in their place. In post-Vedic literature, Soma is a regular name for the moon, which is regarded as being drunk by the gods and so waning, till it is filled up again by the Sun. In both the Rig Veda and Zend Avesta, Soma is the king of plants; in both, it is a medicine which gives health, long life and removes death.

The three species of Asclepias most used in medicine are the *Calotropis procera*, *A. tuberosa* (Pleurisy root) and *A. Incarnata* (Swamp Milkweed).

See under CALATROPIS, PLEURISY ROOT, SWAMP MILKWEED.

¶ *Other Species*.
A. Pulchra (Ehrh.), by many regarded as a variety of *incarnata*, from which it is distinguished by its hairiness, the other being nearly smooth, is indiscriminately used under the same names.

A. syrica (Willd.) (*A. Cornuti*, Decaisne), found abundantly in Syria, cultivated in some parts of Europe.

It is a very common roadside weed in the eastern and central states of North America, where it is called 'Silkweed,' from the silky down which surmounts the seed, being an inch or two in length, and which has been used for making hats and for stuffing beds and pillows. Attempts have been made to use it as a cotton substitute. Both in France and Russia it has had textile use. The fibres of the stem, prepared in the same manner as those of hemp and flax, furnish a very long, fine thread, of a glossy whiteness.

¶ *Medicinal Action and Uses*. The plant is used medicinally in the United States for the anodyne properties of its root and its rhizome and root have been employed successfully, like those of *A. tuberosa*, both in powder and infusion, in cases of asthma and typhus fever attended with catarrh, producing expectoration and relieving cough and

N.O. Asclepiadaceæ

64

pain. It has also been used in scrofula with great success.

¶ *Constituents*. It has a very milky juice, which is used as a domestic application to warts. The juice has a faint smell and sub-acid taste and an acid reaction. It contains a crystalline substance of a resinous character, closely allied to lactucone and called Ascle-pione; also wax-like, fatty matter, caout-chouc, gum, sugar, salts of acetic acid and other salts.

Besides the above-named species, various other species of the genus have been used medicinally.

An indigenous North American species, *A. verticillata* (Linn.), is used in the Southern States as a remedy in snake bites and the bites of venomous insects. Twelve fluid ounces of a saturated decoction are said to cause an anodyne and sudorific effect, followed by a gentle sleep.

From *A. vincetoxicum* (Linn.), 'Tame-Poison,' besides the glucoside Asclepiadin, said closely to resemble emetine in its physio-logical properties, the glucoside Vincetoxin has been isolated. The root of this species sometimes occurs in commercial Senega Root (*Polygala Senega*).

ASH

Synonyms. Common Ash. Weeping Ash
Parts Used. Leaves, bark

¶ *Description*. The Common Ash (*Fraxinus excelsior*, Linn.), a tall, handsome tree, common in Britain, is readily distinguished by its light-grey bark (smooth in younger trees, rough and scaly in older specimens) and by its large compound leaves, divided into four to eight pairs of lance-shaped leaflets, tipped by a single one, an arrange-ment which imparts a light feathery arrange-ment to the foliage. The leaflets have sharply-toothed margins and are about 3 inches long.

In April or May, according to season, and before the appearance of the leaves, the black flower-buds on the previous year's shoots expand into small dense clusters of a greenish white or purplish colour, some of the minute flowers having purple stamens, others pistil only, and some both, but all being devoid of petals and sepals, which, owing to the pollen being wind-borne, are not needed as protection, or as attraction to insect visitors.

After fertilization, the oblong ovary develops into a thick seed-chamber, with a long, strap-shaped wing, which is known as an Ash-key (botanically: a *samara*). The bunches of 'keys' hang from the twigs in

An infusion of its root was formerly recom-mended in dropsical cases and disorders peculiar to women, as well as for promoting perspiration in fevers, measles and other eruptive complaints, but is now much less used.

A. curas-savica (Blood-weed and Redhead) is also called in the West Indies 'Bastard Ipecacuanha.'

It is a native of the West Indies, abound-ing especially in Nevis and St. Kitts.

Both root and expressed juice are emetic, the former in the dose of 20 to 40 grains, the latter in that of a fluid ounce.

They are also cathartic and vermifuge in somewhat smaller doses (*Amer. Journ. Ph.*, XIX, 19). The juice, made into a syrup, is given as a powerful anthelmintic to children in the West Indies. The plant is used by the negroes as an emetic and the root as a purgative.

According to the *Kew Bulletin*, 1897, this plant has insecticidal properties, being espe-cially obnoxious to fleas. The rooms in-fected are thoroughly swept with rough brooms made from the weed and the pests are said to disappear. D. St. Cyr commends it in phthisis (*Ph. Journ.*, 1903, 714).

Fraxinus excelsior (LINN.)
N.O. Oleaceæ

great clusters, at first green and then brown, as the seeds ripen. They remain attached to the tree until the succeeding spring, when they are blown off and carried away by the wind to considerable distances from the parent tree. They germinate vigorously and grow in almost any soil.

The Common Ash and the Privet are the only representatives in England of the Olive tribe: *Oleaceæ*.

There are about fifty species of the genus *Fraxinus*, and cultivation has produced and perpetuated a large number of distinct varieties, of which the Weeping Ash and the Curl-leaved Ash are the best known.

As a timber tree, the Ash is exceedingly valuable, not only on account of the quick-ness of its growth, but for the toughness and elasticity of its wood, in which quality it surpasses every European tree. The wood is heavy, strong, stiff and hard and takes a high polish; it shrinks only moderately in seasoning and bends well when seasoned. It is the toughest and most elastic of our timbers (for which purpose it was used in olden days for spears and bows and is still used for otter-spears) and can be used for more purposes than the wood of other trees.

It is known that Ash timber is so elastic that a joist of it will bear more before it breaks than one of any other tree. It matures more rapidly than Oak and as sapling wood is valuable. Ash timber always fetches a good price, being next in value to Oak and surpassing it for some purposes, being in endless demand in railway and other waggon works for carriage building. From axe-handles and spade-trees to hop-poles, ladders and carts, Ash wood is probably in constant handling on every countryside – for agricultural plenishings it cannot be excelled. It makes the best of oars and the toughest of shafts for carriages. In its younger stages, when it is called Ground Ash, it is much used, as well as for hop-poles (for which it is extensively grown), for walking-sticks, hoops, hurdles and crates, and it matures its wood at so early an age that an Ash-pole 3 inches in diameter is as valuable and durable for any purpose to which it can be applied as the timber of the largest tree. Ash also makes excellent logs for burning, giving out no smoke, and the ashes of the wood afford very good potash.

The finest Ash is that grown in the Midlands, but so little first-class Ash has been of late years obtained in England that in 1901 the Coachbuilders' Association appealed to the President of the Board of Agriculture to try and stimulate landowners to grow more of this valuable timber, as English Ash is better in quality than that imported from other European countries or from America. Any owner of a devastated woodland or other suitable ground may demand a grant of £2 an acre if he is planting pine, and £4 if he is planting hard woods, such as Ash. The supply of standing Ash timber is also becoming limited in America.

Ash is the second most important wood used in aeroplanes, and a study of the spacious afforestation scheme now in force over the Crown Lands of the New Forest reveals the fact that especial trouble has been taken to find suitable homes for the Ash. The great bulk of the wood used in aeroplanes is Spruce from the Pacific Coast.

Ash *bark* is astringent and has been employed for tanning nets.

Both *bark* and the *leaves* have medicinal use and fetch prices which should repay the labour of collecting them, especially the bark.

The bark is collected from the trunk and the root, the latter being preferred.

Ash bark occurs in commerce in quills, which are grey or greenish-grey externally, with numerous small grey or brownish-white warts, the inner surface yellowish or yellowish brown and nearly smooth; fracture smooth, fibrous in the inner layer; odour slight; taste bitter and astringent.

¶ *Constituents*. The bark contains the bitter glucoside Fraxin, the bitter substance Fraxetin, tannin, quercetin, mannite, a little volatile oil, gum, malic acid, free and combined with calcium.

¶ *Medicinal Action and Uses*. Ash bark has been employed as a bitter tonic and astringent, and is said to be valuable as an antiperiodic. On account of its astringency, it has been used, in decoction, extensively in the treatment of intermittent fever and ague, as a substitute for Peruvian bark. The decoction is odourless, though its taste is fairly bitter. It has been considered useful to remove obstructions of the liver and spleen, and in rheumatism of an arthritic nature.

A ley from the ashes of the bark was used formerly to cure scabby and leprous heads.

The *leaves* have diuretic, diaphoretic and purgative properties, and are employed in modern herbal medicine for their laxative action, especially in the treatment of gouty and rheumatic complaints, proving a useful substitute for Senna, having a less griping effect. The infusion of the leaves, 1 oz. to the pint, may be given in frequent doses during the twenty-four hours.

The distilled water of the leaves, taken every morning, was considered good for dropsy and obesity.

A decoction of the leaves in white wine had the reputation of dissolving stone and curing jaundice.

The leaves should be gathered in June, well dried, powdered and kept in well-corked bottles.

The leaves have been gathered to mix with tea and in some parts of the country are used to feed cattle, when grass is scarce in autumn, but when cows eat the leaves or shoots, the butter becomes rank.

The *fruits* of the different species of Ash are regarded as somewhat more active than the bark and leaves. Ash Keys were held in high reputation by the ancient physicians, being employed as a remedy for flatulence. They were also in more recent times preserved with salt and vinegar and sent to table as a pickle. Evelyn tells us: 'Ashen keys have the virtue of capers,' and they were often substituted for them in sauces and salads.

The keys will keep all the year round if gathered when ripe.

In Mexico, the bark and leaves of *F. nigra* (Marsh), the Black Swamp, Water, Hoop or Basket Ash, are similarly employed to those of the Common Ash. In Mexico, also, the bark and leaves of *F. lanceolata* (Borch.), the Green or Blue Ash, are employed as a bitter tonic and the root as a diuretic.

In the United States, the bark of the American White Ash (*F. Americana*, Linn.) (*F. acuminata*, Lam.) finds similar employment. It has numerous small circular depressions externally and a slightly laminate structure.

Gerard tell us:

'The leaves and bark of the Ash tree are dry and moderately hot . . . the seed is hot and dry in the second degree. The juice of the leaves or the leaves themselves being applied or taken with wine cure the bitings of vipers, as Dioscorides saith, "The leaves of this tree are of so greate virtue against serpents as that they dare not so much as touch the morning and evening shadows of the tree, but shun them afar off as Pliny reports."'

There are many old superstitions concerning the tree. The ancient couplets connecting the flowering precedence of the Oak and Ash with the rainfall of the following summer, 'Oak choke, Ash splash,' etc., have no basis on fact.

According to another superstition, if the trunk of a sapling Ash were split and a ruptured child passed through, the sufferer would be cured.

The Ash had the reputation of magically curing warts: each wart must be pricked with a new pin that has been thrust into the tree, the pins are withdrawn and left in the tree, and the following charm is repeated:

'Ashen tree, ashen tree,
Pray buy these warts of me.'

And there was another superstition that if a live shrew mouse were buried in a hole bored in an Ash trunk and then plugged up, a sprig of this Shrew Ash would cure the paralysis supposed to have been caused by a shrew creeping over the sick person's limbs.

ASH, BITTER

Picræna excelsa (SWARTZ)
N.O. Simarubeæ

Synonym. Jamaica Quassia
Habitat. West Indies

¶ *Description.* The Bitter Ash (*Picræna excelsa*, Swartz), a native of the West Indies, a lofty tree somewhat resembling the Ash Tree, the wood of which is the Jamaica Quassia of commerce, is employed in the place of the original *Quassia amara* of Surinam and Trinidad.

¶ *Uses.* It abounds in a peculiar extractive substance of great bitterness which, as a drug, is purely tonic, invigorating the digestive organs with little excitement of the circulation or increase of bodily heat.

The wood is generally sold in small chips, yellowish white, about an inch wide and 1 to 4 inches long and $\frac{1}{8}$ to $\frac{1}{12}$ inch thick. Their taste is extremely bitter, but there is no odour.

Exhausted Quassia chips having hardly any bitterness are sometimes met with in commerce and also chips with greyish markings due to a fungus. Neither of these are, of course, suitable for an infusion.

Sometimes cups turned out of the wood are made. These are sold as Bitter Cups, and water standing in them for a short time acquires the bitterness of the wood.

From Syrup of Quassia, made with molasses, a harmless fly-poison is prepared, with which cloth or filtering-papers are moistened.

Quassia has been used by brewers as a substitute for hops and is in general use by gardeners, mixed with soft soap, for spraying plants affected with green-fly.

¶ *Preparations.* An infusion of Quassia, 2 oz. in a pint of water, affords a valuable and safe injection for seat-worms.

The dose of the fluid extract is 15 to 30 drops; of the tincture, official in the B.Ph. and U.S.Ph., $\frac{1}{2}$ to 1 drachm; of the U.S.Ph. powdered extract the dose is 1 grain. Of the concentrated solution of the B.Ph. the dose is $\frac{1}{2}$ drachm. The dose of the solid extract is $\frac{1}{2}$ to 2 grains.

See QUASSIA.

ASH, MANNA

Fraxinus ornus (LINN.)
N.O. Oleaceæ

Synonym. Flake Manna
Part Used. Concrete exudation

¶ *Description.* A foreign species of Ash (*Fraxinus ornus*, Linn.), the South European Flowering Ash, a small tree indigenous to the coasts of the Mediterranean from Spain to Smyrna, yields from its bark a sugary sap called *Manna*, used in pharmacy.

The tree blossoms early in summer, producing numerous clusters of whitish flowers; in this country it only attains a height of 15 or 16 feet.

To-day, the Manna of commerce is collected exclusively in Sicily, from cultivated trees, exported from Palermo. The trees are grown in plantations, placed about 7 feet apart. When from eight to ten years old, when the trunk is at least 3 inches in diameter, the collection of Manna is begun. In July and August, when the trees have ceased to put forth leaves freely, a vertical series of oblique incisions are made in the bark on alternate sides of the trunk. Dry, warm weather is essential for a good crop of the Manna which exudes. The larger pieces of incrustation that form, and which are collected in September and October, when the heat has begun to moderate, are known as Flake Manna, and this is the best. It is put on the market in long pieces or granulated fragments of a whitish and pale yellow colour, irregular on one side and smoother and curved on the other, rarely more than 1 inch broad and 2 to 3 inches or more long.

The pieces adhering to the stem after the finer pieces have been gathered are scraped off and form part of the small Manna of commerce. The pieces that form on the lowest incisions, or the pieces that are collected on tiles placed under the tree, and known as 'gerace,' are less crystalline, more glutinous, and are in moist adhesive masses of a dark brown colour. These are less esteemed.

¶ *Medicinal Action and Uses*. Manna has a peculiar odour and a sweetish taste.

It was formerly used in medicine as a gentle laxative, but is now chiefly used as a children's laxative or to disguise other medicines.

It is a nutritive and a gentle tonic, usually operating mildly, but in some cases produces flatulence and pain.

It is still largely consumed in South America and is official in the United States Pharmacopœia.

It is generally given dissolved in water or some aromatic infusion, but the best Flake Manna may be administered in substance, in doses of a teaspoonful up to 1 or 2 oz.

Usually it is prescribed with other purgatives, particularly senna, rhubarb, magnesia and the neutral salts, the taste of which it conceals while it adds to the purgative effect.

For infants, a piece about the size of a hazel-nut is dissolved in a little warm water and added to the food. To children, 30 to 60 grams may be given dissolved in warm milk or a mixture prepared with syrup, or syrup of senna and dill water.

Syrups of Manna are prepared with or without other purgatives.

Manna is sometimes used as a pill excipient, especially for calomel.

Under the name of Dulcinol, a mixture of Manna and common salt has been recommended by Steinberg in 1906 as a sweetening agent in diabetes, the dose ½ to 1 oz.

The Codex of the British Pharmacopœia contains a Syrup of Manna to be prescribed as a mild laxative for children, in the proportion of 1 part of Manna to 10 of water.

The Compound Syrup of Manna of the B.P. Codex is stronger than the Syrup of Manna and contains Senna and fennel in addition, the dose being 1 to 4 fluid drachms.

¶ *Constituents*. Manna of the best quality dissolves in about 6 parts of water, forming a clear liquid. It has no bitterness or acridity.

The chief constituent of Manna is a peculiar, crystallizable, sweet principle called Mannite or Manna Sugar, present to the extent of about 70 per cent. It also contains a fluorescent body named Fraxin, which occasionally gives a greenish colour to Manna and on which is thought to depend its purgative property. Some true sugar and a small quantity of mucilage are also present.

Mannite is white, inodorous, crystallizable in semi-transparent needles of a sweetish taste, soluble in 5 parts of cold water, scarcely soluble in cold alcohol, but readily dissolved by alcohol when hot and deposited when cool. Unlike sugar, it is incapable of undergoing vinous fermentation.

¶ *Definition of Manna in Italy*. An Italian Decree-law, dated August 12, 1927, dealing with the repression of fraud and adulteration in the preparation and trade in substances of vegetable origin, states that the name 'Manna' is reserved for the product obtained by incision into the cortex of the flowering or Manna Ash (*F. ornus* or *F. excelsior*). It is forbidden to prepare, sell, or expose for sale or introduce into trade Manna containing milk sugar, starchy matter, or containing foreign substances of whatever nature, other than those bodies which are present naturally as impurities in the normal proportions existing in the various types of Manna.

In Italy, Mannite is prepared for sale in the shape of small cones, resembling loaf sugar in shape, and is frequently prescribed in medicine instead of Manna.

The term 'Manna' is extremely old and is applied to the saccharine exudence of a number of plants, e.g. *Quercus Vallones* and *persica* (Oak Manna); *Alhagi maurorum* (Alhagi Manna); *Tamarix gallica*, var. *mannifera* (Tamarisk Manna); *Larix Europœa* (Briancon Manna).

The Manna of the present day appears to have been unknown before the fifteenth century. In the sixteenth century, it was collected in Calabria, but none is now brought into commerce from this part of Italy.

Although the name Manna, at first applied to the Manna of the Scriptures, has (as stated) also been applied to various saccharine substances of different origin, none of these corresponds in any way to the Manna of Scripture, inasmuch as they are saccharine substances and do not become corrupt in a night.

The Manna of the biblical narrative answers otherwise in its description to the Tamarisk Manna, exuded in June and July from the slender branches of *Tamarisk gallica*, var. *mannifera*, in the form of honey-like drops, which in the cool temperature of the early morning are found in the solid state. This secretion is caused by the puncture of an insect, *Coccus manniparus*. In the valleys of the peninsula of Sinai, this Manna is collected by the Arabs and sold by them to the monks of St. Catherine, who dispose of it to the pilgrims visiting the convent, under the name of 'gazangabin,' which means 'Tamarisk Honey.' It appears to consist of cane sugar, inverted sugar, and dextrin.

A report issued in 1927 by an expedition of entomologists from the Hebrew University of Jerusalem declares that Manna is not an exudation from the Tamarisk tree, as is popularly supposed, but an excretion from the bodies of the coccid insects themselves. Clear, syrup-like drops (the report states) come from the abdomen of the insects and fall to the ground, where they form grains of sugar, ranging from the size of a pinhead to that of a pea. The amount varies with the abundance or scarcity of the winter rains, and the Bedouins assert that during a good season a man can collect nearly 3½ lb. in a day. The expedition, which was led by Dr. Fritz Bodenheimer of the Zionist experimental agricultural station, observed Manna deposits throughout the long stretch of country which was covered by its journey. The report goes on to state that 'modern science, it seems, was equally ignorant of the true nature of manna till now, and it has been revealed by descendants of those wanderers in the wilderness.'

The only substance which in all respects seems to agree with the Manna of the Israelites is that described a few years ago by Mr. A. J. Swann, in his book on *Fighting the Slave Driver in Central Africa*. The Manna which he saw on the plateaux between the lakes Tanganyika and Nyasa occupied by the Ananbwi tribe, Mr. Swann describes as possessing all the characters of the Manna which is said to have fallen for the benefit of the Israelites. In appearance it resembled coriander seed, was white in colour like hoar-frost and sweet to taste, melted in the sun, and if kept overnight was full of worms in the morning. It required to be baked to keep it any length of time. A cake of this Manna was baked and sent to England, but no one seemed able to identify it, though there can be little doubt that it is a small fungus. The baking process would, of course, destroy its structure, and it is evident that to determine its nature, some of the Manna should be sent home in formaldehyde or corrosive sublimate, when it would be quite possible to make out its structure and classification and to describe it, if new. It does not appear to be regular in its occurrence, as travellers have reported its appearance only at long intervals.

ASH, MOUNTAIN

Pyrus Aucuparia (GÆRTN.)
Sorbus Aucuparia (LINN.)
N.O. Rosaceæ

Synonym. Rowan Tree
Parts Used. Bark, fruit

¶ *Description.* The Mountain Ash (*Pyrus Aucuparia*, Gærtn.) is not related to the true Ashes, but has derived its name from the similarity of the leaves.

In comparison to the true Ash, it is but a small tree, rarely more than 30 feet high. It belongs to the order *Rosaceæ* and is distinguished from its immediate relations the Pear, Crab Apple, White Beam and Wild Service Tree by its regularly pinnate, Ash-like leaves. It is generally distributed over the country in its wild state, but is also much cultivated as an ornamental tree.

All parts of the tree are astringent and may be used in tanning and dyeing black. When cut, the Mountain Ash yields poles and hoops for barrels.

Both the bark and fruit have *medicinal* properties.

The fruit is rather globose, with teeth at the apex and two to three seeded cells. They are used medicinally in either the fresh or the dried state.

¶ *Constituents.* The fruit contains tartaric acid *before*, citric and malic acids *after* ripening; two sugars, sorbin and sorbit, the latter after fermentation; parasorbic acid, which is aromatic and is converted into isomeric sorbic acid by heating under pressure with potassa; bitter, acrid and colouring matters. A crystalline saccharine principle, Sorbitol, which does not undergo the vinous fermentation, has also been found in the fruit.

The seeds contain 22 per cent. of fixed oil. It has been claimed that these seeds killed a child, apparently by prussic acid poisoning.

The *bark* has a soft, spongy, yellowish-grey outer layer and an inner thicker portion, with many layers of a light brown colour. It has a bitterish taste, but is odourless.

It is astringent and also yields amygdalin.

¶ *Medicinal Action and Uses.* In herbal medicine, a decoction of the bark is given for diarrhœa and used as a vaginal injection in leucorrhœa, etc.

AMERICAN MOUNTAIN ASH

American Mountain Ash bark is derived from *Pyrus Americana* (D.C.), which has many local names.

It has similar properties to the bark of the European species and was formerly used as a tonic in fevers of supposed malarial type,

The ripe berries furnish an acidulous and astringent gargle for sore throats and inflamed tonsils. For their anti-scorbutic properties, they have been used in scurvy. The astringent infusion is used as a remedy in hæmorrhoids and strangury.

The fruit is a favourite food of birds. A delicious jelly is made from the berries, which is excellent with cold game or wild fowl, and a wholesome kind of perry or cider can also be made from them.

In Northern Europe they are dried for flour, and when fermented yield a strong spirit. The Welsh used to brew an ale from the berries, the secret of which is now lost.

Pyrus Americana (D.C.)

where it was often substituted for cinchona bark.

No analysis of the bark of the American species has been made, though the fruit has been found to yield 4·92 to 6·6 of malic acid.

ASH, PRICKLY

Xanthoxylum Americanum (MILL.)
N.O. Rutaceæ

Synonyms. Toothache Tree. Yellow Wood. Suterberry

Parts Used. Root-bark, berries

¶ *Description.* The Prickly Ash (*Xanthoxylum Americanum*, Mill.; *X. fraxineum*, Willd.; *X. Carolinianum*, Lamb.) is a small North American tree growing in the open air in this country. It has pinnate leaves and alternate branches, which are covered with sharp and strong prickles: the common footstalk is also sometimes prickly, and also the bark.

It belongs to the Yellow Wood family (*Rutaceæ*), which all possess aromatic and pungent properties.

The berries, growing in clusters on the top of the branches, are black or deep blue and enclosed in a grey shell.

The leaves and berries have an aromatic odour similar to that of oil of Lemons, and the berries and bark have a hot, acrid taste.

The *root-bark* and *berries* are used medicinally, being official in the United States Pharmacopœia.

¶ *Constituents.* The barks of numerous species of *Xanthoxylum* and the allied genus *Fagara* have been used medicinally. There are two principal varieties of Prickly Ash in commerce: *X. Americanum* (Northern Prickly Ash) and *Fagara Clava-Herculis* (Southern Prickly Ash), which is supposed to be more active. Although not absolutely identical, the two Prickly Ash barks are very similar in their active constituents. Both

contain small amounts of volatile oil, fat, sugar, gum, acrid resin, a bitter alkaloid, believed to be Berberine and a colourless, tasteless, inert, crystalline body, *Xanthoxylin*, slightly different in the two barks. Both yield a large amount of Ash: 12 per cent. or more. The name Xanthoxylin is also applied to a resinous extractive prepared by pouring a tincture of the drug into water.

The fruits of both the species are used similarly to the barks. Their constituents have not been investigated, but they apparently agree in a general way with those of the bark.

The drug is practically never adulterated. The Northern bark occurs in commerce in curved or quilled fragments about $\frac{1}{24}$ inch thick, externally brownish grey, with whitish patches, faintly furrowed, with some linear-based, two-edged spines about $\frac{1}{4}$ inch long. The fracture is short, green in the outer, and yellow in the inner part. The Southern bark, which is more frequently sold, is $\frac{1}{12}$ inch thick and has conical, corky spines, sometimes $\frac{3}{8}$ inch in height.

Xanthoxylin is included in the United States Pharmacopœia for the preparation of a fluid extract, the dose of which is $\frac{1}{2}$ to 1 drachm.

¶ *Medicinal Action and Uses.* It acts as a stimulant – resembling guaiacum resin and mezereon bark in its remedial action and is greatly recommended in the United States for chronic rheumatism, typhoid and skin diseases and impurity of the blood, administered either in the form of fluid extract or in doses of 10 grains to ½ drachm in the powdered form, three times daily.

The following formula has also become popular in herbal medicine: Take ½ oz. each of Prickly Ash Bark, Guaiacum Raspings, and Buckbean Herb, with 6 Cayenne Pods. Boil in 1½ pint of water down to 1 pint. Dose: a wineglassful three or four times daily.

On account of the energetic stimulant properties of the bark, it produces when swallowed a sense of heat in the stomach, with more or less general arterial excitement and tendency to perspiration and is a useful tonic in debilitated conditions of the stomach and digestive organs, and is used in colic, cramp and colera, in fever, ague, lethargy, for cold hands and feet and complaints arising from a bad circulation.

A decoction made by boiling an ounce in 3 pints of water down to a quarter may be given in the quantity of a pint, in divided doses, during the twenty-four hours. As a counter-irritant, the decoction may be applied on compresses. It has also been used as an emmenagogue.

The powdered bark forms an excellent application to indolent ulcers and old wounds for cleansing, stimulating, drying up and healing the wounds. The pulverized bark is also used for paralytic affections and nervous headaches and as a topical irritant the bark, either in powdered form, or chewed, has been a very popular remedy for toothache in America, hence the origin of a common name of the tree in the States: Toothache Tree.

The berries are considered even more active than the bark, being carminative and antispasmodic, and are used as an aperient and for dyspepsia and indigestion; a fluid extract of the berries being given, in doses of 10 to 30 drops.

Xanthoxylin. Dose, 1 to 2 grains.

Both berries and bark are used to make a good bitter.

The name Prickly Ash has also been given to *Aralia spinosa* (Linn.), the Prickly Elder, or Angelica Tree, the bark, roots and berries of which are used as alteratives.

See ANGELICA TREE.

ASH, WAFER

Ptelea trifoliata (LINN.)
N.O. Rutaceæ

Synonyms. Swamp Dogwood. Shrubby Trefoil. Wingseed. Hop Tree
Part Used. Root-bark

¶ *Description.* The Wafer Ash is a shrub growing 6 to 8 feet high, a native of North America, but cultivated here, having been introduced in 1714. In America it is also called the Swamp Dogwood, Wingseed, and Hop Tree.

The root-bark is employed medicinally, both in herbal medicine and in homœopathy, but it has never been an official drug, though formerly it was employed to a certain extent by physicians in the western United States.

It has a peculiar, somewhat aromatic odour and a bitter, persistently pungent and slightly acrid, but not disagreeable taste.

¶ *Constituents.* The bark contains at least three active constituents, a powerful volatile oil, a salt, acrid resin, and an alkaloid: Berberine. The alkaloid Arginine is also stated to be present in the root.

¶ *Medicinal Action and Uses.* The bark has tonic, antiperiodic and stomachic properties, and has been employed in dyspepsia and debility, and also in febrile diseases, especially in those requiring a mild, non-irritating bitter tonic, as it has a soothing influence upon the mucous membrane and promotes appetite, being tolerated when other tonics cannot be retained.

It is also useful in chronic rheumatism.

The dose of the powdered bark is 10 to 30 grains. The infusion of the bark is taken in tablespoonful doses three or four times daily.

The bark occurs in commerce in quilled or curved pieces, 1½ to 3 inches long and ½ to ¾ inch in diameter, ⅛ to ¾ inch thick, transversely wrinkled, with a whitish brown surface of thin, papery layers, the inner surface being smooth, with faintly projecting medullary layers. It breaks with a short fracture, yellowish white, the papery layer pale buff.

ASPARAGUS

Asparagus officinalis
N.O. Liliaceæ

This well-known table delicacy may be found wild on the sea-coast in the South-west of England, especially near the Lizard, in the Isle of Anglesea, otherwise it is a rare native. In the southern parts of Russia and Poland the waste steppes are covered with this plant, which is there eaten by horses and cattle as grass. It is also common in Greece, and was formerly much esteemed as a vegetable by the Greeks and Romans. It appears to have been cultivated in the time of Cato the Elder, 200 years B.C., and Pliny mentions a species that grew near Ravenna, of which three heads would weigh a pound.

Asparagus is noticed by Gerard in 1597, and in 1670 forced Asparagus was supplied to the London market.

¶ *Medicinal Action and Uses.* The virtues of Asparagus are well known as a diuretic and laxative; and for those of sedentary habits who suffer from symptoms of gravel, it has been found very beneficial, as well as in cases of dropsy. The fresh expressed juice is taken medicinally in tablespoonful doses.

Prussian Asparagus, which is brought to some English markets, is not a species of Asparagus at all, but consists of the spikes of *Ornithogalum pyrenaicum*, which grows abundantly in hedges and pastures (especially in the locality of Bath). *See* STAR OF BETHLEHEM.

Culpepper tells us, 'The decoction of the roots (Asparagus) boiled in wine, and taken, is good to clear the sight, and being held in the mouth easeth the toothache.' He also tells us it helps those sinews that 'are shrunk by cramps and convulsions, and helpeth the sciatica.'

ASPHODEL

Asphodelus Ramosus
N.O. Liliaceæ

Synonyms. White Asphodel. Asphodele Rameux. Royal Staff. Branched Asphodel. King's Spear

Part Used. The roots

Habitat. Middle Europe. The shores of the Mediterranean

¶ *Description.* The plant is about 3 feet high, with large, white, terminal flowers, and radical, long, numerous leaves. It is only cultivated in botanical and ornamental gardens, though it easily grows from seeds or division of roots.

The roots must be gathered at the end of the first year.

The ancients planted the flowers near tombs, regarding them as the form of food preferred by the dead, and many poems refer to this custom. The name is derived from a Greek word meaning *sceptre.*

The roots, dried and boiled in water, yield a mucilaginous matter that in some countries is mixed with grain or potato to make Asphodel bread. In Spain and other countries they are used as cattle fodder, especially for sheep. In Barbary the wild boars eat them greedily.

In Persia, glue is made with the bulbs, which are first dried and then pulverized. When mixed with cold water, the powder swells and forms a strong glue.

Hippocrates, Dioscorides, and Pliny said the roots were cooked in ashes and eaten. The Greeks and Romans used them in several diseases, but they are not employed in modern medicine.

¶ *Constituents.* An acrid principle separated or destroyed by boiling water, and a matter resembling *inuline* have been found. An alcohol of excellent flavour has been obtained from plants growing abundantly in Algeria.

¶ *Medicinal Action and Uses.* Acrid, heating, and diuretic. Said to be useful in menstrual obstructions and as an antispasmodic. The bruised root has been recommended for rapidly dissolving scrofulous swellings.

¶ *Other Species.*

A. luteus, or Yellow Asphodel, Jacob's Staff, is a native of Sicily.

A. fistulosus, or Onion-leaved Asphodel, of Southern France and Crete, is also employed.

BOG OR LACASHIRE ASPHODEL is a common name of *Narthecium ossifragum*. The name of 'bone-breaker' was unfortunately given, because, as it grows on wet moors and mountains, sheep pasturing there frequently suffered from foot rot, and this was attributed to their browsing on the plants.

FALSE ASPHODEL is an American name for *Tofieldia*.

SCOTCH ASPHODEL is a common name of *Tofieldia palustris*.

AUBERGINE. *See* NIGHTSHADE

AURICULA. *See* COWSLIP, PRIMULAS

AVENS
Geum urbanum (LINN.)
N.O. Rosaceæ

Synonyms. Colewort. Herb Bennet. City Avens. Wild Rye. Way Bennet. Goldy Star. Clove Root

Parts Used. Herb, root

Habitat. The Avens (*Geum urbanum*, Linn.), belonging to the order *Rosaceæ*, its genus being nearly related to the *Potentilla* genus, is a common wayside plant in Great Britain, abundant in woods and hedges in England, Ireland and southern Scotland, though becoming scarcer in the north. It is common in the greater part of Europe, Russia and Central Asia

¶ *Description*. It has thin, nearly upright, wiry stems, slightly branched, from 1 to 2 feet in height, of a reddish brown on one side. Its leaves vary considerably in form, according to their position. The radical leaves are borne on long, channelled foot-stalks, and are interruptedly pinnate, as in the Silverweed, the large terminal leaflet being wedge-shaped and the intermediate pairs of leaflets being very small. The upper leaves on the stem are made up of three long, narrow leaflets: those lower on the stems have the three leaflets round and full. The stem-leaves are placed alternately and have at their base two stipules (leaf-like members that in many plants occur at the junction of the base of the leaf with the stem). Those of the Avens are very large, about an inch broad and long, rounded in form and coarsely toothed and lobed. All the leaves are of a deep green colour, more or less covered with spreading hairs, their margins toothed.

The rhizomes are 1 to 2 inches long terminating abruptly, hard and rough with many light brown fibrous roots. The flowers, rather small for the size of the plant, are on solitary, terminal stalks. The corolla is composed of five roundish, spreading, yellow petals, the calyx cleft into ten segments – five large and five small – as in the Silverweed. The flowers, which are in bloom all the summer and autumn, often as late as December, are less conspicuous than the round fruit-heads, which succeed them, which are formed of a mass of dark crimson achenes, each terminating in an awn, the end of which is curved into a hook.

¶ *History*. The plant derives its name of Avens from the Latin *Avencia*, Mediæval Latin, *avantia* or *avence*, a word of obscure origin and which in varieties of spelling has been applied to the plant from very early times.

The botanical name, *Geum*, originated from the Greek *geno*, to yield an agreeable fragrance, because, when freshly dug up, the root has a clove-like aroma. This gives rise to another name, *Radix caryophylata*, or Clove Root, and its corruption, Gariophilata.

Avens had many names in the fourteenth century, such as Assarabaccara, Pesleporis, or Harefoot, and Minarta.

It was called 'the Blessed Herb' (*Herba benedicta*), of which a common name still extant – Herb Bennet – is a corruption, because in former times it was believed that it had the power to ward off evil spirits and venomous beasts. It was worn as an amulet. The *Ortus Sanitatis*, printed in 1491, states: 'Where the root is in the house, Satan can do nothing and flies from it, wherefore it is blessed before all other herbs, and if a man carries the root about him no venomous beast can harm him.' Dr. Prior (*Popular Names of English Plants*) considers the original name to have probably been 'St. Benedict's Herb,' that name being assigned to such as were supposed to be antidotes, in allusion to a legend respecting the saint. It is said that on one occasion a monk presented him with a goblet of poisoned wine, but when the saint blessed it, the poison, being a sort of devil, flew out of it with such force that the glass was shivered to atoms, the crime of the monk being thus exposed. Hemlock is also known as Herb Bennet, probably for the same reason.

Goldy Star of the Earth, City Avens, Wild Rye and Way Bennet are other local names for the plant.

In mediæval days, the graceful trefoiled leaf and the five golden petals of the blossoms symbolized the Holy Trinity and the five wounds of Our Lord, and towards the end of the thirteenth century the plant frequently occurs as an architectural decoration in the carved leafage on the capitals of columns and in wall patterns.

The roots should be dug up in spring; some of the old physicians were so particular on this point that the 25th March was fixed for procuring the root (and it was specified that the soil should be dry). At this time the root was said to be most fragrant. It loses much of its odour in drying, so must be dried with great care, and gradually, then sliced and powdered as required, as they are less likely to lose their properties in this form than when kept in slices.

Externally, the rhizome, when dried, is of a

brownish to a brownish-yellow colour. The fracture is short. Internally, it is of a light purplish-brown when dried. In transverse section, it shows a large pith, a narrow woody ring, with thin bark. The taste of the drug is astringent, slightly bitter and clove-like.

¶ *Constituents*. The principal constituent is a volatile oil, which is mainly composed of Eugenol, and a glucoside, Gein, geum-bitter, tannic acid, gum and resin. It imparts its qualities to water and alcohol, which it tinges red. Distilled with water, it yields 0·04 per cent. of thick, greenish, volatile oil.

The root has been found by Milandi and Moretti to contain one-eleventh of its weight of tannin.

¶ *Medicinal Action and Uses*. Astringent, Styptic, febrifuge, sudorific, stomachic, antiseptic, tonic and aromatic.

In earlier days the roots were not only used medicinally, as at present, but to flavour ale, and to put among linen to preserve from moths and to impart a pleasant odour.

The Augsburg Ale is said to owe its peculiar flavour to the addition of a small bag of Avens in each cask. The fresh root imparts a pleasant clove-like flavour to the liquor, preserves it from turning sour, and adds to its wholesome properties.

A cordial against the plague was made by boiling the roots in wine. Gerard recommends a 'decoction made in wine against stomach ills and bites of venomous beasts.' On account of its stomachic properties, chewing of the root was recommended for foul breath.

Culpepper says:

'It is governed by Jupiter and that gives hopes of a wholesome healthful herb. It is good for the diseases of the chest or breath, for pains and stitches in the sides, it dissolveth inward congealed blood occasioned by falls and bruises and the spitting of blood, if the roots either green or dried be boiled in wine and drunk. The root in the spring-time steeped in wine doth give it a delicate flavour and taste and being drunk fasting every morning comforteth the heart and is a good preservative against the plague or any other poison. It is very safe and is fit to be kept in every body's house.'

¶ In modern herbal medicine Avens is considered useful in diarrhœa, dysenteries, leucorrhœa, sore throat, ague, chills, fresh catarrh, intermittent fevers, chronic and passive hæmorrhages, gastric irritation and headache.

The infusion or decoction is made from ½ oz. of the powdered root or herb to 1 pint of boiling water, strained and taken cold. The infusion is the most grateful, but the decoction may be made much stronger by boiling it down to half.

The simple tincture is made by pouring a pint of proof spirit on an ounce of the bruised root and macerating it for fourteen days and then filtering through paper. Two or three teaspoonsful of this tincture in any watery vehicle, or in a glass of wine, are a sufficient dose.

An excellent *compound tincture* may be made as follows: Take of Avens root 1½ oz.; Angelica root, bruised, and Tormentil root, bruised, of each 1 oz.; Raisins, stoned, 2 oz.; French brandy, 2 pints. Macerate for a month in a warm place. Filter then through paper. Dose, ½ oz.

The same ingredients infused in a quart of wine will form an excellent vinous tincture.

The infusion is considered an excellent cordial sudorific at the commencement of chills and catarrh, cutting short the paroxysm, and the continued use of it has restorative power in weakness, debility, etc.

Its astringency makes it useful in diarrhœa, sore throat, etc. It is taken, strained and cold, in wineglassful doses, three or four times a day.

The infusion is also used in some skin affections. When used externally as a wash, it will remove spots, freckles or eruptions from the face.

Taken as decoction in the spring, Avens acts as a purifier and removes obstructions of the liver.

The powdered root has been used both in America and Europe as a substitute for Peruvian bark and has frequently been found to cure agues when the latter has failed, a drachm of powder being given every two hours.

The dose of the fluid extract of the herb is 1 drachm, of the fluid extract of the root, ½ to 1 drachm. As a tonic, the usual dose of the powdered herb or root is 15 to 30 grains.

As Arnica adulterant, the rhizome is sometimes present in the imported drug.

AVENS (MOUNTAIN)

Dryas octopetala (LINN.)
N.O. Rosaceæ

¶ *Description*. The Mountain Avens (*Dryas octopetala*, Linn.) is a small plant, 2 to 3 inches high, distinguished from all other plants of the order *Rosaceæ* by its oblong deeply-cut leaves, which are white with a woolly down beneath, and by its large, handsome, anemone-like, white flowers, which have eight petals. It blooms in the spring. It

74

is not uncommon in the mountainous parts of the British Isles, especially on limestone.

When cultivated, it likes a sunny spot, not too dry, and prefers a little lime in the soil. It is propagated by layers or seeds, layers being the easiest method.

Although our native species are not striking enough to be made use of by the horticulturist, there are many garden varieties of *Geum* which are easily grown in fairly rich, loamy soil and are mostly propagated by dividing the roots in early autumn or in spring as growth commences. Seeds can be sown in the spring, either in the open or in well-drained pots or shallow boxes in cold frames.

The favourite varieties are the Scarlet Avens of Chile, *Geum coccineum*, the red *G. sylvaticum*, and the yellow-flowered *G. montanum* and *G. elatum* of the Himalayas, and *G. reptans* of the Alps.

AVENS, WATER

Geum rivale (LINN.)
N.O. Rosaceæ

Synonyms. Nodding Avens. Drooping Avens. Cure All. Water Flower. Indian Chocolate
Part Used. Root
Habitat. The Water Avens (*Geum rivale*, Linn.) flourishes freely in the northern parts of Eurọpe, in Canada and Siberia, and in Britain is more common in the northern counties and in Scotland than in the southern counties

It is a lover of moist situations, found chiefly in damp woods and in ditches and among the coarse herbage fringing canals

¶ *Description*. It is a much stouter plant than the Common Avens, the stem 1 foot high or more, scarcely branching and with few leaves, of a simpler form. The lower part of the stem is clothed with bent-back hairs and is very downy above. The radical leaves, in the form of a rosette, as in the Common Avens, are long-stalked, lobed, the terminal leaflet larger, with more numerous segments than in *Geum urbanum*.

The flowers are larger than those of the Common Avens, fewer in number, not a widely-spreading star, but drooping, the petals forming together a compact and bell-like corolla, of a dull purplish hue with darker veins, the calyces brownish, deeply tinged with purple. The awns feathery, not hooked.

¶ *Medicinal Action and Uses*. The Water Avens has similar properties to those of the Common Avens and is employed in the same way, the root having tonic and powerfully astringent action and being beneficial in passive hæmorrhage and diarrhœa.

In the eastern states of North America (where it is called Indian Chocolate, Cure All and Water Flower) it is much used as a popular remedy in pulmonary consumption, simple dyspepsia and diseases of the bowels consequent on disorders of the stomach, and is valued as a febrifuge and tonic.

AZADIRACHTA

Melia Azadirachta
N.O. Meliaceæ

Synonyms. Bead Tree. Pride of China. Nim. Margosa. Neem. Holy Tree. Indian Lilac Tree
Parts Used. The bark of the root and trunk; the seed
Habitat. Widely distributed through Tropics

¶ *Description*. Under the name of Neem it grows luxuriantly in Bengal, where it was known to the author. It grows from 30 .to 50 feet high, leaves bipinnate, large bunches of lilac flowers agreeably perfumed. In Southern France and Spain it is found growing in avenues. It is said to be a native of China. The bark should be new and is a rusty grey colour, inside yellow and foliated, coarsely fibrous, no odour, powerfully bitter and less astringent than the outer coarser bark, if taken from old roots the outer crust must be taken off.

¶ *Constituents*. Margosin, a crystalline principle, and tannic acid.

¶ *Medicinal Action and Uses*. The oil obtained from the fruit is used for burning, that from the bark is used medicinally and is anthelmintic and emetic; it is applied externally for rheumatism. The decoction of Azadirachta is said to be cathartic and in large doses slightly narcotic; it is also supposed to have febrifuge properties; it is used as a remedy for hysteria. The Hindu considers it a stomachic and taps it for toddy. The name Bead Tree is derived from the hard nuts which are used for making rosaries. An ointment to destroy lice is made from the pulp and is also used for scald head and other skin diseases. The oil from the

75

nuts is useful for cramps, obstinate ulcers, etc.

¶ *Dosages and Preparations*. The decoction is made from 2 oz. of bark to 1 pint of water boiled down to ½ pint, one tablespoonful every two or three hours for a dose. This,

or 20 grains of the powdered bark, is an effective dose for worms if followed by a purgative.

¶ *Poisons*. The name Azadarach implies a poisonous plant and the fruit is considered to be so.

BAEL

Aegle Marmelos (CORREA)
N.O. Rutaceæ

Synonyms. Belæ Fructus. Bel. Indian Bael
Part Used. Unripe fruit
Habitat. India

¶ *Description*. Fruit 2½ to 3¼ inches in diameter, globular or ovoid in shape, colour greyish brown, outside surface hard and nearly smooth. Rind about ¼ inch thick and adherent to a light red pulp, in which are ten to fifteen cells, each containing several woolly seeds. It has a faint aromatic odour and mucilagenous taste.

¶ *Constituents*. The chief constituents appear to be mucilage and pectin contained in the pulp of the unripe fruit; the ripe fruit differs in yielding a tannin reaction and possessing a distinct aroma.

¶ *Medicinal Action and Uses*. Fresh half-ripe Bael fruit is mildly astringent and is used in

India for dysentery and diarrhœa; the pulp may be eaten or the decoction administered. The dried fruit does not contain the constituents requisite for the preparation of the decoction. It is said to cure without creating any tendency to constipation.

¶ *Dosages and Preparations*. Decoction Belæ, B.P.C., 1 in 2½: dose, ½ to 2 oz. Fluid extract, ½ to 2 drachms.

¶ *Other Species*. Mangosteen Fruit (*Garania Mangostana*) is sometimes substituted for it, also another species of the order *Rutaceæ*, Wood Apple or Elephant Apple (*Feronia Elephantum*), but neither are as effective as the fruit of the Bael Tree.

BALM

Melissa officinalis (LINN.)
N.O. Labiatæ

Synonyms. Sweet Balm. Lemon Balm
Part Used. Herb
Habitat. A native of South Europe, especially in mountainous situations, but is naturalized in the south of England, and was introduced into our gardens at a very early period

¶ *Description*. The root-stock is short, the stem square and branching, grows 1 to 2 feet high, and has at each joint pairs of broadly ovate or heart-shaped, crenate or toothed leaves which emit a fragrant lemon odour when bruised. They also have a distinct lemon taste. The flowers, white or yellowish, are in loose, small bunches from the axils of the leaves and bloom from June to October. The plant dies down in winter, but the root is perennial.

The genus *Melissa* is widely diffused, having representatives in Europe, Middle Asia and North America. The name is from the Greek word signifying 'bee,' indicative of the attraction the flowers have for those insects, on account of the honey they produce.

¶ *History*. The word Balm is an abbreviation of Balsam, the chief of sweet-smelling oils. It is so called from its honeyed sweetness. It was highly esteemed by Paracelsus, who believed it would completely revivify a man. It was formerly esteemed of great use in all complaints supposed to proceed from a disordered state of the nervous system. The *London Dispensary* (1696) says: 'An essence of Balm, given in Canary wine, every morning

will renew youth, strengthen the brain, relieve languishing nature and prevent baldness.' John Evelyn wrote: 'Balm is sovereign for the brain, strengthening the memory and powerfully chasing away melancholy.' Balm steeped in wine we are told again, 'comforts the heart and driveth away melancholy and sadness.' Formerly a spirit of Balm, combined with lemon-peel, nutmeg and angelica root, enjoyed a great reputation under the name of Carmelite water, being deemed highly useful against nervous headache and neuralgic affections.

Many virtues were formerly ascribed to this plant. Gerard says: 'It is profitably planted where bees are kept. The hives of bees being rubbed with the leaves of bawme, causeth the bees to keep together, and causeth others to come with them.' And again, quoting Pliny, 'When they are strayed away, they do find their way home by it.' Pliny says: 'It is of so great virtue that though it be but tied to his sword that hath given the wound, it stauncheth the blood.' Gerard also tells us: 'The juice of Balm glueth together greene wounds,' and gives the opinion of Pliny and Dioscorides that 'Balm, being applied, doth close up wounds without any perill of inflammation.' The leaves steeped in wine, and the wine drunk, and the leaves applied externally, were considered to be a certain cure for the bites of venomous beasts and the stings of scorpions. It is now recognized as a scientific fact that the balsamic oils of aromatic plants make excellent surgical dressings: they give off ozone and thus exercise anti-putrescent effects. Being chemical hydrocarbons, they contain so little oxygen that in wounds dressed with the fixed balsamic herbal oils, the atomic germs of disease are starved out, and the resinous parts of these balsamic oils, as they dry upon the sore or wound, seal it up and effectually exclude all noxious air.

¶ *Cultivation.* Balm grows freely in any soil and can be propagated by seeds, cuttings or division of roots in spring or autumn. If in autumn, preferably not later than October, so that the offsets may be established before the frosts come on. The roots may be divided into small pieces, with three or four buds to each, and planted 2 feet apart in ordinary garden soil. The only culture required is to keep them clean from weeds and to cut off the decayed stalks in autumn, and then to stir the ground between the roots.

¶ *Medicinal Action and Uses.* Carminative, diaphoretic and febrifuge. It induces a mild perspiration and makes a pleasant and cooling tea for feverish patients in cases of catarrh and influenza. To make the tea, pour 1 pint of boiling water upon 1 oz. of herb, infuse 15 minutes, allow to cool, then strain and drink freely. If sugar and a little lemon-peel or juice be added it makes a refreshing summer drink.

Balm is a useful herb, either alone or in combination with others. It is excellent in colds attended with fever, as it promotes perspiration.

Used with salt, it was formerly applied for the purpose of taking away wens, and had the reputation of cleansing sores and easing the pains of gout.

John Hussey, of Sydenham, who lived to the age of 116, breakfasted for fifty years on Balm tea sweetened with honey, and herb teas were the usual breakfasts of Llewelyn, Prince of Glamorgan, who died in his 108th year. Carmelite water, of which Balm was the chief ingredient, was drunk daily by the Emperor Charles V.

Commercial oil of Balm is not a pure distillate, but is probably oil of Lemon distilled over Balm. The oil is used in perfumery.

Balm is frequently used as one of the ingredients of pot-pourri. Mrs. Bardswell, in *The Herb Garden,* mentions Balm as one of the bushy herbs that are invaluable for the permanence of their leaf-odours, which,

'though ready when sought, do not force themselves upon us, but have to be coaxed out by touching, bruising or pressing. Balm, with its delicious lemon scent, is by common consent one of the most sweetly smelling of all the herbs in the garden. Balm-wine was made of it and a tea which is good for feverish colds. The fresh leaves make better tea than the dry.'

A Refreshing Drink in Fever

' Put *two sprigs of Balm*, and a *little* wood-sorrel, into a stone-jug, having first washed and dried them; peel thin a small lemon, and clear from the white; slice it and put a bit of peel in; then pour in 3 pints of boiling water, sweeten and cover it close.'

' *Claret Cup.* One bottle of claret, one pint bottle of German Seltzer-water, a *small bunch of Balm*, ditto of burrage, one orange cut in slices, half a cucumber sliced thick, a liqueur-glass of Cognac, and one ounce of bruised sugar-candy.

'Process: Place these ingredients in a covered jug well immersed in rough ice, stir all together with a silver spoon, and when the cup has been iced for about an hour, strain or decanter it off free from the herbs, etc.' (Francatelli's *Cook's Guide.*)

A bunch of Balm improves nearly all cups.

BALM OF GILEAD. *See* BALSAM OF GILEAD

BALMONY   Chelone Glabra (LINN.)
                                                 N.O. Scrophulariaceæ

Synonyms. Chelone. Snake-head. Turtle-head. Turtle-bloom. Shellflower. Salt-rheum Weed. Bitter Herb. Chelone Obliqua. Glatte. White Chelone. The Humming-bird Tree
Part Used. The whole fresh herb
Habitat. Eastern United States and Canada

¶ *Description.* This erect little plant, from 2 to 4 feet high, grows sparingly on the margins of swamps, wet woods, and rivers. It is a perennial, smooth herb, bearing opposite, oblong leaves, and short, dense, terminal spikes of two-lipped, white or purplish, cream or rose flowers, the lower lip bearded in the throat and the heart-shaped anthers and filaments woolly. The leaves have a slight, somewhat tea-like odour and a markedly bitter taste. They should be planted in pots to prevent the roots from creeping too far.

The name of the genus Chelone comes from the Greek word meaning a tortoise, from the resemblance of the corolla to a tortoise-head. The whole, fresh plant is chopped, pounded to a pulp, and weighed, and a tincture is prepared with alcohol. The decoction is made with 2 oz. of the fresh herb to a pint.

¶ *Constituents.* The bitter leaves communicate their properties to both water and alcohol. Chelonin is an eclectic medicine prepared from Chelone, and is a brown, bitter powder given as a tonic laxative.

¶ *Medicinal Action and Uses.* The leaves have anti-bilious, anthelmintic, tonic and detergent properties, with a peculiar action on the liver, and are used largely in consumption, dyspepsia, debility and jaundice, in diseases of the liver, and for worms in children, for which the powder or decoction may be used internally or in injection. As an ointment it is recommended for inflamed tumours, irritable ulcers, inflamed breasts, piles, etc.

For long it has been a favourite tonic, laxative and purgative among the aborigines of North America, though their doses render its tonic value doubtful.

¶ *Dosages.* Of decoction, 1 to 2 fluid ounces. Of fluid extract, $\frac{1}{2}$ to 1 drachm. Of the powder, 1 drachm. Of the tincture, 1 to 2 fluid drachms. Of Chelonin, 1 to 2 grains.

BALSAM OF GILEAD

Commiphora Opobalsamum
N.O. Burseraceæ

Synonyms. Balsamum Meccæ var. Judiacum. Balsamum Gileadense. Baume de la Mecque. Balsamodendrum Opobalsamum. Balessan. Bechan. Balsam Tree. Amyris Gileadensis. Amyris Opobalsamum. Balsumodendron Gileadensis. Protium Gileadense. Dossémo

Part Used. The resinous juice
Habitat. The countries on both sides of the Red Sea

¶ *Description.* This small tree, the source of the genuine Balm of Gilead around which so many mystical associations have gathered, stands from 10 to 12 feet high, with wand-like, spreading branches. The bark is of a rich brown colour, the leaves, trifoliate, are small and scanty, the flowers unisexual, small, and reddish in colour, while the seeds are solitary, yellow, and grooved down one side. It is both rare, and difficult to rear, and is so much valued by the Turks that its importation is prohibited. They have grown the trees in guarded gardens at Matarie, near Cairo, from the days of Prosper Alpin, who wrote the *Dialogue of Balm,* and the balsam is valued as a cosmetic by the royal ladies. In the Bible, and in the works of Bruce, Theophrastes, Galen, and Dioscorides, it is lauded.

¶ *History. Balm, Baulm* or *Bawm,* contracted from *Balsam,* may be derived from the Hebrew *bot smin,* 'chief of oils,' or *bâsâm,* 'balm,' and *besem,* 'a sweet smell.' *Opobalsamum* is used by Dioscorides to mean 'the juice flowing from the balsam-tree.'

Pliny states that the tree was first brought to Rome by the generals of Vespasian; while Josephus relates that it was taken from Arabia to Judea by the Queen of Sheba as a present to Solomon. There, being cultivated for its juice, particularly on Mount Gilead, it acquired its popular name. Later, it was called Opobalsamum, its dried twigs Xylo-

balsamum, and its dried fruit Carpobalsamum.

Its rarity, combined with the magic of its name, have caused the latter to be adopted for several other species.

Abd-Allatif, a Damascan physician of the twelfth century, noted that it had two barks, the outer reddish and thin, the inner green and thick, and a very aromatic odour.

The juice exudes spontaneously during the heat of summer, in resinous drops, the process being helped by incisions in the bark. The more humid the air, the greater the quantity collected. When the oil is separated, it is prepared with great secrecy, and taken to the stores of the ruler, where it is carefully guarded. The quantity of oil obtained is roughly one-tenth the amount of juice. It is probable that an inferior kind of oil is obtained after boiling the leaves and wood with water.

The wood is found in small pieces, several kinds being known commercially, but it rapidly loses its odour.

The fruit is reddish grey, and the size of a small pea, with an agreeable and aromatic taste.

In Europe and America it is so seldom found in a pure state that its use is entirely discontinued.

¶ *Constituents.* The liquid balm is turbid, whitish, thick, grey and odorous, and becomes solid by exposure. It contains a resin

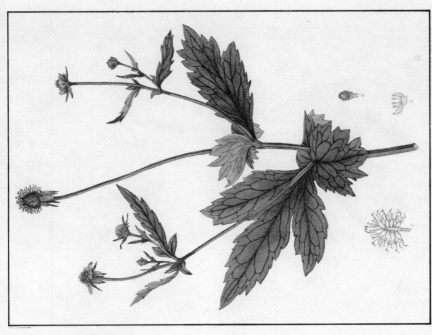
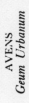

AVENS
Geum Urbanum

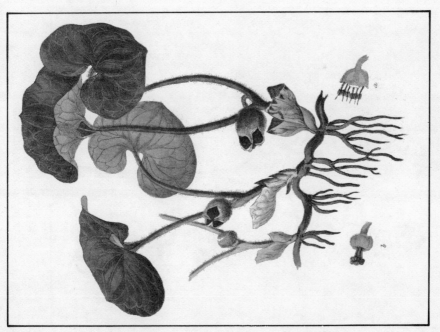

ASARABACCA
Asarum Europæum

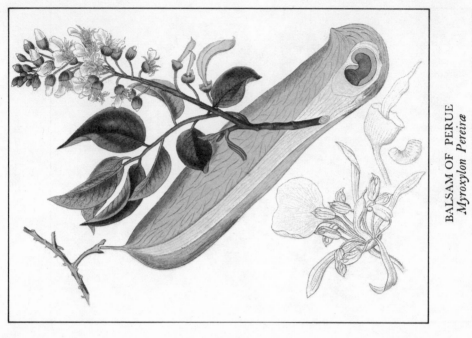

BALSAM OF PERUE
Myroxylon Pereiræ

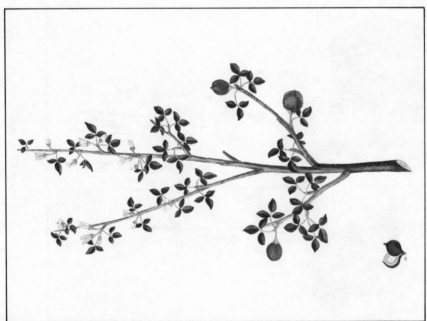

BALSAM OF GILEAD
Commiphora Opobalsamum

soluble in alcohol, and a principle resembling Bassorin.

¶ *Medicinal Action and Uses.* It has been used in diseases of the urinary tracts, but is said to possess no medicinal properties not found in other balsams.

¶ *Other Species.*
Abies Balsamea, Balm of Gilead Fir, or American Silver Fir. The name is applied to this Canadian species, in *Europe*, because of the supposed resemblance of its product, an oleoresinous fluid obtained from punctured blisters in the bark, which is really a true turpentine, known as Canada Balsam or Canada Turpentine. Its odour distinguishes it from Strassburg Turpentine, which is sometimes substituted for it. It is diuretic, and stimulates mucous tissues in small doses. In large doses it is purgative, and may cause nausea.

Populus Candicans is called Balm of Gilead in *America*. The buds are used, and called Balm of Gilead Buds, as are those of *P. Nigra* and *P. balsamifera*, the product of the last being imported into Europe under the name of *Tacomahaca*. They are covered with a fragrant, resinous matter, which may be separated in boiling water, the odour being like incense, and the taste bitter and rather unpleasant. They are stimulant, tonic, diuretic, and antiscorbutic. A tincture of them is useful for complaints of the chest, stomach, and kidneys, and for rheumatism and scurvy. With lard or oil they are useful as an external application in bruises, swellings, and some cutaneous diseases. In ointments they are a little inferior to paraffin as a preventive of rancidity.

The bark of *P. balsamifera* is tonic and cathartic.

¶ *Dosages.* Of solid extract, 5 to 10 grains. Of tincture, 1 to 4 fluid drachms. Of fluid extract, 1 to 2 drachms. Of extract of the bark, 5 to 15 grains.

Dracocephalum Canariense or *Cedronella Triphylla* is known as a garden plant something like Salvia, and called Balm of Gilead for no better reason than that its leaves are fragrant. It is a native of America and the Canaries.

BALSAM OF PERU

Myroxylon Pereiræ (KLOTSCH)
N.O. Leguminosæ

Synonyms. Toluifera Pereira. Myrosperum Pereira
Part Used. Oleoresinous liquid
Habitat. Central America in the forests of San Salvador

¶ *Description.* A large and beautiful tree with a valuable wood like mahogany, and a straight smooth trunk; the last is coarse grey, compact, heavy granulated and a pale straw colour, containing a resin which changes from citron to dark brown; smell and taste balsamic and aromatic. Leaves alternately, abruptly pinnate, leaflets two pairs mostly opposite, ovate, lanceolate with the end blunt, emarginate; every part of the tree including the leaves abounds in a resinous juice. The mesocarp of the fruit is fibrous, and the balsamic juice which is abundant is contained in two distinct receptacles, one on each side. The beans contain Coumarin, the husks an extremely acrid bitter resin, and a volatile oil; a gum resin, quite distinct from the proper balsam, exudes from the trunk of the tree and contains gum resin and a volatile oil; the tree commences to be productive after five or six years, and continues to yield for thirty years; the flower has a fragrance which can be smelt a hundred yards away.

The process of extraction produces three grades of balsam; the title 'Balsam of Peru' is derived from the fact of its being shipped from Peru. There are several fictitious Peruvian balsams found in commerce, but they do not contain the same properties. A white balsam is made from the fruit of *Myroxylon* *Peruviana* or *Pereiræ*, which has a peculiar resinous body and none of the chemical constituents of Balsam of Peru; this is termed Myroxocarpin. Another substance obtained from the same tree and much used in Central America is termed Balsamito; it is an alcoholic extract of the young fruit. This is used as a stimulant, diuretic, anthelmintic and external application to gangrenous ulcers, and to remove freckles. Balsam of Peru is warm and aromatic, much hotter and more stimulating than Balsam of Copaiba and is used for similar complaints. It is specially useful for rheumatic pains and chronic coughs.

¶ *Constituents.* A colourless, aromatic, oily liquid, termed cinnamein, dark resin, peruviol, small quantity of vanillin and cinnamic acid.

¶ *Medicinal Action and Uses.* Stimulant, expectorant, parasiticide. Used in scabies and skin diseases; it destroys the itch acarus and its eggs, and is much to be preferred to sulphur ointment, also of value in prurigo, pruritis and in later stages of acute eczema. It is a good antiseptic expectorant and a stimulant to the heart, increasing blood pressure; its action resembles benzoic acid. It is applied externally to sore nipples and discharges from the ear. Given internally, it lessens mucous secretions, and is of value in bronchorrhœa gleet, leucorrhœa and chronic bronchitis, and asthma. It is also used in soap manufacturing, for its fragrance, and because it makes a soft creamy lather, useful for chapped hands. Balsam of Peru can be applied alone or as an ointment made by melting it with an equal weight of tallow.

¶ *Dose.* 10 to 30 drops, best given in syrup, with the yolk of an egg added, or with gum-arabic.

¶ *Adulterations.* Castor oil, Copaiba, Canada turpentine, etc.

¶ *Other Species.*
MYROXYLON FRUTESCENS.
Habitat. Trinidad.
The pod is used in the island as a carminative, and externally in the form of a tincture. As a lotion for rheumatic pains, the stems yield a balsamic juice.
GUINA-GUINA.
Habitat. Paraguay.
This bark is used in powder and in decoction for wounds and ulcers, and the dried concrete juice of the trunk of the tree is very similar to Balsam of Peru.

BALSAM OF TOLU

Myrospermum Toluiferum
N.O. Leguminosæ

Synonyms. Balsamum Tolutanum. Tolutanischer Balsam. Balsamum Americanum
Part Used. Exudation
Habitat. Many parts of South America, especially New Granada, the high plains and mountains near Carthagena, Tolu, and the Magdalena province of Colombia

¶ *History.* There is still some obscurity about the origin of the different South American balsam-yielding trees. The appearance of the above variety is said to differ but slightly from the Peruvian, but the method of gathering the balsam is quite different. V-shaped cuts are made in the tree, and the liquid is received into calabash cups placed at an angle; these are emptied into flasks of raw hide, conveyed by donkeys to the depôts, and finally shipped in tin or earthen vessels, which occasionally contain large pieces of red brick. On arrival the balsam is soft and sticky, but exposure to the air makes it hard and brittle, more like resin, with a crystalline appearance. In colour it is pale, yellowish red or brown. It has a sweet, aromatic, resinous taste – becoming soft again when chewed – with an odour resembling vanilla or benzoin, especially fragrant when the balsam is burned, but completely changing and resembling the clove-pink if dissolved in a minute portion of liquor potassa.

As the balsam solidifies, its odour becomes more feeble, but the quantity of cinnamic acid increases, and it thus becomes valuable to perfumers as a fixative, an ounce added to a pound of volatile perfume making it much more permanent.

Tolu Balsam is frequently adulterated with turpentines, styrax, colophony, etc., and may

be tested by heating it in sulphuric acid. If pure, it will yield a cherry-red liquid, and will dissolve without any appearance of sulphurous acid.

¶ *Constituents.* About 80 per cent. amorphous resin, with cinnamic acid, a volatile oil, and a little vanillin, benzyl benzoate and benzyl cinnamate. It is freely soluble in chloroform, glacial acetic acid, acetone, ether, alcohol and liquor potassa; scarcely soluble in petroleum-benzine and benzol.

To distinguish it from Balsam of Peru it can be tested with sulphuric acid and water, yielding a grey mass instead of the lovely violet colour of the genuine Peruvian Balsam.

¶ *Medicinal Action and Uses.* Stimulant and expectorant, much used as the basis of cough mixtures. The vapour from the balsam dissolved in ether when inhaled, is beneficial in chronic catarrh and other non-inflammatory chest complaints. The best form is that of an emulsion, made by triturating the balsam with mucilage and loaf sugar, and adding water.

Two parts of Tolu, 3 of Almond oil, 4 of gum-arabic, and 16 of Rose-water, make an excellent liniment for excoriated nipples.

¶ *Preparations.* Tincture, B.P. and U.S.P., $\frac{1}{2}$ to 1 drachm. Syrup, B.P. and U.S.P., $\frac{1}{2}$ to 1 drachm. Lozenges, incense and pastilles are also prepared.

BALSAM, WHITE

Gnaphalium polycephalum
N.O. Asteraceæ

Synonyms. Indian Posy. Sweet-scented Life Everlasting. Old Field Balsam. Gnaphalium Obtusifolium or Blunt-leaved Everlasting. Gnaphalium Connoideum. Fragrant Everlasting. None-so-Pretty. Catsfoot. Silver Leaf
Parts Used. Herb, leaves, flowers
Habitat. Virginia, Pennsylvania and New England

¶ *Description.* Leaves lanceolate; stalk tomentose, panicled; flowers tubular, yellow, glomerate, conical, terminating; stems single,

9 inches high. Corollas yellow, flowering July to August. Leaves have a pleasant aromatic smell and an aromatic, slightly bitter,

astringent, agreeable taste. The *Antennaria Margaritacea* or *Gnaphalium Margaritacea*, or Pearl-flowered Life Everlasting, has the same properties as White Balsam.

¶ *Medicinal Action and Uses.* Astringent. Beneficial for ulcerations of the throat and mouth; warm infusions used to produce diaphoresis; also of service in quinsy, pulmonary complaints, leucorrhœa. Can be used internally and as a local application, likewise used as fomentations to bruises, indolent tumours. An infusion given in diseases of the bowels – hæmorrhages, etc. The fresh juice is reputed anti-venereal and anti-aphrodisiac; the cold infusion vermifugal; the dried flowers are used as a sedative filling for the pillows of consumptives. A tincture is made from whole plant.

See CATSFOOT, CUDWEED, LIFE EVERLASTING, GNAPHALIUM.

BAMBOO BRIER

Aralia nudicaulis (LINN.)
N.O. Araliaceæ

Synonyms. Wild Sarsaparilla. Shot Bush. Wild Liquorice
Part Used. The root
Habitat. United States

¶ *Description.* An indigenous perennial in shady rocky woods, very common in rich soil, rhizome horizontal, creeping several feet in length and more or less twisted; of a yellowish-brown colour externally and about ¼ inch in diameter, has a fragrant odour and a warm, aromatic, sweetish taste.

¶ *Constituents.* Contains 3·05 per cent. of resin, 0·33 per cent. of oil tannin, an acid albumen, mucilage and cellulose.

¶ *Medicinal Action and Uses and Dosage.* As Sarsaparilla.

See ARALIAS; ELDER (AMERICAN DWARF); SARSAPARILLAS; SPIKENARD (AMERICAN).

BANANA. *See* PLANTAIN (FRUIT)

BANEBERRY (POISON)

Actæa spicata (LINN.)
N.O. Ranunculaceæ

Synonyms. Herb Christopher. Bugbane. Toadroot
Part Used. Root
Habitat. It is to be found in copses on limestone in Yorkshire and the Lake District, but is so uncommon as to be regarded by some botanists as almost a doubtful native

The Baneberry, or Herb Christopher, is a rather rare British plant belonging (like the Pæony) to the Buttercup order, but distinguished from all other species in the order by its berry-like fruit. It is considered to have similar anti-spasmodic properties to the Pæony.

¶ *Description.* The black, creeping root-stock is perennial, sending up each year erect stems, growing 1 to 2 feet high, which are triangular and either not branched, or very sparingly so. The foot-stalks of the leaves are long and arise from the root. These divide into three smaller foot-stalks, and are so divided or re-divided that each leaf is composed of eighteen, or even twenty-seven, lobes or leaflets.

The flower-stem arises from the roots and has leaves of the same form, but smaller. The flowers grow in spikes and are of a pure white.

The whole plant is dark green and glabrous (without hairs), or only very slightly downy. It flowers in June and in autumn ripens its fruits, which are egg-shaped berries, ½ inch long, black and shining, many-seeded and very poisonous, well justifying the popular name of Baneberry.

The plant is of an acrid, poisonous nature throughout, and though the root has been used in some nervous cases, and is said to be a remedy for catarrh, it must be administered with great caution.

¶ *Medicinal Action and Uses.* Antispasmodic. The juice of the berries, mixed with alum, yields a black dye.

There are two varieties of this species, one of British origin, only distinguished from the rest of the species by its berries being red, instead of black, and the other an American plant (*Actæa alba*, or White Cohosh) with white berries. Both varieties grow in the writer's garden.

The American species is considered by the natives a valuable remedy against snake-bite, especially of the rattlesnake, hence it is – with several other plants – sometimes known as one of the 'Rattlesnake herbs.'

It is said the name 'Herb Christopher' was also formerly applied to the flowering fern, *Osmunda regalis.*

The name of the genus is from the Greek *acte*, the elder, which these plants resemble as regards the leaves and berries.

Toads seem to be attracted by the smell of the Baneberry, which causes it also to be termed Toadroot, the name arising possibly also from its preference for the damp shady situations in which the toad is found.

It is also called Bugbane, because of its offensive smell, which is said to drive away vermin.

BARBERRY, COMMON

Closely allied to this plant, and at one time assigned to the same genus, is the plant known as Black Cohosh.

See (BLACK) COHOSH.

BARBERRY, COMMON

Berberis vulgaris (LINN.)
N.O. Berberidaceæ

Synonyms. Berbery. Pipperidge Bush. Berberis Dumetorum
Parts Used. Bark, root-bark
Habitat. The Common Barberry, a well-known, bushy shrub, with pale-green deciduous leaves, is found in copses and hedges in some parts of England, though a doubtful native in Scotland and Ireland. It is generally distributed over the greater part of Europe, Northern Africa and temperate Asia. As an ornamental shrub, it is fairly common in gardens

¶ *Description.* The stems are woody, 8 to 10 feet high, upright and branched, smooth, slightly grooved, brittle, with a white pith and covered with an ash-coloured bark.

The leaves of the barren shoots of the year are alternate, 1 to 1½ inch long, shortly petioled, presenting various gradations from leaves into spines, into which they become transformed in the succeeding year. The primary leaves on the woody shoots are reduced to three-forked spines, with an enlarged base. The secondary leaves are in fascicles from the axil of these spines, simple, oval, tapering at the base into a short foot-stalk, the margins finely serrate, with the teeth terminating in small spines.

The flowers are small, pale yellow, arranged in pendulous racemes, produced from the fascicles of leaves, towards the ends of the branches. Their scent is not altogether agreeable when near, but by no means offensive at a distance. Their stamens show remarkable sensibility when touched, springing and taking a position closely applied to the pistil. Insects of various kinds are exceedingly fond of the Barberry flower. Linnæus observed that when bees in search of honey touch the filaments, they spring from the petal and strike the anther against the stigma, thereby exploding the pollen. In the original position of the stamens, lying in the concavity of the petals, they are sheltered from rain, and there remain till some insect unavoidably touches them. As it is chiefly in fine, sunny weather that insects are on the wing, the pollen is also in such weather most fit for the purpose of impregnation, hence this curious contrivance of nature for fertilizing the seeds at the most suitable moment.

The berries are about ½ inch long, oblong and slightly curved; when ripe, of a fine, red colour and pleasantly acidulous.

The leaves are also acid, and have sometimes been employed for the same purposes as the fruit. Gerard recommends the leaves 'to season meat with and instead of a salad.'

Cows, sheep and goats are said to eat the shrub, horses and swine to refuse it, and birds, also, seldom touch the fruit, on account of its acidity; in this respect it approaches the tamarind.

¶ *History.* In many parts of Europe, farmers have asserted that wheat planted within three or four hundred yards of a Barberry bush became infected with rust or mildew, but this belief has not been substantiated by recent observations.

Professor Henslow (*Floral Rambles in Highways and Byways*) writes:

'It was thought by farmers in the middle of the last century that the Barberry blighted wheat if it grew near the hedge. Botanists then ridiculed the idea; but in a sense the farmers were right! What they observed was that if a Barberry bush grew, say, at the corner of a wheatfield the leaves of the wheat became "rusty," i.e. they were streaked with a red colour when close to the bush; and that this "red rust" extended steadily across the field till the whole was rusted. The interpretation was at that time unknown. A fungus attacks the leaves of the Barberry, making orange-coloured spots. It throws off minute spores which do attack the wheat. These develop parasitic threads within the leaf, from which arise the red rust-spores: subsequently dark brown or black spores, consisting of two cells, called wheat-mildew, appear. After a time these throw off red, one-celled spores which attack the Barberry; and so a cycle is completed. Though it was *not* really the bush which blighted the wheat, the latter suffered through its agency as the primary host plant.'

¶ *Uses.* The Barberry used to be cultivated for the sake of the fruit, which was pickled and used for garnishing dishes. The ripe berries can be made into an agreeable, refreshing jelly by boiling them with an equal weight of fine sugar to a proper consistence and then straining it. They were formerly used as a sweetmeat, and in sugar-plums, or comfits. It is from these berries that the delicious *confitures d'epine vinette*, for which Rouen is famous, are commonly prepared.

The roots, boiled in lye, will dye wool yellow, and in Poland they dye leather of a beautiful yellow colour with the bark of the root. The inner bark of the stems will also dye linen of a fine yellow, with the assistance of alum.

Provincially, the plant is also termed Pipperidge Bush, from 'pepon,' a pip, and 'rouge,' red, as descriptive of the scarlet, juiceless fruit.

Berberis is the Arabic name of the fruit, signifying a shell, and many authors believe the name is derived from this word, because the leaves are glossy, like the inside of an oyster-shell.

Among the Italians, the Barberry bears the name of Holy Thorn, because it is thought to have formed part of the crown of thorns made for our Saviour.

¶ *Cultivation.* It is generally propagated by suckers, which are put out in plenty from the roots, but these plants are subject to send out suckers in greater plenty than those which are propagated by *layers*, therefore the latter method should be preferred.

The best time for laying down the branches is in autumn (October), and the young shoots of the same year are the best; these will be well rooted by the next autumn, when they may be taken off and planted where they are designed to remain.

Barberry may also be propagated by ripened *cuttings*, taken also in autumn and planted in sandy soil, in a cold frame, or by *seeds*, sown in spring, or preferably in autumn, 1 inch deep in a sheltered border, when, if fresh from the pulp, or berry, they will germinate in the open in the following spring.

¶ *Parts Used.* Stem-bark and root-bark. The stem-bark is collected by shaving and is dried spread out in trays in the sun, or on shelves in a well-ventilated greenhouse or in an airy attic or loft, warmed either by sun or by the artificial heat of a stove, the door and window being left open by day to ensure a warm current of air. The bark may be also strung on threads and hung across the room.

When dried, the pieces of bark are in small irregular portions, about 2 inches long and ½ inch wide, and of a dark-yellowish grey colour externally, and marked with shallow longitudinal furrows. It frequently bears the minute, black 'fruits' of lichen. The bark is dark yellowish brown on the inner surface, separating in layers of bast fibres.

The bark has a slight odour and a bitter taste, and colours the saliva yellow when chewed.

The root-bark is greyish brown externally and is dried in a similar manner after being peeled off. When dry, it breaks with a short fracture. It contains the same constituents as the stem-bark and possesses similar qualities.

¶ *Constituents.* The chief constituent of Barberry bark is Berberine, a yellow crystalline, bitter alkaloid, one of the few that occurs in plants belonging to several different natural orders. Other constituents are oxyacanthine, berbamine, other alkaloidal matter, a little tannin, also wax, resin, fat, albumin, gum and starch.

¶ *Medicinal Action and Uses.* Tonic, purgative, antiseptic. It is used in the form of a liquid extract, given as decoction, infusion or tincture, but generally a salt of the alkaloid Berberine is preferred.

As a bitter stomachic tonic, it proves an excellent remedy for dyspepsia and functional derangement of the liver, regulating the digestive powers, and if given in larger doses, acting as a mild purgative and removing constipation.

It is used in all cases of jaundice, general debility and biliousness, and for diarrhœa.

¶ *Preparations.* Powdered bark, ¼ teaspoonful several times daily. Fluid extract, ½ to 1 drachm. Solid extract, 5 to 10 grains.

It possesses febrifuge powers and is used as a remedy for intermittent fevers. It also forms an excellent gargle for a sore mouth.

A good lotion for application to cutaneous eruptions has also been made from it.

The berries contain citric and malic acids, and possess astringent and anti-scorbutic properties. They are useful in inflammatory fevers, especially typhus, also in bilious disorders and scurvy, and in the form of a jelly are very refreshing in irritable sore throat, for which also a syrup of Barberries made with water, proves an excellent astringent gargle.

The Egyptians are said still to employ a diluted juice of the berries in pestilential fevers, and Simon Paulli relates that he was cured of a malignant fever by drinking an infusion of the berries sweetened with sugar and syrup of roses.

RECIPES

Barberry Drops

The black tops must be cut off; then roast the fruit before the fire till soft enough to pulp with a silver spoon through a sieve into a china basin; then set the basin in a saucepan of water, the top of which will just fit it, or on a hot hearth, and stir it till it grows thick. When cold, put to every pint 1½ lb. of sugar, the finest double-refined, pounded and sifted through a lawn sieve, which must be covered with a fine linen to prevent its wasting while sifting. Beat the sugar and juice together 3½ hours if a large quantity, but 2½ for less; then drop it on sheets of white, thick paper, the size of the drops sold in the shops. Some fruit is not so sour and then less sugar is necessary. To know if there be enough, mix till well incorporated and then drop; if it runs, there is not enough sugar, and if there is too much it will be rough. A dry room will suffice to dry them. No metal must touch the juice but the point of a knife, just to take the drop off the end of the wooden spoon, and then as little as possible.

To prepare Barberries for Tartlets

Pick Barberries that have no stones, from the stalks, and to every pound weigh ¾ lb. of lump sugar; put the fruit into a *stone* jar, and either set it on a hot hearth or in a saucepan of water, and let them simmer very slowly till soft; put them and the sugar into a preserving-pan, and boil them gently 15 minutes. Use no metal but silver.

Barberries in Bunches

Have ready bits of flat white wood, 3 inches long and ¼ inch wide. Tie the stalks of the fruit on the stick from *within* an inch of one end to beyond the other, so as to make them look handsome. Simmer them in some syrup two successive days, covering them each time with it when cold. When they look clear they are simmered enough. The third day do them like other candy fruit.

Mrs. Beeton (an old edition) says:

'Barberries are also used as a dry sweetmeat, and in sugar-plums or comfits; are pickled with vinegar and are used for various culinary purposes. They are well calculated to allay heat and thirst in persons afflicted with fevers. The berries arranged on bunches of nice curled parsley, make an exceedingly pretty garnish for supper-dishes, particularly for white meats, like boiled fowl à la Béchamel; the three colours, scarlet, green and white contrasting so well, and producing a very good effect.'

BARBERRY, NEPAL

Berberis aristata
N.O. Berberidaceæ

Synonyms. Ophthalmic Barberry. Darlahad
Part Used. Dried stems
Habitat. A shrub indigenous to India and Ceylon

It is known as 'Darlahad,' under which names are included the dried stems of *Berberis lycium* and *B. asiatica*, but only the stem of *B. aristata* is official in the Indian and Colonial Addendum for use in India and the Eastern Colonies, in intermittent fevers.
¶ *Medicinal Action and Uses.* A bitter tonic, antiperiodic and diaphoretic. The chief constituents are those of common Berberia bark, the bitter principle being the alkaloid Berberine, which is present in considerable quantity, together with tannin, resin, gum, starch and other alkaloidal matter. When dried, it occurs in undulating, cylindrical pieces, 1 to 2 inches in diameter. The drug has a faint odour and a bitter taste.

BARBERRY (INDIAN)

Berberis asiatica
N.O. Berberiaceæ

Part Used. Root-bark

The root-bark is light coloured, corky, almost inodorous, with a bitter, mucilaginous taste. It contains much Berberine, and a dark-brown extract is made from it employed in India under the name of 'Rusot.' This extract is sometimes prepared from the wood or roots of different species of Barberry. It has the consistency of opium and a bitter, astringent taste.

For *Berberis aquifolium, see* (MOUNTAIN) GRAPE.

BARLEY

Hordeum distichon (LINN.)
N.O. Graminaceæ

Synonyms. Pearl Barley. Perlatum
Part Used. Decorticated seeds
Habitat. Britain

¶ *Description.* Pearl Barley is the grain without its skin; rounded and polished; this is the official variety. Taste and odour farinaceous. The Scotch, milled, or pot barley is the grain with husks only partly removed. Patent Barley is the ground decorticated grain.

¶ *Constituents.* Pearl Barley contains about 80 per cent. of starch and about 6 per cent. of proteins, cellulose, etc.

¶ *Medicinal Action and Uses.* Pearl Barley is used for the preparation of a decoction which is a nutritive and demulcent drink in febrile conditions and in catarrhal affections of the respiratory and urinary organs: barley water is used to dilute cows' milk for young infants, it prevents the formation of hard masses of curd in the stomach. Malt is produced from barley by a process of steeping and drying which develop a ferment 'diatase'

needed for the production of alcoholic malt liquors, but in the form of Malt Extract it is largely used in medicine. Vinegar is an acid liquid produced by oxidation of fermented malt wort. Malt vinegar is the only vinegar that should be used medicinally.

¶ *Dosage and Preparation.* Barley water. Pearl Barley washed 10 parts, water to 100 parts, boil for 20 minutes, strain. Dose, 1 to 4 oz.

¶ *Adulterants.* Pearl Barley is sometimes treated with french chalk and starch to whiten it and increase the weight.

BARTSIA, RED

Bartsia odontites
N.O. Scrophulariaceæ

Part Used. Herb

This common little plant, which has no old popular name, is an abundant weed in cornfields and by the roadside. It is not very attractive in appearance, its narrow, tapering leaves being of a dingy purplish green and the flowers of a dull rose colour, small and in one-sided spikes, which usually droop at the ends.

A less common species, *Bartsia viscosa*, is found in marshes and damp places; the flowers are yellow, and might be mistaken for Yellow Rattle, from which it may be easily dis-

tinguished by its solitary, unspiked, yellow flowers, and by being covered with clammy down. It grows to a height of 6 to 12 inches, and is very common in many parts of Devon and Cornwall, where it sometimes grows 2 feet high.

BARTSIA LATIFOLIA

Synonyms. Common Bartsia. Red Nettle.

A small annual, with reddish stems, leaves and flowers; partly parasitic on the roots of grasses.

BASIL, BUSH

Ocymum minimum
N.O. Labiatæ

Part Used. Leafy tops

Bush Basil (*Ocymum minimum*) is a low, bushy plant, seldom above 6 inches in height, much smaller than Sweet Basil.

The leaves are ovate, quite entire, the white flowers in whorls towards the top of the branches, smaller than those of Sweet Basil, and seldom succeeded by ripe seeds in England.

There are two varieties, one with black-purple leaves and the other with variable leaves.

Both Bush and Garden Basil are natives of India, from whence it was introduced in 1573. Bush Basil may occasionally live through the winter in this country, though Sweet Basil never does.

Both varieties flower in July and August.

The leafy tops of Bush Basil are used in the same manner as the Sweet Basil for seasoning and in salads.

The leaves of *O. viride*, a native of Western Africa, possess febrifugal properties; and at Sierra Leone, where it bears the name of 'Fever-plant,' a decoction of them, drunk as tea, is used as a remedy for the fevers so prevalent there.

The leaves of *O. canum*, and *O. gratissimum* in India, and of *O. crispum* in Japan, all sweet-scented varieties, are prescribed as a remedy for colds.

O. teniflorum is regarded as an aromatic stimulant in Java; and *O. guineense* is much employed by the negroes as a medicine in cases of bilious fever.

These plants are all free of any deleterious secretions; for the most part they are fragrant and aromatic, and hence they have not only been used as tonics, but are also valuable as kitchen herbs.

In Persia and Malaysia Basil is planted on graves, and in Egypt women scatter the flowers on the resting-places of those belonging to them.

These observances are entirely at variance with the idea prevailing among the ancient Greeks that it represented hate and misfortune. They painted poverty as a ragged woman with a Basil at her side, and thought the plant would not grow unless railing and abuse were poured forth at the time of sowing. The Romans, in like manner, believed that the more it was abused, the better it would prosper.

The physicians of old were quite unable to agree as to its medicinal value, some declaring that it was a poison, and others a precious simple. Culpepper tells us:

'Galen and Dioscorides hold it is not fitting to be taken inwardly and Chrysippus rails at it. Pliny and the Arabians defend it. Something is the matter, this herb and rue will not grow together, no, nor near one another, and we know rue is as great an enemy to poison as any that grows.'

But it was said to cause sympathy between human beings and a tradition in Moldavia still exists that a youth will love any maiden from whose hand he accepts a sprig of this plant. In Crete it symbolizes 'love washed with tears,' and in some parts of Italy it is a love-token.

Boccaccio's story of Isabella and the Pot of Basil, immortalized by Keats, keeps the plant in our memory, though it is now rarely cultivated in this country. It was formerly grown in English herb gardens. Tusser includes it among the Strewing herbs, and Drayton places it first in his poem *Polyolbion*.

'With Basil then I will begin
Whose scent is wondrous pleasing.'

In Tudor days, little pots of Basil were often given as graceful compliments by farmers' wives to visitors. Parkinson says:

'The ordinary Basill is in a manner wholly spent to make sweete or washing waters among other sweet herbs, yet sometimes it is put into nosegays. The Physicall properties are to procure a cheerfull and merry hearte whereunto the seeds is chiefly used in powder.'

¶ *Cultivation*. Basil dies down every year in this country, so that the seeds have to be sown annually. If in a very warm sheltered spot, seeds may be sown in the open, about the last week in April, but they are a long time coming up, and it is preferable to sow in a hot bed, about the end of March, and remove to a warm border in May, planting 10 inches to a foot apart.

Basil flourishes best in a rich soil.

¶ *Part Used Medicinally*. The whole herb, both fresh and dried, gathered in July.

¶ *Medicinal Action and Uses*. Aromatic and carminative. Though generally employed in cooking as a flavouring, Basil has been occasionally used for mild nervous disorders, and for the alleviation of wandering rheumatic pains; the dried leaves, in the form of snuff, are said to be a cure for nervous headaches.

BASIL, SWEET

Part Used. Herb

¶ *Description*. Common or Sweet Basil, which is used in medicine and also for culinary purposes, especially in France, is a hairy, labiate plant, growing about 3 feet

An infusion of the green herb in boiling water is good for all obstructions of the internal organs, arrests vomiting and allays nausea.

The seeds have been reckoned efficacious against the poison of serpents, both taken internally and laid upon the wound. They are also said to cure warts.

In common with other labiates, Basil, both the wild and the sweet, furnishes an aromatic, volatile, camphoraceous oil, and on this account is much employed in France for flavouring soups, especially turtle soup. They also use it in ragoûts and sauces. The leafy tops are a great improvement to salads and cups.

Although it is now comparatively little used in England for culinary purposes, this herb was one of our favourite pot-herbs in older days, and gave the distinctive flavour that once made Fetter Lane sausages famous.

RECIPES

A Recipe for Aromatic Seasoning

'Take of nutmegs and mace one ounce each, of cloves and peppercorns two ounces of each, one ounce of dried bay-leaves, three ounces of *basil*, the same of marjoram, two ounces of winter savory, and three ounces of thyme, half an ounce of cayenne-pepper, the same of grated lemon-peel, and two cloves of garlic; all these ingredients must be well pulverized in a mortar and sifted through a fine wire sieve, and put away in dry corked bottles for use.' (Francatelli's *Cook's Guide*.)

O. Americanum. First recorded in 1789 as found in the West Indies.

The name 'Ocymum' is said by Mathiolus to be derived from the Greek word 'To smell,' because of the powerful aromatic and pungent scent characterizing most of the plants of this genus. Decoctions made from *O. Americanum* are used in cases of chest trouble and dysentery; and an essential oil is also extracted from the plant.

Closely akin to the above-named is the *O. gratissimum* cultivated in China as a culinary herb.

O. canum is used as a tincture made from the leaves in homœopathy.

Ocymum basilium (LINN.)
N.O. Labiatæ

high. The stem is obtusely quadrangular, the labiate flowers are white, in whorls in the axils of the leaves, the calyx with the upper lobe rounded and spreading. The leaves, greyish-green beneath and dotted with dark oil cells, are opposite, 1 inch long and ½ inch broad, stalked and peculiarly smooth, soft and cool to the touch, and if slightly bruised exale a delightful scent of cloves.

There are several varieties, differing in the size, shape, odour and colour of the leaves. The Common Basil has very dark green leaves, the curled-leaved has short spikes of flowers, the narrow-leaved smells like Fennel, another has a scent of citron and another a tarragon scent, one species has leaves of three colours, and another 'studded' leaves.

¶ *History*. The derivation of the name Basil is uncertain. Some authorities say it comes from the Greek *basileus*, a king, because, as Parkinson says, 'the smell thereof is so excellent that it is fit for a king's house,' or it may have been termed royal, because it was used in some regal unguent or medicine. One rather unlikely theory is that it is shortened from *basilisk*, a fabulous creature that could kill with a look. This theory may be based on a strange old superstition that connected the plant with scorpions. Parkinson tells us that 'being gently handled it gave a pleasant smell, but being hardly wrung and bruised would breed scorpions. It is also observed that scorpions doe much rest and abide under these pots and vessells wherein Basil is planted.' It was generally believed that if a sprig of Basil were left under a pot it would in time turn to a scorpion. Superstition went so far as to affirm that even smelling the plant might bring a scorpion into the brain. Culpepper says:

'Being applied to the place bitten by venomous beasts, or stung by a wasp or hornet, it speedily draws the poison to it. – *Every like draws its like*. Mizaldus affirms, that being laid to rot in horse-dung, it will breed venomous beasts. Hilarius, a French physician, affirms upon his own knowledge, that an acquaintance of his, by common smelling to it, had a scorpion breed in his brain.'

In India the Basil plant is sacred to both Krishna and Vishnu, and is cherished in every Hindu house. Probably on account of its virtues, in disinfecting, and vivifying malarious air, it first became inseparable from Hindu houses in India as the protecting spirit of the family.

The strong aromatic scent of the leaves is very much like cloves.

Every good Hindu goes to his rest with a Basil leaf on his breast. This is his passport to Paradise.

BASIL, WILD

Calamintha Clinopodium
N.O. Labiatæ

Synonyms. Hedge Basil. Hedge Calamint
Habitat. The plant is widely distributed throughout the North Temperate Zone, and is common in England and Scotland in dry hedges and the borders of copses, mostly in high situations. In Ireland it is somewhat rare

The Wild Basil, or Hedge Basil (*Calamintha Clinopodium*) (sometimes called Hedge Calamint), is a straggling plant with somewhat weak-looking, though erect stems, rising to a height of a foot or 18 inches, and thickly covered with soft hairs.

¶ *Description*. The shortly - stalked, egg - shaped leaves, 1 to 2 inches long, are placed opposite one another on the four-angled stem, the pairs being some distance apart. They are only slightly toothed at their edges and like the stem are downy with soft hairs.

The flowers, with tubular, lipped corollas of a pinkish colour, are arranged on the stem in several crowded, bristly rings or whorls, at the points from which the leaf-stalks spring, and are in bloom from July to September.

The whole herb is aromatic and fragrant, with a faint Thyme-like odour, and like Calamint has been used to make an infusion for similar complaints.

The name of the species, *Clinopodium*, signifies 'bedfoot.' An old writer says 'the tufts of the plant are like the knobs at the feet of a bed,' but the comparison is not very obvious. By some botanists the plant has been described under the name of *C. vulgare*, but it is now assigned to the genus, *Calamintha*.

BAYBERRY

Myrica cerifera (LINN.)
N.O. Myricaceæ

Synonyms. Wax Myrtle. Myrica. Candle Berry. Arbre à suif. Myricæ Cortex. Tallow Shrub. Wachsgagle
Parts Used. The dried bark of the root. The wax
Habitat. Eastern North America

¶ *Description*. The only species of a useful family that is regarded as official, *Myrica cerifera* grows in thickets near swamps and marshes in the sand-belt near the Atlantic coast and on the shores of Lake Erie. Its height is from 3 to 8 feet, its leaves lanceolate, shining or resinous, dotted on both sides, its flowers unisexual, without calyx or corolla, and its fruit small groups of globular berries, having numerous black grains crusted with greenish-white wax. These are persistent for two or three years. The leaves are very fragrant when rubbed.

The bark as found in commerce is in curved pieces from 1 to 7 inches long, covered with a thin, mottled layer, the cork beneath being smooth and red-brown. The fracture is reddish, granular, and slightly fibrous. The odour is aromatic, and the taste astringent, bitter, and very acrid. It should be separated from the fresh root by pounding, in late autumn, thoroughly dried, and when powdered, kept in darkened, well-closed vessels.

The wax was first introduced into medicinal use by Alexandre in 1722. It is removed from the berries by boiling them in water, on the top of which it floats. It melts at 47° to 49° C. (116·6° to 120·2° F.). It is harder and more brittle than beeswax. Candles made from it are aromatic, smokeless after snuffing, and very brittle. It makes a useful body for surgeon's soap plasters, and an aromatic and softening shaving lather. It has also been used for making sealing-wax. Four-fifths of this wax is soluble in hot alcohol, and boiling ether dissolves more than a quarter of its weight. Four pounds of berries yield about one pound of wax.

¶ Constituents. There has been found in the bark of stem and root volatile oil, starch, lignin, gum, albumen, extractive, tannic and gallic acids, acrid and astringent resins, a red colouring substance, and an acid resembling saponin.

The wax (Myrtle Wax) consists of glycerides of stearic, palmitic and myristic acids, and a small quantity of oleaic acid.

¶ Medicinal Action and Uses. Astringent and stimulant. In large doses emetic. It is useful in diarrhœa, jaundice, scrofula, etc. Externally, the powdered bark is used as a stimulant to indolent ulcers, though in poultices it should be combined with elm. The decoction is good as a gargle and injection in chronic inflammation of the throat, leucorrhœa, uterine hæmorrhage, etc. It is an excellent wash for the gums.

The powder is strongly sternutatory and excites coughing. Water in which the wax has been 'tried,' when boiled to an extract, is regarded as a certain cure for dysentery, and the wax itself, being astringent and slightly narcotic, is valuable in severe dysentery and internal ulcerations.

¶ Dosages. Of powder, 20 to 30 grains. Of decoction, 1 to 2 fluid ounces. Of alcoholic extract, or Myricin, 5 grains.

¶ Other Species.

MURICA GALE, SWEET GALE, ENGLISH BOG MYRTLE, or DUTCH MYRTLE, the badge of the Campbells. The leaves of this species have been used in France as an emmenagogue and abortifacient, being formerly official under the name of Herba Myrti Rabantini, and containing a poisonous, volatile oil. The plant is bitter and astringent, and has been employed in the northern counties as a substitute for hops, and also mingled with bark for tanning, and dyeing wool yellow. The dried berries are put in broth and used as spices. Formerly it was much used in cottage practice, its properties being similar to those of M. cerifera. It is covered with a golden, aromatic dust, and is thus used to drive away insects. The leaves are infused like tea, especially in China, as a stomachic and cordial. See GALE (SWEET).

M. nagi. A glucoside, Myricitrin, resembling quercitrin, has been separated from the yellow colouring matter, or myricetin.

M. cordifolia, of the Cape of Good Hope, yields a wax which is said to be eaten by Hottentots.

M. Pensylvanica has roots with emetic properties.

A Brazilian species yields a waxy-resinous product called Tabocas combicurdo, which is used as a 'pick-me-up.'

BAYBERRY is a synonym for the Wild Cinnamon or Pimenta acris of the West Indies and South America, which yields Bay Rum and oil of Bayberry.

BEAN, KIDNEY

Phaceolus vulgaris
N.O. Leguminaceæ

Part Used. Dried ripe seeds
Habitat. Native of Indies; cultivated all over Europe; also said to be found in ancient tombs in Peru

¶ History. This well-known plant has been cultivated from remote times. Because of the seeds close resemblance to the male testicle, the Egyptians made it an object of sacred worship and forbad its use as food. In Italy at the present day beans are distributed among the poor, on the anniversary of a death. The Jewish high priest is forbidden to eat beans on the day of Atonement.

¶ Constituents. Starch and starchy fibrous matter, phaseoline, extractive albumen mucilage, pectic acid, legumin fatty matter, earthy salts, uncrystallizable sugar, inosite, sulphur.

88

¶ *Medicinal Action and Uses*. When bruised and boiled with garlic Beans have cured otherwise uncurable coughs. If eaten raw they cause painful severe frontal headache, soreness and itching of the eyeball and pains in the epigastrium. The roots are dangerously narcotic.

BEARBERRY

Arctostaphylos Uva-Ursi
N.O. Ericaceæ

Synonyms. Arbutus Uva-Ursi. Uva-Ursi

Part Used. Leaves

Habitat. The Bearberry (*Arctostaphylos Uva-Ursi*, Sprengel), a small shrub, with decumbent, much branched, irregular stems and evergreen leaves, is distributed over the greater part of the Northern Hemisphere, being found in the northern latitudes and high mountains of Europe, Asia and America. In the British Isles, it is common in Scotland, on heaths and barren places in hilly districts, especially in the Highlands, and extends south as far as Yorkshire; it grows also on the hills of the north-west of Ireland. In America it is distributed throughout Canada and the United States as far south as New Jersey and Wisconsin.

It is very nearly related to the Arbutus, and was formerly assigned to the same genus – in Green's *Universal Herbal*, 1832, it will be found under the name *Arbutus Uva-Ursi* – but it differs from Arbutus in having a smooth berry with five one-seeded stones, whereas the Arbutus has a rough fruit, each cell of the ovary being four to five seeded.

The only other British species assigned to the genus, *Arctostaphylos*, the Black Bearberry (*A. alpina*), with black berries, found on barren mountains in northern Scotland, and not at all in England, is the badge of the clan of Ross.

The generic name, derived from the Greek, and the Latin specific name, *Uva-Ursi*, mean the same: the Bear's grape, and may have been given to the plant, either from the notion that bears eat the fruit with relish, or from its very rough, unpleasant flavour, which might have been considered only fit for bears.

¶ *Description*. The much-branched trailing stems are short and woody, covered with a pale brown bark, scaling off in patches, and form thick masses, 1 to 2 feet long. The long shoots rise obliquely upward from the stems for a few inches and are covered with soft hairs.

The evergreen leaves are of a leathery texture, from ½ inch to an inch long, like a spatula in form, being rounded at the apex and tapering gradually towards the base to a very short stalk or petiole. The margin is entire and slightly rolled back and the young leaves fringed with short hairs. The upper surface of the leaf is dark, shining green, the veins deeply impressed, the lower side is of a paler green, with the veins prominent and forming a coarse network. The leaves have no distinctive odour, but they have a very astringent and somewhat bitter taste.

The pretty waxy-looking flowers are in small, closely-crowded, drooping clusters, three to fifteen flowers together, at the ends of the branches of the preceding year, appearing in early summer, May – June, before the young leaves. The corolla, about two-thirds inch across, is urn-shaped, reddish white or white with a red lip, transparent at the base, contracted at the mouth, which is divided into four to five short reflexed, blunt teeth, which are hairy within. There are ten stamens, with chocolate-brown, awned anthers. The berry, which ripens in autumn, is about the size of a small currant, very bright red, smooth and glossy, with a tough skin enclosing an insipid mealy pulp, with five one-seeded stones.

¶ *Parts Used Medicinally*. The dried leaves are the only part of the plant used in medicine. The British Pharmacopœia directs that the leaves should be obtained only from indigenous plants. They should be collected in September and October, only green leaves being selected and dried by exposure to gentle heat.

Leaves must be gathered only in fine weather, in the morning, after the dew has dried, any stained and insect-eaten leaves being rejected. Drying may be done in warm, sunny weather out-of-doors, but in half-shade, as leaves dried in the shade retain their colour better than those dried in direct sun. They may be placed on wire sieves, or frames covered with wire or garden netting, at a height of 3 or 4 feet from the ground to ensure a current of air, and must be taken indoors to a dry room, or shed, before there is any risk of damp from dew or showers. The leaves should be spread in a single layer, preferably not touching, and may be turned during drying.

Failing sun, which in the case of leaves collected like the Bearberry in September and October cannot be relied on, any ordinary shed, fitted with racks and shelves can be used, provided it is ventilated near the roof and has a warm current of air, caused by a coke or anthracite stove. Empty glass-houses can readily be adapted into drying-sheds, especially if heated by pipes and the glass is shaded; ventilation is essential, and there must be no open tank in the house to cause steaming. For drying indoors, a warm, sunny attic or loft may be employed, the window being left open by day, so that there is a current of air and the moist, hot air may escape: the door may also be left open. The leaves can be placed on coarse butter-cloth, stented, i.e. if hooks are placed beneath the window and on the opposite wall, the butter-cloth can be attached by rings sewn on each side of it, and hooked on so that it is stretched taut. The drying temperature should be from 70° to 100° F.

All dried leaves should be packed away at once in wooden or tin boxes, in a dry place, as otherwise they re-absorb moisture from the air.

Dried Bearberry leaves are usually quite smooth, and entirely free from the hairs that are present on the margins of the growing leaves and on the foot-stalks, which drop off during the drying process.

The commercial drug frequently consists of the entire plants, and therefore contains a large quantity of stems, but the latter should not be present, according to the official definition of the United States Pharma-copœia, in greater amount than 5 per cent.

The leaves of other plants have been mistaken for Bearberry leaves, notably those of the Cowberry (*Vaccinium Vitis-idæa*) and of the Box (*Buxus sempervirens*), and have occasionally been used to adulterate the drug, but Bearberry leaves are readily distinguished by the characteristics given, viz. the spatu-late outline, entire margin and rounded apex. Those of the Box have a notch cut out at the apex (emarginate) and have the epidermis loose and separable on the under surface of the leaf, and are, moreover, quite devoid of astringency. The leaves of the Cowberry may be distinguished by the glandular brown dots scattered over their under sur-face and the minute teeth on their margins. They have only a very slight astringent taste.

¶ *Constituents.* The chief constituent of Bearberry leaves is a crystallizable gluco-side named Arbutin. Other constituents are methyl-arbutin, ericolin (an ill-defined gluco-side), ursone (a crystalline substance of resinous character), gallic acid, ellagic acid, a yellow colouring principle resembling quer-cetin, and probably also myricetin. Tannin is present to the extent of 6 to 7 per cent. On incineration, the leaves yield about 3 per cent. of ash.

¶ *Medicinal Action and Uses.* In conse-quence of the powerful astringency of the leaves, *Uva-Ursi* has a place not only in all the old herbals, but also in the modern Pharma-copœias. There are records that it was used in the thirteenth century by the Welsh 'Physicians of Myddfai.' It was described by Clusius in 1601, and recommended for medi-cinal use in 1763 by Gerhard of Berlin and others. It had a place in the London Pharma-copœia for the first time in 1788, though was probably in use long before. It is official in nearly all Pharmacopœias, some of which use the name Arbutus.

The usual form of administration is in the form of an infusion, which has a soothing as well as an astringent effect and marked diuretic action. Of great value in diseases of the bladder and kidneys, strengthening and imparting tone to the urinary passages. The diuretic action is due to the glucoside Arbutin, which is largely absorbed un-changed and is excreted by the kidneys. During its excretion, Arbutin exercises an antiseptic effect on the urinary mucous mem-brane: Bearberry leaves are, therefore, used in inflammatory diseases of the urinary tract, urethritis, cystisis, etc.

Besides the simple infusion (1 oz. of the leaves to 1 pint of boiling water), the com-bination of ½ oz. each of *Uva-Ursi*, Poplar Bark and Marshmallow root, infused in 1 pint of water for 20 minutes is used with advantage.

The tannin in the leaves is so abundant that they have been used for tanning leather in Sweden and Russia.

An ash-coloured dye is said to be obtained from the plant in Scandinavian countries.

The berries are only of use as food for grouse. Cattle, however, avoid the plant.

¶ *Allied Species.* Manzanita, the leaves of *A. glauca* from California, are employed like *Uva-Ursi*.

The leaves of *A. polifolia* from Mexico and *A. tomentosa* (madrona) are also used in medicine.

See ARBUTUS.

BEARSFOOT (AMERICAN)
Polymnia uvedalia (LINN.)
N.O. Compositæ

Synonyms. Uvedalia. Leaf Cup. Yellow Leaf Cup
Part Used. Root
Habitat. New York to Missouri and southward

¶ *Description.* A tall branching plant found growing in very rich soil the root is greyish brown in colour and furrowed, bark thin, brittle and easily scales off, odourless, taste salty and slightly bitter.

¶ *Medicinal Action and Uses.* Anodyne laxative and stimulant, valuable in malarial enlargements of the spleen, swollen glands and dyspepsia caused by the spleen. Of great use applied externally in stimulating the growth of the hair, and is an ingredient of many American hair ointments and lotions.

¶ *Dosage and Preparation.* Fluid extract, dose, 15 to 60 minims.

BEARSFOOT (BRITISH). *See* (BLACK) HELLEBORE (HELLEBORUS FŒTIDUS)

BEDSTRAW, LADY'S
Galium verum (LINN.)
N.O. Rubiaceæ

Synonyms. Our Lady's Bedstraw. Yellow Bedstraw. Maid's Hair. Petty Mugget. Cheese Renning. Cheese Rennet
Habitat. Yellow Bedstraw is abundant on dry banks, chiefly near the sea. Its small, bright yellow flowers are closely clustered together in dense panicles at the tops of the wiry, square, upright stems, which are 1 to 3 feet high, and bear numerous very narrow, almost thread-like leaves, placed six to eight together in whorls. The flowers are in bloom in July and August

The plant is inodorous, but has an astringent, acidulous and bitterish taste.

The common English name of this plant, 'Our Lady's Bedstraw,' is derived from its use in former days, even by ladies of rank, for stuffing beds.[1]

Dr. Fernie tells us that because of its bright yellow blossoms, this herb is also named 'Maid's Hair,' for in Henry VIII's reign 'maydens did wear silken callis to keep in order their hayre made yellow with dye.' It has also been known as 'Petty Mugget,' from the French *petit muguet*, a little dandy.

The plant has the property of curdling milk, hence another of its popular names, 'Cheese Rennet.' It was called 'Cheese Renning' in the sixteenth century, and Gerard says (quoting from Matthiolus, a famous commentator of Dioscorides), 'the people of Thuscane do use it to turne their milks and the cheese, which they make of sheepes and goates milke, might be the sweeter and more pleasant to taste. The people in Cheshire especially about Nantwich, where the best cheese is made, do use it in their rennet, esteeming greatly of that cheese above other made without it.' The rich colour of this cheese was probably originally derived from this plant, thoughi t is now obtained from annatto.

The Highlanders also made special use of Yellow Bedstraw to curdle milk and colour their cheese, and it has been used in Glou-cestershire for the same purpose, either alone or with the juice of the stinging-nettle.

The name of this genus, *Galium*, from the Greek word *gala*, milk, is supposed to have been given from this property of the plants which is shared more or less by most of the group.

¶ *Medicinal Action and Uses. Galium verum* contains the same chemical principles as *G. aparine.*

It is still used to a limited degree as a popular remedy in gravel, stone and urinary diseases.

It was formerly highly esteemed as a remedy in epilepsy and hysteria, and was applied externally in cutaneous eruptions, in the form either of the recently expressed juice, or of a decoction from the fresh plant.

'An ointment,' says Gerard, 'is prepared which is good for anointing the weary traveller.'

Culpepper recommends the decoction to stop inward bleeding and bleeding at the nose, and to heal all inward wounds generally.

The flowering tips, distilled with water, are stated to yield an acid liquor which forms a pleasant summer drink.

The flowers of this species and still more those of *G. elatum*, an allied non-British species, are considered in France a remedy for epilepsy.

The Yellow Bedstraw can furnish a red dye, like its ally, the Madder of the Continent, *Rubia tinctorum*. It has been culti-

---

[1] The origin of the name is more probably from the Christian legend that this was one of the 'Cradle Herbs,' i.e. was in the hay in the manger at Bethlehem. – EDITOR.

vated for the purpose, but with little or no profit, as the roots are too small, though it has been used in the Hebrides for dyeing woollen stuffs red. When attempts have been made to cultivate it, the produce per acre has occasionally exceeded 12 cwt., which is considered an average crop for Madder, but the roots do not yield as much in proportion, and its cultivation has never been undertaken on a very large scale, the crops having been found too small to pay under ordinary circumstances. The same cultivation is necessary as for Madder, the plant requiring a deep, light, but rich loam to succeed well,

and the land must be well trenched and manured before planting. The running roots are to be planted, though it may be raised from seed, a plan that has also sometimes been adopted with Madder.

The stem and leaves of this *Galium* yield a good yellow dye, which has been used to a great extent in Ireland.

Several other species of this genus have roots capable of yielding red or yellow dyes, but none of them have been practically applied, their produce being too small to admit of their successful cultivation as dye plants.

BEDSTRAW (HEDGE)

Galium molugo
N.O. Rubiaceæ

Galium molugo, the Hedge Bedstraw, another closely allied species, with white flowers, very common in this country, has much the same properties as Lady's Bedstraw.

An American species, *G. tinctorum* (Linn.), is closely allied in properties to *G. verum*. It is said to be useful in cutaneous diseases, and the root is employed by the Indians for staining their feathers and other ornaments red.

Besides the above, there are also four other British species, i.e. *G. palustré* (Water Bedstraw), common in watery places; *G. uliginosum* (Rough Marsh Bedstraw), smaller than

the first-mentioned, the stem being rarely more than a foot high, slender and brittle; *G. saxatile* (Heath Bedstraw), a small species with dense panicles of white flowers; *G. tricorué* which is tolerably common in some of the English counties and in the Isle of Wight. The stems of this species are about a foot long and rough, as well as the leaves, with prickles pointing backwards; the flowers grow in threes and the first is reflexed. About seven or eight other species have been described by British botanists; they are, however, of rare occurrence.

See also CLIVERS, CROSSWORT, WOODRUFF.

BEECH

Fagus sylvatica
N.O. Corylaceæ

Synonyms. Buche. Buke. Boke. Bog. Bok. Buk. Hetre. Faggio. Faya. Haya. Fagos
Part Used. The oil of the nuts
Habitat. Europe, including Britain. (Indigenous only in England.) Armenia, Palestine, Asia Minor, Japan

¶ *History*. The common name of the Beech tree, found in varying forms throughout the Teutonic dialects, means, with difference of gender, either 'a book' or 'a beech,' the Runic tablets, or early books, having been made of this wood. *Fagus* is from a Greek word meaning 'to eat,' referring to the edible character of the Beechmast.

The Beech is one of the largest British trees, especially on chalky and sandy soil. In England it may grow to 140 feet in height, or spread to 130 feet in diameter, with a trunk 21 feet in girth. As the wood is brittle and short-grained, it is not well suited for purposes where strength and durability are required. One of the principal objections to it is that it is liable to be perforated by a small beetle. Its chief uses are for panels for carriages, carpenter's planes, stonemason's mallets, wooden bowls, granary shovels, boot-lasts, sabots, and for chair-making, small articles in turnery, also for making charcoal for colour

manufacturers, and gunpowder. On the Continent Beech is used for parquet flooring, wood pavement and bentwood furniture, and very extensively as fuel for domestic heating, as its heating power surpasses that of most other timber.

Owing to the capacity of its root system for assisting in the circulation of air throughout the soil, and by the amount of potash in the leaves, Beech trees conserve the productive capacity of the soil better than any other kind of tree, and improve the growth of other trees when planted with them.

Fences of young Beech trees may be employed with advantage in flower gardens, as their leaves generally remain on the branches during the winter and screen the young plants.

The *nuts* of Beech, called 'mast,' are chiefly used in England as food for park deer. In other countries they are valued for feeding farm animals: in France for feeding swine and fattening domestic poultry, especially turkeys, and pigs which are turned into Beech woods to utilize the fallen mast. Beech mast has even been used as human food in time of distress or famine. Horses, however, should not be fed on it.

Well-ripened mast yields from 17 to 20 per cent. of a non-drying oil – similar to hazel and Cotton-seed oils – and is used in European countries for cooking, as well as for burning, and in Silesia as a substitute for butter. The cake left when the oil has been pressed out may be used as a cattle food.

During the War an attempt was made in Germany to use Beech *leaves* as a substitute for tobacco, and a mixture was served to the army, but proved a failure.

¶ *Constituents.* The *wood ash* of the Beech affords a large proportion of potash. The *oil* of the nuts occupies a position in the fixed oils between the vegetable non-drying and the true drying oils. Like the Cotton-seed oils, it forms more or less elaidin on treatment with nitrous acid or mercuric nitrate, but does not become wholly solidified. *Beech tar* is completely soluble in 95 per cent. acetic acid. Turpentine oil, chloroform and absolute ether do not entirely dissolve it. The petroleum ether is not coloured by copper acetate solution. Choline is present in the seeds.

¶ *Medicinal Uses.* The tar is stimulating and antiseptic, used internally as a stimulating expectorant in chronic bronchitis, or externally as an application in various skin diseases.

The oil is used in the same ways as the other fixed oils of its class.

¶ *Other Species.*

BEECH DROPS (OROBANCHE VIRGINIANA, EPIFAGUS VIRGINIANA, BROOM RAPE, CANCER ROOT), a parasite on Beech tree roots, has a bitter, nauseous, astringent taste, diminished by drying. It is given internally in bowel affections, and is reputed to cure cancer, though this is doubtful. As a local application to wounds or ulcers it will arrest gangrene. It appears to act upon the capillary system like the tincture of muriate of iron.

ALBANY BEECH DROPS (*Pterospora Andromeda*) is a rare plant of North America, valuable as a sedative diaphoretic in typhus, pleurisy and erysipelas.

COPPER-BEECH (*F. sylvatica* var. *purpurea*). The leaves of this species may be used like those of the Red-leaved Hazel for the extraction of anthocyan pigment.

BEETROOTS

N.O. Chenopodiaceæ

Synonyms. Spinach Beet. Sea Beet. Garden Beet. White Beet. Mangel Wurzel
Parts Used. Leaves, root

¶ *Description. Beta vulgaris* (Linn.) is a native of South Europe, extensively cultivated as an article of food and especially for the production of sugar, and presents many varieties.

It is derived from the Sea Beet (*B. maritima*, Linn.), which grows wild on the coasts of Europe, North Africa and Asia, as far as India, and is found in muddy maritime marshes in many parts of England, a tall, succulent plant, about 2 feet high, with large, fleshy, glossy leaves, angular stems and numerous leafy spikes of green flowers, much like those of the Stinking Goosefoot.

The lower leaves, when boiled, are quite equal in taste to Spinach, and the leaf-stalks and midrib of a cultivated form, the Spinach Beet (*B. vulgaris*, var. *cicla*), are sometimes stewed, under the name of Swiss Chard (being the *Poirée à Carde* of the French, with whom it is served as Sea Kale or Asparagus). This white-rooted Beet is also cultivated for its leaves, which are put into soups, or used as spinach, and in France are often mixed with sorrel, to lessen its acidity. It is also largely used as a decorative plant for its large handsome leaves, blood-red or variegated in colour. Its root, though containing almost as much sugar as the red Garden Beet, neither looks so appetizing nor tastes so well.

The Mangel Wurzel, or Mangold, also a variety of the Beet, too coarse for table use, is good for cattle, who thrive excellently upon this diet, both its leaves and roots affording an abundance of valuable and nutritious food.

In its uncultivated form, the root of the Sea Beet is coarse and unfit for food, nor has any use been made of the plant medicinally, but the Garden Beet has been cultivated from very remote times as a salad plant and for general use as a vegetable. It was so appreciated by the ancients, that it is recorded that it was offered on silver to Apollo in his temple at Delphi.

¶ *Constituents.* The root contains about a tenth portion of pure sugar, which is one of the glucoses or fruit sugars and is very wholesome. It is softer than cane sugar and does not crystallize as well as the latter. There is a treacle principle in it, but this renders it all the more nutritious. Cane-sugar has to be converted by the digestive juices into fruit sugar, before the body can absorb it, but the sugar present in the Beet-root is already in the more easily assimilated form, thus making the Beet a valuable food. Its sugar is a force-giver and an energy creator, a source of vitality to the human body. Besides its tenth portion of pure sugar, Beetroot has as much as a third of its weight in starch and gum.

The Beet makes an appetizing vegetable, plain boiled, stewed, or baked and a good pickle; and in Russia forms an appetizing soup – called *Bortsch* – the red root in this case being made to exude all its juice into a rich, white stock.

A pleasant wine can be made from the roots and an equally good domestic ale has also been brewed from Mangolds. A con-siderable amount of alcohol can be obtained by distillation.

Although modern medicine disregards the Beet, of old it was considered to have distinct remedial properties.

¶ *Medicinal Action and Uses*. The juice of the White Beet was stated to be 'of a cleansing, digestive quality,' to open obstruc-tions of the liver and spleen, and, says Cul-pepper, 'good for the headache and swim-mings therein and all affections of the brain.' Also,

'effectual against all venomous creatures and applied upon the temples, it stayeth in-flammations in the eyes; it helpeth burnings, being used without oil and with a little alum put to it is good for St. Anthonys Fire. It is good for all weals, pushes, blisters and blains in the skin: the decoction in water and vine-gar healeth the itch if bathed therewith and cleanseth the head of dandriff, scurf and dry scabs and relieves running sores and ulcers and is much commended against baldness and shedding the hair.'

The juice of the Red Beetroot was recom-mended 'to stay the bloody flux' and 'to help the yellow jaundice,' also the juice 'put into the nostrils, purgeth the head, helpeth the noise in the ears and the toothache.'

The Sugar Beet, or White Beet, is a selected form of the ordinary red-rooted Garden Beet and is now the chief source of our sugar; as food for animals, it has been preferred to turnips and carrots.

About 1760, the Berlin apothecary Marg-graff obtained in his laboratory by means of alcohol, 6·2 per cent. of sugar from a white variety of Beet and 4·5 per cent. from a red variety. At the present day, as a result of careful study of many years, improvement of cultivation, careful selection of seed and suit-able manuring, especially with nitrate of soda, the average Beet worked up contains 7 per cent. of fibre and 92 per cent. of juice. The average yield of its weight in sugar was stated in 1910 to be 12·79 per cent. in Ger-many and 11·6 per cent. in France.

In Great Britain, the cultivation of Beet for sugar was first seriously undertaken in Essex in 1910, as the result of careful consideration during several years and since the War. The Beet Sugar Industry, aided by Government subsidy, can now be regarded as on a per-manent basis. In 1926–7, no less than four-teen factories were handling the Beet crops, mostly in Norfolk, Cambridgeshire, Lincoln-shire and Nottinghamshire, producing large quantities of white refined sugar.

See ARRACHS, BLITES, CLIVERS, GLASSWORTS, GOOSEFOOTS, WORMSEED.

BELLADONNA. *See* (DEADLY) NIGHTSHADE

BENNE

Sesamum Indicum (LINN.)
N.O. Pedaliaceæ

Synonyms. Gingilly. Teel
Parts Used. Leaves, seeds
Habitat. America, Southern States, and India. Cultivated in Africa and Asia

¶ *Description*. An annual plant with branch-ing stem 4 or 5 feet high, leaves opposite, petiolate, shape varies; flower reddish white, single, on short peduncles in axils of leaves; fruit an oblong capsule with small oval yellowish seeds. The genus *Sesamum* com-prises ten or twelve species. In India two species occur wild; it is cultivated in the U.S.A. and in the West Indies; it grows as far north as Philadelphia.

¶ *Constituents*. The seeds by expression yield a fixed oil consisting essentially of the glycerides of oleic and linoleic acids with small preparations of stearin, palmitin and myristin. Sesamin, another constituent of the oil, may be obtained in long crystalline needles melting at 118° F., insoluble in water, light petroleum, ether alkaloids and mineral acids, easily soluble in chloroform, benzine, and glacial acetic acid. Liquid fatty acids are present to about 70 per cent., solid fatty acids 12 to 14 per cent.

¶ *Medicinal Action and Uses*. Sesame oil is used in the preparation of Iodinol and Brominol, which are employed for external, internal or subcutaneous use. The best qualities of the oil are largely used in the manufacture of margarine. Sesame oil may be used as a substitute for Olive oil in making the official liniments, ointments and plasters in India and the African, Eastern, and North America Colonies. The negroes use the seed as food, boiling them for broth and making them into puddings and other dishes. The leaves which abound in gummy matter when mixed with water form a rich bland mucilage used in infantile cholera, diarrhœa, dysentery, catarrh and bladder troubles, acute cystitis and strangury. The oil is said to be laxative and to promote menstruation.

¶ *Dosage*. 1 or 2 full-sized leaves stirred in ½ pint of cold water, or in hot water if the dried leaves are used.

BENZOIN

Styrax benzoin (DRY.)
N.O. Styraceæ

Synonyms. Gum Benzoin. Gum Benjamin. Siam Benzoin. Sumatra Benzoin
Part Used. Resin
Habitat. Siam, Sumatra and Java

¶ *Description*. Benzoin is a balsamic resin. Normally the trees do not produce it or any substance analogous to it, but the infliction of a wound sufficiently severe to injure the cambium results in the formation of numerous oleoresin ducts in which the secretion is produced; it is, therefore, a pathological product. The trunk of the tree is hacked with an axe, and after a time the liquid Benzoin either accumulates beneath the bark or exudes from the incisions. When it has sufficiently hardened it is collected and exported, either in the form of loose pieces (tears) or in masses packed in oblong boxes or in tins; several varieties are known, but Siam and Sumatra Benzoins are the most important. The incisions are made when the tree is seven years old, and in Sumatra each tree yields about 3 lb. annually for ten or twelve years. The first three years' collections give the finest Benzoin; after that the runnings are known as the 'belly,' and finally the tree is cut down and the resin scraped out, this being termed the 'foot.' Siam Benzoin externally is reddish yellow, internally milky white, has an agreeable odour, recalling vanilla, contains benzoic acid but *not* cinnamic acid. Sumatra Benzoin is always in blocks of a dull reddish or greyish-brown colour. Fine qualities have a strong storax-like odour, quite distinct from the vanilla odour of the Siamese variety. Sumatra Benzoin contains cinnamic acid.

¶ *Constituents*. The chief constituent of Siam Benzoin is benzoic acid (up to 38 per cent.), partly free and partly combined with benzoresinol and siaresinotannol; it also contains vanillin and an oily aromatic liquid. When quite pure it should be entirely soluble in alcohol and yield only traces of ash. Sumatra benzoin contains 18 per cent. or more of benzoic acid and about 20 per cent. of cinnamic acid, the latter partly free and partly combined with benzoresinol and sumarisinotannol; it also contains 1 per cent. of vanillin, styrol, styracin, phenyl-prophyl, cinnamate and benzaldehyde, all of which combine to produce its characteristic odour.

¶ *Medicinal Action and Uses*. It is used externally in the form of a tincture, diluted with water as a mild stimulant and antiseptic in irritable conditions of the skin. It acts as a carminative when taken internally, is rapidly absorbed, and mildly expectorant, diuretic and antiseptic to the urinary passages. In the form of Compound Tincture of Benzoin, it is used as an inhalant with steam in laryngitis and bronchitis. It is a preservative of fats, and is used for that purpose in Adips Benzoatus.

¶ *Dosages and Preparations*. Benzoic Acid, B.P., 5 to 15 grains. Compound Tincture of Benzoin, B.P. and U.S.P., ½ to 1 drachm. Compound Tincture of Camphor, B.P. (paregoric) *poison*, ½ to 1 drachm. Tincture of Benzoin, B.P.C., ½ to 1 drachm. Tincture of Benzoin, U.S.P., 15 minims.

BERGAMOT

Monarda didyma
N.O. Rustaceæ

Synonyms. Scarlet Monarda. Oswego Tea. Bee Balm

So far, *Monarda punctata* is considered the only plant indigenous to North America which can be looked upon as a fruitful source of Thymol, though another American swamp plant, closely allied to it, *M. didyma*, the Scarlet Monarda, is said to yield an oil of similar composition, though not to the same degree.

¶ *Description*. This species, on account of its aromatic odour, has become a favourite in our gardens. It has showy, scarlet flowers in large heads or whorls at the top of the stem, supported by leafy bracts, the leaflets of which are of a pale-green colour tinged with red. Its square, grooved and hard stems rise about 2 feet high, and the leaves which it bears in pairs are rather rough on both surfaces.

The whole plant is strongly impregnated with a delightful fragrance; even after the darkly-coloured leaves have died away, the surface rootlets give off the pleasant smell by which the plant has earned its common name 'Bergamot,' it being reminiscent of the aroma of the Bergamot Orange.

It is known in America as 'Oswego Tea,' because an infusion of its young leaves used to form a common beverage in many parts of the United States.

It is also sometimes called 'Bee Balm,' as bees are fond of its blossoms, which secrete much nectar.

It delights in a moist, light soil, and in a situation where the plants have only the morning sun, where they will continue in flower longer than those which are exposed to the full sun. It is a very ornamental plant and readily propagated by its creeping roots and by slips or cuttings, which, if planted in a shady corner in May, will take root in the same manner as the other Mints.

See MINTS, HORSEMINTS.

BETEL

Piper betel (LINN.)
N.O. Peperaceæ

Synonyms. Chavica Betel. Artanthe Hixagona
Part Used. The leaves
Habitat. India, Malaya and Java

¶ *Description.* The Betel plant is indigenous throughout the Indian Malay region and also cultivated in Madagascar, Bourbon and the West Indies. It is a climbing shrub and is trained on poles or trellis in a hot but shady situation. The leaves are pressed together and dried, sometimes being sewn up together in packets for commerce.

¶ *Constituents.* The chief constituent of the leaves is a volatile oil varying in the leaves from different countries and known as Betel oil. It contains two phenols, betel-phenol (chavibetol) and chavicol. Cadinene has also been found. The best oil is a clear yellow colour obtained from the fresh leaves. The

Indians use the leaves as a masticatory (the taste being warm, aromatic and bitter), together with scraped areca nut and lime.

¶ *Medicinal Action and Uses.* The leaves are stimulant, antiseptic and sialogogue; the oil is an active local stimulant used in the treatment of respiratory catarrhs as a local application or gargle, also as an inhalant in diphtheria. In India the leaves are used as a counter-irritant to suppress the secretion of milk in mammary abscesses. The juice of 4 leaves is equivalent in power to one drop of the oil.

¶ *Dosage.* Betel oil, 1 to 2 minims.

BETHROOT

Trillium pendulum (WILLD.)
Trillium erectum (LINN.)
N.O. Liliaceæ

Synonyms. Indian Shamrock. Birthroot. Lamb's Quarters. Wake-Robin. Indian Balm. Ground Lily
Parts Used. The dried root and rhizome. The leaves
Habitat. Middle and Western United States

¶ *Description.* All the seventeen species of the genus are North American plants, distinguished by their possession of three green, persistent sepals and three larger withering petals, of varying colour.

Trillium erectum or *T. pendulum*, perennial, smooth herb, has an erect stem of from 10 to 15 inches in height, bearing three leaves, broad, almost rhomboid, and drooping white flowers, terminal and solitary. Grows in the rich soil of damp and shady woodlands, flowering in May and June.

The official description of the rhizome is 'oblique, globular, oblong or obconical, truncate below, terminated by a small bud surrounded by a sheath of scarious leaf bases, annulated by leaf scars and fissured by stem

scars. It is from 0·6 to 5 cm. in length, and from 0·6 to 3·5 cm. in width, more or less compressed laterally, rootlet scars in several concentric rows on the underside in the upper portions. Externally yellowish to reddish brown; internally of a pale yellow; fracture somewhat uneven with a more or less spongy appearance. Odour distinct; taste bitter and acrid, with a sensation of warmth in the throat, and when chewed causing an increased flow of saliva. Trillium yields not more than 5 per cent. of ash.'

The drug is one of those prepared by the Shakers.

¶ *Constituents.* There have been found in it volatile and fixed oils, tannic acid, saponin, a glucoside resembling convallamarin, an acid crystalline principle coloured brown tinged with purple by sulphuric acid, and light green with sulphuric acid and potassium dichromate, gum, resin, and much starch.

The fluid extract is an ingredient in Compound Elixir of *Viburnum Opulus*.

Professor E. S. Wayne isolated the active principle, calling it Trilline, but the preparation sold under that name has no medicinal value, while the Trilline of Professor Wayne has not been used.

¶ *Medicinal Action and Uses*. Is said to have been in use among the aborigines and early settlers of North America. It is antiseptic, astringent and tonic expectorant, being used principally in hæmorrhages, to promote parturition, and externally, usually in the

form of a poultice, as a local irritant in skin diseases, or to restrain gangrene.

The *leaves*, boiled in lard, are sometimes applied to ulcers and tumours.

The *roots* may be boiled in milk, when they are helpful in diarrhœa and dysentery.

¶ *Dosages*. Of powdered root, a drachm three times a day. Of fluid extract, 30 minims, as astringent and tonic expectorant. Trilline, 2 to 4 grains.

¶ *Other Species*. Most of the genus *Trillium* have medicinal properties, especially *T. erythrocarpum*, *T. grandiflorum*, *T. sessile*, and *T. nivale*.

The acrid species are useful in fevers and chronic affections of the air-passages. Merely smelling the freshly-exposed surface of the red Beth roots will check bleeding from the nose.

BETONY, WOOD

Stachys Betonica (BENTH.)
Betonica officinalis (LINN.)
N.O. Labiatæ

Synonym. Bishopswort
Part Used. Herb
Habitat. It is a pretty woodland plant, met with frequently throughout England, but by no means common in Scotland. Though generally growing in woods and copses, it is occasionally to be found in more open situations, and amongst the tangled growths on heaths and moors

There are five species of *Stachys* growing wild in this country – the once much-valued Betony (*S. Betonica*); the Marsh Stachys, or Clown's Woundwort (*S. palustris*); the true Woundwort (*S. Germanica*), a doubtful native, occurring occasionally on limestone soils in England, but very common on the Continent, where the dense covering of its leaves was at one time in rustic surgery employed in the place of lint for dressing wounds; the low-creeping Field Stachys (*S. arvensis*); and the Hedge Stachys, or Hedge Woundwort (*S. sylvatica*), perhaps the commonest of them all.

¶ *History*. The Wood Betony (*S. Betonica* according to present-day nomenclature, though nemed *Betonica officinalis*, by Linnæus) was held in high repute not only in the Middle Ages, but also by the Greeks, who extolled its qualities. An old Italian proverb, 'Sell your coat and buy Betony,' and 'He has as many virtues as Betony,' a saying of the Spaniards, show what value was placed on its remedial properties. Antonius Musa, chief physician to the Emperor Augustus, wrote a long treatise, showing it was a certain cure for no less than forty-seven diseases.

Throughout the centuries, faith in its virtues as a panacea for all ills was thoroughly ingrained in the popular estimation. It was largely cultivated in the physic gardens, both of the apothecaries and the monasteries, and

may still be found growing about the sites of these ancient buildings. Robert Turner, a physician writing in the latter half of the seventeenth century, recounts nearly thirty complaints for which Betony was considered efficacious, and adds, 'I shall conclude with the words I have found in an old manuscript under the virtues of it: "More than all this have been proved of Betony." '

In addition to its medicinal virtues, Betony was endowed with power against evil spirits. On this account, it was carefully planted in churchyards and hung about the neck as an amulet or charm, sanctifying, as Erasmus tells us, 'those that carried it about them,' and being also 'good against fearful visions' and an efficacious means of 'driving away devils and despair.' An old writer, Apelius, says:

'It is good whether for the man's soul or for his body; it shields him against visions and dreams, and the wort is very wholesome, and thus thou shalt gather it, in the month of August without the use of iron; and when thou hast gathered it, shake the mold till nought of it cleave thereon, and then dry it in the shade very thoroughly, and with its root altogether reduce it to dust: then use it and take of it when thou needst.'

Many extravagant superstitions grew up round Betony, one, of very ancient date, was that serpents would fight and kill each other if placed within a ring composed of it; and others declared that even wild beasts recognized its efficacy, and used it if wounded, and that stags, if wounded with a dart, would search out Betony, and, eating it, be cured.

¶ *Description.* It comes up year after year from a thickish, woody root. The stems rise to a height of from 1 to 2 feet, and are slender, square and furrowed. They bear at wide intervals a few pairs of oblong, stalkless leaves, 2 to 3 inches long, and about ¾ to 1 inch broad, with roughly indented margins; in other plants of this group, the pairs of leaves arise on alternate sides of the stem. The majority of the leaves, however, spring from the root and these are larger, on long stalks and of a drawn-out, heart shape. All the leaves are rough to the touch and are also fringed with short, fine hairs; their whole surface is dotted with glands containing a bitter, aromatic oil.

At the top of the stem are the two-lipped flowers of a very rich purplish-red, arranged in dense rings or whorls, which together form short spikes. Then there is a break and a piece of bare stem, with two or four oblong, stalkless leaves and then more flowers, the whole forming what is termed an interrupted spike, a characteristic peculiarity by which Wood Betony is known from all other labiate flowers. The cup or calyx of each flower is crowned by five sharp points, each representing a sepal. The corolla is a long tube ending in two lips, the upper lip slightly arched, the lower one flat, of three equal lobes. The four stamens lie in two pairs within the arch of the upper lip, one pair longer than the other, and shed their pollen on to the back of bee visitors who come to drink the honey in the tube, and thus unconsciously effect the fertilization of the next flower they visit, by carrying to it this pollen that has been dusted upon them. After fertilization, four brown, smooth three-cornered nutlets are developed. The flowers are in bloom during July and August.

The common name of this plant is said by Pliny to have been first Vettonica, from the Vettones, a people of Spain, but modern authors resolve the word into the primitive or Celtic form of *bew* (a head) and *ton* (good), it being good for complaints in the head. It has sometimes, also, been called Bishopswort, the reason for which is not evident. The name of the genus, *Stachys*, is a Greek word, signifying a spike, from the mode of flowering.

¶ *Part Used Medicinally.* The whole herb, collected from wild plants in July, when at their best, and dried.

Collect only on a fine day, in the morning, but after the dew has been dried by the sun, Cut off the stems shortly above the root (which is no longer used, as in olden days); strip off all discoloured or insect-eaten leaves, and as the stems are fairly firm, tie them up in bunches of about six stalks together, spread out fanwise, so that the air can penetrate to them all, and hang them over strings to dry, either in half-shade, in the open air, or in the drying room. The bunches should be of uniform sizes to facilitate packing when dry. If dried out-of-doors, take in before there is any risk of becoming damp from dew or showers. For drying indoors, a warm, sunny attic or loft may be employed, the window being left open by day, so that there is a current of air, and the moist, hot air may escape: the door may also be left open. The temperature should be from 70° to 100° F. Failing sun, any ordinary shed, fitted with racks and shelves, can be used as a drying room, provided it is ventilated near the roof and has a warm current of air, caused by an ordinary coke or anthracite stove. The important point in drying is rapidity and the avoidance of steaming: the quicker the process of drying, the more even the colour obtained, making the product more saleable.

All dried leaves and herbs should be packed away at once in wooden boxes or tins, in a dry place, as otherwise they re-absorb about 12 per cent. of moisture from the air, and are liable to become mouldy. The herbs should not be pressed down heavily when packing, or they will tend to crumble.

¶ *Medicinal Action and Uses.* Betony was once the sovereign remedy for all maladies of the head, and its properties as a nervine and tonic are still acknowledged, though it is more frequently employed in combination with other nervines than alone. It is useful in hysteria, palpitations, pain in the head and face, neuralgia and all nervous affections. In the *Medicina Britannica* (1666) we read: 'I have known the most obstinate headaches cured by daily breakfasting for a month or six weeks on a decoction of Betony made with new milk and strained.'

As an aromatic, it has also astringent and alterative action, and combined with other remedies is used as a tonic in dyspepsia and as an alterative in rheumatism, scrofula and impurities of the blood.

The weak infusion forms a very acceptable substitute for tea, and in this way is extensively used in many localities. It has somewhat the taste of tea and all the good qualities of it, without the bad ones. To make Betony tea, pour a pint of boiling water on an ounce of the dried herb. A wineglassful of this decoction three times a day proves a benefit against languid nervous headaches.

The dried herb may also be smoked as tobacco, combined with Eyebright and Coltsfoot, for relieving headache.

A pinch of the powdered herb will provoke violent sneezing. The dried leaves formed an ingredient in Rowley's British Herb Snuff, which was at one time quite famous for headaches.

The fresh leaves are said to have an intoxicating effect. They have been used to dye wool a fine yellow.

Gerard tells us, among other uses, that Betony

'preserveth the lives and bodies of men from the danger of epidemical diseases. It helpeth those that loathe and cannot digest their food. It is used either dry or green – either the root or herb – or the flowers, drunk in broth or meat or made into conserve, syrup, water, electuary or powder – as everyone may best frame themselves, or as time or season requires.'

He proceeds to say that the herb cures the jaundice, falling sickness, palsy, convulsions, gout, dropsy and head troubles, and that

'the powder mixed with honey is no less available for all sorts of colds or cough, wheezing, of shortness of breath and consumption,' also that 'the decoction made with mead and Pennyroyal is good for putrid agues,' and made in wine is good as a vermifuge, 'and also removes obstructions of the spleen and liver.' Again,

'the decoction with wine gargled in the mouth easeth the toothache. . . . It is a cure for the bites of mad dogs. . . . A dram of the powder taken with a little honey in some vinegar is good for refreshing those that are wearied by travel. It stayeth bleeding at the nose and mouth, and helpeth those that spit blood, and is good for those that have a rupture and are bruised. The green herb bruised, or the juice, applied to any inward hurt, or outward wound in body or head, will quickly heal and close it up. It will draw forth any broken bone or splinter, thorn or other thing gotten into the flesh, also healeth old sores or ulcers and boils. The root is displeasing both to taste and stomach, whereas the leaves and flowers by their sweet and spicy taste, comfort both in meat and medicine.'

See also WOUNDWORT.

BETONY, WATER. *See* FIGWORT, WATER

BILBERRY

Vaccinium myrtillus (LINN.)
N.O. Vacciniaceæ

Synonyms. Whortleberry. Black Whortles. Whinberry. Trackleberry. Huckleberry. Hurts. Bleaberry. Hurtleberry. Airelle. Vaccinium Frondosum. Blueberries
Parts Used. The ripe fruit. The leaves
Habitat. Europe, including Britain, Siberia and Barbary

¶ *Description. V. myrtillus* grows abundantly in our heathy and mountainous districts; a small branched shrub, with wiry, angular branches, rarely over a foot high, bearing globular wax-like flowers and black berries, which are covered when quite ripe with a delicate grey bloom, hence its name in Scotland, 'Blea-berry,' from an old North Country word, 'blae,' meaning livid or bluish. The name Bilberry (by some old writers 'Bulberry') is derived from the Danish 'bollebar,' meaning *dark berry*. There is a variety with white fruits.

The leathery leaves (in form somewhat like those of the myrtle, hence its specific name) are at first rosy, then yellowish-green, and in autumn turn red and are very ornamental. They have been utilized to adulterate tea.

Bilberries flourish best on high grounds, being therefore more abundant in the north and west than in the south and east of England: they are absent from the low-lying Cambridgeshire and Suffolk, but on the Surrey hills, where they are called 'Hurts,' cover the ground for miles.

The fruit is globular, with a flat top, about the size of a black currant. When eaten raw, they have a slightly acid flavour. When cooked, however, with sugar, they make an excellent preserve. Gerard tells us that 'the people of Cheshire do eate the black whortles in creame and milke as in these southern parts we eate strawberries.' On the Continent, they are often employed for colouring wine.

Stewed with a little sugar and lemon peel in an open tart, Bilberries make a very enjoyable dish. Before the War, immense quantities of them were imported annually from Holland, Germany and Scandinavia. They were used mainly by pastrycooks and restaurant-keepers.

Owing to its rich juice, the Bilberry can be used with the least quantity of sugar in making jam: half a pound of sugar to the pound of berries is sufficient if the preserve is to be eaten soon. The minuteness of the seeds makes them more suitable for jam than currants.

¶ *Constituents.* Quinic acid is found in the leaves, and a little tannin. Triturated with water they yield a liquid which, filtered and assayed with sulphate of iron, becomes a beautiful green, first of all transparent, then giving a green precipitate.

The fruits contain sugar, etc.

¶ *Medicinal Action and Uses.* The *leaves* can be used in the same way as those of *Uva-Ursi.* The *fruits* are astringent, and are especially valuable in diarrhœa and dysentery, in the form of syrup. The ancients used them largely, and Dioscorides spoke highly of them. They are also used for discharges, and as antigalactagogues. A decoction of the leaves or bark of the root may be used as a local application to ulcers, and in ulceration of the mouth and throat.

The fruit is helpful in scurvy and urinary complaints, and when bruised with the roots and steeped in gin has diuretic properties valuable in dropsy and gravel. A tea made of the leaves is also a remedy for diabetes if taken for a prolonged period.

¶ *Dosages.* Of powder of the berries, 4 grammes. Of syrup, 60 grammes to a litre of water. Of fluid extract, ½ to 2 drachms.

¶ *Other Species.* *V. arboreum,* or Farkleberry. This is the most astringent variety, and both berries and root-bark may be used internally for diarrhœa, chronic dysentery, etc. The infusion is valuable as a local application in sore throat, chronic ophthalmia, leucorrhœa, etc.

V. resinosum, V. damusum, and *V. gorymbosum* have properties resembling those of *V. myrtillus.*

The Bog Bilberry (*V. uliginosum*) is a smaller, less erect plant, with round stems and untoothed leaves, greyish green beneath. Both flowers and berries are smaller than those of the common Bilberry. This kind is quite absent in the south and only to be found in mountain bogs and moist copses, in Scotland, Durham and Westmorland.

The berries of both species are a favourite food of birds.

The 'Huckleberry' of North America, so widely appreciated there, is our Bilberry – the name being an obvious corruption of 'Whortleberry.'

RECIPE

Recipe for Bilberry Jam

Put 3 lb. of clean, fresh fruit in a preserving pan with 1½ lb. of sugar and about 1 cupful of water and bring to the boil. Then boil rapidly for 40 minutes. Apple juice, made from windfalls and peelings, instead of the water, improves this jam. To make apple juice, cover the apples with water, stew down, and strain the juice through thick muslin. Blackberries may also be added to this mixture.

If the jam is to be kept long it must be bottled hot in screw-top jars, or, if tied down in the ordinary way, more sugar must be added.

Bilberry juice yields a clear, dark-blue or purple dye that has been much used in the dyeing of wool and the picking of berries for this purpose, as well as for food, constitutes a summer industry in the 'Hurts' districts. Owing to the shortage of the aniline dye-stuffs formerly imported from Germany, Bilberries were eagerly bought up at high prices by dye manufacturers during the War, so that in 1917 and 1918 a large proportion of the Bilberry crop was not available for jam-making, as the dyers were scouring the country for the little blue-black berries.

BINDWEEDS

N.O. Convolvulaciæ

¶ *Uses.* All the Convolvulus family have purgative properties in a greater or less degree. *Convolvulus Scammonia* is used in homœopathy. A tincture is made from the gum resin. The drugs known as Jalap and Scammony are produced from the Jalap Bindweed and the *C. Scammonia.*

There are three kinds of Convolvulus or Bindweed in our native flora: the Field,

Hedge, and the Sea Convolvulus. We have also many southern species growing in our gardens, chief among which are the handsome Morning Glory (*Ipomea purpurea,* Linn.), *C. purpureus,* a native of Asia and America, with large purple flowers, and the pretty little annual, *C. minor,* a native of southern Europe, its cheerful flowers a combination of blue, yellow and white.

BINDWEED, GREATER
Convolvulus sepium

Synonyms. Hedge Convolvulus. Old Man's Night Cap. Hooded Bindweed. Bearbind

Habitat. The Greater Bindweed, or Hedge Convolvulus (*C. sepium*), is a hedge plant found abundantly throughout England and Scotland, but only of local occurrence in Scotland. Like the Field Convolvulus, it is, in spite of the beauty of its flowers, regarded as a pest by both the farmer and the gardener, its roots being long and penetrating in a dense mass that exhausts the soil, and its twining stems extending in masses over all other plants near, and strangling them to a still greater degree than its smaller relative

¶ *Description.* The leaves of this Bindweed are arrow-shaped and large, somewhat thin and delicate in texture. They are arranged singly on alternate sides of the stem, as is the case with all species of Convolvulus, and from their axils spring the flower-stalks, which are square and in every case bear only one large blossom, conspicuous for its snowy whiteness. The flowers are among the largest which this country produces. The calyx is entirely hidden by the two large bracts that enclose it, and which completely hide the flower while in bud, a feature that has gained it also the name of 'Hooded Bindweed,' and has led some botanists to place it in a different genus, *Calystegia*, the name being derived from two Greek words signifying 'beautiful covering.' The specific name, *sepium*, is de-rived from the Latin *sepes*, a hedge, and refers to its place of growth.

The flowers are in bloom from July to September, and like all the other species expand during sunshine and remain closed during dull weather. They do not, however, like those of the Field Convolvulus, close during a shower.

Anne Pratt (*Flowers and their Associations*) notices the fact that while some twining plants follow the apparent course of the sun and turn round the supporting stem from left to right, others, like the large White Bindweed or Convolvulus, twine *contrary* to the sun, from right to left, and never otherwise; even if the gardener turn it in another direction, the plant, if unable to disengage itself and assume its natural bias, will eventually perish.

BINDWEED, JALAP
Convolvulus Jalapa (LINN.)

Synonym. Ipomea purga

Habitat. The Jalap Bindweed (*C. Jalapa*, Linn.), but more often called *Ipomea Jalapa* or *purga*, is a native of South America and Mexico. It derives its name from Xalapa, in Mexico, where it is very abundant. It is freely grown out of doors, however, in the southern countries of Europe, and plants have been grown here in the garden of the Society of Apothecaries and also in Norfolk and Hampshire

¶ *Description.* It is a handsome climbing convolvulaceous plant with crimson flowers and a tuberous root, which is of officinal value. The tubers, varying in size from a walnut to an orange, are dark, umber-brown in colour and much wrinkled. They are imported either whole or sliced.

¶ *Medicinal Action and Uses.* The drug Jalap is prepared from a resin which abounds in the roots. It has a slight smoky odour and the taste is unpleasant, followed by pungent acridity. It has strong cathartic and purgative action, and is used in constipation, pain and colic in the bowels and general intestinal torpor, being combined, in compound powder, with other laxatives, and with carminatives such as ginger, cloves, etc. It accelerates the action of rhubarb.

Jalap forms a safe purge for children, being given in sugar or jam to disguise the taste, and has been used thus with calomel or wormwood as a vermifuge. It proves an excellent purge in rheumatism.

¶ *Preparations.* Powdered root, 3 to 20 grains. Tincture, B.P., ½ to 1 drachm. Pow-dered resin, 2 to 5 grains. Compound powder, B.P., 1 to 2 drachms. Jalapin, 1 to 3 grains.

Other members of this Convolvulus family have economic uses. *C. dissectus*, an American species abounds in prussic acid, the liquor known as *Noyau* being prepared from it with the aid of alcohol, and the oil of Rodium, which is so attractive to rats as to cause them to swarm to it without fear, even if held in the hand of a rat-catcher, is the produce of another Convolvulus, known as *C. Rhodorhiza*.

One of the most important members of the order economically is *C. Batatas*, the tuberous-rooted Bindweed, or SWEET POTATO, the roots of which abound in starch and sugar and form a nourishing food, very valuable in the tropics, where it is largely cultivated. The roots are somewhat in shape like an oblong and ugly potato, often club-shaped, and are of a reddish colour. When cooked, they are excessively sweet, not unlike liquorice, and not attractive in appearance. They are usually of greater size and weight than ordinary potatoes.

Before the introduction of the Potato into Europe, the Sweet Potato was regularly imported as a wholesome article of diet, and was grown in Spain and Portugal, to which it had been brought from the West Indies.

The Potato which Shakespeare mentions twice – in the *Merry Wives of Windsor* and in *Troilus and Cressida* – is the Sweet Potato, and not the more familiar tuber of our days.

BINDWEED, SEA.

Convolvulus Soldanella

Habitat. The Sea Bindweed (*C. Soldanella*) is a very beautiful species growing only on sandy sea-shores, decorating the sloping sides of sand-hills with its large, pale rose-coloured flowers striped with red

¶ *Description.* Its stems are not climbing, being usually buried beneath the sand, the flowers and leaves merely rising above the surface. The leaves are fleshy, roundish or kidney-shaped, about the size of the Lesser Celandine, placed singly on alternate sides of the stem on long foot-stalks. The flowers are produced singly at each side of the stem, on four-sided, winged stalks, and blossom in July, being succeeded by round capsules. The bracts are large, egg-shaped and close to the flower, which is nearly as large as the Great Bindweed, and expands in the morning and in bright weather, closing before night. This species is also frequently assigned to the genus *Calystegia*.

BINDWEED, SYRIAN

Convolvulus Scammonia

Synonym. Scammony

Habitat. The Syrian Bindweed, or Scammony (*C. Scammonia*), can be grown here and will thrive well on dry soil, but we import from Smyrna and Aleppo what is needed for medicinal purposes

¶ *Description.* It has flowers of a very delicate tint of sulphur yellow and leaves of a similar shape to our native species.

The roots are 3 to 4 feet long and from 9 to 12 inches in circumference; tapering, covered with a light grey bark and containing a milky juice. Scammony is a gummy resin, obtained from this milky juice of the root by clearing away the earth from the upper part of the root and cutting off the top obliquely, about 2 inches below where the stalks spring. Then a vessel is fixed in such a position as to receive the exuding juice, which gradually hardens and becomes the Scammony of commerce. The best Scammony is black, resinous and shining when in the lump, but of a whitish-ash colour when powdered, with a strong cheesy smell and a somewhat acrid taste, turning milky when touched by the tongue. It occurs in commerce in irregular pieces 1 to 2 inches or more in diameter.

¶ *Medicinal Action and Uses.* Scammony is a drastic cathartic, closely allied in its operation to Jalap; though not so nauseous, it is more active and irritating, and in inflammatory conditions of the alimentary canal should not be used.

The root itself is seldom used: the resin prepared from it is generally combined with other cathartics to diminish its action and prevent griping.

¶ *Preparations.* Powdered root, 3 to 12 grains. Powdered resin, B.P., 3 to 8 grains. Compound Powder, B.P., 10 to 20 grains.

It appears to have been well known to the Greek and Arabian physicians, who used it for various other purposes as well as for a purgative. The dose is generally from 3 to 12 grains. Seven grains of Scammony resin gradually rubbed well up with 3 oz. milk forms a safe purgative, to which a taste of ginger can be added. It is used as a smart purge for children, especially for those with worms, on account of the smallness of the dose necessary to produce its effect, the slight taste and the energy of its operation.

It is useful as a hydragogue in dropsies. Meyrick considered it a rough and powerful, but very useful purgative of great service in rheumatic and other chronic disorders, reaching the seat of many sources of trouble that an ordinary purge does not affect.

The leaves of the Sea Bindweed abound with a milky juice which has been employed as a purge – in ½ oz. doses. Applied externally, the leaves are reputed to diminish dropsical swelling of the feet. The whole plant used to be gathered fresh, when about to flower, and boiled in ale, with nutmegs and cloves, and the decoction given as a strong purge, which was said to be best adapted to robust constitutions, being very violent in its action. The juice oozing from the stalks and root of the Sea Bindweed hardens into a kind of resin, which is also used as a purge in the same way as Scammony – a closely-related plant of foreign origin, which is much imported for this purpose.

Both the preceding species of Convolvulus also possess the virtues of Scammony. The smallness of their roots prevents the juice being collected in the same way as the foreign

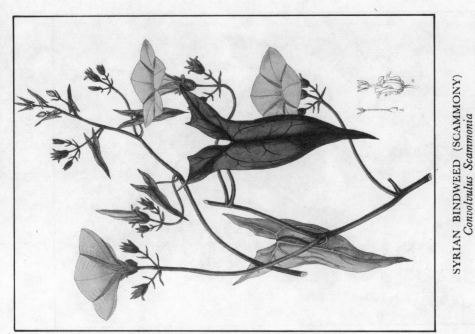

SYRIAN BINDWEED (SCAMMONY)
Convolvulus Scammonia

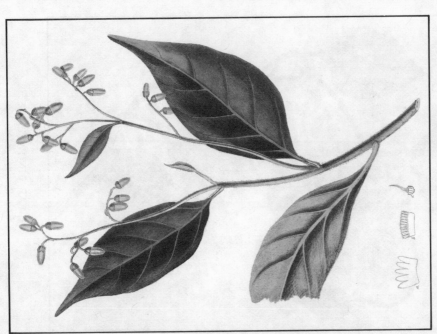

BENZOIN
Styrax Benzoin

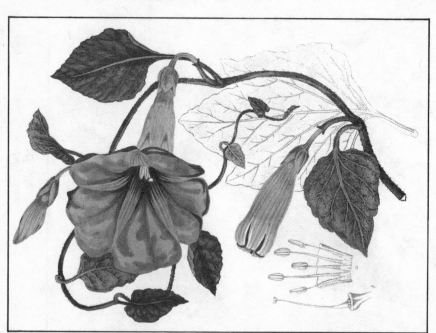

GREATER BINDWEED (CONVOLVULUS)
Convolvulus Sepium

JALAP BINDWEED
Convolvulus Jalapa

species, but an extract made from the expressed juice of the roots or any preparation of them has the same purgative quality, only in less degree. Meyrick states that the root of *C. arvensis* is a rough purgative, and to such constitutions as can bear it, will prove serviceable in jaundice, dropsy and other disorders arising from obstructions of the viscera, the best method of administering it being to bruise the roots and give their expressed juice in strong beer. The juice of the Greater Bindweed, taken in doses of 20 to 30 grains is also a powerful drastic purge, and country people often boil its freshly-gathered roots in ale in the same manner as the Field Bindweed. Though for those of a strong constitution there is no better purge, on account of the nausea which it tends to produce, it is not considered fit for the delicate.

CONVOLVULUS DUARTINUS   Morning Glory

Synonyms. Morning Glory. Ipomœa. Vona-nox

A tincture of the flowers is used for headaches, rheumatism and inflamed eyes.

See (FIELD) CONVOLVULUS.

BIRCH, COMMON   Betula alba (LINN.)
                                                N.O. Betulaceæ

Synonyms. White Birch. Bouleau. Berke. Bereza. Monoecia triandria. *B. pubescens*. *B. verrucosa*
Parts Used. The bark and the leaves
Habitat. Europe, from Sicily to Iceland. Northern Asia

¶ *History*. The name is a very ancient one, probably derived from the Sanscrit *bhurga*, 'a tree whose bark is used for writing upon.' From its uses in boat-building and roofing it is also connected with the A.S. *beorgan*, 'to protect or shelter.'

Coleridge speaks of it as the 'Lady of the Woods.' It is remarkable for its lightness, grace, and elegance, and after rain it has a fragrant odour.

The young branches are of a rich red brown or orange brown, and the trunks usually white, especially in the second species of *B. alba*, *B. verrucosa*. *B. pubescens* is darker, and has downy instead of warted twigs.

The wood is soft and not very durable, but being cheap, and the tree being able to thrive in any situation and soil, growing all over Europe, is used for many humble purposes, such as bobbins for thread mills, herring-barrel staves, broom handles, and various fancy articles. In country districts, the Birch has very many uses, the lighter twigs being employed for thatching and wattles. The twigs are also used in broom making and in the manufacture of cloth. The tree has also been one of the sources from which asphyxiating gases have been manufactured, and its charcoal is much used for gunpowder.

The white epidermis of the bark is separable into thin layers, which may be employed as a substitute for oiled paper and applied to various economical uses. It yields oil of Birch Tar, and the peculiar, well-known odour of russia leather is due to the use of this oil in the process of dressing. It likewise imparts durability to leather, and it is owing to its presence that books bound in russia leather are not liable to become mouldy. The production of Birch Tar oil is a Russian industry of considerable importance. It is also distilled in Holland and Germany, but these oils are appreciably different from the Russian oil. It has the property of keeping away insects and preventing gnatbites when smeared on the hands. It is likewise employed in photography.

When the stem of the tree is wounded, a saccharine juice flows out which is susceptible, with yeast, of vinous fermentation. A beer, wine, spirit and vinegar are prepared from it in some parts of Europe. Birch Wine, concocted from this thin, sugary sap of the tree, collected from incisions made in the trees in March, honey, cloves and lemon peel being added and then the whole fermented with yeast, makes a very pleasant cordial, formerly much appreciated. From 16 to 18 gallons of sap may be drawn from one large tree, and a moderate tapping does no harm.

¶ *Constituents*. Birch *bark* only contains about 3 per cent. of tannic acid, but is extensively used for tanning, wherever there are large birch forests, throughout Northern Europe. As it gives a pale colour to the skin, it is used for the preliminary and the final stages of tanning. It contains betulin and betuls camphor.

The *leaves* contain betulorentic acid.

By destructive distillation, the white epidermis of the bark yields an empyreumatic oil, known variously in commerce as oil of Birch Tar, Oleum Rusci, Oleum Betulinum or Dagget. This is a thick, bituminous, brownish-black liquid, with a pungent, balsamic odour. It contains a high percentage of methylsalicylate, and also creosol and guaiacol. The Rectified Oil (*Oleum Rusci Rectificatum*) is sometimes substituted for oil of Cade.

Birch Tar oil is almost identical with Wintergreen oil. It is not completely soluble in 95 per cent. acetic acid, nor in aniline, but Turpentine oil dissolves it completely.

¶ *Medicinal Action and Uses.* Various parts of the tree have been applied to medicinal uses. The *young shoots* and *leaves* secrete a resinous substance having acid properties, which, combined with alkalies, is said to be a tonic laxative. The *leaves* have a peculiar, aromatic, agreeable odour and a bitter taste, and have been employed in the form of infusion (Birch Tea) in gout, rheumatism and dropsy, and recommended as a reliable solvent of stone in the kidneys. With the *bark* they resolve and resist putrefaction. A decoction of them is good for bathing skin eruptions, and is serviceable in dropsy.

The *oil* is astringent, and is mainly employed for its curative effects in skin affections, especially eczema, but is also used for some internal maladies.

The *inner bark* is bitter and astringent, and has been used in intermittent fevers.

The *vernal sap* is diuretic.

Moxa is made from the yellow, fungous excrescences of the wood, which sometimes swell out from the fissures.

¶ *Dosage.* Of alcoholic extract of the leaves, 25 to 30 grains daily.

¶ *Other Species.*

B. benta (Cherry Birch, Black Birch, Sweet Birch, Mahogany Birch, or Mountain Mahogany) is an American variety, with richly-marked wood suitable for the use of cabinet and pianoforte makers. The liquor is used in Kamschatka without previous fermentation. The cambium, or the layer between the wood and the bast, is eaten in the spring, cut into strips like vermicelli, and the bark is stimulant, diaphoretic, and astringent, in a warm infusion. In decoction or syrup it forms an excellent tonic for dysentery, and is said to be useful in gravel and female obstructions.

B. trophylla is a *syn.* of *Rhus Aromatica*, or Fragrant Sumach.

B. papyracea, or Paper Birch, is largely used for canoe-making in America.

B. nana, or Smooth Dwarf Birch, rarely grows above 3 feet in height. The leaves are said to dye a better yellow than the Common Birch; the seeds are a principal food of ptarmigan in Lapland; Moxa is prepared from it and regarded as an effective remedy in all painful diseases.

BIRTHWORT

Aristolochia longa (LINN.)
N.O. Aristolochiaceæ

Synonym. Long-rooted Birthwort
Part Used. The root
Habitat. Southern Europe and Japan

¶ *Description.* There are several species of the Aristolochias used by herbalists in India. The root is spindle-shaped from 5 cm. to 3 dm. in length, about 2 cm. in thickness, fleshy, very brittle, greyish externally, brownish-yellow inside, bitter and of a strong disagreeable odour when fresh.

¶ *Constituent.* Aristolochine.

¶ *Medicinal Action and Uses.* Said to be useful as an aromatic stimulant in rheumatism and gout and for removing obstructions, etc., after childbirth. Dose, ½ to 1 drachm of the powdered root.

¶ *Other Species.*

Aristolochia, cymbifera from Brazil and Mexico is said to have medicinal properties similar to the official species. Butte affirms it is a depressant to the sensory nerve centres and is useful in neuralgia and pruritis; it was formerly considered alexiteric, antiparalytic, antiperiodic and aphrodisiac.

A. Argentina root is used in that republic as a diuretic and diaphoretic, especially for rheumatism.

A. Indica is used as an emmenagogue, antiarthritic, stomachic, purgative and vermifuge, and in the East Indies is used for similar purposes as the American and European species.

A. Sempervirens is said to be used by the Arabians as a remedy against the poisonous effects of snake-bite.

A. Fœtida in Mexico is used as a stimulant to foul ulcers.

A. serpentaria used in bilious, typhoid and typhus fevers, smallpox, pneumonia, amenorrhœa and fevers of a septicæmic type. It is often given in combination with Peruvian Bark, rendering it more active and preventing ill effects on the stomach. It is also used in North America, as are several other varieties of the species, as an alexiteric and for the bites of mad dogs.

See SNAKEWORT.

BISTORT   Polygonum Bistorta (LINN.)
                                           N.O. Polygonaceæ

Synonyms. Osterick. Oderwort. Snakeweed. Easter Mangiant. Adderwort. Twice Writhen
Part Used. The root-stock, gathered in March, when the leaves begin to shoot, and dried
Habitat. A native of many parts of Northern Europe, occurring in Siberia and in Japan and in Western Asia to the Himalayas. It is common in the north of England and in southern Scotland, growing in moist meadows, though only of local occurrence; in Ireland, it is very rare

¶ *History.* In many places, it can only be regarded as an escape from cultivation, its leaves and young shoots having formerly been widely used in the spring as a vegetable, being still, indeed, in the north of England an ingredient in Herb Pudding, under the name of 'Easter-mangiant,' the latter word a corruption of *mangeant*, i.e. a plant to be eaten at Easter, 'Easter Giant' and 'Easter Ledges' being variations of this name. In Lancashire and Cumberland, the leaves and young shoots were eaten as a green vegetable under the name of Patience Dock and Passions. The roots and leaves had also a great reputation as a remedy for wounds, so that the plant was generally cultivated for medicinal use, as well as for employment as a vegetable.

The name Bistort (Latin *bis* = twice, *torta* = twisted) bears reference to the twice-twisted character of the root-stock, an old local name, 'Twice-Writhen,' being a literal translation of the Latin. Its twisted, creeping nature is also the origin of the names Snakeroot, Adderwort and Snakeweed. It was at one time called Serpentaria, Columbrina, Dracunculus and Serpentary Dragonwort, and has been thought to be the *Oxylanathum Britannicum* and *Limonium* of the ancients.

Externally, the root-stock is black, but internally is coloured red and is rich in tannic and gallic acids, which makes it a powerful astringent and has enabled it to be used in tanning leather, when procurable in sufficient quantity.

The root-stock, as it appears in commerce, is about 2 inches long and $\frac{3}{5}$ inch broad, twice bent, as in the letter S, more or less annulate, bearing a few slender roots, otherwise smooth, reddish brown internally, dark purplish or blackish brown externally, depressed or channelled on the upper surface, convex and with depressed root-scars below; with a thick bark surrounding a ring of small woody wedges, which encloses a pith equal in thickness to the bark.

The drug has an astringent and starchy taste, but no odour.

Besides being one of the strongest vegetable astringents among our native plants, the roots contain much starch, and after being steeped in water and subsequently roasted have been largely consumed in Russia, Siberia and Iceland in time of scarcity and are said after such preparation to be nutritious and a useful article of food, bread having been made of the root-flour of this and another Siberian species of *Polygonum*.

Where established, the Bistort becomes often a noxious weed in low-lying pastures, frequently forming large patches difficult to extirpate on account of its creeping root-stock.

¶ *Description.* A number of tuberous roots are produced from the S-shaped root-stock, from the upper side of which spring directly large oval leaves, with heart-shaped bases, of a bluish-green colour on the upper side and ash-grey, tinged with purple, underneath, both leaf-stalks and blades being about 6 inches long. The upper part of the leaf-stalk is winged. The flower-stalk, 12 to 18 inches high, is very erect, slender, unbranched, and bears leaves smaller than the root-leaves and few in number, broader at their base and on very short stalks. The stems terminate in a dense, cylindrical spike of striking flesh-coloured flowers, which consist of five coloured sepals, eight stamens and an ovary with two to three styles. The flowers are grouped in twos, one flower complete, the other with normal stamens, but only a rudimentary ovary. The styles of the complete flower do not mature and become receptive of pollen from visiting insects, till their stamens have shed their pollen and fallen, cross-fertilization thus being ensured. The flowers are produced in May and June and again in September and October. The fruit is three-seeded, the ripe seeds are small, brown and shining. Birds commonly feed upon the seeds, which can be employed to fatten poultry.

¶ *Cultivation.* The plant may be propagated by division of the root-stock; in early autumn or spring. Bistort is sometimes used to ornament moist parts of the rockery and shady border. When grown in bold masses, it is a handsome and attractive plant.

When it has a corner in the kitchen garden, it is well to pluck it now and then, even when it is not immediately required for culinary purposes, as the plant has a strong tendency to disappear.

¶ *Constituents*. Bistort root has never been carefully analysed, but it is known to contain about 20 per cent. of tannin and a large amount of starch, as well as some gallic acid and gum. Its virtues are extracted by water and its decoction becomes inky black on the addition of a persalt of iron and with gelatine it forms a precipitate. Red colouring matter is also present.

¶ *Medicinal Action and Uses*. Bistort root is one of the strongest astringent medicines in the vegetable kingdom and highly styptic and may be used to advantage for all bleedings, whether external or internal, and wherever astringency is required. Although its use has greatly been superseded by other astringents of foreign origin, it is of proved excellence in diarrhœa, dysentery, cholera and all bowel complaints and in hæmorrhages from the lungs and stomach, and is a most effectual remedy for bleeding from the nose and exceedingly useful in dealing with hæmorrhoids. It is used – as a medicine, injection and gargle – in mucous discharges, as well as for hæmorrhages.

A teaspoonful of the powdered root, in a cupful of boiling water, may be drunk freely as required.

The decoction, often also used, is made from 1 oz. of the bruised root boiled in 1 pint of water. One tablespoonful of this is given every two hours in passive bleedings and for simple diarrhœa. The decoction is also useful as an injection in profuse menstruation and in leucorrhœa and is a useful wash in ulcerated mouth and gums, and as a gargle. It is also used as a lotion to ulcers attended with a discharge.

Bistort is considered valuable for diabetes, given in conjunction with tonics, and has itself tonic action.

The older herbalists considered both the leaves and roots to have 'a powerful faculty to resist poison.' Combined with the bitter flag root (*calamus*), the root was used to cure intermittent fever and ague. Green (*Universal Herbal*, 1832) cites its frequent use in intermittent fever, both alone and with gentian, 3 drachms daily being administered.

It was used, dried, and powdered on cuts and wounds to stop bleeding. The decoction in wine, made from the powder, was drunk freely 'to stay internal bleedings and fluxes,' and was considered 'available against ruptures, burstings and bruises from falls and blows'; also to 'help jaundice, expel the venom of the plague, smallpox, measles or other infectious disease, driving it out by sweating.' A distilled water of the leaves and roots was used to wash any part stung or bitten by a venomous creature, or to wash running sores or ulcers; also as a gargle in sore throat and to harden spongy gums, attended with looseness of teeth and soreness of the mouth. Gerard stated that the root would have this effect, 'being holden in the mouth for a certaine space and at sundry times.' He also states that 'the juice of Bistort put into the nose prevaileth much against the disease called Polybus.'

The root was also employed externally as a poultice.

The powdered leaves were employed to kill worms in children.

In Salmon's *Herbal* the following preparations are given, with their uses: –

1. A liquid juice of the whole plant.
2. A distilled water of the roots and leaves.
3. A powder of the leaves (good to kill worms and for other things.)
4. A powder of the root. (Prevails against malignity of measles and small-pox and expels the poyson of the Plague or Pestilence or of any other infectious disease, driving it out by sweating.)
5. A compound powder of the root (made of equal quantities of Bistort, Pellitory of Spain and burnt Allum made into a paste with a little honey and put in hollow of a tooth or at the side, eases their pain and stops the defluxion of rheum on the part, cleanses the head and brain and causes evacuation of abundance of rheumatic matter.
6. A decoction of the root in wine or water.
7. A decoction compound of the root. (6 oz. Bistort root, 4 oz. Angelica, 4 oz. of Zedoary, 1 oz. of Winter's Cinnamon; all being bruised, infuse in red port wine or Canary, 5 quarts, for 6 hours, then giving it 2 or 3 boils, take it from the fire, strain out the wine from the ingredients, which let settle, then decant the clear from the rest, sweeten with syrup of lemons or syrup of vinegar. This is a notable medicament against Measles, Small-Pox, Calenture, Spotted Fever and even the Plague. It also prevails against any vegetable poison, which is taken inwardly, if timely given.)
8. The diet drink, made of the roots, leaves and seeds.
9. The spiritous tincture.
10. The acid tincture.
11. The oily tincture.
12. The saline tincture.
13. The fixed salt (resists putrefaction).
14. The essence.

¶ *Dosage*. The root is generally administered in *powder*, the dose being from ¼ to ½ drachm in water.

A fluid extract is also prepared from the root, the dose being $\frac{1}{2}$ to 1 drachm.

A decoction is also much employed.

SOME MODERN HERBAL RECIPES IN WHICH BISTORT IS AN INGREDIENT

Infants' Diarrhœa Syrup

1 oz. Bistort root, $\frac{1}{4}$ oz. Cloves, $\frac{1}{2}$ oz. Marshmallow root, $\frac{1}{4}$ oz. Angelica powder, $\frac{1}{4}$ oz. best Ginger powder.

Bruise the root and cloves small. Add $1\frac{1}{2}$ pint boiling water and simmer down to a pint. Then pour boiling mixture upon the powder, mix well and let it simmer for 10 minutes. Allow to get cold, strain and add lump sugar, sufficient to form a syrup, boil up again, skim, and when cold bottle for use.

This may be given to children in a little Raspberry Leaf Tea, 3 to 6 teaspoonfuls daily, according to age of child. If bleeding from bowels, or flux, a tea of Cranesbill is recommended instead of Raspberry Tea. (SKELTON).

Hæmorrhoids

$\frac{1}{2}$ oz. Marshmallow root powder, $\frac{1}{2}$ oz. Bistort root powder, $\frac{1}{2}$ oz. Cranesbill root powder.

Mix the powders thoroughly and then form into a stiff paste with treacle. Preserve in a jar and take a small quantity (about the size of a bean) three times a day. When constipation is present, $\frac{1}{4}$ oz. Turkey rhubarb powder may be added to the other powdered roots. For the blind piles, $\frac{1}{2}$ oz. Barberry bark should be added.

Pile Ointment should be applied at the same time, made as follows: $\frac{1}{2}$ oz. Bistort root, $\frac{1}{2}$ oz. Cranesbill herb, cut up fine.

Simmer gently for an hour with 2 oz. lard and 2 oz. mutton suet. Strain through a coarse cloth and squeeze out as much strength as possible. Add 1 oz. Olive oil and mix well. Allow to cool gradually. This is equally good for Chapped Hands, Sore Lips, etc. (SKELTON.)

Decoction for Piles

1 oz. Marshmallow root, 1 oz. Bistort root, 1 oz. Comfrey root, 1 oz. White Poplar bark, 1 oz. Cranesbill, 1 oz. Yarrow, 2 drachms each Cloves and Cinnamon.

Bruise the roots, add 2 quarts of water and boil 20 minutes, then add the herbs, Cloves and Cinnamon and boil 10 minutes longer. Strain and sweeten with brown sugar.

Dose, a wineglassful four times a day. Also use Celandine (Pilewort) Ointment. (*Medical Herbalist*.)

Gargle for Ulcerated Tonsils

2 drachms Tincture of Bistort root, 2 drachms Tincture of Bloodroot. Add 2 tablespoonsful of warm water.

Use as gargle, or spray the throat.

Compound Bistort Wash

1 drachm Tincture of Bistort, $\frac{1}{2}$ oz. Bayberry powder.

Infuse the powder in 8 oz. of boiling water, let it remain until cold, strain the liquid off clear, add the tincture and use freely morning, noon and night.

In inflamed mucous discharges from the ears, nose, vagina, urethra or any other part, this wash is exceedingly useful. (*National Botanic Pharmacopœia*.)

For Diabetes

Fluid Extract Bistort, Jambul Seed, Pinus Can., Rhus Aromat., Potentilla Tormentilla, of each 2 drachms. The same quantity of Tincture of Hydrastis.

Put the whole into a 12-oz. bottle and fill with distilled water. Dose, 1 tablespoonful every four hours after meals. (*Medical Herbalist*.)

CULINARY USE

Recipe for Bistort Pudding.

The Herb Pudding still eaten in Cumberland and Westmorland, where Bistort is common in moist meadows and is also cultivated, is a very wholesome dish and very suitable in May, when ordinary green vegetables used to be scarce.

The chief constituents are Bistort shoots and Nettles, and the younger and fresher these greens are the more satisfactory is the resultant food. Allow about $1\frac{1}{2}$ lb. of Bistort to 1 lb. of Nettles. A few leaves of Black Currant and Yellow Dock may be added and a sprig of Parsley. Wash the vegetables thoroughly (in salt and water in the last rinsing), then chop them fairly fine. Place them in a bowl and mix in about a teacupful of barley (washed and soaked), half a teacupful of oatmeal, salt and pepper to flavour, and if liked, a bunch of chives mixed. Boil the whole in a bag for about $2\frac{1}{2}$ hours, to allow the barley to get thoroughly cooked. The bag should be tied firmly, for while the greens shrink, the barley swells. Turn out into a very hot bowl, add a lump of butter and a beaten egg: the heat of the turned-out pudding is sufficient to cook the egg.

¶ *Other Species.* About forty species of *Polygonum* are recorded as having been medicinally employed. A number of species yield blue or yellow dyestuffs.

See KNOTGRASS, SMARTWEED, BUCKWHEAT.

BITTER APPLE. *See* APPLE, BITTER

BITTER ROOT

Apocynum androsæmifolium (LINN.)
N.O. Apocynaceæ

Synonyms. Milkweed. Dogsbane. Fly-Trap
Parts Used. The dried rhizome, roots
Habitat. North America

¶ *Description.* The genus *Apocynum* contains only four species, two of which, *Apocynum androsæmifolium* and *A. cannabinum*, or Black Indian Hemp, resemble each other very closely, the roots being distinguished by the thick-walled stone cells, which in the former are found in an interrupted circle near the middle of the bark, and in the latter are absent.

A. androsæmifolium is a perennial herb, 5 or 6 feet in height, branching, and, in common with the other three members of the genus, yielding on incision a milky juice resembling indiarubber when dry.

The leaves are dark green above, paler and downy beneath, ovate, and from 2 to 3 inches long. The flowers are white, tinged with red, having five scales in the throat of the corolla which secrete a sweet liquid, attractive to flies. These scales are very sensitive, and when touched bend inward, imprisoning the insects.

The tough, fibrous bark of all four species is used by the Indians of California as a substitute for hemp, in making twine, bags, fishing-nets and lines, and linen.

The milky root is found in commerce in cylindrical, branched pieces, about a quarter of an inch thick, reddish or greyish brown outside, longitudinally wrinkled, and having a short fracture and small pith. There is scarcely any odour, and the taste is starchy, afterwards bitter and acrid.

¶ *Constituents.* The nature of the active principle is uncertain. A glucoside, Apocynamarin, was separated, but the activity is thought to be due not to the glucoside, but to an intensely bitter principle, Cymarin.

¶ *Medicinal Action and Uses.* One of the digitalis group of cardiac tonics, apocynum, is the most powerful in slowing the pulse, and its action on the vaso-motor system is also very strong. Being rather irritant to mucous membranes, it may cause nausea and catharsis, so that some cannot tolerate it. It is a powerful hydragogue, helpful in dropsies due to heart-failure, and in the ascites of hepatic cirrhosts has been called the 'vegetable trocar.'

It is used as an alterative in rheumatism, syphilis and scrofula.

¶ *Dosage.* 5 to 15 grains.

¶ *Poisons and Antidotes.* The absorption in the gastro-intestinal tract being very irregular, the dosage and patient must be carefully watched and guarded.

¶ *Other Species.*

A. cannabinum, or Black Indian Hemp, Canadian Hemp, American Hemp, Amyroot, Bowman's Root, Indian Physic, Bitter Root, Rheumatism Weed, Milkweed, Wild Cotton, Choctaw Root, is diuretic, expectorant, diaphoretic, emetic, and cathartic. It should not be substituted for *A. androsæmifolium* or vice versa.

It is *not* the Indian Hemp (*Cannabis Indica*) which yields 'hashish.'

A. hypericifolium bears some resemblance to the above.

A. venetum contains an alkaloid, Apocynteine, said to be a cardiac sedative.

BITTER ROOT is also a common name of *Gentiana lutea*, or Yellow Gentian, the well-known bitter, and of *Lewisia rediviva* or *Spathulum*, with a starchy, edible root.

MILKWEED is also a common name of *Asclepias*.

DOG'S BANE is also a common name of *Aconitum Cynoctonum*.

BITTERSWEET. *See* (WOODY) NIGHTSHADE

BLACKBERRY

Rubus fructicosus
N.O. Rosaceæ

Synonyms. Bramble. Bumble-Kite. Bramble-Kite. Bly. Brummel. Brameberry. Scald-head. Brambleberry
Parts Used. Root, leaves
Habitat. In Australia, the Blackberry grows more luxuriantly than in any other part of the world, though it is common everywhere

The Blackberry, or Bramble, growing in every English hedge-row, is too well known to need description. Its blossoms, as well as its fruits, both green and ripe, may be seen on the bush: at the same time, a somewhat unusual feature, not often met with in other plants.

¶ *History.* The name of the bush is derived from *brambel*, or *brymbyl*, signifying prickly. We read of it as far back as the days of Jonathan, when he upbraided the men of Shechem for their ingratitude to his father's house, relating to them the parable of the trees choosing a king, the humble bramble being finally elected, after the olive, fig-tree and vine had refused the dignity. The ancient Greeks knew Blackberries well, and considered them a remedy for gout.

Opinions differ as to whether there is one true Blackberry with many aberrant forms; or many distinct types. Professor Babington divides the British *Rubi* into forty-one species, or more.

Rubus rhamnifolius and *R. coryfolius* furnish the Blackberries of the hedges, in which the calyx of the fruit is reflexed; *R. fructicosus* has also a reflexed calyx, but the leaves are hoary underneath. *R. cœsius* furnishes Dewberries, distinguished by the large size of the grains, which are covered with bloom and few in number, the whole being closely clasped by the calyx. *R. saxatilis*, the Roebuck-berry, and the badge of the McNabs, is an herbaceous species found in mountainous places in the North, and distinguished by its ternate leaves and fruit of few red large grains.

R. chamænorus, the Cloudberry, and badge of the McFarlanes, is also herbaceous, with an erect stem, 6 to 8 inches high, lobed leaves, and a single flower which is succeeded by a large orange-red fruit of an agreeable flavour. The double-flowering *Rubus* of gardens is a variety of *R. fructicosus*. *R. lancinatus*, of which the native country is unknown, is a rampant species with deeply-cut leaves and large black fruit, which are highly ornamental in autumn.

R. odoratus, the American Bramble, is an erect, unbranched shrub, with large five-lobed leaves and rose-coloured flowers.

R. occidentalis, the Virginian raspberry, has pinnate and ternate leaves, white flowers and black fruit. It is well known that the barren shoots of most of our British *Rubi*, from being too flexile to keep upright, bend downwards even from the hedges and thickets, and root their ends in the soil, thus following that mode of increase which in the strawberry is effected by the scion. The loop thus formed was formerly an object of occasional search, being reputed in some counties (and we have known it so in Gloucestershire) as capable of curing hernia or rupture when used aright, to which end the afflicted child is passed backwards and forwards through the arching bramble. The origin of this custom is difficult to trace; but quoting from *Notes and Queries*, the passing of children through holes in the earth, rocks, and trees, once an established rite, is still practised in various parts of Cornwall.

Children affected with hernia are still passed through a slit in an ash sapling before sunrise, fasting; after which the slit portions are bound up, and as they unite so the malady is cured.

It would appear that in Cornwall the bramble-cure is only employed for boils, the sufferer being either dragged or made to crawl beneath the rooted shoot. We have heard of *cows* that were said to be 'mouse-crope,' or to have been walked over by a shrew-mouse (an ancient way of accounting for paralysis), being dragged through the bramble-loop, in which case, if the creature could wait the time of finding a loop large enough, and suffer the dragging process at the end, we should say the case would not be so hopeless as that of our friend's fat pig, who, when she was ailing, 'had a mind to kill her to make sure on her!' (LINDLEY'S *Treasury of Botany*.)

The Blackberry is known in some parts of the country as 'Scaldhead,' either from producing the eruption known as scaldhead in children who eat the fruit to excess – the over-ripe fruit being indigestible – or from the curative effects of the leaves and berries in this malady of the scalp, or from the remedial effects of the leaves, when applied externally to scalds. The leaves are said to be still in use in England as a remedy for burns and scalds; formerly their operation was helped by a spoken charm. Creeping under a Bramble-bush was itself a charm against rheumatism, boils, blackheads, etc. Blackberries were in olden days supposed to give protection against all 'evil runes,' if gathered at the right time of the moon. The whole plant had once a considerable popular reputation both as a medicine and as a charm for various disorders. The flowers and fruit were from very ancient times used to remedy venomous bites; the young shoots, eaten as a salad, were thought – though Gerard cautiously suggests the addition of a little alum – to fasten loose teeth. Gerard and other herbalists regard the bramble as a valuable astringent, whether eaten or applied: its leaves 'heal the eies that hang out,' and are a most useful application for piles; its fruit stops looseness of the bowels and is good for stone, and for soreness in mouth and throat.

¶ *Medicinal Action and Uses.* The bark of the root and the leaves contain much tannin, and have long been esteemed as a capital astringent and tonic, proving a valuable remedy for dysentery and diarrhœa, etc. The root is the more astringent.

¶ *Preparations.* Fluid extract, $\frac{1}{2}$ to 1 drachm. Fluid extract, root, U.S.P., 15 drops. Syrup, U.S.P., 1 drachm.

The fruit contains malic and citric acids, pectin and albumen. If desiccated in a moderately hot oven and then reduced to a powder, it is a reliable remedy for dysentery.

The root-bark, as used medicinally, should appear in thin tough, flexible bands, inodorous, strongly astringent and somewhat bitter. It should be peeled off the root and dried by artificial heat or in strong sun. One ounce, boiled in 1½ pint water or milk down to a pint, makes a good decoction. Half a teacupful should be taken every hour or two for diarrhœa. One ounce of the bruised root, likewise boiled in water, may also be used, the dose being larger, however. The same decoction is said to be useful against whooping-cough in the spasmodic stage.

The leaves are also employed for the same purpose. One ounce of the dried leaves, infused in one pint of boiling water, and the infusion taken cold, a teacupful at a time, makes a serviceable remedy for dysentery, etc.

RECIPES

Blackberry jelly has been used with good effects in cases of dropsy caused by feeble, ineffective circulation, and the London Pharmacopœia (1696) declared the ripe berries of the bramble to be a great cordial, and to contain a notable restorative spirit. Blackberry wine is made by crushing the fruit and adding one quart of boiling water to each gallon of the fruit, allowing to stand for 24 hours, stirring occasionally, and then straining off the liquid. 2 lb. of white sugar are then added to every gallon, and it is kept in a tightly corked cask till the following October.

This makes a trustworthy cordial astringent, used in looseness of the bowels. Another delicious cordial is made from pressing out the juice from the ripe Blackberries, adding 2 lb. of sugar to each quart and ½ oz. of nutmegs and cloves. Boil all together for a short time, allow to get cold and then add a little brandy.

In Crusoe's *Treasury of Easy Medicines* (1771) a decoction of Blackberry leaves is recommended as a fomentation for long-standing ulcers. There is also a popular country notion that the young shoots, eaten as a salad, will fasten loose teeth. A noted hair-dye has been made by boiling the leaves in strong lye, which imparts to the hair a permanent soft black colour.

Blackberry Vinegar

is a wholesome drink that is easily made and can with advantage have its place in the store cupboard for use in winter, being a fine cordial for a feverish cold.

Gather the berries on a fine day, stalk them, put into an earthenware vessel and cover with malt vinegar. Let them stand three days to draw out the juice. Strain through a sieve, drain thoroughly, leaving them to drip through all day. Measure the juice and allow a pound of sugar to each pint. Put into a preserving pan, boil gently for 5 minutes, removing scum as it rises, set aside to cool, and when cold, bottle and cork well.

A teaspoonful of this, mixed with water, will often quench thirst when other beverages fail and makes a delicious drink in fever.

BLACKBERRY, AMERICAN

Rubus villosus (AIT.)
N.O. Rosaceæ

Synonyms. Brombeere. Bramble, or Fingerberry. Or. Nigrobaccus, and R. Cuneifolius
Parts Used. Leaves, root, bark
Habitat. Cultivated in United States of America from a *European species*

¶ *Description.* It is prepared in thin tough flexible bands, outer surface blackish or blackish grey, inner surface, pale brownish, sometimes striped, with whitish tasteless wood adhering. It is inodorous, very astringent (root more so than the leaves) and rather bitter.

¶ *Constituents.* Tannic acid is abundant in it up to 10 per cent., and can be extracted readily by boiling water or dilute alcohol.

¶ *Medicinal Action and Uses.* An astringent tonic for diarrhœa, dysentery, etc. It is

very similar in action to the wild English Blackberry.

¶ *Preparations.* Fluid extract of dried bark of root Rubus, U.S.P., 15 minims.

Syrup of Rubus, U.S.P., 1 fluid drachm.

¶ *Other Species.* Of the genus *Rubus* a large number are indigenous in the United States, where they are called Blackberry, Dewberry, Cloudberry. Most of them are shrubby or suffruticose briers, with astringent roots and edible berries; some have annual stems without prickles, these are called Raspberries.

BLACK CURRANT. *See* CURRANT

BLACK HAW. *See* GUELDER ROSE

BLACK ROOT

Leptandra Virginica (NUTT.)
N.O. Scrophulariaceæ

Synonyms. Veronica Virginica. Veronica purpurea. Pæderota Virginica. Eustachya purpurea and Eustachya alba. Culveris Root. Culver's Physic. Physic Root. Leptandra-Wurzel

Parts Used. The dried rhizome, roots

Habitat. Eastern United States

¶ *Description.* This tall, herbaceous perennial was included by Linnæus in the genus *Veronica*, but was later assigned by Nuttall to the genus *Leptandra*, a nomenclature followed by present-day botanists. It has a simple, erect stem, 3 or 4 feet high or more, smooth and downy, furnished with leaves in whorls and terminating in a long spike of white flowers, 6 to 10 inches long. The leaves, of which there are from four to seven in each whorl, are lanceolate, pointed and minutely serrate, and stand on short footstalks. A variety with purple flowers has been described as a distinct species under the name of *Leptandra purpurea.* The plant flowers in July and August. It grows throughout the United States, in the south, mostly in mountain meadows – in the north in rich woods, and is not unfrequently cultivated. It will grow readily in Britain. The rhizome and roots are nearly odourless, the taste bitter and rather acrid, and are generally used dried. The rhizome is of horizontal growth, nearly cylindrical, somewhat branched, externally dark brown to purplish brown, smooth and faintly longitudinally wrinkled, and showing stem bases at intervals of ½ to 1½ inch. The rootlets, rising from the under portion, are wiry and brittle when dry.

¶ *Constituents.* The roots contain volatile oil, extractive, tannic acid, gum, resin, a crystalline principle, a saccharine principle resembling mannite, and a glucoside re-sembling senegin. Both the crystalline principle and the impure resin obtained by precipitating with water a tincture of the root have been called Leptandrin and is said to be the active principle. The properties are extracted by both water and alcohol.

An ester of *p*-methoxycinnamic acid, a phytosterol verosterol, and some dimethoxycinnamic acid are also obtained.

¶ *Medicinal Action and Uses.* The fresh root is a violent cathartic and may also be emetic. The dried root is milder and less certain. Leptandrin excites the liver gently and promotes the secretion of bile without irritating the bowels or purging. As it is also a tonic for the stomach, it is very useful in diarrhœa, chronic dysentery, cholera infantum, and torpidity of the liver.

The accounts of its use are conflicting, perhaps owing to the difference in the action of the root in its dry and fresh states. There appears to be a risk of the fresh root producing bloody stools and possibly abortion, though a decoction may be useful in intermittent fever. It has been stated that the dried root has been employed with success in leprosy and cachetic diseases, and in combination with cream of tartar, in dropsy.

¶ *Dosages.* 15 to 60 grains. Of the impure resin, 2 to 4 grains. Of the powdered extract, U.S.P., 4 grains. Of the fluid extract, 15 minims as a laxative. Leptandrin, ¼ to 2 grains.

BLADDERWRACK

Fucus vesiculosis (LINN.)
N.O. Fucaceæ

Synonyms. Fucus. Sea-Wrack. Kelp-Ware. Black-Tang. Quercus marina. Cutweed. Bladder Fucus. Fucus (Varech) vesiculeux. Blasentang. Seetang. Meeriche

Parts Used. The dried mass of root, stem and leaves. (The thallus.)

Habitat. North Atlantic Ocean

¶ *Description.* Almost all the more solid *Algæ* were formerly described by the name of *Fucus,* but now it is applied to one genus of *Fucaceæ,* most of the species of which are found only in the northern seas, many being more or less exposed at low water. *Fucus vesiculosis* is found on submerged rocks on both coasts of North America, and in Europe north of the Mediterranean, where it drifts in from time to time through the Strait of Gibraltar.

The perennial frond or thallus is coarse, light yellow or brownish-green in colour, erect, and from 2 to 3 feet in height. It attaches itself to the rocks by branched, root-like, discoid, woody extremities, developed from the base of the stalk. The frond is almost fan-shaped, narrow and strap-shaped at the base, the rest flat and leaf-like in form, wavy, many times divided into two, with erect divisions having a very strong, broad, compressed midrib running to the apex. The margin is entire, the texture tough and leathery, mainly olive brown in colour, the younger portion yellower, shining. Air vesicles developed in the substance of the frond, usually in pairs, one on either side of the midrib and often one at the fork of the divisions, broadly oval, or spherical, attaining when fully grown half an inch in diameter, are the characteristics of this species which have suggested both the English and Latin names.

The fructification is contained in small globose conceptacles with a firm wall lined with numerous jointed hairs and sunk in the surface of large ovoid-oblong or narrower, pointed or blunt, swollen receptacles, filled with a transparent mucous. These attain an inch in length and are situated at the ends of the divisions of the fronds.

The entire living plant is gathered from the rocks about the end of June and dried rapidly in the sun, when it becomes brittle and may be easily reduced to a coarse powder. Care should be taken to turn it frequently, to avoid the development of a putrid odour. If dried by artificial heat, it retains its hygroscopic qualities and does not become brittle. It is in perfect condition only during early and middle summer, and should not be collected when too fully matured, as it quickly undergoes decomposition. When thrown up on the shore by the sea, the seaweed is not suitable for medicinal purposes, as the soaking of the detached plants in sea-water causes the loss of important constituents by diffusion from cells containing protoplasm which has lost its vitality.

As found in commerce, the drug *Fucus* is hard and brittle, forming a much wrinkled mass, blackish or with more or less of a whitish efflorescence or incrustation, but it acquires a cartilaginous consistency when slightly moistened. It has a strong, sea-weed-like odour and a nauseous, saline and mucilaginous taste. Occasionally, from some unexplained cause, it is very astringent. The powder is reddish brown, with numerous fragments of epidermal tissue, with polygonal cells from 0·012 to 0·025 mm. in length.

Bladderwrack is a valuable *manure* for potatoes and other crops and is gathered for this purpose all along the British coast. It is largely used in the Channel Islands, where it is called *Vraic*, the early potatoes from Jersey being grown by seaweed manure. Fresh seaweed contains 20 to 40 lb. of potash to the ton, and dried seaweed 60 to 230, so that its collection and use were strongly recommended to farmers while the War caused a shortage of artificial fertilizers. It may be spread on the land and left for some time before ploughing in, but should not be left in heaps, as rotting liberates the potash, which may be wasted. The seaweed may be dried and burnt to ashes, then sprinkled on the ground as *Kelp*.

The early broccoli from Cornwall is fertilized with wrack, and on the west coast of Ireland, driftweed is almost the only manure used for raising potatoes. In the Channel Islands it is used for producing the smoke for drying bacon and fish, while in the Hebrides, cheeses while drying are covered with the salty ashes, and horses, cattle and sheep have been fed with it.

During the War the French Ministry of War experimented with regard to the value of seaweed as food for horses. A batch of twenty fed on the usual ration of oats and fodder gained eleven kilogrammes *less* in two months than a similar number fed on the same weight of seaweed. Another trial resulted in the cure of some sick horses fed on seaweed, while others fed on oats remained out of health.

In Denmark, a few years ago, the possibility of making *paper* from seaweed was mooted, but the cost of collecting probably proved too serious an obstacle.

It is also possible that considerable quantities of *alcohol* might be obtained from various species.

Many attempts have been made to make kelp-burning successful by finding a use for by-products from destructive distillation in retorts, but the cost of collection, drying and fuel prevents such experiments being financially profitable. There were at one time flourishing kelp industries in the Hebrides, and Lord Leverhulme, the owner of Lewis Isle, sent experts to report on the possibilities, but his death and lack of official support caused the matter to be dropped.

Kelp is prepared from several species of *Fucus* (including Black Wrack, *F. serratus* and Knobbed Wrack, *F. nodosus*, and on the coast of France about a dozen other species) and from the deep-sea tangle, *Laminaria* species, especially *L. digitata*. The latter yield 'drift-wood kelp,' obtainable only when cast up on the shore by gales or other causes. These contain ten times as much iodine as the *Fuci* and are practically now the only kelps used in making iodine. The species of *Fucus* growing within the tidal range and cut at low water are called 'cut-weeds.'

F. vesiculosis is the badge of the M'Neills.

¶ *Constituents.* Bladderwrack contains about 0·1 per cent. of a volatile oil, cellulose, mucilage, mannite, colouring and bitter principles, soda and iodine, and bromine compounds of sodium and potassium. These saline ingredients constitute 14 to 20 per cent. of its ashes, which the dry plant yields in the proportion of 2·5 to 4 per cent., and

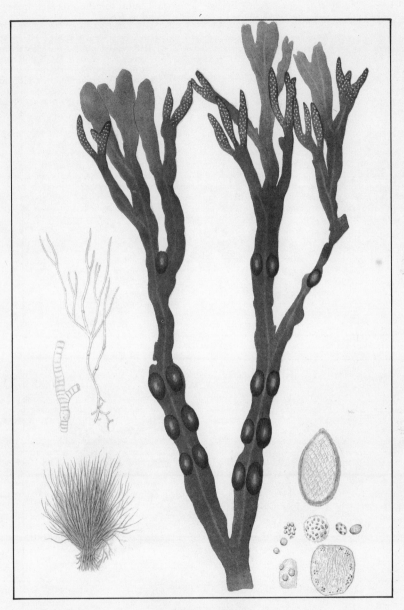

BLADDERWRACK
Fucus Vesiculosis

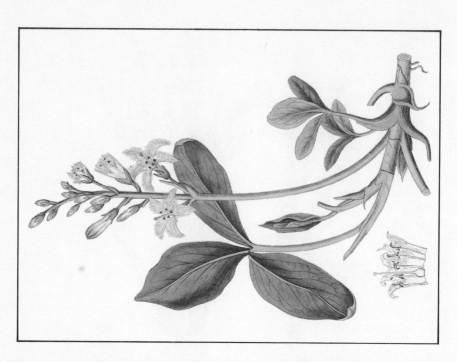

BOGBEAN
Menyanthes Trifoliata

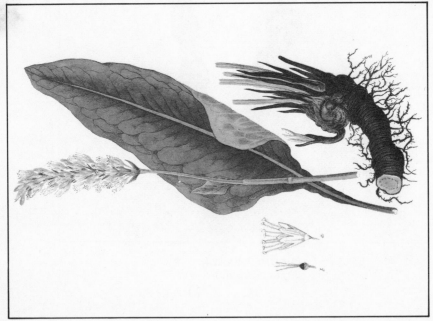

BISTORT
Polygonum Bistorta

also remain in the charcoal resulting from its exposure to heat in closed vessels. The proportions, especially of iodine, vary according to both locality and season. They are most abundant at the end of June. It has been stated that 0·8 per cent. of a sugar named Fucose exists in dried seaweed, and that this yields an alcohol, Fucitol. The air in the vesicles consists of a considerably higher percentage of Oxygen and a lower percentage of Nitrogen than in the outer atmosphere. Its value as a fertilizer is due to its potash.

One hundred pounds of red wrack, dried to a moisture content of 10 per cent., when heated for a short time with weak sulphuric acid and the acidity still further reduced after cooling, may be fermented with brewers' yeast and is then capable of yielding about 6 litres of alcohol on distillation. It is alleged that under industrial conditions this amount might be increased.

Kelp, or dried seaweed, was the original source of iodine, being discovered as such by Courtois in 1812, when investigating the products obtained from the mother-liquors prepared by lixiviating burnt seaweed. Iodine does not occur in nature in the uncombined condition, but is widely, though sparingly, distributed in the form of *iodides* and *iodates*, chiefly of sodium and potassium, in sea-water, some seaweeds, and various mineral and medicinal springs.

Kelp-burning as a source of iodine is a dead industry, owing to a cheaper process of obtaining it from the mother-liquors obtained in the purification of Chile saltpetre, and the use of kelp – an impure carbonate of soda, containing sulphate and chloride of sodium and a little charcoal – as a source of alkalies for soap and glass manufacture has been rendered obsolete by the modern process of obtaining carbonate of soda cheaply from common salt. Unless very recently discontinued, however, the preparation of iodine from kelp is still carried on at Glasgow.

Several methods were employed: (1) the weeds being dried in the sun, burned until formed into a confused mass, and sprinkled with water to break it up into pieces which were treated at chemical works; or (2) the seaweed was heated in large retorts, whereby tarry and ammoniacal liquors pass over and a very porous residue of kelp remained; or (3) the weeds were boiled with sodium carbonate, the liquid filtered and hydrochloric acid added to the filtrate, when alginic acid is precipitated; this is filtered off, the filtrate neutralized by caustic soda and the whole evaporated to dryness and carbonized.

The resulting kelp was then lixiviated with water, which extracts the soluble salts, and the liquid concentrated to crystallize the less soluble salts for removal. The addition of sulphuric acid set chemical processes in action, which finally liberated the iodine from its compounds.

Three tons of Tangle (Laminaria) give a ton of kelp, or 20 tons of cut-weed, or Fucus.

Good drift may yield as much as 10 to 15 lb. of iodine per ton, and cut-weed kelp only 3 to 4 lb. Other constituents vary from 2 to 10 per cent. in different samples.

¶ *Medicinal Action and Uses.* Bladderwrack is not largely used at present, any virtues it may have being due to the iodine contained in it. It has alterative properties, has been used in scrofula, and is thought by some authorities to reduce obesity through stimulating the thyroid gland.

The charcoal derived from Kelp has been used in the treatment of goitre and scrofulous swellings under the name of *Æthiops vegetabilis* or *vegetable ethiops*, introduced by Dr. Russell in 1750, who also used a jelly for similar purposes, both internally and externally. He was also successful in dispersing scrofulous tumours by rubbing in the mucus of the vesicles of Bladderwrack, afterwards washing the parts with sea-water. The charcoal was also helpful in goitre. The iodine from other sources led to the neglect of kelp products.

In 1862 Dr. Duchesne-Duparc found, while experimenting in cases of chronic psoriasis, that weight was reduced without injuring health, and used the drug with success for the latter purpose. Dr. Godfroy experimented on himself, losing five and a quarter pounds in a week after taking before three meals a day an extract made into pills containing 25 grams (3·75 grains). The bromine and iodine stimulated the absorbent glands to increased activity, without causing an atrophied wasting of the glands. Later experiments of Hunt and Seidell indicated that the result is brought about by stimulation of the thyroid gland.

Sea-pod liniment, is the expressed juice and decoction of fresh seaweed as dispensed by sea-side chemists for rheumatism, and the extract, taken continuously in pills or fluid form is reputed to relieve rheumatic pains as well as to diminish fat without harm.

Sea-pod essence is good for rubbing into sprains and bruises, or for applying on wet lint under oiled silk, as a compress, changed as often as hot or dry. It may be preceded by fomentations of the hot decoction.

Embrocation for strengthening the limbs of rickety children can be made from the glutinous substance of the vesicles, bottled in rum.

Fucus or Seaweed wine, from grapes and

dried Fucus, has been praised as a remedy in diseases of the hip and other joints and bones in children.

For external application to enlarged or hardened glands, the bruised weed may be applied as a cold poultice.

¶ *Dosage.* Of charcoal, 10 grains to 2 drachms.

Of extract, 3 to 10 grains, in pills, massed with powdered Liquorice or Marshmallow roots, to reduce swelling and obesity.

Of liquid extract, 1 to 2 fluid drachms. It is the basis of many advertised nostrums. Sodium and potassium iodides are often added to supplement the small proportion of iodine. It is used in mixture form, generally with alkali iodides and sometimes in combination with *Liquor Thyroidei.*

Of decoction, 2 fluid ounces, three times daily.

Of infusion, 1 wineglassful.

Solid extract may be dissolved in diluted alcohol and mixed with *syrup.*

(All doses for combating obesity are gradually increased.)

Of fluid extract, 10 minims.

The Alginic acid obtained from seaweed is used to form an organic compound with iron, which is sold under the trade name of *Algiron* or *Alginoid Iron.* It contains about 11 per cent. of iron and is given in doses of 2 to 10 decigrams (3 to 15 grains).

Fucol is a trade name for a cod-liver oil substitute, said to be obtained from roasted Bladderwrack with a bland oil. It is green in colour, and resembles coffee in odour and taste.

Fucusin tablets are recommended in obesity.

¶ *Other Species.*
F. nodosus, the Knobbed Wrack, has a narrower thallus, without a midrib and single vesicles.

F. serratus, the Black Wrack, has a veined and serrate frond, without vesicles. Both contain the same constituents as Bladderwrack.

F. serratus has been much used in Norway for feeding cattle, being called there 'cowweed.' Linnæus stated that in Gothland the inhabitants boiled it with water, mixed it with a little coarse meal or flour, and fed their hogs with it, for which reason they called the plant 'Swine-tang.' In Sweden the poor people covered their cottages with it and sometimes used it for fuel.

F. siliquosus has a very narrow frond, with short branches and articulated vesicles of a pod-like appearance.

This and the two preceding species are permitted by the French Codex to be employed in the place of *F. vesiculosis.*

F. natans (*Sargassum bacciferum*) is the Gulf-weed of the Atlantic Ocean and is often found in immense masses floating in the sea.

The frond is terrate and has linear and serrate branches and globular vesicles of the size of a pea.

F. vesiculosis was reputed to be the *Antipolyscarcique nostrum* of Count Mattei.

F. canaliculatus is remarkable for its amphibious habits, growing on large boulders and recovering after being baked by the sun into hard brown masses.

F. amylaceus, or Ceylon Moss, abounding in starch and vegetable jelly, is used like carrageen, or Irish moss.

F. Helminthocorton (Corsican Moss or *Gigartina Helminthocorton*) is regarded in Europe as an anthelmintic and febrifuge. It is an ingredient in the trade mixture called Corsican Moss, used in decoction of from 4 to 6 drachms to a pint, the dose being 1 wineglassful three times a day.

Another seaweed, *Agar-agar,* of the East Indies, is sent to China in large quantities for making jellies and for a size used in stiffening silks. An aperient medicine is known by its name. (American.)

Laminaria digitata, sea-girdles or tangles, of Scotland, gives a good substance for bougies. The stems are strong and tenacious, from 2 to 12 inches long and an inch or more wide, drying easily with much shrinkage and becoming firm, only slightly softer than horn, and yet elastic. It may be kept thus for years, and will absorb moisture at any time and swell to the original size, thus being valuable for dilating bougies and tents.

The Laminariaceæ species are very remarkable in many ways. *L. digitata, L. stenophylla,* and *L. saccharina* are the principal ones associated with the kelp industry.

F. crispus is a name of *Chondrus crispus* or *Gigartina mamillosa* (Irish Moss or Carrageen) of European coasts, well known as a demulcent. Dosage, 4 drachms.

BLITES   N.O. Chenopodiaceæ

Habitat. They grow only on seashores, or in saline plains and other places where the soil is impregnated with salt, and are almost exclusively confined to the temperate and tropical regions of the Northern Hemisphere, very few being found in the Southern.

The Sea-blites are members of the genus *Suæda,* the name derived from the Greek word for soda, in which the plants abound.

They are smooth or downy herbaceous, or more frequently shrubby, plants, with alternate, somewhat tapering, fleshy, stalkless leaves, bearing solitary or clustered stalk-less or short-stalked, usually perfect flowers in their axils. Their fruits, utricles, are enclosed in the slightly enlarged or in-flated berry-like calyx, but do not adhere to it.

BLITE, SEA
Suæda fruticosa

Synonym. Shrubby Sea Blite

The Shrubby Sea-Blite is one of our rarer British species. It grows on sandy and shingly beaches, mostly on the east coast, but it is very common in the warmer parts of Europe and also in Northern Africa and Western Asia.

It is a shrubby, erect, branching, evergreen, perennial plant, 2 to 5 feet high, with thick and succulent, semi-cylindrical, bluntish, pale-green leaves, and small stalkless flowers, either solitary, or two or three together.

It is one of the plants burned in Southern Europe for the manufacture of barilla.

BLITE, ANNUAL SEA
Suæda maritima

Suæda maritima (Linn.), the Annual Sea-Blite, is our other British species and is com-mon on muddy seashores. It is a low, straggling plant, smooth, glaucous and red-dish in winter, with slender branches rising 1 to 2 feet; acute, semi-cylindrical, short, fleshy leaves; flowers, 1 to 5 together, styles two. It is in flower from July to October.

Culpepper tells us there are

'two sorts, the white and the red. The white hath leaves somewhat like unto beets, but smaller, rounder and of a whitish-green colour. The red is in all things like the white, but that its leaves and tufted heads are ex-ceedingly red at first and after turn more purplish. . . . They are all of them cooling, drying and binding and useful in fluxes of blood, especially the red.'

He also mentions

'another sort of wild Blites, like the other wild kinds, but having long and spiky heads of greenish seeds, seeming by the thick setting together to be all seed. This sort fishes are delighted with, and it is a good and usual bait, for fishes will bite fast enough at them, if you have but wit enough to catch them when they bite.'

The name Blite has also been applied to several of the *Chenopodiums*.

BLITE, STRAWBERRY
Amaranthus blitus

Synonyms. Strawberry Spinach. Berry-bearing Orache

The Strawberry Blite belongs to the closely allied order *Amaranthaceæ*, and is not strictly a native of Britain, only occasionally appear-ing on rubbish heaps. It is an inconspicuous weed, and to the casual observer would be regarded as an Orache or Goosefoot. Its trailing stems are a foot or so in length, bear-ing more or less oval leaves and numerous green flowers clustered in the leaf axils. The flowers are unisexual and without petals, both kinds of flowers being borne, however, on the same plant. The female flower develops into a juicy crimson capsule, full of ⸢purple juice, having somewhat the appearance of a Wood Strawberry, hence the popular name of the plant. Was formerly much used for colouring in cookery. It flowers in August.

See ARRACHS, BEETROOTS, CHENOPODIUMS, GOOSEFOOTS, GLASSWORTS, SPINACH, WORM-SEED.

(POISON)
BLOODROOT
Sanguinaria Candensis (LINN.)
N.O. Papaveraceæ

Synonyms. Indian Paint. Tetterwort. Red Pucoon. Red Root. Paucon. Coon Root. Snakebite. Sweet Slumber

Parts Used. Root, whole plant

Habitat. United States of America and Canada, found in rich open woods from Canada, south to Florida and west to Arkansas, and Nebraska

¶ *Description.* A perennial plant, one of the earliest and most beautiful spring flowers. In England it will grow freely if cultivated carefully, it has even grown in the open in gravelly dry soil in the author's garden. It has a lovely white flower and produces only a single leaf and a flowering scape about 6 inches high. When the leaf first appears it is wrapped round the flower bud and is a greyish-green colour covered with a downy bloom – Leaves palmate five to nine lobed, 6 to 10 inches long. After flowering the leaves increase in size, the underside paler showing prominent veins. The white flower is wax-like with golden stamens. The seed is an oblong narrow pod about 1 inch long.

The rootstock is thick, round and fleshy, slightly curved at ends, and contains an orange-red juice, and is about 1 to 4 inches long, with orange-red rootlets. When dried it breaks with a short sharp fracture, little smell, taste bitter acrid and persistent, powdered root causes sneezing and irritation of the nose. The root is collected in the autumn, after leaves die down; it must be stored in a dry place or it quickly deteriorates.

¶ *Constituents*. Alkaloids Sanguinarine, Chelerythrine, Protopine and B. homochelidonine; Sanguinarine forms colourless crystals. Chelerythrine is also colourless and crystalline. Protopine (also found in opium) is one of the most widely diffused of the opium alkaloids. The rhizome also contains red resin and an abundance of starch.

¶ *Medicinal Action and Uses*. Emetic, cathartic expectorant and emmenagogue, and of great value in atonic dyspepsia, asthma, bronchitis and croup. (The taste is so nauseating, that it may cause expectorant action.) Of value in pulmonary consump-tion, nervous irritation and helpful in lowering high pulse, and in heart disease and weakness and palpitation of heart of great use. For ringworm apply the fluid extract. Also good for torpid liver, scrofula, dysentery. It is applied to fungoid growths, ulcers, fleshy excrescences, cancerous affections and as an escharotic. Sanguinaria root is chiefly used as an expectorant for chronic bronchitis and as a local application in chronic eczema, specially when secondary to varicose ulcers. In *toxic doses*, it causes burning in the stomach, intense thirst, vomiting, faintness, vertigo, intense prostration with dimness of eyesight.

The root has long been used by the American Indians as a dye for their bodies and clothes and has been used successfully by American and French dyers.

¶ *Preparations and Dosages*. Fluid extract of Sanguinaria, U.S.P., dose 1½ minims. Tincture of Sanguinaria, U.S.P., 15 minims. Powdered root, 10 to 30 grains. Sanguinarin, ¼ to 1 grain. Fluid extract, 10 to 30 drops.

BLUEBELL

Scilla nutans (S. M.)
Hyacinthus nonscriptus (LINN.)

Synonyms. Calverkeys. Culverkeys. Auld Man's Bell. Ring-o'-Bells. Jacinth. Wood Bells. Agraphis nutans, Link
Part Used. Bulb, dried and powdered
Habitat. Abundant in Britain, Western Europe to Spain, eastward to Central France, along the Mediterranean to Italy

¶ *Description*. From the midst of very long, narrow leaves, rising from the small bulb, and overtopping them, rises the flower-stem, bearing the pendulous, bell-shaped blossoms, arranged in a long curving line. Each flower has two small bracts at the base of the short flower-stalk. The perianth is bluish-purple and composed of six leaflets.

The Wild Hyacinth is in flower from early in April till the end of May, and being a perennial and spreading rapidly, is found year after year in the same spot, forming a mass of rich colour in the woods where it grows. The long leaves remain above ground until late in the autumn.

Linnæus first called it *Hyacinthus*, tradition associating the flower with the Hyacinth of the Ancients, the flower of grief and mourning. Hyacinthus was a charming youth whom both Apollo and Zephyrus loved, but Hyacinthus preferred the Sun-God to the God of the West Wind, who sought to be revenged, and one day when Apollo was playing quoits with the youth, a quoit (blown by Zephyrus out of its proper course) killed Hyacinthus. Apollo, stricken with grief, raised from his blood a purple flower, on which the letters *Ai*, *Ai* were traced, so that his cry of woe might for evermore have existence upon earth. As our native variety of Hyacinth had no trace of these mystic letters, our older botanists called it *Hyacinthus non-scriptus*, or 'not written on.' A later generic name, *Agraphis*, is of similar meaning, being a compound of two Greek words, meaning 'not to mark.'

It is the 'fair-hair'd hyacinth' of Ben Jonson, a name alluding to the old myth. We also find it called Jacinth in Elizabethan times. In Walton's *Angler* it is mentioned as Culverkeys.

¶ *Constituents*. The bulbs contain inulin, but are characterized by the absence of starch (which in many other monocotyledons is found in company with inulin). Even if fed on cane-sugar, Bluebell bulbs will not form starch. They also contain a very large quantity of mucilage.

¶ *Medicinal Action and Uses*. Though little used in modern medicine, the bulb has diuretic and styptic properties.

Dried and powdered it has been used as a styptic for leucorrhœa: 'There is hardly a more powerful remedy,' wrote Sir John Hill

(1716–75), warning at the same time that the dose should not exceed 3 grains. He also informs us that a decoction of the bulb operates by urine.

Tennyson speaks of Bluebell juice being used to cure snake-bite.

The flowers have a slight, starch-like scent, but no medicinal uses have been ascribed to them.

The bulbs are poisonous in the fresh state. The viscid juice so abundantly contained in them and existing in every part of the plant has been used as a substitute for starch, and in the days when stiff ruffs were worn was much in request. From its gummy character, it was also employed as bookbinders' gum.

Gerard informs us that it was also used for setting feathers upon arrows. De Candolle (1778–1841) suggested that the abundant mucilage might be put to some economic purpose.

¶ *Dosage.* 3 grains.

¶ *Substitutes.* Many other bulbous plants related to *Scilla* (*Hyacinthus*, *Muscari*, *Gagea*, etc.) have been used as diuretics, and probably contain related, if not identical substances. *See* HYACINTH, SQUILL

BLUE FLAG. *See* IRIS

BLUE MALLOW. *See* MALLOW

BOGBEAN   Menyanthes trifoliata (TOURNEF.)
                           N.O. Gentianaceæ

Synonyms. Buckbean. Marsh Trefoil. Water Trefoil. Marsh Clover
   (Dutch) Bocks. Boonan
   (German) Bocksbohne or Scharbocks-Klee
Part Used. Herb
Habitat. The Buckbean, or Bogbean, grows in spongy bogs, marshes and shallow water throughout Europe, being rather scarce in the south of England, though common in the north and in Scotland

¶ *Description.* It is a green, glabrous plant, with creeping rootstock and procumbent stem, varying in length according to situation, covered by the sheaths of the leaves, which are on long, fleshy, striated petioles, and three-partite, the leaflets being entire and about 2 inches long and 1 broad. It blossoms from May to July, the flowers being borne on long stalks, 6 to 18 inches high, longer than the leaves and clustered together in a thick, short spike, rendering them very conspicuous. The corollas, ¾ inch across, are outwardly rose-coloured and inwardly white and hairy, with reddish stamens. The Buckbean is one of the prettiest of our wild flowers, deserving of cultivation in the garden, where it grows and thrives well, if planted in peat with water constantly round the roots.

¶ *History.* The plant was held to be of great value as a remedy against the once-dreaded scurvy. *Scharbock*, its German name, is a corruption of the Latin *scorbutus*, the old medical name for the disease.

'Bean' is probably an affix from the resemblance of the foliage to that of the beans grown in cottage gardens. Gerard says that the leaves are 'like to those of the garden beane.'

Its specific name, *trifoliata*, carries the same reference to the form of its leaves.

The generic name, *Menyanthes*, is from two Greek words signifying month and flower. It was a name bestowed by Linnæus, and it has been suggested that the plant was so called because it remains in flower for a month; but it is actually often in bloom during *May*, *June* and *July*!

One of the older writers describes its inflorescence as a 'bush of feather-like floures of a white colour, dasht ouer slightly with a wash of light carnation.'

Buckbean has a reputation for preserving sheep from rot, but it is doubtful whether they really touch it, on account of its extreme bitterness.

¶ *Constituents.* The chief constituents are a small quantity of volatile oil and a bitter principle, a glucoside called Menyanthin. The bitterness is imparted to both alcohol and water.

¶ *Medicinal Action and Uses.* Tonic, cathartic, deobstruent and febrifuge. An extract is made from the leaves, which possesses strong tonic properties, and which renders great service in rheumatism, scurvy, and skin diseases. An infusion of 1 oz. of the dried leaves to 1 pint of boiling water is taken in wineglassful doses, frequently repeated. It has also been recommended as an external application for dissolving glandular swellings. Finely powdered Buckbean leaves have been employed as a remedy for ague, being said to effect a cure when other means fail. In large doses, the powder is also purgative. It is used also as a herb tobacco.

The juice of the fresh leaves has proved efficacious in dropsical cases, and mixed with whey has been known to cure gout.

In Halliwell's *Popular Rhymes and Nursery Tales* this rhyme occurs:

'Buckee, Buckee, biddy Bene,
Is the way now fair and clean?
Is the goose ygone to nest,
And the fox ygone to rest?
Shall I come away?'

These curious lines are said by Devonshire children when they go through any passages in the dark, and are said to be addressed to Puck or Robin Goodfellow. Biddy bene = Anglo-Saxon *biddan*, to ask or pray; *bén*, a supplication or entreaty. Buckee is perhaps a corruption of Puck.

Buckbean tea, taken alone or mixed with wormwood, centaury or sage, is said to cure dyspepsia and a torpid liver.

¶ *Preparation*. Fluid extract, 10 to 40 drops.

BOLDO

Peumus Boldus (MOLINA)
N.O. Monimiaceæ

Synonyms. Boldu. Boldus. Boldoa Fragrans
Part Used. The leaves
Habitat. Chile

¶ *Description*. An evergreen shrub growing in the fields of the Andes in Chile, where its yellowish-green fruit is eaten, its bark used for tanning, and its wood utilized in charcoal-making.

Leaves are opposite, sessile, about 2 inches long entire, and colour when dried red brown, coriaceous, prominent midrib, a number of small glands on their surface. Odour peculiar, when crushed very strongly disagreeable, not unlike oil of Chenopodium (wormseed). The leaves contain about 2 per cent. on distillation of an aromatic volatile oil, chemically related to oil of Chenopodium.

A peculiar alkaloid called Boldine has been found in the leaves and when injected hyperdermically, paralyses both motor and sensory nerves, also the muscle fibres. When given internally, in toxic doses, it causes great excitement, exaggerates the reflexes and the respiratory movements, increases diuresis, causes cramp and convulsions ending in death

from centric respiratory paralysis, the heart continuing to beat long after respiration ceases. Of late years Boldine has been largely used in veterinary practice for jaundice.

¶ *Constituents*. Boldo leaves contain about 2 per cent. of volatile oil, in which, in addition to terpenes, terpineol has been detected. They also contain the bitter alkaloid Boldine and the glucoside Boldin or Boldoglucin.

¶ *Medicinal Action and Uses*. Tonic, antiseptic, stimulant. Useful in chronic hepatic torpor. The oil in 5-drop doses has been found useful in genito-urinary inflammation. Has long been recognized in South America as a valuable cure for gonorrhœa.

¶ *Preparations*. Tincture of Boldo, B.P.C., used as a diuretic. Dose, 10 to 40 minims. Fluid extract, ¼ to ½ drachm.

¶ *Other Species*. The Australian tree *Monimia rotundifolia* contains an oil rather similar, which may be safely substituted for Boldo.

BONESET

Eupatorium perfoliatum (LINN.)
N.O. Compositæ

Synonym. Thoroughwort
Part Used. Herb
Habitat. Thoroughwort or Boneset is a very common and familiar plant in low meadows and damp ground in North America, extending from Nova Scotia to Florida

Boneset was a favourite medicine of the North American Indians, who called it by a name that is equivalent to 'Ague-weed,' and it has always been a popular remedy in the United States, probably no plant in American domestic practice having more extensive and frequent use ; it is also in use to some extent in regular practice, being official in the United States Pharmacopœia, though it is not included in the British Pharmacopœia.

¶ *Constituents*. All parts of the plant are active, but the *herb* only is official, the leaves and tops being gathered after flowering

has commenced. They contain a volatile oil, some tannic acid, and Eupatorin, a bitter glucosidal principle, also resin, gum and sugar. The virtues of the plant are yielded both tb water and alcohol.

¶ *Description*. Boneset is a perennial herb, with an erect, stout, cylindrical hairy stem, 2 to 4 feet high, branched at the top. The leaves are large, opposite, united at the base, lance-shaped, 4 to 8 inches long (the lower ones being the largest), tapering to a sharp point, the edges finely toothed, the veins prominent, the blades rough above, downy and resinous and dotted beneath. The leaves serve to distinguish the species at the first glance – they may be considered either as perforated by the stem, *perfoliate* (hence the specific name), or as consisting of two opposite leaves joined at the base, the botanical term for which is *connate*. The flower-heads are terminal and numerous, large and slightly convex, with from ten to twenty white florets, having a bristly pappus, the hairs of which are arranged in a single row. The odour of the plant is slightly aromatic, the taste astringent and strongly bitter. This species shows considerable variety in size, hairiness, form of leaves and inflorescence. It flowers from July to September.

¶ *Medicinal Action and Uses*. Stimulant, febrifuge and laxative. It acts slowly and persistently, and its greatest power is manifested upon the stomach, liver, bowels and uterus.

It is regarded as a mild tonic in moderate doses, and is also diaphoretic, more especially when taken as a warm infusion, in which form it is used in attacks of muscular rheumatism and general cold. In large doses it is emetic and purgative.

Many of the earlier works allude to this species as a diuretic, and therefore of use in dropsy, but this is an error, this property being possessed by *Eupatorium purpureum*, the purple-flowered Boneset, or Gravel Root.

It has been much esteemed as a popular febrifuge, especially in intermittent fever, and has been employed, though less successfully, in typhoid and yellow fevers. It is largely used by the negroes of the Southern United States as a remedy in all cases of fever, as well as for its tonic effects. As a mild tonic it is useful in dyspepsia and general debility, and particularly serviceable in the indigestion of old people. The infusion of 1 oz. of the dried herb to 1 pint of boiling water may be taken in wineglassful doses, hot or cold: for colds and to produce perspiration, it is given hot; as a tonic, cold.

As a remedy in catarrh, more especially in influenza, it has been extensively used and with the best effects, given in doses of a wineglassful, warm every half hour, the patient remaining in bed the whole time; after four or five doses, profuse perspiration is caused and relief is obtained. It is stated that the popular name Boneset is derived from the great value of this remedy in the treatment of a species of influenza which had much prevailed in the United States, and which from the pain attending it was commonly called Break-Bone Fever.

This species of *Eupatorium* has also been employed in cutaneous diseases, and in the expulsion of tapeworm.

See GRAVEL ROOT, EUPATORIUM, and (HEMP) AGRIMONY.

¶ *Preparations*. Powdered herb. Dose 12 to 20 grains.

Fluid extract, ½ to 1 drachm.

Eupatorin. Dose, 1 to 3 grains.

BORAGE

Borago officinalis (LINN.)
N.O. Boraginaceæ

Synonym. Burrage
Parts Used. Leaves and flowers
Habitat. The Common Borage is a hardy annual plant coming originally from Aleppo, but now naturalized in most parts of Europe and frequently found in this country, though mostly only on rubbish heaps and near dwellings, and may be regarded as a garden escape. It has long been grown freely in kitchen gardens, both for its uses as a herb and for the sake of its flowers, which yield excellent honey

¶ *Description*. The whole plant is rough with white, stiff, prickly hairs. The round stems, about 1½ feet high, are branched, hollow and succulent; the leaves alternate, large, wrinkled, deep green, oval and pointed, 3 inches long or more, and about 1½ inch broad, the lower ones stalked, with stiff, one-celled hairs on the upper surfaces and on the veins below, the margins entire, but wavy. The flowers, which terminate the cells, are bright blue and star-shaped, distinguished from those of every plant in this order by their prominent black anthers, which form a cone in the centre and have been described as their beauty spot. The fruit consists of four brownish-black nutlets.

¶ *History*. In the early part of the nineteenth century, the young tops of Borage were still sometimes boiled as a pot-herb, and the young leaves were formerly considered good in salads.

The fresh herb has a cucumber-like fragrance. When steeped in water, it imparts a coolness to it and a faint cucumber flavour, and compounded with lemon and sugar in wine, and water, it makes a refreshing and restorative summer drink. It was formerly always an ingredient in cool tankards of wine and cider, and is still largely used in claret cup.

Our great grandmothers preserved the flowers and candied them.

Borage was sometimes called Bugloss by

the old herbalists, a name that properly belongs to *Anchusa officinalis*, the Alkanet, the Small Bugloss being *Lycopsis arvensis*, and Viper's Bugloss being the popular name for *Echium vulgare*.

Some authorities consider that the Latin name Borago, from which our popular name is taken, is a corruption of *corago*, from *cor*, the heart, and *ago*, I bring, because of its cordial effect.

In all the countries bordering the Mediterranean, where it is plentiful, it is spelt with a double 'r,' so the word may be derived from the Italian *borra*, French *bourra*, signifying hair or wool, words which in their turn are derived from the Low Latin *burra*, a flock of wool, in reference to the thick covering of short hairs which clothes the whole plant.

Henslow suggests that the name is derived from *barrach*, a Celtic word meaning 'a man of courage.'

Gerard says:

'Pliny calls it Euphrosinum, because it maketh a man merry and joyfull: which thing also the old verse concerning Borage doth testifie:

Ego Borago   I, Borage
Gaudia semper ago.   Bring alwaies courage.

Those of our time do use the flowers in sallads to exhilerate and make the mind glad. There be also many things made of these used everywhere for the comfort of the heart, for the driving away of sorrow and increasing the joy of the minde. The leaves and floures of Borage put into wine make men and women glad and merry and drive away all sadnesse, dulnesse and melancholy, as Dioscorides and Pliny affirme. Syrup made of the floures of Borage comforteth the heart, purgeth melancholy and quieteth the phrenticke and lunaticke person. The leaves eaten raw ingender good bloud, especially in those that have been lately sicke.'

According to Dioscorides and Pliny, Borage was the famous Nepenthe of Homer, which when drunk steeped in wine, brought absolute forgetfulness.

John Evelyn, writing at the close of the seventeenth century, tells us: 'Sprigs of Borage are of known virtue to revive the hypochrondriac and cheer the hard student.'

Parkinson commends it 'to expel pensiveness and melanchollie.' Bacon says that it 'hath an excellent spirit to repress the fuliginous vapour of dusky melancholie.' Culpepper finds the plant useful in putrid and pestilential fever, the venom of serpents, jaundice, consumption, sore throat, and rheumatism.'

¶ *Cultivation.* Borage flourishes in ordinary soil. It may be propagated by division of rootstocks in spring and by putting cuttings of shoots in sandy soil in a cold frame in summer and autumn, or from seeds sown in fairly good, light soil, from the middle of March to May, in drills 18 inches apart, the seedlings being thinned out to about 15 inches apart in the rows. If left alone, Borage will seed itself freely and comes up year after year in the same place. Seeds may also be sown in the autumn. Those sown then will flower in May, whereas those sown in the spring will not flower till June.

¶ *Part Used Medicinally.* The leaves, and to a lesser extent, the flowers. Gather the leaves when the plant is coming into flower. Strip them off singly and reject any that are stained and insect-eaten. Pick only on a fine day, when the sun has dried off the dew.

¶ *Constituents.* Borage contains potassium and calcium, combined with mineral acids. The fresh juice affords 30 per cent., the dried herb 3 per cent. of nitrate of potash. The stems and leaves supply much saline mucilage, which when boiled and cooked likewise deposits nitre and common salt. It is to these saline qualities that the wholesome invigorating properties of Borage are supposed to be due. Owing to the presence of nitrate of potash when burnt, it will emit sparks with a slight explosive sound.

¶ *Medicinal Action and Uses.* Diuretic, demulcent, emollient. Borage is much used in France for fevers and pulmonary complaints. By virtue of its saline constituents, it promotes the activity of the kidneys and for this reason is employed to carry off feverish catarrhs. Its demulcent qualities are due to the mucilage contained in the whole plant.

For internal use, an infusion is made of 1 oz. of leaves to 1 pint of boiling water, taken in wineglassful doses.

Externally, it is employed as a poultice for inflammatory swellings.

¶ *Preparation.* Fluid extract. Dose, $\frac{1}{2}$ to 1 drachm.

The flowers, candied and made into a conserve, were deemed useful for persons weakened by long sickness, and for those subject to swoonings; the distilled water was considered as effectual, and also valuable to cure inflammation of the eyes.

The juice in syrup was thought not only to be good in fevers, but to be a remedy for jaundice, itch and ringworm. Culpepper tells us that in his days: 'The dried herb is never used, but the green, yet the ashes thereof boiled in mead or honeyed water, is available in inflammation and ulcers in the mouth or throat, as a gargle.'

BOX

Buxus sempervirens (LINN.)
N.O. Buxaceæ

Synonym. Dudgeon
Parts Used. Wood and leaves
Habitat. Chiefly in limestone districts in western and southern Europe, westward to the Himalayas and Japan, northward to central and western France and in Britain, in some parts of southern and central England

¶ *Description.* Box in its familiar dwarfed state is merely a shrub, but when left to grow naturally it will become a small tree 12 to 15 feet in height, rarely exceeding 20 feet, with a trunk about 6 inches in diameter, covered with a rugged, greyish bark, that of the branches being yellowish. It belongs to the family *Buxaceæ*, a very small family of only six genera and about thirty species, closely related to the Spurge family – *Euphorbiaceæ*. Only this evergreen species has been utilized in medicine.

Its twigs are densely leafy and the leaves are about $\frac{1}{2}$ inch in length, ovate, entire, smooth, thick, coriaceous and dark green. They have a peculiar, rather disagreeable odour and a bitter and somewhat astringent taste. The flowers are in heads, a terminal female flower, surrounded by a number of male flowers. The fruit dehisces explosively, the inner layer of the pericarp separating from the outer and shooting out the seed by folding into a U-shape.

¶ *Constituents.* The *leaves* have been found to contain besides a small amount of tannin and unimportant constituents, a butyraceous volatile oil and three alkaloids: (*i*) Buxine, the important constituent, chiefly responsible for the bitter taste and now regarded as identical with the Berberine of Nectander bark, (*ii*) Parabuxine, (*iii*) Parabuxonidine, which turns turmeric paper deep red. The *bark* contains chlorophyll, wax, resin, argotized tallow, gum, lignin, sulphates of potassium and lime, carbonates of lime and magnesia, phosphates of lime, iron and silica.

¶ *Medicinal Action and Uses.* The *wood* in its native countries is considered diaphoretic, being given in decoction as an alterative for rheumatism and secondary syphilis. Used as a substitute for guaiacum in the treatment of venereal disease when sudorifics are considered to be the correct specifics.

It has been found narcotic and sedative in full doses; emetico-cathartic and convulsant in overdose. The tincture was formerly used as a bitter tonic and antiperiodic and had the reputation of curing leprosy.

A volatile oil distilled from the wood has been prescribed in cases of epilepsy. The oil has been employed for piles and also for toothache.

The leaves, which have a nauseous taste, have sudorific, alterative and cathartic properties being given in powder, in which form they are also an excellent vermifuge.

Various extracts and perfumes were formerly made from the leaves and *bark*. A decoction was recommended by some writers as an application to promote the growth of the hair. The leaves and sawdust boiled in lye were used to dye hair an auburn colour.

Dried and powdered, the leaves are still given to horses for the purpose of improving their coats. The powder is regarded by carters as highly poisonous, to be given with great care. In Devonshire, farriers still employ the old-fashioned remedy of powdered Box leaves for bot-worm in horses.

In former days, Box was the active ingredient in a once-famous remedy for the bite of a mad dog.

Animals in this country will not touch Box, and though camels are said to readily eat the leaves, they are poisoned by them.

The *timber*, though small, is valuable on account of its hardness and heaviness, being the hardest and heaviest of all European woods. It is of a delicate yellow colour, dense in structure with a fine uniform grain, which gives it unique value for the wood-engraver, the most important use to which it is put being for printing blocks and engraving plates. An edge of this wood stands better than tin or lead, rivalling brass in its wearing power. A large amount is used in the manufacture of measuring rules, various mathematical instruments, flutes and other musical instruments and the wooden parts of tools, for which a perfectly rigid and non-expansive material is required, as well as for toilet boxes, pill-rounders and similar articles.

The Boxwood used by cabinet-makers and turners in France is chiefly the root. Gerard tells us:

'The root is likewise yellow and harder than the timber, but of greater beauty and more fit for dagger haftes, boxes and suchlike. Turners and cuttlers do call this wood Dudgeon, wherewith they make Dudgeon-hafted daggers.'

In France, Boxwood has been used as a *substitute for hops* and the branches and leaves of Box have been recommended as by far the best manure for the vine, as it is said no plant by its decomposition affords a greater quantity of vegetable manure.

¶ *Dosage.* As a *purgative*: dose of the powdered leaves, 1 drachm.

As *vermifuge*: 10 to 20 grains of the powdered leaves.

As *sudorific*: 1 to 2 oz. of the wood, in decoction.

¶ *Other Species.* DWARF BOX (*Buxus suffructaca*) possesses similar medicinal properties.

The *American Boxwood* used in herbal medicine as a substitute for Peruvian Bark, being a good tonic, astringent and stimulant, is not this Box but a kind of Dogwood, native to America, *Cornus florida*.

¶ As *Adulterant.* Box bark, which is also bitter and free from tannin, is sometimes substituted for Pomegranate Bark, which is employed as a worm-dispeller.

Box leaves have sometimes been substituted for Bearberry leaves (*Uva-Ursi*), from which they are distinguished by their notched apex.

Box leaves are also sometimes used as adulteration of senna, but are easily detected by their shape and thickness.

The custom of clipping Dwarf Box in topiary gardening is said to have originated with the Romans, a friend of Julius Cæsar having invented it.

BOXWOOD, AMERICAN

Cornus florida (LINN.)
N.O. Cornaceæ

Synonyms. Bitter Redberry. Cornel. New England Boxwood. Dog-Tree. Flowering Dogwood. American Dogwood. Benthamidia florida. Box Tree. Virginian Dogwood. Cornouiller à grandes fleurs. Mon-ha-can-ni-min-schi. Hat-ta-wa-no-min-schi

Part Used. The dried bark of the root

Habitat. The United States, from Massachusetts to Florida

¶ *Description.* An ornamental little tree introduced into English cultivation about 1740, but still uncommon. It grows from 10 to 30 feet in height, with oval, opposite leaves, dark, clear green above and lighter below. The flowers occur in a small bunch surrounded by four large, white, involucral bracts that give the tree the appearance of bearing large white flowers. The name 'Florida' alludes to this effect, and the name 'Cornus,' from *cornu*, 'a horn,' refers to the density of the wood. It flowers so punctually in the third week in May that it sets the time for the Indians' corn-planting. The oval berries are a brilliant red. The bark is blackish, and cut into almost square sections. The inner bark can be utilized to make black ink, half an ounce of bark being mixed with two scruples of sulphate of iron and two scruples of gum-arabic dissolved in sixteen ounces of rainwater. A scarlet pigment can be obtained from the root bark. The wood is heavy and fine-grained, valuable for small articles because it takes an excellent polish. It is cut in autumn and dried before using. The twigs, stripped of their bark, whiten the teeth, and are used as a dentifrice by the Creoles who inhabit Virginia. The juice of the twigs preserves and hardens the gums. A bitter but agreeable drink can be prepared from the fruits infused in eau-de-vie.

In commerce the bark is usually in quilled pieces several inches long and from $\frac{1}{2}$ to 2 inches broad, which may be covered with the greyish-red outer bark or may be deprived of it. They are brittle, and the short fracture shows a mottled red and white colour. There is a slight odour, and the taste is bitter and a little aromatic; when fresh, almost acrid. The powder is a reddish-grey colour.

¶ *Constituents.* The bark has been found to contain tannic and gallic acids, resin, gum, extractive, oil, wax, red colouring matter, lignin, potassa, lime, magnesia, iron, and a neutral, crystalline glucoside called Cornin. Either water or alcohol extracts the virtues of the bark. The flowers are said to have similar properties, and to be sometimes used as a substitute. It is said that the berries, boiled and pressed, yield a limpid oil.

¶ *Medicinal Action and Uses.* Before Europeans discovered America, the Red Indians were using the bark in the same way as Peruvian bark. It is valuable in intermittent fevers, as a weak tonic for the stomach, and antiperiodic, as a stimulant and astringent. As a poultice in anthrax, indolent ulcers, and inflamed erysipelas, it is tonic, stimulant and antiseptic. In the recent state it should be avoided, as it disagrees with stomach and bowels. Cinchona bark or sulphate of quinea often replace it officially. 35 grains of Cornus bark are equal to 30 grains of cinchona bark.

The leaves make good fodder for cattle, and in Italy the oil is used in soups.

The ripe fruit, infused in brandy, is used as a stomachic in domestic practice, and a tincture of the berries restores tone to the stomach in alcoholism. Hippocrates, Dioscorides, and Pliny recommend them in diarrhœa.

¶ *Dosage*. Formerly, 1 to 2 oz. of the powder between paroxysms of intermittent fever. Of fluid extract, 30 minims as a tonic. Of cornin, 2 grains.

¶ *Other Species*. *C. circinata*, or Round-leaved Dogwood, and *C. Amomum* or *C. Sericea* (Silky Cornel or Swamp Dogwood), have similar properties and are sometimes used as substitutes.

C. sanguinea or *C. stolonifera*, a European species, is stated to have cured hydrophobia. A decoction was formerly used for washing mangy dogs, hence its name of Dogberry or Hound's Tree. It also yields an oil that is both edible and good for burning.

A Chilian species has edible berries, with which a drink called *Theca* is prepared. The juice of the leaves, or *Maqui*, is administered in angina.

C. cærulea has an astringent bark.

C. mascula, called in Greece *akenia*, and in Turkey *kizziljiek*, or redwood, yields the red dye used for the fez, and the astringent fruit is good in bowel complaints, and is used in cholera and for flavouring sherbet. The flowers are used in diarrhœa, and the berries were formerly made into tarts called *rob de cornis*.

The dwarf *C. suecica* has small red berries which form part of the Esquimaux' winter food-store. In Scotland they have such a reputation as a tonic for the appetite that the tree is called lus-a-chraois, or Plant of Gluttony.

Dogwood is also a popular name of *Pisicia Erythrina*, which yields a powerful soporific used for toothache. Its chief use is for poisoning birds, fish, or animals, which may be eaten afterwards without ill effect. Fish after eating it may be caught in the hand, stupefied.

BROOKLIME

Veronica beccabunga (LINN.)
N.O. Scrophulariaceæ

Synonyms. Water Pimpernel. Becky Leaves. Cow Cress. Horse Cress. Housewell Grass. Limewort. Brooklembe. Limpwort. Wall-ink. Water-Pumpy. Well-ink
Part Used. Herb
Habitat. Brooklime is found in all parts of Great Britain, being very common and generally distributed, occurring as far north as the Shetlands, and in the Highlands ascending up to 2,800 feet. It is found in Ireland and the Channel Islands

¶ *Description*. It grows abundantly in shallow streams, ditches, the margins of ponds, etc., flourishing in the same situations as Water Cress and Water Mint, throwing out stout, succulent, hollow stems that root and creep along the ground at the base, giving off roots at intervals, and then ascend, bearing pairs of short, stalked, oval-oblong leaves, smooth, about 1½ inch long, slightly toothed on their margin and thick and leathery in texture. The whole plant is very smooth and shiny in appearance, turning blackish in drying. The flowers are rather numerous, in lax, axillary racemes, 2 to 4 inches long, given off in pairs, whereas in Germander, Speedwell, only one flower stem rises from each pair of leaves. They begin to open in May and continue in succession through the greater part of the summer, though are at their best in May and June. The corollas are bright blue, with darker veins and a white eye, the petals oval and unequal. Occasionally a pink form is found.

The flower is adapted for cross-fertilization in the same manner as *Veronica chamædrys*, the stamens and style projecting from the flower and forming an alighting place for insects. The petals are wide open in the sun, but only partly expanded in dull weather. The flowers are much visited by insects, especially by a fly, *Syritta pipians*. The

Honey Bee is also a visitor and some other small wild bees. Two species of beetle and the larva of a moth, *Athalia annulata*, feed on the leaves. The capsule is round, flat, notched and swollen and contains winged, smooth seeds.

The specific name of this plant seems to be derived from the German name, *Bachbunge bach*, signifying a brook, and *bunge*, a bunch. Another source given for the specific name is from the Flemish *beckpunge*, meaning 'mouth smart,' a name suggested by the pungency of its leaves, which were formerly eaten in salads. Dr. Prior tells us that the name Brooklime is in old writers Broklempe or Lympe, from its growing in the *lime* or mud of brooks, the Anglo-Saxon word *lime*, coming from the Latin *limus*, a word that from mud used in the rude buildings of Anglo-Saxon times, has come to be applied to the calcareous stone of which mortar is now made.

¶ *Constituents*. Tannin and a special bitter principle, a pungent volatile oil and some sulphur.

¶ *Medicinal Action and Uses*. Alterative, Diuretic. The leaves and young stems were once in favour as an antiscorbutic, and even now the young shoots are sometimes eaten in spring with those of Watercress, the two plants being generally found growing together. As a green vegetable, Brooklime is also wholesome, but not very palatable.

In earlier days the leaves were applied to wounds, though their styptic qualities appear to be slight. They are sometimes bruised and put on burns.

The juice, with that of scurvy-grass and Seville oranges, formed the 'spring juices' once valued as an antiscorbutic.

The plant has always been a popular simple for scrofulous affections, especially of the skin. An infusion of the leaves is recommended for impurity of the blood, an ounce of them being infused in a pint of boiling water.

In the fourteenth century, Brooklime was used for many complaints, including swellings, gout, etc.

BROOM

Cytisus scoparius (LINN.)
N.O. Leguminosæ

Synonyms. Spartium scoparium (Linn.). Genista scoparius (Lam.). Sarothamnus scoparius (Koch). Broom Tops. Irish Tops. Basam. Bisom. Bizzom. Browme. Brum. Breeam. Green Broom
Part Used. Tops
Habitat. The densely-growing Broom, a shrub indigenous to England and common in this country, grows wild all over temperate Europe and northern Asia, being found in abundance on sandy pastures and heaths. It is sparingly naturalized in sandy soil in North America

It is remarkable as the only native medicinal plant used as an *official* drug that we draw from the important order of the *Leguminosæ*, or pod-bearing tribe. Though now more generally known as *Cytisus scoparius* (Linn.), it has also been named *Spartium scoparium* (Linn.), *Sarothamnus scoparius* (Koch), and *Genista scoparius* (Lam.).

Its long, slender, erect and tough branches grow in large, close fascicles, thus rendering it available for broom-making, hence its English name. The local names of Basam, Bisom, Bizzom, Breeam, Browme, Brum and Green Broom have all been given it in reference to the habit of making brooms of it, and the name of the genus, *Sarothamnus*, to which it was formerly assigned, also points out this use of the plant, being formed from the Greek words signifying 'to sweep' and 'a shrub.' The specific name, *Scoparius*, also, is derived from the Latin *scopa*, a besom. The generic name *Cytisus* is said to be a corruption of the name of a Greek island, Cythnus, where Broom abounded, though it is probable that the Broom known to the ancients, and mentioned by Pliny and by Virgil under the name of *Genista*, was another species, the Spanish Broom, *Spartium junceum*, as the Common Broom is in Greece and not found in Southern and Eastern Europe, being chiefly a native of Western, Northern and Central Europe.

The medicinal use of the brush-like branches of the Broom, under the name Genista, Genesta, or Genestia, is mentioned in the earliest printed herbals, under Passau, 1485, the *Hortus Sanitatis*, 1491, the *Grete Herball*, 1516, and others. It is likewise the Genista figured by the German botanists and pharmacologists of the sixteenth century.

Broom was used in ancient Anglo-Saxon medicine and by the Welsh physicians of the early Middle Ages. It had a place in the London Pharmacopœia of 1618 and is included in the British Pharmacopœia of the present day.

Bartholomew says of Broom:

'Genesta hath that name of bytterness for it is full of bytter to mannes taste. And is a shrub that growyth in a place that is forsaken, stony and untylthed. Presence thereof is witnesse that the ground is bareyne and drye that it groweth in. And hath many braunches knotty and hard. Grene in winter and yelowe floures in somer thyche (the which) wrapped with hevy (heavy) smell and bitter sauer (savour). And ben, netheles, moost of vertue.'

¶ *Description.* It grows to a height of 3 to 5 feet and produces numerous long, straight, slender bright green branches, tough and very flexible, smooth and prominently angled. The leaves are alternate, hairy when young, the lower ones shortly stalked, with three small, oblong leaflets, the upper ones, near the tips of the branches, sessile and small, often reduced to a single leaflet. Professor G. Henslow (*Floral Rambles in Highways and Byways*) says with reference to the 'leaves' of the broom: 'It has generally no leaves, the green stems undertaking their duties instead. If it grows in wet places, it can develop three-foliate leaves.' The large bright yellow, papilionaceous, fragrant flowers, in bloom from April to July, are borne on axillary footstalks, either solitary or in pairs, and are succeeded by oblong, flattened pods, about 1½ inch long, hairy on the edges, but smooth on the sides. They are nearly black when mature. They burst with a sharp report when the seeds are ripe, flinging them to a distance by the spring-like twisting of the valves or sides of the pods. The continuous crackling of the bursting seed-vessels on a hot, sunny July day is readily noticeable. The flowers have a great attraction for bees; they contain no honey, but abundance of pollen.

'In flowers without honey, such as the Broom, there is a curious way of "exploding" to expel the pollen. In the Broom the stigma lies in the midst of the five anthers of the longer stamens, and when a bee visits the flower those of the shorter explode and disperse their pollen on the bee pressing upon the closed edges of the keel petal. "The shock is not enough to drive the bee away . . . The split now quickly extends further . . . when a second and more violent explosion occurs." The style was horizontal with a flattened end below the stigma; but when freed from restraint it curls inwards, forming more than a complete spiral turn. It springs up and strikes the back of the bee with its stigma. The bee then gathers pollen with its mouth and legs.' (From *The Fertilization of Flowers*, by Professor H. Mueller, pp. 195–6.)

¶ *History*. As a heraldic device, the Broom was adopted at a very early period as the badge of Brittany. Geoffrey of Anjou thrust it into his helmet at the moment of going into battle, that his troops might see and follow him. As he plucked it from a steep bank which its roots had knit together, he is reputed to have said: 'This golden plant, rooted firmly amid rock, yet upholding what is ready to fall, shall be my cognizance. I will maintain it on the field, in the tourney and in the court of justice.' Fulke of Anjou bore it as his personal cognizance, and Henry II of England, his grandson, as a claimant of that province, also adopted it, its mediæval name *Planta genista*, giving the family name of Plantagenets to his line. It may be seen on the Great Seal of Richard I, this being its first official, heraldic appearance in England. Another origin is claimed for the heraldic use of the Broom in Brittany. A prince of Anjou assassinated his brother there and seized his kingdom, but being overcome by remorse, he made a pilgrimage to the Holy Land, in expiation of his crime. Every night on the journey, he scourged himself with a brush of 'genets,' or genista, and adopted this plant as his badge, in perpetual memory of his repentance. St. Louis of France continued the use of this token, founding a special order on the occasion of his marriage in the year 1234. The *Colle de Genet*, the collar of the order, was composed alternately

of the fleur-de-lys of France and the Broom-flower, the Broomflower being worn on the coat of his bodyguard of a hundred nobles, with the motto, 'Exaltat humiles,' 'He exalteth the lowly.' The order was held in great esteem and its bestowal regarded as a high honour. Our Richard II received it, and a Broom plant, with open, empty pods, can be seen ornamenting his tomb in Westminster Abbey. In 1368 Charles V of France bestowed the insignia of the Broom pod on his favourite chamberlain, and in 1389 Charles VI gave the same decoration to his kinsmen.

The Broom is the badge of the Forbes. Thus, according to Sandford, it was the bonny broom which the Scottish clan of Forbes wore in their bonnets when they wished to arouse the heroism of their chieftains, and which in their Gaelic dialect they called *bealadh*, in token of its beauty.

'This humble shrub,' writes Baines, 'was not less distinguished than the Rose herself during the civil wars of the fourteenth century.'

Apart from its use in heraldry, the Broom has been associated with several popular traditions. In some parts, it used to be considered a sign of plenty when it bore many flowers. The flowering tops were used for house decoration at the Whitsuntide festival, but it was considered unlucky to employ them for menial purposes when in full bloom. An old Suffolk tradition runs:

'If you sweep the house with blossomed Broom in May
You are sure to sweep the head of the house away.'

And a yet older tradition is extant that when Joseph and Mary were fleeing into Egypt, the plants of the Broom were cursed by the Virgin because the crackling of their ripe pods as they touched them in passing, risked drawing the attention of the soldiers of Herod to the fugitives.

The Broom has been put to many uses. When planted on the sides of steep banks, its roots serve to hold the earth together. On some parts of our coast, it is one of the first plants that grow on the sand-dunes after they have been somewhat consolidated on the surface by the interlacing stems of the mat grasses and other sand-binding plants. It will flourish within reach of sea spray, and, like gorse, is a good sheltering plant for sea-side growth.

Broom is grown extensively as a shelter for game, and also in fresh plantations among more important species of shrubs, to protect them from the wind till fully established. The shrub seldom grows large enough to furnish useful wood, but when its stem acquires sufficient size, it is beautifully veined, and being very hard, furnishes the cabinetmaker with most valuable material for veneering.

The twigs and branches are serviceable not only for making brooms, but are also used for basket-work, especially in the island of Madeira. They are sometimes used in the north of England and Scotland for thatching cottages and cornricks, and as substitutes for reeds in making fences or screens.

The bark of the Common Broom yields an excellent fibre, finer but not so strong as that of the Spanish Broom, which has been employed from very ancient times; it is easily separated by macerating the twigs in water, like flax. From the large quantity of fibrous matter contained, the shoots have been used in the manufacture of paper and cloth.

Tannin exists in considerable amount in the bark, which has been used in former times for tanning leather.

Before the introduction of Hops, the tender green tops were often used to communicate a bitter flavour to beer, and to render it more intoxicating.

Gerard says of the Broom:

'The common Broom groweth almost everywhere in dry pastures and low woods. It flowers at the end of April or May, and then the young buds of the flowers are to be gathered and laid in pickle or salt, which afterwards being washed or boiled are used for sallads as capers be and be eaten with no less delight.'

Broom buds were evidently a favourite delicacy, for they appeared on three separate tables at the Coronation feast of James II. The flowers served the double purpose of an appetizer and a corrective.

Sometimes a bunch of green Broom tied up with coloured ribbons was carried by the guests at rustic weddings instead of rosemary, when that favourite aromatic herb proved scarce.

Withering (*Arrangement of Plants*) stated that the green tops were a good winter food for sheep, preventing rot and dropsy in them.

The blossoms were used for making an unguent to cure the gout, and Henry VIII used to drink a water made from the flowers against the surfeit.

Dodoens (*Herbal*, 1606) recommended a decoction of the tops in dropsy and for 'stoppages of the liver.'

Gerard tells us: 'The decoction of the twigs and tops of Broom doth cleanse and open the liver, milt and kidnies.'

Culpepper considered the decoction of Broom to be good not only for dropsy, but also for black jaundice, ague, gout, sciatica and various pains of the hips and joints.

Some of the old physicians burned the tops to ashes and infused the salts thus extracted in wine. They were known as Salts of Broom (*Sal Genistæ*).

The powdered seeds are likewise administered and sometimes a tincture is employed. Bruised Broom seeds were formerly used infused in rectified spirit, allowed to stand two weeks and then strained. A tablespoonful in a glass of peppermint water was taken daily for liver complaints and ague.

The leaves or young tops yield a green dye.

The seeds have similar properties to the tops, and have also been employed medicinally, though they are not any longer used officially. They have served as a substitute for coffee.

¶ *Cultivation.* Broom is most easily raised from seed, sown broadcast in the open air, as soon as ripe. Seedlings may be transplanted in autumn or spring to their permanent position. Prune directly after flowering, if the shoots have not been gathered for medicinal use, shortening the old shoots to the base of promising young ones.

As their roots strike down deeply into the ground, the plants can be grown in dry, sandy soil, where others will not grow. They do well on rough banks.

Broom may also be increased by layers. Choice garden varieties are generally increased by cuttings inserted in cold frames in September.

¶ *Constituents.* Broom contains two principles on which its activity depends. *Sparteine*, discovered in 1851 by Stenhouse, of which about 0·03 per cent. is present, is a transparent, oily liquid, colourless when fresh, turning brown on exposure, of an aniline-like odour and a very bitter taste. It is but slightly soluble in water, but readily soluble in alcohol and ether. Stenhouse stated that the amount of Sparteine in Broom depends much upon external conditions, that grown in the shade yielding less than that produced in sunny places.

Scoparin, the other principal constituent, is a glucoside, occurring in pale-yellow crystals, colourless and tasteless, soluble in alcohol and hot water. It represents most of the direct diuretic activity of Broom.

Volatile oil, tannin, fat, wax, sugar, etc., are also present. Broom contains a very large quantity of alkaline and earthy matter, on incineration yielding about 3 per cent. of ash, containing 29 per cent. of carbonate of potash.

Sparteine forms certain salts of which the

sulphate (official in the British and the United States Pharmacopœias) is most used in medicine. It occurs in colourless crystals, readily soluble in water.

Oxysparteine'(formed by the action of acid on Sparteine) is used as a cardiac stimulant.

The *flowers* contain volatile oil, fatty matter, wax, chlorophyll, yellow colouring matter, tannin, a sweet substance, mucilage, albumen and lignin. Scoparin and the alkaloid sparteine have been separated from them.

¶ *Part Used Medicinally*. The young, herbaceous tips of the flowering branches are collected in early spring, generally in May, as they contain most alkaloid at the close of the winter. They are used officially both in the fresh and dried state.

Broom Juice (*Succus Scoparii*) is directed to be obtained by pressing out the bruised, *fresh* tops, adding one-third volume of alcohol and setting aside for seven days, filtering before use.

For the expression of the juice the fresh tops may be gathered in June. Broom Juice is official in the British, French, German and United States Pharmacopœias.

Infusion of Broom (*Infusum Scoparii*) is made by infusing the *dried* tops with boiling water for fifteen minutes and then straining. It was introduced in the British Pharmacopœia of 1898, in place of the decoction of Broom of the preceding issues.

The Fluid Extract of Broom of the United States Pharmacopœia is prepared from the powdered dried tops.

The drug, as it appears in commerce, consists of very long, much-branched, tough and flexible twigs, which lie parallel with and close to one another and are about $\frac{1}{25}$ to $\frac{1}{12}$ inch thick, narrowly five-winged, with alternating, slight nodes, dark-green and usually naked; internally, greenish-white.

When fresh, the whole plant has a strong and peculiar odour, especially when bruised, which almost entirely disappears on drying.

The tops are dark green when fresh and dark brownish-green when dried.

The quality of the drug deteriorates with keeping, and this condition can be determined by the partial or complete loss of the slight, peculiar odour of the recently dried drug.

The deep yellow *flowers*, dried, are considerably employed separately, under the name *Flores Genistæ*, or *Flores Scoparii*.

Broom *Seeds* are used sometimes and are as active as the tops. Water and alcohol extract their active properties.

¶ *Medicinal Action and Uses*. Diuretic and cathartic. Broom tops are used in the form of decoction and infusion, often with squill

and ammonium and potassium acetate, as a feeble diuretic, generally in dropsical complaints of cardiac origin. The action is due to the Scoparin contained, whose action on the renal mucous membrane is similar to that of Buchu and Uva-Ursi.

The infusion is made from 1 oz. of the dried tops to a pint of boiling water, taken in wineglassful doses frequently. When acute renal inflammation is present, it should not be given.

Broom Juice, in large doses, is apt to disturb the stomach and bowels and is therefore more often used as an adjuvant to other diuretics than alone.

A compound decoction of Broom is recommended in herbal medicine as of much benefit in bladder and kidney affections, as well as in chronic dropsy. To make this, 1 oz. Broomtops and $\frac{1}{2}$ oz. of Dandelion Roots are boiled in one pint of water down to half a pint, adding towards the last, $\frac{1}{2}$ oz. of bruised Juniper berries. When cold, the decoction is strained and a small quantity of cayenne added. A wineglassful is taken three or four times a day.

The statements of different investigators, both clinical and pharmacological, concerning the effects of the Sparteine in preparations of Broom, have elicited absolutely opposing views on the effect upon the nerves and circulatory system. It is found to produce a transient rise in arterial pressure, followed by a longer period of decreased vascular tension. Small doses slow the heart for a short period of time and then hasten its rate and at the same time increase the volume of the pulse. Those who advocate its employment claim that it is a useful heart tonic and regulator in chronic valvular disease. It has no cumulative action, like Digitalis.

In large doses, Sparteine causes vomiting and purging, weakens the heart, depresses the nerve cells and lowers the blood pressure and has a strong resemblance to the action of Conine (Hemlock) on the heart. In extreme cases, death is caused by impairing the activity of the respiratory organs. Shepherds have long been aware of the narcotic properties of Broom, due to Sparteine, having noticed that sheep after eating it become at first excited and then stupefied, but the intoxicating effects soon pass off.

¶ *Preparations*. Fluid extract, $\frac{1}{2}$ to 1 drachm. Juice, B.P., 1 to 2 drachms. Infusion, B.P., 1 to 2 oz.

¶ *Substitutes*. It is essential that true Broom be carefully distinguished from Spanish Broom (*Spartium junceum*), since a number of cases of poisoning have occurred from the substitution of the dried flowers of Spartium for those of the true Broom.

BROOM, BUTCHER'S

Ruscus aculeatus (LINN.)
N.O. Liliaceæ

Synonyms. Kneeholy. Knee Holly. Kneeholm. Jew's Myrtle. Sweet Broom. Pettigree
Parts Used. Herb and root
Habitat. Butcher's Broom, a low, shrubby, evergreen plant, which occurs not infrequently
in woods and waste and bushy places, especially in the south of England, is sometimes called Knee Holly, though it is in no way allied to the true Holly, being a
member of the Lily tribe. It is, however, entirely different in appearance to the
bulbous plants we regard as the characteristic representatives of this group, it being,
in fact, the only Liliaceous shrub known in this country, and the only representative
of its genus among our flora, the other species of the genus, *Ruscus*, being mostly
native to northern Africa

¶ *Description.* The name Knee Holly appears to have been given it from its rising
to about the height of a man's knee (though
occasionally specimens are found growing
about 3 feet high), and from its having, like
the true Holly, prickly leaves, which are also
evergreen.

There is no other British plant exhibiting
any similarity to the Butcher's Broom. Its
tough, green, erect, striated stems, which are
destitute of bark, send out from the upper
part many short branches, plentifully furnished with very rigid leaves, which are really
a mere expansion of the stem, and terminate
each in a single sharp spine. The small
greenish-white flowers are solitary, growing
from the centre of the leaves and blossom in
the early spring. They are dioecious, i.e.
stamens and pistils are on different plants,
as is also mostly the case with the Holly and
Mistletoe. The corolla is deeply six-cleft, the
stamens, in the one kind of flower, connected
at the base, the style, in the fertile flowers,
surrounded by a nectary. The fertile flowers
are succeeded by scarlet berries as large as
cherries, which are ripe in September, and
remain attached to the plant all the winter
and cause it often to be picked for room
decoration.

Another member of the same family is
Ruscus racemosus or *Alexandrinus*, a favourite
evergreen shrub with the leaf-like branches
unarmed, and the racemes of small flowers
terminal. It is the original of the 'poets'
laurel' so often seen in classic prints. It, too,
has red berries – smaller than those of the
Butcher's Broom.

Other species are *R. androgynous*, a native
of the Canaries, which bears its flowers along
the edges of the so-called leaves; *R. Hypophyllum*, in which the flowers are borne on
the underside of the flattened branches; and
R. Hypoglossum, also from southern Europe,
in which the flowers are on the upper side
under a bract-like branchlet.

The young shoots of Butcher's Broom have
often been eaten like those of the Asparagus, a
plant to which it is closely allied. The matured

branches used to be bound into bundles
and sold to butchers for sweeping their
blocks, hence the name: Butcher's Broom.
It is frequently made into besoms in Italy.
One of the names given the plant, 'Jew's
Myrtle,' points to its use for service during
the Feast of Tabernacles. 'Pettigree' is
another old popular name, the meaning of
which is not clear.

Parkinson tells us that Butcher's Broom
was used to preserve 'hanged meate' from
being eaten by mice, and also for the making
of brooms,

'but the King's Chamber is by revolution of
time turned to the Butcher's stall, for that a
bundle of the stalkes tied together serveth
them to cleanse their stalls and from thence
have we our English name of Butcher's
broom.'

Culpepper says it is

'a plant of Mars, being of a gallant cleansing
and opening quality. The decoction of the
root drank, and a poultice made of the berries
and leaves applied, are effectual in knitting
and consolidating broken bones or parts out
of joint. The common way of using it is to
boil the root of it, and Parsley and Fennel
and Smallage in white wine, and drink the
decoction, adding the like quantity of Grass-
root to them: The more of the root you boil,
the stronger will the decoction be; it works
no ill effects, yet I hope you have wit enough
to give the strongest decoction to the
strongest bodies.'

¶ *Cultivation.* Butcher's Broom is very
hardy, thriving in almost any soil or situation, and is often planted in shrubberies or
edges of woods, on account of its remaining
green after the deciduous trees have shed
their leaves.

Propagation is generally effected by division of the roots in autumn. The shrub may
also be propagated by seed, but quicker
results are obtained by the other method.
When planted under trees it soon spreads
into large clumps.

¶ *Part Used.* The root or rhizome, collected in autumn. The root is thick, striking deep into the ground. When dry, it is brownish grey, 2 to 4 inches long and ⅓ inch in diameter, having somewhat crowded rings and rounded stem scars on the upper surface and many woody rootlets below. If a transverse section be made, a number of vascular bundles in the central portion are to be seen. The root has no odour, but its taste is sweetish at first and then slightly acrid.

The whole herb is also collected, being dried in the same manner as Holly leaves.

¶ *Medicinal Action and Uses.* Diaphoretic, diuretic, deobstruent and aperient. Was much recommended by Dioscorides and other ancient physicians as an aperient and diuretic in dropsy, urinary obstructions and nephritic cases.

A decoction of the root is the usual form of administration, and it is still considered of use in jaundice and gravel. One pint of boiling water to 1 oz. of the twigs, or ½ oz. of the bruised fresh root has also been recommended as an infusion, which may be taken as tea.

In scrofulous tumours, advantage has been realized by administering the root in doses of a drachm every morning.

The decoction, sweetened with honey, is said to clear the chest of phlegm and relieve difficult breathing.

The boughs have been employed for flogging chilblains.

BROOM, DYER'S

Genista tinctoria (LINN.)
N.O. Leguminosæ

Synonyms. Dyer's Greenwood. Dyer's Weed. Woad Waxen
(French) Genêt des Teinturiers
(German) Färberginster
Parts Used. Twigs and leaves
Habitat. The Dyer's Broom (*Genista tinctoria*, Linn.) is a small shrubby plant with narrow, pointed leaves and yellow flowers, growing in meadows, pastures and heaths and on the borders of fields, not uncommon in England, but rare in Scotland. It is wild throughout Europe and established on barren hills and on roadsides in the eastern states of North America. It is also cultivated in greenhouses in the United States, on account of its profusion of yellow papilionaceous flowers

¶ *Description.* The bright green, smooth stems, 1 to 2 feet high, are much branched; the branches erect, rather stiff, smooth or only lightly hairy and free from spines. The leaves are spear-shaped, placed alternately on the stem, smooth, with uncut margins, ½ to 1 inch in length, very smoothly stalked; the margins fringed with hairs.

The shoots terminate in spikes of bright-yellow, pea-like flowers, opening in July. They are ½ to ¾ inch long, on foot-stalks shorter than the calyx. Like those of the Broom, they 'explode' when visited by an insect. The 'claws' of the four lower petals are straight at first, but in a high state of tension, so that the moment they are touched, they curl downwards with a sudden action and the flower bursts open. The flowers are followed by smooth pods, 1 to 1¼ inch long, much compressed laterally, brown when ripe, containing five to ten seeds.

A dwarf kind grows in tufts in meadows in the greater part of England and is said to enrich poor soil.

Cows will sometimes eat the plant, and it communicates an unpleasant bitterness to their milk and even to the cheese and butter made from it.

All parts of the plant, but especially the flowering tops, yield a good yellow dye, and from the earliest times have been used by dyers for producing this colour, especially for wool; combined with woad, an excellent green is yielded, the colour being fixed with alum, cream of tartar and sulphate of lime. In some parts of England, the plant used to be collected in large quantities by the poor and sold to the dyers.

Tournefort (1708) describes the process of dyeing linen, woollen, cloth or leather by the use of this plant, which he saw in the island of Samos. It is still applied to the same purpose in some of the Grecian islands. The Romans employed it for dyeing, and it is described by several of their writers.

The plant is called in French *Genêt des Teinturiers* and in German *Färberginster*. Its English name in the fourteenth century was Wede-wixin, or Woud-wix, which later became Woad Waxen. We find it also called Green Weed and Dyer's Weed.

It has diuretic, cathartic and emetic properties and both flower tops and seeds have been used medicinally, though it has never been an official drug.

The powdered seeds operate as a mild purgative, and a decoction of the plant has been used medicinally as a remedy in dropsy and is stated to have proved effective in gout and rheumatism, being taken in wineglassful doses three or four times a day.

The ashes form an alkaline salt, which has also been used as a remedy in dropsy and other diseases.

In the fourteenth century it was used, as well as Broom, to make an ointment called *Unguentum geneste*, 'goud for alle could goutes,' etc. The seed was also used in a plaster for broken limbs.

A decoction of the plant was regarded in the Ukraine as a remedy for hydrophobia, but its virtues in this respect do not seem to rest on very good evidence.

BROOM, SPANISH

Spartium junceum (LINN.)
N.O. Leguminosæ

Habitat. The Spanish Broom is a small shrub, indigenous in the south of Europe and cultivated as an ornamental plant. The flowers are large, yellow and of an agreeable scent. It is identified with the Spartium of the ancients, which is reputed to have been very violent in action and was said by Gerard and other herbalists 'to cause to vomit with great violence, even as white Hellebor.'

¶ *Medicinal Action and Uses.* The Spanish Broom in its medicinal properties closely resembles the common Broom, but is from five to six times more active. The symptoms produced by overdoses are vomiting and purging, with renal irritation. The seeds have been used to a considerable extent in dropsy, in the form of a tincture. The flowers yield a yellow dye.

The dried flowers of Spanish Broom are readily differentiated, those of the true Broom having a small bell-shaped calyx with two unequal lobes, the upper of which is bi-dentate and the lower minutely tridentate, while in *Spartium junceum*, the calyx is deeply cleft to the base on one side only.

By macerating the twigs a good fibre is obtained, which is made into thread in Languedoc, and its cord and a coarse sort of cloth in Dalmatia.

The name *Spartium* is from the Greek word denoting 'cardage,' in allusion to the use of the plant.

Coronilla scorpioides (Koch) has been used medicinally as substitute for Broom.

Coronilla is the herbage of various species of the genus of that name, natives of Europe and some naturalized in North America.

The drug, at least that from *Coronilla scorpioides* (Koch), contains the glucoside *Coronillin*, a yellow powder. The action and uses of the drug are very similar to those of Broom.

The leaflets are said to produce a dye like indigo by proper fermentation, and are also reported as a laxative.

See also GORSE and LABURNUM.

BROOM-CORN

Sorghum vulgare (PERS.)
N.O. Graminacæ

Synonyms. Sorghum Seeds. Sorghum Saccharatum (Moench). Guinea Corn
Part Used. Seeds
Habitat. Spain, Italy and south of Europe. Cultivated in the United States of America

¶ *Description.* Known as Millet or Guinea Corn. Is cultivated in the same way as oats or barley in northern Europe; the seeds are small, round and white, the plant is cane-like and similar to Indian Corn, but producing large heads of the small grain. Sorghum is generally classified under two varieties, saccharine and non-saccharine. The saccharine sorghums are not used for producing sugar owing to the difficulty of crystallization.

¶ *Medicinal Action and Uses.* It yields a very white flour which is used for making bread, and the grain is used for feeding cattle, horses and poultry. The grain is diuretic and demulcent if taken as a decoction. The plant is extensively cultivated in America for the manufacture of brooms and brushes.

The decoction of 2 oz. of seeds to 1 quart of water, boiled down to 1 pint, is used in urinary and kidney complaints.

In the semi-arid districts of western America it is reported that cattle have been poisoned by eating the green sorghum of the second growth; possibly due to hydrocyanic acid in the leaves.

BRYONY, BLACK (*POISON*)

Tamus communis (LINN.)
N.O. Dioscoreaceæ

Synonym. Blackeye Root
Part Used. Root

Black Bryony belongs to a family of twining and climbing plants which generally spring from large tubers, some of which are cultivated for food, as the Yam, which forms an important article of food in many tropical countries. Great Britain only furnishes one species of this tribe, *Tamus communis*, which, from its powerful, acrid and cathartic qualities, ranks as a dangerous irritant poison.

It is a very common plant in woods and hedges, with weak stems twining round anything within reach, and thus ascending or creeping among the trees and bushes to a considerable distance.

¶ *Description*. The leaves are heart-shaped, pointed, smooth and generally shining as if they had been varnished. Late in autumn they turn dark purple or bright yellow, making a very showy appearance. In winter, the stems die down, though the root is perennial.

The flowers are small, greenish-white, in loose bunches and of two kinds, barren and fertile on different plants, the latter being succeeded by berries of a red colour when ripe.

The large, fleshy root is black on the outside and exceedingly acrid, and, although an old cathartic medicine, is a most dangerous remedy when taken internally. It is like that of the yam, thick and tuberous and abounding in starch, but too acrid to be used as food in any manner.

The young shoots are said to be good eating when dressed like Asparagus; the Moors eat them boiled with oil and salt, after they have been first soaked in hot water.

Gerard says of this plant:

'The wild black Briony resembleth the white Briony vine, but has not clasping tendrils and is easier to be losed. The root is black without and of a pale yellow colour within, like Box. It differs from white Briony only in that the root is of a yellow box colour on the inside, and the fruit or berries are black when they come to ripeness.'

As to the colour of the berries, Gerard is at fault: they are bright red. Other writers have also made the same mistake. The root is nearly cylindrical, 1 to 1½ inch in diameter, 3 to 4 inches long or more, and black.

¶ *Medicinal Action and Uses*. Rubifacient, diuretic. The expressed juice of the fresh root, mixed with a little white wine, has been used as a remedy for gravel, being a powerful diuretic, but it is not given internally now, and is not included in the British Pharmacopœia. Death in most painful form is the result of an overdose, while the effect of a small quantity, varying not with the age only, but according to the idiosyncrasies of the patient, leaves little room for determining the limit between safety and destruction. The expressed juice of the root, with honey, has also been used as a remedy for asthmatic complaints, but other remedies that are safer should be preferred.

The berries act as an emetic, and children should be cautioned against eating them.

As an external irritant, Black Bryony has, however, been used with advantage, and it was formerly much employed. The scraped pulp was applied as a stimulating plaster, and in gout, rheumatism and paralysis has been found serviceable in many instances.

A tincture made from the *root* proves a most useful application to unbroken chilblains, and also the *fruits*, steeped in gin, are used for the same remedy.

Black Bryony is a popular remedy for removing discoloration caused by bruises and black eyes, etc. The fresh root is scraped to a pulp and applied in the form of a poultice.

For sores, old writers recommend it being made into an ointment with 'hog's grease or wax, or other convenient ointment.'

The generic name *Tamus* is given to the plant from the belief that it is the same as that referred to in the works of Pliny under the name of *Uva Taminia*.

The Greeks use the young suckers like Asparagus, which they much resemble.

T. cretica is a native of Greece and the Greek Archipelago.

¶ *Preparation*. Tincture, 1 to 5 drops.

BRYONY, EUROPEAN WHITE (*POISON*)

Bryonia alba (LINN.)
N.O. Cucurbitaceæ

Synonyms. Black-berried White Bryony. European White Bryony
Part Used. Root

The Black-berried White Bryony is a plant very similar in general appearance to *Bryonia dioica*, having also palmate rough leaves and similar unisexual flowers, which are succeeded, however, by globular *black* berries.

The root is very similar to that of *Bryonia dioica* and contains the same substances, but it is stated also to contain a glucoside *Brein*, which causes the drug to produce a somewhat different physiological effect.

The tincture is used by homœopathists, and is said to be one of the best diuretics in medicine. It is an excellent remedy in gravel and all other obstructions and disorders of the urinary passages, and has also been used for relieving coughs and colds of a feverish, bronchial nature.

¶ *Preparation*. Fluid extract, ⅙ to 1 drachm. Bryonin, ¼ to 2 grains.

BRYONY, WHITE (*POISON*)

Bryonia dioica (LINN.)
N.O. Cucurbitaceæ

Synonyms. English Mandrake. Wild Vine. Wild Hops. Wild Nep. Tamus. Ladies' Seal. Tetterbury
(*French*) Navet du diable
Part Used. Root
Habitat. The Cucumber tribe has a single representative among our wild plants in the Red-berried, common or White Bryony. This is a vine-like plant growing in woods and hedges, and exceedingly common in the south of England, rarer in the Midland counties, and not often found in the north of England. It is of frequent occurrence in central and southern Europe

¶ *Description.* The stems climb by means of long tendrils springing from the side of the leaf stalks, and extend among the trees and shrubs often to the length of several yards during the summer, dying away after ripening their fruit. They are angular and brittle, branched mostly at the base, and are, as well as the somewhat vine-shaped leaves, very rough to the touch, with short, prickle-like hairs – a general character of the exotic plants of this order.

The leaves are stalked, with the stalk curved, shorter than the blade, which is divided into five lobes, of which the middle one is the longest – all five are slightly angular.

The flowers, which bloom in May, are small, greenish, and produced, generally three or four together, in small bunches springing from the axils of the leaves. Stamens and pistils are never found in the same flower, nor are the flowers which have them individually ever met with on the same plant in this species, whence the name *dioica*, signifying literally 'two dwellings.' The male flowers are in loose, stalked bunches, 3 to 8 flowers in a bunch, or cyme, the stamens having one-celled, yellow anthers. The fertile flowers, easily distinguished from the barren by the presence of an ovary beneath the calyx, are generally either stalkless (sessile) or with very short stalks – two to five together. The corollas in each case consist of five petals, cohering only at the base. The outer green calyx is widely bell-shaped and five-toothed.

The berries, which hang about the bushes after the stem and leaves are withered, are almost the size of peas when ripe, a pale scarlet in colour. They are filled with juice of an unpleasant, fœtid odour and contain three to six large seeds, greyish-yellow, mottled with black, and are unwholesome to eat.

The whole plant is rather succulent, bright green and somewhat shining.

The name of the genus, *Bryonia*, derived from the Greek *bryo*, I shoot, or sprout, appears to have reference to the vigorous and active growth of its annual stems, which pro-

ceed from the perennial roots, and so rapidly cover other shrubs, adhering to them with their tendrils. *Bryonia dioica* is the only British representative of the genus.

¶ *History.* Under the name of Wild Nep it was known in the fourteenth century as an antidote to leprosy.

It produces a large, tuberous rootstock, which is continuous with a thick, fleshy root which attains an enormous size. Gerard says of it:

'The Queen's chief surgeon, Mr. William Godorous, a very curious and learned gentleman, shewed me a root hereof that waied half an hundredweight, and of the bignes of a child of a yeare old.'

This large, fleshy, pale-coloured root used often to be seen suspended in herb shops, occasionally trimmed into a rude human form. Green (*Universal Herbal*, 1832) tells us:

'The roots of Bryony grow to a vast size and have been formerly by imposters brought into a human shape, carried about the country and shown for Mandrakes to the common people. The method which these knaves practised was to open the earth round a young, thriving Bryony plant, being careful not to disturb the lower fibres of the root; to fix a mould, such as is used by those who make plaster figures, close to the root, and then to fill in the earth about the root, leaving it to grow to the shape of the mould, which is effected in one summer.'

The plant is still sometimes called Mandrake in Norfolk.

In this fleshy root is found a somewhat milky juice, very nauseous and bitter to the taste. It is of a violently purgative and cathartic nature, and was a favourite medicine with the older herbalists, well known to and much used by the Greeks and Romans, prescribed by Galen and Dioscorides, and afterwards by Gerard, but is now seldom employed by regular practitioners, though sometimes by the homœopathists, though they mostly use another variety of Bryony that is not indigenous to this country. The French call the root *Navet du Diable* (Devil's

Turnip), from its violent and dangerous action.

Withering says a decoction made by boiling one pound of the fresh root in water is 'the best purge for horned cattle,' and it has been considered a sovereign remedy for horse grip.

Gerard declared the root to be profitable for tanners to thicken their hides with.

Bartholomew's *Anglicus* tells us that Augustus Cæsar used to wear a wreath of Bryony during a thunderstorm to protect himself from lightning.

Culpepper says it is a 'furious martial plant,' but good for many complaints; among others, 'stiches in the side, palsies, cramps, convulsions,' etc.

The acrid and cathartic properties of the root are shared in some measure by all parts of the plant: the berries are emetic and even poisonous. They have been used for dyeing. The young shoots in the spring are considered to be inert, and have sometimes been boiled and eaten as greens without harm resulting. Among animals, goats alone are said to eat this plant.

The extracts made from some exotic species of this tribe, as the Squirting Cucumber (*Momordica elaterium*) and the Colocynth (*Cucumis colocynthis*), afford useful medicine.

¶ *Part Used.* The root is collected in the autumn and used both in the fresh and dry state. When fresh, it is of a dirty yellow or yellowish-white colour, externally marked at close intervals with prominent transverse corky ridges, which often extend half round the root and give it the appearance of being circularly wrinkled. Internally, it is whitish, succulent and fleshy, with a nauseous odour – which disappears in great measure on drying – and a bitter, acrid taste. The juice which exudes on cutting the root is milky, owing to the presence of numerous minute starch grains. The root is usually simple, like a carrot or parsnip, but sometimes is forked into two.

When sold dry, Bryony root appears in circular, brittle pieces, ¼ to ⅛ inch thick, about 2 inches in diameter, the thin bark greyish-brown and rough, longitudinally wrinkled, the central portion whitish or greyish, showing numerous round wood bundles arranged in concentric rays, with projecting radiating lines. The taste is disagreeably bitter, but there is no odour.

The large size, tapering shape, transverse corky ridges and nauseously bitter taste of Bryony root are distinctive. Small specimens may resemble Horseradish root, but that is cylindrical and smooth and has a pungent taste.

¶ *Medicinal Action and Uses.* Irritative, hydragogue, cathartic. Its chief use was as a hydragogue cathartic, but is now superseded by Jalap. Its use as a purgative has been discontinued as dangerous, on account of its powerful and highly irritant nature.

It was formerly given in dropsy and other complaints. It is of so acrid a character that, if applied to the skin, it produces redness and even blisters. It has been used for cataplasms, and praised as a remedy for sciatica, rheumatism and lumbago.

It is still considered useful in small doses for cough, influenza, bronchitis and pneumonia, and has also been recommended for pleurisy and whooping-cough, relieving the pain and allaying the cough.

It has proved of value in cardiac disorders caused by rheumatism and gout, also in malarial and zymotic diseases.

In case of poisoning by Bryony, the stomach must be evacuated and demulcent drinks given. The body temperature must be maintained by the use of blankets and hot bottles.

See APPLE, BITTER; and CUCUMBER, SQUIRTING.

BUCHU

Barosma betulina (BART. and WENDL.)
N.O. Rutaceæ

Synonym. Diosma betulina
Part Used. Leaves
Habitat. A small shrubby plant chiefly found in the south-west region of Cape Colony.

The standard Buchus of commerce are obtained from three species: *Barosma betulina*, known as 'shorts'; *B. crenulata*, known 'ovals' and 'shortbroads,' and *B. serratifolia*, known as 'longs.' The leaves of the first-named are most valued and constitute the *foliæ buchu* of the British Pharmacopœia.

The Hottentots use several species, all under the common name of 'Bucku.' The leaves have a rue-like smell, and are used by the natives to perfume their bodies.

Buchu leaves are collected while the plant is flowering and fruiting, and are then dried and exported from Cape Town. The bulk of the Buchu exported to London from South Africa eventually finds its way to America, where it is used in certain proprietary medicines.

¶ *Description.* The leaves of *B. betulina* (short Buchu) are of a pale green colour, ½ to ¾ inch long, ½ inch or less wide, leathery and glossy, with a blunt, strongly-curved tip and finely-toothed margin, with round oil glands scattered through the leaf. Frequently the small flowers, with five whitish petals, and the brownish fruits may be found mixed with the drug. The leaves have a strongly aromatic taste and a peppermint-like odour.

¶ *Constituents.* The principal constituents of Buchu leaves are volatile oil and mucilage, also diosphenol, which has antiseptic properties, and is considered by some to be the most important constituent of Buchu; its absence from the variety known as 'Long Buchu' has led to the exclusion of the latter leaves from the British Pharmacopœia.

The Cape Government exercises strict control over the gathering of Buchu leaves, and has lately made the terms and conditions more onerous, in order to prevent the wholesale destruction of the wild plants, no person being permitted to pick or buy Buchu without a licence. Cultivation experiments with Buchu have been made from time to time by private persons, and during the war experiments were conducted at the National Botanic Gardens, Kirstenbosch (near Cape Town), the result of which (given in the *South African Journal of Industries*, 1919, 2, 748) indicate that, under suitable conditions, the commercial cultivation of Buchu should prove a success, *B. betulina*,

the most valuable kind, being the species alone to be grown. The plant is particularly adapted to dry conditions, and may be cultivated on sunny hillsides where other crops will not succeed.

It is doubtful whether the cultivation of Buchu could be conducted satisfactorily outside South Africa. *B. betulina* was introduced to this country in 1790, but does not appear to be in cultivation at the present time, except as a greenhouse plant. This and *B. serratifolia* are grown in Kew Gardens.

¶ *Medicinal Action and Uses.* In gravel, inflammation and catarrh of the bladder it is specially useful. The infusion (B.P.) of 1 oz. of leaves to 1 pint of boiling water is taken in wineglassful doses three or four times a day.

¶ *Other Preparations.* Fluid extract: dose, ½ to 1 drachm. Tincture, B.P.: dose, ½ to 1 drachm. Solid extract: dose, 5 to 15 grains. Barosmin: dose, 2 to 3 grains.

Buchu has long been known at the Cape as a stimulant tonic and remedy for stomachic troubles, where it is infused in Brandy and known as Buchu Brandy. Its use was learnt from the Hottentots.

It was introduced into official medicine in Great Britain in 1821 as a remedy for cystitis, urethritis, nephritis and catarrh of the bladder.

BUCKBEAN. *See* BOGBEAN

BUCKTHORNS
BUCKTHORN (COMMON)

N.O. Rhamnaceæ

Synonyms. Highwaythorn. Waythorn. Hartsthorn. Ramsthorn
Part Used. Berries

Three species of the genus *Rhamnus* (the name derived from the Greek *rhamnos*, a branch) are possessed of the same medicinal properties in varying degrees.

The Common or Purging Buckthorn, a much-branched shrub, usually about 6 feet high, but sometimes as much as 10 or 12 feet, is indigenous to North Africa, the greater part of Europe and North Asia. Though found throughout England in woods and thickets and near brooks, it is practically confined to a calcareous soil, except in a few counties, such as Bucks., Herts., Oxon. and Wilts. In Scotland it occurs only in a single locality.

¶ *Description.* The main stem is erect, the bark smooth, of a blackish-brown colour, on the twigs ash-coloured. The smaller branches generally terminate in a stout thorn or spine, hence the ordinary name of Buckthorn, and the older names by which the shrub has been known: Highwaythorn and Waythorn. Gerard calls it Ram or Hart's

Thorn. The leaves grow in small bunches on footstalks, mostly opposite towards the base of the young shoots, though more generally alternate towards the apex. They are egg-shaped and toothed on the edges, the younger ones with a kind of soft down. In the axils of the more closely arranged leaves, developed from the wood of the preceding year, are dense branches of small greenish-yellow flowers, about one-fifth inch across, which are followed by globular berries about the size of a pea, black and shining when ripe, and each containing four hard, dark-brown seeds.

Goats, sheep and horses browse on this shrub, but cows refuse it. Its blossoms are very grateful to bees.

¶ *Part Used.* The *berries* are the part used medicinally, collected when ripe and from which an acrid, nauseous, bitter juice is obtained by expression. From this juice, with the addition of sugar and aromatics, syrup of Buckthorn (*Succus Rhamni*) is prepared.

When freshly gathered in the autumn, the

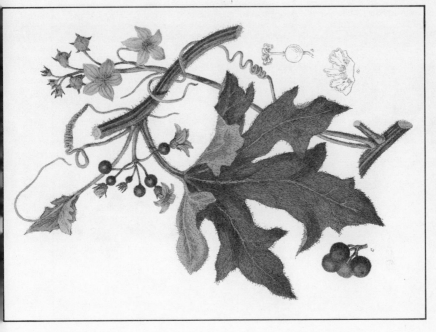

EUROPEAN WHITE BRYONY
Bryonia Alba

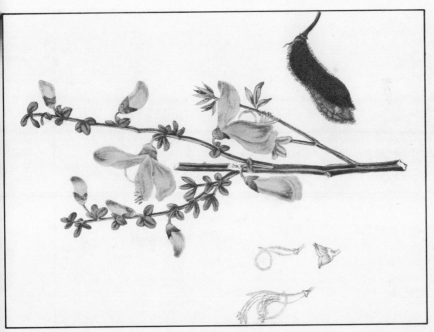

BROOM
Cytisus Scoparius

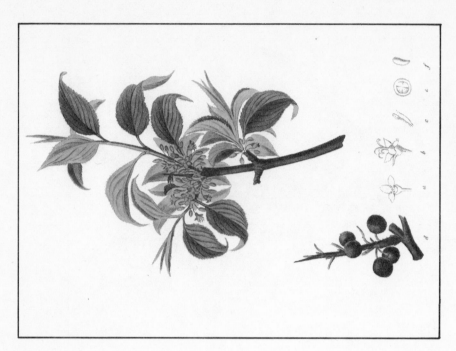

ALDER BUCK'THORN
Rhamnus Frangula

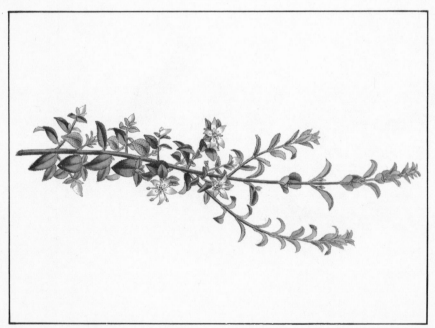

BUCHU
Barosma Betulina

berries are about ⅓ inch in diameter, with the remains of a calyx beneath. The fruit is collected for use chiefly in the counties of Herts., Bucks. and Oxon, and is usually expressed in the locality where it is grown, by the collectors themselves, who sell the juice to the wholesale druggists, generally more or less diluted with water, the admixture being generally about 6 parts water to 1 of juice.

From the dried berries, a series of rich but fugitive colours is obtained; the berries used to be sold under the name of 'French berries' and imported with those of *Rhamnus infectorius* from the Levant. If gathered before ripe, the berries furnish a yellow dye, used formerly for staining maps or paper. When ripe, if mixed with gum-arabic and lime-water, they form the pigment 'Sap or bladder green,' so well known to water-colour painters. The bark also affords a yellow dye.

¶ *Cultivation.* Buckthorn is seldom cultivated, the berries being collected from the wild shrubs, but it can be easily raised from seed in autumn, soon after the berries are ripe, usually about September, but if left too late the berries soften and will not bear carriage well. The shrub may also be propagated like any other hardy deciduous tree or shrub by cuttings or layers: if the young shoots be laid in autumn, they will have struck roots by the following autumn, when they may be separated and either planted in a nursery for a year or two, or at once planted in permanent quarters. Buckthorn is not so suitable for hedges as the hawthorn.

¶ *Constituents.* Buckthorn berry juice contains Rhamnocathartin (which is yellow and uncrystallizable), Rhamnin, a peculiar tannic acid, sugar and gum. The fresh juice is coloured red by acids and yellow by alkalies, and has a bitter taste and nauseous odour. Its specific gravity should be between 1·035 and 1·070, but it is seldom sold pure. The ripe berries yield on expression 40 to 50 per cent. of juice of a *green* colour, which on keeping turns, however, gradually to a reddish or purplish brown colour, on account of the acidification of the saccharine and mucilaginous matter.

¶ *Medicinal Action and Uses.* Laxative and cathartic.

Buckthorn was well known to the Anglo-Saxons and is mentioned as Hartsthorn or Waythorn in their medical writings and glossaries dating before the Norman Conquest. The Welsh physicians of the thirteenth century prescribed the juice of the fruit of Buckthorn boiled with honey as an aperient drink.

The medicinal use of the berries was familiar to all the writers on botany and materia medica of the sixteenth century, though Dodoens in his *Herbal* wrote: 'They be not meat to be administered but to the young and lusty people of the country which do set more store of their money than their lives.'

Until late in the nineteenth century, syrup of Buckthorn ranked, however, among favourite rustic remedies as a purgative for children, prepared by boiling the juice with pimento and ginger and adding sugar, but its action was so severe that, as time went on, the medicine was discarded. It first appeared in the London Pharmacopœia of 1650, where, to disguise the bitter taste of the raw juice, it was aromatized by means of aniseed, cinnamon, mastic and nutmeg. It was still official in the British Pharmacopœia of 1867, but is no longer so, being regarded as a medicine more fit for animals than human beings, and it is now employed almost exclusively in veterinary practice, being commonly prescribed for dogs, with equal parts of castor oil as an occasional purgative.

The flesh of birds eating the berries is stated to be purgative.

There used to be a superstition that the Crown of Thorns was made of Buckthorn.

BUCKTHORN (ALDER)

Rhamnus Frangula (LINN.)

Synonyms. Black Dogwood. Frangula Bark
Part Used. Bark
Habitat. The Alder Buckthorn is a slender shrub, widely distributed over Europe and northern Asia, and found in woods and thickets throughout England, though rare in Scotland

In place of the violently-acting juice of the berries of the Common Buckthorn, a fluid extract prepared from the bark of the closely allied and milder Alder Buckthorn or Black Alder (*Rhamnus Frangula*, Linn.) has been proved a very satisfactory substitute. Frangula bark is official both in the United States and the British Pharmacopœia. Its use has been, however, somewhat neglected and the much advertized Cascara Sagrada (*R. pur-* shianus) has greatly taken its place, though it is a less agreeable aperient.

¶ *Description.* It is generally about the same size as the Common Buckthorn, but is distinguished from it by its less bushy and more tree-like habit, by the absence of thorns on its branches and by its larger and entire, not toothed, feather-veined leaves, which are all arranged alternately on the stem, none opposite to one another. The flowers are produced not only from the wood of the preceding year, but also on the shoots of the current year, and have a five-parted calyx, while that of the Common Buckthorn is four-cleft. They bloom in May and are of an inconspicuous green. Their fruit, which is ripe in September, is not unlike that of the Common Buckthorn, but the berry has only two, or at most three, roundish, angular seeds, instead of four. Bees are likewise constant visitors of the flowers of this species, and goats eat the leaves voraciously.

It grows as a rule in leaf-mould in woods comparatively free from lime.

The bark and leaves of the Alder Buckthorn yield a yellow dye much used in Russia; when mixed with salts of iron it turns black. The berries, when unripe, afford a good green colour, readily taken by woollen stuffs; when ripe, they give various shades of blue and grey.

After removal of the bark from the stem and branches, the wood of this shrub is used for making charcoal, yielding a very light, inflammable kind, and being on that account preferred to that of almost any other tree by gunpowder makers, who name it 'Black Dogwood.' In Germany, for the same reason, it is called *Pulverholz* ('powder-wood').

¶ *Cultivation.* Frangula bark is usually collected from wild shrubs, but this Buckthorn can readily be cultivated. The seeds should be sown as soon as ripe, not kept till the following spring. The seedlings should be kept free from weeds, and in the autumn planted in the nursery in rows 2 feet asunder and 1 foot distant in the rows. Stock may also be increased by layers and cuttings, though propagation by seedling plants is preferable.

¶ *Part Used Medicinally.* The dried bark collected from the young trunk and moderately-sized branches in early summer and kept at least one year before being used. It is stripped from the branches and dried either on sunny days, out of doors, in half-shade, or by artificial heat, on shelves or trays, in a warm, well-ventilated room.

The dried bark varies considerably in appearance, according to the age of the branch or stem from which it has been taken. Young bark, which is to be preferred, occurs in narrow, single or double quills and is of papery texture, about $\frac{1}{25}$ inch thick. It is of a greyish or blackish-brown colour outside,

with numerous small, whitish corky warts. When gently scraped, the inner layers are seen to be crimson in colour. The inner surface of the bark is smooth, of a pale, yellowish brown and very finely striated. The fracture is short. Older bark is rougher externally, thicker and usually in single quills or channelled pieces.

The bark is nearly inodorous; its taste is pleasant, sweetish and slightly bitter. When masticated, it colours the saliva yellow.

¶ *Constituents.* The chemical constituents of Frangula Bark, especially those to which the laxative properties are due, are but imperfectly known. A yellow, crystalline glucoside, Frangulin has been isolated from it. Emodin is present in old bark; this principle is also present in rhubarb root; it is allied to Chrysophane, and is said to result from the glucosic fermentation of Frangulin or Frangulic acid, and to its presence the drug owes its purgative action. Possibly other glucosides are also present and contribute to the laxative action, but the evidence in favour of this assumption is not conclusive. Two resins, resinous bitter matter and a little tannic acid are likewise present in the bark.

¶ *Medicinal Action and Uses.* Tonic, laxative, cathartic.

Dried, seasoned bark from one to two years old alone should be used, as the freshly-stripped bark acts as an irritant poison on the gastro-intestinal canal. The action of the bark becomes gradually less violent when kept for a length of time and more like that of rhubarb.

It is used as a gentle purgative in cases of chronic constipation and is principally given in the form of the fluid extract, in small doses, repeated three or four times daily, a decoction of 1 oz. of the bark in 1 quart of water, boiled down to a pint, may also be taken in tablespoonful doses.

¶ *Preparation.* Fluid extract, $\frac{1}{2}$ to 2 drachms.

This milder English Buckthorn acts likewise as a tonic to the intestine and is especially useful for relieving piles.

Lozenges of the Alder Buckthorn are dispensed under the name of 'Aperient Fruit Lozenges.'

The juice of the berries, though little used, is aperient without being irritating.

Country people used to take the bark boiled in ale for jaundice.

BUCKTHORN (CALIFORNIAN)

Synonyms. Sacred Bark. Cascara Sagrada
Part Used. Bark

The Californian Buckthorn (*Rhamnus purshianus*), known more commonly as Cascara Sagrada, is a nearly-allied shrub growing in the United States, from northern Idaho westward to the Pacific Ocean. The drug prepared from its bark is now more commonly employed than those prepared from the two previously described species.

The bark is collected in spring and early summer, when it is easily peeled from the wood, and is dried in the shade.

Since, as is the case with *R. Frangula*, it is considered that the action of the bark becomes milder and less emetic by keeping, matured bark, three years old, is preferred for pharmaceutical purposes.

¶ *Description.* As imported, the drug mostly occurs in quills or incurved pieces of varying lengths and sizes, smooth or nearly so externally, covered with a greyish-white layer, which is usually easily removed, and frequently marked with spots or patches of adherent lichens. Beneath the surface it is violet-brown, reddish-brown or brownish, and internally a pale yellowish-brown and nearly smooth. It has no marked odour, but a nauseous, bitter taste.

It is frequently also imported in flattened packets, consisting of small pieces of the bark compressed into a more or less compact mass.

The fluid extract is made by maceration and percolation with diluted alcohol and evaporation.

¶ *Constituents.* The chemical constituents of the bark are but imperfectly known. It has been proved to contain Emodin and an allied substance possibly identical with the Frangula-Emodin of Alder Buckthorn bark. Fat, starch, glucose, a volatile odorous oil, malic and tannic acids are also present. The assertion has been made that the bark contains glucosides which yield on hydrolysis Chrysophanic acid, but the evidence on this point is conflicting.

¶ *Medicinal Action and Uses.* Cascara Sagrada is a mild laxative, acting principally on the large intestine. It is considered suitable for delicate and elderly persons, and may with advantage be given in chronic constipation, being generally administered in the form of the fluid extract.

It acts also as a stomachic tonic and bitter, in small doses, promoting gastric digestion and appetite.

¶ *Preparations.*
Fluid extract, B.P., 5 drops to 1 drachm.
Fluid extract, U.S.P., 15 drops.
Fluid extract, tasteless, ¼ to 1 drachm.
Fluid extract, aromatic, U.S.P., 15 drops.
Aromatic syrup, B.P., ½ to 2 drachms.
Powder extract, 2 to 10 grains.
Rhamnin, 2 to 6 grains.

In veterinary practice, Cascara Sagrada is also much used and is probably the best mild purgative remedy for dogs with chronic constipation, as the dose does not require to be increased by repetition and the tone of the bowels is improved by the drug.

BUCKTHORN (SEA)

Synonym. Sallow Thorn

The Sea Buckthorn (*Hippophæ rhamnoides*), a thorny shrub with narrow willow-like leaves growing on sandhills and cliffs on the East Coast, and called also 'Sallow Thorn,' is in no way related to these medicinally employed Buckthorns, but belongs to a different natural order: *Elæagnaceæ.* Its fruit, an orange-coloured berry, is made (in Tartary) into a pleasant jelly, because of its acid flavour, and is used in the countries bordering on the Gulf of Bothnia as an ingredient to a fish sauce. The name *Hippophæ* has been variously derived either as meaning 'giving light to a horse,' because of a supposed power to cure equine blindness, or as signifying 'shining underneath,' an allusion to the silvery underside of the leaf. The stems, roots and foliage are said to impart a yellow dye.

Henslow relates that in some parts of Europe the berries are considered poisonous, and a story is told by Rousseau of a person who saw him eating them, and, though believing them to be poisonous, had too much respect for the great man to caution him against the supposed danger! A decoction of them is said to be useful in cutaneous eruptions. The colour may be extracted by hot water and used as a dye for woollen stuffs, but it is not very brilliant when so obtained. This plant runs very much at the root, and by its long suckers often assists in binding loose sandy dunes on which it grows.

Some of the plants of this order (*Elæagnaceæ*) are said to possess narcotic properties.

BUCKWHEAT
Polygonum fagopyrum
N.O. Polygonaceæ

Synonyms. Brank. Beechwheat. Le Blé noir. Sarrasin. Buchweizen. Heidekorm. French Wheat. Saracen Corn
Part Used. The fruit
Habitat. A native of Northern or Central Asia. Largely cultivated in the United States

¶ *Description.* The Buckwheat is not really a native plant, and when found apparently wild in this country, it is only on cultivated land, where it is grown as food for pheasants, which are very partial to it. One of its local names, 'French Wheat,' points to the recognition of the fact that it is a foreign grain.

It is a native of Central Asia, cultivated in China and other Eastern countries as a bread-corn and was first brought to Europe from Asia by the Crusaders, and hence in France is called 'Saracen Corn.'

It is a herbaceous plant, with a knotted stem a foot or two in height, round and hollow, generally green, but sometimes tinged with red, lateral branches growing out of the joints, which give off alternately from opposite sides, heart-shaped, or somewhat arrow-shaped leaves, and from July to September, spreading panicles of numerous light fresh-coloured flowers, which are perfumed. They are dimorphic, i.e. there are two forms of flowers, one with long styles and short stamens, the other with short styles and long stamens and are very attractive to bees. It is frequently cultivated in the Middle United States of America and also in Brabant as food for bees, and an immense quantity of Buckwheat honey is also collected in Russia. It gives a particularly pleasant flavour to honey.

The nut (so-called 'seed') has a dark brown, tough rind, enclosing the kernel or seed, and is three-sided in form, with sharp angles, resembling the triangular Beech-nut, hence the name of the plant, Buckwheat, a corruption of *Boek-weit*, the Dutch form of the name, adopted with its culture from the Dutch, meaning 'Beech-wheat' (German *Buchweizen*), a translation of the Latin name *Fagopyrum* (Latin *fagus*, a beech).

By some botanists, the Buckwheat is separated from the *Polygonums*, receiving the name *Fagopyrum esculentum* (Moench).

The nut contains a floury endosperm, and though rarely employed in this country as human food is extensively cultivated for that purpose in Northern Europe, North America (where it also goes by the name of Indian Wheat) and in India and the East.

Buckwheat flour is occasionally used for bread, but more frequently employed for cakes, which when baked have an agreeable taste, with a darkish, somewhat violet colour and are a national dish throughout America in the winter. They are baked on gridirons and eaten with maple syrup as breakfast cakes. The meal of Buckwheat is also baked into crumpets, which are popular among Dutch children and are said to be nutritious and easily digested.

By the Hindus, Buckwheat, which is extensively cultivated in the Himalayas, is eaten on 'bart' or fast days, being one of the lawful foods for such occasions. *Polygonum cymosum* (Meism.), the Chinese perennial

Buckwheat, and *P. Tartaricum* (Ge·), the Tartary or Rough Buckwheat, also constitute an important source of flour in the East. In Japan, Buckwheat is called *Soba*, and its flour is prepared in various ways; kneaded with hot water to make a dough, *Soba-neri*; a kind of macaroni, *Soba-kiri*; and so on. The grains, steamed and dried, are eaten, boiled or made into bread or *Manju*, a small cake. Its young leaves are eaten as a vegetable and its stalks are used to feed cattle.

In the Russian Army, Buckwheat groats are served out as part of the soldiers' rations and cooked with butter, tallow or hemp-seed oil. In Germany it forms an ingredient in pottage, puddings and other food.

Beer may be brewed from the grain, and by distillation it yields an excellent spirit, in Danzig much used in the preparation of cordial waters.

The blossoms may be used for dyeing a brown colour.

¶ *Cultivation.* It is sown in May or June and ripens rapidly, thriving in the poorest soil. The flowers appear about July and the seeds ripen in October, but so tender are the plants that a single night's frost will destroy a whole crop. As a grian, Buckwheat is chiefly cultivated in England to supply food for pheasants and to feed poultry, which devour the seeds with avidity and thrive on it – hence one of its local names: Fat Hen. Mixed with bran, chaff or grain, its seeds are sometimes given to horses, either whole or broken. When used as food for cattle, the hard angular rind must first be removed. The meal is considered specially good for fattening pigs: 8 bushels of Buckwheat have been said to go as far as 12 bushels of barleymeal and a bushel of the seeds to go further than 2 bushels of oats, though all farmers do not quite agree as to the superior food value of Buckwheat. If it is given to pigs at first in too large quantities, they will show symptoms of intoxication. As compared with the principal cereal grains, it is poor in nitrogenous substances and fat, its nutritious properties are greatly inferior to wheat, though as a food it ranks much higher than rice; but the rapidity and the ease with which it can be grown renders it a fit crop for very poor, badly-tilled land which will produce scarcely anything else, its culture, compared with that of other grain, being attended with little expense.

When grown by the preservers of game as a food for pheasants, it is often left standing, as it affords both food and shelter to the birds during the winter. With some farmers it is the practice to sow Buckwheat for the purpose only of ploughing it into the ground as a *manure* for the land. The best time for ploughing it in is when it is in full blossom, allowing the land to rest till it decomposes.

Whilst green, it serves as food for sheep and oxen, and mixed with other provender it may also with advantage be given to horses. If sown in April, two green crops may be procured during the season.

The best mode of harvesting this grain is said to be by pulling it out of the ground like flax, stripping off the seeds with the hand and collecting these into aprons or cloths tied round the waist.

In the United States, Buckwheat is sown at the end of June or beginning of July, the amount of seed varying from 3 to 5 pecks to the acre. The crop matures rapidly and continues blooming till the frosts set in, so that at harvest, which is usually set to occur just before this period, the grain is in various stages of ripeness. There, after cutting, it is allowed to lie in swaths for a few days and then set up in shocks. Threshing is done on the field in most cases.

It grows so quickly that it will kill off any weeds.

¶ *Constituents.* The leaves have been found by Schunch to contain a crystalline colouring principle (1 part in a thousand) identical with the Rutin or Rutic acid previously discovered by Weiss in the leaves of the common Rue and probably existing in the leaves of the Holly.

The seeds contain starch, sugar, gum, and various matters soluble in alcohol. A small amount of the glucoside Indican has been found.

¶ *Medicinal Action and Uses.* Astringent, acrid.

An infusion of the herb has been used in erysipelas, and a poultice made of the flour and buttermilk for restoring the flow of milk in nurses.

The breakfast cakes are very heating, and in many people cause severe itching,[1] felt chiefly after removing the clothing at night, with an eruption of vesicles. The fæces may become so glutinous that expulsion is difficult.

¶ *Other Species.*

The FALSE BUCKWHEAT, or Arrow-leaved Tear Thumb, is *Polygonum sagittarum* (Linn.), a North American plant that has become naturalized in County Kerry, Ireland.

It is an annual, with a rough stem, 6 inches to 2 feet high, bearing turned-back prickles. The leaves are oblong-ovate to arrow-shaped and the flowers white, in bloom from July to October.

It has been used with success in nephritic colic, relieving the pains caused by gravel.

The CLIMBING BUCKWHEAT, or Black Bindweed, also called Bearbind and Cornbind, is *Polygonum Convolvulus* (Linn.), a troublesome climbing cornfield weed, which occurs indifferently in all soils.

Its stems are 1 to 3 feet long, angular, twining or trailing, bearing leaves 1 to 3 inches long, from heart-shaped to arrow-shaped. The flowers are very small, in loose axillary spikes, about four together, greenish-white, often tinged with red, and are insect-pollinated, containing nectar secreted in glands near the base of the stamens. The fruits are three-angled, bearing a resemblance to those of Buckwheat.

It is largely distributed by the seeds being sown with those of the crop among which it has grown. Spraying as for Charlock (with solutions of copper-, iron- or ammonium sulphate) will largely destroy this weed in cereals. It may be injurious to animals, owing to mechanical injury from the seeds when fed with corn; horses are said to have been killed in this way.

See BISTORT

BUGLE, COMMON

Ajuga reptans (LINN.)
N.O. Labiatæ

Synonyms. Carpenter's Herb. Sicklewort. Middle Comfrey
Part Used. Herb
Habitat. It is abundantly distributed throughout Britain in damp, shady pastures and woods

The Bugle and the Self-Heal, nearly related plants (both, with their two-lipped corollas, belonging to the important order *Labiatæ*), for many centuries stood in equally high estimation as valuable vulneraries or wound herbs.

There are three Bugles in the British flora – the common creeping form (*Ajuga reptans*), the erect Bugle (*A. pyramidalis*), a rare Highland species, and the Yellow Bugle or Ground Pine (*A. Chamæpitys*), which likewise has its reputation as a curative herb.

¶ *Description.* It is a perennial, to be found in flower from the end of April to the beginning of July and well marked by its solitary, tapering flower-stalks, 6 to 9 inches high, and its creeping scions or runners. These are long shoots, sometimes a couple of feet or more long, sent out from the rootstock. At intervals upon them are pairs of

---

[1] The Buckwheat used in America to-day is so refined that these symptoms are not liable to occur. – EDITOR.

leaves, and at the same point rootlets are given off below, which enter the earth. As winter approaches, the runners die, but at every point where the leaf-pairs and the rootlets were formed, there is a dormant plant waiting to develop fully in the spring, a Bugle plant thus being the centre of quite a colony of new young plants, quite independently of setting its seeds, which as a matter of fact do not always ripen, the plant propagating itself more largely by its creeping scions.

The erect flower-stalk sent up from the root-stock is square, pale green, often purplish above, with the leaves opposite in pairs, the lower leaves on stalks, the upper leaves stalkless, oblong and obtuse in form, toothed or almost entire at the margin, having many-celled hairs on both surfaces, the margins also fringed with hairs. The runners are altogether smooth, but the stems are smooth only on two sides and downy on the other two.

The flowers are of a purplish blue, crowded into a spike formed of about six or more rings of whorls, generally six flowers in a whorl. The upper leaves or bracts interspersed between the whorls are also tinged with the same colour, so that ordinarily the whole of the upper portion of the plant has a bluish appearance. A white variety is sometimes found, the upper leaves then being of the normal green colour.

The flowers are adapted by their lipped formation for cross-fertilization by bees, a little honey being found at the base of the long tube of the corolla. The upper lip is very short and the lower three-cleft. The stamens project. The flowers have practically no scent. After fertilization, small blackish seeds are formed, but many of the ovules do not mature.

The rather singular names of this plant – both popular and botanical – are not very easy to account for. It has been suggested that 'Bugle' is derived from *bugulus*, a thin, glass pipe used in embroidery, the long, thin tube of the corolla being thought to resemble this bead bugle. It is more likely to be a corruption of the Latin name *Ajuga*, the generic name which Linnæus was the first to apply to this plant, from a belief that this or some closely-allied species was the one referred to by Pliny and other writers by a very similar name, a name probably corrupted from *Abija*, in turn derived from the Latin word *abigo*, to drive away, because the plant was thought to drive away various forms of disease. In former days it was held to possess great curative powers. Prior, writing in the seventeenth century, tells us: 'It is put in

drinkes for woundes and that is the cause why some doe commonly say that he that hath Bugle and Sanicle will scarce vouchsafe the chirugeon a bugle.' The early writers speak of the plant as the Abija, Ajuga, Abuga and Bugula, and the common English name, Bugle, is clearly a corruption of one or other of these forms.

¶ *Part Used Medicinally*. The whole herb, gathered in May and early June, when the leaves are at their best, and dried.

¶ *Medicinal Action and Uses*. Bitter, astringent and aromatic.

In herbal treatment, an infusion of this plant is still considered very useful in arresting hæmorrhages and is employed in coughs and spitting of blood in incipient consumption and also in some biliary disorders, a wineglassful of the infusion – made from 1 oz. of the dried herb to 1 pint of boiling water – being given frequently.

In its action, it rather resembles digitalis, lowering the pulse and lessening its frequency; it allays irritation and cough, and equalizes the circulation and has been termed 'one of the mildest and best narcotics in the world.' It has also been considered good for the bad effects of excessive drinking.

Green (*Universal Herbal*, 1832) gives as his opinion that

'the leaves may be advantageously used in fluxes and disorders of that kind as they do not, like many other plants of the same value, produce costiveness, but rather operate as gentle laxatives.'

He states that a decoction of the herb has been employed for quinsy on the Continent, where the herb has been more employed as a remedy than in this country.

The roots have by some authorities been considered more astringent than the rest of the plant.

Culpepper had a great opinion of the value of the Bugle and says,

'if the virtues of it make you fall in love with it (as they will if you be wise) keep a syrup of it to take inwardly, and an ointment and plaster of it to use outwardly, always by you. The decoction of the leaves and flowers in wine dissolveth the congealed blood in those that are bruised inwardly by a fall or otherwise and is very effectual for any inward wounds, thrusts or stabs in the body or bowels; and is an especial help in wound drinks and for those that are liver-grown, as they call it. It is wonderful in curing all ulcers and sores, gangrenes and fistulas, if the leaves, bruised and applied or their juice be used to wash and bathe the place and the same made into lotion and some honey and gum added, cureth the worse sores. Being also taken inwardly or outwardly applied, it helpeth those that have broken any bone or have any member out of joint. An ointment made with the leaves of Bugle, Scabious and Sanicle bruised and boiled in hog's lard until the herbs be dry and then strained into a pot for such occasions as shall require, it is so efficacious for all sorts of hurts in the body, that none should be without it.'

See SELF-HEAL.

BUGLE, YELLOW

Ajuga chamæpitys (SCHREB.)
N.O. Labiatæ

Synonym. European Ground Pine
Habitat. It is a native of many parts of Europe, the Levant and North Africa, is common in sandy and chalky fields in Kent, Surrey and Essex, but otherwise is a scarce plant in England
Part Used. Leaves

¶ *Description*. Both in foliage and blossom it is very unlike its near relative, the Common Bugle, forming a bushy, herbaceous plant, 3 to 6 inches high, the four-cornered stem, hairy and viscid, generally purplish red, being much branched and densely leafy. Except the lowermost leaves, which are lance-shaped and almost undivided, each leaf is divided almost to its base into three very long, narrow segments, and the leaves being so closely packed together, the general appearance is not altogether unlike the long, needle-like foliage of the pine, hence the plant has received a second name – Ground Pine. The flowers are placed singly in the axils of leaf-like bracts and have bright yellow corollas, the lower lip spotted with red. They are in bloom during May and June.

The whole plant is very hairy, with stiff hairs, which consist of a few long joints. It has a highly aromatic and turpentiny odour and taste.

¶ *Uses*. Ground Pine has stimulant, diuretic and emmenagogue action and is considered by herbalists to form a good remedy, combined with other suitable herbs, for gout and rheumatism and also to be useful in female disorders, an infusion of 1 oz. of the dried herb to 1 pint of boiling water being recommended, taken in tablespoonful doses, frequently repeated.

The herb was formerly regarded almost as a specific in gouty and rheumatic affections, the young tops, dried and reduced to powder being employed. It formed an ingredient of the once famous Portland Powder.

It likewise operates powerfully by urine, removing obstructions and is serviceable in dropsy, jaundice and ague, reputed great cures having been performed by its use, either in infusion, or powder.

BUGLEWEED

Lycopus Virginicus (LINN.)
N.O. Labiatæ

Synonyms. Water Bugle. Sweet Bugle. Virginian Water Horehound. Gipsyweed
Part Used. Herb
Habitat. An American plant. It is a very common weed in North America, growing in low, damp, shady ground and flowering from July to September

¶ *Description*. Though a Labiate, it does not actually belong to the same genus as the British Bugles, but has certain points in common. From the perennial, creeping root, the quadrangular, smooth stem rises to a height of from 6 to 24 inches, bearing pairs of opposite leaves on short stalks, those on the upper part being toothed and lance-shaped, the lower ones wedge-shaped and with entire margins. The leaves are destitute of hairs and gland-dotted beneath. The flowers are in clusters in the axils of the leaves; the calyx has four broad, blunt teeth and the corolla is four-lobed, purplish in colour, with only two fertile stamens.

¶ *Part Used*. The whole herb is used. It is slightly aromatic, with a mint-like odour and is used, fresh, when in flower, for the preparation of a tincture and a fluid extract, until recent years official in the United States Pharmacopœia. It is also used dried for making an infusion.

¶ *Constituents*. It contains a peculiar bitter principle, insoluble in ether, another soluble in ether, the two forming more than 10 per cent. of the whole solid extract, also tannin and a volatile oil.

¶ *Medicinal Action and Uses*. Sedative, astringent and mildly narcotic. Used in coughs, bleeding from the lungs and consumption. The infusion made from 1 oz. of the dried herb to 1 pint of boiling water is taken in wineglassful doses, frequently, the fluid extract in doses of 10 to 30 drops, and the dry extract, Lycopin, in doses of 1 to 4 grains.

BUGLOSS, VIPER'S

Echium vulgare (LINN.)
N.O. Boraginaceæ

Synonym. Blueweed
Part Used. Herb

Viper's Bugloss is a showy plant covered with prickly hairs. It grows on walls, old quarries and gravel pits, and is common on calcareous soils. The name Bugloss, which is of Greek origin, signifies an Ox's Tongue, and was applied to it from the roughness and shape of the leaves.

¶ *Description.* The stems grow from 2 to 3 feet high and are covered with bristly hairs, as are also the leaves, which are 4 or 5 inches long, lanceolate, sessile, quite entire and rough on both sides. The stem is often spotted with red and sometimes the leaves also. The root-leaves form a tuft nearly 18 inches to 2 feet across. They are petioled. The flowers are in curved spikes, numerous, those of each spike pointing one way and closely wedged together. On their first opening they are bright rose-coloured and turn to a brilliant blue. They are in bloom throughout June and July, and are much visited by bees. The corollas are irregularly tubular and funnel-shaped. A variety is occasionally found with white flowers. The fruit consists of four small nutlets. The roots are biennial and descend to a great depth in the loose soil in which the plant generally grows.

Lycopsis arvensis, the Common or Small Bugloss, has small wheel-shaped flowers and wavy toothed leaves, which have also rigid hairs with a bulbous base.

Viper's Bugloss was said of old to be an expellent of poisons and venom, and to cure the bites of a viper, hence its name. Coles tells us in his *Art of Simples*:

'Viper's Bugloss hath its stalks all to be speckled like a snake or viper, and is a most singular remedy against poyson and the sting of scorpions.'

Its seeds are also thought to resemble snake heads, thus specifying it as a cure for the bites of serpents. Its generic name *Echium* is derived from *Echis,* a viper.

Parkinson says of it:

'the water distilled in glasses or the roote itself taken is good against the passions and tremblings of the heart as also against swoonings, sadness and melancholy.'

¶ *Medicinal Action and Uses.* Diuretic, demulcent and pectoral. The leaves, especially those growing near the root, make a good cordial on infusion, which operates by perspiration and alleviates fevers, headaches and nervous complaints, relieving inflammatory pains. The infusion is made of 1 oz. of the dried leaves to a pint of boiling water, and is given in wineglassful to teacupful doses, as required.

A decoction of the seeds in wine, we are told by old writers, 'comforts the heart and drives away melancholy.'

BULLACE

Prunus insititia (LINN.)
N.O. Rosaceæ

Synonyms. Bully-bloom (for the flowers). Bullies, Bolas, Bullions and Wild Damson (for the fruit)
(*French*) Sibarelles
Parts Used. Fruit, wood and bark
Habitat. Common in England in thickets, woods and hedges, though more rare in Scotland and probably not wild north of the Forth and Clyde. Common in South-East Europe and in Northern and Central Asia

¶ *Description.* A tall shrub, sometimes developing into a small tree about 15 feet high. Resembles the Blackthorn or Sloe (*Prunus spinosa*), but is less thorny and has straight, not crooked branches, covered by brown, not black bark, only a few of the old ones terminating in spines, the younger ones downy. It has also larger leaves than the Blackthorn, downy underneath, alternate, finely-toothed, on short, downy foot-stalks, and flowers, white like those of the Blackthorn, but larger, with broader petals, borne in less crowded clusters and not on the naked branches, but expanding just after the leaves have begun to unfold.

The globular, fleshy fruit, marked with a faint suture, has generally a black skin, covered with a thin bluish bloom, and is similar to the Sloe, but larger, often an inch across, and drooping from its weight, not erect as the Sloe. Occasionally yellow varieties are found.

¶ *Constituents.* The volatile oil expressed from the seeds contains benzaldehyde and hydrocyanic acid. These substances are also present in the young leaves and flowers.

¶ *Medicinal Action and Uses.* The bark of the root and branches is considerably styptic. An infusion of the flowers, sweetened with sugar, has been used as a mild purgative for children.

The wood, branches, fruit and entire plant are used throughout France for the same properties as those of the Sloe, the bark of which is used as a febrifuge and the gin, prepared from the fruit on account of its astringency, as a good remedy in cases of diarrhœa.

In this country, the fruit is gathered for 'Bullace Wine,' and is also made into excellent pies and puddings and a good preserve is made by mixing the pulp with three times its weight of sugar.

There are several varieties of the Bullace in cultivation, and they frequently appear on the market as 'Damsons.' Both Bullace and Damson originate from the same source, *P. domestica*, the only difference being that the former is round and the latter oval. All cultivated Bullaces are immense bearers; the following are the best known:

ROYAL BULLACE. Fruit large, 1¼ inch in diameter. Skin bright grass-green, mottled with red on the side next to the sun and becoming yellowish-green as it ripens, with a thin, grey bloom on the surface. Flesh green, separating from the stone, briskly flavoured with sufficient sweetness to make it an agreeable late fruit. Ripe in early October.

WHITE BULLACE. Fruit small, round. Skin pale yellowish-white, mottled with red next the sun. Flesh firm, juicy, sub-acid, adhering to the stone, becoming sweetish when quite ripe in end of October and beginning of November. Often sold in London as 'White Damsons.'

ESSEX BULLACE. Skin green, becoming yellowish as it ripens. Flesh juicy and not so acid as the common Bullace. Ripens end of October and beginning of November. Fruit an inch or more in diameter, larger than the common White Bullace.

BURDOCK

Arctium lappa (LINN.)
N.O. Compositæ

Synonyms. Lappa. Fox's Clote. Thorny Burr. Beggar's Buttons. Cockle Buttons. Love Leaves. Philanthropium. Personata. Happy Major. Clot-Bur

Parts Used. Root, herb and seeds (fruits)

Habitat. It grows freely throughout England (though rarely in Scotland) on waste ground and about old buildings, by roadsides and in fairly damp places

The Burdock, the only British member of its genus, belongs to the Thistle group of the great order, *Compositæ*.

¶ *Description.* A stout handsome plant, with large, wavy leaves and round heads of purple flowers. It is enclosed in a globular involucre of long stiff scales with hooked tips, the scales being also often interwoven with a white, cottony substance.

The whole plant is a dull, pale green, the stem about 3 to 4 feet and branched, rising from a biennial root. The lower leaves are very large, on long, solid foot-stalks, furrowed above, frequently more than a foot long, heart-shaped and of a grey colour on their under surfaces from the mass of fine down with which they are covered. The upper leaves are much smaller, more egg-shaped in form and not so densely clothed beneath with the grey down.

The plant varies considerably in appearance, and by some botanists various sub-species, or even separate species, have been described, the variations being according to the size of the flower-heads and of the whole plant, the abundance of the whitish cotton-like substance that is sometimes found on the involucres, or the absence of it, the length of the flower-stalks, etc.

The flower-heads are found expanded during the latter part of the summer and well into the autumn: all the florets are tubular, the stamens dark purple and the styles whitish. The plant owes its dissemination greatly to the little hooked prickles of its involucre, which adhere to everything with which they come in contact, and by attaching themselves to coats of animals are often carried to a distance.

'They are Burs, I can tell you, they'll stick
    where they are thrown,'

Shakespeare makes Pandarus say in *Troilus and Cressida*, and in *King Lear* we have another direct reference to this plant:

'Crown'd with rank Fumiter and Furrow-
    weeds,
With Burdocks, Hemlocks, Nettles, Cuckoo-
    flowers.'

Also in *As You Like It*:

ROSALIND. How full of briers is this working-day world!

CELIA. They are but *burs*, cousin, thrown upon thee in holiday foolery. If we walk not in the trodden paths, our very petticoats will catch them.

The name of the genus, *Arctium*, is derived from the Greek *arktos*, a bear, in allusion to the roughness of the burs, *lappa*, the specific name, being derived from a word meaning 'to seize.'

Another source derives the word *lappa*

from the Celtic *llap*, a hand, on account of its prehensile properties.

The plant gets its name of 'Dock' from its large leaves; the 'Bur' is supposed to be a contraction of the French *bourre*, from the Latin *burra*, a lock of wool, such is often found entangled with it when sheep have passed by the growing plants.

An old English name for the Burdock was 'Herrif,' 'Aireve,' or 'Airup,' from the Anglo-Saxon *hœg*, a hedge, and *reafe*, a robber – or from the Anglo-Saxon verb *reafian*, to seize. Culpepper gives as popular names in his time: Personata, Happy Major and Clot-Bur.

Though growing in its wild state hardly any animal except the ass will browse on this plant, the stalks, cut before the flower is open and stripped of their rind, form a delicate vegetable when boiled, similar in flavour to Asparagus, and also make a pleasant salad, eaten raw with oil and vinegar. Formerly they were sometimes candied with sugar, as Angelica is now. They are slightly laxative, but perfectly wholesome.

¶ *Cultivation.* As the Burdock grows freely in waste places and hedgerows, it can be collected in the wild state, and is seldom worth cultivating.

It will grow in almost any soil, but the roots are formed best in a light, well-drained soil. The seeds germinate readily and may be sown directly in the field, either in autumn or early spring, in drills 18 inches to 3 feet apart, sowing 1 inch deep in autumn, but less in spring. The young plants when well up are thinned out to 6 inches apart in the row.

Yields at the rate of 1,500 to 2,000 lb. of dry roots per acre have been obtained from plantations of Burdock.

¶ *Parts Used Medicinally.* The dried root from plants of the first year's growth forms the official drug, but the leaves and fruits (commonly, though erroneously, called seeds) are also used.

The roots are dug in July, and should be lifted with a beet-lifter or a deep-running plough. As a rule they are 12 inches or more in length and about 1 inch thick; sometimes, however, they extend 2 to 3 feet, making it necessary to dig by hand. They are fleshy, wrinkled, crowned with a tuft of whitish, soft, hairy leaf-stalks, grey-brown externally, whitish internally, with a somewhat thick bark, about a quarter of the diameter of the root, and soft wood tissues, with a radiate structure.

Burdock root has a sweetish and mucilaginous taste.

Burdock leaves, which are less used than the root, are collected in July. For drying, follow the drying of Coltsfoot leaves. They have a somewhat bitter taste.

The seeds (or fruits) are collected when ripe. They are brownish-grey, wrinkled, about $\frac{1}{4}$ inch long and $\frac{1}{16}$ inch in diameter. They are shaken out of the head and dried by spreading them out on paper in the sun.

¶ *Constituents.* Inulin, mucilage, sugar, a bitter, crystalline glucoside – Lappin – a little resin, fixed and volatile oils, and some tannic acid.

The roots contain starch, and the ashes of the plant, burnt when green, yield carbonate of potash abundantly, and also some nitre.

¶ *Medicinal Action and Uses.* Alterative, diuretic and diaphoretic. One of the best blood purifiers. In all skin diseases, it is a certain remedy and has effected a cure in many cases of eczema, either taken alone or combined with other remedies, such as Yellow Dock and Sarsaparilla.

The *root* is principally employed, but the leaves and seeds are equally valuable. Both root and seeds may be taken as a decoction of 1 oz. to $1\frac{1}{2}$ pint of water, boiled down to a pint, in doses of a wineglassful, three or four times a day.

The anti-scorbutic properties of the root make the decoction very useful for boils, scurvy and rheumatic affections, and by many it is considered superior to Sarsaparilla, on account of its mucilaginous, demulcent nature; it has in addition been recommended for external use as a wash for ulcers and scaly skin disorders.

An infusion of the *leaves* is useful to impart strength and tone to the stomach, for some forms of long-standing indigestion.

When applied externally as a poultice, the leaves are highly resolvent for tumours and gouty swellings, and relieve bruises and inflamed surfaces generally. The bruised leaves have been applied by the peasantry in many countries as cataplasms to the feet and as a remedy for hysterical disorders.

From the *seeds*, both a medicinal tincture and a fluid extract are prepared, of benefit in chronic skin diseases. Americans use the seeds only, considering them more efficacious and prompt in their action than the other parts of the plant. They are relaxant and demulcent, with a limited amount of tonic property. Their influence upon the skin is due largely to their being of such an oily nature: they affect both the sebaceous and sudoriferous glands, and probably owing to their oily nature restore that smoothness to the skin which is a sign of normal healthy action.

The infusion or decoction of the seeds is employed in dropsical complaints, more especially in cases where there is co-existing derangement of the nervous system, and is considered by many to be a specific for all affections of the kidneys, for which it may with advantage be taken several times a day, before meals.

¶ *Preparations.* Fluid extract, root, $\frac{1}{2}$ to 2 drachms. Solid extract, 5 to 15 grains. Fluid extract, seed, 10 to 30 drops.

Culpepper gives the following uses for the Burdock:

'The Burdock leaves are cooling and moderately drying, wherby good for old ulcers and sores. . . . The leaves applied to the places troubled with the shrinking in the sinews or arteries give much ease: a juice of the leaves or rather the roots themselves given to drink with old wine, doth wonderfully help the biting of any serpents; the root beaten with a little salt and laid on the place suddenly easeth the pain thereof, and helpeth those that are bit by a mad dog: . . .

the seed being drunk in wine 40 days together doth wonderfully help the sciatica: the leaves bruised with the white of an egg and applied to any place burnt with fire, taketh out the fire, gives sudden ease and heals it up afterwards. . . . The root may be preserved with sugar for consumption, stone and the lax. The seed is much commended to break the stone, and is often used with other seeds and things for that purpose.'

It was regarded as a valuable remedy for stone in the Middle Ages, and called Bardona. As a rule, the recipes for stone contained some seeds or 'fruits' of a 'stony' character, as gromel seed, ivy berries, and nearly always saxifrage, i.e. 'stone-breaker.' Even date-stones had to be pounded and taken; the idea being that what is naturally 'stony' would cure it; that 'like cures like' (Henslow).

BURNET, GREAT

Sanguisorba officinalis (LINN.)
N.O. Rosaceæ

Synonyms. Garden Burnet. Common Burnet
Parts Used. Herb, root
Habitat. Grows in moist meadows and shady places, chiefly in mountainous districts, almost all over Europe. In Britain it is not uncommon, but is rare in Ireland

Closely related to the *Alchemillas*, belonging to the same subdivision, *Sanguisorbidæ*, of the order Rosaceæ and having similar medicinal properties to *Alchemilla vulgaris*, are the Burnets, *Sanguisorba officinalis* and *Poterium sanguisorba*.

It is a tall and not inelegant plant, with pinnate leaves on long stalks, bearing thirteen sharply serrate leaflets and branched stems, 2 feet high or more, sparsely clothed with leaves, and oblong heads of deep purple-brown flowers, which have four-toothed, coloured, membraneous calyces. The root is black and long. The plant has no odour.

It is cultivated to a considerable extent in Germany for fodder, and has been grown here with that view, but is not in esteem among English farmers. It will grow tolerably on very poor land, but is not a very valuable fodder plant.

An Italian proverb says: 'The salad is neither good nor good-looking when there is no pimpernel.' This pimpernel is our Common Burnet and must not be confused with the plant known by that name which has poisonous properties. The roots are perennial and should be divided in early spring. It likes a dry and chalky soil.

¶ *Parts Used Medicinally.* The herb and root, the herb gathered in July, and the root dug in autumn.

Culpepper says of 'The Great Wild Burnet':

'This is an herb the Sun challenges dominion over, and is a most precious herb, little inferior to Betony; the continual use of it preserves the body in health and the spirits in vigour, for if the Sun be the preserver of life under God, his herbs are the best in the world to do it by. . . . Two or three of the stalks, with leaves put into a cup of wine, especially claret, are known to quicken the spirits, refresh and cheer the heart, and drive away melancholy: It is a special help to defend the heart from noisome vapours, and from infection of the pestilence, the juice thereof being taken in some drink, and the party laid to sweat thereupon.'

He also recommends it for wounds, both inwardly and outwardly applied.

¶ *Cultivation.* Burnet may be cultivated. It prefers a light soil. Sow seeds in March and thin out to 9 inches apart. Propagation may also be effected by division of roots, in the autumn, that they may be well-established before the dry summer weather sets in. The flowers should be picked off when they appear, the stem and leaves only of the herb being used.

¶ *Medicinal Action and Uses.* Astringent and tonic. Great Burnet was formerly in high repute as a vulnerary, hence its generic name, from *sanguis*, blood, and *sorbeo*, to staunch. Both herb and root are administered internally in all abnormal discharges: in diarrhœa, dysentery, leucorrhœa, it is of the utmost service; dried and powdered, it has been used to stop purgings.

The whole plant has astringent qualities, but the root possesses the most astringency.

A decoction of the whole herb has, however, been found useful in hæmorrhage and is a tonic cordial and sudorific; the herb is also largely used in Herb Beer.

BURNET, LESSER

Pimpinella saxifraga (LINN.)
N.O. Umbelliferæ

Synonyms. Salad Burnet. Burnet Saxifrage. Pimpinella sanguisorba
Parts Used. Root, herb
Habitat. The Salad Burnet is common in dry pastures and by the wayside, especially on chalk and limestone, but is rarer in Scotland and Ireland than in England

The Lesser or Salad Burnet is not unlike the Great Burnet in habit, but it is much smaller and more slender. It was known by older writers as *Pimpinella sanguisorba*, Pimpinella being a corruption of *bipennula*, from the two pinnate leaves. *Pimpinella* is now reserved for the name of a genus belonging to the order Umbelliferæ, and the Salad Burnet is assigned to the genus *Poterium*, which name is derived from the Greek *poterion*, a drinking-cup, from the use to which the leaves of the Salad Burnet were applied in the preparation of the numerous beverages with which the *poterion* was filled in ancient times. The leaves when bruised smell like cucumber and taste somewhat like it, and it was used to cool tankards in the same manner as Borage, and was also added to salads and cups.

Hooker places both the Great Burnet and the Salad or Lesser Burnet in the same genus, *Poterium*, rejecting the generic name of *Sanguisorba*, assigned to the former by Linnæus.

¶ *Description.* Its leaflets are more numerous, five to ten pairs, and shorter than those of the Great Burnet. The flowers in each head bear crimson tufted stigmas, the lower ones thirty to forty stamens, with very long, drooping filaments. Both the flower and leaf-stalks are a deep-crimson colour.

Turner (*Newe Herball,* 1551), in his description of the plant, tells us that

'it has two little leives like unto the wings of birdes, standing out as the bird setteth her wings out when she intendeth to flye. Ye Dutchmen call it Hergottes berdlen, that is God's little berde, because of the colour that it hath in the topp.'

The great Burnet and the Salad Burnet both flower in June and July.

The Salad Burnet forms much of the turf on some of the chalk downs in the southern counties. It is extremely nutritious to sheep and cattle, and was formerly extensively cultivated as a fodder plant on calcareous soils, but is now little grown in that way. Cattle do not seem to like it as well as clover when full grown, but when kept closely cropped sheep are fond of it. It has the advantage of keeping green all the winter in dry barren pastures, affording food for sheep when other green crops are scarce. The results of cultivation have, however, not been very satisfactory, except on poor soil, although it contains a larger amount of nutritive matter than many grasses.

In the herb gardens of older days, Salad Burnet always had its place. Bacon recommends it to be set in alleys together with wild thyme and water mint, 'to perfume the air most delightfully, being trodden on and crushed.'

¶ *Cultivation.* It is easily propagated by seeds, sown in autumn, soon after they are ripe. If the seeds be permitted to scatter, the plants will come up plentifully, and can be transplanted into an ordinary or rather poor soil, at about a foot distant each way. If kept clear from weeds, they will continue some years without further care, especially if the soil be dry. Propagation may also be effected by division of roots in spring or autumn.

When used for salad, the flower-stalks should be cut down if not required for seed. The leaves, for salad use, should be cut young, or may be tough.

¶ *Part Used Medicinally.* The whole herb, as in the Great Burnet, gathered in July and dried in the same manner.

¶ *Medicinal Action and Uses.* The older herbalists held this plant in greater repute than it enjoys at the present day. Pliny recommended a decoction of the plant beaten up with honey for divers complaints.

Dodoens recommended it as a healer of wounds,

'made into powder and dronke with wine, wherin iron hath bene often quenched, and so doth the herbe alone, being but only holden in a man's hande as some have written. The leaves stiped in wine and dronken, doth comfort and rejoice the hart, and are good against the trembling and shaking of the same.'

Parkinson grew Burnet in his garden and

the early settlers in America introduced it from the Mother Country.

'It gives a grace in the drynkynge,' says Gerard, referring to this use of it in cool tankards. We are also told that it affords protection against infection,

'a speciall helpe to defend the heart from noysome vapours and from the infection of the Plague or Pestilence, and all other contagious diseases for which purpose it is of great effect, the juice thereof being taken in some drink.'

and that

it is a capital wound herb for all sorts of wounds, both of the head and body, either inward or outward, used either in juice or decoction of the herb, or by the powder of the herb or root, or the water of the distilled herb, or made into an ointment by itself or with other things to be kept.'

It is still regarded as a styptic, an infusion of the whole herb being employed as an astringent. It is also a cordial and promotes perspiration.

Turner advised the use of the herb, infused in wine or beer, for the cure of gout and rheumatism.

See LADIES' MANTLE, PARSLEY PURT.

BURNET SAXIFRAGE. *See* (LESSER) BURNET

BURNING BUSH
Dictamnus albus
N.O. Rutaceæ

Synonyms. Fraxinella. Bastard. False or White Dittany
Part Used. The root
Habitat. Germany. France. Alsace. Spain. Austria. Italy. Asia Minor

¶ *Description.* The members of this small genus are plants about 2 feet high, bearing flowers in a long, pyramidal, loose spike, varying in colour from pale purple to white. It prefers to grow in woods in warm places. The whole plant, especially when rubbed, gives out an odour like lemon-peel, and when bruised this grows more like that of a fine balsam, strongest in the pedicels of the flowers. It is due to an essential oil, which gives off an inflammable vapour in heat or in dry, cloudy weather, which also congeals as resinous wax, exuding from rusty-red glands in the flowers. This accounts for the fact that the atmosphere surrounding it will often take fire if approached by a lighted candle, without injuring the plant.

The fragrant leaves and handsome flowers cause it to be frequently cultivated in gardens.

The prepared root-bark is whitish, almost odourless, and rolled in pieces from 1 to 2 inches long.

¶ *Constituents.* The acrid and resinous principles have not been analysed.

¶ *Medicinal Action and Uses.* The drug is very little used to-day, though it is an ingredient in 'Orvieton,' 'Solomon's Opiate,' 'Guttète Powder,' 'Balm of Fioraventi,' 'Eau generale,' 'Hyacinth Mixture,' etc. It is recommended in nervous complaints and intermittent fevers, and used to be given in scrofulous and scorbutic diseases. It is a cordial and stomachic. The *distilled water* is used as a cosmetic. An infusion of the *leaves* is regarded as a substitute for tea. The *powder* is combined with that of peppermint for use in epilepsy.

¶ *Dosage.* Of powdered root, 4 to 8 grammes, or double the quantity in infusion.

¶ *Other Species.*
Several drugs bear the name of Dictamnus, such as Dictamnus of Barbados, or Arrowroot des tilles.

The leaves of a plant growing in Crete and Candy were used by the Ancients for wounds, and it is still known as Dictamnus or Dittany of Crete, being *Origanum Dictamnus* of the Labiatæ family.

BURR MARIGOLD. *See* AGRIMONY, WATER

BURRA GOOKEROO
Pedalium Murex (LINN.)
Tribulus terrestes (LINN.)
N.O. Pedaliaceæ

Synonyms. Burra Gokhru
Part Used. Seeds
Habitat. India

¶ *Description.* Fruits brown, two-celled with four narrow and long seeds. Taste mucilaginous. Odourless.

¶ *Medicinal Action and Uses.* Diuretic, demulcent, aphrodisiac.

Used for impotence in males, nocturnal emissions, gonorrhœa, gleet and incontinence of urine.

Infusion, 1 in 20, is taken three times daily. Fluid extract, 10 to 30 drops.

BUTCHER'S BROOM. *See* BROOM

BUTTER SNAKEROOT. *See* SNAKEROOT.

BUTTERBUR

Petasites vulgaris (DESF.)
N.O. Compositæ

Synonyms. Langwort. Umbrella Plant. Bog Rhubarb. Flapperdock. Blatterdock. Capdockin. Bogshorns. Butter-Dock
Part Used. Root

The Butterbur, a plant nearly allied to the Coltsfoot – being the *Tussilago petasites* of Linnæus – is found in wet ground, lowlying, marshy meadows and by riversides, but is usually local.

¶ *Description.* It has a fleshy, stout root-stock, extensively creeping, which, like the Coltsfoot, sends up the flowers before the leaves appear. The flower-heads are, however, not produced singly, on separate stalks, but in crowned clusters in a dense spike, with many bracts interspersed, at the summit of a round, thick flower-stalk, 4 inches to a little over a foot in height, which first appears at the end of February or beginning of March, and is generally of a purplish hue.

There are two kinds of flowers – the male or stamen-bearing and the female or seed-producing – as a rule on different spikes, the female flowers being in denser, longer spikes than the male flowers, which are in shorter, loose clusters. Occasionally a few female flowers are found on the male spikes, and a few male flowers on the female spikes. The corollas are pale reddish purple or flesh-coloured, bell-shaped in the male flowers, and containing abundant nectar, but only thread-like in the female flowers, which contain no nectar, and are succeeded by the white feathery pappus, which crowns the seeds.

In April, as the flowers begin to decay, the leaves appear. They are on stout hollowed channelled foot-stalks, and when full grown very large – the largest leaves of any plant in Great Britain – the blade sometimes attaining 3 feet in diameter. It is roundish, heart-shaped at the base, scalloped at the edges, with the portion between the projections finely toothed. The leaves are white and cobwebby with down both above and below when young, but when mature, most of the covering disappears from the upper surface, though the leaves still remain grey and more or less downy beneath.

The name of the genus, *Petasites*, is derived from *petasos*, the Greek word for the felt hats worn by shepherds, and familiar to us in representations of Mercury, in reference to the large size of the leaves, which could be used as a head-covering. No other vegetation can live where these leaves grow, for they exclude light and air from all beneath, and where the plant abounds, it has been described as 'the most pernicious of all the weeds which this country produces.'

The name Butterbur is supposed to have been given it because formerly these large leaves were used to wrap butter in during hot weather. 'Lagwort' is an old name we sometimes find for it, in reference to the leaves delaying their appearance till after the flowers have faded, though once the leaf-shoots make a start, they grow with almost tropical luxuriance.

'The early flowering of this rank weed,' Hooker writes, 'induces the Swedish farmers to plant it near their beehives. Thus we see in our gardens the bees assembled on its affinities, *P. alba* and *P. fragrans*, at a season when scarcely any other flowers are expanded.'

In Germany an old name for the plant was *Pestilenzenwurt*, but one finds really very little either of evil or good assigned by the older writers to the Butterbur as compared with most other herbs. The old German name was given it, not as suggesting the plant was provocative of pestilence, but as an indication of its value as a remedy in time of such calamity (Henslow).

Anne Pratt says the former name of this plant was the 'plague-flower,' as it gained a successful reputation among the few remedies during the time of that malady. Lyte, in his *Herbal*, 1578, calls it 'a soveraigne medicine against the plague', and remarks of its leaves that 'one of them is large enough to cover a small table, as with a carpet,' and they are often 2 feet in width. Under its ample foliage, the poultry in farm meadows, shelter themselves from the rain, or find a cool retreat from the noonday sun. The Swedish farmers plant it in great quantities near their beehives, as bees are attracted by its flowers.

The seeds in some parts of the country have been used for love divination.

'The seeds of butterdock must be sowed by a young unmarried woman half an hour before sunrise on a Friday morning, in a lonesome place. She must strew the seeds gradually on the grass, saying these words:

I sow, I sow!
Then, my own dear,
Come here, come here,
And mow and mow!

The seed being scattered, she will see her future husband mowing with a scythe at a short distance from her. She must not be frightened, for if she says, "Have mercy on me," he will immediately vanish! This method is said to be infallible, but it is looked upon as a bold, desperate, and presumptuous undertaking!'

¶ *Part Used.* The rhizome, or root-stock, which is blackish on the outside and whitish internally, and has a bitter and unpleasant taste, due to the resinous, bitter juice it contains.

¶ *Medicinal Action and Uses.* Butterbur root is medicinally employed as a heart stimulant, acting both as a cardiac tonic and also as a diuretic. It has been in use as a remedy in fevers, asthma, colds and urinary complaints, a decoction being taken warm in wineglassful doses, frequently repeated.

Both Butterbur and Coltsfoot are specific homœopathic remedies for severe and obstinate neuralgia in the small of the back and the loins, a medicinal tincture being prepared in each case.

Gerard writes of the Butterbur:

'The roots dried and beaten to powder and drunke in wine is a soveraigne medicine against the plague and pestilent fevers, because it provoketh sweat and driveth from the heart all venim and evill heate; it killeth worms. The powder of the roots cureth all naughty filthy ulcers, if it be strewed therein.'

Culpepper says:

'It is a great strengthener of the heart and cheerer of the vital spirits: . . . if the powder thereof be taken in wine, it also resisteth the force of any other poison . . . the decoction of the root in wine is singularly good for those that wheeze much or are short-winded. . . . The powder of the root taketh away all spots and blemishes of the skin.'

Another species known as the Winter Heliotrope, or Sweet-scented Coltsfoot (*P. fragrans*), flourishes in warm districts like South Devon, where it is abundant. It is even more spreading and luxuriant in growth than our native Coltsfoot, but as it flowers in the poorest soil and clothes waste land with its handsome foliage, it is certainly welcome *outside* the garden, and is even frequently planted in shrubberies. The fragrant flowers, which have the scent of vanilla and are like Butterbur in appearance, are freely borne in the depth of winter. The leaves appear in the spring and in favourable situations remain green till the young leaves appear in the succeeding season.

See COLTSFOOT.

BUTTERCUP, BULBOUS

Ranunculus bulbosus (LINN.)

N.O. Ranunculaceæ

Parts used. Juice and Herb

Synonyms. St. Anthony's Turnip. Crowfoot. Frogsfoot. Goldcup
(French) Jaunet

The Bulbous Buttercup or Crowfoot is perhaps the commonest of the *Ranunculus* family, covering the meadows in May with dazzling yellow, being one of the earliest of the varieties to flower, owing to the nourishment stored up in the bulbs.

The specific name *bulbosus* refers to the bulb-like swelling at the base of the stem, roundish and white, flattened a little both at the top and bottom, somewhat resembling a small turnip – hence one of the popular names for this plant: St. Anthony's Turnip. It is, however, not a true bulb, only 'bulb-like.'

This is the 'Cuckow buds of yellow hue' of Shakespeare, and in France it is called the *jaunet* from the brilliance of its blossoms. Frogs-foot (from the form of its leaves) and Goldcup, from the shape and colour of its flowers, are other English names it bears.

The Bulbous Buttercup has some superficial resemblance to the Upright Crowfoot and the Creeping Crowfoot, but is distinguished not only by its bulb and by the fact that it never throws out runners, but by the fact that its sepals are turned back in the fully-expanded blossom, so as to touch the stem that supports the flower.

The stems are furrowed slightly, not merely round, as in *Ranunculus acris*. The upper leaves are composed of long, narrow segments, the lower ones broadened out into very distinct masses.

When once established it is not easily eradicated.

¶ *Medicinal Action and Uses.* Like most of the Crowfoots, the Bulbous Buttercup possesses the property of inflaming and blistering the skin, particularly the roots, which are said to raise blisters with less pain and greater safety than Spanish Fly, and have been applied for that purpose, especially to the joints, in gout. The juice, if applied to the nostrils, provokes sneezing and cures certain cases of headache. The leaves have been used to produce blisters on the wrists in rheumatism, and when infused in boiling water, as a poultice, at the pit of the stomach.

A tincture made with spirits of wine will cure shingles very expeditiously, it is stated, both the outbreak of the small pimples and the accompanying sharp pains between the ribs, 6 to 8 drops being given three or four times daily. For sciatica, the tincture has been employed with good effect.

The roots on being kept lose their stimulating quality, and are even eatable when boiled. Pigs are remarkably fond of them, and will go long distances to get them.

The herb is too acrid to be eaten alone by cattle, but possibly mixed with grasses it may act as a stimulus.

It is recorded that two obstinate cases of nursing soremouth have been cured with an infusion made by adding 2 drachms of the recent root, cut into small pieces, to 1 pint of hot water; when cold, a tablespoonful was given three or four times a day, and the mouth was frequently washed with a much stronger infusion.

Its action as a counter-irritant is both uncertain and violent, and may cause obstinate ulcers. The beggars of Europe sometimes use it to keep open sores for the purpose of exciting sympathy.

See also CROWFOOT, CELANDINE, SPEARWORT (LESSER).

BUTTERNUT

Juglans cinerea (LINN.)
N.O. Juglandaceæ

Synonyms. White Walnut. Oilnut
Part Used. Bark of the root
Habitat. New Brunswick and mountains of Georgia

¶ *Description.* The leaves possess much the same properties as the Black Walnut. The inner bark of the root is the best for medicinal use and should be collected in May or June; it is generally found in quills, curved strips or chips from $\frac{1}{8}$ to $\frac{1}{2}$ inch thick, deep brown in colour all through, outer surface smooth and a little warty, inner surface smooth and striate with fragments and thin stringy fibre, short fracture, weak and fibrous, odour slightly aromatic, taste bitter (astringent and acrid). The powdered drug is dark brown.

¶ *Constituents.* A bitter extractive, a large proportion of oily matter, a volatilizable acid and juglandic acid.

¶ *Medicinal Action and Uses.* Butternut is a mild cathartic like rhubarb; it does not constipate and is often used as a habitual laxative, also for dysentery and hypatic congestions. It has been employed as a vermifuge and is recommended for syphilis and old ulcers. The expressed oil of the fruit removes tapeworm. The fruit when halfgrown is made into pickles and when matured is a valuable article of diet. The bark is used for dyeing wool a dark brown colour but is inferior to that of the black walnut for this purpose. It is said to be rubefacient when applied to the skin.

¶ *Preparations.* Fluid extract, 1 to 2 drachms. Solid extract, 5 to 10 grains. Juglandin, 2 to 5 grains.

(*POISON*)
CABBAGE TREE

Andira inermis
N.O. Leguminosæ

Synonyms. Vouacapoua inermis. Bastard Cabbage Tree. Worm Bark. Yellow Cabbage Tree. Jamaica Cabbage Tree
Part Used. Bark
Habitat. Jamaica and other West Indian Islands. Senegambia

¶ *Description.* A leguminous tree, growing very tall and branching towards the top, called Cabbage Tree because it forms a head in growing; it has a smooth grey bark which, cut into long pieces, is the part utilized for medicine. It is thick, fibrous, scaly, and of an ashy brownish colour externally, covered with lichens – the inside bark is yellow and contains a bitter sweet mucilage, with an unpleasant smell. In Europe the bark of another species, *Avouacouapa retusa*, has been utilized. It grows in Surinam, is a more powerful vermifuge than *Vouacapoua inermis* and does not as a rule produce such injurious after-effects. In the dried state it is without odour, but has a very bitter taste; when powdered it has the colour of cinnamon.

¶ *Constituents.* Jamaicine-Andirin aglucoside, an inodorous, bitter, acrid resin.

¶ *Medicinal Action and Uses.* Narcotic, vermifuge. Cabbage Tree bark used in large doses may cause vomiting, fever and delirium, especially if cold water is drunk just before or after taking it. In the West Indies it is largely employed as a vermifuge to expel worm – *ascaris lumbrecoides* – but if used incautiously death has been known to occur. The powder purges like jalap.

¶ *Dosages.* Usually given in decoction, though the powder, syrup and extract are all used. Dose of powder, 20 to 30 grains. Fluid extract, $\frac{1}{4}$ to 1 drachm.

¶ *Antidote.* Lime-juice or Castor oil.

¶ *Other Species.* Andira retusa, a Brazilian species, has purple flowers, the odour of oranges and a slight aroma. The fruit is said to smell like tonka beans.

CACAO

Theobroma cacao (LINN.)
N.O. Sterculiaceæ

Synonyms. Cocoa. Chocolate Tree
Part Used. The seeds
Habitat. Tropical America. Cultivated in Ceylon, Java, etc.

¶ *Description and History*. Cacao was named *Theobroma* by Linnæus, the word meaning 'food of the gods,' so called from the goodness of its seeds. Mexicans named the pounded seeds 'Chocolate.' The tree is handsome, 12 to 16 feet high; trunk about 5 feet long; wood light and white coloured; bark brown; leaves lanceolate, bright green, entire; flowers small reddish, almost odourless; fruit yellowy red, smooth; rind flesh-coloured; pulp white; when seeds are ripe they rattle in the capsule when shaken; each capsule contains about twenty-five seeds; if separated from the capsule they soon become infertile, but if kept therein they retain their fertility for a long time. The tree bears its leaves, flowers and fruit (like the orange tree) all the year round, but the usual season for gathering the fruit is June and December. In Mexico during the time of the Aztec kings the small seeds were utilized as coins, twelve approximating to the value of 1*d*., the smallest actual coin in use then being worth about 6*d*. The seeds were necessary for small transactions. The method is still in use in some parts of Mexico. The tree is generally cultivated on large estates under the shade of other trees, such as the banana, and develops the pods continuously. When ripe they are cut open and the beans or nuts surrounded by their sweetish acid pulp are allowed to ferment so that they may be more easily separated from the shell. The beans are then usually dried in the sun, though sometimes in a steam drying shed.

¶ *Constituents*. The seeds contain about 2 per cent. of theobromine and 40 to 60 per cent. of solid fat. The shells contain about 1 per cent. of theobromine, together with mucilage, etc.

¶ *Medicinal Action and Uses*. Cocoa is prepared by grinding the beans into a paste between hot rollers and mixing it with sugar and starch, part of the fat being removed. Chocolate is prepared in much the same way, but the fat is retained. Oil of Theobroma or cacao butter is a yellowish white solid, with an odour resembling that of cocoa, taste bland and agreeable; generally extracted by expression. It is used as an ingredient in cosmetic ointments and in pharmacy for coating pills and preparing suppositories. It has excellent emollient properties and is used to soften and protect chapped hands and lips. Theobromine, the alkaloid contained in the beans, resembles caffeine in its action, but its effect on the central nervous system is less powerful. Its action on muscle, the kidneys and the heart is more pronounced. It is used principally for its diuretic effect due to stimulation of the renal epithelium; it is especially useful when there is an accumulation of fluid in the body resulting from cardiac failure, when it is often given with digitalis to relieve dilatation. It is also employed in high blood pressure, as it dilates the blood-vessels. It is best administered in powders or cachets.

¶ *Dosage*. Theobromine, 5 to 10 grains.

CACTUS. *See* (NIGHT-BLOOMING) CEREUS

CAJUPUT

Melaleuca leucadendron (LINN.)
N.O. Myrtaceæ

Synonyms. Cajeput. White Tea Tree. Swamp Tea Tree. White Wood
Part Used. The oil
Habitat. East Indies, Tropical Australia. Imported from Macassar, Batavia, Singapore, Queensland and N.S. Wales

¶ *Description*. The tree has a long flexible trunk with irregular ascending branches, covered with a pale thick, lamellated bark, it is soft and spongy and from time to time throws off its outer layer in flakes; leaves entire, linear, lanceolate, ash colour, alternate on short foot-stalks; flowers sessile, white, on a long spike. The leaves have a very aromatic odour and the oil is distilled from the fresh leaves and twigs, and is volatile and stimulating with an aroma like camphor,

rosemary, or cardamom seeds; taste bitter, aromatic and camphoraceous. Traces of copper have been found in it, hence the greenish tint; it should be stored in dark or amber-coloured bottles in a cool place. Cajuput oil is obtained from *Melaleuca leucadendron*, Roxburgh, and the *minor*, Smith, but several other species of *Melaleuca leucadendron* are utilized, such as *M. hypericifolia*, *M. veridifolia*, *M. lalifolia*, and others. The Australian species *M. Decussata* and *M.*

Erucifolia are also used. The oil is fluid, clear, inflammable, burns without residue, highly volatile. The trace of copper found may be due to the vessels in which the oil is prepared, but it is doubtless sometimes added in commerce to produce the normal green tinge when other species have been used which do not impart it naturally.

¶ *Constituents*. The principal constituent of oil is cineol, which should average 45 to 55 per cent. Solid terpineol is also present and several aldehydes such as valeric, butyric and benzoic.

¶ *Medicinal Action and Uses*. Antispasmodic, diaphoretic, stimulant, antiseptic, anthelmintic. Highly stimulant, producing a sensation of warmth when taken internally, increasing the fullness and rapidity of the pulse and sometimes producing profuse perspiration. Used as a stimulating expectorant in chronic laryngitis and bronchitis, as an antiseptic in cystisis and as an anthelmintic for round worms, also used in chronic rheumatism. Applied externally, it is stimulant and mildly counter-irritant and is usually applied diluted with 2 parts of olive oil or turpentine ointment. Used externally for psoriasis and other skin affections.

¶ *Adulterants*. The oils of Rosemary and Turpentine, impregnated with Camphor and coloured, are said to be used. Spirit of Cajeput, B.P., 5 to 20 minims. Oil, U.S.P., 3 to 10 minims. Oil, B.P., $\frac{1}{2}$ to 3 minims.

(*POISON*)
CALABAR BEAN

Physostigma venenosum (EALF.)
N.O. Leguminosæ

Synonyms. Ordeal Bean. Chop Nut
Part Used. The seeds
Habitat. West Africa, Old Calabar. Has been introduced into India and Brazil

¶ *Description*. The plant came into notice in 1846 and was planted in the Edinburgh Botanical Gardens, where it grew into a strong perennial creeper. It is a great twining climber, pinnately trifoliate leaves, pendulous racemes of purplish bean-like flowers; seeds are two or three together in dark brown pods about 6 inches long and kidney-shaped, thick, about 1 inch long, rounded ends, roughish but a little polished, and have a long scar on the edge where adherent to the placenta. The seeds ripen at all seasons, but are best and most abundant during the rainy season in Africa, June till September. The natives of Africa employ the bean as an ordeal owing to its very poisonous qualities. They call it *esere*, and it is given to an accused person to eat. If the prisoner vomits within half an hour he is accounted innocent, but if he succumbs he is found guilty. A draught of the pounded seeds infused in water is said to have been fatal to a man within an hour.

¶ *Constituents*. The chief constituent is the alkaloid physostigmine (eserine), with which are calabarines, eseridine, and eseramine. Eseridine is not employed medicinally.

¶ *Medicinal Action and Uses*. Chiefly used for diseases of the eye; it causes rapid contraction of the pupil and disturbed vision. Also used as a stimulant to the unstriped muscles of the intestines in chronic constipation. Its action on the circulation is to slow the pulse and raise blood-pressure; it depresses the central nervous system, causing muscular weakness; it has been employed internally for its depressant action in epilepsy, cholera, etc., and given hypodermically in acute tetanus. Physostigmine Salicylas is preferred for the preparation of eyedrops.

¶ *Preparation of Doses*. Extract of Calabar Bean, B.P.: dose, $\frac{1}{4}$ to 1 grain. Extract of Physostigma, U.S.P.: dose, $\frac{1}{8}$ grain. Tincture of Calabar Bean, B.P.C.: dose, 5 to 15 minims. Tincture of Physostigma, U.S.P.: dose, 15 minims. Physostigmine Eyedrops, B.P.C. Physostigmine eye ointment, B.P.C. Fluid extract, 1 to 3 drops.

¶ *Poisons and Antidotes*. In case of poisoning by the beans the stomach should be evacuated and atropine injected until the pulse quickens. With poisoning by physostigmine the stomach should be washed out with 0·2 per cent. of potassium permanganate and atropine and strychnine administered hypodermically,

CALAMINT

Calamintha officinalis (MOENCH)
N.O. Labiatæ

Synonyms. Mill Mountain. Mountain Balm. Basil Thyme. Mountain Mint
Part Used. Herb

¶ *Description*. Calamint belongs to a genus closely related to both the Thymes and to Catnep and Ground Ivy.

It is an erect, bushy plant with square stems, rarely more than a foot high, bearing pairs of opposite leaves, which, like the stems, are downy with soft hairs. The flowers bloom in July and August, and are

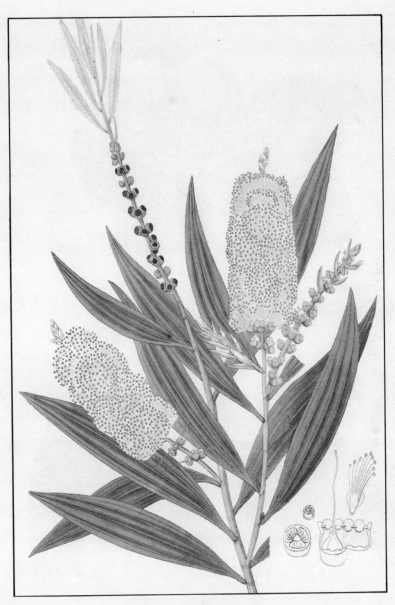

CAJUPUT
Melaleuca Leucadendron

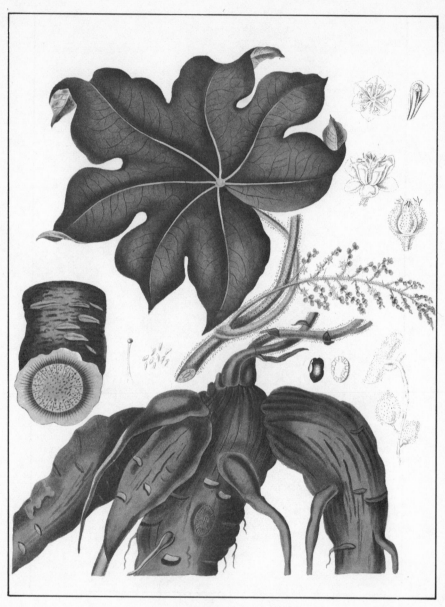

CALUMBA
Jateorhiza Calumba

somewhat inconspicuous, drooping gracefully before expansion: the corollas are of a light purple colour.

The plant grows by waysides and in hedges, and is not uncommon, especially in dry places. It may be cultivated as a hardy perennial, propagated by seeds sown outdoors in April, by cuttings of side shoots in cold frames in spring, or by division of roots in October and April.

¶ *Constituents*. It contains a camphoraceous, volatile, stimulating oil in common with the other mints. This is distilled by water, but its virtues are better extracted by rectified spirit.

¶ *Medicinal Actions and Uses*. Diaphoretic, expectorant, aromatic. The whole herb has a sweet, aromatic odour and an infusion of the dried leaves, collected about July, when in their best condition and dried in the same way as Catmint tops, makes a pleasant cordial tea, which was formerly much taken for weaknesses of the stomach and flatulent colic. It is useful in hysterical complaints, and a conserve made of the young fresh tops has been used, for this purpose.

Culpepper says that it 'is very efficacious in all afflictions of the brain,' that it 'relieves convulsions and cramps, shortness of breath or choleric pains in the stomach or bowels,' and that 'it cures the yellow jaundice.' He also recommends it, taken with salt and honey, for killing worms:

'It relieves those who have the leprosy,

taken inwardly, drinking whey after it, or the green herb outwardly applied, and that it taketh away black and blue marks in the face, and maketh black scars become well coloured, if the green herb (not the dry) be boiled in wine and laid to the place or the place washed therewith.'

He also considers it 'helpful to them that have a tertian ague,' and beneficial in all disorders of the gall and spleen

Gerard says, 'the seede cureth the infirmities of the hart, taketh away sorrowfulnesse which commeth of melancholie, and maketh a man merrie and glad.'

The LESSER CALAMINT (*Calamintha nepeta*) is a variety of the herb possessing almost superior virtues, with a stronger odour, resembling that of Pennyroyal, and a moderately pungent taste somewhat like Spearmint, but warmer. It is scarcely distinct from *C. officinalis*, and by some botanists is considered a sub-species. The leaves are more strongly toothed, and it bears its flowers on longer stalks. Both this and the Common Calamint seem to have been used indifferently in the old practice of medicine under the name of Calamint.

The name of the genus, *Calamintha*, is derived from the Greek *Kalos* (excellent because of the ancient belief in its power to drive away serpents and the dreaded basilisk – the fabled king of the serpents, whose very glance was fatal.

See BASIL and BASIL THYME.

CALAMUS AROMATICUS. *See* SEDGE

CALISAYA

Cinchona calisaya (WEDD.)
N.O. Rubiaceæ

Synonyms. Jesuit's Powder. Yellow Cinchona
Part Used. Bark
Habitat. Tropical valleys of the Andes, Bolivia and Southern Peru

¶ *Description*. Cinchona is an important genus and comprises a large number of evergreen trees and shrubs, flowers white and pinkish arranged in panicles, very fragrant. Not all the species yield cinchona or Peruvian bark. The most important is called Calisaya or yellow bark. Its great value as a tonic and febrifuge depends on an alkaloid, *quina* (Quinine). This substance chiefly exists in the cellular tissue outside the liber in combination with kinic and tannic acids. Calisaya yields the largest amount of this alkaloid of any of the species – often 70 to 80 per cent. of the total alkaloids contained in the bark which is not collected from trees growing wild, but from those cultivated in plantations. The bark for commerce is classified under two headings: the druggist's bark, and the manufacturer's at a low price. The great bulk

of the trade is in Amsterdam, and the bark sold there mainly comes from Java. That sold in London from India, Ceylon and South America. Mature Calisaya bark has a scaly appearance, which denotes maturity and high quality. It is very bitter, astringent and odourless.

¶ *Constituents*. The bark should yield between 5 and 6 per cent. of total alkaloids, of which not less than half should consist of quinine and cinchonidin. Other constituents are cinchonine, quinidine, hydrocinchonidine, quinamine, homokinchonidine, hydroquinine; quinic and cinchotannic acids, a bitter amorphous glucocide, starch and calcium-oxalate.

¶ *Medicinal Action and Uses. See* PERUVIAN BARK.

153

¶ *Preparations and Dosages*. Decoction of Cinchona, B.P., ½ to 2 fluid ounces. Elixir of Cinchona or Elixir of Calisaya, B.P.C., ½ to 1 fluid drachm. Tincture of Cinchona, B.P.C., ½ to 1 fluid drachm. Cinchona wine, B.P.C., ½ to 1 fluid ounce.

(*POISON*)
CALOTROPIS

Calotropis procera (R. BR.) and gigantea
N.O. Asclepiadaceæ

  Synonyms. Mudar Yercum
  Parts Used. Bark, root-bark
  Habitat. Native of Hindustan, but widely naturalized in the East and West Indies and Ceylon

¶ *Description*. The dried root freed from its outer cork layer and called Mudar. It occurs in commerce in short quilled pieces about ⅛ to 1/10 of an inch thick and not over 1½ inch wide. Deeply furrowed and reticulated, colour greyish buff, easily separated from periderm. Fracture short and mealy, taste bitter, nauseous, acrid; it has a peculiar smell and is mucilaginous; official in India and the Colonial addendum for the preparation of a tincture.

¶ *Constituents*. A yellow bitter resin; a black acid resin; Madaralbum, a crystalline colourless substance; Madarfluavil, an amber-coloured viscid substance; and caoutchouc, and a peculiar principle which gelatinizes on being heated, called Mudarine. Lewin found a neutral principle, Calatropin, a very active poison of the digitalis type. In India the author's husband experimented with it for paper-making, the inner bark yielding a fibre stronger than Russian hemp. The acrid juice hardens into a substance like gutta-percha. It has long been used in India for abortive and suicidal purposes. Mudar root-bark is very largely used there as a treatment for elephantiasis and leprosy, and is efficacious in cases of chronic eczema, also for diarrhœa and dysentery.

¶ *Preparations*. Tincture of Calatropis, ½ to 1 fluid drachm. Powder, 3 to 12 grains.

¶ *Antidotes*. As an antidote to poisoning, atropine may be administered. In severe cases the stomach pump may be used and chloral or chloroform administered. Amyl nitrite may also be useful.

See ASCLEPIAS, PLEURISY ROOT, SWAMP MILKWEED.

CALUMBA

Jateorhiza calumba (MIERS)
N.O. Menispermaceæ

  Synonyms. Cocculus Palmatus. Colombo
  Part Used. The dried root sliced transversely.
  Habitat. Forests of Eastern Africa. Indigenous to Mozambique, where it is abundant in the forests

¶ *Description*. A diœcious climbing plant with a perennial root, consisting of several tuberous portions, flowers small and inconspicuous; the root is dug in dry weather, in March, but only the fusiform offsets are used; the old root is rejected and the brightest, least worm-eaten and well-shaped pieces are preferred. The root and powder, if kept any length of time, are liable to be attacked by worms; the colour of the freshly prepared powder is greenish, later on it turns brown and when moistened very dark; it quickly absorbs moisture from the air and is apt to decompose, so only a small quantity should be prepared at a time. Odour aromatic, taste very bitter, rind more so than the central pith, which is somewhat mucilaginous. It is rarely adulterated since the price has been lowered.

¶ *Constituents*. Columbamine, Jateorhizine and Palmatine, three yellow crystalline alkaloids closely allied to berberine; also a colourless crystalline principle, Columbine, and an abundance of starch and mucilage.

¶ *Medicinal Action and Uses*. A bitter tonic without astringency, does not produce nausea, headache, sickness or feverishness as other remedies of the same class. It is best given as a cold infusion; it is a most valuable agent for weakness of the digestive organs. In pulmonary consumption it is useful, as it never debilitates or purges the bowels. The natives of Mozambique use it for dysentery. It allays the sickness of pregnancy and gastric irritation. In Africa and the East Indies it is cultivated for dyeing purposes.

¶ *Preparations*. Calumba is generally combined with other tonics. For flatulence, ½ oz. of Calumba, ½ oz. of ginger, 1 drachm of senna, added to 1 pint of boiling water, is taken three times daily in wineglassful doses.

Calumba can be safely combined with salts of iron and alkalies, as it does not contain tannic or gallic acid. The powdered root, 10 to 15 grains. The solid extract, 2 grains. The powdered extract, 2 grains. The fluid extract, 10 to 30 minims. The infusion, B.P., ½ to 1 drachm. The tincture, B.P. and U.S.P., ½ to 1 drachm. The concentrated solution, B.P., ½ to 1 drachm.

CAMELLIA. *See* TEA

CAMPANULA. *See* RAMPION

CAMPHOR Cinnamonum camphora (T. NEES and EBERM.)
N.O. Lauraceæ

Synonyms. Laurel Camphor. Gum Camphor
Part Used. Gum
Habitat. China, Japan, and adjacent parts of East Asia. Formosa official in the U.S.P.
Dryobalanops aromatica is indigenous to Borneo and Sumatra

¶ *Description.* Camphor is a white crystalline substance, obtained from the tree *Cinnamonum camphora*, but the name has been given to various concrete odorous volatile products, found in different aromatic plants. The commercial Camphor comes only from *C. camphora* and *Dryobalanops camphora* (fam. *Dipterocarpacæa*). The first gives our official Camphor, the latter the Borneo Camphor, which is much valued in the East, but unknown in Europe and America. *C. camphora* is an evergreen tree looking not unlike our linden; it grows to a great size, is many-branched, flowers white, small and clustered, fruit a red berry much like cinnamon. While the tree grows in China, etc., it can be cultivated successfully in sub-tropical countries, such as India and Ceylon, and it will thrive in Egypt, Formosa, Madagascar, Canary Islands and southern parts of Europe, California, Florida, and also in Argentina. It grows so slowly that the return financially is a long investment. Some growers think that Camphor cannot be taken from the trees till they are fifty years old. In Japan and Formosa the drug comes from the root, trunk and branches of the tree by sublimation, but there is less injury done to the tree in the American plantations, as it is taken there from the leaves and twigs of the oldest trees. A Camphor oil exudes in the process of extracting Camphor, which is valued by the Chinese, used for medicinal purposes. Two substances are found in commerce under the name of oil of Camphor: one is the produce of *C. cinnamonum*, and is known as Formosa or Japanese oil of Camphor; the other as East Indian oil of Camphor, from the *D. aromatica*, but this oil is not found in European or American trade. It is less volatile than the other, and has a distinctive odour; it is highly prized by the Chinese, who use it for embalming purposes and to scent soap. The Chinese attribute many virtues to it. It is mentioned by Marco Polo in the thirteenth century and Camoens in 1571, who called it the 'balsam of disease.' During the last few years large quantities have come into the American and European markets as Japanese oil; it varies in quality and colour from a thin watery oil to a thick black one. It is imported in tin cans and varies greatly in the amount of Camphor it contains, some cans having had all the solid principle extracted before importation. The odour is peculiar, like sassafras, and distinctly camphoraceous; this oil is said to be used in Japan for burning, making varnish and for Chinese inks, as a diluent for artists' colours; it has a capacity for dissolving resins that oil of Turps has not. The properties in the oil are much the same as in Camphor, but it is more stimulant and very useful in complaints of stomach and bowels, in spasmodic cholera and flatulent colic. It is also used as a rubefacient and sedative liniment, and if diluted with Olive oil or soap is excellent for local rheumatism, sprains, bruises, and neuralgia; dose, 2 or 3 minims. There is an erroneous idea that Camphor acts as a preventive to infectious diseases. It is very acrid and in large doses very poisonous, and should be used cautiously in certain heart cases. It is a well-known preventive of moths and other insects, such as worms in wood; natural history cabinets are often made of it, the wood of the tree being occasionally imported to make cabinets for entomologists. The Dryobalanops oil of Camphor is said to be found in trees too young to produce Camphor, and is said to be the first stage of the development of Camphor, as it is found in the cavities of the trunk, which later on become filled with Camphor. Its chief constituent is an oil called Borneene. The *D. aromatica* tree, found in Sumatra and Borneo, grows to an enormous height, often over 100 feet, and trunk 6 or 7 feet in diameter. The Camphor of the older trees exists in concrete masses, in longitudinal cavities, in the heart of the tree, $1\frac{1}{2}$ feet long at certain distances apart. The only way of finding out if Camphor has formed in the tree is by incision. This Camphor is chiefly used for funeral rites, and any that is exported is bought by the Chinese at a high price, as they use it for embalming, it being less volatile than ordinary Camphor. Another Camphor called N'gai, obtained from the *Blumea Balcamferi* (*Compositæ*), differs chemically from the Borneo species, being lævogyrate, and is converted by boiling nitric acid, to a substance considered identical with stearoptene of *Chrysanthemum parthenium*. This plant grows freely in the author's garden, and is known in Great Britain as Double-flowered Bush Fever-Few.

¶ *Medicinal Action and Uses.* Camphor has a strong, penetrating, fragrant odour, a bitter, pungent taste, and is slightly cold to the touch like menthol leaves; locally it is an irritant, numbs the peripheral sensory nerves, and is slightly antiseptic; it is not readily absorbed by the mucous membrane, but is easily absorbed by the subcutaneous tissue; it combines in the body with glucuronic acid, and in this condition is voided by the urine. Experiments on frogs show a depressant action to the spinal column, no motor disturbance, but a slow increasing paralysis; in mankind it causes convulsions, from the effect it has on the motor tract of the brain; it stimulates the intellectual centres and prevents narcotic drugs taking effect, but in cases of nervous excitement it has a soothing and quieting result. Authorities vary as to its effect on blood pressure; some think it raises it, others take an opposite view; but it has been proved valuable as an excitant in cases of heart failure, whether due to diseases or as a result of infectious fevers, such as typhoid

and pneumonia, not only in the latter case as a stimulant to circulation, but as preventing the growth of pneumococci. Camphor is used in medicine internally for its calming influence in hysteria, nervousness and neuralgia, and for serious diarrhœa, and externally as a counter-irritant in rheumatisms, sprains, bronchitis, and in inflammatory conditions, and sometimes in conjunction with menthol and phenol for heart failure; it is often given hypodermically, 3 to 5 grains dissolved in 20 to 30 minims of sterile Olive oil – the effect will last about two hours. In nervous diseases it may be given in substance or in capsules or in spirit; dose 2 to 5 grains. Its great value is in colds, chills, and in all inflammatory complaints; it relieves irritation of the sexual organs.

¶ *Preparations and Dosages.* Spirit of Camphor, B.P., 5 to 20 drops. Tincture of Camphor Comp., B.P. (Paregoric), ½ to 1 drachm. Camphor water, B.P., 1 to 2 oz. Liniment of Aconite, B.P. Liniment of Belladonna, B.P. Liniment of Camphor Comp., B.P. Liniment of Opium, B.P. Liniment of Soap, B.P. Liniment of Mustard, B.P. Liniment of Turpentine, B.P. Liniment of Turpentine and Acetic Acid, B.P. Spirit of Camphor, B.P., 5 to 20 drops. Tincture of Camphor Comp., B.P.

CAMPION. *See* CORNCOCKLE

CANADIAN HEMP. *See* HEMP, CANADIAN

CANCHALAGUA. *See* CENTAURY, CHILIAN

CANDYTUFT, BITTER

Iberis amara
N.O. Cruciferæ

Parts Used. Leaves, stem, root, seeds
Habitat. Found in various parts of Europe and in English and Scotch cornfields, specially in limestone districts

¶ *Description.* This plant is an erect, rather stiff, very bitter annual, 6 to 12 inches high; flowers milky white, forming a terminal flat corymb; leaves oblong, lanceolate, acute, toothed; pod nearly orbicular, the long style projecting from notch at top; it flowers with the corns.

¶ *Medicinal Action and Uses.* A tincture made from the ripe seeds is much used in homœopathy, but the plant is more generally used by American herbalists. All parts of the plant are used, leaves, stem, root and seeds,

more particularly the latter. It has always been used for gout, rheumatism and kindred ailments, and is now usually combined with other plants for the same diseases in their acute form, and as a simple to allay excited action of the heart, especially when it is enlarged. For asthma, bronchitis and dropsy it is considered very useful.

¶ *Dosage.* 1 to 3 grains of the powdered seeds. In overdoses or too large ones it is said to produce giddiness, nausea and diarrhœa.

CANELLA. *See* (WHITE) CINNAMON

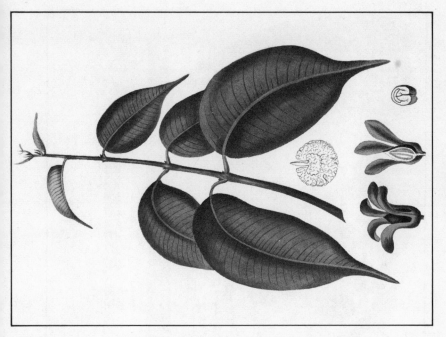

CAMPHOR
Cinnamomum Camphora

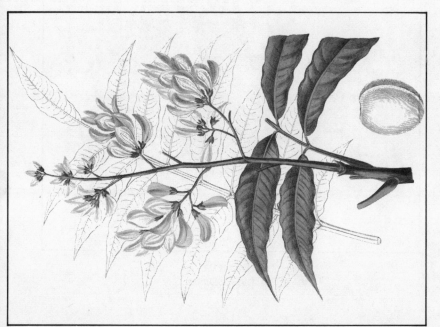

CABBAGE TREE
Andira Inermis

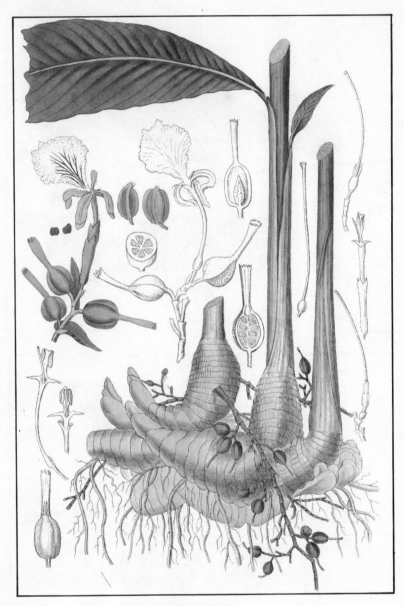

CARDAMOM
Elettaria Cardamomum

CAPSICUM. *See* CAYENNE

CARAWAY
Carum Carvi (LINN.)
N.O. Umbelliferæ

Synonym. Caraway Seed
Part Used. Fruit
Habitat. The plant is distributed throughout the northern and central parts of Europe and Asia, though where it occurs in this country it is only considered a naturalized species, having apparently escaped from cultivation

Caraway is another member of the group of aromatic, umbelliferous plants characterized by carminative properties, like Anise, Cumin, Dill and Fennel. It is grown, however, less for the medicinal properties of the fruits, or so-called 'seeds,' than for their use as a flavouring in cookery, confectionery and liqueurs.

¶ *Description.* It is a biennial, with smooth, furrowed stems, growing $1\frac{1}{2}$ to 2 feet high, bearing finely cut leaves, and umbels of white flowers which blossom in June. The fruits – which are popularly and incorrectly called seeds – and which correspond in general character to those of the other plants of this large family, are laterally compressed, somewhat horny and translucent, slightly curved, and marked with five distinct, pale ridges. They evolve a pleasant, aromatic odour when bruised, and have an agreeable taste.

The leaves possess similar properties and afford an oil identical with that of the fruit. The tender leaves in spring have been boiled in soup, to give it an aromatic flavour.

¶ *History.* The roots are thick and tapering, like a parsnip, though much smaller and are edible. Parkinson declared them, when young, to be superior in flavour to Parsnips. Mixed with milk and made into bread, they are said to have formed the 'Chara' of Julius Cæsar, eaten by the soldiers of Valerius. Caraway was well known in classic days, and it is believed that its use originated with the ancient Arabs, who called the 'seeds' *Karawya*, a name they still bear in the East, and clearly the origin of our word Caraway and the Latin name *Carvi*, although Pliny would have us believe that the name Carvi was derived from Caria, in Asia Minor, where according to him the plant was originally found. In old Spanish the name occurs as *Alcaravea*.

Caraway is frequently mentioned by the old writers. Dioscorides advised the oil to be taken by pale-faced girls. In the Middle Ages and in Shakespeare's times it was very popular.

'The seed,' says Parkinson, 'is much used to be put among baked fruit, or into bread, cakes, etc., to give them a rellish. It is also made into comfites and taken for cold or wind in the body, which also are served to the table with fruit.'

In *Henry IV*, Squire Shallow invites Falstaff to 'a pippin and a dish of caraways.' The custom of serving roast apples with a little saucerful of Caraway is still kept up at Trinity College, Cambridge, and at some of the old-fashioned London Livery Dinners, just as in Shakespeare's days – and in Scotland to this day a saucerful is put down at tea to dip the buttered side of bread into and called 'salt water jelly.'

The scattering of the seed over cakes has long been practised, and Caraway-seed cake was formerly a standing institution at the feasts given by farmers to their labourers at the end of the wheat-sowing. The little Caraway comfits consist of the seeds encrusted with white sugar. In Germany, the peasants flavour their cheese, cabbage, soups, and household bread with Caraway, and in Norway and Sweden, polenta-like, black, Caraway bread is largely eaten in country districts.

The oil extracted from the fruits is used as an ingredient of alcoholic liquors: both the Russians and the Germans make from Caraway a liqueur, 'Kummel,' and Caraway enters into the composition of *l'huile de Venus* and other cordials.

A curious superstition was held in olden times about the Caraway. It was deemed to confer the gift of retention, preventing the theft of any object which contained it, and holding the thief in custody within the invaded house. In like manner it was thought to keep lovers from proving fickle (forming an ingredient of love potions), and also to prevent fowls and pigeons from straying. It is an undoubted fact that tame pigeons, who are particularly fond of the seeds, will never stray if they are given a piece of baked Caraway dough in their cote.

¶ *Cultivation. Preparation for Market.* Caraway does best when the seeds are sown in the autumn, as soon as ripe, though they may be sown in March. Sow in drills, 1 foot apart, the plants when strong enough, being thinned out to about 8 inches in the rows. The ground will require an occasional hoeing to keep it clean and assist the growth of the plants. From an autumn-sown crop, seeds will be produced in the following summer, ripening about August.

When the fruit ripens, the plant is cut and the Caraways are separated by threshing. They can be dried either on trays in the sun, or by very gentle heat over a stove, shaking occasionally.

There are several varieties, the English, the Dutch and the German (obtained from plants extensively cultivated in Moravia and Prussia), and other varieties imported from Norway, Finland, Russia and the Morocco ports.

¶ *Habitat.* One marked peculiarity about Caraway is that it is indigenous to all parts of Europe, Siberia, Turkey in Asia, Persia, India and North Africa, and yet it is cultivated only in a few comparatively restricted areas. It grows wild in many parts of Canada and the United States, but is nowhere grown there as a field or garden crop. Its cultivation is restricted to relatively small areas in England, Holland, Germany, Finland, Russia, Norway and Morocco, where it constitutes one of the chief agricultural industries within its narrow confines. It has so far received comparatively little attention in England, where it is grown only in Essex, Kent and Suffolk, upon old grassland broken up for the purpose. Holland cultivates the main crop, producing and exporting far larger quantities than any other country. It is cultivated most extensively there in the provinces of Gröningen and North Holland, in which more than half the acreage is found. In the whole country about 20,000 acres are devoted to this crop, each acre yielding about 1,000 lb., whereas while Caraway is grown commercially throughout Germany, Austria, France and parts of Spain, the character and amounts produced are very variable, and the yield per acre varies only from 400 to 700 lb., and these countries do not produce much more than they require for home consumption. Morocco produces a grade of Caraway that comes regularly into the English and American markets, but is somewhat inferior in quality. Dutch Caraway is preferred among consumers in the United States, and the bulk used there comes from Holland.

During the last year or two there has been a scarcity of Caraway, owing partly to the fact that the extensive area of land in Holland usually employed for the cultivation of the plant was devastated by floods towards the close of 1915. Much Dill seed is now being sold in its place. Quite lately, a small grower reported that she had netted £5 from growing Caraway on a corner of what otherwise would have been waste ground.

¶ *Constituents.* The seeds contain from 4 to 7 per cent. of volatile oil, according to the variety of Caraway fruit from which obtained, that distilled from home-grown fruits being considered the best. Caraway grown in more northerly latitudes is richer in essential oil than that grown in southern regions, and if grown in full sun a greater percentage and a richer oil is obtained.

The oil is distilled chiefly from Dutch, Norwegian and Russian fruits. The Dutch are small and dark brown in colour. English fruits, of which only a small quantity is produced, are of a brighter tint.

The chief constituent of the oil is a hydrocarbon termed Carvene, also found in oils of Dill and Cumin, and an oxygenated oil, Carvol, a mobile liquid (isomeric with the menthol of Spearmint).

From 6 lb. of the unbruised seeds, 4 oz. of the pure essential oil can be expressed.

The exhausted seed, after the distillation of the oil, contains a high percentage of protein and fat, and is used as a cattle food.

¶ *Medicinal Action and Uses.* Both fruit and oil possess aromatic, stimulant and carminative properties. Caraway was widely employed at one time as a carminative cordial, and was recommended in dyspepsia and symptoms attending hysteria and other disorders. It possesses some tonic property and forms a pleasant stomachic. Its former extensive employment in medicine has much decreased in recent years, and the oil and fruit are now principally employed as adjuncts to other medicines as corrective or flavouring agents, combined with purgatives. For flatulent indigestion, however, from 1 to 4 drops of the essential oil of Caraway given on a lump of sugar, or in a teaspoonful of water, will be found efficacious. Distilled Caraway water is considered a useful remedy in the flatulent colic of infants, and is an excellent vehicle for children's medicine. When sweetened, its flavour is agreeable.

One ounce of the bruised seeds infused for 6 hours in a pint of cold water makes a good Caraway julep for infants, from 1 to 3 teaspoonful being given for a dose.

The bruised seeds, pounded with the crumb of a hot new loaf and a little spirit to moisten, was an old-fashioned remedy for bad earache. The powder of the seeds, made into a poultice, will also take away bruises.

CARDAMOMS

Elettaria Cardamomum (MATON)
N.O. Zingiberaceæ (Scitamineæ)

Synonyms. Amomum Cardamomum. Alpinia Cardamomum. Matonia Cardamomum. Cardamomum minus. Amomum repens. Cardamomi Semina. Cardamom Seeds. Malabar Cardamums. Ebil. Kakelah seghar. Capalaga. Gujatatti elachi. Ilachi. Ailum

Part Used. The dried, ripe seeds

Habitat. Southern India

¶ *Description.* The large perennial herb yielding Cardamom seeds is known in its own country as 'Elattari' or 'Ilachi,' while 'Cardamomum' was the name by which some Indian spice was known in classical times.

It has a large, fleshy rhizome, and the alternate, lanceolate leaves are blades from 1 to $2\frac{1}{2}$ feet long, smooth and dark green above, pale, glaucous green and finely silky beneath. The flowering stems spread horizontally near the ground, from a few inches to 2 feet long, and bear small, loose racemes, the small flowers being usually yellowish, with a violet lip. The fruits are from $\frac{2}{5}$ to $\frac{4}{5}$ of an inch long, ovoid or oblong, bluntly triangular in section, shortly beaked at the apex, pale yellowish grey in colour, plump, and nearly smooth. They are three-celled, and contain in each cell two rows of small seeds of a dark, reddish-brown colour. These should be kept in their pericarps and only separated when required for use. Though only the seeds are official, the retention of the pericarp is an obstacle to adulteration, while it contains some oil and forms a good surface for grinding the seeds. The value is estimated by the plumpness and heaviness of the fruits and the soundness and ripeness of the seeds. Unripe seeds are paler and less plump. The unbroken fruits are gathered before they are quite ripe, as the seeds of fruits which have partially opened are less aromatic, and such fruits are less valued. The seeds have a powerful, aromatic odour, and an agreeable, pungent, aromatic taste, but the pericarps are odourless and tasteless.

There is some confusion as to the different kinds, both botanically and commercially, different writers distinguishing them in varied ways.

The official Cardamums in the United States are stated to be *only* those produced in India, chiefly in Malabar and Mysore, but in Britain the seeds corresponding most closely to the official description are recognized, in spite of their names, as being imported from Ceylon.

The Cardamom is a native of Southern India, and grows abundantly in forests 2,500 to 5,000 feet above sea-level in North Canara, Coorgi and Wynaad, where it is also largely cultivated. It flowers in April and May and the fruit-gathering lasts in dry weather for three months, starting in October. The methods of cultivating and preparing vary in different districts.

In the Bombay Presidency the fruits are washed by women with water from special wells and pounded soap nut (a kind of acacia). They are dried on house-roofs, the stalks clipped, and sometimes a starchy paste is sprinkled over them, in addition to the bleaching.

Bombay ships about 250,000 lb. annually to the London market. They were formerly known by their shapes as *shorts*, *short-longs*, and *long-longs*, but the last are now rarely seen. One hundred parts of the fruit yield on an average 74 parts of seeds and 26 of pericarp. The powdered seeds may be distinguished from the powdered fruit by the absence of the tissues of the pericarp.

The seeds are about $\frac{1}{5}$ of an inch long, angular, wrinkled, and whitish inside. They should be powdered only when wanted for use, as they lose their aromatic properties.

In Great Britain and the United States Cardamums are employed to a small extent as an ingredient of curry powder, and in Russia, Sweden, Norway, and parts of Germany are largely used for flavouring cakes and in the preparation of liqueurs, etc. In Egypt they are ground and put in coffee, and in the East Indies are used both as a condiment and for chewing with betel. Their use was known to the ancients.[1] In France and America the oil is used in perfumery.

¶ *Constituents.* The seeds contain volatile oil, fixed oil, salt of potassium, a colouring principle, starch, nitrogenous mucilage, ligneous fibre, an acrid resin, and ash. The volatile oil contains terpenes, terpineol and cineol. Good 'shorts' yield about 4·6 per cent. It is colourless when fresh, but becomes thicker, more yellow, and less aromatic. It is very soluble in alcohol and readily soluble in four volumes of 70 per cent. alcohol, forming a clear solution.

Its specific gravity is 0·924 to 0·927 at 25° C. (77° F.). It is not used medicinally, but solely for pharmaceutical purposes, being employed as a flavouring in the compound

---

[1] There are constant references to Cardamom Seeds in *The Arabian Nights.* – EDITOR.

spirit and compound elixir of Cardamums, and in other elixirs and mixtures. It is largely adulterated, owing to the high price of the seeds and the small percentage of volatile oil found in them.

¶ *Medicinal Action and Uses.* Carminative, stimulant, aromatic, but rarely used alone; chiefly useful as an adjuvant or corrective.

The seeds are helpful in indigestion and flatulence, giving a grateful but not fiery warmth. When chewed singly in the mouth the flavour is not unpleasant, and they are said to be good for colic and disorders of the head.

In flavouring they are combined with oils of Orange, Cinnamon, Cloves, and Caraway.

The substitution of glycerine for honey in the 1880 United States' formula for compound tincture increased its stability.

¶ *Dosages.* 15 to 30 grains of the powdered seeds. Of tincture, $\frac{1}{2}$ to 1 fluid drachm. Of compound tincture, B.P., $\frac{1}{2}$ to 1 fluid drachm. Fluid extract, 5 to 30 drops.

¶ *Adulterations.* Various unofficial Cardamums are included, the product of other species. Orange seeds and unroasted grains of coffee are also admixed. The oil is said to be no longer distilled from *Elettaria cardamomum.* It is often factitious, and composed of oils of Cajuput, Nutmeg, etc.

¶ *Other Species.*

MADRAS CARDAMUMS, exported from Madras and Pondicherry.

ALEPPY CARDAMUMS, exported from Aleppy and Calicut, are also recognized in Britain, the former being paler and 'short-longs' and the latter 'shorts.'

CEYLON WILD CARDAMOMS are the fruits of *E. cardamomum* var. *major*, imported from Ceylon, and sometimes called Long Wild Natives. They are cultivated in Kandy, and

sometimes called in the East, Grains of Paradise, but they are not the product known by that name in Europe and America.

ROUND or SIAM CARDAMUMS are probably those referred to by Dioscorides, and called *Amomi uva* by Pliny. They are the fruits of *A. cardamomum* and *A. globosum*, growing in Java, Siam, and China, etc., and are nearly the size of a cherry. In their natural clusters they are the *amomum racemosum* or *amome en grappe* of the French, and in Southern Europe are sometimes used in the same way as the official kinds.

BENGAL CARDAMOMS, from *A. subulatum*, are sometimes called Winged Bengal Cardamums, Morung elachi, or Buro elachi. They are oblong or oval, and about an inch long.

NEPAL CARDAMUMS, of unknown origin, are like the Bengal species, but usually stalked, and have a long, tubular calyx.

WINGED JAVA CARDAMOMS, from *A. maximum*, growing in the Malay islands, are about an inch long, and when soaked in water show from 4 to 13 ragged wings on each side. They are feebly aromatic, and are usually sent abroad from the London markets.

KORARIMA CARDAMOMS, from *A. kararima*, have recently become known.

MADAGASCAR CARDAMUMS, of *A. angustifolium*, have pointed, ovate flattened capsules. The flavour of the seeds resembles the official variety.

BASTARD CARDAMUMS, from *A. Xanthioides*, looks like the real kind, but is greenish in colour, and tastes like crude camphor.

Cardamomum Siberiense (Star Aniseed), Annis de Sibérie of the seventeenth century, and *badiane* of the French, is from *Illicium verum*, the fruit of which is chiefly used in preparing a volatile oil resembling the official oil of Anise.

CARDOONS. *See* ARTICHOKE

CAROBA

Jacaranda procera (SPRENG.)
N.O. Bignoniaceæ

Synonyms. Carob Tree. Carobinha. Bignonia Caroba. Jacaranda Caroba. Caaroba
Part Used. The leaves
Habitat. South America

¶ *Description.* The genus *Jacaranda* includes several species which are used medicinally in South America, and especially in Brazil. The trees are small, and the leaves thick, tough, and lanceolate, about $2\frac{1}{2}$ inches long, odourless, and slightly bitter in taste.

¶ *Constituents.* There has been found in the leaves Caroba balsam, caroborelinic acid, carobic acid, steocarobic acid, carobon, and crystalline substance, carobin.

¶ *Medicinal Actions and Uses.* The value of the *Jacaranda* active principles has been proved in syphilis and venereal diseases, being widely used by the aborigines of Brazil and other South American countries. The leaves have also been tried in epilepsy for their soothing influence.

¶ *Dosage.* From 15 to 60 grains.

¶ *Other Species.*
CAROB-TREE, or *Ceratonia siliqua*, is a small

tree of the Mediterranean coasts.[1] Beyond its name it has no connexion with Caroba. It furnishes the St. John's Bread which probably corresponds to the husks of the Prodigal Son parable, and the seed which is said to have been the original jewellers' carat weight.

The Spaniards call it Algaroba, and the Arabs Kharoub, hence Carob or Caroub Pods, Beans, or Sugar-pods. It is also called Locust Pods. These pods are much used in the south of Europe for feeding domestic animals and, in times of scarcity, as human food. Being saccharine, they are more heat-giving than nourishing. The seeds or beans were used as fodder for British cavalry horses during the Spanish campaign of 1811–12.

South American varieties are *Prosopis dulcis* and *P. siliquastrum* of the Leguminosæ family.

CARROT

Daucus carota (LINN.)
N.O. Umbelliferæ

Synonyms. Philtron (Old Greek). Bird's Neat
Part Used. Whole herb
Habitat. A native wild plant common everywhere in the British Islands

Both the Carrot and Parsnip are striking examples of the effect of cultivation on wild plants. The roots of the wild variety are small and woody, while those of the cultivated kind are fleshy and succulent and grow to a considerable size.

¶ *History.* The Carrot was well known to the ancients, and is mentioned by Greek and Latin writers under various names, being, however, not always distinguished from the Parsnip and Skirret, closely allied to it. The Greeks – Professor Henslow tells us – had three words: *Sisaron*, first occurring in the writings of Epicharmus, a comic poet (500 B.C.); *Staphylinos*, used by Hippocrates (430 B.C.) and *Elaphoboscum*, used by Dioscorides (first century A.D.), whose description of the plant applies accurately to the modern Carrot. Pliny says:

'There is one kind of wild *pastinaca* which grows spontaneously; by the Greeks it is known as *staphylinos*. Another kind is grown either from the root transplanted or else from seed, the ground being dug to a very considerable depth for the purpose. It begins to be fit for eating at the end of the year, but it is still better at the end of two; even then, however, it preserves its strong pungent flavour, which it is found impossible to get rid of.'

In speaking of the medical virtue of the first species (which is evidently the Carrot, the second variety presumably the Parsnip), he adds, 'the cultivated has the same as the wild kind, though the latter is more powerful, especially when growing in stony places.'

The name *Carota* for the garden Carrot is found first in the writings of Athenæus (A.D. 200), and in a book on cookery by Apicius Cælius (A.D. 230). It was Galen (second century A.D.) who added the name *Daucus* to distinguish the Carrot from the Parsnip, calling it *D. pastinaca*, and *Daucus* came to be the official name in the sixteenth century, and was adopted by Linnæus in the eighteenth century.

From the time of Dioscorides and Pliny to the present day, the Carrot has been in constant use by all nations. It was long cultivated on the Continent before it became known in this country, where it was first generally cultivated in the reign of Queen Elizabeth, being introduced by the Flemings, who took refuge here from the persecutions of Philip II of Spain, and who, finding the soil about Sandwich peculiarly favourable for it, grew it there largely. As vegetables were at that time rather scarce in England, the Carrot was warmly welcomed and became a general favourite, its cultivation spreading over the country. It is mentioned appreciatively by Shakespeare in *The Merry Wives of Windsor*. In the reign of James I, it became the fashion for ladies to use its feathery leaves in their head-dresses. A very charming, fern-like decoration may be obtained if the thick end of a large carrot be cut off and placed in a saucer of water in a warm place, when the young and delicate leaves soon begin to sprout and form a pretty tuft of verdant green, well worth the slight trouble entailed.

Its root is small and spindle-shaped, whitish, slender and hard, with a strong aromatic smell and an acrid, disagreeable taste, very different to the reddish, thick, fleshy, cultivated form, with its pleasant odour and peculiar, sweet, mucilaginous

---

[1] One species of *Jacarande* tree grows in Palermo, and the exquisite blue flowers when in bloom about the middle of June are an arresting sight, much more suggestive of 'Love in the Mist' than the plant which actually bears that name. – EDITOR.

flavour. It penetrates some distance into the ground, having only a few lateral rootlets.

¶ *Description*. The stems are erect and branched, generally about 2 feet high, tough and furrowed. Both stems and leaves are more or less clothed with stout, coarse hairs. The leaves are very finely divided, the lowest leaves considerably larger than the upper; their arrangement on the stem is alternate, and all the leaves embrace the stem with the sheathing base, which is so characteristic of this group of plants, the Umbelliferæ, to which the Carrot belongs. The blossoms are densely clustered together in terminal umbels, or flattened heads, in which the flower-bearing stalks of the head all arise from one point in rays, like the ribs of an umbrella, each ray again dividing in the case of the Carrot, to form a secondary umbel, or umbellule of white flowers, the outer ones of which are irregular and larger than the others. The wild Carrot is in bloom from June to August, but often continues flowering much longer. The flowers themselves are very small, but from their whiteness and number, they form a conspicuous head, nearly flat while in bloom, or slightly convex, but as the seeds ripen, the umbels contract, the outer rays, which are to begin with 1 to 2 inches long, lengthening and curving inwards, so that the head forms a hollow cup – hence one of the old popular names for the plant: Bird's Nest. The fruit is slightly flattened, with numerous bristles arranged in five rows. The ring of finely-divided and leaf-like bracts at the point where the umbel springs is a noticeable feature.

The Carrot is well distinguished from other plants of the same order by having the central flower of the umbel, or sometimes a tiny umbellule, of a bright red or deep purple colour, though there is a variety, *D. maritimus*, frequent on many parts of the sea coast in the south of England, which differs in having somewhat fleshy leaves and in being destitute of the central purple flower. In this case, all the flowers of the head have often a somewhat pinkish tinge. There was a curious superstition that this small purple flower of the Carrot was of benefit in epilepsy.

¶ *Parts Used Medicinally*. The whole herb, collected in July; the seeds and root. The whole herb is the part now more generally in use.

¶ *Medicinal Action and Uses*. Diuretic, Stimulant, Deobstruent. An infusion of the whole herb is considered an active and valuable remedy in the treatment of dropsy, chronic kidney diseases and affections of the bladder. The infusion of tea, made from one ounce of the herb in a pint of boiling water, is taken in wineglassful doses. Carrot tea, taken night and morning, and brewed in this manner from the whole plant, is considered excellent for lithic acid or gouty disposition. A strong decoction is very useful in gravel and stone, and is good against flatulence. A fluid extract is also prepared, the dose being from $\frac{1}{2}$ to 1 drachm.

The *seeds* are carminative, stimulant and very useful in flatulence, windy colic, hiccough, dysentery, chronic coughs, etc. The dose of the seeds, bruised, is from one-third to one teaspoonful, repeated as necessary. They were at one time considered a valuable remedy for calculus complaints. They are excellent in obstructions of the viscera, in jaundice (for which they were formerly considered a specific), and in the beginnings of dropsies, and are also of service as an emmenagogue. They have a slight aromatic smell and a warm, pungent taste. They communicate an agreeable flavour to malt liquor, if infused in it while in the vat, and render it a useful drink in scorbutic disorders.

Old writers tell us that a poultice made of the *roots* has been found to mitigate the pain of cancerous ulcers, and that the *leaves*, applied with honey, cleanse running sores and ulcers. An infusion of the root was also used as an aperient.

¶ *Cultivation*. The root of the Carrot consists of Bark and Wood: the bark of the Garden Carrot is the outer red layer, dark and pulpy and sweet to the taste; the wood forms the yellow core, gradually becoming hard, stringy and fibrous. The aim of cultivation, therefore, is to obtain a fleshy root, with the smallest part of wood. This depends on soil and the quality and kind of seed.

For its successful cultivation, Carrot needs a light, warm soil, which has been well manured in the previous season. The most suitable soil is a light one inclining to sand, a somewhat sandy loam or dry, peaty land being the best, but even heavy ground, properly prepared, may be made to produce good Carrots. Formerly the cultivation of the Carrot was almost entirely confined to the light lands of Norfolk and Suffolk.

The ground should be well prepared some months in advance; heavy ground should be lightened by the addition of wood ash, road scrapings, old potting soil and similar materials. It is essential that the soil be in such a state as to allow the roots to penetrate to their full length without interruption. Previous to sowing the seed, the soil should be lightly forked over, and, if possible, be

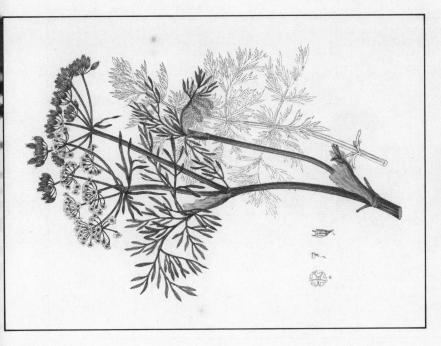

CARAWAY
Carum Carvi

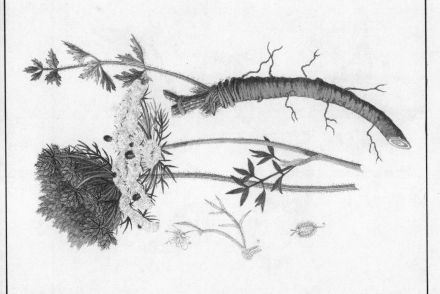

CARROT
Daucus Carota

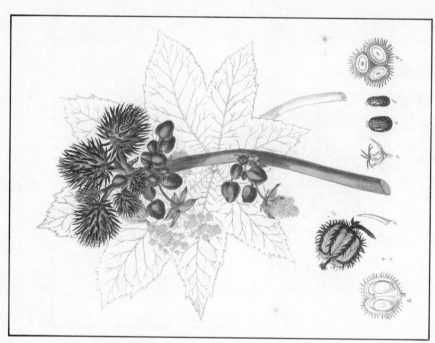

CASTOR OIL PLANT
Ricinus Communis

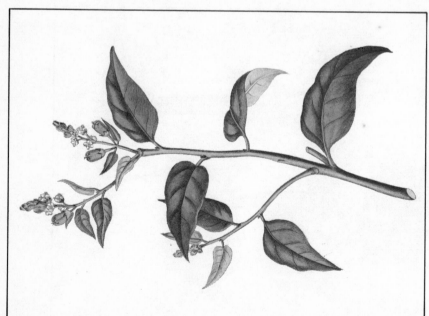

CASCARILLA
Crown Eleuteria

given a dressing of leaf soil or well decayed vegetable matter, but no fresh manure must be dug into the top spit of ground intended for Carrots and Parsnips, as it may cause the roots to become forked. The crops will, however, benefit by about an ounce of super-phosphate to the square yard, raked in before sowing, or by a light dressing of soot.

Sowing of the main crop should be done in calm weather about the middle of March or early in April. The seeds frequently adhere to one another by means of the forked hairs which surround them. These hairs can be removed by rubbing through the hands or a fine chaff sieve. The seeds should then be mixed with about twice the bulk of dry earth, sand or sifted ashes (about one bushel of seeds to 4 or 5 lb. of sand). When the ground is thoroughly prepared and has been firmly trodden, draw flat-bottomed drills from north to south, $\frac{1}{2}$ inch deep and 3 inches wide. Distribute the seed along the row evenly and thinly and cover lightly. Carrots can hardly be covered too lightly, $\frac{1}{2}$ inch of fine soil is quite enough, and for ordinary use they may be sown in drills one foot apart, but if extra large roots are desired, more room must be given between the rows. As soon as the young plants are large enough to handle they may be thinned to 6 inches or 8 inches apart. The thinning may be at first to a distance of 3 inches, and then a final thinning later, the second thinnings being used as young Carrots for culinary purposes. Frequent dustings of soot will greatly benefit the crop. Light hoeings between the rows to keep the crop free from weeds is all that is necessary during the period of growth. Partial shade from other crops is often found beneficial.

Scarlet Immediate is the best sort for general purposes.

Main-crop Carrots are generally taken up about the last week in October, or early in November, by three-pronged forks, and stored in sand in a dry place, where they can be kept till the following March or April. Some of the roots dug in the autumn can be replanted in February, about 2 feet apart, with the crown or head a few inches below the surface. Leaves and flowers will spring from them, and the seeds produced will ripen in the autumn.

By making successional sowings, good crops of small roots will be always available. In gardens, Carrots are grown in succession of crops from the latter part of February to the beginning of August. For early Carrots sow on a warm border in February: such a sowing, if made as soon as the state of ground allows, will assure early Carrots just when fresh and quickly-grown vegetables are most highly prized. They will be off in time to leave the ground ready for other crops.

After a good dressing of soot has been given, Carrots may be sown again, and even then it leaves the room vacant for winter greens or cabbage for use next spring. Sowing as late as July is generally successful in most districts. Main crops are often sown too early, especially on cold soils. Carrots are liable to attacks of grubs and insects, the upper part of the root being also attacked by the grub of a kind of fly, the best remedy being late sowing, to avoid the period at which these insects are evolved from the egg. Dusting with ashes and a little soot or lime wards off both birds and slugs from the young tender growths.

Carrots are a valuable product for the farmer in feeding his cattle, and for this purpose are raised in large quantities. The produce of an acre of Carrots in Suffolk is on an average 350 bushels per acre, but sometimes much more. In the Channel Islands and Brittany, much larger crops of Carrots and Parsnips are obtained than are yielded in England, the soil being deeply trenched by a spade or specially-constructed plough. Far more Carrots are grown in France, Germany and Belgium for fodder than here. Horses are remarkably fond of Carrots, and when mixed with oats, Carrots form a very good food for them; with a small quantity of oats or other corn, a horse may be supported on from 20 to 30 lb. of Carrots daily. In Suffolk, Carrots were formerly given as a specific for preserving and restoring the wind of horses, but they are not considered good for cattle if fed too long on them. They may also with advantage be given both to pigs and poultry, and rabbits are especially fond of them. The kinds grown for farm purposes are generally larger than those in the kitchen garden and are known as Red Carrots, the more delicate Orange Carrot being the variety used in cooking. Some farmers sow the seeds on the top of the drills, which is said to be an improvement over the gardener, who makes his Carrot-bed on the flat in the ordinary way. This ridge system gives good results, the Carrots being clean and well-shaped and free from grubs. The farmers reckon about 2 lb. of seed for an acre for drills, and 5 or 6 lb. if sown broadcast. For ordinary garden purposes, one ounce of seed is reckoned to be sufficient for about 600 feet sown in drills.

¶ *Chemical Constituents.* The juice of the Carrot when expressed contains crystallizable and uncrystallizable sugar, a little starch, extractive gluten, albumen, volatile oil (on which the medicinal properties of the root depend and which is fragrant, aromatic and stimulating), vegetable jelly or pectin, saline matter, malic acid and a peculiar crystallizable, ruby-red neutral principle, without odour or taste, called Carotin.

Carrots contain no less than 89 per cent. of water; their most distinguishing dietical substance is sugar, of which they contain about 4·5 per cent.

Owing to the large percentage of carbohydrate material contained by Carrots, rabbits fed for some days on Carrots alone, are found to have an increased amount of glycogen stored in the liver, carbohydrate being converted into glycogen in the body.

Sir Humphry Davy ascertained the nutritive matter of Carrots to amount to 98 parts in 1,000, of which 95 are sugar, and three are starch. Weight for weight, they stand third in nourishing value on the list of roots and tubers, potatoes and parsnips taking first and second places. Carrots, containing less water and more nourishing material than green vegetables, have higher nutritive qualities than turnips, swedes, cabbage, sprouts, cauliflower, onions and leeks. Moreover, the fair proportion of sugar contained in their composition adds to their nourishing value.

In the interesting collection of the Food Collection at Bethnal Green Museum, prepared by Dr. Lankester, we learn that the maximum amount of work produceable by a pound of Carrots is that it will enable a man to raise 64 tons one foot high, so that it would appear to be a very efficient force-producer. From 1 lb. of Carrots we can obtain 1 oz. and 11 grains of sugar, while out of the 16 oz. fourteen are water. When we consider that in an average man of 11 stone or 154 lb. weight, about 111 of these are water, we see what a large supply is needful to repair waste and wear and tear.

¶ *Medicinal and General Uses.* The chief virtues of the Carrot lie in the strong antiseptic qualities they possess, which prevent all putrescent changes within the body.

Carrots were formerly of some medicinal repute as a laxative, vermifuge, poultice, etc., and the seeds have been employed as a substitute for caraways.

At Vichy, where derangements of the liver are specially treated, Carrots in one form or the other are served at every meal, whether in soup or as vegetables, and considerable efficacy of cure is attributed to them.

In country districts, raw Carrots are still sometimes given to children for expelling worms, and the boiled roots, mashed to a pulp, are sometimes used as a cataplasm for application to ulcers and cancerous sores.

Carrot sugar, got from the inspissated juice of the roots, may be used at table, and is good for the coughs of consumptive children.

A good British wine may be brewed from the root of the Carrot, and a very tolerable bread prepared from the roots, dried and powdered. The pectic acid contained can be extracted from the root and solidifies into a wholesome, appetizing jelly.

In Germany, a substitute and adulteration for coffee has been made of Carrots chopped into small pieces, partially carbonized by roasting and then ground.

In France and Germany a spirit is distilled from the Carrot, which yields more spirit than the potato. The refuse after making the spirit is good for feeding pigs.

Attempts have also been made to extract sugar from Carrots, but the resulting thick syrup refuses to crystallize, and in competition with either cane sugar or that obtained from the beetroot, it has not proved commercially successful.

Carrots are also used in winter and spring in the dairy, to give colour and flavour to butter, and a dye similar to woad has been obtained from the leaves.

RECIPES

Carrot Jam

Wash and grate some carrots; boil until reduced to a thick pulp. To 1 lb. of this pulp add 9 oz. sugar, the juice and grated rind of 2 lemons, and 3 oz. margarine. Boil the mixture well for 45 minutes to 1 hour. The result is a useful and inexpensive jam, which can be made for 6d. to 8d. a lb. (according to the price of the lemons), if all materials have to be bought, and for considerably less by those who have home-grown carrots available.

Preserved Young Carrots

Turn the carrots in their own shape, and as you do so, them turn into hot water; when all are ready, put them in a stewpan with water enough to cover them; add fresh butter in the proportion of an ounce to the pound of carrots, and salt to season; boil the carrots in this till half done, and then arrange them neatly in tin boxes; fill up with their own liquor, solder down, boil for ½ hour, and put them away in the cool.

CARROT, WILD

Daucus carota (LINN.)
N.O. Umbelliferæ

Synonyms. Birds' Nest and Bees' Nest
Parts Used. Whole herb, seeds, root
Habitat. Britain, near the sea in greatest abundance, and in waste places throughout Europe, Russian Asia, America, and is even found in India

¶ *Habitat*. Probably originally a native of the sea-coasts of Southern Europe degenerated into its present wild state, but of very ancient cultivation. The name 'Carrot' is Celtic, and means 'red of colour,' and *Daucus* from the Greek *dais* to burn, signifying its pungent and stimulating qualities.

The Carrot was in ancient times much valued for its medicinal properties; the Wild Carrot, which is found so plentifully in Britain, both in cultivated lands and by waysides, thriving more especially by the sea, is superior, medicinally, to the cultivated kind.

¶ *Description*. Its root is small and spindle-shaped, whitish, slender and hard, with a strong aromatic smell and an acrid, disagreeable taste, very different to the reddish, thick, fleshy, cultivated form, with its pleasant odour and peculiar, sweet, mucilaginous flavour. It penetrates some distance into the ground, having only a few lateral rootlets.

The stems are erect and branched, generally about 2 feet high, tough and furrowed. Both stems and leaves are more or less clothed with stout, coarse hairs. The leaves are very finely divided, the lowest leaves considerably larger than the upper; their arrangement on the stem is alternate, and all the leaves embrace the stem with the sheathing base, which is so characteristic of this group of plants, the Umbelliferæ, to which the Carrot belongs. The blossoms are densely clustered together in terminal umbels, or flattened heads, in which the flower-bearing stalks of the head all arise from one point, in rays, like the ribs of an umbrella, each ray again dividing in the case of the Carrot, in like manner to form a secondary umbel, or umbellule of white flowers, the outer ones of which are irregular and larger than the others. The Wild Carrot is in bloom from June to August, but often continues flowering much longer. The flowers themselves are very small, but from their whiteness and number, they form a conspicuous head, nearly flat while in bloom, or slightly convex, but as the seeds ripen, the umbels contract, the outer rays, which are to begin with 1 to 2 inches long, lengthening and curving inwards, so that the head forms a hollow cup – hence one of the old popular names for the plant – Birds' Nest. The fruit is slightly flattened, with numerous bristles arranged in five rows. The ring of finely-divided and leaf-like bracts at the point where the umbel springs is a noticeable feature.

The Carrot is well distinguished from other plants of the same order by having the central flower of the umbel, or sometimes a tiny umbellule, of a bright red or deep purple colour, though there is a variety, *Daucus maritimus*, frequent in many parts of the sea-coast in the south of England, which differs in having somewhat fleshy leaves and no central purple flower. In this case, all the flowers of the head have usually a somewhat pinkish tinge. There was a curious superstition that this small purple flower of the Carrot was of benefit for mitigating epilepsy.

¶ *Constituents*. The medicinal properties of the seeds are owing to a volatile oil which is colourless or slightly tinged with yellow; this is procured by distilling with water. They also yield their virtues by infusion to water at 212° F.; boiling dissipates them. No thorough analysis has been made.

¶ *Medicinal Action and Uses*. Diuretic, stimulant, deobstruent. An infusion of the whole herb is considered an active and valuable remedy in the treatment of dropsy, chronic kidney diseases and affections of the bladder. The infusion, made from 1 oz. of the herb in a pint of boiling water, is taken in wineglassful doses. Carrot tea, taken night and morning, and brewed in this manner from the whole front, is considered excellent for a gouty disposition. A strong decoction is very useful in gravel and stone, and is good against flatulence. A fluid extract is also prepared, the dose being from ½ to 1 drachm.

The seeds are carminative, stimulant and very useful in flatulence, windy colic, hiccough, dysentery, chronic coughs, etc. The dose of the seeds, bruised, is from one-third to one teaspoonful, repeated as necessary. They were at one time considered a valuable remedy for calculus complaints. They are excellent in obstructions of the viscera, in jaundice (for which they were formerly considered a specific), and in the beginnings of dropsies, and are also of service as an emmenagogue. They have a slight aromatic smell and a warm, pungent taste. They communicate an agreeable flavour to malt liquor, if infused in it while working in the vat, and render it a useful drink in scorbutic disorders.

Old writers tell us that a poultice made of the roots has been found to mitigate the pain of cancerous ulcers, and that the leaves, applied with honey, cleanse running sores and ulcers. An infusion of the root was also used as an aperient.

CASCARA, AMARGA

Picramnia antidesma (s. w.)
N.O. Simarubacæa

Synonyms. Mountain Damson Bark. Simaruba Honduras Bark
Parts Used. Bark, root-bark
Habitat. Jamaica and South Guiana

¶ *Description.* A native of the West Indies and yields the drug known as Simaruba bark. The tree grows to a considerable height and thickness and has alternate spreading branches; the bark on the old trees is black and furrowed, on the younger trees smooth grey, in places spotted with big patches of yellow; the wood is hard, white and without any special taste; it has numerous leaves alternately on the branches, each leaf has several pinnæ, nearly elliptical, upper side smooth deep green, under side whitish, short foot-stalks, flowers male and female on different trees, colour yellow in long panicles. The bark is rough scaly and poor; inside when fresh is a good yellow colour, but when dry paler; it has very little smell and taste and though very bitter is not disagreeable. Macerated in water or rectified spirits it gives a yellow tincture; makes a better and stronger infusion in cold water than in boiling water; the decoction is transparent yellow when hot, but when cooled is turbid and brownish red in colour. The bark was brought from Guiana in 1713 as a remedy for dysentery. In France in 1718 to 1825 an epidemic flux was cured by the bark and this established its medicinal use in Europe.

¶ *Constituents.* A bitter tonic credited with specific alternative properties. It belongs to an undetermined species of picrammia and contains a bitter sweet amorphous alkaloid.

¶ *Medicinal Action and Uses.* Purgative, tonic, diaphoretic. A very valuable bitter tonic, useful in diarrhœa, dysentery, and in some forms of indigestion; in large doses it is said to act as an emetic. It restores tone to the intestines, allays spasmodic motions, promotes a healthy secretion. Big doses cause vomiting and nausea – should not be used in dysentery attended with fever. In dysentery with weak indigestion it is often preferred to chamonilee.

¶ *Dosage.* The infusion taken in wineglassful doses every four to six hours.

¶ *Other Species.*
Simaruba versicolor, a Brazilian species, has similar properties; the fruits and barks are also used as anthelmintics, and an infusion of the bark is used for snake-bite. The plant is so bitter that insects will not attack it – on which account the powdered bark has been used to kill vermin.

S. alauca, a native of Cuba, gives a glutinous juice which has been found useful in some forms of skin disease.

CASCARA SAGRADA. *See* BUCKTHORN, CALIFORNIAN

CASCARILLA

Croton Eleuteria (J. BENN.)
N.O. Euphorbiaceæ

Synonyms. Sweetwood Bark. Sweet Bark. Bahama Cascarilla. Elutheria. Clutia Eleuteria. Cascarillæ Cortex. Cortex Thuris. Aromatic Quinquina. False Quinquina
Part Used. The dried bark
Habitat. The Bahama Islands

¶ *History.* The name *Croton* comes from a Greek word meaning 'a tick,' and *Eleuteria* from the name of one of the Bahama Islands, Eleuthera, near Providence Island.

¶ *Description.* It is a small tree rarely reaching 20 feet in height, with scanty, alternate, ovate-lanceolate leaves, averaging 2 inches long, closely-scaled below, giving a metallic silver-bronze appearance, with scattered, white scales above. The flowers are small, with white petals, and very fragrant, appearing in March and April. The scented bark is fissured, and pale yellowish brown. It is imported from Nassau, in New Providence.

The quills of dried bark average 2 inches in length, and $\frac{3}{8}$ inch in thickness. They are often furrowed in both directions, so that they appear to be chequered. The outer, thin, corky layer is white, often covered with a fine lichen (*Verrucaria albissima*). The second layer is brownish, and sometimes shows through. The bark is hard and compact, breaking with a short, resinous fracture. The taste is nauseating, warm and bitter, and the odour agreeable and aromatic, especially when burned, resembling weak musk, so that it is used in fumigating pastilles, and sometimes mixed with tobacco, though in the latter case some regard it as being liable to cause giddiness and symptoms of intoxication.

The *leaves* can be infused for a digestive tea, and the bark yields a good, black dye.

¶ *Constituents.* There have been found in the *bark* albumen, tannin, cascar illin (a bitter, crystallizable principle, soluble in alcohol, ether, and hot water), red colouring matter, fatty matter with a sickly odour, volatile oil, gum, wax, resin, starch, pectic acid, potassium chloride, a salt of calcium, and lignin.

The *oil* contains an alcohol, two sesquiterpenes, a free acid consisting of liquid cascarillic acid and a mixture of solid palmitic and stearic acids, eugenol, a terpene (differing from pinene), cymene, and possibly some *l*-limonene. Betaine has also been found.

¶ *Medicinal Action and Uses.* An aromatic, bitter tonic, with possibly narcotic properties. It is used in dyspepsia, intermittent and low fevers, diarrhœa and dysentery. It is a stimulant to mucous membranes, and in chronic bronchitis is used as an expectorant; while it is valuable in atonia dyspepsia, flatulence, chronic diarrhœa, nocturnal pollutions, debility and convalescence. Added to cinchona, it will arrest vomiting caused by that drug.

¶ *Dosages.* Of Cascarilla powdered Bark, 20 to 30 grains. Of Infusum Cascarillæ (B.P. 1 oz. to ½ pint), 1 to 2 fluid ounces. Of Tinctura Cascarillæ, ½ to 2 fluid drachms. Of fluid extract, ½ to 1 fluid drachm. Tincture, B.P., ½ to 1 drachm.

¶ *Other Species.*
Cascarilla is also the name of *Quina morada*, the bark of *Pogonopus febrifugus*, used in the Argentine Republic as a substitute for cinchona bark. An alkaloid, Moradeine, and a blue fluorescent substance, Moradin, have been separated from it.

Croton Cascarilla, the Wild Rosemary of the West Indies, was at first thought to be the source of the Cascarilla of commerce.

C. Pseudo-China, or Copalchi Bark, of Mexico, also known as Copalche Bark or *C. niveus*, resembles *C. Eleuteria* so closely that it can be mistaken for it. It is used in the same way. A second variety, more bitter, may be a product of *C. suberosus*.

It has also been mistaken for a variety of cinchona.

C. micans is thought to have similar properties.

White, red, and black Cascarillas are also found in commerce, differing in form and properties, but these are other names for varieties of quinquina.

CASHEW NUT

Anacardium occidentale (LINN.)
N.O. Anacardiaceæ

Synonym. Cassavium pomiferum
Part Used. Nut
Habitat. Jamaica, West Indies, and other parts of tropical America

¶ *Description.* A medium-sized tree, beautiful, and not unlike in appearance the walnut tree, with oval blunt alternate leaves and scented rose-coloured panicles of bloom — the tree produces a fleshy receptacle, commonly called an apple, at the end of which the kidney-shaped nut is borne; the end of it which is attached to the apple, is much bigger than the other. The outer shell is ashy colour, very smooth, the kernel is covered with an inner shell, and between the two shells is found a thick inflammable caustic oil, which will raise blisters on the skin and be dangerously painful if the nuts are cracked with the teeth.

¶ *Constituents.* Two peculiar principles have been found: Anacardic Acid and a yellow oleaginous liquid Cardol.

¶ *Medicinal Action and Uses.* The oil must be used with great caution, but has been successfully applied to corns, warts, ringworms, cancerous ulcers and even elephantiasis, and has been used in beauty culture to remove the skin of the face in order to grow a new one. The nuts are eaten either fresh or roasted, and contain a milky juice which is used in puddings. The older nuts are roasted and salted and the dried and broken kernels are sometimes imported to mix with old Madeira as they greatly improve its flavour. In roasting great care must be taken not to let the fumes cover the face or hands, etc., as they cause acute inflammation and external poisoning. Ground and mixed with cocoa the nuts make a good chocolate. The fruit is a reddy yellow and has a pleasant sub-acid stringent taste; the expressed juice of the fruit makes a good wine, and if distilled, a spirit much better than arrack or rum. The fruit itself is edible, and its juice has been found of service in uterine complaints and dropsy. It is a powerful diuretic. The black juice of the nut and the milky juice from the tree after incision are made into an indelible marking-ink; the stems of the flowers also give a milky juice which when dried is hard and black and is used as a varnish. A gum is also found in the plant having the same qualities as gum-arabic; it is imported from South America under the name of Cadjii gum, and used by South American bookbinders, who wash their books with it to keep away moths and ants. The caustic oil found in the layers of the fruit is sometimes rubbed into the floors of houses in India to keep white ants away.

¶ *Other Species.*

The Oriental *Anacardium* or Cashew Nut (*Semecarpus anacardium*), a native of India, has similar qualities to the West Indian Cashew, and is said to contain an alkaloid called Chuchunine.

Ammonium anarcadate. This is the Ammonium compound of beta and delta resinous acids of *A. occidentale* (Cashew Nut), and is used as a hair-dye, but cannot be used with acids, acid salts, or acetate of lead.

CASSAVA. *See* MANDIOCA

CASSIA (CINNAMON)

Cinnamomum cassia (BLUME)
N.O. Lauraceæ

Synonyms. Bastard Cinnamon. Chinese Cinnamon. Cassia lignea. Cassia Bark. Cassia aromaticum. Canton Cassia

Part Used. The dried bark

Habitat. Indigenous to China. Cochin-China and Annam. Also cultivated in Sumatra, Ceylon, Japan, Java, Mexico and South America

¶ *Description.* As its name of Bastard Cinnamon implies, the product of this tree is usually regarded as a substitute for that of the *Cinnamomum zeylanicum* of Ceylon, which it closely resembles. The cultivated trees are kept as coppices, and numerous shoots, which are not allowed to rise higher than 10 feet, spring from the roots. Their appearance when the flame-coloured leaves and delicate blossoms first appear is very beautiful. The fruit is about the size of a small olive. The leaves are evergreen, oval-oblong blades from 5 to 9 inches long. The trees are at their greatest perfection at the age of ten to twelve years, but they continue to spread and send up new shoots. The bark may be easily distinguished from that of cinnamon, as it is thicker, coarser, darker, and duller, the flavour being more pungent, less sweet and delicate, and slightly bitter. The stronger flavour causes it to be preferred to cinnamon by German and Roman chocolate makers. The fracture is short, and the quills are single, while pieces of the corky layer are often left adhering. The best and most pungent bark is cut from the young shoots when the leaves are red, or from trees which grow in rocky situations. The bark should separate easily from the wood, and be covered inside with a mucilaginous juice, though the flavour of the spice is spoiled if this is not carefully removed. The wood without the bark is odourless and is used as fuel. When clean, the bark is a little thicker than parchment, and curls up while drying in the sun. It is imported in bundles of about 12 inches long, tied together with strips of bamboo and weighing about a pound. It is the kind almost universally kept in American shops.

The dried, unripe fruits, or *Chinese Cassia*
Buds, have the odour and taste of the bark, and are rather like small cloves in appearance. They have been known in Europe as a spice since the Middle Ages, being then probably used in preparing a spiced wine called Hippocras. Now they are employed in confectionery and in making Pot-Pourri. The importation of the buds into the U.S.A. in 1916 was 197,156 lb., and of Cassia and Cassia leaves 7,487,156 lb.

¶ *Constituents.* Cassia bark yields from 1 to 2 per cent. of volatile oil, somewhat resembling that of cinnamon. It should be kept from the light in well-stoppered, amber-coloured bottles. It is cheaper and more abundant than the Ceylon variety, and is the only official oil of Cinnamon in the United States Pharmacopœia and German Pharmacopœia. It is imported from Canton and Singapore. Its value depends on the percentage of cinnamic aldehyde which it contains. It is heavier, less liquid, and congeals more quickly than the Ceylon oil.

There are also found in it cinnamyl acetate, cinnamic acid, phenylpropyl acetate and orthocumaric aldehyde, tannic acid and starch.

Ceylon cinnamon, if tested with one or two drops of tincture of iodine to a fluid ounce of a decoction of the powder, is but little affected, while with Cassia a deep blue-black colour is produced. The cheaper kinds of Cassia can be distinguished by the greater quantity of mucilage, which can be extracted by cold water.

Eighty pounds of the freshly-prepared bark yield about 2·5 oz. of the lighter of the two oils produced, and 5·5 of the heavier.

An oil was formerly obtained by distilling the leaves after maceration in sea water, and this was imported into Great Britain.

¶ *Medicinal Action and Uses.* Stomachic, carminative, mildly astringent, said to be emmenagogue and capable of decreasing the secretion of milk. The tincture is useful in uterine hæmorrhage and menorrhagia, the doses of 1 drachm being given every 5, 10, or 20 minutes as required. It is chiefly used to assist and flavour other drugs, being helpful in diarrhœa, nausea, vomiting, and to relieve flatulence.

The oil is a powerful germicide, but being very irritant is rarely used in medicine for this purpose. It is a strong local stimulant, sometimes prescribed in gastro-dynia, flatulent colic, and gastric debility.

¶ *Dosages.* Of oil, 1 to 3 minims. Of powder, 10 to 20 grains.

¶ *Poisons and Antidotes.* It was found that 6 drachms of the oil would kill a moderately sized dog in five hours, and 2 drachms in forty hours, inflammation of the gastro-intestinal mucous membrane being observed.

¶ *Other Species, Substitutes and Adulterations.* The powder cinnamon is often adulterated with sugar, ground walnut shells, galanga rhizome, etc.

The oil sometimes contains resin, petroleum, or oil of Cloves. *Saigon cinnamon* was recognized by the United States Pharmacopœia in 1890. It comes from French Cochin-China, its botanical origin being uncertain. It is also known as Annam Cinnamon, China Cinnamon, and God's Cinnamon.

C. inners gives the Wild Cinnamon of Japan. It is also found in Southern India, where the buds are more mature, and are employed medicinally by the Indians in dysentery, diarrhœa and coughs. The bark is used as a condiment.

C. lignea includes several inferior varieties from the Malabar Coast.

C. Sintok comes from Java and Sumatra.

C. obtusifolium, from East Bengal, Assam, Burmah, etc., is perhaps not distinct from *C. Zeylanicum.*

C. Culilawan and *C. rubrum* come from the Moluccas, Amboyna, and have a flavour of cloves.

C. Loureirii grows in Cochin-China and Japan.

C. pauciflorum is found from Silhet and Khasya.

C. Burmanni is said to yield Massoi Bark, which is also a product of *Massora aromatica.*

The bark of *C. Tamala* as well as the above species gives the inferior *Cassia Vera.*

C. inserta is slightly known.

C. nitidum has aromatic leaves, which, when dried, are said to have been the 'folia Malabathri.'

Martinique and Cayenne contribute three varieties, from trees introduced from Ceylon and Sumatra. Other kinds are known as Black Cinnamon, Isle of France Cinnamon, and Santa Fé Cinnamon.

Oil of Cassia is now recognized in the United States Pharmacopœia under the name of oil of Cinnamon.

CASTOR OIL PLANT

Ricinus communis (LINN.)
N.O. Euphorbiaceæ

Synonyms. Palma Christi. Castor Oil Bush
Part Used. Seeds
Habitat. By cultivation it has been distributed through not only all tropical and subtropical regions, but also in many of the temperate countries of the globe

The valuable purgative known as Castor Oil is the fixed oil obtained from the seeds of the Castor Oil plant. Besides being used medicinally, the oil is also employed for lubricating purposes, burning and for leather dressing. The Chinese are said to have some mode of depriving it of its medicinal properties so as to render it suitable for culinary purposes.

The Castor Oil plant is a native of India, where it bears several ancient Sanskrit names, the most ancient and most usual being *Eranda,* which has passed into several other Indian languages.

It is very variable in habit and appearance, the known varieties being very numerous, and having mostly been described as species. In the tropical latitudes most favourable to its growth, it becomes a tree 30 to 40 feet high;

in the Azores and the warmer Mediterranean countries – Algeria, Egypt, Greece and the Riviera – it is of more slender growth, attaining an average height of only 10 to 15 feet, and farther north in France, and in this country, where it is cultivated as an ornamental plant on account of its large and beautiful foliage, it is merely a shrubby, branched annual herb, rarely more than 4 to 5 feet high, with thick, hollow, herbaceous stems, which are cylindrical, smooth and shiny, with a purplish bloom in the upper part.

¶ *Description.* The handsome leaves are placed alternately on the stem, on long, curved, purplish foot-stalks, with drooping blades, generally 6 to 8 inches across, sometimes still larger, palmately cut for three-fourths of their depth into seven to eleven lance-shaped, pointed, coarsely toothed segments. When fully expanded, they are of a blue-green colour, paler beneath and smooth; when young, they are red and shining.

The flowers are male and female on the same plant, and are produced on a clustered, oblong, terminal spike. The male flowers are placed on the under portion of the spike; they have no corolla, only a green calyx, deeply cut into three to five segments, enclosing numerous, much branched, yellow stamens. The female flowers occupy the upper part of the spike and have likewise no corolla. The three narrow segments of the calyx are, however, of a reddish colour, and the ovary in their centre is crowned by deeply-divided, carmine-red threads (styles). The fruit is a blunt, greenish, deeply-grooved capsule less than an inch long, covered with soft, yielding prickles in each of which a seed is developed. The seeds of the different cultivated varieties differ much in size and in external markings, but average seeds are of an oval, laterally compressed form. The smaller, annual varieties yield small seeds; the tree forms, large seeds. They have a shining, marble-grey and brown, thick, leathery outer coat, within which is a thin, dark-coloured, brittle coat. A large, distinct, leafy embryo lies in the middle of a dense, oily tissue (endosperm). The seeds contain a toxic substance which make them actively poisonous, so much so that *three* large seeds have been known to kill an adult.

The following letter, taken from *The Chemist and Druggist* (February 19, 1921), corroborates the statement as to the 'toxic substance' in this plant:

CASTOR-OIL SEEDS DANGER

SIR, – On looking through my *C. & D.* I noticed your illustration of three ancient gentlemen "conferring at the Home Office as to whether Castor Oil should be put on the list of dangerous drugs," etc. Let me say that I think it very well might be, and I shall tell you why. In 1874, when I was in Squire's, Oxford Street, an assistant there was reading for his Minor examination, and as I had just come from Dr. Muter's school I used to bring up sometimes from the stockroom below samples of leaves, roots, seeds, etc., and show them to this assistant to see if he could tell what they were. One day I brought up some Castor Oil seeds, and asked if he knew what they were. He did not know, so I told him they were Castor Oil seeds. He said "I think it would be a good idea to make an emulsion of these and take it instead of the oil." I told him to shell them first, as there was a poisonous principle under the shell. He did so. I do not think he used more than six of the seeds, and when he had made the emulsion, which looked very nice, he drank it all. Within ten minutes he disappeared out of the shop unexpectedly, and an hour or two afterwards someone went up to his bedroom and found him lying there unconscious. It was not then known what was wrong with him; but three West-End doctors near at hand were called in, and thinking he had taken some irritant poison they treated him with opiate injections, etc., as he had been severely purged and vomiting. I had gone off duty that afternoon at five o'clock, and when I came back at eleven there was considerable commotion among the assistants. They told me what had happened, and I was able to tell them exactly what the assistant had done, as until then they did not know. He lay for nearly a fortnight before he was able to resume work, and during that time he scarcely took any food, but one of the assistants made him jellies with gelatin and the juice of lemons and oranges, as well as other light articles of diet. I guess it – the emulsion – had acted very much in the same way as a few drops of croton oil would have done had it been made into an emulsion – as an irritant poison. I therefore think some caution is needed in dealing with Castor Oil seeds, if not particularly with the oil itself. On old-fashioned Castor Oil bottles the labels stated that it was "cold-drawn" oil. This, no doubt, would be because if heat were used in expressing the oil some of the poisonous principle would be dissolved by it. The coarser varieties of Castor Oil, I think, are all more active than the fine oils, and this may likely be due to some of the poisonous element being expressed by the greater pressure used in making the cruder oil. Perhaps this note may serve as a caution to someone else who might be tempted to try an emulsion of Castor Oil seeds.

Yours truly,
R. THOMSON

Elgin.

In the South of England the plant ripens its seeds in favourable situations, and it has been known to come to maturity as far north as Christiania in Norway.

¶ *History.* It was known to Herodotus, who calls it *Kiki*, and states that it furnishes an oil much used by the Egyptians, in whose ancient tombs seeds of *Ricinus* are met with. At the period when Herodotus wrote (the fourth century B.C.), it would appear to have been already introduced into Greece, where it is cultivated to the present day under the same ancient name. The *Kikajon* of the Book of Jonah, rendered by the translators of the

English Bible, 'gourd,' is believed to be the same plant. Kiki is also mentioned by Strabo as a production of Egypt, the oil from which is used for burning in lamps and for unguents. Theophrastus and Dioscorides, in the first century, describe the plant, Dioscorides giving an account of the process for extracting the oil and saying that it is not fit for food, but is used externally in medicine, and stating that the seeds are extremely purgative. Pliny, about the same time, also speaks of it as a drastic purgative.

We read of it being employed medicinally in Europe during the early Middle Ages: it is recorded that it was cultivated by Albertus Magnus, Bishop of Ratisbon, in the middle of the thirteenth century, but later it fell into disuse, though Gerard (1597) was familiar with it under the name of *Ricinus* or Kik: the oil, he says, is called *Oleum cicinum* and used externally in skin diseases. As a garden plant, it was well known in this country in the time of Turner (1551). In the eighteenth century, its cultivation in Europe as a medicinal plant had, however, practically ceased, and the small supplies of the seeds and oil required for European medicine were obtained from Jamaica. The name 'Castor' was indeed originally applied about this period to the plant in Jamaica, where it seems to have been called 'Agnus Castus,' though it bears no resemblance to the South European plant properly so called. The botanical name is from the Latin *Ricinus* (a dog-tick), from the form and markings of the seed.

¶ *Cultivation.* The various varieties of *Ricinus*, which are perennial in their native countries, are generally annuals in England, though sometimes they may be preserved through the winter.

Plants are readily grown from seed, which should be sown on a hot bed early in March. When the plants come up, each should be planted in a separate small pot, filled with light soil and plunged into a fresh hot bed. The young plants are kept under glass till early in June, when they are hardened and put out.

Ricinus (Bronze King) and *R. Africanus* are two good garden varieties for this country, which if given good soil and kept well supplied with water, grow to a large size and make a fine effect in the garden.

¶ *Preparation for Market.* The seeds are collected when ripe: as the capsules dry, they open and discharge the seeds.

The oil is obtained from the seeds by two principal methods – *expression* and *decoction.* The latter process is largely used in India, where the oil on account of its cheapness and abundance, is extensively employed for illu-

minating, as well as for other domestic and medicinal purposes.

The oil exported from Calcutta to Europe is prepared by shelling and crushing the seed between rollers. The crushed mass is then placed in hempen cloths and pressed in a screw or hydraulic press. The oil which exudes is mixed with water and heated till the water boils and the mucilaginous matter in the oil separates as a scum. It is next strained, then bleached in the sunlight and stored for exportation.

In France, the oil is obtained by macerating the bruised seeds in alcohol, but the process is expensive and the product inferior.

There are two modes of extracting the oil by *expression*: (1) without heat, when it is termed 'cold drawn Castor Oil,' this process being largely carried out in Italy, Marseilles, Belgium, Hull and London; (2) with heat, the process generally adopted in America.

Italian Castor Oil, which is of an excellent quality, is pressed from seeds grown chiefly in the neighbourhood of Verona and Legnago. Two varieties of *Ricinus* are cultivated in these localities, the black-seeded Egyptian and the red-seeded American; the latter yields the larger percentage, but the oil is not so pale in colour. All the Castor Oil pressed in Italy, however, is not pressed from Italian seed, but some seeds are imported from India into Italy – as also into this country.

In the north of Italy, the fresh seeds are alone used, and after they have been crushed and the seed coats very carefully removed with a winnowing machine and by hand, the blanched seeds are put into small hempen bags, which are arranged in superposed layers in a powerful hydraulic press, with a sheet of iron heated to 90° F. between each layer, so as to enable the oil to flow readily; they are finally submitted to pressure in a room, which in the winter is heated to a temperature of about 70°. The oil which first flows is of the finest quality, but an inferior oil is subsequently obtained by pressing the mass at a somewhat higher temperature. The peeled seeds yield about 40 per cent. of oil. After expression, the oil is usually bleached by exposure to sunlight or by chemical means.

In America, where the oil is obtained by expression with heat, the manufacture is conducted on an extensive scale in California. There the seeds are submitted to a dry heat in a furnace for an hour or so, by which they are softened and prepared to part easily with their oil. They are then pressed in a large powerful screwpress, and the oily matter which flows out is mixed with an equal proportion of water, and boiled to purify it from mucilaginous and albuminous matter. After boiling about an hour, it is allowed to cool, the water is drawn off and the oil is transferred to zinc tanks or clarifiers capable of holding from 60 to 100 gallons. In these it stands about eight hours, bleaching in the sun, after which it is ready for storing. By this method, 100 lb. of good seeds yield about five gallons of pure oil.

Of these three varieties of extraction, the Italian or cold drawn is considered the best – the East Indian, the poorest, as the mode of purifying by heating with water is considered very imperfect. The former owes its freedom from acridity and unpleasant taste partly to the removal of the seed coats before pressing, and partly to the low temperature used during the manufacture.

¶ *Constituents.* The seeds contain 50 per cent. of the fixed oil, which is a viscid fluid, almost colourless when pure, possessing only a slight odour and a mild, yet highly nauseous and disagreeable taste. Its specific gravity is high for an oil, being 0·96, a little less than that of water, and it dissolves freely in alcohol, ether and glacial acetic acid. It contains Palmitic and several other fatty acids, among which there is one – Ricinoleic acid – peculiar to itself. This occurs in combination with glycerine, constituting the greater part of the bulk of the oil. The oil is decomposed by the fat-splitting ferments of the intestinal canal liberating this irritant Ricinoleic acid, to which the purgative action is considered in all probablity to be due.

Both the seeds themselves and the cake left after the expression of the oil are violently purgative, a property which is due to the presence of the highly toxic albumin Ricin. The seeds are never employed in this country on account of their violent action. Ricin exhibits its highest toxicity when injected into the blood. It is of interest to note that the work upon which is based the whole science of Serum therapeutics was carried out by Ehrlich with Ricin. He found that by injecting gradually increasing doses, immunity was established, a condition which he attributed to the formation of an antibody and termed Antiricin.

¶ *Medicinal Action and Uses.* Castor Oil is regarded as one of the most valuable laxatives in medicine. It is of special service in temporary constipation and wherever a mild action is essential, and is extremely useful for children and the aged. It is used in cases of colic and acute diarrhœa due to slow digestion, but must not be employed in cases of chronic constipation, which it only aggravates whilst relieving the symptoms. It acts in about five hours, affecting the entire length of the bowel, but not increasing the flow of bile, except in very large doses. The mode of its action is unknown. The oil will purge when rubbed into the skin, or injected. It is also used for expelling worms, after other special remedies have been administered.

The only serious objections to the use of Castor Oil are its flavour and the sickness often produced by it. The nauseous taste may be disguised by administering it covered by Lemon oil, Sassafras oil and other essential oils, or floating on Peppermint or Cinnamon water, or coffee, or shaken up with glycerine, or given in fresh or warmed milk, the dose varying from 1 to 4 teaspoonsful. Probably the best way, however, is to administer it in capsules. Small repeated doses may be given in the intestinal colic of children.

It may also be made into an emulsion with the yolk of an egg or mucilage; or with orange-wine or gin.

Castor Oil forms a clean, light-coloured soap, which dries and hardens well and is free from smell. It has been recommended for medicinal use. The inferior qualities of the oil are frequently employed in India for soap-making.

Externally, the oil has been recommended for various cutaneous complaints, such as ringworm, itch, etc. The fresh leaves are used by nursing mothers in the Canary Islands as an external application, to increase the flow of milk.

The oil varies much in activity – the East Indian is the more active, but the Italian has the least taste.

Castor Oil is an excellent solvent of pure alkaloids and such solutions of Atropine, Cocaine, etc., as are used in ophthalmic surgery. It is also dropped into the eye to remove the after-irritation caused by the removal of foreign bodies.

'Castor Oil is finding increasing uses in the industrial world. It figures largely in the manufacture of the artificial leather used in upholstery; it furnishes a colouring for butter, and from it is produced the so-called 'Turkey-red' oil used in the dyeing of cotton textures. It is an essential component in some artificial rubbers, in various descriptions of celluloid, and in the making of certain waterproof preparations, and one of the largest uses is in the manufacture of transparent soaps. It also furnishes sebacic acid, which is employed in the manufacture of candles, and caprylic acid, which enters into the composition of varnishes, especially suitable for the polishing of high-class furniture and carriage bodies. One of its minor uses is in the manufacture of fly-papers.'– 'West India Committee Circular.' (Quoted in *The Chemist and Druggist.*)

'THE CLEANING OF PICTURES. – Lecturing in London, on November 15, on the preservation and restoration of pictures, Professor A. P. Lawrie, while not prepared to give a final opinion as to the safest methods of cleaning, suggested that where alcohol was used Castor Oil should be laid on the surface with a soft brush, and then a mixture of Castor Oil and alcohol dabbed on with a soft brush, and removed by diluting with turpentine and sopping up with a large dry brush. Where alcohol was not a sufficiently powerful solvent, copaiba balsam emulsified with ammonia might be used, a preparation of copaiba balsam thinned with a little turpentine being laid on first.' (*Chemist and Druggist*, November 25, 1922.)

Combined with citron ointment, it is used as a topical application in common leprosy.

CATECHU, PALE

CATECHU PALLIDUM

Synonyms. Terra Japonica. Gambier
Habitat. Singapore and other places of the Eastern Archipelago

Uncaria Gambier (ROXB.)
N.O. Rubiaceæ

CATECHU, BLACK

Synonym. Cutch.
Habitat. Burma, India

Catechu nigrum
Acacia catechu (WILLD.)
N.O. Leguminosæ

Pale Catechu is an extract made from the leaves and young shoots of *Uncaria Gambier* (Roxb.), a member of the order Rubiaceæ, not an Acacia. It occurs in commerce in dark or pale-brown cubes with a dull, powdery fracture, or sometimes in lozenge form.

Black Catechu occurs in black, shining pieces or cakes.

Both substances are sold under the name of Catechu.

¶ *Medicinal Action and Uses.* Both the dark and the pale Catechu are employed in medicine, the former is more astringent, the latter, being sweeter, is less disagreeable.

It depends almost entirely for its virtues upon the tannic acid it contains and is hence employed as an astringent to overcome relaxation of mucous membranes in general.

An infusion can be employed to stop nose-bleeding, and is also employed as an injection for uterine hæmorrhage, leucorrhœa and gonorrhœa.

Externally, it is applied in the form of powder, to boils, ulcers and cutaneous eruptions, and also used for the same purposes mixed with other ingredients, in an ointment.

A small piece, held in the mouth and allowed slowly to dissolve, is an excellent remedy in relaxation of the uvula and simple pharyngitis.

In powder, applied to spongy gums, it often proves of use and has been recommended as a dentifrice with powdered charcoal, myrrh, etc.

The pharmaceutical preparations are: Powdered Catechu, dose 5 to 15 grains; Compound Powder of Catechu, B.P., dose 10 to 40 grains; Tincture of Catechu, B.P., dose $\frac{1}{2}$ to 1 drachm; Comp. Tincture, U.S.P., dose 1 drachm. Catechu Lozenges are also official preparations in both the British and United States Pharmacopœias.

Like *Acacia arabica*, the wood-extract of this species has, however, a larger field in the tanning industry than in medicine. The Pale Catechu (*Gambier Catechu*) is largely used in the arts, for dyeing purposes, yielding a colour known as 'Cutch Brown.'

Cutch is subject to the most extensive *adulteration*, though this exists chiefly in the tanning grades. The chief adulterants are Than (an extract obtained by boiling the bark of *Buceras oliverii*), dried blood, ashes, sand, clay and starch, and their detection is provided for in the official tests.

See ACACIA

CATMINT

Synonym. Catnep
Parts Used. Leaves, herb
Habitat. Catmint or Catnep, a wild English plant belonging to the large family *Labiatæ*, of which the Mints and Deadnettles are also members, is generally distributed throughout the central and the southern counties of England, in hedgerows, borders of fields, and on dry banks and waste ground, especially in chalky and gravelly soil. It is less common in the north, very local in Scotland and rare in Ireland, but of frequent occurrence in the whole of Europe and temperate Asia, and also common in North America, where originally, however, it was an introduced species

Nepeta cataria (LINN.)
N.O. Labiatæ

¶ *Description.* The root is perennial and sends up square, erect and branched stems, 2 to 3 feet high, which are very leafy and covered with a mealy down. The heart-shaped, toothed leaves are also covered with a soft, close down, especially on the under sides, which are quite white with it, so that the whole plant has a hoary, greyish appearance, as though it had had dust blown over it.

The flowers grow on short footstalks in dense whorls, which towards the summit of the stem are so close as almost to form a spike. They are in bloom from July to September. The individual flowers are small, the corollas two-lipped, the upper lip straight, of a whitish or pale pink colour, dotted with red spots, the anthers a deep red colour. The calyx tube has fifteen ribs, a distinguishing feature of the genus *Nepeta*, to which this species belongs.

¶ *History*. The plant has an aromatic, characteristic odour, which bears a certain resemblance to that of both Mint and Pennyroyal. It is owing to this scent that it has a strange fascination for cats, who will destroy any plant of it that may happen to be bruised. There is an old saying about this plant:

'If you set it, the cats will eat it,
If you sow it, the cats don't know it.'

And it seems to be a fact that plants transplanted are always destroyed by cats unless protected, but they never meddle with the plants raised from seed, being only attracted to it when it is in a withering state, or when the peculiar scent of the plant is excited by being bruised in gathering or transplanting.

In France the leaves and young shoots are used for seasoning, and it is regularly grown amongst kitchen herbs for the purpose. Both there and in this country, it has an old reputation for its value as a medicinal herb. Miss Bardswell, in *The Herb Garden*, writes of Catmint:

'Before the use of tea from China, our English peasantry were in the habit of brewing Catmint Tea, which they said was quite as pleasant and a good deal more wholesome. Ellen Montgomery in *The Wide, Wide World* made Catmint Tea for Miss Fortune when she was ill. It is stimulating. The root when chewed is said to make the most gentle person fierce and quarrelsome, and there is a legend of a certain hangman who could never screw up his courage to the point of hanging anybody till he had partaken of it. Rats dislike the plant particularly, and will not approach it even when driven by hunger.'

This dislike of rats for Catmint might well be utilized by growing it round other valuable crops as a protective screen.

Closely allied to the Catmint is the Ground Ivy (*Nepeta glechoma*, Benth.), named *Glechoma hederacea* by Linnæus.

¶ *Cultivation*. Catmint is easily grown in any garden soil, and does not require moisture in the same way as the other Mints. It may be increased by dividing the plants in spring, or by sowing seeds at the same period. Sow in rows, about 20 inches apart, thinning out the seedlings to about the same distance apart as the plants attain a considerable size. They require no attention, and will last for several years if the ground is kept free from weeds. The germinating power of the seeds lasts five years.

Catmint forms a pretty border plant, especially in conjunction with Hyssop, the soft blues blending pleasingly, and it is also a suitable plant for the rock garden.

¶ *Part Used Medicinally*. The flowering tops are the part utilized in medicine and are harvested when the plant is in full bloom in August.

¶ *Medicinal Action and Uses*. Carminative, tonic, diaphoretic, refrigerant and slightly emmenagogue, specially antispasmodic, and mildly stimulating.

Producing free perspiration, it is very useful in colds. Catnep Tea is a valuable drink in every case of fever, because of its action in inducing sleep and producing perspiration without increasing the heat of the system. It is good in restlessness, colic, insanity and nervousness, and is used as a mild nervine for children, one of its chief uses being, indeed, in the treatment of children's ailments. The infusion of 1 oz. to a pint of boiling water may be taken by adults in doses of 2 tablespoonsful, by children in 2 or 3 teaspoonsful frequently, to relieve pain and flatulence. An injection of Catnep Tea is also used for colicky pains.

The herb should always be *infused*, boiling will spoil it. Its qualities are somewhat volatile, hence when made it should be covered up.

The tea may be drunk freely, but if taken in very large doses when warm, it frequently acts as an emetic.

It has proved efficacious in nervous headaches and as an emmenagogue, though for the latter purpose, it is preferable to use Catnep, not as a warm tea, but to express the juice of the green herb and take it in tablespoonful doses, three times a day.

An injection of the tea also relieves headache and hysteria, by its immediate action upon the sacral plexus. The young tops, made into a conserve, have been found serviceable for nightmare.

Catnep may be combined with other agents of a more decidedly diaphoretic nature. Equal parts of warm Catnep tea and Saffron are excellent in scarlet-fever and small-pox, as well as colds and hysterics. It will relieve painful swellings when applied in the form of a poultice or fomentation.

Old writers recommended a decoction of the herb, sweetened with honey for relieving a cough, and Culpepper tells us also that 'the

juice drunk in wine is good for bruises,' and that 'the green leaves bruised and made into an ointment is effectual for piles,' and that 'the head washed with a decoction taketh away scabs, scurf, etc.'

See MINTS

CATNEP. *See* CATMINT

CATSFOOT

Antennaria dioca (GÆERTN.)
N.O. Compositæ

Synonyms. Life Everlasting. Mountain Everlasting. Gnaphalium dioicum (Linn.). Cudweed
Part Used. Whole herb
Habitat. Europe, Asia, America to the Arctic regions, abundant in Great Britain, often to the coast level

¶ *Description.* This plant derives its name from the antennæ of a butterfly which the pappus hairs of the Staminate florets resemble.

It is the only British species, a small perennial with tufted or creeping leafly stalks and almost simple flowering stems, from 2 to 5 inches high. Lower leaves obovate or oblong, upper ones linear, white underneath or on both sides. Flowers early summer white and pinky, diœcious. In the males, inner bracts of the involucre have broad white petal-like tips, the females inner bracts narrow and white at tips, florets filiform with long protruding pappus to the achenes. Taste astringent, odour pleasant and strongest in the female heads, male plant has white membraneous scales, and the female rose-coloured. Gerard alludes to it as 'Live for ever,' and says:

'When the flower hath long flourished and is waxen old, then comes there in the middest of the floure a certain brown yellow thrumme, such as is in the middest of the daisie, which floure being gathered when it is young may be kept in such manner (I meane in such freshness and well-liking) by the space of a whole year after in your chest or elsewhere, wherefore our English women have called it "Live Long," or "Live-for-

ever," which name doth aptly answer this effects.'

Another variety of Cudweed was called 'Herbe Impious' or 'Wicked Cudweed,' a variety

'like unto the small Cudweed, but much larger and for the most part those floures which appear first are the lowest and basest; and they are over topt by other floures, which come on younger branches, and grow higher as children seeking to overgrow or overtop their parents (as many wicked children do) for which cause it hath been called "Herbe Impious." '

¶ *Medicinal Action and Uses.* Discutient and used for its astringent properties, as a cure for quinsy, and mumps; said to be efficacious for bites of poisonous reptiles, and for looseness of bowels.

¶ *Constituents.* Resin, volabile oil tanin and a bitter principle.

¶ *Doses. For a mouthwash:* 1 oz. Cudweed, 1 oz. Raspberry Leaves, 1 oz. Tincture of Myrrh. *As an infusion:* 1 oz. herb to pint boiling water is given internally in wineglassful doses and applied externally, as a gargle and as a fomentation. *Fluid extract:* Dose, $\frac{1}{2}$ to 1 drachm.

CAULOPHYLLUM. *See* (BLUE) COHOSH

CAYENNE

Capsicum minimum (ROXB.)
N.O. Solanaceæ

Synonyms. African Pepper. Chillies. Bird Pepper
Part Used. Fruit, ripe and dried
Habitat. Zanzibar – but now grown in most tropical and sub-tropical countries

¶ *Description.* Cayenne or Capsicum derives its name from the Greek, 'to bite,' in allusion to the hot pungent properties of the fruits and seeds. Cayenne pepper was introduced into Britain from India in 1548, and Gerard mentioned it as being cultivated in

his time. The plant was described by Linnæus under the name of *C. frutescens* proper. This species appeared in Miller's *Garden Dictionary* in 1771. It is a shrubby perennial plant 2 to 6 feet high. Branches angular, usually enlarged and slightly purple at the nodes; petioles medium; peduncles slender, often in pairs, and longer than the fruit; calyx cup-shaped, clasping base of fruit which is red, ovate, and long; seeds small and flat, from ten to twenty-nine. The cuticle of the pericarp is uniformly striated and in this particular is distinct from other species. Taste very pungent and smell characteristic. It is difficult to determine the source of true powdered Capsicum, as the colour is affected by light, so that it should always be kept in dark receptacles. African pepper is generally light brownish-yellow colour and very pungent; its pungency appears to depend on a principle called Capsicin. Cayenne is sometimes adulterated with oxide of red lead, which may be detected by digesting in dilute nitric acid. Other adulterants are coloured sawdust which can be found by the aid of the microscope. The British Pharmacopœia requires that capsicum should yield not more than 6 per cent. of ash, and this test detects the presence of most adulterants.

¶ *Constituents.* Capsaicin, a red colouring matter, oleic, palmitic and stearic acids.

¶ *Medicinal Action and Uses.* A powerful local stimulant, with no narcotic effect, largely used in hot climates as a condiment, and most useful in atony of the intestines and stomach. It should not be used in ordinary gastric catarrh. For persons addicted to drink it seems to be useful possibly by reducing the dilated blood-vessels and thus relieving chronic congestion. It is often added to tonics and is said to be unequalled for warding off diseases. Herbalists use it largely in pill form and powdered. Externally it is a strong rubefacient and acts gently with no danger of vesication; is applied as a cataplasm or as a liniment; it can be mixed with 10 to 20 per cent. of cotton-seed oil. The powder or the tincture is beneficial for relaxed uvula. A preparation in use in the West Indies called Mandram, for weak digestion and loss of appetite, is made of thinly sliced and unskinned cucumbers, shallots, chives, or onions, lemon or lime juice, Madeira, and a few pods of bird pepper well mashed up in the liquids. It can be used as a chutney.

¶ *Doses. For a gargle:* ½ drachm of powder to 1 pint of boiling water, or ½ fluid ounce of the tincture to 8 fluid ounces of rose water. If the throat is very sensitive it can be given in *pill form* – generally made with 1 to 10 grains powder. *The infusion* is made with 2 drachms to ½ pint boiling water taken in ½ fluid ounce doses. The tincture is used as a paint for chilblains.

See PAPRIKA

CEDAR, YELLOW

Thuja occidentalis (LINN.)
N.O. Coniferæ

Synonyms. Tree of Life. Arbor Vitæ. American Arbor Vitæ. Cedrus Lycea. Western Arbor Vitæ. False White Cedar. Hackmatack. Thuia du Canada. Lebensbaum
Part Used. The recently-dried, leafy young twigs
Habitat. North America, from Pennsylvania northward

¶ *Description.* The tallest of this species of Conifer rarely grows above 30 feet high. These trees have regular, graceful conical forms that make them valuable as highhedge trees, and they also take easily any other shape to which they may be clipped. The leaves are of two kinds on different branchlets, one awl-shaped and the other short and obtuse. Both have a small, flattened gland, containing a thin, fragrant turpentine. They are persistent, and overlap in four rows. The flowers are very small and terminal, and the cones nodding, first ovoid and then spreading, with blunt scales arranged in three rows.

The name Thuja is a latinized form of a Greek word meaning 'to fumigate,' or *thuo* ('to sacrifice'), for the fragrant wood was burnt by the ancients with sacrifices. The tree was described as 'arbor vitæ' by Clusius, who saw it in the royal garden of Fontainebleau after its importation from Canada. It was introduced into Britain about 1566.

In America the wood is much used for fencing and palings, as a light roofing timber, and, as it is both durable and pliable, for the ribs and bottom of bark boats, and also for limekilns, bowls, boxes, cups, and small articles of furniture.

The fresh branches are much used in Canada for besoms, which have a pleasing scent. The odour is pungent and balsamic, and the taste bitter, resembling camphor and terebinth.

The trees grow well on the western coast hills of Britain, and the wood is soft, finely grained, and light in texture.

¶ *Constituents.* The bitter principle, Pinipicrin, and the tannic acid, said to be identical with Pinitannic acid, occur also in *Pinus sylvestris.* Thuja also contains volatile oil, sugar, gelatinous matter, wax, resin, and Thujin. The last is a citron-yellow, crystallizable colouring principle, soluble in alcohol. It has an astringent taste, is inflammable, and can be split up into glucose,

Thujigenin and Thujetin (*probably identical with Quercitin*).

The leaves and twigs are said to yield also a camphor-like essential oil, sp. gr. 0·925, boiling point 190°–206° C., easily soluble in alcohol and containing pinene, fenchone, thujone, and perhaps carvone.

A yellow-green volatile oil can be distilled from the leaves and used as a vermifuge.

¶ *Medicinal Action and Uses.* Aromatic, astringent, diuretic. The twigs may produce abortion, like those of savin, by reflex action on the uterus from severe gastro-intestinal irritation. Both fenchone and thujone stimulate the heart muscle. The decoction has been used in intermittent fevers, rheumatism, dropsy, coughs, scurvy, and as an emmenagogue. The leaves, made into an ointment with fat, are a helpful local application in rheumatism. An injection of the tincture into venereal warts is said to cause them to disappear. For violent pains the Canadians have used the cones, powdered, with four-fifths of Polypody, made into a poultice with lukewarm water or milk and applied to the body, with a cloth over the skin to prevent scorching.

¶ *Dosage.* Of fluid extract, ¼ drachm, three to six times a day, as stimulating expectorant and diuretic. The infusion of 1 oz. to a pint of boiling water is taken cold in tablespoonful doses.

¶ *Poisons.* The oil, resembling camphor, may produce convulsions in warm-blooded and paralysis in cold-blooded animals. Sixteen drops of the oil, taken by a girl of fifteen, caused unconsciousness, followed by spasms and convulsions, with subsequent stomachic irritation. It causes great flatulence and distension of the stomach.

¶ *Other Species.*
CHINESE ARBOR VITÆ (*Thuja orientalis* or *Biota orientalis*), a native of China and Japan, has the same properties. The young branches yield a yellow dye, and the wood withstands conditions of humidity well.

T. articulata, of Northern Africa, yields the resin known as Sandarac, formerly used as a drug, and for ointments and plasters. At present it is used as varnish and incense, and the powder, or Pounce, is used to prevent ink spreading on paper after letters have been scratched out. It is occasionally adulterated with mastic, rosin, etc. A false sandarac consists largely of colophony.

Sandarac is said to be used in India for hæmorrhoids and diarrhœa and the tincture for friction in cases of low spirits.

The Australian sandarac, from *C. robusta*, is very similar.

WHITE CEDAR is a common name of *Cupressus thujoides*.

RED CEDAR OF BRITISH COLUMBIA, the Giant Arbor Vitæ, is next to the Douglas Fir in importance in British Columbia, where it attains its greatest height of 100 feet. It is the best wood to use for shingles.

RED CEDAR, or *Juniperus virginiana*, resembles savin, but is less energetic. Externally it is an irritant, and an ointment prepared from the fresh leaves is used as a substitute for savin cerate in discharge from blisters. The volatile oil has been used for abortion and has caused death, preceded by burning in the stomach, vomiting, convulsions, coma, and gastro-intestinal inflammation. It is used in perfumery, and is a principal constituent of extract of white rose.

Small excrescences called cedar apples are sometimes found on the branches, and used as an anthelmintic. Dosage: from 10 to 20 grains three times a day.

To obtain Cedrene camphor the oil must be cooled until coagulated and the crystalline portion separated by expression.

HAITIAN CEDAR yields an oil resembling that of *J. virginiana*, but having a higher specific gravity.

HACKMATACK is also the name of *Larix americana*.

CEDAR OF LEBANON (*Cedrus libani*) and its two varieties,

INDIAN CEDAR or DEODAR (*C. deodara*) and AFRICAN CEDAR (*C. Atlantica*), or satinwood, yield an oil which, when distilled, is called Libanol. The oil of the last resembles oil of santal, and is good for phthisis, bronchitis, blennorrhagia, and also for eruptions on the skin, in the form of 25 per cent. ointment with vaseline. Dosage: capsules up to 45 grains per day.

Cedrela odorata of the West Indies yields a volatile oil that is said to be a powerful insecticide. The wood is used for making cigar boxes. Another cedar of the same family of Cedrelaceæ or Meliaceæ is AUSTRALIAN RED CEDAR (*C. tooma*) or Red Cedar of Queensland, yielding Cedar Gum, containing 68 per cent. arabin, and 6 per cent. metarabin, but no resin.

NEW ZEALAND CEDAR (*Libocedrus bidwillii*) and also CALIFORNIAN WHITE CEDAR (*L. decurrens*) possess some of the same properties.

PRICKLY CEDAR (*J. oxycedrus*) (*syn.* Large, Brown-fruited Juniper), of the Mediterranean coasts, yields Oil of Cade by destructive distillation of the wood. It has been used from remote ages for the skin diseases of animals, and more recently in medicine for psoriasis and chronic eczema. It is a good parasiticide in psora and favus.

It is also made into ointments and soaps, and a glycerite is prepared.

On the very rare occasions of its internal use, its action resembles oil of tar. Dosage: 1 to 3 minims.

J. phœnicia is used in Europe to adulterate savin.

See PINES

CEDRON

Simaba Cedron (PLANCH.)
N.O. Simarubaceæ

Synonym. Cedron seeds
Part Used. Seeds
Habitat. Columbia and Central America

¶ *Description.* A small tree, a native of New Grenada, remarkable for the properties of its seed. It has large pinnated leaves with over twenty narrow elliptical leaflets and large panicles of flowers, 3 to 4 feet long; the fruit is about the size of a swan's egg, and contains only one fruit, four of the cells being barren. The Cedron of commerce is not unlike a large blanched almond – it is often yellowish, hard and compact, but can be easily cut, it is intensely bitter, not unlike quassia in taste and has no odour. The Cedron of commerce is obtained from the seed. Cedron has always been used in Central America as a remedy for snake-bite, and first came into notice in Britain in 1699.

¶ *Medicinal Action and Uses.* It has been found of considerable value in New Grenada as a febrifuge in intermittent fever, and is also recommended as an antiperiodic. There is almost a superstitious belief in its efficacy in eradicating poison, and the natives always carry some of the seeds on their person. For snake-bites, a small quantity is scraped off, mixed with water and applied to the wound, and then about 2 grains are put into brandy or into water and taken internally. Every part of the plant, including the seed, is intensely bitter.

¶ *Constituents.* A crystalline substance called Cedrin was separated by Lowry, but this has been disputed.

¶ *Dosages.* Of the crude drug, 5 to 15 grains. Of powdered seeds, 1 to 10 grains.

The infusion, which is taken in tablespoonful doses, is made with 1 oz. of the herb to 1 pint of boiling water. Hyperdermically, Cedrin has been given, $\frac{1}{15}$ of a grain.

The powdered bark is used to kill vermin.

¶ *Other Species.* The *Simaruba versicolor* has similar properties.

CELANDINE, GREATER

Chelidonium majus (LINN.)
N.O. Papaveraceæ

Synonyms. Common Celandine. Garden Celandine
Part Used. Herb
Habitat. Found by old walls, on waste ground and in hedges, nearly always in the neighbourhood of human habitations

¶ *Description.* At first glance, the four petals arranged in the form of a cross make it appear a member of the order *Cruciferæ*, but it is not related to these plants, belonging to the same family as the Poppies (*Papaveraceæ*) and has, like these flowers, a dense mass of stamens in the centre of its blossoms.

The Celandine is a herbaceous perennial. The root is thick and fleshy. The stem, which is slender, round and slightly hairy, grows from $1\frac{1}{2}$ to 3 feet high and is much branched; at the points where the branches are given off, it is swollen and jointed and breaks very easily.

The whole plant abounds in a bright, orange-coloured juice, which is emitted freely wherever the stems or leaves are broken. This juice stains the hands strongly and has a persistent and nauseous taste and a strong, disagreeable smell. It is acrid and a powerful irritant.

The yellowish-green leaves, which are much paler, almost greyish below, are very thin in texture, drooping immediately on gathering. They are graceful in form and slightly hairy, 6 to 12 inches long, 2 to 3 inches wide, deeply divided as far as the central rib, so as to form usually two pairs of leaflets, placed opposite to one another, with a large terminal leaflet. The margins (i.e. edges) of the leaflets are cut into by rounded teeth.

The flowers drop very quickly when picked. They are arranged at the ends of the stems in loose umbels. They blossom throughout the summer, being succeeded by narrow, long pods, containing blackish seeds.

¶ *History.* This plant is undoubtedly the true Celandine, having nothing in common with the Lesser Celandine except the colour of its flowers. It was a drug plant in the Middle Ages and is mentioned by Pliny,

178

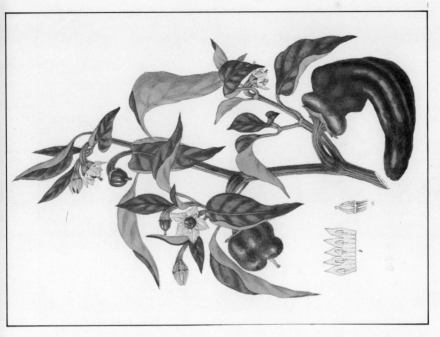

CAYENNE
Capsicum Minimum

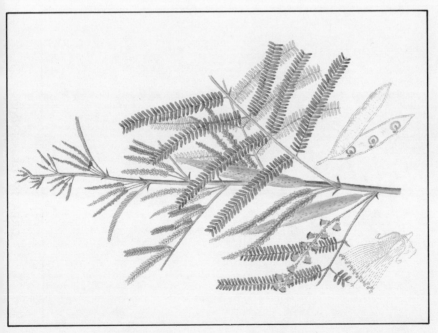

BLACK CATECHU
Acacia Catechu

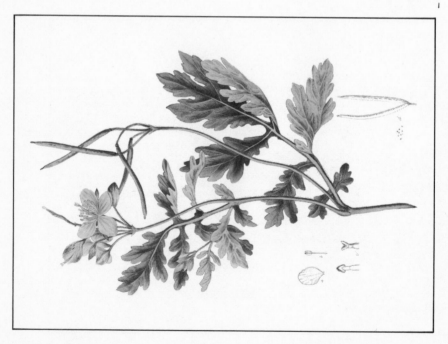

CENTAURY

GREATER CELANDINE
Chelidonium Majus

to whom we owe the tradition that it is called Chelidonium from the Greek *chelidon* (a swallow), because it comes into flower when the swallows arrive and fades at their departure. (The English name Celandine is merely a corruption of the Greek word.) Its acrid juice has been employed successfully in removing films from the cornea of the eye, a property which Pliny tells us was discovered by swallows, this being a double reason why the plant should be named after these birds.

Gerard says:

'the juice of the herbe is good to sharpen the sight, for it cleanseth and consumeth away slimie things that cleave about the ball of the eye and hinder the sight and especially being boiled with honey in a brasen vessell, as Dioscorides teacheth.'

It is one of the twenty-four herbs mentioned in Mercer's *Herbal*.

In the fourteenth century, a drink made with Celandine was supposed to be good for the blood. Clusius, the celebrated Dutch botanist, considered that the juice, dropped into small green wounds, effected rapid cure, and when dropped into the eye would take away specks and stop incipient suffusions. The old alchemists held that it was good to 'superstifle the jaundice,' because of its intense yellow colour.

¶ *Part Used*. The whole herb, collected in the wild state, from May to July, when in flower, and dried. Likewise, the fresh juice.

¶ *Constituents*. The alkaloids Chelidonine and Chelerythrin, the latter narcotic and poisonous; also the two nearly allied alkaloids, Homochelidonine A, and Homocheli-donine B. In addition, Protopine and Sanguinarine, and a body named Chelidoxanthin, a neutral bitter principle.

¶ *Medicinal Action and Uses*. Alterative, diuretic, purgative. It is used in jaundice, eczema, scrofulous diseases, etc., the infusion of 1 oz. of the dried herb to a pint of boiling water being taken in wineglassful doses. The infusion is a cordial and greatly promotes perspiration. The addition of a few aniseeds in making a decoction of the herb in wine has been held to increase its efficacy in removing obstructions of the liver and gall.

A fluid extract is also prepared, the dose being ½ to 1 drachm. Eight to 10 drops of the tincture made from the whole herb, or of the fresh juice, given as a dose three times a day in sweetened water, is considered excellent for overcoming torpid conditions of the liver. In the treatment of the worst forms of scurvy it has been given with benefit.

The orange-coloured, acrid juice is commonly used fresh to cure warts, ringworm and corns, but should not be allowed to come into contact with any other part of the skin.

In milk, it is employed as an eye-lotion, to remove the white, opaque spots on the cornea. Mixed with sulphur, it was formerly used to cure the itch.

An ointment made of the roots and lard boiled together, also of the leaves and flowers, has been used with advantage for piles.

Celandine is a very popular medicine in Russia, where it is said to have proved effective in cases of cancer.

It is still used in Suffolk as a fomentation for toothache.

CELANDINE, LESSER

Ranunculus ficaria (LINN.)
N.O. Ranunculaceæ

Synonyms. Small Celandine. Figwort. Smallwort. Pilewort
Part Used. Herb
Habitat. The Lesser Celandine, one of the very earliest of spring flowers, its cheery, starlike blossoms lighting up our hedges even before winter is quite spent, is distributed throughout Europe, Western Asia, and North Africa, in these islands, growing up the hillsides in Wales to a height of 2,400 feet. It grows in moist corners of fields and places near watersides, but is found also on drier ground, if shady, being one of the few plants that thrive beneath the shade of trees, where its glossy foliage frequently forms a dense carpet

Wordsworth, whose favourite flower this was (in recognition of which the blossoms are carved on his tomb), fancifully suggests that the painter who first tried to picture the rising sun, must have taken the idea of the spreading pointed rays from the Celandine's 'glittering countenance.' The burnishing of the golden petals gives a brilliant effect to the flowers, which burst into bloom about the middle of February, a few days only after their bright, shining leaves. The leaves are on long stalks, arising from a short, prostrate stem, and are very variable, the first being heart-shaped, the later ones bluntly cut into, somewhat like the ivy. They often have dark markings.

The blossoms shut up before rain, and even in fine weather do not open before nine o'clock, and by 5 p.m. have already closed for the night. The Celtic name of the plant, *Grian* (i.e. the sun), refers to this habit. The petals are green on the underside, and directly the flowers close they become inconspicuous.

Throughout March and April, this cheerful little plant is in full bloom, but as the spring passes into summer, the flowers pale somewhat, and the whole plant looks rather sickly, the warmth of the lengthening days withdrawing from it the needed moisture. By the end of May, no flowers are to be seen, and all the plant above ground withers and dies, the virtue being stored up in the fibres of the root, which swell into the form of tubers. If the plant is dug up, late in the summer or autumn, these tubers are seen hanging in a bunch, a dozen or more together, looking like figs, hence the plant's specific Latin name *ficaria*, from *ficus* (a fig). By these tubers, the plant is increased, as they break off readily, each tuber, like a potato, producing a new plant. To eradicate this plant from any ground, it is necessary to remove the roots bodily, for if the plants are dug into the soil, they work their way up to the surface again, the stems branching as they grow upward from the tubers, and at every branch producing fresh tubers.

The early awakening of the plant is due to these fully-stored tubers, which lie quiescent all the summer and autumn, but all necessary materials being at hand, leaves and flowers are quickly pushed upwards directly the depth of the winter has passed.

Although the Lesser Celandine has been placed by some botanists in a distinct genus, when it is called *Ficaria verna*, it is more generally assigned to the Buttercup or Crowfoot genus, *Ranunculus*. The name of this genus, first employed by Pliny, alludes to the damp and marshy localities preferred by the plants of the family, *Rana*, being the Latin for a frog, whose native haunts are those of the majority of this group of plants. The Lesser Celandine is distinguished from the Buttercup by having nine or ten, even sometimes a dozen narrow petals, instead of five, and only three sepals (the outer, generally green leaves of the flower), which fall off on opening, instead of the usual five, which remain after the flower has expanded, in the other species of *Ranunculus*. The flowers rise singly from the root, on long, slender, leafless stalks and are about 1 inch in diameter. There are a number of stamens. The fruits are not unlike those of the Buttercups, being dry and distinct, set together in a globular head, somewhat like a grain of corn and whitish in colour, but comparatively few fertile seeds are produced.

The flowers would originally appear to have been designed with the object of attracting insects for their fertilization, the bright-coloured, burnished petals having honey sacs at their base, but the flowers can face colder days than the insects can, for whom the honey has been provided, blooming when few of the insects have emerged, with the result that comparatively few become fertilized in this country and not many seeds are produced. The plant, therefore, has recourse to another method of reproduction, independent of all external aid. At the point where the upper leaves join the stem are to be seen little objects like minute round tumours, which grow about the size of a grain of wheat. In the early summer, when the leaves and stems are dying down, these grains become loose and drop to the ground. Each is capable of producing a new plant. A heavy rain will sometimes wash them from the plants in every direction. Kerner, in his *Natural History of Plants*, tells us that

'a sudden downpour of rain in a region abundantly overgrown with Lesser Celandine is sufficient to float away numbers of the tubers, and heap them up on the borders of irrigation channels when the rain disperses. In such places the quantity of tubers which have floated together is often so large that one can hardly gather them in one's hands. In this way arose the idea that the tubers had fallen from heaven with the rain and the myth of a rain of potatoes.'

This fact probably accounts, also, for the 'rains of wheat' sometimes vouched for by country people in various parts. These bulbils (i.e. little bulbs) are only produced on those plants whose fruits have failed to set.

The root of the Lesser Celandine is perennial.

Seedlings do not flower in their first year, but collect and store up material to start their accustomed course at the end of the ensuing winter.

The whole plant is glabrous.

It is called the Lesser Celandine to distinguish it from the Greater Celandine, to which it has neither relationship nor similarity, except in the colour of its flowers, though the older herbalists applied the name to both plants indiscriminately. The confusion of names existed in Gerard's time, for he published a list of all the plants in cultivation in his garden on Holborn Hill – towards the close of the sixteenth century – and introduced in it, under the same name, both this and the Greater Celandine (*Chelidonium majus*), which certainly is in bloom when the swallows arrive, and continues to flower the whole summer, and so would have more right to the name Celandine than this species, which blossoms long before they come, and dies down months before they leave our shores.

A figure of the Lesser Celandine – under the name of *Erdöpffel* – appears in an old German Herbal of 1533, Rhodion's *Kreutterbuch*, evidence that this plant was well known to the herbalists of the Middle Ages.

It is also called 'Small-wort.'

The old English name of Pilewort is due to the fact that it has long been considered a cure for piles, one of the reasons assigned for this resting on the strange doctrine of signatures. We are told by an old writer: 'If you dig up the root of it you will perceive the perfect image of the disease commonly called the piles.' Gerard writes of it:

'It presently, as Galen and Dioscorides affirm (though this perhaps refers to the Greater Celandine) exulcerateth or blistereth the skin: it maketh rough and corrupt nails to fall away. The juice of the roots mixed with honie and drawn up into the nosthrils purgeth the head of foul and filthy humours. The later age use the roots and graines for the piles . . . there be also who think that if the berbe be but carried about one that hath the piles, the pain forthwith ceaseth.'

Culpepper, writing fifty years later, tells us:

'It is certain by good experience that the decoction of the leaves and roots doth wonderfully help piles and hæmorrhoids; also kernels by the ears and throat called the King's Evil, or any other hard wens or tumours.'

He had such faith in the virtues of this little plant that he further tells us, with more definite belief than Gerard: 'The very herb borne about one's body next the skin helps in such diseases though it never touch the place grieved.'

The young leaves, the substance of which is soft and mucilaginous, have sometimes been boiled and eaten as a vegetable in Sweden, but have not the reputation of being very palatable, either thus treated or raw as a salad.

Linnæus advised farmers to eradicate the plant from their land on account of it being disliked by cattle (though wood-pigeons eat it with avidity), also for its injurious effect on other herbs in the meadow, but there seems little ground for this assumption, as although the tissues of most plants in this order contain acrid juices to a high degree, the acrimony of the Lesser Celandine is of a very mild character. A dressing of coal or wood ash is said to effectually destroy the whole plant.

¶ *Part Used.* The whole herb is collected in the wild state, while in flower in March and April, and dried.

¶ *Constituents.* Nothing is known definitely concerning the constituents of Pilewort; the fresh plant, however, probably contains traces of an acrid principle resembling or identical with Anemonin.

¶ *Medicinal Action and Uses.* Astringent. This herb is an old remedy for piles, for which it has recently been re-introduced into the British Pharmacopœia, and is considered almost a specific.

Internally, the infusion of 1 oz. in a pint of boiling water is taken in wineglassful doses, and will in most cases be sufficient to effect a cure.

It is also used externally as an ointment, made from the bruised herb with fresh lard, applied locally night and morning, or in the form of poultices, fomentations, or in suppositories.

A most excellent ointment has been recommended for external abscesses, etc., made from Pilewort, Elder-buds, House-leek, and leaves of the Broad Plantain, prepared in the early spring, when the Pilewort is in flower.

The roots are highly valued as a medicine in Cochin-China.

RECIPES

The following old-time recipes connected with this herb occur in *A Plain Plantain* (R. G. Alexander):

For a Sore Throat

'Take a pinte of whitewine, A good handful of Sallendine, and boile them well together; put to it A piece of the best Roach Allome, sweeten it with English honey, and use it.'

A Marvellous Precious Water

'Take Gallingall (Galingale), Cloves, Cubibs, Ginger, Mellilote, Cardamonia, Maces, Nutmegs, one dram; of the juice of Salendine, 8 drams; mingle all these made in powder with the said juice and a pint of Aquavitæ, and 3 pints of Whitewine; putt itt into A Stillitory of Glass; and the next day still it with An easy fire.

'This water is of an excellent Virtue Agst A Consumption or any other Disease that proceeds from Rheume Choller or Fleagnie.'

All the species of *Ranunculus*, except the Water Crowfoot, are acrid, and before the introduction of Cantharides (Spanish Fly), many, especially *R. sceleratus*, were used as vesicatories. They are said to act with less pain and without any action on the urinary passages, but their action is supposed to be uncertain, and they are accused of frequently leaving ill-conditioned ulcers. Since the introduction of Cantharides, their employment has therefore fallen into disuse. Formerly it was not at all uncommon for beggars to produce sores about their bodies by the medium of various species of *Ranunculus*, for the sake of getting alms, afterwards curing these sores by applying fresh Mullein leaves to heal them.

Pliny tells us that

'they raise blisters like those caused by fire, hence the plant is used for the removal of leprous spots. They form an ingredient in all caustic preparations.'

See BUTTERCUP and CROWFOOT

CELERY (WILD)

Apium graveolens (LINN.)
N.O. Umbelliferæ

Synonyms. Smallage. Wild Celery
Parts Used. Ripe seeds, herb and root
Habitat. Levant, South Europe, and cultivated in Great Britain, etc.

¶ *Description*. Odour characteristic and agreeable. Taste, aromatic, warm, and slightly pungent.

¶ *Constituents*. Celery seed contains two oils – one heavy, the other lighter; it also contains apiol, but not so much as is found in parsley.

¶ *Medicinal Action and Uses*. Carminative, stimulant, diuretic, tonic, nervine, useful in hysteria, promoting restfulness and sleep, and diffusing through the system a mild sustaining influence. Good combined with Scutellaria for nervous cases with loss of tone. On this account it is recommended to eat the *cultivated* fresh root as well as taking the oil or fluid extract. Is said to be very good for rheumatism, when it is often combined with Coca, Damiana, etc. Dose: fluid extract, 3 to 7 drops every four hours.

CENTAURY

Erythræa centaurium (PERS.)
N.O. Gentianaceæ

Synonyms. Centaury Gentian. Century. Red Centaury. Filwort. Centory. Christ's Ladder. Feverwort
Parts Used. Herb and leaves
Habitat. The plant is a native of Europe and North Africa. Though common in this country in dry pastures and on chalky cliffs, it cannot be easily reared in a garden, and for its medicinal use is, therefore, collected in the wild state

¶ *Description*. The Red Centaury (*Erythræa centaurium*, Pers.) is an annual, with a yellowish, fibrous, woody root, the stem stiff, square and erect, 3 to 12 inches in height, often branching considerably at the summit. The leaves are of a pale green colour, smooth and shiny, their margins undivided. The lowest leaves are broader than the others, oblong or wedge-shaped, narrowed at the base, blunt at the end and form a spreading tuft at the base of the plant, while the stalkless stem-leaves are pointed and lance-shaped, growing in pairs opposite to one another at somewhat distant intervals on the stalk, which is crowned by flat tufts (corymbs) of rose-coloured, star-like flowers, with five-cleft corollas. The stamens are five in number: the anthers have a curious way of twisting themselves round after they have shed their pollen, this being one of the distinctive points between the plants of this genus and those of the genus *Gentiana*, with which it has much in common, having by some earlier botanists been assigned to that genus, under the name of *Gentiana centaurium*, or Centaury Gentian. The flowers open only in fine weather and not after mid-day: Gerard chronicles their love of light, saying that they 'in the day-time and after the sun is up, do open themselves and towards evening do shut up again.' A variety is sometimes found with white corollas.

Centaury varies a great deal according to its situation, and some botanists enumerate several distinct species, namely: *E. pulchella* (Dwarf Centaury), a minute plant, 2 to 8 inches high, with an exceedingly slender stem and a few stalked flowers (often only one); this is found on the sandy seashore, especially in the West of England, and has been picked at Newquay, Cornwall; *E. littoralis* (Dwarf Tufted Centaury), a stunted plant, with broad leaves, and flowers crowded into a kind of head; this occurs on turfy sea-cliffs, and *E. latifolia* (Broad-leaved Centaury), which has even broader leaves than the last, and bears its flowers in forked tufts, the main stem being divided into three branches. There are other minute differences, for which the student may consult more scientific works.

Besides the English species, others from the south of Europe, the Azores, etc., with yellow or pink flowers, are occasionally grown in gardens.

¶ *History*. The name of the genus to which it is at present assigned, *Erythræa*, is derived from the Greek *erythros* (red), from the colour of the flowers. The genus was formerly called *Chironia*, from the Centaur Chiron, who was famous in Greek mythology for his skill in medicinal herbs, and is supposed to have cured himself with it from a wound he had accidentally received from an arrow poisoned with the blood of the hydra. The English name Centaury has the same origin. The ancients named the plant *Fel Terræ*, or Gall of the Earth, from its extreme bitterness. The old English name of Felwort is equivalent in meaning to this, and is applied to all the plants of the Gentian family. It is also thought to be the 'Graveolentia Centaurea' of Virgil, to which Lucretius gives the more significant epithet of *tristia*, in reference to this same intense bitterness. As this bitterness had a healing and tonic effect attributed to it, we sometimes find the Centaury called Febrifuga and Feverwort. It is known popularly also as Christ's Ladder, and the name Centaury has become corrupted in Worcestershire to 'Centre of the Sun.'

We find a reference to it in *Le Petit Albert*. Fifteen magical herbs of the Ancients are given:

'The eleventh hearbe is named of the Chaldees, Isiphon . . . of Englishmen, Centory . . . this herbe hath a marvellous virtue, for if it be joined with the blood of a female lapwing, or black plover, and put with oile in a lamp, all that compass it about shall believe themselves to be witches, so that one shall believe of another that his head is in heaven and his feete on earth; and if the aforesaid thynge be put in the fire when the starres shine it shall appear yt the sterres runne one agaynste another and fyghte.' (English translation, 1619.)

Also in a translation of an old mediæval Latin poem of the tenth century, by Macer, there is mention of Centaury (with other herbs) as being powerful against 'wykked sperytis.'

Of all the bitter appetizing wild herbs which serve as excellent simple tonics, the Centaury is the most efficacious, sharing the antiseptic virtues of the Field Gentian and the Buckbean.

¶ *Part Used*. The whole herb, collected in July, when just breaking into flower and dried. The plant has a slight odour, which disappears when dried.

The Field Gentian is dried in the same manner.

¶ *Constituents*. Centaury contains a bitter principle, Erythro-centaurin, which is colourless, crystalline, non-nitrogenous, reddened by sunlight; a bitter glucoside, Erytaurin; Valeric acid, wax, etc.

¶ *Medicinal Action and Uses*. Aromatic, bitter, stomachic and tonic. It acts on the liver and kidneys, purifies the blood, and is an excellent tonic.

The dried herb is given in infusion or powder, or made into an extract. It is used extensively in dyspepsia, for languid digestion with heartburn after food, in an infusion of 1 oz. of the dried herb to 1 pint of water. When run down and suffering from want of appetite, a wineglassful of this infusion – Centaury Tea – taken three or four times daily, half an hour before meals, is found of great benefit. The same infusion may also be taken for muscular rheumatism.

Culpepper tells us that

'the herbe is so safe that you cannot fail in the using of it, only give it inwardly for inward diseases, use it outwardly for outward diseases. 'Tis very wholesome, but not very toothsome.'

He says:

'it helps those that have the dropsy, or the green-sickness, being much used by the Italians in powder for that purpose. It kills worms . . . as is found by experience. . . . A dram of the powder taken in wine, is a wonderful good help against the biting and poison of an adder. The juice of the herb with a little honey put to it, is good to clear the eyes from dimness, mists and clouds that offend or hinder sight. It is singularly good both for green and fresh wounds, as also for old ulcers and sores, to close up the one and cleanse the other, and perfectly to cure them both, although they are hollow or fistulous; the green herb, especially, being bruised and laid thereto. The decoction thereof dropped into the ears, cleanses them from worms . . . and takes away all freckles, spots, and marks in the skin, being washed with it.'

The Saxon herbalists prescribed it largely for snake-bites and other poisons, and it was long celebrated for the cure of intermittent fevers, hence its name of Feverwort.

The herb formed the basis of the once

famous Portland Powder, which was said to be a specific for gout.

Centaury is given with Barberry Bark for jaundice. It has also been much employed as a vermifuge, and a decoction of the plant is said to destroy body vermin.

The green herb, bruised, is reputed to be good as an application to wounds and sores.

CENTAURY, CHILIAN

Erythræa chilensis
N.O. Gentianaceæ

Synonym. Canchalagua
Part Used. The herb
Habitat. Chile

¶ *Description.* A small, herbaceous plant, with branched stems and pink or yellow flowers, widely used in Chile as a mild tonic.

¶ *Medicinal Action and Uses.* Stimulant, bitter, tonic. Useful in dyspepsia and indigestion. An infusion may be made of 1 oz. to 1 pint of boiling water.

¶ *Dosage.* Of infusion – a wineglassful. Of fluid extract – ½ to 1 drachm.

¶ *Other Species*
Erythræa acaulis, a native of Southern Algeria, has roots that yield a yellow dye.

Sabatia angularis, or American Centaury, is a simple bitter used as a tonic and antiperiodic, in doses of 1 drachm of fluid extract or decoction of the whole plant. It has been found to contain a small proportion of Erythrocentaurin. The root of *S. Elliottii* is used in a similar manner in the south-eastern United States, and the whole plant of *S. campestris* in the south-western. *S. Elliottii* is known as the Quinine Flower, its properties resembling quinine.

CEREUS, NIGHT BLOOMING

Cereus grandiflorus (LINN.)
N.O. Cactaceæ

Synonyms. Vanilla Cactus. Sweet-scented Cactus. Large-flowered Cactus
Parts Used. The flowers, young and tender stems
Habitat. Tropical America, Mexico, West Indies, and Naples

¶ *Description.* A fleshy, creeping, rooting shrub, stems cylindrical, with five or six not very prominent angles, branching, armed with clusters of small spines, in radiated forms. Flowers, terminal and lateral from the clusters of spines, very large, 8 to 12 inches in diameter, expanding in the evening and only lasting for about six hours, exhaling a delicious vanilla-like perfume. Petals are white, spreading, shorter than the sepals, which are linear, lanceolate, outside brown, inside yellow. Fruit ovate, covered with scaly tubercles, fleshy and of a lovely orange-red colour, seeds very small and acid. The flower only lasts in bloom about six hours and does not revive; when withered, the ovary enlarges, becomes pulpy and forms an acid juicy fruit, something like a gooseberry. The plant was brought to the notice of the medical profession by Dr. Scheile, but it aroused little interest till a homœopathic doctor of Naples, R. Rubini, used it as a specific in heart disease. The flowers and young stems should be collected in July and a tincture made from them whilst fresh. The plant contains a milky acrid juice.

¶ *Constituents.* No special analysis seems yet to have been made; the chief constituents are resins, the presence of the alleged alkaloid cactine not having been confirmed.

¶ *Medicinal Action and Uses.* Diuretic Sedative, Cardiac. Cereus has been used as a cardiac stimulant and as a partial substitute for digitalis. In large doses it produces gastric irritation, slight delirium, hallucinations and general mental confusion. It is said to greatly increase the renal secretion. It does not appear to weaken the nervous system. It has a decided action on the heart and frequently gives prompt relief in functional or organic disease. It has been found of some service in hæmoptysis, dropsy and incipient apoplexy.

¶ *Dosages and Preparations.* Liquid extract of Cereus, B.P.C.: dose, 1 to 10 minims. Tincture of Cereus, B.P.C.: dose, 2 to 30 minims.

¶ *Other Species.*
Cactus bomplandi, a cardiac stimulant not now used. *Cereus cæspitosus.* An alkaloid separated from this variety, called Pectenine, produces tetanus convulsions in animals. *C. pilocereus* gives an alkaloid which produces central paralysis with great cardiac depression in frogs and death by cardiac arrest in warm-blooded animals.

C. flagelliformis and *C. divaricatus* are said to have anthelmintic properties.

Opuntias decumana and other species are often substituted for *C. grandiflorus*, but are of little use. *C. giganteus*, the Suwarron or Saguaro of the Mexicans, is the largest, and most striking species of the genus. The fruits are 2 to 3 inches long, oval and green, having a broad scar at the top caused by the flowers falling away when the fruits are ripe. They burst into three or four pieces, which curve back to resemble a flower. Inside they contain small black seeds embedded in a crimson pulp, which the Pimos and Papagos Indians make into an excellent preserve. They also eat the ripe fruit as a food and gather it by means of a forked stick tied to the end of a long pole.

Opuntia vulgaris (Prickly Pear), of the Cactus tribe, is cultivated in the south of Europe, and much esteemed by the Spaniards, who consume large quantities. In homœopathy a tincture is made from the flowers and wood for spleen troubles and diarrhœa.

O. cochinellifera, the Cochineal Insect Cactus, is a native of Mexico, but cultivated in the West Indies and other places. There are two kinds of *O. grana* – finagrana and sylvestre. The substance which envelops the insect is pulverulent in the first species and flocculent in the second. It has not yet been decided whether they are different species of coccus or whether the difference is in the plant.

CHAMOMILES
N.O. Compositæ

Habitat. There are a number of species of Chamomile spread over Europe, North Africa and the temperate region of Asia, but in Great Britain we have four growing wild: the sweet-scented, true Chamomile (*Anthemis nobilis*); the Fœtid Chamomile or Stinking Mayweed (*A. cotula*), which has what Gerard calls 'a naughty smell'; the Corn Chamomile (*A. arvensis*), which flowers rather earlier and is noticeable because its ray florets are empty and wholly for show and possess no sort of ovary or style; and fourthly, the Yellow Chamomile, with yellow instead of white rays, which is found sometimes on ballast heaps, but is not a true native

CHAMOMILE, COMMON
Anthemis nobilis (LINN.)

Synonyms. Manzanilla (Spanish). Maythen (Saxon)
Parts Used. Flowers and herb

Chamomile is one of the oldest favourites amongst garden herbs and its reputation as a medicinal plant shows little signs of abatement. The Egyptians reverenced it for its virtues, and from their belief in its power to cure ague, dedicated it to their gods. No plant was better known to the country folk of old, it having been grown for centuries in English gardens for its use as a common domestic medicine to such an extent that the old herbals agree that 'it is but lost time and labour to describe it.'

¶ *Description.* The true or Common Chamomile (*Anthemis nobilis*) is a low-growing plant, creeping or trailing, its tufts of leaves and flowers a foot high. The root is perennial, jointed and fibrous; the stems, hairy and freely branching, are covered with leaves which are divided into thread-like segments, the fineness of which gives the whole plant a feathery appearance. The blooms appear in the later days of summer, from the end of July to September, and are borne solitary on long, erect stalks, drooping when in bud. With their outer fringe of white ray-florets and yellow centres, they are remarkably like the daisy. There are some eighteen white rays arranged round a conical centre, botanically known as the receptacle, on which the yellow, tubular florets are placed; the centre of the daisy is, however, considerably flatter than that of the Chamomile.

All the Chamomiles have a tiny, chaffy scale between each two florets, which is very minute and has to be carefully looked for, but which all the same is a vital characteristic of the genus *Anthemis*. The distinction between *A. nobilis* and other species of *Anthemis* is the shape of these scales, which in *A. nobilis* are short and blunt.

The fruit is small and dry, and as it forms, the hill of the receptacle gets more and more conical.

The whole plant is downy and greyish-green in colour. It prefers dry commons and sandy soil, and is found wild in Cornwall, Surrey, and many other parts of England.

Small flies are the chief insect-visitors to the flowers.

¶ *History.* The fresh plant is strongly and agreeably aromatic, with a distinct scent of apples – a characteristic noted by the Greeks, on account of which they named it 'ground-apple' – *kamai* (on the ground) and *melon* (an apple) – the origin of the name Chamomile. The Spaniards call it 'Manzanilla,' which signifies 'a little apple,' and give the same name to one of their lightest sherries, flavoured with this plant.

When walked on, its strong, fragrant scent will often reveal its presence before it is seen. For this reason it was employed as one of the aromatic strewing herbs in the Middle Ages, and used often to be purposely planted in green walks in gardens. Indeed, walking over the plant seems specially beneficial to it.

'Like a camomile bed –
The more it is trodden
The more it will spread,'

The aromatic fragrance gives no hint of its bitterness of taste.

The Chamomile used in olden days to be looked upon as the 'Plant's Physician,' and it has been stated that nothing contributes so much to the health of a garden as a number of Chamomile herbs dispersed about it, and that if another plant is drooping and sickly, in nine cases out of ten, it will recover if you place a herb of Chamomile near it.

¶ *Parts Used Medicinally.* The whole plant is odoriferous and of value, but the quality is chiefly centred in the flower-heads or capitula, the part employed medicinally, the herb itself being used in the manufacture of herb beers.

Both single and double flowers are used in medicine. It is considered that the curative properties of the single, wild Chamomile are the more powerful, as the chief medical virtue of the plant lies in the central disk of yellow florets, and in the cultivated double form the white florets of the ray are multiplied, while the yellow centre diminishes. The powerful alkali contained to so much greater extent in the single flowers is, however, liable to destroy the coating of the stomach and bowels, and it is doubtless for this reason that the British Pharmacopœia directs that the 'official' dried Chamomile flowers shall be those of the double, cultivated variety.

The double-flowered form was already well known in the sixteenth century. It was introduced into Germany from Spain about the close of the Middle Ages.

Chamomile was largely cultivated before the war in Belgium, France and Saxony and also in England, chiefly in the famous herb-growing district of Mitcham. English flower-heads are considered the most valuable for distillation of the oil, and during the war the price of English and foreign Chamomile reached an exorbitant figure.

The 'Scotch Chamomile' of commerce is the Single or Wild Chamomile, the yellow tubular florets in the centre of the head being surrounded by a variable number of white, ligulate or strap-shaped ray florets. The 'English Chamomile' is the double form, with all or nearly all the florets white and ligulate. In both forms the disk or receptacle is solid and conical, densely covered with chaffy scales, and both varieties, but especially the single, have a strong aromatic odour and a very bitter taste.

¶ *Cultivation and Preparation for Market.* Chamomile requires a sunny situation. The single variety, being the wild type, flourishes in a rather dry, sandy soil, the conditions of its natural habits on wild, open common-land, but the double-flowered Chamomile needs a richer soil and gives the heaviest crop of blooms in moist, stiffish black loam.

Propagation may be effected by seed, sown thinly in May in the open and transplanting when the seedlings are large enough to permanent quarters, but this is not to be recommended, as it gives a large proportion of single-flowered plants, which, as stated above, do not now rank for pharmaceutical purposes as high as the double-flowered variety, though formerly they were considered more valuable.

The usual manner of increasing stock to ensure the double-flowers is from 'sets,' or runners of the old plants. Each plant normally produces from twelve to fourteen sets, but may sometimes give as many as from twenty-five to fifty. The old plants are divided up into their sets in March and a new plantation formed in well-manured soil, in rows 2½ feet apart, with a distance of 18 inches between the plants. Tread the small plants in firmly, it will not hurt them, but make them root better. Keep them clean during the summer by hand-weeding, as hœing is apt to destroy such little plants. They will require no further attention till the flowers are expanded and the somewhat tedious process of picking commences.

In autumn, the sets may be more readily rooted by placing a ring of good light soil about 2 or 3 inches from the centre of the old plant and pressing it down slightly.

¶ *Chemical Constituents.* The active principles are a volatile oil, of a pale blue colour (becoming yellow by keeping), a little Anthemic acid (the bitter principle), tannic acid and a glucoside.

The volatile oil is yielded by distillation, but is lost in the preparation of the extract. Boiling also dissipates the oil.

¶ *Medicinal Action and Uses.* Tonic, stomachic, anodyne and antispasmodic. The official preparations are a decoction, an infusion, the extract and the oil.

The infusion, made from 1 oz. of the flowers to 1 pint of boiling water and taken in doses of a tablespoonful to a wineglass, known popularly as Chamomile Tea, is an old-fashioned but extremely efficacious remedy for hysterical and nervous affections in women and is used also as an emmenagogue. It has a wonderfully soothing, sedative and absolutely harmless effect. It is considered a preventive and the sole certain remedy for nightmare. It will cut short an attack of delirium tremens in the early stage. It has sometimes been employed in intermittent fevers.

Chamomile Tea should in all cases be prepared in a covered vessel, in order to prevent the escape of steam, as the medicinal value of the flowers is to a considerable extent impaired by any evaporation, and the infusion should be allowed to stand on the flowers for 10 minutes at least before straining off.

Combined with ginger and alkalies, the cold infusion (made with ½ oz. of flowers to 1 pint of water) proves an excellent stomachic in cases of ordinary indigestion, such as flatulent colic, heartburn, loss of appetite, sluggish state of the intestinal canal, and also in gout and periodic headache, and is an appetizing tonic, especially for aged persons, taken an hour or more before a principal meal. A strong, warm infusion is a useful emetic. A concentrated infusion, made eight times as strong as the ordinary infusion, is made from the powdered flowers with oil of chamomile and alcohol and given as a stomachic in doses of ½ to 2 drachms, three times daily.

Chamomile flowers are recommended as a tonic in dropsical complaints for their diuretic and tonic properties, and are also combined with diaphoretics and other stimulants with advantage.

An official tincture is employed to correct summer diarrhœa in children. Chamomile is used with purgatives to prevent griping, carminative pills being made from the essential essence of the flowers. The extract, in doses of 10 to 15 grains, combined with myrrh and preparations of iron, also affords a powerful and convenient tonic in the form of a pill. The fluid extract of flowers is taken in doses of from ½ to 1 drachm; the oil, B.P. dose, ½ to 3 drops.

Apart from their employment internally, Chamomile flowers are also extensively used by themselves, or combined with an equal quantity of crushed poppy-heads, as a poultice and fomentation for external swelling, inflammatory pain or congested neuralgia, and will relieve where other remedies have failed, proving invaluable for reducing swellings of the face caused through ab-

scesses. Bags may be loosely stuffed with flowers and steeped well in boiling water before being applied as a fomentation. The antiseptic powers of Chamomile are stated to be 120 times stronger than sea-water. A decoction of Chamomile flowers and poppy-heads is used hot as fomentation to abscesses – 10 parts of Chamomile flowers to 5 of poppy capsules, to 100 of distilled water.

The *whole herb* is used chiefly for making herb beers, but also for a lotion, for external application in toothache, earache, neuralgia, etc. One ounce of the dried herb is infused in 1 pint of boiling water and allowed to cool. The herb has also been employed in hot fomentations in cases of local and intestinal inflammation.

Culpepper gives a long list of complaints for which Chamomile is 'profitable,' from agues and sprains to jaundice and dropsy, stating that 'the flowers boiled in lye are good to wash the head,' and tells us that bathing with a decoction of Chamomile removes weariness and eases pain to whatever part of the body it is employed. Parkinson, in his *Earthly Paradise* (1656), writes:

'Camomil is put to divers and sundry users, both for pleasure and profit, both for the sick and the sound, in bathing to comfort and strengthen the sound and to ease pains in the diseased.'

Turner says:

'It hath floures wonderfully shynynge yellow and resemblynge the appell of an eye . . . the herbe may be called in English, golden floure. It will restore a man to hys color shortly yf a man after the longe use of the bathe drynke of it after he is come forthe oute of the bathe. This herbe is scarce in Germany but in England it is so plenteous that it groweth not only in gardynes but also VIII mile above London, it groweth in the wylde felde, in Rychmonde grene, in Brantfurde grene. . . . Thys herbe was consecrated by the wyse men of Egypt unto the Sonne and was rekened to be the only remedy of all agues.'

The dried flowers of *A. nobilis* are used for blond dyeing, and a variety of Chamomile known as Lemon Chamomile yields a very fine essential oil.

CHAMOMILE, GERMAN

Matricaria chamomilla (LINN.)
N.O. Compositæ

Synonym. Wild Chamomile
Part Used. Flowers

The German Chamomile, sometimes called the Wild Chamomile, has flower-heads about ¾ inch broad, with about fifteen white, strap-shaped, reflexed ray florets and numerous tubular yellow, perfect florets. It is frequent in cornfields and so remarkably like the Corn

Chamomile (*Anthemis arvensis*) that it is often difficult to distinguish it from that plant, but it is not ranked among the true Chamomiles by botanists because it does not possess the little chaffy scales or bracts between its florets; also the conical receptacle, or disk, on which the florets are arranged is hollow, not solid, like that of the Corn Chamomile. It may also be distinguished from *A. cotula* and *Matricaria inodora*, the Mayweeds, by the lapping-over scales of its involucre surrounding the base of the flower-head not being chaffy at the margin, as in those species. It has a strong smell, somewhat like that of the official Common Chamomile (*A. nobilis*), but less aromatic, whereas the Corn Chamomile which it so closely resembles is scentless.

¶ *Constituents.* The flowers of the German Chamomile, though aromatic, have a very bitter taste. They contain a volatile oil, a bitter extractive and little tannic acid.

¶ *Medicinal Action and Uses.* Carminative, sedative and tonic. The infusion of ½ oz. of the dried flowers to 1 pint of boiling water may be given freely in teaspoonful doses to children, for whose ailments it is an excellent remedy. It acts as a nerve sedative and also as a tonic upon the gastro-intestinal canal. It proves useful during dentition in cases of earache, neuralgic pain, stomach disorders and infantile convulsions. The flowers may also be used externally as a fomentation.

¶ *Preparations.* Fluid extract: dose, ¼ to 1 drachm.

CHAMOMILE, STINKING

Anthemis cotula (LINN.)
N.O. Compositæ

Synonyms. Mayweed. Maruta Cotula. Dog Chamomile. Maruta Fœtida. Dog-Fennel
Part Used. Whole herb

Stinking Chamomile or Stinking Mayweed (*Anthemis cotula*), an annual, common in waste places, resembles the true Chamomile, having large solitary flowers on erect stems, with conical, solid receptacles, but the white florets have no membraneous scales at their base. It is distinguished from the other Chamomiles and closely allied genera by its fœtid odour, which Gerard calls 'a *naughty smell.*' This disagreeable smell, and the resemblance to fennel of its much-cut leaves, gains it its other name of 'Dog's Fennel.' The whole plant, not only the flowers, has this intense odour and is penetrated by an acrid juice that often will blister the hand which gathers it. Writers on toxicology have classed this plant amongst the vegetable poisons.

¶ *Medicinal Action and Uses.* Tonic, antispasmodic, emmenagogue and emetic.

The whole herb is used (for drying, *see* FEVERFEW). Like true Chamomile, a strong decoction will produce vomiting and sweating. In America it is used in country districts as a sudorific in colds and chronic rheumatism. The infusion made from 1 oz. of the dried herb in a pint of boiling water and taken warm in wineglassful doses has been used with success in sick headache and in convalescence from fevers. It was formerly used in scrofula and hysteria and externally in fomentations. A weaker infusion taken to a moderate extent acts as an emetic.

See FEVERFEW (CORN) and PELLITORY

CHASTE TREE

Agnus castus
N.O. Verbenaceæ

Part Used. The ripe berries
Habitat. Shores of the Mediterranean

¶ *Description.* A deciduous shrub of free spreading habit, young shoots covered with a fine grey down; leaves opposite, composed of five to seven radiating leaflets borne on a main stalk 1 to 2½ inches long, leaflets linear, lance-shaped, toothed, dark green above, grey beneath with a very close felt; stalks of leaflets ¼ inch or less long; flowers fragrant, produced in September or October, in whorls on slender racemes 3 to 6 inches long, sometimes branched; the berries somewhat like peppercorns, dark purple, half-covered by their sage-green calyces, yellowish

within, hard, having an aromatic odour; taste warm, peculiar. The seeds were once held in repute for securing chastity, and the Athenian matrons in the sacred rites of Ceres used to string their couches with the leaves.

¶ *Medicinal Action and Uses.* The fresh ripe berries are pounded to a pulp and used in the form of a tincture for the relief of paralysis, pains in the limbs, weakness, etc.

¶ *Other Species.* Vitex trifolia, the three-leaved Chaste Tree, has similar properties.

CHAULMOOGRA

Taraktogenos kurzii (KING)
N.O. Bixaceæ

Synonyms. Chaulmugra. Chaulmogra
Part Used. The oil from the seeds

¶ *Description*. Seeds are ovoid, irregular and angular, 1 to 1¼ inches long, ½ inch wide, skin smooth, grey, brittle; kernel oily and dark brown. A fatty oil is obtained by expression, known officially as Gynocardia oil in Britain, as Oleum Chaulmoogræ in the U.S.A.

¶ *Constituents*. The oil contains chaulmoogric acid and palmitic acid, and the fatty oil has been found to yield glycerol, a very small quantity of phytosterol and a mixture of fatty acids.

¶ *Medicinal Action and Uses*. Employed internally and externally in the treatment of skin diseases, scrofula, rheumatism, eczema, also in leprosy, as a counter-irritant for bruises, sprains, etc., and sometimes applied to open wounds and sores. Also used in veterinary practice. Dose of oil, 5 or 10 to 60 minims. Gynocardia Ointment, I.C.A.

¶ *Other Species*. The seeds of *Gynocardia odorata* have been erroneously given as the source of the oil.

Some of the commercial oil on the market probably comes from the allied species *Hydnocarpus*.

CHEKEN

Eugenia cheken (MOL.)
N.O. Myrtaceæ

Synonyms. Arryan. Myrtus Chekan
Part Used. Leaves
Habitat. Chile

¶ *Description*. The flowers grow in the axils of the leathery leaves, white with a four-parted calyx, four petals and numerous stamens; the berry is crowned by the calyx, one or two-celled, containing one or two seeds. The leaves nearly sessile, oval, 1 inch long, smooth, slightly wrinkled, aromatic, astringent, and bitter.

¶ *Constituents*. Volatile oil, tannin and four principles, viz. Chekenon, Chekenin, Chekenetin, and Cheken bitter, an amorphous, soluble bitter substance. The virtues of the leaves appear to be in the volatile oil they contain and in their tannin.

¶ *Medicinal Action and Uses*. Most useful in the chronic bronchitis of elderly people and in chronic catarrh of the respiratory organs. Dose: Fluid extract, 1 to 2 fluid drachms.

CHENOPODIUMS

N.O. Chenopodiaceæ

Synonyms. Goosefoots. Wormseeds. Spinach. Glassworts. Sea Beets

The *Chenopodiaceæ*, or Goosefoot order, is a large family of homely and more or less succulent herbs – common weeds in most temperate climates, usually growing on the seashore and on salt marshes and on waste or cultivated ground.

The tribe derives its distinctive name from the Greek words, *chen* (a goose) and *pous* (a foot), in allusion to the supposed resemblance borne by the leaves of most of its members to the webbed feet of the goose. The leaves are entire, lobed or toothed, often more or less triangular in shape.

The minute flowers – which are wind fertilized – are without petals, bisexual and borne in dense axillary or terminal clusters or spikes. The small fruit is membraneous and one-seeded, often enclosed by the persistent calyx, which frequently is inflated.

Most of these plants contain large quantities of iron in the form of digestible organic compounds and many of the species provide soda in abundance.

Ten species of *Chenopodium* occur in Britain, one of which, *C. Bonus-Henricus*, has been much cultivated as a pot-herb, under the name of English Mercury and All Good. The Garden Orache and the Arrach, the Sea Beet and the Glassworts are other native plants belonging to this large family, which has about 600 members.

The seeds of *C. Quinoa* (Linn.), of the Andean region of South America, there constitute the staple and principal food of millions of the native inhabitants.

Quinoa is a perennial, indigenous to the high tableland of the Cordilleras, where, at the conquest by the Spaniards, it was the only farinaceous grain used as food. The plant is from 4 to 6 feet high and has many angular branches, dull glaucous leaves, of a triangular outline on long, narrow stalks, and flowers forming large, compact, branched heads and succeeded by minute, strong, flat seeds, of a black, white or red colour.

The Quinoa has been introduced into Europe, but though large crops have been grown in France, the grain has an unpleasant acrid taste and will hardly be used as human food when anything better can be got, though the leaves make a pleasant vegetable, like spinach.

But in Peru, Chile and Bolivia, Quinoa is largely cultivated for its nutritious seeds, which are produced in great abundance and are made into soup and bread, and when fermented with millet, make a kind of beer. They are called 'Little Rice.'

The seeds are prepared by boiling in water, like rice or oatmeal, a kind of gruel being the result, which is seasoned with Chile pepper and other condiments; or the grains are slightly roasted, like coffee, boiled in water and strained, the brown-coloured broth thus prepared being seasoned as in the first process. This second preparation is called Carapulque, and is said to be a favourite dish with the ladies of Lima, but, as already stated, in whatever way prepared, Quinoa is unpalatable to strangers, though it is probably a nutritious article of food, due to the amount of albumen it contains.

Two varieties are cultivated, one producing very pale seeds, called the White or Sweet variety, which is that used as food, and a dark-red fruited one, called the Red Quinoa. Both kinds contain an amaroid (or bitter substance), in specially large amounts in the bitter variety, which is reputed anthelmintic and emetic. By repeated washings, the substance is removed and the seeds can then be used as a food, like the 'sweet' variety.

A sweetened decoction of the fruit is used medicinally, as an application to sores and bruises, and cataplasms are also made from it.

The grain is said to be excellent for poultry and the plant itself to form good green food for cattle.

See ARRACHS, BEETS, BLITES, CLIVERS, GLASSWORTS, GOOSEFOOTS, SPINACH AND WORMSEED

(*POISON*)
CHERRY LAUREL

Prunus laurocerasus (LINN.)
N.O. Rosaceæ

Part Used. The leaves
Habitat. Asia Minor; cultivated in Europe

¶ *Description.* A small evergreen tree rising 15 to 20 feet, with long, spreading branches which, like the trunk, are covered with a smooth blackish bark. Leaves oval, oblong, petiolate, from 5 to 7 inches in length, acute, finely toothed, firm, coriaceous, smooth, beautifully green and shiny, with oblique nerves and yellowish glands at the base. Flowers small, white, strongly odorous, disposed in simple axillary racemes. Fruit an oval drupe, similar in shape and structure to a blackcherry; the odour of hydrocyanic acid may be detected in almost all parts of the tree and especially in the leaves when bruised.
¶ *Constituents.* Prulaurasin (laurocerasin) is the chief constituent of the leaves. This has been obtained in long, slender, acicular, bitter crystals, closely resembling amygdalin, but not identical with it. The leaves yield an average of 0·1 per cent. of hydrocyanic acid, young leaves yielding more than the old.
¶ *Medicinal Action and Uses.* Sedative, narcotic. The leaves possess qualities similar to those of hydrocyanic acid, and the water distilled from them is used for the same purpose as that medicine. Of value in coughs, whooping-cough, asthma, and in dyspepsia and indigestion.
¶ *Dosage.* Cherry Laurel Water, B.P., ½ to 2 fluid drachms.

CHERRY STALKS

Prunus avium and Other Species (LINN.)
N.O. Rosaceæ

Part Used. Fruit stalks
Habitat. Britain, Clermond Ferrand in France, and other parts of the Continent

¶ *Description.* The fruit stalks of all species are used, their distinctive characteristics are stalks 1¾ inch long, very thin and enlarged at one end.

¶ *Medicinal Action and Uses.* Astringent, tonic. Used in bronchial complaints, anæmia, and for looseness of bowels, in the form of an infusion or decoction. ½ oz. of the stalks to a pint of water.

CHERRY, WILD

Prunus serotina (EHRL.)
N.O. Rosaceæ

Synonyms. Virginian Prune. Black Cherry
Parts Used. Bark of root, trunk and branches
Habitat. North America generally, especially in Northern and Central States

¶ *Description.* This tree grows from 50 to 80 feet high, and 2 to 4 feet in diameter. The bark is black and rough and separates naturally from the trunk. Wood polishes well, as it is fine-grained and compact, hence it is much used by cabinet-makers. Leaves deciduous, 3 to 5 inches long, about 2 inches wide, on petioles which have two pairs of reddish glands; they are obovate, acuminate, with incurved short teeth, thickish and smooth and glossy on upper surface; flowers bloom in May, and are white, in erect long terminal racemes, with occasional solitary flowers in the axils of the leaves. Fruit about the size of a pea, purply-black, globular drupe, edible with bitterish taste, is ripe in August and September. The tree is most abundant and grows to its full size in the south-western States. The root-bark is of most value, but that of the trunk and branches is also utilized. This bark must be freshly collected each season as its properties deteriorate greatly if kept longer than a year. It has a short friable fracture and in commerce it is found in varying lengths and widths 1 to 8 inches, slightly curved, outer bark removed, a reddish-fawn colour. These fragments easily powder. It has the odour of almonds, which almost disappears on drying, but is renewed by maceration. Its taste is aromatic, prussic, and bitter. It imparts its virtues to water or alcohol, boiling impairs its medicinal properties.

¶ *Constituents.* Starch, resin, tannin, gallic acid, fatty matter, lignin, red colouring matter, salts of calcium, potassium, and iron, also a volatile oil associated with hydrocyanic acid by distillation of water from the bark.

¶ *Medicinal Action and Uses.* Astringent, tonic, pectoral, sedative. It has been used in the treatment of bronchitis of various types. Is valuable in catarrh, consumption, nervous cough, whooping-cough, and dyspepsia.

¶ *Dosages.* Syrup, B.P. and U.S.P., 1 to 4 drachms. Tincture, B.P., ½ to 1 drachm. Infusion, U.S.P., 2 oz. Fluid extract, ½ to 1 drachm. Prunin, 1 to 3 grains.

¶ *Adulterant.* A spurious cherry bark has been noted which may be distinguished by the fact that no hydrocyanic acid is found when macerated with water.

CHERRY, WINTER

Physalis alkekengi (LINN.)
N.O. Solonaceæ

Synonyms. Alkekengi officinale. Coqueret. Judenkirsche. Schlutte. Cape Gooseberry. Strawberry Tomato
Parts Used. The fruits and the leaves
Habitat. Europe. China and Cochin-China. An escape in the United States

¶ *Description.* The name of *Physalis* is derived from the Greek *phusa* (a bladder), for the five-cleft calyx greatly increases in size after the corolla falls off, thus enclosing the fruit in a large, leafy bladder. The plant bears smooth, dark-green leaves and yellowish-white flowers. The fruit is a round, red berry, about the size of a cherry, containing numerous flat seeds, kidney-shaped. It will grow freely in any garden, but sufficient is found growing wild for medicinal purposes.

The leaves and capsules are the most bitter parts of the plant. The epicarp and calyx include a yellow colouring matter which has been used for butter.

The berries are very juicy, with a rather acrid and bitter flavour. In Germany, Spain and Switzerland they are eaten freely, as are other edible fruits. By drying they shrink, and fade to a brownish-red.

¶ *Constituents.* Physalin, a yellowish, bitter principle, has been isolated by extracting an infusion of the plant with chloroform. Lithal is sold as an extract of the berries to which lithium salt has been added. The fruit contains citric acid.

¶ *Medicinal Action and Uses.* The berries are aperient and diuretic, are employed in gravel, suppression of urine, etc., and are highly recommended in fevers and in gout. Ray stated that a gouty patient had prevented returns of the disorder by taking eight berries at each change of the moon. Dioscorides claimed that they would cure epilepsy. The country people often use them both for their beasts and for themselves, and especially for the after-effects of scarlet fever.

The leaves and stems are used for the malaise that follows malaria, and for weak or anæmic persons they are slightly tonic. A strong dose causes heaviness and constipation, but sometimes they have cured colic followed by diarrhœa.

While not so prompt in its action as sulphate of quinine, the powder is a valuable febrifuge.

The leaves, boiled in water, are good for soothing poultices and fomentations.

¶ *Dosage*. From 6 to 12 berries, or ½ an oz. of the expressed juice.

¶ *Other Species*.

P. viscosa (Ground Cherry or Yellow Henbane) can be used in a similar manner.

CHESTNUT, HORSE

Synonym. Hippocastanum vulgare (Gærtn.)
Parts Used. Bark and fruit

The Horse Chestnut, *Æsculus hippocastanum*, which has also been known as *Hippocastanum vulgare* (Gærtn.), is an entirely different tree from the Sweet Chestnut, to which it is not even distantly related, and is of much more recent importation to English soil. It is a native of northern and central parts of Asia, from which it was introduced into England about the middle of the sixteenth century

The name *Æsculus* (from *esca*, food) was applied originally to a species of oak, which, according to Pliny, was highly prized for its acorns, but how it came to be transferred to the Horse Chestnut is very uncertain; perhaps, as Loudon suggests, it was given ironically, because its nuts bear a great resemblance, externally, to those of the Sweet Chestnut, but are unfit for food. *Hippocastanum* (the specific name of the common sort) is a translation of the common name, which was given – Evelyn tells us – 'from its curing horses brokenwinded and other cattle of coughs.' Some writers think that the prefix 'horse' is a corruption of the Welsh *gwres*, meaning hot, fierce, or pungent, e.g. 'Horse-chestnut' = the bitter chestnut, in opposition to the mild, sweet one.

The tree is chiefly grown for ornamental purposes, in towns and private gardens and in parks, and forms fine avenues, which in the spring, when the trees are in full bloom, present a beautiful sight.

¶ *Description*. The trunk of the tree is very erect and columnar, and grows very rapidly to a great height, with widely spreading branches. The bark is smooth and greyish-green in colour: it has been used with some success in dyeing yellow. The wood, being soft and spongy, is of very little use for timber. It is often used for packing-cases.

The sturdy, many-ribbed boughs and thick buds of the Horse Chestnut make it a conspicuous tree even in winter. The buds are protected with a sticky substance: defended by fourteen scales and gummed together, thus no frost or damp can harm the

P. somnifera is a narcotic. The leaves are used in India, steeped in warm castor-oil, as an application to carbuncles and other inflammatory swellings. The seeds are used to coagulate milk. Kunth states that the leaves have been found with Egyptian mummies.

The plant sold in pots as Winter Cherry is *Solanum pseudo-capsicum*.

Æsculus hippocastanum
N.O. Sapindaceæ

leaf and flower tucked safely away within each terminal bud, which develops with startling rapidity with the approach of the first warm days after the winter. The bud will sometimes develop the season's shoot in the course of three or four weeks. The unfolding of the bud is very rapid when the sun melts the resin that binds it so firmly together.

The large leaves are divided into five or seven leaflets, spreading like fingers from the palm of the hand and have their margins finely toothed. All over the small branches may be found the curious marks in the shape of minute horse-shoes, from which, perhaps, the tree gets its name. They are really the leaf scars. Wherever a bygone leaf has been, can be traced on the bark a perfect facsimile of a horse-shoe, even to the seven nail markings, which are perfectly distinct. And among the twigs may be found some with an odd resemblance to a horse's foot and fetlock.

The flowers are mostly white, with a reddish tinge, or marking, and grow in dense, erect spikes. There is also a dull red variety, and a less common yellow variety, which is a native of the southern United States, but is seldom seen here.

The fruit is a brown nut, with a very shining, polished skin, showing a dull, rough, pale-brown scar where it has been attached to the inside of the seed-vessel, a large green husk, protected with short spines, which splits into three valves when it falls to the ground and frees the nut.

¶ *Cultivation*. The Horse Chestnut is generally raised from the nuts, which are collected in the autumn and sown in the early spring. The nuts should be preserved in sand during the winter, as they may become mouldy and rot. If steeped in water, they will germinate more quickly. They will grow a foot the first summer and require little care, being never injured by the cold of this climate. They thrive in most soils and situations, but do best in a good, sandy loam.

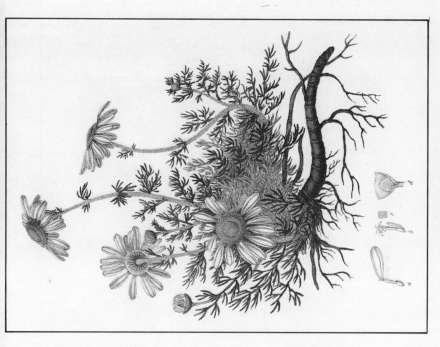

COMMON CHAMOMILE
Anthemis Nobilis

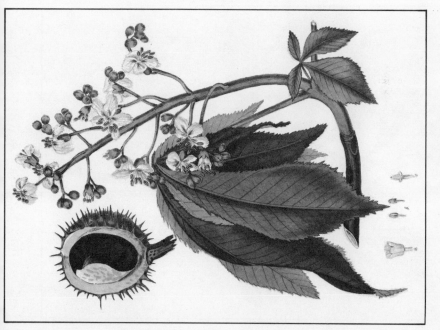

HORSE CHESTNUT
Æsculus Hippocastanum

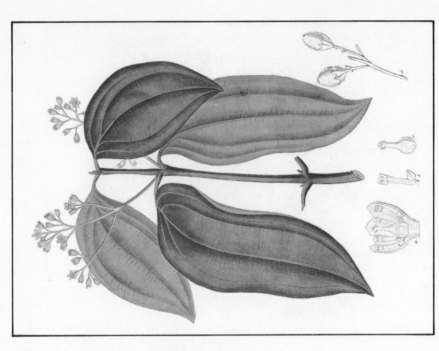

CINNAMON
Cinnamomum Zeylanicum

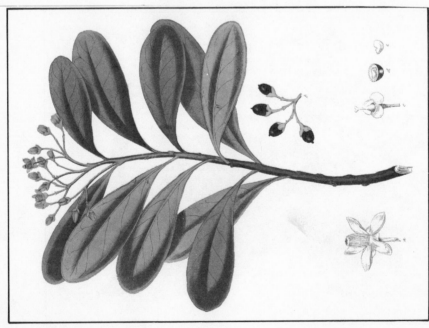

WHITE CINNAMON (CANELLA)
Canella Alba

¶ *Part Used Medicinally.* The bark and the fruit, from both of which a fluid extract is made. The bark is stripped in the spring and dried in the sun, or by slight artificial heat, and when dry, occurs in commerce in flattened pieces, 4 to 5 inches long and about 1 to 1½ inch broad – about 1 to 1¼ inch thick, greyish-brown externally, showing corky elongated warts, and on the inner surface pinkish-brown, finely striated longitudinally. The bark is odourless, but has a bitter astringent taste.

¶ *Medicinal Action and Uses.* The bark has tonic, narcotic and febrifuge properties and is used in intermittent fevers, given in an infusion of 1 oz. to the pint, in tablespoonful doses, three or four times daily. As an external application to ulcers, this infusion has also been used with success.

The fruits have been employed in the treatment of rheumatism and neuralgia, and also in rectal complaints and for hæmorrhoids.

¶ *Preparations.* Fluid extract, fruit, 5 to 20 drops. Fluid extract, bark, ½ to 2 drachms.

Horse Chestnuts as Fodder

In Eastern countries considerable use is made of Horse Chestnuts for feeding horses and cattle, and cattle are said to eat them with relish, though pigs will not touch them. The method of utilizing them is to first soak them in lime-water, which deprives them of the well-known bitter flavour inherent in the nuts, and then to grind them to a meal and mix them with the ordinary provender.

¶ *Constituents.* Analysis has shown that the nuts contain 3·04 per cent. water; 2·66 per cent. ash; 10·99 crude protein; oil, 5·34 per cent.; and 73·97 per cent. carbohydrates. Experiments conducted at Wye College proved that the most satisfactory way to prepare the Horse Chestnuts as food for animals was to soak partly crushed nuts in cold water overnight, then boil them for half an hour or so

and strain off the water. The nuts were then dried, partially husked and reduced to a meal, which, though slightly bitter, had a pleasant taste and appearance. The meal was fed to a calf, a sheep and two pigs. The calf received up to 5 lb. of the meal per day and made good increase in live weight, and the sheep suffered no ill effects, but the pig refused to eat the food containing the meal. It is concluded that Horse Chestnuts are not poisonous to any of the farm animals experimented with, within the limits of what they can be induced to eat, and that they form a highly nutritious food. Chestnut meal is a fairly concentrated food, and contains about 14 per cent. of starch, it being calculated that 1 lb. of Horse Chestnut meal would be equivalent to 1 lb. 1 oz. of feeding barley, 1 lb. 4 oz. of oats, 1 lb. 8 oz. of bran, and 3 lb. 5 oz. of good meadow hay.

Experiments made during the Great War proved that for every ton of Horse Chestnuts which are harvested, half a ton of grain can be saved for human consumption, and thus the Horse Chestnuts, though totally unfit for human food, can be utilized indirectly to increase the national food supply.

The genus *Pavia* is so closely allied as to be now generally grouped with the *Æsculus.* The Red Buckeye (*Æ. pavia*) is a handsome small tree with dense and large foliage, together with bright red flowers in large loose clusters in early summer. Sometimes it rises from 15 to 20 feet high, but some of its varieties are only low-spreading or trailing shrubs. The Yellow Buckeye (*Æ. flava*) is common, and sometimes 40 feet high. It has somewhat the habit of the Red Horse Chestnut (*Æ. rubicunda*), but has smoother leaves. The DWARF HORSE CHESTNUT (*Æ. parviflora*) is a handsome shrub, 6 to 10 feet high, flowering in later summer. Its foliage is much like that of other *Æsculi*, and its small, white, fragrant flowers are in long, erect plume-flowers.

CHESTNUT, SWEET

Castanea vesca (GÆRTN.)
N.O. Cupuliferæ

Synonyms. Fagus Castanea. Sardian Nut. Jupiter's Nut. Husked Nut. Spanish Chestnut

Parts Used. Leaves and fruit

The Sweet Chestnut (*Castanea vesca* or *Fagus castanea*) has been with some reason described as the most magnificent tree which reaches perfection in Europe.

It grows so freely in this country that it has been by some authorities considered a true native, its claim resting chiefly upon the use of what was for centuries supposed to be Chestnut timber in very ancient buildings, such as the roof of Westminster Hall and the

Parliament House of Edinburgh. It is now, however, recognized that the wood of Chestnut loses all virtue of durability when over fifty years old, and though the tree is of very quick growth, the beams in question could not have been grown in fifty years, so it has been proved that they are of Durmast Oak, which closely resembles Chestnut both in grain and colour.

It is now generally accepted that the Chestnut is really a native of sunnier skies than ours, but was probably introduced into England by the Romans. Before then it was introduced into Europe from Sardis, in Asia Minor, whence the fruit was called the 'Sardian Nut.' From Italy and Greece it seems to have spread itself over the greater part of temperate Europe, ripening its fruit and sowing itself wherever the vine flourishes.

In France, Italy and Spain it attains a great size. Theophrastus called it the 'Eubœan Nut' from Eubœa, now Negropont, where it was very abundant.

The famous Tortworth Chestnut, in Gloucestershire, was a landmark in the boundary records compiled in the reign of John, and was already known as the Great Chestnut of Tortworth in the days of Stephen. This enormous tree at 5 feet from the ground measured over 50 feet in circumference in 1720, and was still flourishing some years ago. Many of the trees forming the vast Chestnut forests on the slopes of Mount Etna are said to be even larger. In the Mediterranean region the Chestnut flourishes luxuriantly.

¶ *Description.* The tree grows very erect when planted among others, is firmly set and massive, the trunk columnar, tapering little, upstanding to the summit. When standing alone, it spreads its branches firmly on every side. Its bark is dark grey in colour, thick and deeply furrowed: the furrows run longitudinally, but in age tend to twist, often then presenting almost the appearance of thick strands in a great cable.

The handsome, narrow leaves are large and glossy, somewhat leathery in texture, 7 to 9 inches in length, about 2½ inches broad, tapering to a point at each end, the margins with distant, sharp-pointed, spreading teeth, arranged alternately on the twig. They remain on the trees late in autumn, turning to a golden colour, and are then very beautiful, especially as they are not so liable to be insect-eaten as are the leaves of the oak. They make useful litter.

The flowers appear after the leaves, in late spring or early summer, and are arranged in long catkins of two kinds. Some of the catkins bear only male flowers, each with eight stamens, and these mature first, the ripe pollen having a rather sickly odour. Other catkins have both kinds of flowers, the majority of them being pollen-bearing, but having also, near the twig from which they spring, the female or fruit-producing flowers in clusters, two or three flowers together in a four-lobed prickly involucre, which later grows completely together and becomes the thick, leathery hull which covers the ripening seeds. The fruit hangs in clusters of these forbidding-looking burs – the brown nuts, which are roundish in shape, drawn up to a point and flattened on one side, being thus enclosed in a kind of casket protected by spines.

¶ *Uses.* In this country, as a rule not more than one of these nuts matures, and as they rarely come to great perfection, nearly all of those used are imported, mostly from Spain, whence they are also called Spanish Chestnuts. The larger and better sorts, called Marones, are the produce of Italy, France, Switzerland and southern Germany, in which countries, especially in southern France and Italy, it forms an important article of diet, constituting in Italy a considerable proportion of the food of the peasantry.

They make an excellent stuffing for turkey, also roast pheasant; which is one of the few forms in which they are eaten here, apart from simply being roasted. Evelyn spoke of them as 'delicacies for princes and a lusty and masculine food for rusticks, and able to make women well-complexioned,' and then not unnaturally lamented that in England they are chiefly given to swine.

The meal of the Chestnut has also been used for whitening linen cloth and for making starch. The best kind, the Marones, contain 15 per cent. sugar, and by expression yield a thick syrup, from which in turn a very usable sugar can be derived. This variety in France forms the favourite sweetmeat: *Marons glacés.*

Chestnut makes excellent timber. Though in old age the wood is brittle and liable to crack, when in a *growing* stage, having very little sap wood, it contains more timber of a durable quality than an oak of the same dimensions, and young chestnuts have proved more durable than oak for woodwork that has to be partly in the ground, such as stakes and fences. It is used for many other purposes, such as pit-props and wine-barrels, and formerly Chestnut timber was used indiscriminately with oak for the construction of houses, mill-work and household furniture. In hop-growing districts it is in great demand for poles, and a coppice of prime chestnut is worth over £50 per acre. It makes excellent underwood and is quick growing. We read of an abbot in the reign of Henry II having a grant made to him of 'tithes of Chestnuts in the Forest of Dean,' and in modern days extensive plantings of Chestnuts have been made in the same great forest.

The usual method of *propagation* is by well-selected nuts, but if the tree is grown with the object of fruit-bearing, grafting is the best method. This is done in foreign countries and the method has been adopted in Devonshire. The grafted trees – called

CHICKWEED

marronniers by the French – are, however, unfit for timber. The most suitable soil for Chestnut trees is a sandy loam, with a dry bottom, but they will grow in any soil, provided the subsoil be dry.

The Chestnut takes its name, *Castanea*, from a town of the name of Castanis in Thessaly, near where the tree grew in great abundance. It has the same name in different forms in all the European languages.

¶ *Part Used Medicinally*. The leaves, picked in June and July when they are in best condition and dried. They have also been used in the fresh state.

Chestnut leaves have no odour, but an astringent taste.

¶ *Medicinal Action and Uses*. In some places Chestnut leaves are used as a popular remedy in fever and ague, for their tonic and astringent properties.

Their reputation rests, however, upon their efficacy in paroxysmal and convulsive coughs, such as whooping-cough, and in other irritable and excitable conditions of the respiratory organs. The infusion of 1 oz. of the dried leaves in a pint of boiling water is administered in tablespoonful to wineglassful doses, three or four times daily.

Culpepper says:

'if you dry the chestnut, both the barks being taken away, beat them into powder and make the powder up into an electuary with honey,

it is a first-rate remedy for cough and spitting of blood.'

RECIPES

Chestnut Soup

Scald, peel and scrape 50 large chestnuts; put these into a stewpan with 2 oz. of butter, an onion, 4 lumps of sugar, and a little pepper and salt, and simmer the whole over a slow fire for three-quarters of an hour; then bruise the chestnuts in a mortar; remove the pulp into a stewpan, add a quart of good brown gravy, and having rubbed the purée through a Tammy, pour it into a stewpan; make it hot and serve with fried crusts.

Chestnut Pudding

Put 12 oz. of chestnut farina into a stewpan, and add 6 oz. of pounded sugar, a spoonful of vanilla sugar, a pinch of salt, 4 oz. of butter, and a pint of milk; stir this over the fire till it thickens, and then quicken the motion of the spoon until the paste leaves the sides of the stewpan; it must then be removed from the fire, and the yolks of 6 eggs incorporated therewith; then mix in gently the 6 whites whipped firm, and use this preparation to fill a plain mould spread inside with butter; place it on a baking-sheet, and bake it in an oven of moderate heat for about an hour; when done, turn it out on its dish, pour some diluted apricot jam round it, and serve.

CHICKWEED

Stellaria media (CYRILL.)
N.O. Caryophylleæ

Synonyms. Starweed. Star Chickweed. Alsine media (Linn.). Passerina
(*French*) Stellaire
(*German*) Augentrosgräs
Part Used. Herb
Habitat. It has been said that there is no part of the world where the Chickweed is not to be found. It is a native of all temperate and north Arctic regions, and has naturalized itself wherever the white man has settled, becoming one of the commonest weeds

From the Groundsel, we naturally from association of ideas turn to the Chickweed, though it is in no way *botanically* allied to the Groundsel.

Several plants have been named Chickweed, one of them a plant belonging to the Purslane family and four species of Cerastium – the Mouse Ear Chickweeds – but the name especially belongs to the plant in question, *Stellaria media*, the ubiquitous garden weed, of which our caged birds are as fond as they are of Groundsel, a taste shared by young chickens, to whose diet it makes a wholesome addition.

Chickweed is a most variable plant. Gerard enumerates no less than thirteen species, but the various forms are nowadays merely considered deviations from the one type.

Hooker gives three varieties which have been named by other botanists as separate species.

¶ *Description*. The stem is procumbent and weak, much branched, often reaching a considerable length, trailing on the ground, juicy, pale green and slightly swollen at the joints. Chickweed is readily distinguished from the plants of the same genus by the line of hairs that runs up the stem on one side only, which when it reaches a pair of leaves is continued on the opposite side. The leaves are succulent, egg-shaped, about ½ inch long and ¼ inch broad, with a short point, pale green and quite smooth, with flat stalks below, but stalkless above. They are placed on the stem in pairs. The small white star-like flowers are situated singly in the axils of the upper leaves. Their petals are narrow and deeply cleft, not longer than the sepals. They open about nine o'clock in the morning and are said to remain open just twelve hours in bright weather, but rain prevents them expanding, and after a heavy shower they become pendent instead of having their faces turned up towards the sun, though in the course of a few days rise again. The flowers are already in bloom in March and continue till late in the autumn. The seeds are contained in a little capsule fitted with teeth which close up in wet weather, but when ripe are open and the seeds are shaken out by each movement of the plant in the breeze, this being one of the examples of the agency of the wind in the dispersal of seeds, which is to be seen in similar form in the capsules of poppy, henbane, campion and many other common plants.

The Chickweed is also an instance of what is termed the 'Sleep of Plants,' for every night the leaves approach each other, so that their upper surfaces fold over the tender buds of the new shoots, and the uppermost pair but one of the leaves at the end of the stalk are furnished with longer leafstalks than the others, so that they can close upon the terminating pair and protect the tip of the shoot.

The young leaves when boiled can hardly be distinguished from spring spinach, and are equally wholesome. They may also be used uncooked with young Dandelion leaves to form a salad.

The custom of giving Chickweed to birds is a very old one, for Gerard tells us:

'Little birds in cadges (especially Linnets) are refreshed with the lesser Chickweed when they loath their meat, whereupon it was called of some "Passerina." '

Both wild and caged birds eat the seeds as well as the young tops and leaves. Pigs like Chickweed, and also rabbits; cows and horses will eat it; sheep are indifferent to it, but goats refuse to touch it.

¶ *Part Used Medicinally*. The whole herb, collected between May and July, when it is in the best condition, and dried in the same manner as Groundsel. It is used both fresh and dried.

¶ *Medicinal Action and Uses*. Demulcent, refrigerant. It is held in great repute among herbalists, used mostly in the form of an ointment.

The fresh leaves have been employed as a poultice for inflammation and indolent ulcers with most beneficial results. A poultice of Chickweed enclosed in muslin is a sure remedy for a carbuncle or an external abscess. The water in which the Chickweed is boiled should also be used to bathe the affected part.

Gerard tells us that

'the leaves of Chickweed boyled in water very soft, adding thereto some hog's grease, the powder of Fenugreeke and Linseed, and a few roots of Marsh Mallows, and stamped to the forme of Cataplasme or pultesse, taketh away the swelling of the legs or any other part . . . in a word it comforteth, digesteth, defendeth and suppurateth very notably.'

He says that 'the leaves boyled in vinegar and salt are good against mangines of the hands and legs, if they be bathed therewith.'

Combined with Elecampane, Chickweed has also been recommended as a specific for hydrophobia, and the juice, taken internally, for scurvy.

The plant chopped and boiled in lard makes a fine green cooling ointment, good for piles and sores, and cutaneous diseases. It has also been employed as an application for ophthalmia.

A decoction made with the fresh plant is good for constipation, and an infusion of the dried herb is efficacious in coughs and hoarseness. The dose of the fluid extract is 10 to 60 drops.

Culpepper calls it 'a fine, soft, pleasing herb, under the dominion of the Moon,' and goes on to tell us that

'It is found to be as effectual as Purslain to all the purposes whereunto it serveth, except for meat only. The herb bruised, or the juice applied, with cloths or sponges dipped therein to the region of the liver, and as they dry to have fresh applied, doth wonderfully temper the heat of the liver, and is effectual for all impostumes and swellings whatsoever; for all redness in the face, wheals, pushes, itch or scabs, the juice being either simply used, or boiled in hog's grease; the juice or distilled water is of good use for all heat and redness in the eyes . . . as also into the ears. . . . It helpeth the sinews when they are shrunk by cramps or otherwise, and extends and makes them pliable again, by using the following methods, viz.: Boil a handful of Chickweed and a handful of dried red-rose leaves, but not distilled, in a quart of muscadine, until a fourth part be consumed; then put to them a pint of oil of trotters, or sheep's feet; let them boil a good while, still stirring them well, which being strained, anoint the grieved part therewith warm against the fire, rubbing it well with your hand, and bind also some of the herb, if you choose, to the place, and with God's blessing it will help in three times dressing.'

Chickweed water is an old wives' remedy for obesity.

CHICORY
Cichorium intybus (LINN.)
N.O. Compositæ

Synonyms. Succory. Wild Succory. Hendibeh. Barbe de Capucin
Part Used. Root
Habitat. Wild Chicory or Succory is not uncommon in many parts of England and Ireland, though by no means a common plant in Scotland. It is more common on gravel or chalk, especially on the downs of the south-east coast, and in places where the soil is of a light and sandy nature, when it is freely to be found on waste land, open borders of fields and by the roadside, and is easily recognized by its tough, twig-like stems, along which are ranged large, bright blue flowers about the size and shape of the Dandelion. Sir Jas. E. Smith, founder of the Linnean Society, says of the tough stems: 'From the earliest period of my recollection, when I can just remember tugging ineffectually with all my infant strength at the tough stalks of the wild Succory, on the chalky hills about Norwich. . . .'

¶ *Description*. It is a perennial, with a tap root like the Dandelion. The stems are 2 to 3 feet high, the lateral branches numerous and spreading, given off at a very considerable angle from the central stem, so that the general effect of the plant, though spreading, is not rich and full, as the branches stretch out some distance in each direction and are but sparsely clothed with leaves of any considerable size. The general aspect of the plant is somewhat stiff and angular.

The lower leaves of the plant are large and spreading – thickly covered with hairs, something like the form of the Dandelion leaf, except that the numerous lateral segments or lobes are in general direction about at a right angle with the central stem, instead of pointing downwards, as in similar portions of the leaf of the Dandelion. The terminal lobe is larger and all the segments are coarsely toothed. The upper leaves are very much smaller and less divided, their bases clasping the stems.

The flowerheads are numerous, placed in the axils of the stem-leaves, generally in clusters of two or three. When fully expanded, the blooms are rather large and of a delicate tint of blue: the colour is said to specially appeal to the humble bee. They are in blossom from July to September. However sunny the day, by the early afternoon every bloom is closed, its petal-rays drawing together. Linnæus used the Chicory as one of the flowers in his floral Clock at Upsala, because of its regularity in opening at 5 a.m. and closing at 10 a.m. in that latitude. Here it closes about noon and opens between 6 and 7 in the morning.

¶ *History*. It has been suggested that the name *Succory* came from the Latin *succurrere* (to run under), because of the depth to which the root penetrates. It may, however, be a corruption of Chicory, or *Cichorium*, a word of Egyptian origin, which in various forms is the name of the plant in practically every European language. The Arabian physicians called it 'Chicourey.' *Intybus*, the specific name of the Chicory, is a modification of another Eastern name for the plant – *Hendibeh*. The Endive, an allied but foreign species (a native of southern Asia and northern provinces of China) derives both its common and specific names from the same word. The Endive and the Succory are the only two species in the genus *Cichorium*. There is little doubt that the Cichorium mentioned by Theophrastus as in use amongst the ancients was the wild Chicory, since the names by which the wild plant is known in all the languages of modern Europe are merely corruptions of the original Greek word, while there are different names in the different countries for the Garden Endive.

Succory was known to the Romans and eaten by them as a vegetable or in salads, its use in this way being mentioned by Horace, Virgil, Ovid, and Pliny.

On the Continent, Chicory is much cultivated, not only as a salad and vegetable, but also for fodder and more especially for the sake of its root, which though woody in the wild state, under cultivation becomes large and fleshy, with a thick rind, and is employed extensively when roasted and ground, for blending with coffee.

In this country Chicory has been little grown. There was an attempt in 1788 to introduce its cultivation here as fodder, it being grown largely for that purpose in France, especially for sheep, but it would seem not to have met with success and has not been grown as a farm crop, though it furnishes abundance of good fodder at a time when green food is scarce, growing very quickly, two cuttings being possible in the first year and three in subsequent years, the produce being said to be superior on the whole to Lucerne. Although this plant, being succulent, seldom dries well for hay in this country, it seems valuable as fresh food for horses, cows and sheep: rabbits are fond of it. There has been an attempt since the war to re-introduce the cultivation of Chicory, and it has been successfully grown at the experimental farm of the University College of North Wales at Bangor, and at Kirton, Lincolnshire, for the first time for forty years, was reported in March, 1917, to be yielding 20 tons per acre.

When grown for a forage crop, it should be sown during the last week in May, or first week in June, in drills about 15 inches apart, the plants being afterwards singled to from 6 inches to 8 inches in the row. About 5 lb. of seed will be needed for the acre. If sown too early the plant is likely to bolt. So grown, the crop of leaves can be cut in autumn to be fed to stock of all kinds, such as poultry, rabbits, cows, etc., and in following years, if the crop is kept clean, the foliage may be mown off three or four times. So grown it should of course never be allowed to seed.

On the Continent, especially in Belgium, the young and tender roots are boiled and eaten with butter like parsnips, and form a very palatable vegetable.

¶ *Uses.* The leaves are used in salads, for which they are much superior to Dandelion. They may be cut and used from young plants, but are generally blanched, as the unblanched leaves are bitter. This forced foliage is termed by the French *Barbe de Capucin* and forms a favourite winter salad, much eaten in France and Belgium. A particularly fine strain is known as *Witloof*, in Belgium, where smallholders make a great feature of this crop and excel in its cultivation. The young blanched heads also form a good vegetable for cooking, similar to Sea Kale.

Enormous quantities of the plant are cultivated on the Continent, to supply the grocer with the ground Chicory which forms an ingredient or adulteration to coffee. In Belgium, Chicory is sometimes even used as a drink without admixture of coffee. For this purpose, the thick cultivated root is sliced, kiln-dried, roasted and then ground. It differs from coffee in the absence of volatile oil, rich aromatic flavour, caffeine and caffeotannic acid, and in the presence of a large amount of ash, including silica. When roasted, it yields 45 to 65 per cent. of soluble extractive matter. Roasted Coffee yields only 21 to 25 per cent. of soluble extract, this difference affording a means of approximately determining the amount of Chicory in a mixture.

When infused, Chicory gives to coffee a bitterish taste and a dark colour. French writers say it is *contra-stimulante*, and serves to correct the excitation caused by the principles of coffee, and that it suits bilious subjects who suffer from habitual constipation, but is ill-adapted for persons whose vital energy soon flags, and that for lymphatic or bloodless persons its use should be avoided.

¶ *Cultivation.* Chicory is a hardy perennial and will grow in almost any soil. For use as a salad, the plant may be easily cultivated in the kitchen garden. Sow the seed in May or June, in drills about 1 inch deep, about 12 inches apart, and thin out the young plants to 6 or 8 inches apart in the rows; when well up, water in very dry weather.

For blanching, dig up in October as many as may be needed, and after cutting off the leaves, it is well to let the roots be exposed to the air for a fortnight or three weeks; they should then be planted in deep boxes or pots of sand or light soil, leaving 8 inches between the soil and the top of the box. A cover of some sort is put on the box to exclude the light, and the box put into a warm place, either in a warm green-house, under the stage, or, being so hardy, they may be successful in a moderately warm cellar and shed, from which frost is excluded. Deprived of light, the young oncoming leaves become blanched and greatly elongated, and in this state are cut and sent to the market. If light is totally debarred, as it should be, the produce will be of a beautiful creamy white colour, soft and nearly destitute of the bitter flavour present when the plants are grown in the open air.

The fresh root is bitter, with a milky juice which is somewhat aperient and slightly sedative, suiting subjects troubled with bilious torpor, whilst, on good authority, the plant has been pronounced useful against pulmonary consumption.

A decoction of 1 oz. of the root to a pint of boiling water, taken freely, has been found effective in jaundice, liver enlargements, gout and rheumatic complaints, and a decoction of the plant, fresh gathered, has been recommended for gravel.

Syrup of Succory is an excellent laxative for children, as it acts without irritation.

An infusion of the herb is useful for skin eruptions connected with gout.

The old herbalists considered that the leaves when bruised made a good poultice for swellings, inflammations and inflamed eyes, and that 'when boiled in broth for those that have hot, weak and feeble stomachs doe strengthen the same.' Tusser (1573) considered it – together with Endive – a useful remedy for ague, and Parkinson pronounced Succory to be a 'fine, cleansing, jovial plant.'

Chicory when taken too habitually, or freely, causes venous passive congestion in the digestive organs within the abdomen and a fullness of blood in the head. If used in excess as a medicine it is said to bring about loss of visual power in the retina.

From the flowers a water was distilled to allay inflammation of the eyes. With violets, they were used to make the confection, 'Violet plates,' in the days of Charles II.

The seeds contain abundantly a demulcent oil, whilst the petals furnish a glucoside which is colourless unless treated with alkalies, when it becomes of a golden yellow. The leaves have been used to dye blue.

SWINE'S CHICORY (*Arnoseris pusilla*, Gærtn.), also known as Lamb's Succory, is a cornfield weed belonging to a closely related genus. All its leaves are radical, and it has small heads of yellow flowers on leafless, branched flower-stalks. It has no therapeutic uses.

To obtain roots of a large size, the ground must be rich, light and well manured.

¶ *Part Used Medicinally.* The root. When dried – in the same manner as Dandelion – it is brownish, with tough, loose, reticulated white layers surrounding a radiate, woody column. It often occurs in commerce crowned with remains of the stem. It is inodorous and of a mucilaginous and bitter taste.

¶ *Constituents.* A special bitter principle, not named, inulin and sugar.

¶ *Medicinal Action and Uses.* Chicory has properties similar to those of Dandelion, its action being tonic, laxative and diuretic.

CHIMAPHILA. *See* PIPSISSIWA, PYROLA, WINTERGREEN

CHINA [1]

Smilax China (LINN.)
N.O. Liliaceæ

Habitat. China, Japan and East Indies

¶ *Description.* A climbing shrub with tuberous roots, stems prickly, leaves stalked and veined, with a tendril on each side of the leaf stalks. The flowers have globular heads, sessile in the axils of the leaves, Tubers cylindrical, irregular, 4 to 6 inches long, 2 inches thick, slightly flattened, having short knotty branches, with a rust-coloured shiny bark, sometimes smooth, may be wrinkled, internally pale fawn colour, mealy, small resin cells, no odour, taste indifferent, afterwards slightly bitter and acrid, not unlike ordinary sarsaparilla.

¶ *Medicinal Action and Uses.* Alterative, diaphoretic, tonic. China Smilax is used for the same purposes and has much the same properties as the official Sarsaparilla. In large doses it causes nausea and vomiting, especially valuable in weakened and depraved conditions due to a poisoned state of the blood, it is a useful alterative in old syphilitic cases and in chronic rheumatism; it is also used for certain skin diseases. It was

introduced into China in A.D. 1535, when it was considered an infallible remedy for gout; in that country the roots are eaten as a food. With alum the root gives a yellow dye and with sulphate of iron a brown colour.

The name Smilax was used by the Greeks to denote a poisonous tree, but some authorities consider it is derived from 'Smile,' meaning cutting or scratching, having reference to the rough prickly nature of the plant.

¶ *Preparations.* The compound syrup is mostly used to form a vehicle for the administration of mercury and iodide of potassium. Dose, ½ to 1 drachm.

The smoke from sarsaparilla has been highly recommended for asthma.

¶ *Other Species.* The rootstocks of *Smilax Pseudo-China* are made into a sort of beer in South Carolina. They are also used to fatten pigs. In Persia the young shoots of some of these species are eaten as asparagus.

See SARSAPARILLA.

CHIRETTA

Swertia chirata (BUCH.-HAM.)
N.O. Gentianaceæ

Synonyms. Chirata. Indian Gentian. Indian Balmony
Part Used. Herb
Habitat. Northern India, Nepal

¶ *Description.* This plant first came into notice in Britain in 1829, and in 1839 was admitted to the Edinburgh Pharmacopœia. It is an annual, about 3 feet high; branching stem; leaves smooth entire, opposite, very acute, lanceolate; flowers numerous; peduncles yellow; one-celled capsule. The whole

herb is used and collected when flower is setting for seed and dried.

¶ *Constituents.* Two bitter principles, Ophelic acid and Chiratin, the latter in larger proportion.

¶ *Medicinal Action and Uses.* The true Chiretta has a yellowish pith, is extremely

[1] The China used in homœopathy is not to be confused with this plant. In homœopathy China is the name given to Peruvian bark. – EDITOR.

bitter and has no smell, an overdose causes sickness and a sense of oppression in the stomach. It acts well on the liver, promoting secretion of bile, cures constipation and is useful for dyspepsia. It restores tone after illness.

¶ *Dosages and Preparations.* Dried plant, 5 to 30 grains. Infusion of Chiretta, B.P., ½ to 1 fluid drachm. Fluid extract, ½ to 1 drachm. Solid extract, 4 to 8 grains.

¶ *Other Species.* In Indian bazaars where Chiretta is much more used than in Eng-

land, the name Chirata is given to many kinds of Gentian-like plants. The one that is most in use among them is *Ophelia augustifolia*, the hill Chirata. It can easily be recognized by the stem being hollow, without pith and lower part of stem square. Another adulterant is *Andrographis paniculata*, also a native of India, one of the *Acanthaceæ*; this in the dried state looks more like a bundle of broomtops, but is used a great deal in India as it has two valuable bitter tonic principles, Andrographolide and Halmeghin.

CHIVES

Allium schœnoprasum (LINN.)
N.O. Liliaceæ

Synonyms. Cives
(*French*) Ail civitte
(*Old French*) Petit poureau
Part Used. Herb
Habitat. The Chive is the smallest, though one of the finest-flavoured of the Onion tribe, belonging to the botanical group of plants that goes under the name of *Allium*, which includes also the Garlic, Leek and Shallot. Though said to be a native of Britain, it is only very rarely found growing in an uncultivated state, and then only in the northern and western counties of England and Wales and in Oxfordshire. It grows in rocky pastures throughout temperate and northern Europe. De Candolle says: 'This species occupies an extensive area in the northern hemisphere. It is found all over Europe from Corsica and Greece to the south of Sweden, in Siberia as far as Kamschatka and also in North America. The variety found in the Alps is the nearest to the cultivated form.' Most probably it was known to the Ancients, as it grows wild in Greece and Italy. Dodoens figures it and gives the French name for it in his days: '*Petit poureau*,' relating to its rush-like appearance. In present day French it is commonly called '*Ail civitte*.' The Latin name of this species means 'Rush-Leek.'

¶ *Description.* The plant is a hardy perennial. The bulbs grow very close together in dense tufts or clusters, and are of an elongated form, with white, rather firm sheaths, the outer sheath sometimes grey.

The slender leaves appear early in spring and are long, cylindrical and hollow, tapering to a point and about the thickness of a crowsquill. They grow from 6 to 10 inches high.

The flowering stem is usually nipped off with cultivated plants (which are grown solely for the sake of the leaves, or 'grass'), but when allowed to rise, it seldom reaches more than a few inches to at most a foot in height. It is hollow and either has no leaf, or one leaf sheathing it below the middle. It supports a close globular head, or umbel, of purple flowers; the numerous flowers are densely packed together on separate, very slender little flower-stalks, shorter than the flowers themselves, which lengthen slightly as the fruit ripens, causing the heads to assume a conical instead of a round shape. The petals of the flowers are nearly half an inch long; when dry, their pale-purple colour, which has in parts a darker flush, changes to rose-colour. The anthers (the pollen-bearing part of the flower) are of a bluish-purple colour. The seed-vessel, or capsule, is a

little larger than a hemp seed and is completely concealed within the petals, which are about twice its length. The small seeds which it contains are black when ripe and similar to Onion seeds.

The flowers are in blossom in June and July, and in the most cold and moist situations will mature their seeds, though rarely allowed to do so under cultivation.

¶ *Cultivation.* The Chive will grow in any ordinary garden soil. It can be raised by seed, but is usually propagated by dividing the clumps in spring or autumn. In dividing the clumps, leave about six little bulbs together in a tiny clump, which will spread to a fine clump in the course of a year, and may then be divided. Set the clumps from 9 inches to a foot apart each way. For a *quick return*, propagation by division of the bulb clumps is always to be preferred.

The green from the clumps can be cut three or four times in the season. When required for use, each clump may be cut in turn, fairly close to the ground. The leaves will soon grow again and be found more tender each time of cutting. By carefully cropping, the 'grass' can be obtained quite late in the season, until the early frosts come, when it withers up and disappears through the winter, pushing up again in the first warm days of February. For early crops, a little 'grass' can be forced on the clumps by placing cloches or a 'light' over them.

Beyond weeding between the clumps, no further care or attention is needed after division. Beds should be re-planted at least once in three or four years.

If it is desired to produce seed, grow two plantations, one for producing 'grass' for use, and the other to be left to flower and set seed, as you cannot get the two crops – 'grass' and seed, off the one set of plants.

¶ *Uses.* The Chive contains a pungent volatile oil, rich in sulphur, which is present in all the Onion tribe and causes their distinctive smell and taste.

It is a great improvement to salads – cut fresh and chopped fine – and may be put not only into green salads, but also into cucumber salad, or sprinkled on sliced tomatoes.

Chives are also excellent in savoury omelettes, and may be chopped and boiled with potatoes that are to be mashed, or chopped fresh and sprinkled, just before serving, on mashed potatoes, both as a garnish and flavouring. They may also be put into soup, either dried, or freshly cut and finely chopped, and are a welcome improvement to home-made sausages, croquettes, etc., as well as an excellent addition to beefsteak puddings and pies.

Chives are also useful for cutting up and mixing with the food of newly-hatched turkeys.

Parkinson mentions Chives as being cultivated in his garden, among other herbs.

CHRYSANTHEMUM. *See* PELLITORY

CICELY, SWEET   Myrrhis odorata (SCOP.)
                                 N.O. Umbelliferæ

Synonyms. British Myrrh. Anise. Great (Sweet) Chervil. Sweet Chervil. Smooth Cicely. Sweet Bracken. Sweet-fern. Sweet-Cus. Sweet-Humlock. Sweets. The Roman Plant. Shepherd's Needle. Smoother Cicely. Cow Chervil

Parts Used. The whole plant and seeds

Habitat. Mountain pastures from the Pyrenees to the Caucasus. In Britain, in the hilly districts of Wales, northern England and Scotland

¶ *Description.* The name *Myrrhis odorata* is derived from the Greek word for perfume, because of its myrrh-like smell.

It is a native of Great Britain, a perennial with a thick root and very aromatic foliage, on account of which it was used in former days as a salad herb, or boiled, when the root, leaves, and seed were all used. The leaves are very large, somewhat downy beneath, and have a flavour rather like Anise, with a scent like Lovage. The first shoots consist of an almost triangular, lacey leaf, with a simple wing curving up from each side of its root. The stem grows from 2 to 3 feet high, bearing many leaves, and white flowers in early summer appear in compound umbels. In appearance it is rather like Hemlock, but is of a fresher green colour. The fruit is remarkably large, an inch long, dark brown, and fully flavoured. The leaves taste as if sugar had been sprinkled over them. It is probable that it is not truly a wild plant, as it is usually found near houses, where it may very probably be cultivated in the garden. Sweet Cicely is very attractive to bees; in the north of England it is said that the seeds are used to polish and scent oak floors and furniture. In Germany they are still very generally used in cookery. The old herbalists describe the plant as 'so harmless you cannot use it amiss.' The roots were supposed to be not only excellent in a salad, but when boiled and eaten with oil and vinegar, to be 'very good for old people that are dull and without courage; it rejoiceth and comforteth the heart and increaseth their lust and strength.'

¶ *Medicinal Action and Uses.* Aromatic, stomachic, carminative and expectorant. Useful in coughs and flatulence, and as a gentle stimulant for debilitated stomachs. The fresh root may be eaten freely or used in infusion with brandy or water. A valuable tonic for girls from 15 to 18 years of age. The roots are antiseptic, and a decoction is used for the bites of vipers and mad dogs. The distilled water is said to be diuretic, and helpful in pleurisy, and the essence to be aphrodisiac. The decoction of roots in wine is also said to be effective for consumption, in morning and evening doses of 4 to 8 oz., while the balsam and ointment cure green wounds, stinking ulcers, and ease the pain of gout.

The medicinal properties resemble those of the American variety.

Chervil, or *Scandix Cerefolium* (fam. Umbelliferæ), a native of southern Europe and the Levant, is used only in cookery, and used in the French bouquet of herbs known as 'fines herbes.'

American Sweet Cicely (fam. Apicceæ) or

Ozmorrhiza longistylis. This plant grows in various parts of the United States, on low-lying, moist lands, flowering in May and June. The root has a sweet smell and taste, resembling aniseed, and yields its properties to water or diluted alcohol.

CINERARIA MARITIMA

Senecio maritima (LINN.)
N.O. Compositæ

Synonym. Dusty Miller
Part Used. Juice of the leaves
Habitat. Shores of the Mediterranean. Also found on the maritime rocks of Holyhead

¶ *Description.* The word 'Cineraria' means ashy grey, a mixture of black and white colouring resulting in the beautiful colour of the plant which grows sparsely in the author's garden at Chalfont St. Peter. This plant is perennial, propagated by cuttings, layers, or seeds. It belongs to the groundsel or ragwort family, of which there are nearly 900 different species known to botanists.

The species takes its name from *Senex* (an old man) in allusion to the white hairy pappus which crowns the achenes. The leaves are about 6 inches long, 2 inches wide, pinnately divided; flowers yellow.

¶ *Medicinal Action and Uses.* The fresh juice is said to remove cataract. A few drops of the fresh juice are dropped into the eye.
See GROUNDSEL, LIFE ROOT, RAGWORT

CINNAMON

Cinnamomum zeylanicum (NEES.)
N.O. Lauraceæ

Synonym. Laurus Cinnamomum
Part Used. Bark
Habitat. Ceylon, but grows plentifully in Malabar, Cochin-China, Sumatra and Eastern Islands. Has also been cultivated in the Brazils, Mauritius, India, Jamaica, etc.

¶ *Description.* Grows best in almost pure sand, requiring only 1 per cent. of vegetable substance; it prefers a sheltered place, constant rain, heat and equal temperature. The Dutch owned the monopoly of the trade of the wild produce, and it was not cultivated until 1776, owing to Dutch opposition and the belief that cultivation would destroy its properties.

Cinnamon is now largely cultivated. The tree grows from 20 to 30 feet high, has thick scabrous bark, strong branches, young shoots speckled greeny orange, the leaves petiolate, entire, leathery when mature, upper side shiny green, underside lighter; flowers, small white in panicles; fruit, an oval berry like an acorn in its receptacle, bluish when ripe with white spots on it, bigger than a blackberry; the root-bark smells like cinnamon and tastes like camphor, which it yields on distillation. Leaves, when bruised, smell spicy and have a hot taste; the berry tastes not unlike Juniper and has a terebine smell; when ripe, bruised, and boiled it gives off an oily matter which when cool solidifies and is called cinnamon suet.

The commercial Cinnamon bark is the dried inner bark of the shoots.

Cinnamon has a fragrant perfume, taste aromatic and sweet; when distilled it only gives a very small quantity of oil, with a delicious flavour.

¶ *Constituents.* 0 to 10 per cent. of volatile oil, tannin, mucilage and sugar.

¶ *Medicinal Action and Uses.* Carminative, astringent, stimulant, antiseptic; more powerful as a local than as a general stimulant; is prescribed in powder and infusion, but is usually combined with other medicines. It stops vomiting, relieves flatulence, and given with chalk and astringents is useful for diarrhœa and hæmorrhage of the womb.

¶ *Preparations and Dosages.* Cinnamon Water, B.P., 1 to 2 fluid ounces. Tincture of Cinnamon, B.P., $\frac{1}{2}$ to 1 drachm. Oil, B.P., $\frac{1}{2}$ to 3 drops. Comp. Powd. Arom., B.P., 10 to 40 grains. Spirit, B.P., 5 to 20 drops.

¶ *Other Species.*
Cinnamon Cassia is often substituted for it; it possesses much the same qualities and constituents but is inferior. *See* CASSIA.

C. Culiawan. Native of Amboyna; the bark has the flavour of cloves.

C. iners. Native of Malabar; seeds useful for fevers and dysentery; bark employed as a condiment.

C. nitidum. Dried leaves are said to furnish the aromatic called 'folid Malabathri.'

CINNAMON, WHITE

Canella alba (MURRAY)
N.O. Canellaceæ

Synonyms. Canella. White Wood. Wild Cinnamon. Canellæ Cortex
Part Used. The bark, deprived of its corky layer and dried
Habitat. The West Indies and Florida

¶ *Description.* A straight tree, from 10 to 50 feet in height, branched only at the top. The bark is whitish and the leaves alternate, oblong, thick, and of a dark, shining, laurel green. The flowers are small, and seldom open. They are of a violet colour, and grow in clusters at the tops of the branches. The fruit is an oblong berry containing four kidney-shaped seeds, and turns from green to blue and then to a glossy black. The wild pigeons of Jamaica eat the fruit, and their flesh is flavoured by them. The whole tree is aromatic, and if the flowers are dried, then softened again in warm water, they have a fragrance resembling musk. Canella was first introduced into Britain in 1600. The Spaniards, on seeing it in America, thought it was a species of cinnamon, and brought it to Europe as 'white cinnamon.'

The corky layer of the bark can be gently beaten off, and the inner bark is dried, and exported chiefly from the Bahamas.

In commerce the bark is found in quills or twisted pieces, of a pale orange-brown, with characteristic markings, scars, or spots. The fracture is short, granular, and whitish. The odour is agreeable, resembling cloves and cinnamon, and the taste is pungent, bitter, and acrid.

The negroes and Caribs use it as a condiment or spice, and it is sometimes added by smokers to their tobacco to remove the unpleasant odour and make their rooms fragrant.

¶ *Constituents*. A volatile oil, gum, starch, canellin, bitter extractive, resin, albumen, mannite, etc. The oil has a pungent, aromatic taste, and contains eugenol, cineol, and terpenes. There is no tannin.

¶ *Medicinal Action and Uses*. An aromatic bitter, useful in enfeebled conditions of the stomach, and often given with other medicines. It was formerly given in scurvy. The powder is used with aloes as a stimulating purgative.[1] It is often sold as a substitute for winter's bark, but it contains no tannic acid, or oxide of iron, both of which are present in the other.

¶ *Dosage*. 10 to 40 grains of the powder.

¶ *Other Species*.

¶ *C. axillaris* of Brazil. Thought by some authorities to be the source of Malambo bark and Matias bark.

CINQUEFOIL. *See* FIVE-LEAF GRASS

CLARY, COMMON

Salvia Sclarea (LINN.)
N.O. Labiatæ

Synonyms. Clarry. Orvale. Toute-bonne. Clear Eye. See Bright. Eyebright
Parts Used. The herb and leaves, both fresh and dry
Habitat. Middle Europe

Common Clary, like the Garden Sage, is not a native of Great Britain, having first been introduced into English cultivation in the year 1562. It is a native of Syria, Italy, southern France and Switzerland, but will thrive here upon almost any soil that is not too wet, though it will rot frequently upon moist ground in the winter.

Gerard, in 1597, describes and figures several varieties of Clary, under the names of *Horminum* and *Gallitricum*. He describes it as growing 'in divers barren places almost in every country, especially in the fields of Holborne neare unto Grayes Inne . . . and at the end of Chelsea.' It must have become acclimatized very quickly if it was found 'in divers barren places' before the close of the sixteenth century, less than forty years after its introduction into the country.

Salmon, in 1710, in *The English Herbal*, gives a number of varieties of the Garden Clary, which he calls *Horminum Hortense*, in distinction to *Horminum Sylvestre*, the Wild Clary, subdividing it into the Common Clary (*H. commune*), the True Garden Clary of Dioscorides (*H. sativum verum Dioscorides*), the Yellow Clary (*Calus Jovis*), and the Small or German Clary (*H. humile Germanicum* or *Gallitricum alterum Gerardi*). It is interesting

to note that this last variety, being termed *Gerardi*, indicates that Gerard classified this species when it was first brought over from the Continent, evidently taking great pains to trace its history, giving in his *Herball* its Greek name and its various Latin ones. That Clary was known in ancient times is shown by the second variety, the True Garden Clary, being termed *Dioscoridis*.

¶ *Description*. The Common Garden Clary is a biennial plant, its square, brownish stems growing 2 to 3 feet high, hairy and with few branches. The leaves are arranged in pairs, almost stalkless, and are almost as large as the hand, oblong and heart-shaped, wrinkled, irregularly toothed at the margins and covered with velvety hairs. The flowers are in a long, loose, terminal spike, on which they are set in whorls. The lipped corollas, similar to the Garden Sage, but smaller, are of a pale blue or white. The flowers are interspersed with large coloured, membraneous bracts, longer than the spiny calyx. Both corollas and bracts are generally variegated with pale purple and yellowish-white. The seeds are blackish brown, 'contained in long, toothed husks,' as an old writer describes the calyx. The whole plant possesses a very strong, aromatic scent, somewhat resembling

[1] This is a descendant of the Hiera Piera of Galen. – EDITOR.

that of Tolu, while the taste is also aromatic, warm and slightly bitter.

¶ *History.* According to Ettmueller, this herb was first brought into use by the wine merchants of Germany, who employed it as an adulterant, infusing it with Elder flowers, and then adding the liquid to the Rhenish wine, which converted it into a Muscatel. It is still called in Germany *Muskateller Salbei* (Muscatel Sage).

Waller (1822) states it was also employed in this country as a substitute for Hops, for sophisticating beer, communicating considerable bitterness and intoxicating property, which produced an effect of insane exhilaration of spirits, succeeded by severe headache. Lobel says:

'Some brewers of Ale and Beere doe put it into their drinke to make it more heady, fit to please drunkards, who thereby, according to their several dispositions, become either dead drunke, or foolish drunke, or madde drunke.'

In some parts of the country, a wine has been made from the herb in flower, boiled with sugar, which has a flavour not unlike Frontiniac.

Though employed in ancient times and in the Middle Ages for its curative properties, it seems to have fallen into disuse as a medicinal plant, though revived to a certain extent towards the end of the nineteenth century.

The English name Clary originates in the Latin specific name *sclarea*, a word derived from *clarus* (clear). This name Clary was gradually modified into 'Clear Eye,' one of the popular names and generally explained from the fact that the seeds have been employed for clearing the sight, being so mucilaginous that a decoction from them placed in the eye would 'clear' it from any small foreign body, the presence of which might have caused irritation.

Although the Garden Clary has much fallen into disuse as a medicine, there is a big trade done in it now, mainly in France, for the extraction of its oil as a perfume fixer, and there is undoubtedly a big future ahead for it for this purpose, not only on the Continent, but also in this country.

¶ *Uses.* The leaves are used to adulterate digitalis. The dried root and the seeds were formerly used in domestic medicine.

¶ *Cultivation.* Clary is propagated by seed, which should be sown in the spring. When fit to move, the seedlings should be transplanted to an open piece of ground, a foot apart each way, if required in large quantities. After the plants have taken root, they will require no further care but to be kept free of weeds. The winter and spring following, the leaves will be in perfection. As the plant is a biennial only, dying off the second summer, after it has ripened its seeds, there should be young plants annually raised for use.

¶ *Constituents.* Salvia Sclarea yields an oil with a highly aromatic odour, resembling that of ambergris. It is known commercially as Clary Oil, or Muscatel Sage, and is largely used as a fixer of perfumes. Pinene, cineol, and linalol have been isolated from this oil.

French Oil of Clary has a specific gravity of 0·895 to 0·930, and is soluble in two volumes of 80 per cent. alcohol. German oil of Clary has a specific gravity of 0·910 to 0·960, and is soluble in two volumes of 90 per cent. alcohol.

¶ *Medicinal Action and Uses.* Antispasmodic, balsamic, carminative, tonic, aromatic, aperitive, astringent and pectoral.

It has mostly been employed in disordered states of the digestion, as a stomachic, and has also proved useful in kidney diseases.

The seeds when soaked in water for a few minutes form a thick mucilage, which is efficacious in removing particles of dust from the eye. Gerard says:

'It purgeth them exceedingly from the waterish humerous rednesse, inflammation, and drives other maladies or all that happens unto the eies and takes away the paine and smarting thereof, especially being put into the eies one seed at a time and no more.'

Culpepper tells us:

'For tumours, swellings, &c., make a mucilage of the seeds and apply to the spot. This will also draw splinters and thorns out of the flesh. . . . For hot inflammation and boils before they rupture, use a salve made of the leaves boiled with hot vinegar, honey being added later till the required consistency is obtained.'

He recommends a powder of the dry roots taken as snuff to relieve headache, and 'the fresh leaves, fried in butter, first dipped in a batter of flour, egges, and a little milke, serve as a dish to the table that is not unpleasant to any and exceedingly profitable.'

The juice of the herb drunk in ale and beer, as well as the ordinary infusion, has been recommended as very helpful in all women's diseases and ailments.

In Jamaica, where the plant is found, it was much in use among the negroes, who considered it cooling and cleansing for ulcers, and also used it for inflammations of the eyes. A decoction of the leaves boiled in coco-nut oil was used by them to cure the stings of scorpions. Clary and a Jamaican species of

Vervain form two of the ingredients of an aromatic warm bath sometimes prescribed there with benefit.

For violent cases of hysteria or wind colic, a spirituous tincture has been found of use, made by macerating in warm water for fourteen days, 2 oz. of dried Clary leaves and flowers, 1 oz. of Chamomile flowers, ½ oz. bruised Avens root, 2 drachms of bruised Caraway and Coriander seeds, and 3 drachms of bruised Burdock seeds, adding 2 pints of proof spirit, then filtering and diluting with double quantity of water – a wineglassful being the dose.

Other Species

CLARY, WILD ENGLISH   Salvia Verbenaca

    Synonyms. Vervain Sage. Oculus Christi
    Parts Used. Leaves and seeds

    Salvia Verbenaca, the Wild English Clary, or Vervain Sage, is a native of all parts of Europe and not uncommon in England in dry pastures and on roadsides, banks and waste ground, especially near the sea, or on chalky soil. It is a smaller plant than the Garden Clary, but its medicinal virtues are rather more powerful.

¶ *Description.* The perennial root is woody, thick and long, the stem 1 to 2 feet high, erect and with the leaves in distant pairs, the lower shortly stalked, and the upper ones stalkless. The radical leaves lie in a rosette and have foot-stalks 1½ to 4 inches long, their blades about the same length, oblong in shape, blunt at their ends and heart-shaped at the base, wavy at the margins, which are generally indented by five or six shallow, blunt lobes on each side, and their surfaces much wrinkled. The whole plant is aromatic, especially when rubbed, and is rendered conspicuous by its long spike of purplish-blue flowers, first dense, afterwards becoming rather lax. The whorls of the spike are six-flowered, and at the base of each flower are two heart-shaped, fringed, pointed bracts. The calyx is much larger than the corolla. The plant is in bloom from June to August.

The seeds are smooth, and like the Garden Clary produce a great quantity of soft, tasteless mucilage, when moistened. Because, if put under the eyelids for a few moments, the tears dissolve this mucilage, which envelopes any dust and brings it out safely, old writers called this plant 'Oculus Christi,' or 'Christ's Eye.'

¶ *Medicinal Action and Uses.* 'A decoction of the leaves,' says Culpepper, 'being drank, warms the stomach, also it helps digestion and scatters congealed blood in any part of the body.'

This Clary was thought to be more efficacious to the eye than the Garden variety.

'The distilled water strengthening the eyesight, especially of old people,' says Culpepper, 'cleaneth the eyes of redness waterishness and heat: it is a gallant remedy for dimness of sight, to take one of the seeds of it and put it into the eyes, and there let it remain till it drops out of itself, the pain will be nothing to speak on: it will cleanse the eyes of all filthy and putrid matter; and repeating it will take off a film which covereth the sight.'

See SAGE.

(*POISON*)
CLEMATIS

Clematis recta
N.O. Ranunculaceæ

    Synonyms. Upright Virgin's Bower. Flammula Jovis
    Parts Used. The roots, stems
    Habitat. Europe

¶ *Description.* A perennial plant, stem about 3 feet high, leafy, striated, herbaceous, greenish or reddish; leaves large opposite, leaflets five to nine pubescent underneath, petioled; flowers, white in upright stiff terminal umbels, peduncles several times ternate; seeds dark brown, smooth, orbicular, much compressed, tails long yellowish, plumose; time for collecting when beginning to flower.

The leaves and flowers have an acrid burning taste, the acridity being greatly diminished by drying.

¶ *Medicinal Action and Uses.* The leaves and flowers when bruised irritate the eyes and throat giving rise to a flow of tears and coughing; applied to the skin they produce inflammation and vesication, hence the name Flammula Jovis. They are diuretic and diaphoretic, and are useful locally and internally in syphilitic, cancerous and other foul ulcers. Best suited to fair people; much used by homœopathists for eye affections, gonorrhœal symptoms and inflammatory conditions.

¶ *Dosages.* 1 to 2 grains of the extract a day. 30 to 40 grains of the leaves in infusion a day.

¶ *Antidotes.* Camphor moderates the too violent effects of the drug. Bryonia is said to appease the toothache caused by clematis.

¶ *Other Species.*

Clematis flammula (Sweet-scented Virgin's Bower) is cultivated in gardens, together with *C. Vitalba* (Travellers' Joy) and *C. Virginia* (Common Virgin's Bower). *C. Viorna* (Leather Flower) and *C. crispa* has been sometimes used in place of *C. recta*. *C. flammula* is said to contain an alkaloid, Clematine, a violent poison. From the bruised roots and stems of *C. vitalba*, boiled for a few minutes in water and then digested for a while in sweet oil, a preparation is made used as a cure for itch; this variety is also said to contain Clematine.

CLIVERS

Galium aparine (LINN.)
N.O. Rubiaceæ

Synonyms. Cleavers. Goosegrass. Barweed. Hedgeheriff. Hayriffe. Eriffe. Grip Grass. Hayruff. Catchweed. Scratweed. Mutton Chops. Robin-run-in-the-Grass. Loveman. Goosebill. Everlasting Friendship

Part Used. Herb

Habitat. It is abundant as a hedgerow weed, not only throughout Europe, but also in North America, springing up luxuriantly about fields and waste places

The natural order Rubiaceæ, to which the Madder (*Rubia tinctoria*) and our common wild plants, the Clivers, the Bedstraws and Sweet Woodruff belong, comprises upwards of 3,000 species. Many of these are of the highest utility to man, both as food and medicine; among the former the coffee-tree, *Coffea Arabica*, is perhaps of the first importance. The valuable drug quinine is furnished by several species of *Cinchona*, a South American genus, and drugs of similar properties are derived from other plants of the same tribe, while Ipecacuanha is the powdered root of another member of this order, growing in the forests of Brazil. Many species growing in tropical climates are moreover noted for the beauty and fragrance of their flowers.

Our British representatives are of a very different character, being all herbaceous plants, with slender, angular stems, bearing leaves arranged in whorls, or rosettes and small flowers.[1] From the star-like arrangement of their leaves, all these British species have been assigned to the tribe *Stellatæ* of the main order Rubiaceæ. All the members of this tribe, numbering about 300, grow in the cold and temperate regions of the Northern Hemisphere.

Of the fifteen British representatives of the tribe *Stellatæ*, eleven bear the name of *Galium* (the genus of the Bedstraws), and perhaps the commonest of these is the annual herb *Galium aparine*, familiarly known as Clivers or Goosegrass, though it rejoices in many other popular names in different parts of the country.

The angles of its quadrangular stalks and leaves are covered with little hooked bristles, which attach themselves to passing objects, and by which it fastens itself in a ladder-like manner to adjacent shrubs, so as to push its way upwards through the dense vegetation of the hedgerows into daylight, its rough, weak stems then struggling over and through all the other wayside plants, often forming matted masses.

The narrow, lance-shaped *leaves* [1] – about ½ inch long and ¼ inch broad – are arranged in *rosettes or whorls, six or eight together*, and are rough all over, both margins and surface, the prickles pointing backwards. The flowers, two or three together, spring from the axils of the leaves and are small and star-like, either white or greenish-white. They are followed by little globular seed-vessels, about ⅛ inch in diameter, covered with hooked bristles and readily adhering, like the leaves, to whatever they touch. By clinging to the coat of any animal that touches them, the dispersal of the seeds is ensured.

Most of the plant's popular names are connected with the clinging nature of the herb. Some of its local names are of very old origin, being derived from the Anglo-Saxon 'hedge rife,' meaning a taxgatherer or robber, from its habit of plucking the sheep as they pass near a hedge. The old Greeks gave it the name *Philanthropon*, from its habit of clinging. The specific name of the plant, *aparine*, also refers to this habit, being derived from the Greek *aparo* (to seize). Clite, Click, Clitheren, Clithers are no doubt various forms of Cleavers, and Loveman is merely an Anglicized version of *Philanthropon*. Its frequent name, Goosegrass, is a reference to the fact that geese are extremely fond of the herb. It is often collected for the purpose of giving it to poultry. Horses, cows and sheep will also eat it with relish.

The seeds of Clivers form one of the best

[1] Professor Henslow explains that though the *Galiums* look as if they possessed whorls of six *leaves*, in reality each whorl consists of only *two* real leaves, one of which may usually be recognized by having a bud or shoot arising from its *axil*, the other four are *stipules*, two belonging to each leaf. – EDITOR.

substitutes for coffee; they require simply to be dried and slightly roasted over a fire, and so prepared, have much the flavour of coffee. They have been so used in Sweden. The whole plant gives a decoction equal to tea.

We learn from Dioscorides that the Greek shepherds of his day employed the stems of this herb to make a rough sieve, and it is rather remarkable that Linnæus reported the same use being made of it in Sweden, in country districts, as a filter to strain milk; the stalks are still used thus in Sweden.

The plant is inodorous, but has a bitterish and somewhat astringent taste.

The roots will dye red, and if eaten by birds will tinge their bones.

¶ *Part Used Medicinally.* The whole plant, root excepted, gathered in May and June, when just coming into flower.

¶ *Chemical Constituents.* Chlorophyll, starch and three distinct acids, viz. a variety of tannic acid, which has been named galitannic acid, citric acid and a peculiar acid named rubichloric acid.

¶ *Medicinal Action and Uses.* Diuretic, tonic, alterative, aperient.

In old Herbals it is extolled for its powers, and it is still employed in country districts, both in England and elsewhere, as a purifier of the blood, the tops being used as an ingredient in rural 'spring drinks.'

Fluid extract: dose, $\frac{1}{2}$ to 1 drachm.

Modern herbalists and homœopaths still recognize the value of this herb, and as an alterative consider it may be given to advantage in scurvy, scrofula, psoriasis and skin diseases and eruptions generally. The expressed juice is recommended, in doses of 3 oz. twice a day, but as it is a rather powerful diuretic, care should be taken that it is not given where a tendency to diabetes is manifested. Its use, however, is recommended in dropsical complaints, as it operates with considerable power upon the urinary secretion and the urinary organs. It is given in ob-

structions of these organs, acting as a solvent of stone in the bladder.

The dried plant is often infused in hot water and drunk as a tea, 1 oz. of the dried herb being infused to 1 pint of water. This infusion, either hot or cold, is taken frequently in wine-glassful doses.

The same infusion has a most soothing effect in cases of insomnia, and induces quiet, restful sleep.

A wash made from Clivers is said to be useful for sunburn and freckles, a decoction or infusion of the fresh herb being used for this purpose, applied to the face by means of a soft cloth or sponge.

The herb has a special curative reputation with reference to cancerous growths and allied tumours, an ointment being made from the leaves and stems wherewith to dress the ulcerated parts, the expressed juice at the same time being used internally.

Clivers was also used as an ointment for scalds and burns in the fourteenth century, under the name of Heyryt, Cosgres, Clive and Tongebledes (Tonguebleed), the latter doubtless from its roughness due to the incurved hooks all over the plant.

It was later used for colds, swellings, etc., the whole plant being rather astringent, and on account of this property being of service in some bleedings, as well as in diarrhœa. Clivers tea is still a rural remedy for colds in the head.

The crushed herb is applied in France as a poultice to sores and blisters.

Gerard writes of Clivers as a marvellous remedy for the bites of snakes, spiders and all venomous creatures, and quoting Pliny, says: 'A pottage made of Cleavers, a little mutton and oatmeal is good to cause lankness and keepe from fatnesse.'

Culpepper recommends Clivers for earache.

See CHENOPODIUMS, BEDSTRAW, WOODRUFF MADDER, CROSSWORT.

CLOVER, RED

Trifolium pratense (LINN.)
N.O. Leguminosæ

Synonyms. Trefoil. Purple Clover
Part Used. Blossoms
Habitat. Abundant in Britain, throughout Europe, Central and Northern Asia from the Mediterranean to the Arctic Circle and high up into the mountains

¶ *Description.* A perennial, but of short duration, generally abundant on meadow land of a light sandy nature, where it produces abundant blossom, forming an excellent mowing crop. Not of great value as a bee plant – the bees not working it for so long as they will the white variety.

Several stems 1 to 2 feet high, arising from the one root, slightly hairy; leaves ternate, leaflets ovate, entire, nearly smooth, ending in long point often lighter coloured in centre, flowers red to purple, fragrant, in dense terminal ovoid or globular heads.

¶ *Medicinal Action and Uses.* The fluid extract of *Trifolium* is used as an alterative

and antispasmodic. An infusion made by
1 oz. to 1 pint of boiling water may with advantage be used in cases of bronchial and
whooping-cough. Fomentations and poul-

tices of the herb have been used as local
applications to cancerous growths.

¶ *Dosages*. 1 drachm of fluid extract, 1 to
2 drachms of infusion.

CLOVES

Eugenia caryophyllata (THUMB.)
N.O. Myrtaceæ

Synonym. Eugenia Aromatica
Part Used. Undeveloped flowers
Habitat. Molucca Islands, Southern Philippines

¶ *Description*. A small evergreen tree,
pyramidal, trunk soon divides into large
branches covered with a smooth greyish bark;
leaves large, entire, oblong, lanceolate (always
bright green colour), which stand in pairs on
short foot-stalks, when bruised very fragrant.
Flowers grow in bunches at end of branches.

At the start of the rainy season long greenish
buds appear; from the extremity of these the
corolla comes which is of a lovely rosy peach
colour; as the corolla fades the calyx turns
yellow, then red. The calyces, with the
embryo seed, are at this stage beaten from the
tree and when dried are the cloves of commerce. The flowers have a strong refreshing
odour. If the seeds are allowed to mature,
most of the pungency is lost. Each berry has
only one seed. The trees fruit usually about
eight or nine years after planting. The whole
tree is highly aromatic. The spice was introduced into Europe from the fourth to the
sixth century.

The finest cloves come from Molucca and
Pemba, where the trees grow better than anywhere else, but they are also imported from
the East and West Indies, Mauritius and
Brazil.

In commerce the varieties are known by
the names of the localities in which they are
grown. Formerly Cloves were often adulterated, but as production increased the price
lowered and fraud has decreased. Cloves
contain a large amount of essential oil,
which is much used in medicine. When of
good quality they are fat, oily, and dark
brown in colour, and give out their oil when
squeezed with the finger-nail. When pale
colour and dry, they are of inferior quality
and yield little oil. Clove stalks are some-

times imported, and are said to be stronger
and more pungent even than the Cloves.

Clove trees absorb an enormous amount
of moisture, and if placed near water their
weight is visibly increased after a few
hours; dishonest dealers often make use
of this knowledge in their dealings, and the
powdered stems are often sold as pure
powdered Cloves.

¶ *Constituents*. Volatile oil, gallotannic acid;
two crystalline principles – Caryophyllin,
which is odourless and appears to be a
phylosterol, Eugenin; gum, resin, fibre.

¶ *Medicinal Action and Uses*. The most
stimulating and carminative of all aromatics; given in powder or infusion for nausea,
emesis, flatulence, languid indigestion and
dyspepsia, and used chiefly to assist the
action of other medicines. The medicinal
properties reside in the volatile oil. The oil
must be kept in dark bottles in a cool place.
If distilled with water, salt must be added to
raise the temperature of ebullition and the
same Cloves must be distilled over and over
again to get their full essence.

The oil is frequently adulterated with
fixed oil and oil of Pimento and Copaiba. As
a local irritant it stimulates peristalsis. It is
a strong germicide, a powerful antiseptic, a
feeble local anæsthetic applied to decayed
teeth, and has been used with success as
a stimulating expectorant in phthisis and
bronchial troubles. Fresh infusion of Cloves
contains astringent matter as well as the
volatile oil. The infusion and Clove water
are good vehicles for alkalies and aromatics.

¶ *Dosages*. Fluid extract, 5 to 30 drops. Oil
extract, 1 to 5 drops. Infusion, B.P., $\frac{1}{2}$ to
1 oz.

CLUB MOSS. *See* MOSS

(POISON)
COCA, BOLIVIAN

Erythroxylon Coca (LAMK.)
N.O. Linaceæ

Synonyms. Cuca. Cocaine
Part Used. Leaves
Habitat. Bolivia and Peru; cultivated in Ceylon and Java

¶ *Description*. Small shrubby tree 12 to 18
feet high in the wild state and kept down
to about 6 feet when cultivated. Grown from

seeds and requires moisture and an equable
temperature. Starts yielding in eighteen
months and often productive over fifty years.

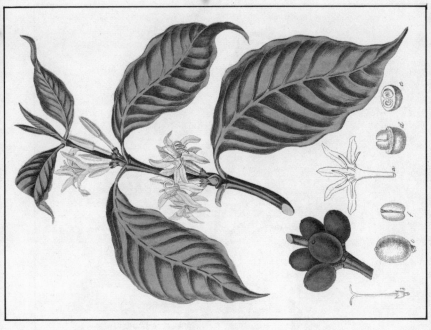

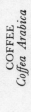

COFFEE
Coffea Arabica

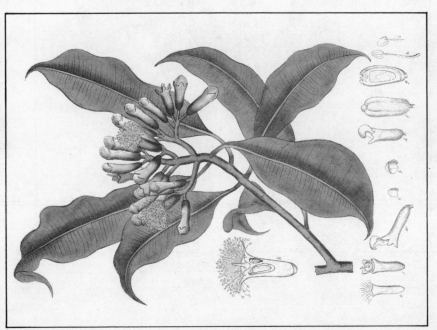

CLOVES
Eugenia Caryophyllata

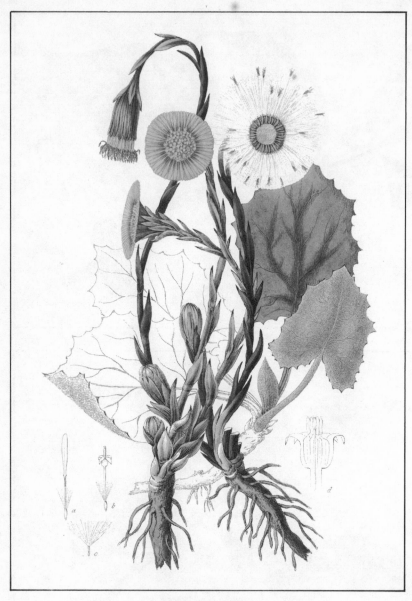

COLTSFOOT
Tussilago Farfara

The leaves are gathered three times a year, the first crop in spring, second in June, and third in October; must always be collected in dry weather. There are two varieties in commerce, the *Huanuco Coca*, or *Erythroxylon Coca*, which comes from Bolivia and has leaves of a brownish-green colour, oval, entire and glabrous, with a rather bitter taste, and Peruvian Coca, the leaves of which are much smaller and a pale-green colour. Coca leaves deteriorate very quickly in a damp atmosphere, and for this reason the alkaloid is extracted from the leaves in South America before *exportation*. The Coca shrubs of India and Ceylon were originally cultivated from plants sent out there from Kew Gardens and grown from seeds.

¶ *Constituents.* Coca leaves contain the alkaloids Cocaine, Annamyl Cocaine, and Truxilline or Cocamine. As a rule the Truxillo or Peruvian leaves contain more alkaloid than the Bolivian, though the latter are preferred for medicinal purposes. Java Coca contains tropacocaine and four yellow crystalline glucosides in addition to the other constituents.

¶ *Medicinal Action and Uses.* The actions of Coca depend principally on the alkaloid Cocaine, but the whole drug is said to be more stimulating and to have a mild astringency. In Peru and Bolivia the leaves are extensively chewed to relieve hunger and fatigue, though the habit eventually ruins the health. Coca leaves are used as a cerebral and muscle stimulant, especially during convalescence, to relieve nausea, vomiting and pains of the stomach without upsetting the digestion. A tonic in neurasthenia and debilitated conditions. The danger of the formation of the habit, however, far outweighs any value the drug may possess, and use of Coca in any form is attended with grave risks. Cocaine is a general protoplasmic poison, having a special affinity for nervous tissue; it is a powerful local anæsthetic, paralysing the sensory nerve fibres. To obtain local cutaneous anæsthesia the drug is injected hypodermically. Applied to the eye it dilates the pupil and produces complete local anæsthesia. It is a general excitant of the central nervous system and the brain, especially the motor areas, producing a sense of exhilaration and an incitement to effort; large doses cause hallucinations, restlessness, tremors and convulsions. Those acquiring the Cocaine habit suffer from emaciation, loss of memory, sleeplessness and delusions.

¶ *Preparations and Dosages.* Elixir Coca, B.P.C., 1 to 4 fluid drachms. Extract of Coca, B.P.C., 2 to 10 grains. Liquid extract of Coca, B.P., ½ to 1 fluid drachm. Fluid extract of Coca, U.S.P., 30 minims. Tincture of Coca, B.P.C., ½ to 1 fluid drachm. Coca Wine, B.P.C., 2 to 4 fluid drachms. Wine of Coca, U.S.P., 4 fluid drachms. Cocaine, P.B., $\frac{1}{30}$ to ½ grain.

¶ *Adulterants.* Coca leaves have sometimes been adulterated with those of Jaborandi.

¶ *Poisoning Antidotes.* Cocaine rarely enters the system through the alimentary canal, therefore the use of a stomach pump, emetics or chemical antidotes is not usual; strong coffee should be given as a stimulant by mouth or rectum and measures taken to prevent cardiac failure.

(*POISON*)
COCCULUS, INDICUS

Anamirta paniculata (COLEBR.)
N.O. Menispermaceæ

Synonyms. Levant Nut. Fish Berry
Part Used. Dried fruit
Habitat. India, Ceylon, Malabar

¶ *Description.* A poisonous climbing plant with ash-coloured corky bark, leaves stalked, heart-shaped, smooth, underside pale with tufts of hair at the junctions of the nerves and at the base of the leaves; the flowers are pendulous panicles, male and female blooms on different plants; fruit round and kidney shaped, outer coat thin, dry, browny, black and wrinkled, inside a hard white shell divided into two containing a whitish seed, crescent shaped and very oily.

¶ *Constituents.* The chief constituent is the bitter, crystalline, poisonous substance, picrotoxin; the seed also contains about 50 per cent. of fat.

¶ *Medicinal Action and Uses.* The powdered berries are sometimes used as an ointment for destroying lice; the entire fruits are used to stupefy fish, being thrown on the water for that purpose. Picrotoxin is a powerful convulsive poison used principally to check night sweats in phthisis by its action in accelerating respiration, but it is not always successful. It was at one time used to adulterate beers, increasing their reputation as intoxicants; it is an antidote in Morphine poisoning.

¶ *Preparations.* Fluid extract, ¼ to 1 drop. Picrotoxin, B.P.

COCILLANA BARK

Guarea rusbyi (BRIT.)
N.O. Meliaceæ

Synonyms. Sycocarpus Rusbyi. Guarea trichiliodes
Part Used. Bark
Habitat. Cuba

¶ *Description*. A large Bolivian tree; flowers in axillary clusters; bark ashy grey on the older trees on account of lichen growths; the inner bark is generally thicker than the outer; fracture, coarse fibrous splinters; odour musk like; taste distinctive, astringent and nauseous; leaves pinnate and of peculiar growth; as the lower leaflets fall young ones grow at the end of the same leaf-stalk, which elongates, the lower outer portion becomes woody with an outer bark and a thin pith inside and grows into a branch.

¶ *Medicinal Action and Uses*. The bark causes vomiting, and often prostration and nausea. In action very like ipecacuanha, but a more stimulating expectorant. Used with success in the treatment of bronchitis and pulmonary complaints.

¶ *Preparations*. Fluid extract: dose, 5 to 20 drops.

COCKLEBUR

Xanthium spinosum (LINN.)
N.O. Annuals in group of Ambroiseceæ of the Compositæ

Synonym. Spiny Clot Burr
Part Used. The whole plant
Habitat. South Europe and naturalized in America near sea-coast, Central Asia northwards to the Baltic and many other parts of the globe

¶ *Description*. Xanthic flowers belong to a type which are yellow in colour and can become white or red but never blue. These plants are spread as weeds or cultivated over a great part of the world. Stem annual, from 1 to 3 feet high, much branched and many spined; these are straw-coloured and divided about ¼ inch from their base into three slender branches, diverging and sharp. Leaves lanceolate, acute, tapering to short leaf-stalks with two lobes at base; underside is covered with a thick white down. Flowers small, monœcious; those at apex sterile, while the fertile ones are at the base of the branchlets. Fruit, a rough burr with a short beak at the apex and covered densely with hooked prickles.

¶ *Medicinal Action and Uses*. A valuable and sure specific in the treatment of hydrophobia. An active styptic, local and general. Fluid extract, 1 to 2 drachms. 10 grains of the powdered plant, four times daily.

¶ *Other Species. Xanthium Strumarium*, a coarse erect annual, 1 to 2 feet high; leaves on long stalks, large broadly heart-shaped, coarsely toothed or angular on both sides. Flower heads, greenish yellow, terminal clusters on short racemes, upper ones male, lower female, forming when in fruit ovoid burrs covered with hooked prickles. The short stout conical beaks erect or curved inwards. It is not a British plant, though is sometimes found there and in Ireland.

COFFEE

Coffea Arabica (LINN.)
N.O. Rubiaceæ

Synonym. Caffea
Parts Used. Seeds, leaves, caffeine
Habitat. South-west point of Abyssinia, and cultivated throughout the tropics

¶ *Description and History*. The name Coffee is derived from Caffa, a province of Abyssinia. In its wild state the tree grows to a height of 30 feet, but in cultivation it is kept shorter to expedite picking; it has evergreen leaves, smooth and shiny on the upper side, dark green under and paler, 6 inches long, 2½ inches wide; flowers in dense clusters at base of leaves, white and very decorative, but only lasting in bloom two days; berries red and fleshy, like small cherries, each berry two-seeded, convex on one side, flat on the other with a long furrowed line running lengthways and covered with a thin parchment which has to be winnowed or milled before roasting, after the outer pulp has been removed by a machine. The roasting develops the volatile oil and peculiar acid to which the aromas and flavours are due. The Coffee shrub was introduced into Arabia early in the fifteenth century from Abyssinia, and for two centuries Arabia supplied the world's Coffee; at the end of the seventeenth century the Dutch introduced the plant into Batavia, and from there a plant was presented to Louis XIV in 1714. All the Coffee now imported from Brazil has been imported from that single plant. The European use of Coffee dates from the sixteenth century when it was introduced into Constantinople, and a century later in 1652 the first Coffee shop was opened in London. In 1858 the quantity imported into the United Kingdom was over sixty million pounds. In Turkey the consumption is enormous, and so necessary is it considered that the refusal to supply a reasonable amount to a Turk's wife is considered a legal cause for divorce.

¶ *Constituents of Roasted Coffee.* Oil, wax, caffeine, aromatic oil, tannic acid, caffetannic acid, gum, sugar, protein.

¶ *Medicinal Action and Uses.* An active brain stimulant, which produces sleepless-ness, hence its great value in narcotic poisoning; in acute cases is injected into the rectum. Very valuable in cases of snake-bite, helping to ward off the terrible coma. It also exerts a soothing action on the vascular system, preventing a too rapid wasting of the tissues of the body; these effects are not only due to the volatile oil but to the caffeine it contains. The Malays infuse the leaves, which contain even more caffeine than the berries. Caffeine is valuable for heart disease, ascites and pleuritic effusion and combines well with digitalis; also valuable in cases of inebrity; is a powerful diuretic, but loses its effect with use.

¶ *Dose.* Preparation Caffeine, 1 to 5 grains.

COHOSH, BLACK

Cimicifuga racemosa (NUTT.)
N.O. Ranunculaceæ

Synonyms. Black Snake Root. Rattle Root. Squaw Root. Bugbane
Part Used. Root
Habitat. A native of North America, where it grows freely in shady woods in Canada and the United States. It is called Black Snake Root to distinguish it from the Common Snake Root (*Aristolochia serpentaria*)

¶ *Description.* The seeds are sent annually to Europe, and should be sown as soon as the season will permit. It flowers in June or early in July, but does not perfect seed in England, though it thrives well in moist, shady borders and is perfectly hardy. It is a tall, herbaceous plant, with feathery racemes of white blossoms, 1 to 3 feet long, which being slender, droop gracefully. The fruits are dry.

The plant produces a stout, blackish rhizome (creeping underground stem), cylindrical, hard and knotty, bearing the remains of numerous stout ascending branches. It is collected in the autumn, after the fruit is formed and the leaves have died down, then cut into pieces and dried. It has only a faint, disagreeable odour, but a bitter and acrid taste.

The straight, stout, dark brown roots which are given off from the under surface of the rhizome are bluntly quadrangular and furrowed. In the dried drug, they are brittle, broken off usually quite close to the rhizome. In transverse section, they show several wedge-shaped bundles of porous, whitish wood. A similar section of the rhizome shows a large dark-coloured, horny pith, surrounded by a ring of numerous pale wedges of wood, alternately with dark rays, outside which is a thin, dark, horny bark.

¶ *Constituents.* The chief constituent of Cimicifuga root is the amorphous resinous substance known as Cimicifugin, or Macrotin, of which it contains about 18 per cent., but the bitter taste is due to a crystalline principle named Racemosin. The drug also contains two resins, together with fat, wax starch, gum, sugar and an astringent substance.

¶ *Medicinal Action and Uses.* Astringent, emmenagogue, diuretic, alterative, expectorant. The root of this plant is much used in America in many disorders, and is supposed to be an antidote against poison and the bite of the rattlesnake. The fresh root, dug in October, is used to make a tincture.

In small doses, it is useful in children's diarrhœa.

In the paroxyms of consumption, it gives relief by allaying the cough, reducing the rapidity of the pulse and inducing perspiration. In whooping-cough, it proves very effective.

The infusion and decoction have been given with success in rheumatism.

In infantile disorders, it is given in the form of syrup. It is said to be a specific in St. Vitus' Dance of children. Overdoses produce nausea and vomiting.

¶ *Preparations.* Fluid extract, U.S.P., 15 to 30 drops. Fluid extract, B.P., 5 to 30 drops. Tincture, U.S.P., 1 drachm. Tincture, B.P., 15 to 60 drops. Cimicifugin, 1 to 6 grains. Powdered extract, U.S.P., 4 grains.

See BANEBERRY.

COHOSH, BLUE

Caulophyllum thalictroides (MICH.)
N.O. Berberidaceæ

Synonyms. Pappoose Root. Squawroot. Blueberry Root
Part Used. Root
Habitat. United States and Canada

¶ *Description.* A handsome perennial plant, growing in low rich, moist, soil in swamps and near running streams, smooth and glaucous, and bears in May and June a panicle of small yellowish green flowers and one or two seeds about the size of a large pea, which ripen in August. These are sometimes roasted and boiled in water, and given as a decoction resembling coffee.

The berries are dry and mawkish; the root is a hard thick, irregular, knotty, contorted caudex, one to several inches long, with long slender radicles up to 8 inches long, externally yellowy brown, internally whitish to yellow, with a central pith running longitudinally; taste, sweetish-bitter, then acrid and pungent, with a slightly (pungent) fragrant odour; yields its properties to alcohol, water or glycerine.

¶ *Constituents.* Gum, starch, salts, extractive, phosphoric acid, soluble resin, greenish-yellow colouring matter, and a body analogous to Saponin.

¶ *Medicinal Action and Uses.* Emmenagogue, antispasmodic, diuretic, diaphoretic and anthelmintic. Said to be successfully used in rheumatism, dropsy, epilepsy, hysteria and uterine inflammation, specially for chronic cases. It is sometimes combined with *Mitchella repens* and *Eupatoria aromatica*. In use it is preferable to Ergot, expediting delivery, where delay results from debility, fatigue or want of uterine nervous energy.

¶ *Doses. Decoction or Infusion.* 1 oz. of root to 1 pint of boiling water, macerated for ½ hour. Dose, 2 to 4 fluid ounces three or four times a day.

Tincture. 3 oz. of finely powdered root to 1 pint of alcohol, allowed to soak for two weeks, then well shaken and filtered. Dose, ½ fluid drachm to 2 fluid drachms. Fluid extract, 10 to 30 drops. Solid extract, 5 to 10 grains. Caulophyllum, 2 to 5 grains.

COLCHICUM. *See* (MEADOW) SAFFRON

COLE SEED. *See* MUSTARD

COLOCYNTH. *See* (BITTER) APPLE

COLTSFOOT

Tussilago Farfara (LINN.)
N.O. Compositæ

Synonyms. Coughwort. Hallfoot. Horsehoof. Ass's Foot. Foalswort. Fieldhove. Bullsfoot. Donnhove
(*French*) Pas d'âne
Parts Used. Leaves, flowers, root
Habitat. Coltsfoot grows abundantly throughout England, especially along the sides of railway banks and in waste places, on poor stiff soils, growing as well in wet ground as in dry situations. It has long-stalked, hoof-shaped leaves, about 4 inches across, with angular teeth on the margins. Both surfaces are covered, when young, with loose, white, felted woolly hairs, but those on the upper surface fall off as the leaf expands. This felty covering easily rubs off and before the introduction of matches, wrapped in a rag dipped in a solution of saltpetre and dried in the sun, used to be considered an excellent tinder

¶ *Description.* The specific name of the plant is derived from *Farfarus,* an ancient name of the White Poplar, the leaves of which present some resemblance in form and colour to those of this plant. There is a closer resemblance, however, to the leaves of the Butterbur, which must not be collected in error; they may be distinguished by their more rounded outline, larger size and less sinuate margin.

After the leaves have died down, the shoot rests and produces in the following February a flowering stem, consisting of a single peduncle with numerous reddish bracts and whitish hairs and a terminal, composite, yellow flower, whilst other shoots develop leaves, which appear only much later, after the flower stems in their turn have died down. These two parts of the plant, both of which are used medicinally, are, therefore, collected separately and usually sold separately.

The root is spreading, small and white, and has also been used medicinally.

An old name for Coltsfoot was *Filius ante*

patrem (the son before the father), because the star-like, golden flowers appear and wither before the broad, sea-green leaves are produced.

The seeds are crowned with a tuft of silky hairs, the *pappus*, which are often used by goldfinches to line their nests, and it has been stated were in former days frequently employed by the Highlanders for stuffing mattresses and pillows.

The underground stems preserve their vitality for a long period when buried deeply, so that in places where the plant has not been observed before, it will often spring up in profusion after the ground has been disturbed. In gardens and pastures it is a troublesome weed, very difficult to extirpate.

¶ *Parts Used.* The leaves, collected in June and early part of July, and, to a slighter extent, the flower-stalks collected in February.

¶ *Constituents.* All parts of the plant abound in mucilage, and contain a little tannin and a trace of a bitter amorphous glucoside. The flowers contain also a phytosterol and a dihydride alcohol, Faradial.

¶ *Medicinal Action and Uses.* Demulcent, expectorant and tonic. One of the most popular of cough remedies. It is generally given together with other herbs possessing pectoral qualities, such as Horehound, Marshmallow, Ground Ivy, etc.

The botanical name, *Tussilago*, signifies 'cough dispeller,' and Coltsfoot has justly been termed 'nature's best herb for the lungs and her most eminent thoracic.' The smoking of the leaves for a cough has the recommendation of Dioscorides, Galen, Pliny, Boyle, and other great authorities, both ancient and modern, Linnæus stating that the Swedes of his time smoked it for that purpose. Pliny recommended the use of both roots and leaves. The leaves are the basis of the British Herb Tobacco, in which Coltsfoot predominates, the other ingredients being Buckbean, Eyebright, Betony, Rosemary, Thyme, Lavender, and Chamomile flowers. This relieves asthma and also the difficult breathing of old bronchitis. Those suffering from asthma, catarrh and other lung troubles derive much benefit from smoking this Herbal Tobacco, the use of which does not entail any of the injurious effects of ordinary tobacco.

A decoction is made of 1 oz. of leaves, in 1 quart of water boiled down to a pint, sweetened with honey or liquorice, and taken in teacupful doses frequently. This is good for both colds and asthma.

Coltsfoot tea is also made for the same purpose, and Coltsfoot Rock has long been a domestic remedy for coughs.

A decoction made so strong as to be sweet and glutinous has proved of great service in scrofulous cases, and, with Wormwood, has been found efficacious in calculus complaints.

The flower-stalks contain constituents similar to those of the leaves, and are directed by the British Pharmacopœia to be employed in the preparation of Syrup of Coltsfoot, which is much recommended for use in chronic bronchitis.

In Paris, the Coltsfoot flowers used to be painted as a sign on the doorpost of an apothecarie's shop.

Culpepper says:

'The fresh leaves, or juice, or syrup thereof, is good for a bad dry cough, or wheezing and shortness of breath. The dry leaves are best for those who have their rheums and distillations upon their lungs causing a cough: for which also the dried leaves taken as tobacco, or the root is very good. The distilled water hereof simply or with elder-flowers or nightshade is a singularly good remedy against all agues, to drink 2 oz. at a time and apply cloths wet therein to the head and stomach, which also does much good being applied to any hot swellings or inflammations. It helpeth St. Anthony's fire (erysypelas) and burnings, and is singular good to take away wheals.'

One of the local names for Coltsfoot, viz. Donnhove, seems to have been derived from *Donn*, an old word for horse, hence *Donkey* (a little horse). Donnhove became corrupted to Tun-hoof as did Hay-hove (a name for Ground Ivy) to ale-hoof.

The plant is so dissimilar in appearance at different periods that both Gerard and Parkinson give two illustrations: one entitled 'Tussilago florens, Coltsfoot in floure,' and the other, 'Tussilaginous folia, the leaves of Coltsfoot,' or 'Tussilago herba sine flore.'

'Coltsfoot hath many white and long creeping roots, from which rise up naked stalkes about a spanne long, bearing at the top yellow floures; when the stalke and seede is perished there appeare springing out of the earth many broad leaves, green above, and next the ground of a white, hoarie, or grayish colour. Seldom, or never, shall you find leaves and floures at once, but the floures are past before the leaves come out of the ground; as may appear by the first picture, which setteth forth the naked stalkes and floures; and by the second, which port-traiteth the leaves only.'

Pliny and many of the older botanists thought that the Coltsfoot was without leaves, an error that is scarcely excusable, for, notwithstanding the fact that the flowers appear in a general way before the leaves, small leaves often begin to make their appearance before the flowering season is over.

Pliny recommends the dried leaves and roots of Coltsfoot to be burnt, and the smoke drawn into the mouth through a reed and swallowed, as a remedy for an obstinate cough, the patient sipping a little wine between each inhalation. To derive the full benefit from it, it had to be burnt on cypress charcoal.

COLUMBINE

Aquilegia vulgaris (LINN.)
N.O. Ranunculaceæ

Synonym. Culverwort (Saxon)
Parts Used. Leaves, root, seeds

The Columbine, though a wild flower in this country, found occasionally in woods and copses, and in open clearings (generally on a calcareous soil), is more familiar as a garden plant.

¶ *Description.* From its branching and fibrous root, which is blackish and rather stout, springs a large tuft of leaves, dark and bluish green on the upper surfaces and greyish beneath. These lowest leaves are on long foot-stalks and are large, having a terminal group of three leaflets, and below them on each side another group of three leaflets. The stem-leaves get gradually smaller, the higher they grow up the stem, the uppermost being without stalks and merely three-lobed. The flower stems are 1 to 2 feet high, erect and slender, often reddish in colour, branching into a loose head of flowers, which are 1½ to 2 inches in diameter and drooping. The only variety in which the flowers are not drooping is *Aquilegia parviflora*, which Ledebour describes with the flowers perfectly erect.

When growing wild, the flowers are usually blue or dull purple, occasionally white. The Columbine may be distinguished from all other British flowers, by having each of its five petals terminated in an incurved, horn-like spur. The petals are tubular and dilated at the other extremity.

The flowers are perfumed like hay.

The plant is in blossom throughout May and June. Its fruit is composed of five carpels, cylindrical in form, with pointed ends, like a cluster of little pea-pods, each carpel (or seed vessel) containing many smooth, dark-coloured seeds, which are freely shed when ripe, so that the parent plant is generally the centre of a little colony of seedlings.

The generic name of *Aquilegia* is derived from the Latin *aquila* (an eagle), the spurs of the flowers being considered to resemble an eagle's talons. The popular name, Columbine, is from the Latin *columba* (a dove or pigeon), from the idea that the flowers resemble a flight of these birds. A still older name, *Culverwort*, has the same reference *wort* being the Saxon word for a plant and *culfre* meaning a pigeon.

The Columbine is a favourite old-fashioned garden-flower, being mentioned by Tusser (1580) among a list of flowers suitable 'for windows and pots'; Parkinson, in 1629, speaks of the many varieties grown in gardens.

It was one of the badges of the House of Lancaster and also of the family of Derby. The flower is referred to in *Hamlet* and in one of Ben Jonson's poems:

'Bring cornflag, tulip and Adonis flower,
Fair Oxeye, goldylocks and columbine.'

¶ *Medicinal Action and Uses.* Astringent. It has been employed on the continent, but according to Linnæus, with very unsatisfactory results, children having sometimes been poisoned by it when given in too large doses. It is no longer used.

Culpepper tells us:

'The leaves of Columbine are successfully used in lotions for sore mouths and throats. . . . The Spaniards used to eat a piece of the root thereof in a morning fasting many days together, to help them when troubled with stone. The seed taken in wine with a little saffron removes obstructions of the liver and is good for the yellow jaundice.'

COLUMBO, AMERICAN

Frasera Carolinensis (WALT.)
N.O. Gentianaceæ

Synonyms. American Calumba. American Colombo. Radix Colombo Americanæ. Frasera Walteri. Frasera Canadensis. Faux Colombo
Part Used. The dried root
Habitat. Middle and Southern United States and west of the Alleghanies

¶ *Description. Frasera Carolinensis* is chiefly known as an occasional substitute for Calumba Root, or *Jateorrhiza Columba*, a native of Mozambique. The English name is derived from the African *Kalumb*.

It is a plant of from 4 to 9 feet in height,

with a smooth, erect stem, bearing lanceolate leaves in whorls, and yellowish-white flowers in terminal panicles. The roots are triennial, horizontal, long, and yellow. They should be collected in the autumn of the second or the spring of the third year, and cut into transverse slices before being dried. When sliced longitudinally they have been put on the market as American Gentian, and when fresh, their properties closely resemble *Gentiana Lutea*, the European Yellow Gentian. The sliced root as found in the market has a reddish-brown epidermis, yellow cortex and spongy centre. The taste is slightly bitter and saccharine. It may be distinguished from true Colombo Root by the absence of concentric circles, and the smaller, thicker slices.

¶ *Constituents*. The root contains a peculiar acid, bitter extractive, gum, pectin, glucose, wax, resin, fatty matter, and yellow colouring matter.

It may be distinguished from Calumba by the absence of starch (though it contains tannin), and by its change of colour when treated with sulphate of iron, remaining unchanged by tincture of iodine or galls. It has not the pectine of gentians.

¶ *Medicinal Uses*. Tonic, cathartic, emetic, stimulant. When dried it is a simple bitter that may be used in a similar way to gentian. In its fresh state it is cathartic and emetic.

¶ *Dosages*. Of powder, 1 to 3 grains. Of infusion of 1 fluid ounce to 1 pint of boiling water – 2 fluid ounces a day.

¶ *Other Species*.
Coscinium fenestratum is the Columbo wood or false Columbo of Ceylon.

COMBRETUM

Combretum sundaicum (MIF.)
N.O. Combretaceæ Myrobalans

Synonym. Jungle Weed
Parts Used. Roasted leaves, stalks
Habitat. Malay Peninsula and Sumatra, and the tropical regions of both Hemispheres

¶ *Description*. Leaves odourless, taste astringent.
¶ *Medicinal Action and Uses*. The leaves and stalks roasted have long been used in China in the form of a decoction, as a cure for the opium habit, the daily dose of opium is added to a decoction of the leaves and the patient is given 1 fluid ounce of the mixture every four hours.

¶ *Constituents*. Combretum contains a large proportion of tannic acid and traces of a glucoside.

COMFREY

Symphytum officinale (LINN.)
N.O. Boraginaceæ

Synonyms. Common Comfrey. Knitbone. Knitback. Consound. Blackwort. Bruisewort. Slippery Root. Boneset. Yalluc (Saxon). Gum Plant. Consolida. Ass Ear
Parts Used. Root, leaves
Habitat. A native of Europe and temperate Asia; is common throughout England on the banks of rivers and ditches, and in watery places generally

This well-known showy plant is a member of the Borage and Forget-me-not tribe, *Boraginaceæ*.

The plant is erect in habit and rough and hairy all over. There is a branched rootstock, the roots are fibrous and fleshy, spindle-shaped, an inch or less in diameter and up to a foot long, smooth, blackish externally, and internally white, fleshy and juicy.

¶ *Description*. The leafy stem, 2 to 3 feet high, is stout, angular and hollow, broadly winged at the top and covered with bristly hairs. The lower, radical leaves are very large, up to 10 inches long, ovate in shape and covered with rough hairs which promote itching when touched. The stem-leaves are decurrent, i.e. a portion of them runs down the stem, the body of the leaf being continued beyond its base and point of attachment with the stem. They decrease in size the higher they grow up the stem, which is much branched above and terminated by one-sided clusters of drooping flowers, either creamy yellow, or purple, growing on short stalks. These racemes of flowers are given off in pairs, and are what is known as scorpoid in form, the curve they always assume suggesting, as the word implies, the curve of a scorpion's tail, the flowers being all placed on one side of the stem, gradually tapering from the fully-expanded blossom to the final and almost imperceptible bud at the extremity of the curve, as in the Forget-me-Not. The corollas are bell-shaped, the calyx deeply five-cleft, narrow to lance-shaped, spreading, more downy in the purple-flowered type. The fruit consists of four shining nutlets, perforated at the base, and adhering to the receptacle by their base. Comfrey is in bloom throughout the greater part of the summer, the first flowers opening at the end of April or early May.

The creamy yellow-flowered form is stated by Hooker to be *Symphytum officinale* proper, and the purple flowered he considered a variety and named it *S. officinale*, var *patens*. The botanist Sibthorpe makes a definite species of it under the name *patens*.

There is another species, *S. tuberosum*, found in wet places from North Wales, Stafford and Lincoln northwards into Scotland, and most common in the south of Scotland, though absent from Ireland.

In this form, the stem is scarcely branched and but slightly winged, the bases of the leaves being hardly at all continued down the stem. Though also covered with hairs, the latter are not so bristly. The root-stock is short and horizontal, with slender root fibres. This is a much smaller plant, the stem rarely more than a foot high, rather slender and leafy. The lower radical leaves are much as in *S. officinale* in form, but with longer footstalks. The flowers, creamy-yellow in colour, though about the same size as those of *S. officinale*, are in much smaller masses.

The Common Comfrey is abundantly met with in England, but is rare in Scotland; the tuberous Comfrey is commonly found in Scotland, but is seldom met with in England, the northern counties of England and North Wales being its extreme southern limit, so that except in the narrow zone of country common to both, there will be no possibility of mistaking the one species for the other.

The variety of *S. officinale*, with a purplish flower, is more common in many parts of the Continent than in England. The purple and yellowish flowers are not found mixed where the plants grow wild: the difference in colour is permanent in plants raised from seed.

[In the water-meadows which form such a well-known feature in South Wilts, especially in the valleys round about Salisbury, Common Comfrey is abundant, and the flowers vary in colour from creamy-white to a pretty rose-pink; while the purple sort is the commonest. – *Note by a Wiltshire writer*.]

A variety with flowers of a rich blue colour, *S. Asperimum*, Prickly Comfrey, was introduced into this country from the Caucasus in 1811 as a fodder plant. This species is the largest of the genus, rising to 5 feet and more, with prickly stems and bold foliage, the leaves very large and oval, the hairs on them having bulbous bases. It was extensively recommended as a green food for most animals, it being claimed for it that it contained a considerable amount of flesh-forming substances, and was, moreover, both preventative and curative of foot and mouth disease in cattle. It has the advantage of producing large crops, two at least in a season, if cut before the flowers quite expand, and in favourable circumstances even more, so that 40 to 50 tons of green food per acre might be reckoned on. At the time of its introduction, a number of farmers and smallholders planted it. It was found, however, that though horses, cattle and pigs would eat it, they never took kindly to it as a forage. Horses in time of scarcity will eat it in small quantities in the green state, though do not care for it dried. It is a useful food in the green state for pigs of all ages, but it takes a little time for them to get used to it. Its feeding value, however, has been proved to be not so very much more than that of grass, and though it grows luxuriantly in all moist situations, where the soil is pretty good, it is not adapted for either dry or poor land.

The following is the result of an analysis of *S. Asperimum*, by Professor Voelcker:

	LEAVES		STEM	
	In Natural State	Calculated Dry	In Natural State	Calculated Dry
Water	88·400	—	94·74	—
Flesh-forming substances	2·712	23·37	·69	13·06
Non-nitrogenized substances:				
Heat and fat-producing matters	6·898	59·49	3·81	72·49
Inorganic matters (ash)	1·990	17·14	·76	14·45
	100·00	100·00	100·00	100·00

On comparison the above figures will show this plant to be almost equal to some of our more important green-food crops; and certainly if we take into consideration the quantity of its produce, there are few plants capable of yielding so much green food as the Comfrey. Dr. Voelcker says that 'the amount of flesh-forming substances is considerable. The juice of this plant contains much gum and mucilage, and little sugar.'

Formerly country people cultivated Comfrey in their gardens for its virtue in wound healing, and the many local names of the plant testify to its long reputation as a vulnerary herb – in the Middle Ages it was a famous remedy for broken bones. The very name, Comfrey, is a corruption of *con firma*, in allusion to the uniting of bones it was thought to effect, and the botanical name, *Symphytum*, is derived from the Greek *symphyo* (to unite).

¶ *Cultivation.* Comfrey thrives in almost any soil or situation, but does best under the shade of trees.

Propagation may be effected either by seed or by division of roots in the autumn: the roots are very brittle, and the least bit of root will start growing afresh. They should be planted about 2½ feet apart each way, and will need no further care except to keep them clear from weeds.

As a green crop they will yield largely if well-rotted manure be dug between the rows when dressing for winter.

As an ornamental plant, Comfrey is often introduced into gardens, from which it is very difficult to eradicate it when it has once established itself, a new plant arising from any severed portion of the root.

¶ *Parts Used Medicinally.* The root and leaves, generally collected from wild plants.

Comfrey leaves are sometimes found as an adulteration to Foxglove leaves, which they somewhat resemble, but may be distinguished by the smaller veins not extending into the wings of the leaf-stalk, and by having on their surface isolated stiff hairs. They are also more lanceolate than Foxglove leaves.

¶ *Constituents.* The chief and most important constituent of Comfrey root is mucilage, which it contains in great abundance, more even than Marshmallow. It also contains from 0·6 to 0·8 per cent. of Allantoin and a little tannin. Starch is present in a very small amount.

¶ *Medicinal Action and Uses.* Demulcent, mildly astringent and expectorant. As the plant abounds in mucilage, it is frequently given whenever a mucilaginous medicine is required and has been used like Marshmallow for intestinal troubles. It is very similar in its emollient action to Marshmallow, but in many cases is even preferred to it and is an ingredient in a large number of herbal preparations. It forms a gentle

remedy in cases of diarrhœa and dysentery. A decoction is made by boiling ½ to 1 oz. of crushed root in 1 quart of water or milk, which is taken in wineglassful doses, frequently.

For its demulcent action it has long been employed domestically in lung troubles and also for quinsy and whooping-cough. The root is more effectual than the leaves and is the part usually used in cases of coughs. It is highly esteemed for all pulmonary complaints, consumption and bleeding of the lungs. A strong decoction, or tea, is recommended in cases of internal hæmorrhage, whether from the lungs, stomach, bowels or from bleeding piles – to be taken every two hours till the hæmorrhage ceases, in severe cases, a teaspoonful of Witch Hazel extract being added to the Comfrey root tea.

A modern medicinal tincture, employed by homœopaths, is made from the root with spirits of wine, 10 drops in a tablespoonful of water being administered several times a day.

Comfrey leaves are of much value as an external remedy, both in the form of fomentations, for sprains, swellings and bruises, and as a poultice, to severe cuts, to promote suppuration of boils and abscesses, and gangrenous and ill-conditioned ulcers. The whole plant, beaten to a cataplasm and applied hot as a poultice, has always been deemed excellent for soothing pain in any tender, inflamed or suppurating part. It was formerly applied to raw, indolent ulcers as a glutinous astringent. It is useful in any kind of inflammatory swelling.

Internally, the leaves are taken in the form of an infusion, 1 oz. of the leaves to 1 pint of boiling water.

Fluid extract: dose, ½ to 2 drachms.

The reputation of Comfrey as a vulnerary has been considered due partly to the fact of its reducing the swollen parts in the immediate neighbourhood of fractures, causing union to take place with greater facility. Gerard affirmed: 'A salve concocted from the fresh herb will certainly tend to promote the healing of bruised and broken parts.' Surgeons have declared that the powdered root, if dissolved in water to a mucilage, is far from contemptible for bleedings and fractures, whilst it hastens the callus of bones under repair. Its virtues as a vulnerary are now attributed to the Allantoin it contains. According to Macalister (*British Medical Journal*, Jan. 6, 1912), Allantoin in aqueous solution in strengths of 0·3 per cent. has a powerful action in strengthening epithelial formations, and is a valuable remedy not only in external ulceration, but also in ulcers of the stomach and duodenum. Comfrey Root is used as a source of this cell proliferant Allantoin, employed in the dealing of chronic wounds, burns, ulcers, etc., though Allantoin is also made artificially.

The following is from the *Chemist and Druggist* of August 13, 1921:

'Allantoin is a fresh instance of the good judgment of our rustics, especially of old times, with regard to the virtues of plants. The great Comfrey or consound, though it was official with us down to the middle of the eighteenth century, never had a very prominent place in professional practice; but our herbalists were loud in its praise and the country culler of simples held it almost infallible as a remedy for both external and internal wounds, bruises, and ulcers, for phlegm, for spitting of blood, ruptures, hæmorrhoids, etc. For ulcers of the stomach and liver especially, the root (the part used) was regarded as of sovereign virtue. It is precisely for such complaints as these that Allantoin, obtained from the rhizome of the plant, is now prescribed. One old *Syrupus de Symphyto* was a rather complicated preparation. Gerard has a better formula, also a compound, which he highly recommends for ulcers of the lungs. The old Edinburgh formula is the simplest and probably the best: Fresh Comfrey leaves and fresh plantain leaves, of each lb.ss.; bruise them and well squeeze out the juice; add to the dregs spring water lb.ij.; boil to half, and mix the strained liquor with the expressed juice; add an equal quantity of white sugar and boil to a syrup.'

Culpepper says:

'The great Comfrey ("great" to distinguish it from the "Middle Comfrey" – another name for the Bugle) restrains spitting of blood. The root boiled in water or wine and the decoction drank, heals inward hurts, bruises, wounds and ulcers of the lungs, and causes the phlegm that oppresses him to be easily spit forth. . . . A syrup made thereof is very effectual in inward hurts, and the distilled water for the same purpose also, and for outward wounds or sores in the fleshy or sinewy parts of the body, and to abate the fits of agues and to allay the sharpness of humours. A decoction of the leaves is good for those purposes, but not so effectual as the roots. The roots being outwardly applied cure fresh wounds or cuts immediately, being

bruised and laid thereto; and is specially good for ruptures and broken bones, so powerful to consolidate and knit together that if they be boiled with dissevered pieces of flesh in a pot, it will join them together again.'

He goes on to describe its curative effect on hæmorrhoids and continues:

'The roots of Comfrey taken fresh, beaten small and spread upon leather and laid upon any place troubled with the gout presently gives ease: and applied in the same manner it eases pained joints and tends to heal running ulcers, gangrenes, mortifications, for which it hath by often experience been found helpful.'

The young leaves form a good green vegetable, and are not infrequently eaten by country people. When fully grown they become, however, coarse and unpleasant in taste. They have been used to flavour cakes and other food.

In some parts of Ireland, Comfrey is eaten as a cure for defective circulation and poverty of blood, being regarded as a perfectly safe and harmless remedy.

Comfrey roots, together with Chichory and Dandelion roots, are used to make a well-known vegetation 'Coffee,' that tastes practically the same as ordinary coffee, with none of its injurious effects.

A strong decoction has been used on the Continent for tanning leather, and in Angora a sort of glue is got from the common Comfrey, which is used for spinning the famous fleeces of that country.

In that inimitable little book by Russell George Alexander, called *A Plain Plantain*, in which he quotes from an old MS. inscribed 'Madam Susanna Avery, Her Book, May ye 12th Anno Domini 1688,' we find the following reference to Comfrey: 'From the French *conserve*, Latin *conserva* – healing: *conserves* – to boil together; to heal. A Wound Herb.' 'The roots,' says a sixteenth-century writer, 'heal all inwarde woundes and burstings,' and Baker (*Jewell of Health*, 1567) says: 'The water of the Greater Comferie druncke helpeth such as are bursten, and that have broken the bone of the legge.' In cookery, the leaves gathered young may be used as a substitute for Spinach; the young shoots have been eaten after blanching by forcing them to grow through heaps of earth.

See BORAGE.

COMPASS PLANT. *See* CUP PLANT

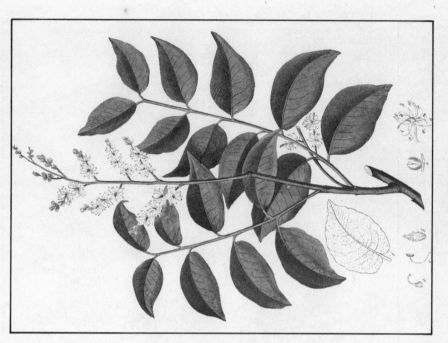

COPAIBA
Copaifera Langsdorffii

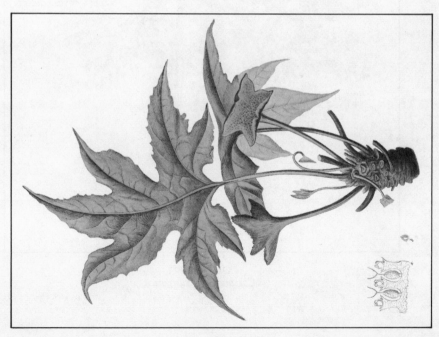

CONTRAYERVA
Dorstenia Contrayerva

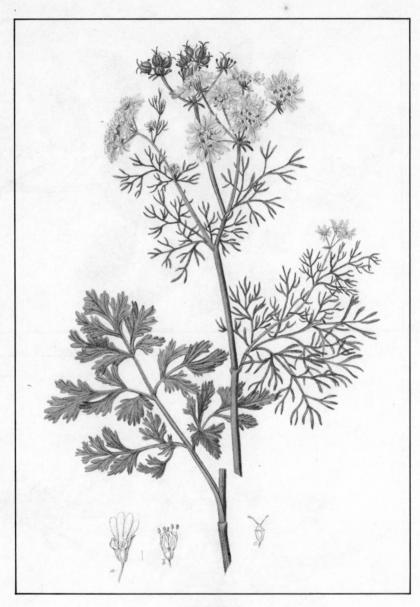

CORIANDER
Coriandrum Sativum

CONDURANGO

Gonolobus Condurango (NICHOLS)
N.O. Asclepiadaceæ

Synonyms. Condurango Blanco. Marsdenia Condurango
Part Used. Bark
Habitat. Ecuador, South America

¶ *Description.* The product of an asclepiadaceous vine about 30 feet long and 2 feet in diameter. The bark is beaten with a mallet to separate it from the stem when it has been sun-dried. In commerce it occurs in quilled pieces 2 to 4 inches long and ½ inch in diameter. External surface, pale greyish brown to dark brown, nearly smooth, more or less scaly and roughened, with numerous warts or lenticels, the scales soft with sometimes a brownish-black fungus on them; inner side whity brown and longitudinally striate; fracture short, fibrous, granular; odour slightly aromatic, specially in the fresh drug; taste bitter and aromatic; yields not more than 12 per cent. of ash.
¶ *Constituents.* A large quantity of tannin, a glucoside and an alkaloid resembling strychnine in its action.

¶ *Medicinal Action and Uses.* Diuretic, stomachic, alterative. Has been regarded as a potential remedy for cancer and is useful in the early stages, but has no effect in the progress of the disease. There are many varieties of the plant, and the species experimented with in cancer is the *Condurango blanco*, which may be considered a genuine *C. Cortex.* It is largely used in South America as an alterative in chronic syphilis and is of great benefit.
It increases the circulation.

¶ *Dose.* Fluid extract, ½ to 1 drachm.

¶ *Caution.* Overdoses produce convulsions, ending in paralysis, vertigo and disturbed sight.

CONTRAYERVA

Dorstenia Contrayerva (LINN.)
N.O. Urticaceæ

Synonyms. Dorstenia Houstoni (LINN.)
Part Used. Root
Habitat. Native of Mexico, West Indies and Peru

¶ *Description.* Name derived from a Spanish-American word signifying counterpoison or antidote. It is probable that the root sold as Contrayerva is derived from several species of Dorstenia, others being *Dorstenia Houstoni* and *D. Drabena*, the former growing near Campeachy, the latter near Vera Cruz. The official root is the product of *D. Brasiliensis* and comes from Brazil. The commercial root is oblong, 1 or 2 inches long, thickness varies, hard rough solid, outside reddish brown, paler inside, odour aromatic, taste warm, bitter, pungent, rootlets not as strong as main tubes. The root properties are extracted by alcohol and boiling water, and makes a very mucilaginous decoction.
¶ *Constituents.* Cajupine and contrayerbine.

¶ *Medicinal Action and Uses.* Stimulant, tonic, and diaphoretic; given in cases of low fevers, typhoid, dysentery, diarrhœa, and other illnesses needing a stimulant.

¶ *Dose.* ½ drachm of powdered root, or 1 oz. to 1 pint infused in boiling water.

CONVOLVULUS, FIELD

Convolvulus arvensis (LINN.)
N. O. Convolvulaceæ

Synonyms. Cornbind. Ropebind. Withywind. Bearwind. Jack-run'-in'-the-Country. Devil's Garters. Hedge Bells
Parts Used. Root, root resin

Although the blossoms of the Field Convolvulus (*C. arvensis*) are some of the prettiest and daintiest of our native wild-flowers, the plant which bears them ranks among the most troublesome of weeds to the farmer, not only creeping up his hedges, but strangling his corn and spreading over everything within its reach. In North America it has intruded as a most unwelcome immigrant, persistently covering the ground with its trailing stems.
Its roots run very deeply into the ground and extend over a large area. It is, therefore, extremely difficult to extirpate, for the long roots are brittle and readily snap, and any portion left in the ground will soon grow as vigorously as ever and send up shoots to the surface, so that in a very brief time it is again spreading over the ground and climbing over everything in its way.
Its delicate creeping stems grow with great rapidity, either when found on banks, trailing along the ground amidst the grass, or climbing wherever they find a support. Their ends swing slowly and continuously in circles and twine round anything with

which they may happen to come in contact. It has been found that a Bindweed stem in favourable circumstances will make a complete revolution in about 1¾ hours, which explains the rapidity of its growth.

The generic name of the plant is derived from the Latin *convolvo* (to intertwine), and is descriptive of its general growth, for it does not, like many climbers, support itself by tendrils, but the whole plant twists itself tightly round the object that supports it – ordinarily a stalk of corn, or some other plant or object of similar size: it is never found twining round anything of bulky dimensions, such as gate-posts, etc. Its English name, Bindweed, is similarly given it for its habit of twining round and matting together all other plants near it. The Latin specific name, *arvensis*, is derived from *arvum* (a cornfield), because this species of Convolvulus, though commonly enough met with in waste places, is one of the characteristic flowers of the cornfield.

Professor Henslow remarks that this Field Convolvulus invariably twines round some stalk or object of small diameter.

¶ *Description.* It is a perennial and has a long period of blooming, generally beginning to flower about the first week of June, and being found in blossom throughout the summer and autumn months. The leaves are arrow-shaped in form, but often very variable, the extremity of the leaf being in some cases far more acute than in others, and the lobes at the base more elongated. They are placed singly along the stem at very regular intervals.

From the axils of the leaves – the points at which their stalks join the main stem – spring the flower-stalks, one to each leaf all up the stem. These flower-stalks often fork into two smaller ones, each bearing a bud. One of these lesser stalks is almost invariably smaller than the other, bearing a bud in an earlier stage of development, so that although the buds occur in pairs on the flower-stem, the flowers never expand at the same time, but always appear singly. At the junction of the flower-stalk and the main stem are a pair of very small scale-like bracts.

The flowers have trumpet-shaped corollas which vary a great deal in colour – in some plants they are almost white, whilst in others the normal pink becomes almost crimson. On the underside are five dark pink rays. In the bud the petals are folded into five pleats, the outermost part of the fold being these deep pink rays. At the bottom of the flower are what appear to be the mouths of five tubes, or pipes, running downwards, the tubes being formed by the flattened filaments of the stamens being joined to the corolla tube and yet projecting ridge-like into the flower. Flowers with tubes like these are known as 'revolver flowers,' because of the resemblance to the barrels of a revolver: the Gentians are another example. These tubes lead to the nectar which is contained in five small sacs, one at the base of each tube. To get to the honey an insect has to thrust its proboscis down each tube in turn, but whilst doing so, he knocks against the pollen in the anther placed just above it, and by carrying that pollen to the next flower it effects its cross-fertilization. In spite of this arrangement, it is a strange and unexplained fact that the flowers seldom set seeds, though the open corollas are visited by many insects, attracted by the nectar and by the faint perfume of vanilla that characterizes it. The failure to set seed is, however, quite compensated for by the vitality of its widely spreading, much branched roots, on which it chiefly depends for its propagation.

The Convolvulus is very sensitive to weather conditions, always closing in rain, to open again with the return of sunshine. It also closes at night. Its blossoms give a deep yellow or orange tint to water, which is heightened by alum and alkalies.

It is found wild throughout Europe, in Siberia, China, Persia and India, in North America where it has been introduced, and in Chile.

See also BINDWEEDS (JALAP), SCAMMONY, WILD

COOLWORT

Tiarella Cordifolia (LINN.)
N.O. Saxifrageæ

Synonyms. Foam Flower. Mitrewort
Part Used. Whole herb
Habitat. North America from Canada to Virginia

¶ *Description.* Perennial, forms a neat little edging with tiny white spiræa-like flowers, buds tinged pink, grows in the author's garden, and, given air and sunlight, in a light rich soil thrives well. It has simple leaves, spotted and veined deep red; basal leaves turn a rich red orange. Needs dividing every second year. Seeds are few, sub-globose. Taste slightly stringent, odourless.

¶ *Medicinal Action and Uses.* Tonic, diuretic. Of value in gravel and other diseases of the bladder, and as a tonic in indigestion and dyspepsia; corrects acidity and aids the liver.

¶ *Dose.* For an infusion or decoction, 1 oz. to the pint of water; take freely 4 oz. of the infusion two or three times daily till conditions improve.

COPAIBA

Copaifera Langsdorffii (DESF.)
N.O. Leguminosæ

Synonyms. Copaiva. Balsam Copaiba. Copaiba officinalis
Part Used. Oleoresin
Habitat. Brazil and north of South Africa

¶ *Description*. An oleoresin obtained from a South American species of Copaiba, by an incision in the trunk. It was first noticed in England in 1625, in a work published by Purchas. There are many species in South America, all yielding Copaiba; a single tree is said to yield about 40 litres. The first yield is clear, colourless and very thin, but in contact with the air its consistency soon becomes thicker and yellower. It is most largely collected from Para and Maranhão in Brazil, and is brought to this country in small casks and barrels; large quantities also come from Maracaibo in Venezuela, and it is also exported from Angostura, Cayenne, Rio Janeiro and some of the West Indian Islands. The variety that comes from Venezuela is more viscid and darker in colour.

¶ *Constituents*. Volatile oil, resin. Amorphous resin acids and resenes.

Copaiba is a clear transparent liquid of the consistency of olive oil, pale yellow with a peculiar but not unpleasant odour, taste bitterish, hot and nauseous; the substance it most closely resembles is turpentine. As it contains no benzoic acid, it cannot properly be called a resin.

¶ *Medicinal Action and Uses*. Stimulant, diuretic, carminative, laxative; in large doses purgative, causing nausea, vomiting, strangury, bloody urine and fever. A good remedy for chronic catarrh and bronchitis, as it assists expectoration and is antiseptic; is given with advantage in leucorrhœa, chronic cystitis, diarrhœa and hæmorrhoids. It is chiefly used in gonorrhœa (though not advocated for chronic cases), often combined with cubebs and sandal. It has also been recommended externally for chilblains. Both the volatile oil and resin are greatly altered when expelled in the urine, and when precipitated by nitric acid might be mistaken for albumen; it is considered a valuable hydragogue diuretic in obstinate dropsy.

It creates an irritant action on the whole mucous membrane, imparts a peculiar odour to the urine and breath, causes an eruption resembling measles attended with irritation and tingling; it is the *resin*, not the oleoresin, that is used as a diuretic.

¶ *Preparations and Dosages*. Oil, B.P., 5 to 20 drops. For obstinate dropsy, 15 to 20 grains three times daily. Usually taken in pill or capsule form (10 to 15 minims), or in the form of an emulsion.

CORIANDER

Coriandrum sativum (LINN.)
N.O. Umbelliferæ

Parts Used. Fruit and fresh leaves
Habitat. Coriander, an umbelliferous plant indigenous to southern Europe, is found occasionally in Britain in fields and waste places, and by the sides of rivers. It is frequently found in a semi-wild state in the east of England, having escaped from cultivation

¶ *Description*. It is an annual, with erect stems, 1 to 3 feet high, slender and branched. The lowest leaves are stalked and pinnate, the leaflets roundish or oval, slightly lobed. The segments of the uppermost leaves are linear and more divided. The flowers are in shortly-stalked umbels, five to ten rays, pale mauve, almost white, delicately pretty. The seed clusters are very symmetrical and the seeds fall as soon as ripe. The plant is bright green, shining, glabrous and intensely foetid.

Gerard described it as follows:

'The common kind of Coriander is a very striking herb, it has a round stalk full of branches, two feet long. The leaves are almost like the leaves of the parsley, but later on become more jagged, almost like the leaves of Fumitorie, but a great deal smaller and tenderer. The flowers are white and grow in round tassels like Dill.'

The inhabitants of Peru are so fond of the taste and smell of this herb that it enters into almost all their dishes, and the taste is often objectionable to any but a native. Both in Peru and in Egypt, the leaves are put into soup.

The seeds are quite round like tiny balls. They lose their disagreeable scent on drying and become fragrant – the longer they are kept, the more fragrant they become.

Coriander was originally introduced from the East, being one of the herbs brought to Britain by the Romans. As an aromatic stimulant and spice, it has been cultivated and used from very ancient times. It was employed by Hippocrates and other Greek physicians.

The name Coriandrum, used by Pliny, is

derived from *koros*, (a bug), in reference to the fœtid smell of the leaves.

Pliny tells us that 'the best (Coriander) came from Egypt,' and from thence no doubt the Israelites gained their knowledge of its properties.

The Africans are said to have called this herb by a similar name (*goid*), which Gesenius derives from a verb (*gadad*), signifying 'to cut,' in allusion to the furrowed appearance of the fruit.

It is still much used in the East as a condiment, and forms an ingredient in curry powder.

In the northern countries of Europe, the seeds are sometimes mixed with bread, but the chief consumption of Coriander seed in this country is in flavouring certain alcoholic liquors, for which purpose it is largely grown in Essex. Distillers of gin make use of it, and veterinary surgeons employ it as a drug for cattle and horses. The fruit is the only part of the plant that seems to have any medical or dietetical reputation.

Confectioners form from the seeds little, round pink and white comfits for children.

It is included in the British Pharmacopœia, but it is chiefly used to disguise unpleasant medicine.

A power of conferring immortality is thought by the Chinese to be a property of the seeds.

Turner says (1551): ' "Coriandre layd to wyth breade or barly mele is good for Saynt Antonyes fyre" (the erysipelas: so called because it was supposed to have been cured by the intercession of St. Anthony). Coriander cakes are seldom made now.'

¶ *Cultivation.* Coriander likes a warm, dry, light soil, though it also does well in the somewhat heavy soil of Essex.

Sow in mild, dry weather in April, in shallow drills, about $\frac{1}{2}$ inch deep and 8 or 9 inches apart, and cover it evenly with the soil. The seeds are slow in germinating. The seeds may also be sown in March, in heat, for planting out in May.

As the seeds ripen, about August, the disagreeable odour gives place to a pleasant aroma, and the plant is then cut down with sickles and when dry the fruit is threshed out.

The best land yields on an average 15 cwt. per acre. It is grown to a small extent in the Eastern counties, but more especially in Essex. It is also cultivated in various parts of Continental Europe, and in northern Africa, Malta and India.

¶ *Parts Used.* The fruit, and sometimes – for salads and soups – the fresh leaves.

The fruit (so-called seeds) are of globular form, beaked, finely ribbed, yellowish-brown $\frac{1}{8}$ inch in diameter, with five longitudinal ridges, separable into two halves (the mericarps), each of which is concave internally and shows two broad, longitudinal oil cells (vittæ). The seeds have an aromatic taste and, when crushed, a characteristic odour.

¶ *Constituents.* Coriander fruit contains about 1 per cent. of volatile oil, which is the active ingredient. It is pale yellow or colourless, and has the odour of Coriander and a mild aromatic taste. The fruit yields about 5 per cent. of ash and contains also malic acid, tannin and some fatty matter.

Coriander fruit of the British Pharmacopœia is directed to be obtained from plants cultivated in Britain, the fruit before being submitted to distillation being brushed or bruised.

The English-grown are said to have the finest flavour, though the Russian and German are the richest in oil. The Mogadore are the largest and brightest, but contain less oil, and the Bombay fruit, which are also large, are distinguished by their oval shape and yield the least oil of any.

¶ *Medicinal Action and Uses.* Stimulant, aromatic and carminative. The powdered fruit, fluid extract and oil are chiefly used medicinally as flavouring to disguise the taste of active purgatives and correct their griping tendencies. It is an ingredient of the following compound preparations of the Pharmacopœia: confection, syrup and tincture of senna, and tincture and syrup of Rhubarb, and enters also into compounds with angelica, gentian, jalap, quassia and lavender. As a corrigent to senna, it is considered superior to other aromatics.

If used too freely the seeds become narcotic.

Coriander water was formerly much esteemed as a carminative for windy colic.

¶ *Preparations.* Powdered fruit: dose, 10 to 60 grains. Fluid extract, 5 to 30 drops. B.P.: dose, $\frac{1}{2}$ to 3 drops.

RECIPE

'Lucknow' Curry Powder

1 oz. ginger, 1 oz. Coriander seed, 1 oz. cardamum seed, $\frac{1}{4}$ oz. best Cayenne powder, 3 oz. turmeric.

Have the best ingredients powdered at the druggist's into a fine powder and sent home in different papers. Mix them *well before the fire*, then put the mixture into a widemouthed bottle, cork well, and keep it in a dry place. – (From an old Family Cookerybook in the author's possession.)

CORKWOOD TREE

Duboisia myoporoides
N.O. Solanaceæ

Synonym. Duboisia
Part Used. Leaves
Habitat. New South Wales and Queensland, Australia; New Caledonia

¶*Description.* A tall glabrous shrub or small tree; flowers, axillary clusters, white with two-lipped calyx; corolla, funnel-shaped; limb, five parted; five stamens within the corolla (two long and two short); one rudimentary ovary, two many-ovalled compartments and fruit berry-like; leaves, inodorous and bitter taste. Another species, *Duboisia Hoopwoodii*, contains an acrid liquid alkaloid, Piturine, which is said to be identical with nicotine; it is largely used by the natives of Central Australia rather in the same way that the Indians use Coca leaves. It is obtained from the leaves and twigs, which are collected while the flowers are in bloom in August; the natives smoke and chew it for its stimulating effect, which enables them to work at high pressure without food.

¶ *Constituents.* Alkaloidal sulphates, mainly hyoscyamine and hyoscine.

¶ *Medicinal Action and Uses.* Sedative, hypnotic and mydriatic (of variable strength), which augments the activity of the respiratory. system. Its alkaloid, Sulphate of Duboisia, is sometimes used as a substitute for atropine. The homœopaths use the tincture and the alkaloid for paralysis and eye affections; a red spot interfering with vision is an indication for its use. It is antidoted by coffee and lemon-juice.

CORN COCKLE

Agrostemna Githago
Lychnis Githago
N.O. Caryophyllaceæ

Synonyms. Corn Pink. Corn Campion. Ray. Nigella. Zizany. Darnel. Tare. Gith. Lychnis. Githage. Agrostemma. Pseudo-melanthium. Lolium
Part Used. Seeds

¶ *Description.* A well-known Corn weed, with large entire purple petals.

'An annual herb of the Pink family; one of the Campions. The tall, slender stem, 2 to 4 feet high, has a dense coat of white hairs. The narrow, lance-shaped leaves, 4 to 5 inches in length, are produced in pairs and their stalkless bases meet around the stem. The large solitary flowers have very long stalks which issue from the axils of the leaves. They are 1½ and 2 inches broad, with purple petals which have pale streaks ("honey guides"), showing the way to the mouth of the tube. There are no scales round the mouth. But the striking feature of the flower which distinguishes it from the Campions is the woolly calyx with its five strong ridges and five long green teeth that far exceed the length of the petals; in the open flower they take their place between the petals, and seem to serve as preliminary alighting perches for the butterflies and moths by which the flowers are pollinated. Nectar is secreted at the bottom of the tube, whose depth makes the flower unsuitable for bees. The flower is at first male, the anthers shedding their pollen before the stigmas are mature; they are so disposed at the mouth of the tube that the nectar-seekers push their faces among them and pick up pollen. On visiting a flower that is a day or two older and has become female, the stigmas occupying the mouth are in the way to receive it by a similar process. Sometimes, smaller flowers are produced in addition, which are entirely female, for the stamens are not developed. The flowers bloom from June to August, and are succeeded by a large, oval capsule, opening by five teeth, and containing about 2 dozen large black seeds. *The seeds contain an irritant poison*, and sometimes cause trouble through being eaten by domestic animals, and by getting into milling corn and thence into the family loaf.' – (*Trees and Flowers of the Countryside.*)

Corn Cockle is *not used* in alopathic medicine to-day, but according to Hill, if used long enough, it was considered a cure for dropsy and jaundice.

In homœopathy a trituration of the seeds has been found useful in paralysis and gastritis.

CORNFLOWER

Centaurea Cyanus (LINN.)
N.O. Compositæ

Synonyms. Bluebottle. Bluebow. Hurtsickle. Blue Cap
(*French*) Bluet
Part Used. Flowers

Centaurea Cyanus, the Cornflower, with its star-like blossoms of brilliant blue, is one of our most striking wild-flowers, though it is always looked on as an unwelcome weed by the farmer, for not only does it by its presence withdraw nourishment from the ground that is needed for the corn, but its tough stems in former days of hand-reaping were wont to blunt the reaper's sickle, earning it the name of 'Hurt Sickle' :

'Thou blunt'st the very reaper's sickle and so
In life and death becom'st the farmer's foe.'

The Latin name, *Cyanus*, was given the Cornflower after a youthful devotee of the goddess Flora (Cyanus), whose favourite flower it was, and the name of the genus is derived from the Centaur, Chiron, who taught mankind the healing virtue of herbs.

It has long been cultivated as a garden plant, in several colours as well as white. *C. montana*, a perennial form, is frequent in gardens.

¶ *Description*. In the wild condition it is fairly common in cultivated fields and by roadsides. The stems are 1 to 3 feet high, tough and wiry, slender, furrowed and branched, somewhat angular and covered with a loose cottony down. The leaves, very narrow and long, are arranged alternately on the stem, and like the stem are covered more or less with white cobwebby down that gives the whole plant a somewhat dull and grey appearance. The lower leaves are much broader and often have a roughly-toothed outline. The flowers grow solitary, and of necessity upon long stalks to raise them among the corn. The bracts enclosing the hard head of the flower are numerous, with tightly overlapping scales, each bordered by a fringe of brown teeth. The inner disk florets are small and numerous, of a pale purplish-rose colour. The bright blue ray florets, that form the conspicuous part of the flower, are large, widely spread, and much cut into.

¶ *Part Used Medicinally*. The flowers are the part used in modern herbal medicine and are considered to have tonic, stimulant and emmenagogue properties, with action similar to that of Blessed Thistle.

A water distilled from Cornflower petals was formerly in repute as a remedy for weak eyes. The famous French eyewash, 'Eau de Casselunettes,' used to be made from them. Culpepper tells us that the powder or dried leaves of the Bluebottle is given with good success to those that are bruised by a fall or have broken a vein inwardly. He also informs us that, with Plantain, Horsetail, or Comfrey,

'it is a remedy against the poison of the scorpion and resisteth all venoms and poisons. The seeds or leaves (or the distilled water of the herb) taken in wine is very good against the plague and all infectious diseases, and is very good in pestilential fevers: the juice put into fresh or green wounds doth quickly solder up the lips of them together, and is very effectual to heal all ulcers and sores in the mouth.'

The expressed juice of the petals makes a good blue ink; if expressed and mixed with alum-water, it may be used in water-colour drawing. It dyes linen a beautiful blue, but the colour is not permanent.

The dried petals are used by perfumers for giving colour to pot-pourri.

See KNAPWEED, SCABIOUS TEAZLE

CORN, INDIAN

Zea Mays (LINN.)
N.O. Gramineæ

Synonym. Maize
Part Used. Seeds
Habitat. South America; also cultivated in other parts of America, in the West Indian Islands, Australia, Africa, India, etc., and now in France

¶ *Description*. A monœcious plant. Male flowers in terminal racemes; spikelets, two-flowered glumes nearly equal, herbaceous, terminating in two sharp points; females, axillary in the sheaths of the leaves. The spikes or ears proceed from the stalls at various distances from the ground, and are closely enveloped in several thin leaves, forming a sheath called the husk; the ears consist of a cylindrical substance, a pith called the cob; on this the seeds are ranged in eight rows, each row having thirty or more seeds. From the eyes or germs of the seeds proceed individual filaments of a silky appearance and bright green colour; these hang from the point of the husk and are called 'the silk.' The use of these filaments or stigmata is to receive the farina which drops from the flowers, and without which the flowers would produce no seed. As soon as this has been effected, the tops and 'the silk' dry up. The maize grains are of varying colour – usually yellow, but often ranging to black.

¶ *Constituents*. Starch, sugar, fat, salts, water, yellow oil, maizenic acid, azotized matter, gluten, dextrine, glucose, cellulose, silica, phosphates of lime and magnesia, soluble salts of potassa and soda.

¶ *Medicinal Action and Uses*. Diuretic and mild stimulant. A good emollient poultice for ulcers, swellings, rheumatic pains. An infusion of the parched corn allays nausea and vomiting in many diseases. Cornmeal makes a palatable and nutritious gruel and is an excellent diet for convalescents.

¶ *Preparations*. A liquid extract is official in U.S.A. and B.P.C.

¶ *Other Species*. There is only one distinct species, but there are several varieties resulting from difference of soil, culture and climate. Five of these have been described by Stendel – and all are natives of South America. Some of the finest cobs have been raised in Australia, and the plant is also extensively grown in many parts of Africa and India for consumption. Maize is easily digested by the human body, and when cooked as porridge is called by the Americans 'Mush.' Hominy, samp and cerealine are all starchy preparations of split maize. Corn-bread contains much more nourishment than wheaten bread, and is suitable for those suffering from kidney or liver diseases. Maizend or cornflour is prepared from the grains and represents only the fat-forming and heat-producing constituents of the grain without mineral salts. It contains only 18 grains of proteids to the pound. Mexicans of to-day are very skilful in making fermented liquors from maize. One preparation called 'Chicka' resembles beer and cider, and a spirituous liquor called 'Pulque de Mahis,' made from the juice of the stalk of the maize, forms an important article of commerce.

See CORN SILK

CORN SALAD

Valerianella olitoria (MOENCH)
N.O. Caryophylleæ.

Synonyms. Lamb's Lettuce. Valerian locusta (Linn.). White Pot Herb. Lactuca agnina (*French*) Loblollie. Mâche. Doucette. Salade de Chanoine. Salade de Prêtre

Part Used. Herb

Closely allied to the Valerians are the members of the genus *Valerianella* (the name signifying 'little Valerian'), the chief representative of which, *V. olitoria* (Moench), the Lamb's Lettuce or Corn Salad, was named by Linnæus, *Valeriana Locusta*. At one time the plant was classed with the lettuces and called *Lactuca agnina*, either, as old writers tell us, from appearing about the lambing season, or because it is a favourite food of lambs. The young leaves in spring and autumn are eaten as a salad and are excellent.

This little plant is a common weed in waste ground and cultivated land, especially corn fields, having been long cultivated in gardens and at present found in an apparently wild state. Gerard says: 'We know the Lamb's Lettuce as Loblollie; and it serves in winter as a salad herb among others none of the worst.' He tells us that the Dutch called it 'White Pot Herb' (probably in distinction from the 'Black Pot Herb' (Alexander's *Smyrnium olusatrum*), and that foreigners using it while in England led to its cultivation in our gardens. It is now not much grown here, and is much more known on the Continent, and has long been a favourite salad plant in France, under the name of *Mâche, Doucette* and *Salade de Chanoine*, and also as *Salade de Prêtre*, from its being generally eaten in Lent.

¶ *Description*. It is now common and generally distributed throughout Great Britain, a small, annual, bright-green plant, with succulent stems, 6 to 12 inches high, generally forking from the very base, or at least within the lowest quarter of their height. The first leaves, springing from the root, are 1 to 3 inches long, bluntly lance-shaped, scarcely-stalked, generally decaying early. The stem leaves are quite stalkless, often stem-clasping. The flowers are minute and are greenish-white in appearance, arranged in close, rounded, terminal heads, surrounded by narrow bracts, the tiny corolla is pale lilac, but so small that the heads of flowers do not give the appearance of any colour.

¶ *Cultivation*. When cultivated in gardens, Lamb's Lettuce may be sown in rows all through the autumn, winter and early spring, so as to produce a constant succession of crops. A small portion of garden earth sown with the seeds in August, will supply an excellent portion of the salad throughout the winter. The younger the leaves, the better they taste in salad.

¶ *Medicinal Action and Uses*. This herb was in request by country folk in former days as a spring medicine, and a homœopathic medicinal tincture is made from the fresh root.

Several other species are found in this country, either indigenous or introduced accidentally with the seeds of the plants described, but they are not common. Some botanists assign these species to the genus *Fedia*, the name of which is of uncertain derivation.

CORN SILK

Zea Mays (LINN.)
N.O. Graminaceæ

Part Used. Flower pistils
Habitat. Sub-tropical countries of the world, and cultivated in warm climates

¶ *Description*. The stigmas (fine soft, yellowish threads) from the female flowers of maize from 4 to 8 inches long and of a light green, purplish red, yellow or light brown colour, stigmas bifid; the segments very slender, frequently unequal, nearly odourless, faintly sweetish taste.

¶ *Constituents.* Maizenic acid is present in the dried corn silk; also fixed oil, resin, chlorophyl, sugar-gum extractive albuminoids phlobaphine salt, cellulose and water.

¶ *Medicinal Action and Uses.* A mild stimulant, diuretic and demulcent, useful in acute and chronic cystitis and in the bladder irritation of uric acid and phosphatic gravel; has also been employed in gonorrhœa. In action like Holy Thistle.

¶ *Preparations and Dosages.* Infusion (1 in 10), 2 fluid ounces. Fluid extract of maize stigmas, B.P.C., 1 to 2 fluid drachms. Syrup of maize stigmas, B.P.C., 2 to 4 fluid drachms. Mazenic is given in doses of $\frac{1}{8}$ grain.

See CORN (INDIAN)

CORSICAN MOSS. *See* MOSS

COSTMARY

Tanacetum balsamita (LINN.)
N.O. Compositæ

Synonyms. Alecost. Balsam Herb. Costmarie. Mace. Balsamita
(*French*) Herbe Sainte-Marie
Part Used. Leaves.

Closely allied to the Tansy is another old English herb – Costmary (*Tanacetum balsamita*, Linn.). The whole of this plant emits a soft balsamic odour – pleasanter and more aromatic than that of Tansy – to which fact it owes its name of *balsamita*, and we find it referred to by Culpepper and others as the 'Balsam Herb.' In some old herbals it appears as *Balsamita mas*, Maudlin, *Achillea ageratum*, being *Balsamita fœmina*.

It is a native of the Orient, but has now become naturalized in many parts of southern Europe and was formerly to be found in almost every garden in this country, having been introduced into England in the sixteenth century – Lyte, writing in 1578, said it was then 'very common in all gardens.' Gerard, twenty years later, says 'it groweth everywhere in gardens,' and Parkinson mentions it among other sweet herbs in his garden, but it has now so completely gone out of favour as to have become a rarity, though it may still occasionally be found in old gardens, especially in Lincolnshire, where it is known as 'Mace.'

In distinction to the feathery leaves of its near relative, the Tansy, the somewhat long and broad leaves of Costmary are entire, their margins only finely toothed. The stems rise 2 to 3 feet from the creeping roots and bear in August, at their summit, heads of insignificant yellowish flowers in loose clusters, which do not set seed in this country.

¶ *Cultivation.* The plant will thrive in almost every soil or situation, but will do best on dry land.

Propagation is effected by division of the roots in early spring, or in autumn, planting 2 feet apart, in a dry, warm situation. As the roots creep freely, the plants will probably spread over the intervening spaces in a couple of years and need dividing and transplanting every second or third year.

Grown in the shade, Costmary goes strongly to leaf, but will not flower.

¶ *Medicinal Action and Uses.* On account of the aroma and taste of its leaves, Costmary was much used to give a spicy flavouring to ale – whence its other name, Aletcost. Markham (*The Countrie Farmer*, 1616) says that 'both Costmarie' and Avens 'give this savour.'

The fresh leaves were also used in salads and in pottage, and dried are often put into pot-pourri, as they retain their aroma. Our great-grandmothers used to tie up bundles of Costmary with Lavender 'to lye upon the toppes of beds, presses, etc., for sweet scent and savour.'

The name Costmary is derived from the Latin *costus* (an Oriental plant), the root of which is used as a spice and as a preserve, and 'Mary,' in reference to Our Lady. In the Middle Ages, the plant was widely associated with her name and was known in France as *Herbe Sainte-Marie.*

It was at one time employed medicinally in this country, having somewhat astringent and antiseptic properties, and had a place in our Pharmacopœia until 1788, chiefly as an aperient, its use in dysentery being especially indicated.

Green's *Universal Herbal* (1532) stated, 'A strong infusion of the leaves to be good in disorders of the stomach and head,' and much celebrated for its efficacy as an emmenagogue.

Salmon (1710), among other uses, recommends the juice of the herb as a diuretic and 'good in cases of Quotidien Ague,' and continues:

'The powder of the leaves is a good stomatick and may be taken from $\frac{1}{2}$ to 1 dram morning and night. I commend it to such as are apt to have the gout to fly upwards into the stomach. It is astringent, resists poison and the bitings of venomous beasts and kills

226

worms in human bodies. The oil by insolation or boiling in Olive oil warms and comforts preternatural coldness, discusses swellings and gives ease in gout, sciatica and other like pains. The Cataplasm draws out the fire in Burnings, being applied before they are blistered. The spirituous tincture helps a weak and disaffected liver, strengthens the nerves, head and brain.'

Culpepper speaks of its being 'astringent to the stomach' and

'strengthening to the liver and all other inward parts; and taken in whey works more effectually. Taken fasting in the morning it is very profitable for pains in the head that are continual, and to stay, dry up, and consume all thin rheums or distillations from the head into the stomach, and helps much to digest raw humours that are gathered therein. . . . It is an especial friend and help to evil, weak and cold livers. The seed is familiarly given to children for the worms, and so is the infusion of the flowers in white wine given them to the quantity of two ounces at a time.'

And before Culpepper's days, Gerard had said:

'The Conserve made with leaves of Cost-maria and sugar doth warm and dry the braine and openeth the stoppings of the same; stoppeth all catarrhes, rheumes and distillations, taken in the quantitie of a beane.'

We find this plant mentioned in a very composite old recipe 'for a Consumption,' called 'Aqua Composita,' in which it is spelt 'Coursemary.' Also in an 'Oyntment,' for 'bruises, dry itches, streins of veins and sinews, scorchings of gunpowder, the shingles, blisters, scabs and vermine.'

An ointment made by boiling the herb in olive oil with Adder's Tongue and thickening the strained liquid with wax and resin and turpentine was considered to be very valuable for application to sores and ulcers.

Achillea ageratum (Linn.), the Maudlin or Sweet Milfoil, a native of Italy and Spain, introduced into England in 1570, an aromatic plant with a sweet smell and a bitter taste, and yellow, tansy-like flowers, was used by the earlier herbalists for the same purposes as Costmary. Culpepper speaks of it growing in gardens and having the same virtues as Costmary, but by the time of Linnæus its use was obsolete. Both Costmary and Maudlin were much used to make 'sweete washing water.'

See TANSY

COTO

Part Used. The bark
Habitat. Bolivia

¶ *Description.* A bark bearing this name came into the London drug market about 1893. The bark of a rubiaceous plant (*Palicourea densiflors*), known as Coto, is employed in Brazil for rheumatism, but it is not known if this is the true Bolivian plant; the outer surface is irregular, of a cinnamon brown colour. It is sold in pieces of 4 to 6 inches long, 3 inches wide and about 1 inch thick, and is sometimes covered with an adherent corry surface, free from lichens. The inner cross-sections of the bark are covered with yellowish spots, the odour is aromatic and much stronger if bruised, taste hot and biting; in powdered form the smell is very pungent. This description conforms with the barks sold in the American markets, but other barks are used under the same name, the chief being Paracote bark; this has an agreeable spicy taste, but is not so strong-smelling or tasting, and has deep white furrows on the surface.

¶ *Constituents.* Coto bark contains a volatile alkaloid, a pungent aromatic volatile oil, a

Botanical source unknown
Possibly N.O. Lauraceæ

light brown soft resin, and a hard brown resin, starch, gum, sugar, tannin, Cal. Oxalate and three acids, acetic, butyric and formic.

¶ *Medicinal Action and Uses.* Antiseptic, astringent. Coto bark is irritating to the skin applied externally. If taken internally it gives constant violent pain and vomiting. Its chief use is in diarrhœa, but it has a tendency to produce inflammation, so must be used with great caution; it is said to lessen peristaltic action. Paracota bark resembles it in action, but is much less powerful. In Japan, paracota bark has been successfully employed for cholera by hypodermic injection of 3 grains of paracotoin. The value of cotoin in diarrhœa is established, and it is also used for catarrhal diarrhœa and for diarrhœa in tubercular ulceration of typhoid fever. Has also a specific action on the alimentary canal, dilating the abdominal vessels and hastening absorption.

¶ *Preparations and Dosages.* Cotoin, 1 to 3 grains. Fluid extract, 5 to 15 drops. Powdered coto, 2 to 15 grains.

COTTON ROOT

Gossypium herbaceum (LINN.)
N.O. Malvaceæ

Part Used. Bark of root and of other cultivated species

Habitat. Asia Minor, and cultivated in U.S.A. and Egypt, India, Mediterranean

¶ *Description. Gossypium herbaceum* is the indigenous species in India, and yields the bulk of the cotton of that country. It is also grown in the south of Europe, and other countries bordering on the Mediterranean, Persia, etc. The seeds are woolly and yield a very short stapled cotton, while *G. Barbadense* gives the Sea Island, or long-stapled cotton, this latter being indigenous to America. The two varieties are recognized in the U.S.A. *G. Barbadense*, the best species, was introduced from the Bahamas in 1785 and only grows in the low islands and sea-coast of Georgia and South Carolina. The upland Georgian, Bowed or short-stapled cotton, which forms the bulk of American cotton, is the produce of the upland or inner districts of the Southern States. Its staple is only about 1¼ inch long, and it adheres firmly to the seed, which is covered with short down. Egyptian cotton and Bourbon are likewise referrable to this species.

G. herbaceum is a biennial or triennial plant with branching stems 2 to 6 feet high, palmate hairy leaves, lobes lanceolate and acute, flowers with yellow petals, and a purple spot in centre, leaves of involucre serrate, capsule when ripe splits open and shows a loose white tuft surrounding the seeds and adhering firmly to outer coating; it requires warm weather to ripen its seeds, which they do not do north of Virginia.

The crushed seeds give a fixed, semi-drying oil used in making soap, etc. The flowering time ends in September, and a month or so earlier the tops are cut off in order to ripen and send the sap back to the capsules. The pods are about the size of a walnut, and are collected by hand as they ripen; the cotton is also separated by hand and packed in bales.

In the Levant the seeds are often used as food. An acre may be expected to produce 240 to 300 lb. of cotton.

The herbaceous part of the plant contains much mucilage and has been utilized as a demulcent. Cotton seeds have been used in the Southern States for intermittent fever with great success. The root and stem-bark deteriorates with age, so only newly harvested material should be used. The root-bark of commerce consists of thin flexible bands of quilled pieces covered with a browny yellow periderm, odour not strong, taste slightly acid.

¶ *Constituents.* A peculiar acid resin, odourless and insoluble in water, absorbing oxygen when exposed, then changes to a red colour. The bark also contains sugar, gum, tannin, fixed oil, chlorophyll.

¶ *Medicinal Action and Uses.* Mainly used as an abortifacient in place of ergot, being not so powerful but safer; it was used largely in this way by the slaves in the south. It not only increases the contractions of the uterus in labour, but also is useful in the treatment of metrorrhagia, specially when dependent on fibroids; useful also as an ecbolic; of value in sexual lassitude. A preparation of cotton seed increases milk of nursing mothers.

¶ *Preparations.* Boil 4 oz. of the inner bark of the root in 1 quart of water down to 1 pint: dose, 1 full wineglass (4 oz.) every thirty minutes. Fluid extract, U.S.D., 1 to 2 drachms. Gossipium, 1 to 5 grains. Solid extract, 15 to 20 grains. Liquid extract of cotton root bark, B.P.C., ½ to 1 fluid drachm. Tinc. Gossipii, B.P.C., ½ to 1 fluid drachm. Decoction of cotton root bark, B.P.C., ½ to 2 fluid ounces (as an emmenagogue or to check hæmorrhages).

COUCHGRASS. *See* GRASSES

COWHAGE

Mucuna pruriens (LINN.)
N.O. Leguminosæ

Synonyms. Dolichos pruriens. Stizolobium pruriens. Mucuna prurita. Setæ Siliquæ Hirsutæ. Cowage. Cowitch. Couhage. Kiwach.

(*French*) Cadjuet. Pois velus. Pois à gratter. Liane à gratter. Pois pouilleux. Œil de bourrique

(*German*) Kratzbohnen. Kuhkratze

Parts Used. The hairs of the pod, seeds

Habitat. Tropical regions, especially East and West Indies

¶ *Description.* The name of the genus, *Mucuna*, is that of a Brazilian species mentioned by Marggraf in 1648, and *pruriens* refers to the itching caused on the skin by the

hairs. The popular name, variously spelt, is from the Hindustani.

Travellers in the tropics know the plants well on account of their annoying seed-pods,

228

covered with stinging hairs which are easily shaken off, and cause great irritation. They are found in Asia, America, Africa, and the Fiji Islands.

M. pruriens is a leguminous climbing plant, with long, slender branches, alternate, lanceolate leaves on hairy petioles, 6 to 12 inches long, with large, white flowers, growing in clusters of two or three, with a bluish-purple, butterfly-shaped corolla.

The pods or legumes, hairy, thick, and leathery, averaging 4 inches long, are shaped like violin sound-holes, and contain four to six seeds. They are of a rich dark brown colour, thickly covered with stiff hairs, about $\frac{1}{10}$ inch long, which are the official part. In commerce they are found in a loose mass mixed with pieces of the pericarp.

When young and tender, the legumes are cooked and eaten in India.

¶ *Constituents.* The hairs are usually filled with air, but sometimes contain granular matter, with tannic acid and resin. No tincture or decoction is effective.

¶ *Medicinal Action and Uses.* A mechanical anthelmintic. The hairs, mixed with syrup, molasses, or honey, pierce the bodies of intestinal worms, which writhe themselves free from the walls, so that a brisk cathartic will bring them away. It is usually a safe remedy, but enteritis has sometimes followed its use.

It has little effect upon tape-worm, but is good for *Ascaris lumbricoides* and in slightly less degree for the smaller *Oxyuris vermicularis*.

In the form of an ointment, Mucuna has been used as a local stimulant in paralysis and other affections, acting like Croton oil. A decoction of the *root or legumes* is said to have been used in dropsy as a diuretic and for catarrh, and in some parts of India an infusion is used in cholera.

It is a good medium for the application of such substances as muriate of morphia. In the proportion of 7 to 8 grains of cowhage to an ounce of lard, it should be rubbed in for from 10 to 20 minutes. It brings out flat, white pimples, which soon disappear. Oil relieves the heat and irritation caused on the skin.

The seeds are said to be aphrodisiac.

¶ *Dosage.* For an adult, a tablespoonful, and for a child a teaspoonful, for three consecutive mornings, after which a brisk cathartic should be given.

¶ *Other Species.*

M. urens,[1] or *Dolichos urens* (*M. prurita*), the seeds of which, called Horse-eye beans, round and brownish, are used as a substitute for Calabar beans. Some authorities regard this East Indian variety as a distinct species, being larger than *M. pruriens*.

COWSLIP

Primula veris (LINN.)
N.O. Primulaceæ

Synonyms. Herb Peter. Paigle. Peggle. Key Flower. Key of Heaven. Fairy Cups. Petty Mulleins. Crewel. Buckles. Palsywort. Plumrocks. Mayflower. Password. Artetyke. Drelip. Our Lady's Keys. Arthritica
(*Anglo-Saxon*) Cuy lippe
(*Greek*) Paralysio

Many of the Primrose tribe possess active medicinal properties. Besides the Cowslip and the Primrose, this family includes the little Scarlet Pimpernel (*Anagallis*), as truly a herald of warm summer weather as the Primrose is of spring, the Yellow Loosestrife and the Moneywort (*Lysimachia vulgaris* and *Nummularia*), the handsome Water Violet (*Hottonia*) and the nodding *Cyclamen* or Sowbread, all of which have medicinal value to a greater or lesser degree. Less important British members of the group are the Chaffweed (*Centunculus minimus*), one of the smallest among British plants, the Chickweed Wintergreen (*Trientalis*), the Sea Milk-wort (*Glaux maritima*), which has succulent salty leaves and has been used as a pickle, and the Common Brookweed or Water Pimpernel (*Samolus*).

The botanical name of the order, *Primulaceæ*, is based on that of the genus *Primula*, to which belong not only those favourite spring flowers of the country-side, the Primrose, Cowslip, and their less common relative the Oxlip, but also the delicately-tinted greenhouse species that are such welcome pot plants for our rooms in mid-winter.

Linnæus considered the Primrose, Cowslip and Oxlip to be but varieties of one species, but in this opinion later botanists have not followed him, though in all essential points they are identical.

¶ *Description.* Quite early in the spring, the Cowslip begins to produce its leaves. At first, each is just two tight coils, rolled backwards and lying side by side; these slowly unroll and a leaf similar to that of a Primrose, but shorter and rounder, appears. All the

---

[1] The pulverized bean of *M. urens* (Horse-eye), macerated in alcohol, is used in homœopathy for hæmorrhoids. – EDITOR

leaves lie nearly flat on the ground in a rosette, from the centre of which rises a long stalk, crowned by the flowers, which spring all from one point, in separate little stalks, and thus form an 'umbel.' The number of the flowers in an umbel varies very much in different specimens.

We quote the following from *Familiar Wild Flowers*:

'It is a curious fact that the inflorescence of the Primrose is as truly umbellate as that of the Cowslip, though in the former case it can only be detected by carefully tracing the flower stems to their base, when all will be found to spring from one common point. In some varieties of the Primrose the umbel is raised on a stalk, as in the Cowslip. This form is sometimes called Oxlip; it is by some writers raised to the dignity of an independent position as a true and distinct species. . . . Primrose roots may at times be met with bearing both forms, one or more stalked umbels together with a number of the ordinary type of flower.'

The sepals of the flowers are united to form pale green crinkled bags, from which the corolla projects, showing a golden disk about ½ inch across with scalloped edges, the petals being united into a narrow tube within the calyx. On the yellow disk are five red spots, one on each petal.

'In their gold coats spots you see,
These be rubies fairy favours
In those freckles lie their savours.'

The *Midsummer Night's Dream* refers to the old belief that the flower held a magic value for the complexion.

The origin of Cowslip is obscure: it has been suggested that it is a corruption of 'Cow's Leek,' *leek* being derived from the Anglo-Saxon word *leac*, meaning a plant (comp. Houseleek).

In old Herbals we find the plant called Herb Peter and Key Flower, the pendent flowers suggesting a bunch of keys, the emblem of St. Peter, the idea having descended from old pagan times, for in Norse mythology the flower was dedicated to Freya, the Key Virgin, and was thought to admit to her treasure palace. In northern Europe the idea of dedication to the goddess was transferred with the change of religion, and it became dedicated to the Virgin Mary, so we find it called 'Our Lady's Keys' and 'Key of Heaven,' and 'Keyflower' remains still the most usual name.

The flowers have a very distinctive and fresh fragrance and somewhat narcotic juices, which have given rise to their use in making the fermented liquor called Cowslip Wine, which had formerly a great and deserved reputation and is still largely drunk in country parts, being much produced in the Midlands. It is made from the 'peeps,' i.e. the yellow petal rings, in the following way: A gallon of 'peeps' with 4 lb. of lump sugar and the rind of 3 lemons is added to a gallon of cold spring water. A cup of fresh yeast is then included and the liquor stirred every day for a week. It is then put into a barrel with the juice of the lemons and left to 'work.' When 'quiet,' it is corked down for eight or nine months and finally bottled. The wine should be perfectly clear and of a pale yellow colour and has almost the value of a liqueur. In certain children's ailments, Cowslip Wine, given in small doses as a medicine, is particularly beneficial.

Young Cowslip leaves were at one time eaten in country salads and mixed with other herbs to stuff meat, whilst the flowers were made into a delicate conserve. Cowslip salad from the petals, with white sugar, is said to make an excellent and refreshing dish.

Children delight in making Cowslip Balls, or 'tosties,' from the flowers. The umbels are picked off close to the top of the main flower-stalk and about fifty to sixty are hung across a string which may be stretched for convenience between the backs of two chairs. The flowers are then pressed carefully together and the string tied tightly so as to collect them into a ball. Care must be taken to choose only such heads or umbels in which all the flowers are open, as otherwise the surface of the ball will be uneven.

¶ *Part Used Medicinally.* The yellow corolla is alone needed, no stalk or green part whatever is required, only the yellow part, plucked out of the green calyx.

¶ *Constituents.* The roots and the flowers have somewhat of the odour of Anise, due to their containing some volatile oil identical with Mannite. Their acrid principle is Saponin.

¶ *Medicinal Action and Uses.* Sedative, antispasmodic.

In olden days, Cowslip flowers were in great request for homely remedies, their special value lying in strengthening the nerves and the brain, and relieving restlessness and insomnia. The Cowslip was held good 'to ease paines in the head and is accounted next with Betony, the best for that purpose.'

Cowslip Wine made from the flowers, as above described, is an excellent sedative. Also, 1 lb. of the freshly gathered blossom, infused in 1½ pint of boiling water and simmered down with loaf sugar to a fine yellow syrup, taken with a little water is admirable for giddiness from nervous debility or from previous nervous excitement, and this syrup was formerly given against palsy.

In earlier times, the Cowslip was considered beneficial in all paralytic ailments, being, as we have seen, often called Palsy Wort or Herba paralysis. The root was also called in old Herbals *Radix arthritica*, from its use as a cure for muscular rheumatism.

In *A Plain Plantain* (Russell G. Alexander) we .read:

'Cowslip water was considered to be good for the memory, and Cowslips of Jerusalem for mitigating "hectical fevers." Mrs. Raffald (*English Housekeeper*, 1778) gives a recipe for the wine. "For the future," says the poet Pope, in one of his letters, "I'll drown all high thoughts in the Lethe of Cowslip Wine" (which is pleasantly soporific). Our Lady's Cowslip is *Gagea lutea*.'

The old writers give a long list of ills that may be remedied by application of the roots or leaves of the plant; the juice of the flowers 'takes off spots and wrinkles from the face and other vices of the skin,' the water of the flowers being 'very proper medicine for weakly people.'

Turner says:

'Some weomen we find, sprinkle ye floures of cowslip w^t whyte wine and after still it and wash their faces w^t that water to drive wrinkles away and to make them fayre in the eyes of the worlde rather than in the eyes of God, Whom they are not afrayd to offend.'

Formerly an ointment was made from the flowers as a cosmetic. Culpepper says:

'Our city dames know well enough the ointment or distilled water of it adds to beauty or at least restores it when lost. The flowers are held to be more effectual than the leaves and the roots of little use. An ointment being made with them taketh away spots and wrinkles of the skin, sunburnings and freckles and promotes beauty; they remedy all infirmities of the head coming of heat and wind, as vertigo, false apparitions, phrensies, falling sickess, palsies, convulsions, cramps, pains in the nerves, and the roots ease pains in the back and bladder. The leaves are good in wounds and the flowers take away trembling. Because they strengthen the brains and nerves and remedy palsies, the Greeks gave them the name *Paralysio*. The flowers preserved or conserved and a quantity the size of a nutmeg taken every morning is a sufficient dose for inward diseases, but for wounds, spots, wrinkles and sunburnings an ointment is made of the leaves and hog's lard.'

A later writer, Hill (1755), tells us that when boiled in ale, the powdered roots were taken with success by country folk for giddiness, wakefulness and similar nervous troubles for which the syrup made from the flowers was also taken.

The usual dose of the dried and powdered flowers is 15 to 20 grains.

From Hartman's *Family Physitian*, 1696:
'Another way to make Cowslip Wine
'Having boil'd your Water and Sugar together, pour it boiling hot upon your Cowslips beaten, stir them well together, and let them stand in a Vessel close cover'd till it be almost cold; then put into it the Yest beaten with the Juice of Lemons; let it stand for two days, then press it out with as much speed as you can, and put it up into a Cask, and leave a little hole open, for the working; when it hath quite done working stop it up close for a Month or Six Weeks, then Bottle it. Cowslip Wine is very Cordial, and a glass of it being drank at night Bedward, causes sleep and rest. . . .'

The Bird's-eye Primrose (*Primula farinosa*) is a plant of mountain slopes and pastures, and may be met with on the mountain ranges of Europe and Asia. It is not uncommon in the northern counties of England, though much less common in Scotland.

Gerard, in his *Herball*, says:

'These plants grow very plentifully in moist and squally grounds in the North parts of England, as in Harwood, neere to Blackburne in Lancashire, and ten miles from Preston in Aundernesse; also at Crosby, Ravensnaith, and Craig-close in Westmorland. They likewise grow in the meadows belonging to a village in Lancashire neere Maudsley called Harwood, and at Hasketh, not far from thence, and in many other places of Lancashire, but not on this side Trent' (Gerard writes as a Londoner) 'that I could ever have certain knowledge of. Lobel reporteth, That Doctor Penny, a famous Physition of our London Colledge, did find them in these Southerne Parts.'

Specimens of the Bird's-eye Primrose growing in the North of Scotland, in Caithness and the Orkney Islands, and in other localities bordering on the sea, vary from the typical form of the plant in being of stouter habit and much smaller, in having leaves of broader proportions and flowers of a deeper purple; and some botanists are inclined to distinguish this variety by creating it an independent species, and calling it the Scotch Bird's-eye (*P. Scotica*), while others are content to consider it but a variety from the type, and label it *P. farinosa*, var. *Scotica*.

All the hardy varieties of Primula, whether Primrose, Cowslip, Polyanthus or Auricula, may be easily propagated by dividing the roots of old plants in autumn. New varieties are raised from seed, which should be sown as soon as ripe, in leaf-mould, and pricked out into beds when large enough.

Among the many splendid flowers that are grown in our greenhouses none shows more improvement under the fostering hand of the British florist than the Chinese Primula, which originally had small, inconspicuous flowers, but now bears trusses of magnificent blooms ranging from the purest white to the richest scarlet and crimson. The Star Primulas, which have attained an even greater popularity in late years, are considered perhaps even more elegant, being looser in growth and carrying their plentiful blossoms in more graceful, if not more beautiful trusses. Both varieties are among the most beautiful of our winter-flowering plants, the toothed and lobed, somewhat heart-shaped leaves being extremely handsome with their crimson tints.

Seeds of these greenhouse Primulas should be sown in the spring in gentle heat, the soil used being very fine and pleasantly moist. The seedlings must be pricked off and potted out as necessary, with a view to ensuring sturdy, healthy growth.

P. obconica is a slightly varying type of these greenhouse Primulas, the leaves approaching more the shape of those of the common Primrose; the plants are exceedingly floriferous and graceful, the full trusses of delicate lilac flowers are borne on tall slender stems and care must be used in the handling of it, as the leaves sometimes cause an eruption like eczema. Homœopaths make a tincture from this species.

The broad, thick leaves of the Auricula (*P. auricula*), a frequent garden plant in this country, though not native to Great Britain, are used in the Alps as a remedy for coughs.

In its native state the Auricula is said to be either yellow or white. It is the skill of the gardener which has brought it to its present purple and brown. It was formerly known as Mountain Cowslip, or Bear's Ears.

See PRIMROSE, PRIMULAS

COW-WHEAT

Melampyrum pratense (LINN.)
N.O. Scrophulariaceæ

Synonyms. Horse Floure. Triticum vaccinium
Part used. Herb

The Cow-wheat (*Melampyrum pratense*, Linn.) is an annual, with slender, branched stems, about a foot high, bearing stalkless, narrow, tapering, smooth leaves in distant pairs, each pair at right angles to those that are next to it, and long-tubed, pale yellow flowers, which are placed in the axils of the upper leaves in pairs, all turning one way. The corolla is four times as long as the calyx, and the lower lip longer than the upper, standing sharply out instead of hanging downwards as in most labiate flowers. The colour is somewhat between the delicate pale yellow of the primrose and the rich bright yellow of the buttercup. The plant is in flower from June to September.

Cow-wheat is said to afford fodder for cattle, though not cultivated in this country for that purpose. Linnæus states that when cows are fed in fields where the Meadow Cow-wheat is abundant, the butter yielded by their milk is peculiarly rich and of a brilliant yellow colour, but in England the plant grows more frequently in the undergrowth of woods and thickets than in meadows, abounding in nearly all copses and woods throughout Great Britain.

The name of Cow-wheat is said to be derived from an extraordinary notion prevalent in some country districts among the peasantry of the Middle Ages, that the small seeds were capable of being converted into wheat, a supposition probably originating in the sudden appearance of the plants among corn, on land that had been recently cleared of wood.

Another reason for the meaning of *Melampyrum* is given in Lindley's *Treasury of Botany*, i.e. it refers to an ancient belief that the seeds, when *mixed with grains of wheat* and ground into flour *tended to make the bread black*.

The seeds, which bear some little resemblance to wheat, are generally eaten by swine, though they will not touch the herb. Cows and sheep are extremely fond of the plant, and Dr. Prior explains the name of the plant on the score that though its seed resembles wheat, it is only fit for cows. In old Herbals, we find it named 'Horse Floure' and also *Triticum vaccinium*. The generic name is derived from the Greek *melas* (black) and *pyros* (wheat), because the seeds made bread black when mixed with them.

Dodonæus tells us that 'the seeds of this herb taken in meate or drinke troubleth the braynes, causing headache and drunkennesse.'

See TOAD-FLAX, SNAPDRAGON

CRAMP BARK. *See* GUELDER ROSE

CRANESBILL ROOT, AMERICAN

Geranium maculatum (LINN.)
N.O. Geraniaceæ

Synonyms. Alum Root. Spotted Cranesbill. Wild Cranesbill. Storksbill. Alum Bloom. Wild Geranium. Chocolate Flower. Crowfoot. Dove's-foot. Old Maid's Nightcap. Shameface

Parts Used. Dried rhizome, leaves

Habitat. Flourishes in low grounds and woods from Newfoundland to Manitoba, south to Georgia, Missouri and in Europe

¶ *Description.* A perennial, grows from 1 to 2 feet high. The entire plant is erect and unbranched, more or less covered with hairs; the leaves deeply parted, each division again cleft and toothed, flowering April to June, colour pale to rosy purple, petals veined and woolly at base, fruit a beaked capsule, divided into five cells, each cell containing one seed, the root stocks 2 to 4 inches long, thick with numerous branches for the next growth, outside brown, white and fleshy inside when fresh, when dried it turns to a darkish purple inside; no odour, taste strongly astringent, contains much tannin which is most active just before the plant flowers. This is the time the root should be collected for drying.

¶ *Constituents.* Tannic and gallic acid, also starch, sugar, gum, pectin and colouring matter.

¶ *Medicinal Action and Uses.* Styptic, astringent, tonic. Used for piles and internal bleeding. Excellent as an injection for flooding and leucorrhœa, and taken internally for diarrhœa, children's cholera, chronic dysentery; a good gargle.

The leaves are also used and give the greatest percentage of tannin and should be collected before the plant seeds.

¶ *Dosages.* 15 to 30 grains. Infusion, 1 oz. herb to 1 pint water. Fluid extract, ½ to 1 drachm. Geranin, 1 to 3 grains.

¶ *Other Species.*
The English herb *Geranium dissectum* has similar properties.

CRAWLEY ROOT ·

Corallorhiza odontorhiza (NUTT.)
N.O. Orchidaceæ

Synonyms. Dragon's Claw. Coral Root. Chicken Toe

Part Used. The root

Habitat. Indigenous to the United States, from Maine to Carolina westward

¶ *Description.* This parasitic plant has been used by herbalists for centuries. It grows in rich woods at the roots of trees.

It is singular and leafless, with much-branched and toothed coral-like root-stocks, the root being a collection of fleshy, articulated tubers, the scape about 14 inches high, fleshy, smooth, striate, with a few long purplish-brown long sheaths, the flowers, 10 to 20, greenish brown in colour, on a long spike, blooming from July to October, with a large, reflexed, ribbed, oblong capsule.

The root is the official part; it is small and dark, with a strong nitrous smell and a slightly bitter mucilaginous astringent taste, the fracture is short and presents under the microscope a frosted granular appearance.

¶ *Medicinal Action and Uses.* Crawley Root is one of the most certain, quick and powerful diaphoretics, but its scarcity and high price prevents it being more generally used. It promotes perspiration without producing any excitement in the system, so is of value in pleurisy, typhus fever and other inflammatory diseases. In addition to being a powerful diaphoretic, its action has a sedative effect. It has been found efficacious in acute erysipelas, cramps, nightsweats, flatulence and hectic fevers generally, and combines tonic, sedative, diaphoretic and febrifuge properties without weakening the patient, its valuable properties being most marked in low stages of fever.

¶ *Dosage.* 20 to 30 grains of powdered root given in very hot water every two or three hours. The powder should be kept in well-stoppered bottles as it is subject to deterioration from insects.

Combined with the resin of Blue Cohosh, it is an excellent remedy for amenorrhœa, dismenorrhœa, afterbirth pains, suppression of lochia and for febrile conditions of the parturient period, and combined with extract of Leptandra or Podophyllum resin, it acts well on the bowels and liver, and if mixed with Dioscorea is excellent for bilious and flatulent colic.

Fluid extract, 15 to 30 drops.

¶ *Other Species.*
It is considered that the varieties *Corallorhiza multiflora, C. Wisteriana, C. verna* and *C. innata* possess similar properties.

233

CROSSWORT

Galium cruciata (SCOPOLI)
N.O. Rubiaceæ

Parts Used. Herb, leaves

¶ *Description.* The Crosswort (*Galium cruciata*, Scopoli), like *G. verum*, has yellow flowers, but they are not so showy, being only in short clusters of about eight together, in the axils of the upper whorls of leaves and of a dull, pale yellow. The stems are slender and scarcely branched, 1 to 2 feet long, and bear soft and downy leaves, oblong in shape, arranged four in a whorl, hence the name Crosswort.

¶ *Medicinal Action and Uses.* This species, though now practically unused, was considered a very good wound herb for both inward and outward wounds. A decoction of the leaves in wine was also used for obstructions in the stomach or bowels and to stimulate appetite. It was also recommended as a remedy for rupture, rheumatism and dropsy.

We have only one representative in Great Britain of the genus *Rubia* (name from Latin *ruber*, red), from which this large natural order takes its name, namely the Wild Madder (*R. peregrina*, Linn.), common in bushy places in the south-west of England.

It is a long, straggling, perennial plant, many feet in length, with remarkably rough stems and leaves, the latter glossy above and growing in whorls of four to six, their margins recurved and bearing prickles, which are also present on the angles of the stem and the midribs of the leaves, the plant being otherwise smooth.

The flowers, in bloom from June to August, are yellowish-green and grow in loose panicles. They are followed by black berries, about as large as currants, which remain attached to the plant till late in winter.

The properties of this native Wild Madder are not made use of, although it yields a good dye, said to be but little inferior to that of the cultivated species, *R. tinctorum*, the Dyer's Madder, formerly a plant of much greater importance than it is now, owing to the researches of chemical science having discovered an easier source of the important dye it yields.

See BEDSTRAW, CLIVERS, MADDER.

CROTON

Croton tiglium (WILLD.)
N.O. Euphorbiaceæ

Synonyms. Tiglium Seeds. Klotzsch
Part Used. The oil from ripe seeds

¶ *Description.* A small tree or shrub with a few spreading branches bearing alternate petiolate leaves which are ovate, acuminate, serrate, smooth, dark green on upper surface, paler beneath and furnished with two glands at base. Flowers in erect terminal racemes, scarcely as long as the leaf, the lower female, upper male, straw-coloured petals. Fruit a smooth capsule of the size of a filbert, three cells, each containing a single seed; these seeds resemble castor beans in size and structure, oblong, rounded at the extremities with two faces; the kernel or endosperm is yellowish brown and abounds in oil. The oil is obtained by expression from the seeds previously deprived of the shell.

¶ *Constituents.* Croton oil consists chiefly of the glycerides of stearic, palmitic, myristic, lauric and oleic acids; there are also present in the form of glycerin ethers the more volatile acids as formic, acetic, isobutyric and isovalerianic acids. The active principle is believed to be Crotonic acid, which is freely soluble in alcohol.

¶ *Medicinal Action and Uses.* A powerful drastic purgative, in large doses apt to excite vomiting and severe griping pains capable of producing fatal effects. It acts with great rapidity, frequently evacuating the bowels in less than an hour. The dose is very small; a drop placed on the tongue of a comatose patient will generally operate. It is chiefly employed in cases of obstinate constipation, often being successful where other drugs have failed. Applied externally, it produces inflammation of the skin attended with pustular eruption, and has been used as a counter-irritant in rheumatism, gout, neuralgia, bronchitis, etc. It should be diluted with three parts of olive oil, soap liniment or other vehicle and applied as a liniment. Must always be used with the greatest care and should never be given to children or pregnant women.

¶ *Preparations and Dosage.* Dose of the oil, $\frac{1}{2}$ to 1 minim on a lump of sugar. Collodium Crotons, B.P.C., a powerful counter-irritant and vesicant. Liniment of Croton oil, B.P., seldom used owing to the painful inflammation which may be produced.

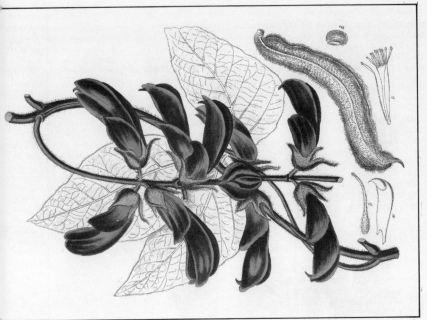

COWHAGE
Mucuna Pruriens

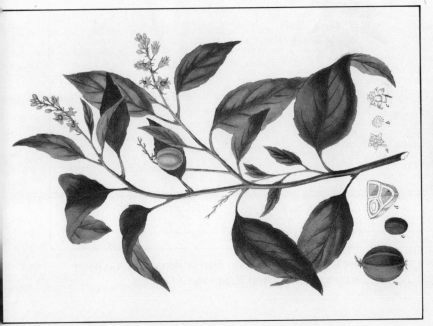

CROTON TREE
Croton Tiglium

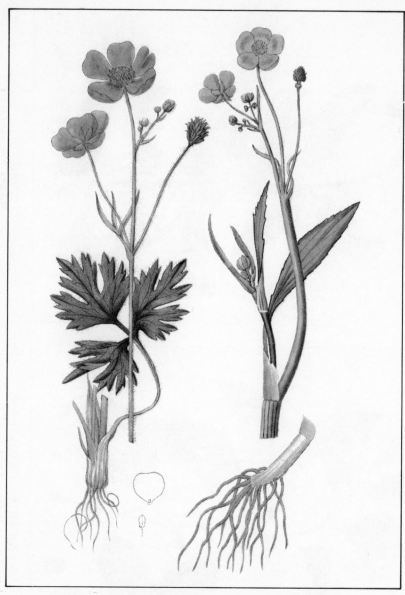

UPRIGHT MEADOW CROWFOOT AND LESSER SPEARWORT
Ranunculus Acris and *Ranunculus Flammula*

CROWFOOT, CELERY-LEAVED

Ranunculus sceleratus (LINN.)
N.O. Ranunculaceæ

Synonym. Marsh Crowfoot
Part Used. Whole plant
Habitat. The Celery-leaved Crowfoot is widely spread throughout Britain, growing in watery places and muddy ditches, flowering during July and August

¶ *Description.* The root is annual. The plant itself is of a pale, shining, yellowish-green colour, juicy and very glabrous except the flower-stalks and upper part of the stem, which are occasionally hairy. The flowers are numerous, small and of a palish yellow.

This species is easily distinguished by its broad, shining, lower leaves, which are on long stalks, the blades palmate, and cut into three divisions, which are notched and toothed. The stem is thick, hollow, furrowed and bears small sessile leaves, divided into three narrow parts, hardly toothed at all. The small, pale yellow flowers, about ¼ inch across, are succeeded by smooth, oblong seed-heads.

¶ *Medicinal Action and Uses.* One of the most virulent of native plants: bruised and applied to the skin, it raises a blister and creates a sore by no means easy to heal. When chewed, it inflames the tongue and produces violent effects. Even the distilled water is intensely acrimonious, and as it cools, deposits crystals which are insoluble, and have the curious property of being inflammable. Yet if the plant be boiled and the water thrown away, it is said to be not unwholesome, the peasants of Wallachia eating it thus as a vegetable. When made into a tincture, given in small diluted doses, it proves curative of stitch in the side and neuralgic pains between the ribs.

See BUTTERCUP CELANDINE.

CROWFOOT, UPRIGHT MEADOW

Ranunculus acris (LINN.)
N.O. Ranunculaceæ

Synonyms. Gold Cup. Grenouillette
Part Used. Whole herb
Habitat. This Buttercup is a native of meadows and pastures in all the northern parts of Europe, and is very common in England, flowering in June and July

The Upright Meadow Crowfoot, a familiar plant in our hay-fields, is recognized at once from all other Buttercups or Crowfoots by its tall flower-stalks not being furrowed, and its fruit-base, or receptacle, not being hairy. The stems are hollow, round, more or less covered with soft, silky hairs and very freely branching towards their summits, where they are terminated by numerous golden-yellow flowers.

¶ *Description.* The leaves vary a good deal in form, according to their position on the plant: the lower leaves are on long petioles (foot-stalks) and are comprised of numerous wide-spreading and deeply divided segments; the upper leaves are small, composed of few segments, simple in form and few in number. The root is perennial, though the plant itself dies down each autumn, and has many long, white fibres.

The petals of the flower are bright, shining yellow; the calyx is composed of five greenish-yellow spreading sepals. The centre of the flower, as in other Buttercups, is a clustering mass of stamens round the smooth, green immature seed-vessels, which develop into a round head of numerous small bodies called achenes.

Most of the Crowfoots are known to be acrid and some even to be poisonous, but this plant receives its Latin specific name of *acris* from its supposed intensity of acridity, for all parts of it are intensely acrid. It has been stated that even pulling it up and carrying it some little distance, has produced considerable inflammation in the palm of the hand, and that cattle will not readily eat it in the green state, and if driven by hunger to feed on it, their mouths become sore and blistered. According to Linnæus, sheep and goats eat it, but cattle, horses and pigs refuse it. When made into hay, it loses its acrid quality, but then seems to be too hard and stalky to yield much nourishment. The notion that the butter owes its yellow colour to the prevalence of buttercups in the meadows, is quite groundless – it is the richness of the pasture that communicates this colour to the butter and not these flowers, which the cattle seldom or never touch willingly.

Miss Pratt (*Familiar Wild Flowers*) states:

'Instances are common in which the wanderer in the meadow has lain down to sleep with a handful of these flowers beside him, and has awakened to find the skin of his cheek pained and irritated to a high degree, by the acrid blossoms having lain near it.'

Poetically, the associations of this plant

are numerous. Gay tells us in *The Shepherd's Oracle* that it was worn by lovers at betrothal time, and its golden colour was dedicated to Hymen in classical history. In France, it is termed the *grenouillette*, a name similar in meaning to its Latin generic name *Ranunculus*, a reference to the moist meadows in which it usually grows. In the astrological Herbals it was deemed a plant of Mars, on account of its acrid, fiery nature. Old authors say:

'this fiery and hot-spirited herb is not fit to be given inwardly, but that an ointment of the leaves and flowers will raise a blister, and may be applied to the nape of the neck to draw rheum from the eyes,'

and that mixed with a little mustard it raises a blister as perfectly as the Spanish Fly.

¶ *Medicinal Action and Uses.* The juice of the leaves takes away warts, and bruised together with the roots will act as a caustic. In violent headaches where pain is confined to one part, a plaster made of them often affords instant relief, and they have been used in gout with great success.

The fresh leaves formed part of a famous cure for cancer, practised by a Mr. Plunkett in 1794.

Thornton, in his *Herbal* of 100 years ago, says if a decoction of the plant be poured on ground containing worms, 'they will be forced to rise from their concealment.'

CUBEBS

Piper cubeba (LINN.)
N.O. Piperaceæ

Synonym. Tailed Pepper
Part Used. The dried, full-grown, unripe fruit
Habitat. Java, Penang, and other parts of East Indies

¶ *Description.* A climbing perennial plant, with diœcious flowers in spikes. The fruit is a globose, pedicelled drupe. It is extensively grown in the coffee plantations, well shaded and supported by the coffee trees. Odour aromatic and characteristic; taste strongly aromatic and pungent and somewhat bitter. Commercial Cubebs are often adulterated with other fruits containing a volatile oil, but with very different properties. There is no evidence that the plant was known to the ancients, though it was probably brought into Europe by the Arabians, who doubtless employed the fruit as pepper.

¶ *Constituents.* 10 to 18 per cent. of volatile oil, also resins, amorphous cubebic acid and colourless crystalline cubebin. By extraction with ether yields about 22 per cent. of oleoresin.

¶ *Medicinal Action and Uses.* Stimulant, carminative, much used as a remedy for gonorrhœa, after the first active inflammatory symptoms have subsided; also used in leucorrhœa, cystitis, urethritis, abscesses of the prostate gland, piles and chronic bronchitis.

¶ *Preparations and Dosages.* Infusion: 1 oz. of Cubebs to 1 pint of water is sometimes used as an injection in discharge from the vagina. In the treatment of gonorrhœa it is usually given in *capsule* form combined with copaiba, etc. Powdered fruit: dose, $\frac{1}{2}$ to 1 drachm. Oil, 5 to 30 drops. Fluid extract, $\frac{1}{4}$ to 1 drachm.

Cubebs should be freshly prepared as the oil evaporates; the powder is often adulterated with pimento. The crushed fruit should turn crimson with the addition of sulphuric acid and give a mace-like smell; this experiment will detect any adulteration.

CUCKOO-PINT

Arum maculatum
N.O. Araceæ

Synonyms. Lords and Ladies. Arum. Starchwort. Adder's Root. Bobbins. Friar's Cowl. Kings and Queens. Parson and Clerk. Ramp. Quaker. Wake Robin
Part Used. Root

The Arum family, *Aroideæ*, which numbers nearly 1,000 members, mostly tropical, and many of them marsh or water plants, is represented in this country by a sole species, *Arum maculatum* (Linn.), familiarly known as Lords and Ladies, or Cuckoo-pint.

¶ *Description.* The flowering organs are contained in a sheath-like leaf called a spathe, within which rises a long, fleshy stem, or column called the spadix, bearing closely arranged groups of stalkless, primitive flowers. At the base are a number of flowers

each consisting of a pistil only. Above these is a belt of sterile flowers, each consisting of only a purplish anther. Above the anther is a ring of glands, terminating in short threads. The spadix is then prolonged into a purple, club-like extremity.

The bright leaves, conspicuous by their glossiness and purple blotches, and their halbert-like shape, are some of the first to emerge from the ground on the approach of spring, and may then be noticed under almost every hedge in shady situations; the pale green spathe is a still more striking object when it appears in April and May.

In autumn, the lowest ring of flowers form a cluster of bright scarlet, attractive berries, which remain long after the leaves have withered away, and on their short, thick stem alone mark the situation of the plant. In spite of their very acrid taste, they have sometimes been eaten by children, with most injurious results, being extremely poisonous. One drop of their juice will cause a burning sensation in the mouth and throat for hours. In the case of little children who have died from eating the berries, cramp and convulsions preceded death if no medical aid had been obtained.

The Arum has large tuberous roots, somewhat resembling those of the Potato, oblong in shape, about the size of a pigeon's egg, brownish externally, white within and when fresh, fleshy yielding a milky juice, almost insipid to the taste at first, but soon producing a burning and pricking sensation. The acridity is lost during the process of drying and by application of heat, when the substance of the tuber is left as starch. When baked, the tubers are edible, and from the amount of starch, nutritious. This starch of the root, after repeated washing, makes a kind of arrowroot, formerly much prepared in the Isle of Portland, and sold as an article of food under the name of Portland Sago, or Portland Arrowroot, but now obsolete. For this purpose, it was either roasted or boiled, and then dried and pounded in a mortar, the skin being previously peeled.

Arum starch was used for stiffening ruffs in Elizabethan times, when we find the name Starchwort among the many names given to the plant. Gerard says:

'The most pure and white starch is made of the rootes of the Cuckoo-pint, but most hurtful for the hands of the laundresse that have the handling of it; for it chappeth, blistereth, and maketh the hands rough and rugged and withall smarting.'

This starch, however, in spite of Gerard's remarks, forms the Cyprus Powder of the Parisians, who used it as a cosmetic for the skin, and Dr. Withering says of this cosmetic formed from the tuber starch, that 'it is undoubtedly a good and innocent cosmetic'; and Hogg (*Vegetable Kingdom*, 1858) reported its use in Italy to remove freckles from the face and hands.

In parts of France, a custom existed of turning to account the mucilaginous juice of the plant as a substitute for soap, the stalks of the plant when in flower being cut and soaked for three weeks in water, which was daily poured off carefully and the residue collected at the bottom of the pan, then dried and used for laundry work.

Withering quotes Wedelius for the supposition that it was this plant, under the name of Chara, on which the soldiers of Cæsar's army subsisted when encamped at Dyrrhachium.

A curious belief is recorded by Gerard as coming from Aristotle, that when bears were half-starved with hibernating and had lain in their dens forty days without any nourishment, but such as they get by 'sucking their paws,' they were completely restored by eating this plant.

The roots, according to Gilbert White, are scratched up and eaten by thrushes in severe snowy seasons, and the berries are devoured by several kinds of birds, particularly by pheasants. Pigs which have eaten the fresh tubers suffered, but none died, though it acts as an irritant and purgative. As the leaves when bruised give out a disagreeable odour, they are not spontaneously eaten by animals, who quickly refuse them.

¶ *Constituents.* The fresh tuber contains a volatile, acrid principle and starch, albumen, gum, sugar, extractive, lignin and salts of potassium and calcium. Saponin has been separated, also a brownish, oily liquid alkaloid, resembling coniine in its properties, but less active.

Arum leaves give off prussic acid when injured, being a product of certain glucosides contained, called cyanophoric glucosides.

¶ *Collection and Uses.* The tubers for medicinal use should be dug up in autumn, or in early spring, before the leaves are fully developed. If laid in sand in a cellar, they can be preserved in sound condition for nearly a year.

When not needed for use in the fresh state, they can be dried slowly in very gentle heat and sliced. The dried slices are reduced to powder and kept in the cool, in stoppered bottles.

The fresh root when beaten up with gum, is recommended as a good pill mass, retaining all the medicinal properties.

The Arum had formerly a great reputation as a drug, in common with all other plants containing acrid or poisonous principles.

The dried root was recommended as a diuretic and stimulant, but is no longer employed. The *British Domestic Herbal* describes a case of alarming dropsy treated most successfully with a medicine composed of Arum and Angelica, which cured in about three weeks.

The juice of the fresh tuber is purgative,

but too violently so to be safely administered, and its use for this purpose has now been abandoned. Other uses of the tuber are, however, advocated in herbal medicine. Preparations were once official in the Dublin Pharmacopœia, and are also recommended by Homœopathy. A homœopathic tincture is prepared from the plant, and its root, which proves curative in diluted doses for a chronic sore throat with swollen mucous membranes and hoarseness, and likewise for a feverish sore throat.

An ointment made by stewing the fresh sliced tuber with lard is stated to be an efficient cure for ringworm, though the fresh sliced tuber applied to the skin produces a blister. The juice of the fresh plant when incorporated with lard has also been applied locally in the treatment of ringworm.

The AMERICAN ARUM (*Arum triphyllum*, Linn.), Dragon Root, has similar characters and properties to the above.

Synonym. Wild Turnip. Jack-in-the-Pulpit.

It is very common in eastern North America, in moist places, where it is known as Indian Turnip, Wild Turnip, Jack-in-the-Pulpit, Devil's Ear, Pepper Turnip, Wake Robin, etc.

It grows 1 to 3 feet high; a green spathe, broadly striped with brown purple, arches over and encloses the spadix. The corm is smaller than the English species, ½ to 2 inches broad and about half as high. It is very acrid when fresh, but loses this property when cooked, or partially when dried.

For the drug market it is collected in the early spring, transversely sliced and dried, and is employed in both herbal and homœopathic treatment.

It has acrid, stimulant, diaphoretic and expectorant properties, and is said to be useful when taken immediately after eating, to assist digestion and promote assimilation. It is considered a stimulant to the lungs in consumption, asthma and chronic forms of lung complaints, and to be of great value in hoarseness, coughs, asthma, rheumatism and lung diseases.

Owing to its acrimony, it is usually given in powder in honey or syrup, or mixed with fine sugar.

In the absolutely fresh state, both English and American Arums are violent irritants to the mucous membrane, producing when chewed, intense burning to the mouth and throat, and if taken internally, causing violent gastro-enteritis, which may end in death.

Dose. Powdered root 10 to 30 grains.

The ITALIAN ARUM drug of Southern Europe is derived from the Mediterranean

A. Italicum (Mill.), which is found also in the Isle of Wight. It has the same poisonous properties.

That of Asia Minor, with similar properties, is *A. dioscorides*, Sib.

In *A. Italicum* and some of the other species, the spadix which supports the flowers disengages a quantity of heat, sufficient to be felt by the hand that touches it. Lamarck mentions an extraordinary degree of heat evolved by *A. maculatum* about the time when the sheath is about to open.

The DRAGON ARUM of the ancients was probably *Amorphophallus campanulatus* (Pol.) of the East Indies, whose corm-like rhizome gives rise yearly to one enormous leaf and an equally gigantic inflorescence. Its dirty red and yellow colour and fœtid smell attract numbers of carrion flies, by which it is fertilized; they are often so deceived as to lay their eggs on the spadix.

The Arrow poison, *Maschi*, of Guiana, is supposed to come from a species of Arum.

On account of their starch, the rhizomes and tubers of many other species of this family are used as foods, or the starches are extracted. Even those which are poisonous may be thus employed, since cooking usually destroys their toxicity.

The most important, edible product is the corm of *Calocasia antiquorum* (Schott) (syn. *Caladium*, or *A. esculentum*, Linn.), Taro, which is one of the most largely used of tropical foods. Other species are similarly used. It abounds in starch and is much used as an article of food by the natives of Hawaii and other Pacific Islands. In the natural state, both the foliage and roots of Taro have all the pungent acrid qualities that mark the genus to which the plant belongs, but these are so dissipated by cooking that they become mild and palatable with no peculiar flavour more than belongs to good bread. The islanders bake the root in ovens in the same way as Bread Fruit, then beat it into a mass like dough, called *Poe*.

In India, a liniment is made of the root of *Calocasia macrorhiza* and Gingilie oil, and used by the native practitioners for frictions to cure intermittent fevers.

In South America, *A. Indicum*, the *Mankuchoo* and *Manguri* of Brazil, is much cultivated about the huts of the natives for its esculent stem and pendulous tubers.

Arum Arrowroot is derived from *A. Dracunculus* (Linn.), being something like Tapioca.

The root of *A. montanum* is used in India to poison tigers. The roots of *A. lyratum* furnish an article of diet to the natives of the Circar mountains. They require, however,

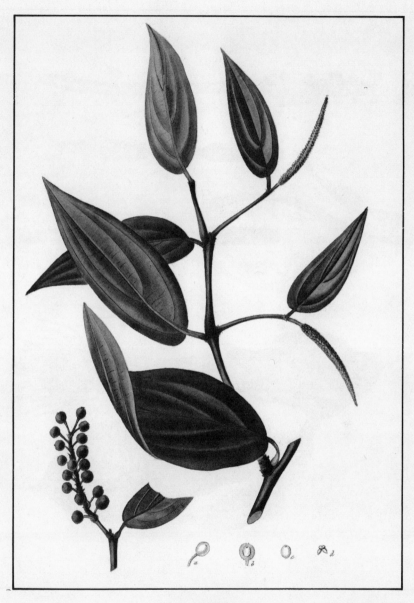

CUBEBS
Piper Cubeba

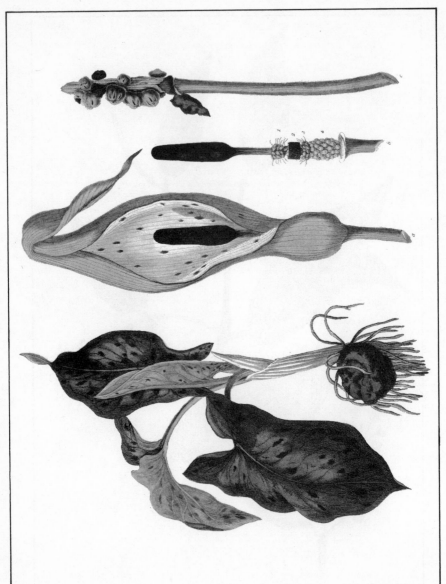

CUCKOO-PINT
Arum Maculatum

to be carefully boiled several times, and dressed in a particular manner, to divest them of a somewhat disagreeable taste.

A. Dracunculus is sometimes cultivated in gardens for the sake of its large pedate leaves, its spotted stem and handsome purple spadix. It is well, however, to advise those

intending to add this plant to their gardens that though its lurid and striking spadix forms a handsome feature in a border yet its odour is decidedly strong and unpleasant, resembling that of putrid meat, a fact which is evidently perceived by insects who swarm to it, especially in hot weather.

CUCUMBER

Cucumis sativa (LINN.)
N.O. Cucurbitaceæ

Synonym. Cowcumber
Part Used. The whole fruit peeled and unpeeled, raw and cooked
Habitat. Native of East Indies. First cultivated in Britain about 1573

¶ *Description.* In the East this trailing annual plant has been extensively cultivated from some 3,000 years and spread westward. It was known to the Greeks (the Greek name being *sikuos*) and to the Romans. According to Pliny, the Emperor Tiberius had it on his table daily, summer and winter. Pliny describes the Italian fruit as very small, probably like our gherkin; the same form is figured in Herbals of the sixteenth century, but states, 'if hung in a tube while in blossom, the Cucumber will grow to a most surprising length.' In Bible history, the Israelites in the wilderness complained to Moses that they missed the luxuries they had in Egypt, 'Cucumbers and Melons,' and Hasselquist in his travels (middle of eighteenth century) states: 'they still form a great part of the food of the lower-class people in Egypt, serving them for meat, drink and physic.' Isaiah, speaking of the desolation of Judah, says: 'The daughter of Zion is left as a cottage in a vineyard, as a lodge in a garden of cucumbers.' The Cucumber of the Scriptures is, however, by some authorities considered to be a wild form of *Cucumis melo*, the melon.

The Cucumber has been long known in England, where it was common in the time of Edward III (1327), then fell into disuse and was forgotten till the reign of Henry VIII, but not generally cultivated here till the middle of the seventeenth century. It is too well known to need description.

¶ *Constituents.* The dietary value of Cucumber is negligible, there being upwards of 96 per cent. water in its composition.

¶ *Medicinal Action and Uses.* Cucumber *seeds* possess similar properties to those of the allied Pumpkin (*Cucurbita Pepo*, Linn.), which are distinctly diuretic, but mainly employed as a very efficient tæniacide, 1 to 2 oz. of the seed, thoroughly ground and made into an electuary with sugar, or into an emetic with water, being taken fasting, followed in from 1 to 2 hours by an active purge. The resin has been given in doses of 15 grains.

Cucumber seeds are much smaller than Pumpkin seeds, relatively narrower and thicker and with almost no marginal groove. The emulsion made by bruising Cucumber seeds and rubbing them up with water was formerly thought to possess considerable virtue and was much used in catarrhal affections and diseases of the bowels and urinary passages.

As a cosmetic, Cucumber is excellent for rubbing over the skin to keep it soft and white. It is cooling, healing and soothing to an irritated skin, whether caused by sun, or the effects of a cutaneous eruption, and Cucumber juice is in great demand in various forms as a cooling and beautifying agent for the skin. Cucumber soap is used by many women, and a Cucumber wash applied to the skin after exposure to keen winds is extremely beneficial. This lotion is made as follows:

Cucumber Lotion

Peel 1 or 2 large Cucumbers, cut them into slices, and place them in a double boiler, which should be closely covered. Cook them slowly until they are soft. Then put the pieces into a fine linen bag and squeeze them until all the juice has been extracted. Add to the extracted juice one-fourth of rectified spirits of wine (or whisky) and one-third of Elder-flower water. Shake the mixture well and pour into small bottles ready for use.

Another Cucumber Lotion for Sunburn

Chop up a Cucumber and squeeze out the juice with a lemon-squeezer. Mix this with a quantity of glycerine and rose-water mixed together in equal parts.

Cucumber juice is used in the preparation of Glycerine and Cucumber creams. After expression and clarification, it is treated with alcohol, benzoin or salicylic acids being added as preservatives.

Emollient ointments prepared from the Cucumber were formerly considerably employed in irritated states of the skin, but they have been largely superseded by non-fatty cosmetics. The most frequently used preparation of Cucumber at the present time is the cosmetic preparation known as *Cucumber Jelly*, which is used as a soothing application in roughness of the skin, etc. It consists of a jelly of tragacanth, quince seeds or some similar mucilaginous drug, flavoured with Cucumber juice, which imparts to the preparation a characteristic odour.

The lotion sold in the shops as *Glycerine and Cucumber* sometimes contain Cucumber juice, but more frequently this is conspicuous by its absence.

The French make an ointment of Cucumber, using it like cold cream, called 'Pomade aux Concombres,' made with Cucumber juice, lard, veal suet, Balsam of Tolu in alcohol, and rose-water.

OTHER CUCUMBER OINTMENT RECIPES

1. Take 7 lb. green Cucumbers, 24 oz. pure lard and 15 oz. veal suet. Grate the washed Cucumbers to a pulp, express and strain the juice. Cut the suet into small pieces, heat over a water bath till melted, then add the lard and when melted, strain through muslin into an earthen vessel capable of holding a gallon and stir until thickening commences, when one-third of the juice is to be added and the whole beaten with a spatula till the odour has been almost wholly extracted. Decant the portion which separates, then add, consecutively, the remaining two-thirds of the juice and decant similarly. Then close the jar closely and place in a water bath till the fatty matter entirely separates from the juice. The green coagulum floating on the surface is now removed and the jar put in a cool place that the ointment may solidify. Then separate the crude ointment from the liquid on which it floats, melt again, strain and put up in closely-sealed glass jars. A layer of rose-water on its surface will aid preservation.

2. Incorporate 1 part of distilled Spirit of Cucumbers with 7 parts of benzoinated lard. The spirit is made by distilling a mixture of 1 part of grated Cucumbers with 3 parts of diluted alcohol, returning the first 2 parts or distillates which come over. This spirit is permanent and ointment or cream made from it keeps well.

Cucumber Milk is made of the following ingredients: 1 oz. soap, 1 oz. olive oil, 1 oz. wax, 1 oz. spermaceti, 1 lb. almonds, 4½ pints freshly expressed Cucumber juice, 1 pint extract of Cucumber, 2 lb. alcohol.

¶ *Use in Perfumery.* The peculiarly refreshing odour of Cucumber has found application in perfumery. Various products belonging under this head requiring the odour of Cucumber – it being used in blending certain bouquet perfumes – this plant is to be included among the aromatic plant in a wider sense.

Extract of Cucumber may be prepared as follows:

To 8 lb. Cucumbers, take 5 quarts of alcohol. The Cucumbers are peeled, cut into thin slices and macerated in the warm alcohol. If the odour is not strong enough in the alcohol after some days, it is poured over some more fresh slices, the macerated residue is expressed and at the end of the operation all the liquors are united and filtered.

Concentrated Cucumber perfume is made by the repeated extraction of the freshly sliced fruit with strong alcohol and subsequent concentration by distillation in vacuo. It is naturally very expensive.

¶ *Other Species.*

The SIKKIM CUCUMBER (*C. sativa*, var. *sikkimensis*) is a large-fruited form, reaching 15 inches long by 6 inches thick, grown in the Himalayas. The fruit, produced abundantly, is reddish brown, marked with yellow and is eaten both raw and cooked.

The WEST INDIAN GHERKIN is *C. anguria*, a plant with slender vines and very abundant, small, egg-shaped green fruit, covered with warts and prickles. It is the principal ingredient in West Indian pickles and is also used there in soups and frequently eaten green, but is far inferior to the common Cucumber.

C. flexuosum is the SNAKE CUCUMBER: it grows to a great length and may be used either raw or pickled.

The Squirting Cucumber, *Ecballium Elaterium*, furnishes the drug Elaterium.

The fruits of *C. trigonis* (Roxb.), 'Karit,' *C. Hardwickii*, Royle (the Hill Colocynth of India), and *C. prophetarum* (Linn.) of Arabia (the last-named containing the bitter substance *prophetin*, which occurs also in Elaterium) are largely employed as purgatives.

A less bitter variety of Karit is said to be eaten after the removal of its bitter principle by maceration in water.

C. myriocarpus (Naud.), a small gourd of South Africa, is used by the Kaffirs as an emetic in the form of the fruit-pulp, 20 grains being found to produce nausea and purgation after several hours. Larger quantities produce vomiting with some blood and considerable salivation. Its active principle has been called Myriocarpin.

The INDIAN CUCUMBER, or Cucumber Root, is the rhizome of *Medeola virginiana*

(Linn.) a member of the order *Liliaceæ*, reputed to be hydragogue and diuretic and therefore used in dropsies. In its fresh state it is somewhat Cucumber-like in taste.

The Bitter Cucumber is another name for Colocynth (*Citrullus colocynthis*, Schrader).

The Cucumber Tree, so called from the resemblance of the young fruits to small cucumbers, is *Magnolia virginiana*, var. *acuminata* (Linn.), the Mountain Magnolia. It has shortly acuminate leaves and yellowish-green flowers, 3 to 4 inches across, with a peculiar bluish tinge. The wood of the tree is yellow and is used for bowls. The bark was formerly official, with that of other species of Magnolia, in the United States Pharmacopœia, employed for its tonic, stimulant and diaphoretic properties and, like other bitters, employed in the treatment of malarial fever and considered a valuable remedy for rheumatism. Dose of the recently-dried bark is ½ to 1 drachm, frequently repeated; of the tincture, 1 fluid drachm.

CUCUMBER, SQUIRTING

Echallium Elaterium
N.O. Cucurbitaceæ

Synonyms. Momordica Elaterium. Wild Cucumber
Habitat. Europe, cultivated in Britain

¶ *Description.* A perennial plant but in Britain an annual, with a large fleshy root from which rise several round, thick stems, branching and trailing like the Common Cucumber but without tendrils; leaves heart-shaped, rough; flower-stalks auxillary; male flowers in clusters with bell-shaped, yellow green veined corollas, females solitary; fruit a small elliptical greenish gourd covered with soft triangular prickles. The fruits forcibly eject their seeds together with a mucilaginous juice, a phenomenon due to endormosis. The plant flowers in July. The fruit is collected just before it ripens and is left until it matures and ejects the seeds and juice; this must not be artificially hastened or the product will be injured; the juice is then dried in flakes and sent to the market as Elaterium. The flakes often bear the impress of the muslin on which they were dried.

¶ *Constituents.* Elaterin; a green resin, starch, lignin, and saline matter.

¶ *Medicinal Action and Uses.* A powerful hydragogue cathartic, and in large doses excites nausea and vomiting. If administered too frequently it operates with great violence on both the stomach and bowels, producing inflammation and possibly fatal results. It also increases the flow of urine, and is of some use in the treatment of dropsy, especially when œdema is due to disease of the kidney. There is a case on record of a French doctor who suffered severely from carrying some of the seeds in his hat from the Jardin des Plante to his Paris lodging.

¶ *Preparations and Dosages.* It must be used with the greatest caution; because of its variability Elaterium should not be employed, preference always being given to the official Elaterin. Elaterium, $\frac{1}{16}$ to $\frac{1}{2}$ grain. Elacterin, $\frac{1}{40}$ to $\frac{1}{16}$ grain. Compound powder of Elacterin = Elaterin in fine powder, 1 part milk, sugar in fine powder 39 parts; dose, 1 to 4 grains.

¶ *Poisons and Antidotes.* As for Bitter Apple.

See (BITTER) APPLE.

CUDBEAR

Rocella tinctoria
N.O. Lichenes

Habitat. Maritime rocks of Madeira. The Azores, Canary and Cape de Verde Islands

Cudbear is a purplish-red powder prepared from a species of the *Rocella tinctoria*, *Lecanora Acharius* and other lichens. It is an alcoholic or agueous preparation of a deep red colour, which is lightened by the addition of acids and changed to a purplish red by alkalies. It yields about 35 per cent. of ash, mostly sodium chloride.

¶ *Action and Uses.* Employed for colouring purposes as a dye. Cudbear is very difficult to extract, so the liquid preparations are rarely uniform in colour, and for this reason powdered Cudbear is generally used. The powder is made from an ammoniacal infusion of the lichen evaporated to dryness and then reduced to powder. In pharmacy it is sometimes used as a test for alkalies and acids.

R. tinctoria is the lichen from which Litmus is obtained. The lichen is boiled with water, containing chalk in suspension, and then concentrated in vacuum; it is then dried, freed from impurities and put in large vats together with the liquor and ammonia. It is kept at 25° to 30° F. for two or three months and then dried and powdered.

CUDWEED
Graphalium uliginosum
N.O. Compositæ

Synonyms. Cotton Weed. March Everlasting
Part Used. Herb
Habitat. Marshy places in most parts of Europe

¶ *Description.* Stalk branched, diffused; flowers crowded, termina tiny; leaves elliptical, tapering into a long foot-stalk, slightly downy and greenish above, whitish and more downy underneath. The ends of the branches crowded with numerous heads of nearly sessile flowers which appear in August.

¶ *Medicinal Action and Uses.* Quinsy, gargle astringent, infusion 1 oz. to 1 pint boiling water taken internally in wineglassful; also used as a gargle.

Fluid extract: *Dose*, ½ to 1 drachm.

See CATSFOOT, EVERLASTING PLANT, GRAPHALIUM (WHITE) BALSAM.

CUMIN
Cuminum cyminum (LINN.)
N.O. Umbelliferæ

Synonym. Cumino aigro (Malta)
Part Used. Fruit
Habitat. Cumin, besides being used medicinally, was in the Middle Ages one of the commonest spice of European growth. It is a small annual, herbaceous plant, indigenous to Upper Egypt, but from early times was cultivated in Arabia, India, China, and in the countries bordering on the Mediterranean

¶ *Description.* Its stem is slender and branched, rarely exceeding 1 foot in height and somewhat angular. The leaves are divided into long, narrow segments like Fennel, but much smaller and are of a deep green colour, generally turned back at the ends. The upper leaves are nearly stalkless, but the lower ones have longer leaf-stalks. The flowers are small, rose-coloured or white, in stalked umbels with only four to six rays, each of which are only about ⅓ inch long, and bloom in June and July, being succeeded by fruit – the so-called seeds – which constitute the Cumin of pharmacy. They are oblong in shape, thicker in the middle, compressed laterally about ⅕ inch long, resembling Caraway seeds, but lighter in colour and bristly instead of smooth, almost straight, instead of being curved. They have nine fine ridges, overlapping as many oil channels, or *vittæ*. The odour and taste are somewhat like caraway, but less agreeable.

¶ *History.* Cumin is mentioned in Isaiah xxviii. 25 and 27, and Matthew xxiii. 23, and in the works of Hippocrates and Dioscorides. From Pliny we learn that the ancients took the ground seed medicinally with bread, water or wine, and that it was accounted the best of condiments. The seeds of the Cumin when smoked, were found to occasion pallor of the face, whence the expression of Horace, *exsangue cuminum*, and Pliny tells us that the followers of the celebrated rhetorician Porcius Latro employed it to produce a complexion such as bespeaks application to study.

Cumin also symbolized cupidity among the Greeks: Marcus Aurelius was so nicknamed because of his avarice, and misers were jocularly said to have eaten Cumin.

In the thirteenth and fourteenth centuries, when it was much in use as a culinary spice, its average price in England per lb. was 2*d.*, equivalent to 1*s.* 4*d.* at the present day.

Cumin has now gone out of use in European medicine, having been replaced by Caraway seed, which has a more agreeable flavour, but it is still used to some extent in India, in native medicine. Its principal employment is in veterinary medicine and as an ingredient in curry powder, for which purposes it is imported from Bombay and Calcutta, Morocco, Sicily and Malta. It is commonly sold in Malta, where they call it *cumino aigro* (hot Cumin), to distinguish it from Anise, which they term *cumino dulce*, or sweet Cumin.

¶ *Cultivation.* Although we get nearly all our supplies from the Mediterranean, it would be perfectly feasible to grow Cumin in England, as it will ripen its fruit as far north as Norway. It is, however, rarely cultivated here, and seeds are generally somewhat difficult to obtain.

They should be sown in small pots, filled with light soil and plunged into a very moderate hot bed to bring up the plants. These should be hardened gradually in an open frame and transplanted into a warm border of good soil, preserving the balls of earth which adhere to the roots in the pots. Keep clean of weeds and the plants will flower very well and will probably perfect their seeds if the season should be warm and favourable.

The plants are threshed when the fruit is ripe and the 'seeds' dried in the same manner as Caraway.

¶ *Constituents.* The strong aromatic smell and warm, bitterish taste of Cumin fruits are due to the presence of a volatile oil which is separated by distillation of the fruit with water, and exists in the proportion of 2 to 4 per cent. It is limpid and pale yellow in colour, and is mainly a mixture of cymol or cymene and cuminic aldehyde, or cyminol, which is its chief constituent.

The tissue of the fruits contains a fatty oil with resin, mucilage and gum, malates and albuminous matter, and in the outer-seed coat there is much tannin. The yield of ash is about 8 per cent.

¶ *Medicinal Action and Uses.* Stimulant, antispasmodic, carminative. The older herbalists esteemed Cumin superior in comforting carminative qualities to Fennel or Caraway, but on account of its very disagreeable flavour, its medicinal use at the present day is almost confined to veterinary practice, in which it is employed as a carminative.

Formerly Cumin had considerable repute as a corrective for the flatulency of languid digestion and as a remedy for colic and dyspetic headache. Bruised and applied externally in the form of a plaster, it was recommended as a cure for stitches and pains in the side caused by the sluggish congestion of indolent parts, and it has been compounded with other drugs to form a stimulating liniment.

Bay-salt and Cumin-seeds mixed, is a universal remedy for the diseases of pigeons, especially scabby backs and breasts. The proportions of the remedy are: ¼ lb. Bay-salt, ¼ lb. Common Salt, 1 lb. Fennel-seeds, 1 lb. Dill-seeds, 1 lb. Cumin-seeds, 1 oz. Assafœtida; mix all with a little wheaten flour and some fine-worked clay; when all are well beaten together, put into two earthen pots and bake them in the oven. When cold, put them on the table in the dove-cote; the pigeons will eat it and thus be cured.

CUP MOSS. *See* MOSS

CUP PLANT

Silphium perfoliatum
N.O. Compositæ

Synonyms. Indian Cup Plant. Ragged Cup
Part Used. Root
Habitat. Western States of America, Oregon, Texas

¶ *Description.* The chief features of the genus are the monæcious radiate heads, the ray florets strap-shaped and pistil bearing, the disc florets tubular and sterile, and the broad flat achenes, surrounded by a wing notched at the summit and usually terminating in two short awn-like teeth which represent the pappus. Its distinctive character is rhizome, cylindrical, crooked, rough, small roots, and transversed section shows large resin cells. Taste, persistent, acrid. The most interesting of the species is the Compass plant, so named from its tendency to point to the North. This plant is also known by the names of Pilot plant, Polar plant, Rosin and Turpentine weed, and like the Cup plant of another species, *Silphium Læve*, with tuberous roots, which are a native food in the Columbia valley, is cultivated in English gardens. The Cup plant derives its name from the cup-like appearance of the winged stalks of its opposite leaves which are united.

¶ *Medicinal Action and Uses.* Tonic, diaphoretic, alterative. Found useful in liver and spleen maladies, also in fevers, internal bruises, debility, ulcers, and a general alterative restorative. Gum is a stimulant and antispasmodic.

¶ *Dose.* 4 oz. of powdered root in decoction. Powder itself in 20-grain doses.

¶ *Other Species.*
S. Ginniferum or Rosin weed is said to be stimulating and antispasmodic, and yields resinous secretions like mastic; this resin is diuretic and imparts to the urine an aromatic odour. Its root is a good expectorant in pulmonary and catarrhal diseases and the Compass plant is said to be emetic.

See ROSIN WEED

CURARE. *See* NUX VOMICA

CURRANT, BLACK

Ribes nigrum (LINN.)
N.O. Saxifragaceæ

Synonyms. Quinsy Berries. Squinancy Berries
Parts Used. Fruit, leaves, bark, roots
Habitat. Europe

¶ *Description.* The Black Currant is occasionally found wild in damp woods as far north as the middle of Scotland, but is considered to be a true native only in Yorkshire and the Lake District – when found apparently wild in other parts of the country, its presence is due to the agency of birds. It is easily distinguished at all seasons by the strong perfume of its buds and leaves.

This shrub shows the only instance of a process by which double flowers may become single, by changing petals into stamina. It has a solitary, one-flowered peduncle at the base of the raceme, and its leaves are dotted underneath.

It was not so popular originally as the Red and White Currants, for Gerard describes the fruit as being 'of a stinking and somewhat loathing savour.'

The berries are sometimes put into brandy like Black Cherries. The Russians make wine of them, with or without honey or spirits, while in Siberia a drink is made of the leaves, which, when young, make common spirits resemble brandy. An infusion of them is like green tea, and can change the flavour of black tea. Goats eat the leaves, and bears especially like the berries, which are supposed to have medicinal properties not possessed by others of the genus.

¶ *Medicinal Uses.* Diuretic, diaphoretic, febrifuge.

The *juice* can be boiled to an extract with sugar, when it is called *Rob*, and is used for inflammatory sore throats. Excellent lozenges are also prepared from it.

The infusion of the *leaves* is cleansing and diuretic, while an infusion of the *young roots* is useful in eruptive fevers and the dysenteric fevers of cattle.

The *raw juice* is diuretic and diaphoretic, and is an excellent beverage in febrile diseases.

A *decoction of the bark* has been found of value in calculus, dropsy, and hæmorrhoidal tumours.

RECIPES

Black Currant Jelly

is deservedly prized for its usefulness in colds and is both laxative and cooling. It should not be made with too much sugar or its medicinal properties will be impaired. For a sore throat, take a tablespoonful of the jam or jelly; put it in a tumbler and fill the tumbler with boiling water. This 'Black Currant Tea' has a soothing, demulcent effect, taken several times in the day and drunk while hot.

A delicious *wine* can be made from the fruit. The following is a recipe from an old Cookery Book:

Black Currant Wine, very fine

To every 3 quarts of juice, put the same of water, unboiled; and to every 3 quarts of the liquor, add 3 lb. of very pure, moist sugar. Put it in a cask, preserving a little for filling up. Put the cask in a warm, dry room, and the liquor will ferment itself. Skim off the refuse, when the fermentation shall be over, and fill up with the reserved liquor. When it has ceased working, pour 3 quarts of brandy to 40 quarts of wine. Bung it close for nine months, then bottle it and drain the thick part through a jelly-bag, until it be clear, and bottle that. Keep it ten or twelve months.

Black Currant Cheese

is delicious and is made by putting equal parts of stalked currants and loaf sugar into a pan; place over low heat and stir until the sugar has dissolved, then bring slowly to the boil, stirring all the time. Remove all scum and simmer for an hour, stirring often. Rub the fruit through a hair sieve, return the puree to the pan, and stir until it boils, then put it into small pots and cover like jam.

CURRANT, RED

Ribes rubrum (LINN.)
N.O. Grossulariaceæ

Synonyms. Ribs. Risp. Reps
Part Used. The fruits, especially the juice
Habitat. Central and Northern Europe, and United States, Siberia and Canada

¶ *Description.* This plant is equally at home in hedges and ditches, trained against the wall of a house, or as a shrub cultivated in gardens. It has straggling stems, three to five lobed leaves, yellowish-green flowers, and fruit in pendulous racemes. The smooth berries are always red in the wild state, but cultivation has added the white and champagne or flesh-coloured varieties. The White and Red Dutch Currants are regarded as the best. The English name was given because the berries were like the Corinth or Zante Grape, the currant of the shops. There are between thirty and forty kinds of currant recognized in catalogues. The fruit is a favourite for tarts and jellies, and being a very hardy plant, is within the reach of all. The juice is a pleasant acid in punch, and was a favourite ingredient in the coffee-houses of Paris, where the sweetened juice is still preferred as a beverage, to syrup of almonds.

¶ *Constituents.* The juice is said to contain citric acid, malic acid, sugar, vegetable jelly and jam.

¶ *Medicinal Action and Uses.* Refrigerant, aperient, antiscorbutic. The juice forms a refreshing drink in fever, and the jelly, made from equal weights of fruit and sugar, when eaten with 'high' meats, acts as an anti-putrescent. The wine made from white 'red' currants has been used for calculous affections.

In some cases the fruit causes flatulence and indigestion. It has frequently given much help in forms of visceral obstruction. The jelly is antiseptic, and will ease the pain of a burn and prevent the formation of blisters, if applied immediately. Some regard the leaves as having emmenagogue properties.

¶ *Poison and Antidotes*. In common with other acidulous fruits, they must be turned out of an open tin *immediately* into a glass or earthenware dish, or the action of the acid combining with the surrounding air will begin to engender a deadly metallic poison.

CYCLAMEN, IVY-LEAFED

Cyclamen hederæfolium
N.O. Primulaceæ

Synonym. Sowbread
Part Used. Tuberous root-stock used fresh when the plant is in flower

The Cyclamens at first glance do not appear to have much similarity with Primulas, but certain structural points in common have caused them to be grouped in the same family.

There are eight members of the genus, distributed over Southern Europe, North Africa and Western Asia, one of which, *Cyclamen hederæfolium*, the Ivy-leaved Cyclamen or Sowbread, has been occasionally found in Kent and Sussex, but is generally considered to have been introduced accidentally, being really a native of Italy. Its large, tuberous root-stock, in common with that of *C. Europæum* and of others found in the south of Europe, is intensely acrid, a quality that has caused its employment as a purgative.

¶ *Description*. It occurs rarely in hedge-banks and copses, flowering in September. The tuber, 1 to 3 inches in diameter, is turnip-shaped, brown in colour and fibrous all over. The nodding rose-coloured or white flowers, which appear before the leaves, are placed singly on fleshy stalks, 4 to 8 inches high. The corolla tube is short, thickened at the throat, the lobes are bent back and are about an inch in length and red at the base. As the fruit ripens, the flower-stalk curls spirally and buries it in the earth. The name of the genus is derived from the Greek *cyclos* (a circle), either from the reflexed lobes of the corolla, or from the spiral form of the fruit-stalk. The leaves, appearing after the flowers, are somewhat heart-shaped, five to nine angled, in the manner of ivy leaves, dark green, with a white mottled border, often purple beneath, and spring straight from the root on longish stalks or petioles. They continue growing all the winter and spring till May, when they begin to decay, and in June are entirely dried up.

The apparently inappropriate name of this beautiful little plant, Sowbread, arises from its tuberous roots having afforded food for wild swine.

The favourite greenhouse Cyclamens, flowering in the winter months, are varieties of a Persian species, *C. Perscum*, introduced into European horticulture in the middle of the eighteenth century.

¶ *Part Used Medicinally*. The tuberous root-stock, used fresh, when the plant is in flower.

¶ *Constituents*. Besides starch, gum and pectin, the tuber yields chemically cyclamin or arthanatin, having an action like saponin.

¶ *Medicinal Action and Uses*. A homœopathic tincture is made from the fresh root, which applied externally as a liniment over the bowels causes purging.

Old writers tell us that Sowbread baked and made into little flat cakes has the reputation of being 'a good amorous medicine,' causing the partaker to fall violently in love.

Although the roots are favourite food of swine, their juice is stated to be poisonous to fish.

Powdered root: dose, 20 to 40 grains.

The fresh tubers bruised and formed into a cataplasm make a stimulating application to indolent ulcers.

An ointment called 'ointment of arthainta' was made from the fresh tubers for expelling worms, and was rubbed on the umbilicus of children and on the abdomen of adults to cause emesis and upon the region over the bladder to increase urinary discharge.

DAFFODIL

Narcissus Pseudo-narcissus
N.O. Amaryllidaceæ

Synonyms. Narcissus. Porillon. Daffy-down-dilly. Fleur de coucou. Lent Lily
Parts Used. Bulb, leaves, flowers
Habitat. Europe, including Britain

¶ *Description*. The Common Daffodil, a representative of the Ajax group, grows wild in most European countries. Its green, linear leaves about a foot long, and golden, terminal flowers, are familiar in moist woods and country gardens.

The bulbs should be gathered during the winter, and the flowers when in full bloom, in dry weather, and dried quickly. The bulbs and not the flowers of other species are used.

¶ *Constituents.* Professor Barger has given the following notes on the alkaloid of *Narcissus Pseudo-narcissus.* 'In 1910 Ewins obtained from the bulbs a crystalline alkaloid, to which he gave the name of *narcissine,* and on analysis found the formula to be $C16H17ON$.' He notes that the alkaloid is characterized by great stability and cannot easily be decomposed. Ringer and Morshead found the alkaloid from resting bulbs acted like pilocarpine, while that from the flowering bulbs resembled atropine. Laidlaw tested Ewins' alkaloid on frogs and cats, but found no action similar to pilocarpine or atropine. 0·125 gram given by mouth to a cat caused vomiting, salivation and purgation. In 1920 Asahtna, Professor of Chemistry in the Tokyo College of Pharmacy, showed that narcissine is identical with lycorine isolated from *Lycoris radiata¸* in 1899. The name narcissine has therefore been dropped. Lycorine is quite common in the N.O. Amaryllidaceæ. It was found in *Buphane disticha* by Tutin in the Mellome Research Laboratory in 1911 (*Journ. Chem. Soc. Transactions* 99, page 1,240). It is generally present in quite small quantities, at most 0·1 to 0·18 per cent. of the fresh material. Chemically, lycorine or narcissine has some resemblance to hydrastine, and like it, contains a dioxymethylene group.

¶ *Medicinal Action and Uses.* The following is a quotation from Culpepper:

'Yellow Daffodils are under the dominion of Mars, and the roots thereof are hot and dry in the third degree. The roots boiled and taken in posset drink cause vomiting and are used with good success at the appearance of approaching agues, especially the tertian ague, which is frequently caught in the springtime. A plaster made of the roots with parched barley meal dissolves hard swellings and imposthumes, being applied thereto; the juice mingled with honey, frankincense, wine, and myrrh, and dropped into the ears is good against the corrupt and running matter of the ears; the roots made hollow and boiled in oil help raw ribed heels; the juice of the root is good for the morphew and the discolouring of the skin.'

It is said by Galen to have astringent properties. It has been used as an application to wounds. For hard imposthumes, for burns, for strained sinews, stiff or painful joints, and other local ailments, and for 'drawing forth thorns or stubs from any part of the body' it was highly esteemed.

The Daffodil was the basis of an ancient ointment called Narcissimum.

The powdered flowers have been used as an emetic in place of the bulbs, and in the form of infusion or syrup, in pulmonary catarrh.

¶ *Dosages.* Of powder, from 20 grains to 2 drachms as an emetic. Of extract, 2 to 3 grains.

¶ *Poison and Antidotes.* It may be noted that Henry states that lycorine or narcissine in warm-blooded animals acts as an emetic, causing eventually collapse and death by paralysis of the central nervous system.

There have been several cases of poisoning by Daffodil bulbs which have been eaten in mistake for onions. In one case the points observed were: (1) the speedy action of the poison; (2) the fact that the high temperature did not destroy the toxicity of the poison; and (3) the relatively small quantity of Daffodil bulbs which caused the trouble.

¶ *Other Species.*
The bulbs of *N. poeticus, N. odorus,* and *N. jonquilla* possess similar acrid and emetic properties.

See NARCISSUS.

DAHLIAS

Dahlia Variabilis
N.O. Compositæ

Synonym. Georgina

The Dahlia is named after Dr. Dahl, a pupil of Linnæus, but is also known, especially on the Continent, by the name 'Georgina.' It is a native of Mexico, where it grows in sandy meadows at an elevation of 5,000 feet above the sea, and from whence the first plants introduced to England were brought by way of Madrid, in 1789, by the Marchioness of Bute. These having been lost, others were introduced, in 1804, by Lady Holland. These, too, perished, so fresh ones were obtained from France, when the Continent was thrown open by the Peace of 1814.

¶ *Constituents.* The Inulin obtained in Dandelion and Chicory is also present in Dahlia tubers under the name of Dahlin. After undergoing a special treatment, Dahlia tubers and Chicory will yield the pure Lævulose that is sometimes called Atlanta Starch or Diabetic Sugar, which is frequently prescribed for diabetic and consumptive patients, and has been given to children in cases of wasting illness.

There was a very considerable business done in this product before the War by certain German firms. In a paper read at the Second International Congress of the Sugar Industry, held at Paris in 1908, it was stated that pure Lævulose is preferably made by the inversion of Inulin with dilute acids, and that the older process of preparation from invert sugar or molasses does not yield a pure product. The first step in the technical production of Lævulose is in the preparation of Inulin, and Dahlia tubers or Chicory root, which contain 6 to 12 per cent. of Inulin are the most suitable material. Chicory root can readily be obtained in quantity, and Dahlia plants, if cultivated for the purpose, should yield in a few years a plentiful supply of cheap raw material.

For extraction of the Inulin, the roots or tubers are sliced, treated with milk of lime and steamed. The juice is then expressed and clarified by subsidence and filtration, the clear liquid being run into a revolving cooler until flakes are produced. These flakes are separated by a centrifugal machine, washed and decolorized, and the thus purified product finally treated with diluted acid, and so converted into Lævulose. This solution of Lævulose is neutralized and evaporated to a syrup in a vacuum pan.

Lævulose can be produced in this manner from Chicory roots and Dahlia tubers at an enormous reduction of price from the older methods of preparing it from molasses or sugar, the resultant product being moreover of absolute purity. Its sweet and pleasant taste are likely to make it used not only for diabetic patients, but also in making confectionery and for retarding crystallization of sugar products. It can also readily be utilized in the brewing and mineral water industries.

The research staff of one of the Scottish Universities during the War developed a process of extracting a valuable and much needed drug for the Army from Dahlia tubers, and was using as much material for the purpose as could be spared by growers.

DAISY, COMMON

Bellis perennis (LINN.)
N.O. Compositæ

Synonyms. Bruisewort. (*Scotch*) Bairnwort. (*Welsh*) Llygad y Dydd (Eye of the Day)
Parts Used. Root, leaves

The Common Daisy, which flowers from the earliest days of spring till late in the autumn, and covers the ground with its flat leaves so closely that nothing can grow beneath them, needs no detailed description.

It had once, in common with the Ox-Eye Daisy, a great reputation as a cure for fresh wounds, used as an ointment applied externally, and against inflammatory disorders of the liver, taken internally in the form of a distilled water of the plant.

The flowers and leaves are found to afford a certain amount of oil and ammoniacal salts.

Gerard mentions the Daisy, under the name of 'Bruisewort,' as an unfailing remedy in 'all kinds of paines and aches,' besides curing fevers, inflammation of the liver and 'alle the inwarde parts.'

In 1771 Dr. Hill said that an infusion of the leaves was 'excellent against Hectic Fevers.' The Daisy was an ingredient of an ointment much used in the fourteenth century for wounds, gout and fevers.

A strong decoction of the roots has been recommended as an excellent medicine in scorbutic complaints, it being stated, however, that the use of it must be continued for a considerable length of time before its effects will appear.

The taste of the leaves is somewhat acrid, notwithstanding which it has been used in some countries as a pot-herb. On account of the acrid juice contained in the leaves, no cattle will touch it, nor insects attack it.

The roots, too, have a penetrating pungency, containing some tannic acid, and there was once a popular superstition (to which Bacon refers) that if they be boiled in milk and the liquid given to puppies, the animals will grow no bigger.

According to some old writers, the generic name is derived from the Latin *bellus* (pretty or charming), though others say its name is from a dryad named Belidis. The common name is a corruption of the old English name 'day's-eye,' and is used by Chaucer in that sense:

'Well by reason men it call maie
The Daisie, or else the Eye of the Daie.'

In Scotland it is the 'Bairnwort,' testifying to the joy of children in gathering it for daisy-chains.

There is a common proverb associated with the flower and its abundance in spring and early summer: 'When you can put your foot on *seven* daisies summer is come.'

DAISY, OX-EYE

Chrysanthemum leucanthemum (LINN.)
N.O. Compositæ

Synonyms. Great Ox-eye. Goldens. Marguerite. Moon Daisy. Horse Gowan. Maudlin Daisy. Field Daisy. Dun Daisy. Butter Daisy. Horse Daisy. Maudlinwort. White Weed. Leucanthemum vulgare. (*Scotch*) Gowan

Parts Used. Whole herb, flowers, root

The Ox-Eye Daisy is a familiar sight in fields. In Somersetshire there is an old tradition connecting it with the Thunder God, and hence it is sometimes spoken of as the 'Dun Daisy.'

It is to be found throughout Europe and Russian Asia. The ancients dedicated it to Artemis, the goddess of women, considering it useful in women's complaints. In Christian days, it was transferred to St. Mary Magdalen and called Maudelyn or Maudlin Daisy after her. Gerard terms it Maudlinwort.

The genus derives its name from the Greek words *chrisos* (golden) and *anthos* (flower), and contains only two indigenous species, this and the Corn Marigold, in which the whole flower is yellow, not only the central disc of florets, as in the Daisy. The specific name of the Ox-Eye signifies 'white flower,' being like the generic name, Greek in origin. The old northern name for the Daisy was Baldur's Brow, and this, with many other species of Chrysanthemum became dedicated to St. John.

¶ *Description.* The plant generally grows from 1 to 2 feet high. The root is perennial and somewhat creeping; the stems, hard and wiry, furrowed and only very slightly branched. The leaves are small and coarsely toothed; those near the root are somewhat rounder in form than those on the stem, and are on long stalks, those on the stem are oblong and stalkless.

By the middle of May, the familiar yellow-centred white flower-heads commence to bloom, and are at their best till about the close of June, though isolated specimens may be met with throughout the summer, especially where undisturbed by the cutting of the hay, as on railway banks, where the plant flourishes well. Beneath each flower-head is a ring of green sheathing bracts, the involucre. These not only protect and support the bloom, but doubtless prevents insects trying to bite their way to the honey from below. They, as well as the rest of the plant, are permeated with an acrid juice that is obnoxious to insects.

The young leaves are said to be eaten in salads in Italy. According to Linnæus, horses, sheep and goats eat the plant, but cows and pigs refuse it on account of its acridity.

¶ *Part Used Medicinally.* The whole herb, collected in May and June, in the wild state, and dried. Also the flowers.

The taste of the dried herb is bitter and tingling, and the odour faintly resembles that of valerian.

¶ *Medicinal Action and Uses.* Antispasmodic, diuretic, tonic. Ox-Eye Daisy has been successfully employed in whooping-cough, asthma and nervous excitability.

As a tonic, it acts similarly to Chamomile flowers, and has been recommended for nightsweats. The flowers are balsamic and make a useful infusion for relieving chronic coughs and for bronchial catarrhs. Boiled with the leaves and stalks and sweetened with honey, they make an excellent drink for the same purpose. In America, the root is also employed successfully for checking the night-sweats of pulmonary consumption, the fluid extract being taken, 15 to 60 drops in water.

Externally, it is serviceable as a lotion for wounds, bruises, ulcers and some cutaneous diseases.

Gerard writes:

'Dioscorides saith that the floures of Oxeie made up in a seare cloth doe asswage and washe away cold hard swellings, and it is reported that if they be drunke by and by after bathing, they make them in a short time well-coloured that have been troubled with the yellow jaundice.'

Culpepper tells us that it is 'a wound herb of good respect, often used in those drinks and salves that are for wounds, either inward or outward' . . . and that it is 'very fitting to be kept both in oils, ointments, plasters and syrups.' He also tells us that the leaves bruised and applied reduce swellings, and that

'a decoction thereof, with wall-wort and agrimony, and places fomented or bathed therewith warm, giveth great ease in palsy, sciatica or gout. An ointment made thereof heals all wounds that have inflammation about them.'

Country people used formerly to take a decoction of the fresh herb in ale for the cure of jaundice.

DAMIANA

Turnera aphrodisiaca (WILLD.)
N.O. Turneraceæ

Part Used. Leaves
Habitat. Mexico, South America, Texas, West Indies

¶ *Description.* A small shrub; leaves smooth and pale green on upper side, underneath glabrous, with a few hairs on the ribs, ovo-lanceolate, shortly petiolate with two small glands at base; flowers yellow, rising singly from axils of the leaves; capsule one-celled, splitting into three pieces; smell aromatic; taste characteristic, bitterish, aromatic and resinous.

¶ *Constituents.* A greenish volatile oil, smelling like chamomile, amorphous bitter principle Damianin, resins and tannin.

¶ *Medicinal Action and Uses.* Mild purgative, diuretic, tonic, acting directly on the reproductive organs, stimulant, hypochondriastic, aphrodisiæ.

¶ *Preparations.* Fluid extract, ½ to 1 drachm. Solid extract, 5 to 10 grains. Often combined with Nux Vomica, Phosphorus, etc.

¶ *Other Species.*
Turnera opifera leaves are used as an infusion and given as an astringent and tonic by the natives of Brazil, also *T. ulmifolia* for its tonic and expectorant properties.

Aplopappus discoideus was formerly sold as Damiana, but can easily be detected, as the leaves are distinctly lanceolate, with only two or three teeth on either side.

DAMIANA, FALSE

Aplopappus laricifolius
N.O. Compositæ

Synonyms. Aplopappus. Bigelovia Veneta
Part Used. The leaves
Habitat. Chili

¶ *Description.* The U.S.D. refers to *Aplopappus discoideus* as False Damiana. Gray refers to it as Bigelovia Veneta.

¶ *Constituents.* A volatile oil, also a fatty oil which has the smell of the plant, brown acid, resin, tannin. The resin is peculiar in containing other resins.

¶ *Medicinal Action and Uses.* It is used as a stimulant in flatulent dyspepsia and chronic inflammation with hæmorrhage of the lower bowel. It is very useful in dysentery and in genito-urinary catarrh and as a stimulant expectorant; the tincture is useful for slowly healing ulcers.

¶ *Preparations and Dosages.* A strong decoction is made by 1 part to 5 of water. 1 tablespoonful as a dose every two hours. Dose of the fluid extract, 5 to 20 minims.

DAMSON. *See* BULLACE
DANDELION

Taraxacum officinale (WEBER)
N.O. Compositæ

Synonyms. Priest's Crown. Swine's Snout
Parts Used. Root, leaves

The Dandelion (*Taraxacum officinale*, Weber; *T. Densleonis*, Desf; *Leontodon taraxacum*, Linn.), though not occurring in the Southern Hemisphere, is at home in all parts of the north temperate zone, in pastures, meadows and on waste ground, and is so plentiful that farmers everywhere find it a troublesome weed, for though its flowers are more conspicuous in the earlier months of the summer, it may be found in bloom, and consequently also prolifically dispersing its seeds, almost throughout the year.

¶ *Description.* From its thick tap root, dark brown, almost black on the outside though white and milky within, the long jagged leaves rise directly, radiating from it to form a rosette lying close upon the ground, each leaf being grooved and constructed so that all the rain falling on it is conducted straight to the centre of the rosette and thus to the root, which is, therefore, always kept well watered. The maximum amount of water is in this manner directed towards the proper region for utilization by the root, which but for this arrangement would not obtain sufficient moisture, the leaves being spread too close to the ground for the water to penetrate.

The leaves are shiny and without hairs, the margin of each leaf cut into great jagged teeth, either upright or pointing somewhat backwards, and these teeth are themselves cut here and there into lesser teeth. It is this somewhat fanciful resemblance to the canine teeth of a lion that (it is generally assumed) gives the plant its most familiar name of Dandelion, which is a corruption of the French *Dent de Lion*, an equivalent of this name being found not only in its former specific Latin name *Dens leonis* and in the Greek name for the genus to which Linnæus assigned it, *Leontodon*, but also in nearly all the languages of Europe.

There is some doubt, however, as to whether it was really the shape of the leaves that provided the original notion, as there is really no similarity between them, but the leaves may perhaps be said to resemble the angular jaw of a lion fully supplied with teeth. Some authorities have suggested that the yellow flowers might be compared to the golden teeth of the heraldic lion, while others say that the whiteness of the root is the feature which provides the resemblance. Flückiger and Hanbury in *Pharmacographia*, say that the name was conferred by Wilhelm, a surgeon, who was so much impressed by the virtues of the plant that he likened it to *Dens leonis*. In the *Ortus Sanitatis*, 1485, under 'Dens Leonis,' there is a monograph of half a page (unaccompanied by any illustration) which concludes:

'The *Herb* was much employed by Master Wilhelmus, a surgeon, who on account of its virtues, likened it to "eynem lewen zan, genannt zu latin Dens leonis" (a lion's tooth, called in Latin *Dens leonis*).'

In the pictures of the old herbals, for instance, the one in Brunfels' *Contrafayt Kreuterbuch*, 1532, the *leaves* very much resemble a lion's tooth. The root is not illustrated at all in the old herbals, as only the herb was used at that time.

The name of the genus, *Taraxacum*, is derived from the Greek *taraxos* (disorder), and *akos* (remedy), on account of the curative action of the plant. A possible alternative derivation of *Taraxacum* is suggested in *The Treasury of Botany*:

'The generic name is possibly derived from the Greek *taraxo* ("I have excited" or "caused") and *achos* (pain), in allusion to the medicinal effects of the plant.'

There are many varieties of Dandelion leaves; some are deeply cut into segments, in others the segments or lobes form a much less conspicuous feature, and are sometimes almost entire.

¶ The shining, purplish flower-stalks rise straight from the root, are leafless, smooth and hollow and bear single heads of flowers. On picking the flowers, a bitter, milky juice exudes from the broken edges of the stem, which is present throughout the plant, and which when it comes into contact with the hand, turns to a brown stain that is rather difficult to remove.

Each bloom is made up of numerous strap-shaped florets of a bright golden yellow. This strap-shaped corolla is notched at the edge into five teeth, each tooth representing a petal, and lower down is narrowed into a claw-like tube, which rests on the single-chambered ovary containing a single ovule. In this tiny tube is a copious supply of nectar, which more than half fills it, and the presence of which provides the incentive for the visits of many insects, among whom the bee takes first rank. The Dandelion takes an important place among honey-producing plants, as it furnishes considerable quantities of both pollen and nectar in the early spring, when the bees' harvest from fruit trees is nearly over. It is also important from the bee-keeper's point of view, because not only does it flower most in spring, no matter how cool the weather may be, but a small succession of bloom is also kept up until late autumn, so that it is a source of honey after the main flowers have ceased to bloom, thus delaying the need for feeding the colonies of bees with artificial food.

Many little flies also are to be found visiting the Dandelion to drink the lavishly-supplied nectar. By carefully watching, it has been ascertained that no less than ninety-three different kinds of insects are in the habit of frequenting it. The stigma grows up through the tube formed by the anthers, pushing the pollen before it, and insects smearing themselves with this pollen carry it to the stigmas of other flowers already expanded, thus insuring cross-fertilization. At the base of each flower-head is a ring of narrow, green bracts – the involucre. Some of these stand up to support the florets, others hang down to form a barricade against such small insects as might crawl up the stem and injure the bloom without taking a share in its fertilization, as the winged insects do.

The blooms are very sensitive to weather conditions: in fine weather, all the parts are outstretched, but directly rain threatens, the whole head closes up at once. It closes against the dews of night, by five o'clock in the evening, being prepared for its night's sleep, opening again at seven in the morning, though as this opening and closing is largely dependent upon the intensity of the light, the time differs somewhat in different latitudes and at different seasons.

When the whole head has matured, all the florets close up again within the green, sheathing bracts that lie beneath, and the bloom returns very much to the appearance it had in the bud. Its shape being then somewhat reminiscent of the snout of a pig, it is termed in some districts 'Swine's Snout.' The withered, yellow petals are, however, soon pushed off in a bunch, as the seeds, crowned with their tufts of hair, mature, and one day, under the influence of sun and wind, the 'Swine's Snout' becomes a large gossamer ball, from its silky whiteness a very noticeable feature. It is made up of myriads of *plumed seeds* or *pappus*, ready to be blown off when quite ripe by the slightest breeze, and forms the 'clock' of the children, who by blowing at it till all the seeds are released, love to tell themselves the time of day by the number of puffs necessary to disperse every seed. When all the seeds have flown, the receptacle or disc on which they were placed remains bare, white, speckled and surrounded by merely the drooping remnants of the sheathing bracts, and we can see why the plant received another of its popular names, 'Priest's Crown,' common in the Middle Ages, when a priest's shorn head was a familiar object.

Small birds are very fond of the seeds of the Dandelion and pigs devour the whole plant greedily. Goats will eat it, but sheep and cattle do not care for it, though it is said to increase the milk of cows when eaten by them. Horses refuse to touch this plant, not appreciating its bitter juice. It is valuable food for rabbits and may be given them from April to September, forming excellent food in spring and at breeding seasons in particular.

The young leaves of the Dandelion make an agreeable and wholesome addition to spring salads and are often eaten on the Continent, especially in France. The full-grown leaves should not be taken, being too bitter, but the young leaves, especially if blanched, make an excellent salad, either alone or in combination with other plants, lettuce, shallot tops or chives.

Young Dandelion leaves make delicious sandwiches, the tender leaves being laid between slices of bread and butter and sprinkled with salt. The addition of a little lemon-juice and pepper varies the flavour. The leaves should always be torn to pieces, rather than cut, in order to keep the flavour.

John Evelyn, in his *Acetaria*, says: 'With thie homely salley, Hecate entertained Theseus.' In Wales, they grate or chop up Dandelion *roots*, two years old, and mix them with the leaves in salad. The seed of a special broad-leaved variety of Dandelion is sold by seedsmen for cultivation for salad purposes. Dandelion can be blanched in the same way as endive, and is then very delicate in flavour. If covered with an ordinary flower-pot during the winter, the pot being further buried under some rough stable litter, the young leaves sprout when there is a dearth of saladings and prove a welcome change in early spring. Cultivated thus, Dandelion is only pleasantly bitter, and if eaten while the leaves are quite young, the centre rib of the leaf is not at all unpleasant to the taste. When older, the rib is tough and not nice to eat. If the flower-buds of plants reserved in a corner of the garden for salad purposes are removed at once and the leaves carefully cut, the plants will last through the whole winter.

The young leaves may also be boiled as a vegetable, spinach fashion, thoroughly drained, sprinkled with pepper and salt, moistened with soup or butter and served very hot. If considered a little too bitter, use half spinach, but the Dandelion must be partly cooked first in this case, as it takes longer than spinach. As a variation, some grated nutmeg or garlic, a teaspoonful of chopped onion or grated lemon peel can be added to the greens when they are cooked. A simple vegetable soup may also be made with Dandelions.

The dried Dandelion leaves are also employed as an ingredient in many digestive or diet drinks and herb beers. Dandelion Beer is a rustic fermented drink common in many parts of the country and made also in Canada. Workmen in the furnaces and potteries of the industrial towns of the Midlands have frequent resource to many of the tonic Herb Beers, finding them cheaper and less intoxicating than ordinary beer, and Dandelion stout ranks as a favourite. An agreeable and wholesome fermented drink is made from Dandelions, Nettles and Yellow Dock.

In Berkshire and Worcestershire, the flowers are used in the preparation of a beverage known as Dandelion Wine. This is made by pouring a gallon of boiling water over a gallon of the flowers. After being well stirred, it is covered with a blanket and allowed to stand for three days, being stirred again at intervals, after which it is strained and the liquor boiled for 30 minutes, with the addition of $3\frac{1}{2}$ lb. of loaf sugar, a little ginger sliced, the rind of 1 orange and 1 lemon sliced. When cold, a little yeast is placed in it on a piece of toast, producing fermentation. It is then covered over and allowed to stand two days until it has ceased 'working,' when it is placed in a cask, well bunged down for two months before bottling. This wine is suggestive of sherry slightly flat, and has the deserved reputation of being an excellent tonic, extremely good for the blood.

The roasted roots are largely used to form Dandelion Coffee, being first thoroughly cleaned, then dried by artificial heat, and slightly roasted till they are the tint of coffee, when they are ground ready for use. The roots are taken up in the autumn, being then most fitted for this purpose. The prepared powder is said to be almost indistinguishable from real coffee, and is claimed to be an improvement to inferior coffee, which is often an adulterated product. Of late years, Dandelion Coffee has come more into use in this country, being obtainable at most vegetarian restaurants and stores. Formerly it used occasionally to be given for medicinal purposes, generally mixed with true coffee to give it a better flavour. The ground root was sometimes mixed with chocolate for a similar purpose. Dandelion Coffee is a natural beverage without any of the injurious effects that ordinary tea and coffee have on the nerves and digestive organs. It exercises a stimulating influence over the whole system, helping the liver and kidneys to do their work and keeping the bowels in a healthy condition, so that it offers great advantages to dyspeptics and does not cause wakefulness.

¶ *Parts Used Medicinally.* The root, fresh and dried, the young tops. All parts of the plant contain a somewhat bitter, milky juice (latex), but the juice of the root being still more powerful is the part of the plant most used for medicinal purposes.

¶ *History.* The first mention of the Dandelion as a medicine is in the works of the Arabian physicians of the tenth and eleventh centuries, who speak of it as a sort of wild Endive, under the name of *Taraxacon.* In this country, we find allusion to it in the Welsh medicines of the thirteenth century. Dandelion was much valued as a medicine in the times of Gerard and Parkinson, and is still extensively employed.

Dandelion roots have long been largely used on the Continent, and the plant is cultivated largely in India as a remedy for liver complaints.

The root is perennial and tapering, simple or more or less branched, attaining in a good soil a length of a foot or more and $\frac{1}{2}$ inch to an inch in diameter. Old roots divide at the crown into several heads. The root is fleshy and brittle, externally of a dark brown, internally white and abounding in an inodorous milky juice of bitter, but not disagreeable taste.

Only large, fleshy and well-formed roots should be collected, from plants *two* years old, not slender, forked ones. Roots produced in good soil are easier to dig up without breaking, and are thicker and less forked than those growing on waste places and by the roadside. Collectors should, therefore, only dig in good, free soil, in moisture and shade, from meadow-land. Dig up in wet weather, but not during frost, which materially lessens the activity of the roots. Avoid breaking the roots, using a long trowel or a fork, lifting steadily and carefully. Shake off as much of the earth as possible and then cleanse the roots, the easiest way being to leave them in a basket in a running stream so that the water covers them, for about an hour, or shake them, bunched, in a tank of clean water. Cut off the crowns of leaves, but be careful in so doing not to leave any scales on the top. Do not cut or slice the roots, or the valuable milky juice on which their medicinal value depends will be wasted by bleeding.

¶ *Cultivation.* As only large, well-formed roots are worth collecting, some people prefer to grow Dandelions as a crop, as by this means large roots are insured and they are more easily dug, generally being ploughed up. About 4 lb. of seed to the acre should be allowed, sown in drills, 1 foot apart. The crops should be kept clean by hoeing, and all flower-heads should be picked off as soon as they appear, as otherwise the grower's own land and that of his neighbours will be smothered with the weed when the seeds ripen. The yield should be 4 or 5 tons of fresh roots to the acre in the second year. Dandelion roots shrink very much in drying, losing about 76 per cent. of their weight, so that 100 parts of fresh roots yield only about 22 parts of dry material. Under favourable conditions, yields at the rate of 1,000 to 1,500 lb. of dry roots per acre have been obtained from second-year plants cultivated.

Dandelion root can only be economically collected when a meadow in which it is abundant is ploughed up. Under such circumstances the roots are necessarily of different ages and sizes, the seeds sowing themselves in successive years. The roots then collected, after washing and drying, have to be sorted into different grades. The largest, from the size of a lead pencil upwards, are cut into straight pieces 2 to 3 inches long, the smaller side roots being removed; these are sold at a higher price as the finest roots. The smaller roots fetch a less price, and the trimmings are generally cut small, sold at a lower price and used for making Dandelion Coffee. Every part of the root is thus used. The root before being dried should have every trace of the leaf-bases removed as their presence lessens the value of the root.

In collecting cultivated Dandelion advantage is obtained if the seeds are all sown at one time, as greater uniformity in the size of the root is obtainable, and in deep soil free from stones, the seedlings will produce elongated, straight roots with few branches, especially if allowed to be somewhat crowded, on the same principles that coppice trees produce straight trunks. Time is also saved in digging up the roots which can thus be sold at prices competing with those obtained as the result of cheaper labour on the Continent. The edges of fields when room is allowed for the plough-horses to turn, could easily be utilized if the soil is good and *free from stones* for both Dandelion and Burdock, as the roots are usually much branched in stony ground, and the roots are not generally collected until October when the harvest is over. The roots gathered in this month have stored up their food reserve of Inulin, and when dried present a firm appearance, whilst if collected in spring, when the food reserve in the root is used up for the leaves and flowers, the dried root then presents a shrivelled and porous appearance which renders it unsaleable. The medicinal properties of the root are, therefore, necessarily greater in proportion in the spring. Inulin being soluble in hot water, the solid extract if made by boiling the root, often contains a large quantity of it, which is deposited in the extract as it cools.

The roots are generally dried whole, but the largest ones may sometimes be cut transversely into pieces 3 to 6 inches long. Collected wild roots are, however, seldom large enough to necessitate cutting. Drying will probably take about a fortnight. When finished, the roots should be hard and brittle enough to snap, and the inside of the roots white, not grey.

The roots should be kept in a dry place after drying, to avoid mould, preferably in tins to prevent the attacks of moths and beetles. Dried Dandelion is exceedingly liable to the attacks of maggots and should not be kept beyond one season.

Dried Dandelion root is $\frac{1}{2}$ inch or less in thickness, dark brown, shrivelled, with wrinkles running lengthwise, often in a spiral direction; when quite dry, it breaks easily with a short, corky fracture, showing a very thick, white bark, surrounding a wooden column. The latter is yellowish, very porous, without pith or rays. A rather broad but indistinct cambium zone separates the wood from the bark, which latter exhibits numerous well-defined, concentric layers, due to the milk vessels. This structure is quite characteristic and serves to distinguish Dandelion roots from other roots like it. There are several flowers easily mistaken for the Dandelion when in blossom, but these have either *hairy* leaves or *branched* flower-stems, and the roots differ either in structure or shape.

Dried Dandelion root somewhat resembles Pellitory and Liquorice roots, but Pellitory differs in having oil glands and also a large radiate wood, and Liquorice has also a large radiate wood and a sweet taste.

The root of Hawkbit (*Leontodon hispidus*) is sometimes substituted for Dandelion root. It is a plant with hairy, not smooth leaves, and the fresh root is *tough*, breaking with difficulty and rarely exuding much milky juice. Some kinds of Dock have also been substituted, and also Chicory root. The latter is of a paler colour, more bitter and has the laticiferous vessels in radiating lines. In the United States it is often substituted for Dandelion. Dock roots have a prevailing yellowish colour and an astringent taste.

During recent years, a small form of a Dandelion root has been offered by Russian firms, who state that it is sold and used as Dandelion in that country. This root is always smaller than the root of *T. officinale*, has smaller flowers, and the crown of the root has often a tuft of brown woolly hairs between the leaf bases at the crown of the root, which are never seen in the Dandelion plant in this country, and form a characteristic distinction, for the root shows similar concentric, horny rings in the thick white bark as well as a yellow porous woody centre. These woolly hairs are mentioned in Greenish's *Materia Medica*, and also in the British Pharmaceutical Codex, as a feature of Dandelion root, but no mention is made of them in the *Pharmacographia*, nor in the British Pharmacopœia or United States Pharmacopœia, and it is probable, therefore, that Russian specimens have been used for describing the root, and that the root with brown woolly hairs belongs to some other species of *Taraxacum*.

¶ *Chemical Constituents.* The chief constituents of Dandelion root are Taraxacin, a crystalline, bitter substance, of which the yield varies in roots collected at different seasons, and Taraxacerin, an acrid resin, with Inulin (a sort of sugar which replaces starch in many of the Dandelion family, *Compositæ*), gluten, gum and potash. The root contains no starch, but early in the year contains much uncrystallizable sugar and lævulin, which differs from Inulin in being soluble in cold water. This diminishes in quantity during the summer and becomes Inulin in the autumn. The root may contain as much as 24 per cent. In the fresh root, the Inulin is present in the cell-sap, but in the dry root it occurs as an amorphodus, transparent solid, which is only slightly soluble in cold water, but soluble in hot water.

There is a difference of opinion as to the best time for collecting the roots. The British Pharmacopœia considers the autumn dug root more bitter than the spring root, and that as it contains about 25 per cent. insoluble Inulin, it is to be preferred on this account to the spring root, and it is, therefore, directed that in England the root should be collected between September and February, it being considered to be in perfection for Extract making in the month of November.

Bentley, on the other hand, contended that it is more bitter in March and most of all in July, but that as in the latter month it would generally be inconvenient for digging it, it should be dug in the spring, when the yield of Taraxacin, the bitter *soluble* principle, is greatest.

On account of the variability of the constituents of the plant according to the time of year when gathered, the yield and composition of the extract are very variable. If gathered from roots collected in autumn, the resulting product yields a turbid solution with water; if from spring-collected roots, the aqueous solution will be clear and yield but very little sediment on standing, because of the conversion of the Inulin into Lævulose and sugar at this active period of the plant's life.

In former days, Dandelion Juice was the favourite preparation both in official and domestic medicine. Provincial druggists sent their collectors for the roots and expressed the juice while these were quite fresh. Many country druggists prided themselves on their Dandelion Juice. The most active preparations of Dandelion, the Juice (*Succus Taraxaci*) and the Extract (*Extractum Taraxaci*), are made from the bruised fresh root. The Extract prepared from the fresh root is sometimes almost devoid of bitterness. The dried root alone was official in the United States Pharmacopœia.

The leaves are not often used, except for making Herb-Beer, but a medicinal tincture is sometimes made from the entire plant gathered in the early summer. It is made with proof spirit.

When collecting the seeds care should be taken when drying them in the sun, to cover them with coarse muslin, as otherwise the down will carry them away. They are best collected in the evening, towards sunset, or when the damp air has caused the heads to close up.

The tops should be cut on a dry day, when quite free of rain or dew, and all insect-eaten or stained leaves rejected.

¶ *Medicinal Action and Uses.* Diuretic, tonic and slightly aperient. It is a general stimulant to the system, but especially to the urinary organs, and is chiefly used in kidney and liver disorders.

Dandelion is not only official but is used in many patent medicines. Not being poisonous, quite big doses of its preparations may be taken. Its beneficial action is best obtained when combined with other agents.

The tincture made from the tops may be taken in doses of 10 to 15 drops in a spoonful of water, three times daily.

It is said that its use for liver complaints was assigned to the plant largely on the doctrine of signatures, because of its bright yellow flowers of a bilious hue.

In the hepatic complaints of persons long resident in warm climates, Dandelion is said to afford very marked relief. A broth of Dandelion roots, sliced and stewed in boiling water with some leaves of Sorrel and the yolk of an egg, taken daily for some months, has been known to cure seemingly intractable cases of chronic liver congestion.

A strong decoction is found serviceable in stone and gravel: the decoction may be made by boiling 1 pint of the sliced root in 20 parts of water for 15 minutes, straining this when cold and sweetening with brown sugar or honey. A small teacupful may be taken once or twice a day.

Dandelion is used as a bitter tonic in atonic dyspepsia, and as a mild laxative in habitual constipation. When the stomach is irritated and where active treatment would be injurious, the decoction or extract of Dandelion administered three or four times a day, will often prove a valuable remedy. It has a good effect in increasing the appetite and promoting digestion.

Dandelion combined with other active remedies has been used in cases of dropsy and for induration of the liver, and also on the Continent for phthisis and some cutaneous diseases. A decoction of 2 oz. of the herb or root in 1 quart of water, boiled down to a pint, is taken in doses of one wineglassful every three hours for scurvy, scrofula, eczema and all eruptions on the surface of the body.

¶ *Preparations and Dosages.* Fluid extract, B.P., ½ to 2 drachms. Solid extract, B.P., 5 to 15 grains. Juice, B.P., 1 to 2 drachms. Leontodin, 2 to 4 grains.

Dandelion Tea

Infuse 1 oz. of Dandelion in a pint of boiling water for 10 minutes; decant, sweeten with honey, and drink several glasses in the course of the day. The use of this tea is efficacious in bilious affections, and is also much approved of in the treatment of dropsy.

Or take 2 oz. of freshly-sliced Dandelion root, and boil in 2 pints of water until it comes to 1 pint; then add 1 oz. of compound tincture of Horseradish. Dose, from 2 to 4 oz. Use in a sluggish state of the liver.

Or 1 oz. Dandelion root, 1 oz. Black Horehound herb, ½ oz. Sweet Flag root, ¼ oz. Mountain Flax. Simmer the whole in 3 pints of water down to 1½ pint, strain and take a wineglassful after meals for biliousness and dizziness.

For Gall Stones

1 oz. Dandelion root, 1 oz. Parsley root, 1 oz. Balm herb, ½ oz. Ginger root, ½ oz. Liquorice root. Place in 2 quarts of water

and gently simmer down to 1 quart, strain and take a wineglassful every two hours.

For a young child suffering from jaundice: 1 oz. Dandelion root, ½ oz. Ginger root, ½ oz. Caraway seed, ½ oz. Cinnamon bark, ¼ oz. Senna leaves. Gently boil in 3 pints of water down to 1½ pint, strain, dissolve ½ lb. sugar in hot liquid, bring to a boil again, skim all impurities that come to the surface when clear, put on one side to cool, and give frequently in teaspoonful doses.

A Liver and Kidney Mixture

1 oz. Broom tops, ½ oz. Juniper berries, ½ oz. Dandelion root, 1½ pint water. Boil ingredients for 10 minutes, then strain and add a small quantity of cayenne. Dose, 1 tablespoonful, three times a day.

A Medicine for Piles

1 oz. Long-leaved Plantain, 1 oz. Dandelion root, ½ oz. Polypody root, 1 oz. Shepherd's Purse. Add 3 pints of water, boil down to half the quantity, strain, and add 1 oz. of tincture of Rhubarb. Dose, a wineglassful three times a day. Celandine ointment to be applied at same time.

In Derbyshire, the juice of the stalk is applied to remove warts.

DATURA. *See* THORNAPPLE

DEER'S TONGUE

Liatris odoratissima (WILLD.)
N.O. Orchidaceæ

Synonyms. Vanilla Leaf. Wild Vanilla. Trilissia odorata
Part Used. Leaves
Habitat. North America; cultivated in England

¶ *Description.* Herbaceous perennial plant, composite, distinguished by a naked receptacle, oblong, imbricated, involucre, and a feathery pappus, fleshy basal leaves obolanceolate, terminating in a flattened stalk. Leaves of stem clasping at base. The leaves are used to flavour tobacco. Their perfume is largely due to Coumarin, which can be seen in crystals on the upper side of the smooth spatulate leaves. Most of the species are used medicinally.

¶ *Medicinal Action and Uses.* Demulcent, febrifuge, diaphoretic.

¶ *Other Species.*
Liatris spicata has a warm bitterish taste and used as a local application for sore throat in the treatment of gonorrhœa.

L. squarrosa, called 'the rattlesnake' because the roots are used to cure rattlesnake bite, a handsome plant with very long narrow leaves, and large heads of lovely purple flowers.

L. scariosa also used for snake-bite and recognized by the involucral scales which are margined with purple.

DELPHINIUM. *See* LARKSPUR, STAVESACRE

DEVIL'S BIT. *See* SCABIOUS

DILL

Peucedanum graveolens (BENTH.)
N.O. Compositæ

Synonyms. Anethum graveolus. Fructus Anethi
Part Used. Dried ripe fruit

Dill is a hardy annual, a native of the Mediterranean region and Southern Russia. It grows wild among the corn in Spain and Portugal and upon the coast of Italy, but rarely occurs as a cornfield weed in Northern Europe.

The plant is referred to in St. Matthew xxiii., 23, though the original Greek name, *Anethon*, was erroneously rendered *Anise* by English translators, from Wicklif (1380) downwards.

Dill is commonly regarded as the Anethon of Dioscorides. It was well known in Pliny's days and is often mentioned by writers in the Middle Ages. As a drug it has been in use from very early times. It occurs in the tenth-century vocabulary of Alfric, Archbishop of Canterbury.

The name is derived, according to Prior's *Popular Names of English Plants*, from the old Norse word, *dilla* (to lull), in allusion to the carminative properties of the drug.

Lyte (*Dodoens*, 1578) says Dill was sown in all gardens amongst worts and pot-herbs.

In the Middle Ages, Dill was also one of the herbs used by magicians in their spells, and charms against witchcraft.

In Drayton's *Nymphidia* are the lines:

'Therewith her Vervain and her Dill,
That hindereth Witches of their Will.'

Culpepper tells us that

'Mercury has the dominion of this plant, and therefore to be sure it strengthens the brain. . . . It stays the hiccough, being boiled in wine, and but smelled unto being tied in a cloth. The seed is of more use than the leaves, and more effectual to digest raw and vicious humours, and is used in medicines that serve to expel wind, and the pains proceeding therefrom. . . .'

¶ *Description.* The plant grows ordinarily from 2 to 2½ feet high and is very like fennel, though smaller, having the same feathery leaves, which stand on sheathing foot-stalks, with linear and pointed leaflets. Unlike fennel, however, it has seldom more than one stalk and its long, spindle-shaped root is only annual. It is of very upright growth, its stems smooth, shiny and hollow, and in midsummer bearing flat terminal umbels with numerous yellow flowers, whose small petals are rolled inwards. The flat fruits, the so-called seeds, are produced in great quantities. They are very pungent and bitter in taste and very light, an ounce containing over 25,000 seeds. Their germinating capacity lasts for three years. The whole plant is aromatic.

The plant was placed by Linnæus in a separate genus, *Anethum*, whence the name *Fructus Anethi*, by which Dill fruit goes in medicine. It is now included in the genus *Peucedanum.*

¶ *Cultivation.* This annual is of very easy culture. When grown on a large scale for the sake of its fruits, it may be sown in drills, 10 inches apart, in March or April, 10 lb. of the seed being drilled to the acre, and thinned out to leave 8 to 10 inches room each way, Sometimes the seed is sown in autumn as soon as ripe, but it is not so advisable as spring sowing. Careful attention must be given to the destruction of weeds. The crop is considered somewhat exhaustive of soil fertility.

¶ *Harvesting.* Mowing starts as the lower seeds begin, the others ripening on the straw. In dry periods, cutting is best done in early morning or late evening, care being taken to handle with the least possible shaking to prevent loss. The loose sheaves are built into stacks of about twenty sheaves, tied together. In hot weather, threshing may be done in the field, spreading the sheaves on a large canvas sheet and beating out. The average yield is about 7 cwt. of Dill fruits per acre.

The seeds are finally dried by spreading out on trays in the sun, or for a short time over the moderate heat of a stove, shaking occasionally.

Dill fruits are oval, compressed, winged, about one-tenth inch wide, with three longitudinal ridges on the back and three dark lines or oil cells (*vittæ*) between them and two on the flat surface. The taste of the fruits somewhat resembles caraway. The seeds are smaller, flatter and lighter than caraway and have a pleasant aromatic odour. They contain a volatile oil (obtained by distillation) on which the action of the fruit depends. The bruised seeds impart their virtues to alcohol and to boiling water.

¶ *Constituents.* Oil of Dill is of a pale yellow colour, darkening on keeping, with the odour of the fruit and a hot, acrid taste. Its specific gravity varies between 0·895 and 0·915. The fruit yields about 3·5 per cent. of the oil, which is a mixture of a paraffin hydrocarbon and 40 to 60 per cent. of d-carvone, with d-limonene. Phellandrine is present in the English and Spanish oils, but not to any appreciable extent in the German oil.

In spite of the difference in odour between Dill and Caraway oils, the composition of the two is almost identical, both consisting nearly entirely of limonene and carvone. Dill oil, however, contains less carvone than caraway oil.

English-distilled oils usually have the highest specific gravity, from 0·910 to 0·916, and are consequently held in the highest esteem.

¶ *Uses.* As a sweet herb, Dill is not much used in this country. When employed, it is for flavouring soups, sauces, etc., for which purpose the young leaves only are required. The leaves added to fish, or mixed with pickled cucumbers give them a spicy taste.

Dill vinegar, however, forms a popular household condiment. It is made by soaking the seeds in vinegar for a few days before using.

The French use Dill seeds for flavouring cakes and pastry, as well as for flavouring sauces.

Perhaps the chief culinary use of Dill seeds is in pickling cucumbers: they are employed in this way chiefly in Germany where pickled cucumbers are largely eaten.

¶ *Medicinal Action and Uses.* Like the other umbelliferous fruits and volatile oils, both Dill fruit and oil of Dill possess stimulant, aromatic, carminative and stomachic properties, making them of considerable medicinal value.

Oil of Dill is used in mixtures, or administered in doses of 5 drops on sugar, but its most common use is in the preparation of Dill Water, which is a common domestic remedy for the flatulence of infants, and is a useful vehicle for children's medicine generally.

¶ *Preparations.* Dill water, 1 to 8 drachms. Oil, 1 to 5 drops.

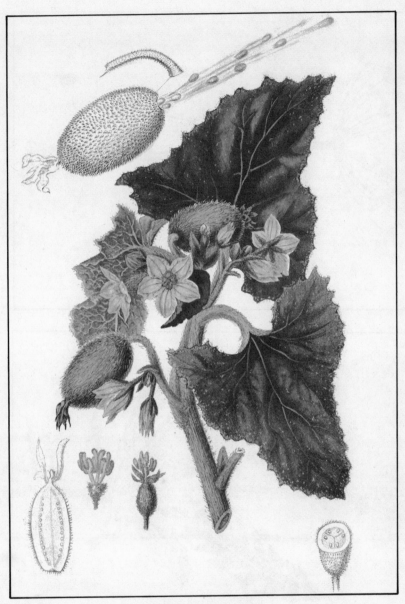

SQUIRTING CUCUMBER
Echallium Elaterium

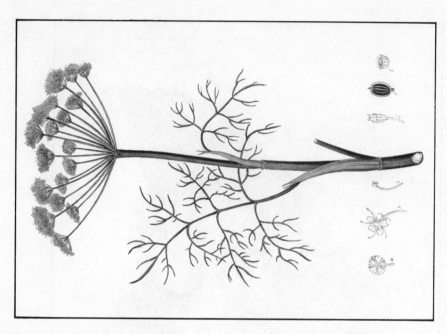

DILL
Peucedanum Graveolens

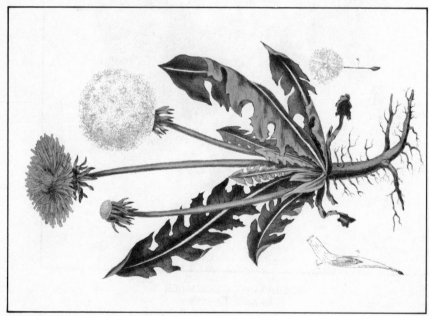

DANDELION
Taraxacum Officinale

Oil of Dill is also employed for perfuming soaps.

The British Pharmacopœia directs that only the fruits from English-grown plants shall be employed pharmaceutically, and it is grown in East Anglia for that purpose. The Dill fruits of commerce are imported from central and southern Europe, the plant being largely cultivated in Germany and Roumania.

Considerable quantities of Dill fruit are imported from India and Japan – they are the fruits of a species of *Peucedanum* that has been considered by some botanists entitled to rank as a distinct species, *P. Sowa* (Kurz), but is included by others in the species, *P. graveolens*. Indian dill is widely grown in the Indies under the name of 'Soyah,' its fruit and leaves being used for flavouring pickles. Its fruits are narrower and more convex than European dill, with paler, more distinct ridges and narrower wings.

The oils from both Japanese and Indian dill differ from European dill oil, in having a higher specific gravity (0·948 to 0·968), which is ascribed to the presence of dill apiol, and in containing much less carvone than the European oil. It should not be substituted for the official oil.

African dill oil is produced from plants grown from English imported seed. The fruits are slightly larger than the English fruits and a little paler in colour, their odour closely resembling the English. The yield of oil is slightly larger than that of English fruits, and it is considered that if the fruits can be produced in Cape Colony, they should form a most useful source of supply.

SOME OLD-FASHIONED FENNEL AND DILL RECIPES

A Sallet of Fennel

'Take young Fennel, about a span long in the spring, tye it up in bunches as you do Sparragrass; when your Skillet boyle, put in enough to make a dish; when it is boyled and drained, dish it up as you do Sparragrass; pour on butter and vinegar and send it up.' (From *The Whole Body of Cookery Dissected*, 1675, by William Tabisha.)

Fennel and Gooseberry Sauce

'Brown some butter in a saucepan with a pinch of flour, then put in a few cives shred small, add a little Irish broth to moisten it, season with salt and pepper; make these boil, then put in two or three sprigs of Fennel and some Gooseberries. Let all simmer together till the Gooseberries are soft and then put in some Cullis.' (From *Receipt Book* of Henry Howard, Cook to the Duke of Ormond, 1710.)

Dill and Collyflower Pickle

'Boil the Collyflowers till they fall in pieces; then with some of the stalk and worst of the flower boil it in a part of the liquer till pretty strong. Then being taken off strain it; and when settled, clean it from the bottom. Then with Dill, gross pepper, a pretty quantity of salt, when cold add as much vinegar as will make it sharp and pour all upon the Collyflower.' (From *Acetaria*, a book about Sallets, 1680, by John Evelyn.)

To Pickle Cucumbers in Dill

'Gather the tops of the ripest dill and cover the bottom of the vessel, and lay a layer of Cucumbers and another of Dill till you have filled the vessel within a handful of the top. Then take as much water as you think will fill the vessel and mix it with salt and a quarter of a pound of allom to a gallon of water and poure it on them and press them down with a stone on them and keep them covered close. For that use I think the water will be best boyl'd and cold, which will keep longer sweet, or if you like not this pickle, doe it with water, salt and white wine vinegar, or (if you please) pour the water and salt on them scalding hot which will make them ready to use the sooner.' (From *Receipt Book* of Joseph Cooper, Cook to Charles I, 1640.)

DITA BARK

Alstonia scholaris (R. BR.)
N.O. Apocyneæ

Synonyms. Devil's Bit. Pali-mara. Bitter Bark. Australian Fever Bush. Devil Tree.
Habitat. India, Moluccas, Philippines

¶ *Description.* The genus of *Alstonia* takes its name from Alston, a Professor of botany in Edinburgh. Grows 50 to 80 feet high, has a furrowed trunk, oblong stalked leaves 6 inches long, 2 to 4 inches wide, in whorls round stem, upper surface glossy, under one white, and marked with nerves running at right-angles to midrib; taste bitter, but no odour. *A. constricta*, belonging to the same order, is also recognized by the British Pharmacopœia; the bark is quite dissimilar, however, and contains different alkaloids, slightly aromatic odour, taste very bitter, used for same purposes, mainly as a febrifuge in malarial fever, tonic and astringent, with much the same properties as Peruvian bark.
¶ *Constituents.* The strongest alkaloids in *A. scholaris* bark are Ditamine, Echitanine,

the latter in character resembling ammonia; other constituents are echierin, echicaoutin, echitin, and echitein – these are crystalline – and *Echiretin amorphous*.

Constituents of *A. constricta* bark, alstonine and porphyrine, is colourless and amorphous; also contains porphyrosine and alstonidine.

¶ *Medicinal Action and Uses*. Though Alstonia is used in India and Eastern Colonies for malarial conditions, its efficacy in this respect is not to be compared with cinchona bark, though it does not produce the bad effects cinchona does. It is also employed as a bitter tonic, vermifuge, and as a cure for chronic diarrhœa and bowel complaints, both varieties are used.

¶ *Preparation*. Dita bark: 1 part in 20 for B.P. infusion, ½ to 1 fluid ounce; 1 part in 8 Alcohol Tinc., B.P., ½ to 1 fluid drachm. Dose, 2 to 4 grains.

¶ *Other Species*. The *A. spectabilis*, a habitat of Java, contains the same alkaloid as Dita bark, with the addition of a crystalline alkaloid, Alstonamine.

DOCKS
N.O. Polygonaceæ

The name *Dock* is applied to a widespread tribe of broad-leaved wayside weeds, having roots possessing astringent qualities united in some with a cathartic principle, rendering them valuable as substitutes for Rhubarb, a plant of the same family.

Although now, in common with the Sorrels, assigned to the genus *Rumex*, the Docks were formerly ranked as members of the genus *Lapathum*, this name being derived from the Greek word, *lapazein* (to cleanse), an allusion to the medicinal virtues of these plants as purgatives, the word still surviving in the name of one of the species, *Rumex Hydrolapathum*.

All the Docks resemble our Garden Rhubarb more or less, both in their general characteristics and in possessing much tannin. Most of them furnish rumicin, or crysophanic acid, which is useful in chronic scrofulous disorders.

The young leaves and shoots of several species of Dock may be eaten as pot-herbs, but are not very palatable, and have a slight laxative effect. 'Sour Docks' were considered formerly a good accompaniment to boiled beef, either hot or cold, but this was a popular name, not for the ordinary kinds of Docks, but for the closely allied Sorrel or Sorrel Dock (*Rumex acetosa*), whose herbage has a somewhat acid flavour. This, with its French variety, *R. scutatus*, has been much cultivated as a pot-herb.

PATIENCE DOCK
Rumex alpinus

Synonyms. Herb Patience. Monk's Rhubarb. Passion's Dock

This, although not considered a native plant, grows wild in some parts of the country, mostly by roadsides and near cottages, being originally a garden escape. It is a large plant, about 6 feet high, with very large, long, pointed leaves on thick hollow footstalks. The long stout root was also formerly used medicinally for its slight astringent qualities. It was considered good for jaundice.

It has a gentle laxative action. There are about ten or eleven kinds of native Docks.

ROUND-LEAVED DOCK
Rumex obtusifolius

Synonyms. Common Wayside Dock. Butter Dock

¶ *Description*. It is a large and spreading plant, its stout stems 2 to 3 feet high, the leaves 6 to 12 inches long, with rather slender foot-stalks, the margins waved and the end or apex of the leaf rounded. The flowers are small, green and numerous, arranged in whorled spikes at the ends of the stem. In this, as in all the Docks, the flowers contain both stamens and pistils – the nearly-related Sorrels, on the contrary, having their stamens and pistils on different plants. This Dock is so coarse that cattle refuse to touch it. It is a troublesome weed, all the more because it prefers growing on good land, not thriving in poor soil. Its broad foliage serves also to lodge the destructive turnip fly. The leaves are often applied as a rustic remedy to burns and scalds and used for dressing blisters, serving also as a popular cure for Nettle stings.

The cure was accompanied by the words:

'Nettle in, Dock;
Dock in, Nettle out;
Dock rub Nettle out,'

and is the origin of the saying: 'In Dock, out Nettle', to suggest inconstancy.

A tea made from the root was formerly given for the cure of boils. The plant is frequently called Butter Dock, because its cool leaves have often been used in the country for wrapping up butter for the market.

SHARP-POINTED DOCK

¶ *Description.* A common plant like the Common Dock, but handsomer, and distinguished by its sharp-pointed leaves being narrower and longer. It grows about 3 feet high, having erect, round, striated stems and small greenish flowers, turning brown when ripe. The root has been used in drinks and decoctions for scurvy and as a general blood cleanser, and employed for outward application to cutaneous eruptions, in the form of an ointment, made by beating it up with lard.

Both the Round-leaved Dock and the

Sharp-pointed Dock, together with the BLOODY-VEINED DOCK (*Rumex sanguineus*) (which is very conspicuous on account of its veins and footstalks abounding in a blood-coloured juice), make respectively with their astringent roots a useful infusion against bleedings and fluxes, also with their leaves, a decoction curative of several chronic skin diseases.

THE YELLOW DOCK (*Rumex crispus*), the RED DOCK (*R. aquaticus*) and the GREAT WATER DOCK (*R. Hydrolapathum*) are, however, the species more generally used medicinally.

YELLOW DOCK

Synonym. Curled Dock

¶ *Description.* The leaves are crisped at their edges. It grows freely in our roadside ditches and waste places. The roots are 8 to 12 inches long, about ½ inch thick, fleshy and usually not forked. Externally they are of a rusty brown and internally whitish, with fine, straight, medullary rays and a rather thick bark. It has little or no smell and a rather bitter taste. The stem is 1 to 3 feet high and branched, the leaves, 6 to 10 inches long.

¶ *Medicinal Action and Uses.* The Yellow Dock is applicable to all the purposes for which the other species are used. The root has laxative, alterative and mildly tonic action, and can be freely used as a tonic and laxative in rheumatism, bilious complaints and as an astringent in piles, bleedings of the lungs, etc. It is largely prescribed for diseases of the blood, from a spring eruption, to scurvy, scrofula and chronic skin diseases. It is also useful in jaundice and as a tonic to the stomach and the system generally. It has an action on the bowels very similar to that of Rhubarb, being perhaps a little less active, but operating without [pain or uneasiness.

Rumicin is the active principle of the Yellow Dock, and from the root, containing Chrysarobin, a dried extract is prepared officially, of which from 1 to 4 grains may be given for a dose in a pill. This is useful

for relieving a congested liver, as well as for scrofulous skin diseases.

A syrup can be made by boiling ½ lb. crushed root in a pint of syrup, which is taken in teaspoonful doses. The infusion – administered in wineglassful doses – is made by pouring 1 pint of boiling water on 1 oz. of the powdered root. A useful homœopathic tincture is made from the plant before it flowers, which is of particular service to an irritable tickling cough of the upper air-tubes and the throat. It is likewise excellent for dispelling any obstinate itching of the skin. It acts like Sarsaparilla for curing scrofulous skin affections and glandular swellings.

To be applied externally for cutaneous affections, an ointment may be made by boiling the root in vinegar until the fibre is softened and then mixing the pulp with lard.

The seeds have been given with advantage in dysentery, for their astringent action.

The Yellow Dock has also been considered to have a positive effect in restraining the inroads made by cancer in the human system, being used as an alterative and tonic to enfeebled condition caused by necrosis, cancer, etc. It has been used in diphtheria.

¶ *Preparations.* Fluid extract, 30 to 60 drops. Solid extract, 5 to 15 grains. Rumin, 3 grains.

The roots are collected in March, being generally ploughed up.

RED DOCK

Synonym. Water Dock

The Red Dock, or Water Dock (*Rumex aquaticus*), has properties very similar to those of the Yellow Dock. It is frequent in fields, meadows and ditches. Its rootstock is top-shaped, the outer surface blackish or dark brown, the bark porous and the pith composed of honeycomb-like cells, with a short zone of woody bundles separated by rays. It has an astringent and somewhat

sweet taste, but no odour. The stem is 1 to 3 feet high, very stout; the leaves similar to those of the Yellow Dock, having also crisped edges, but being broader, 3 to 4 inches across.

¶ *Medicinal Action and Uses.* This Dock has alterative, deobstruent and detergent action. Its powers as a tonic are, perhaps, rather more marked than the previous species. For internal use, it is given in an infusion, in wineglassful doses. Externally, it is used as an application for eruptive and scorbutic diseases, ulcers and sores, being employed for cleansing ulcers in affections of the mouth, etc. As a powder, it has

GREAT WATER DOCK

The Great Water Dock (*Rumex Hydrolapathum*), the largest of all the Docks, 5 to 6 feet high, is frequent on river banks. It is a picturesque plant with several erect, furrowed stems arising from its thick, blackish root, each of which are branched in the upper part, and bear numerous green flowers in almost leafless whorls. The leaves are exceedingly large – 1 to 3 feet long, dull green, not shiny, lance-shaped and narrow, tapering at both ends, the lower ones heart-shaped at the base. It is much like *Rumex acutus*, but larger.

This Dock, also, has some reputation as an antiscorbutic, and was used by the ancients. The root is strongly astringent, and powdered makes a good dentifrice. It is this species that is said to be the *Herba Britannica* of Pliny. This name does not denote British origin – the plant not being confined to the British Isles – but is said to be derived from three Teutonic words: *brit* (to tighten), *tan* (a tooth), and *ica* (loose), thus expressing its power of bracing up loose teeth and spongy gums.

Miss Rohde (*Old English Herbals*) says:

'It is interesting to find that Turner identifies the *Herba Britannica* of Dioscorides and Pliny (famed for having cured the soldiers of Julius Cæsar of scurvy in the Rhine country) with *Polygonum bistorta*, which he observed plentifully in Friesland, the scene of Pliny's observations. This herb is held by modern authorities to be *Rumex aquaticus* (Great Water Dock).'

As a stomach tonic the following decoction was formerly much in use: 2 oz. of the root sliced were put into 3 pints of water, with

cleansing and detergent effect upon the teeth.

The root of this and all other Docks is dried in the same manner as the Yellow Dock. ¶ *Preparation*. Fluid extract, 30 to 60 drops.

Rumex Hydrolapathum

a little cinnamon or liquorice powder, and boiled down to a quart and a wineglassful taken two or three times a day. The astringent qualities of the root render it good in case of diarrhœa, the seeds (as with the other Docks) having been used for the same purpose. The green leaves are reputed to be an excellent application for ulcers of the eyes.

Culpepper says of the Docks:

'All Docks are under Jupiter, of which the Red Dock, which is commonly called Bloodwort, cleanseth the blood and strengthens the liver, but the Yellow Dock root is best to be taken when either the blood or liver is affected by choler. All of them have a kind of cooling, drying quality: the Sorrel being most cool and the Bloodworts most drying. The seed of most kinds, whether garden or field, doth stay laxes and fluxes of all sorts, and is helpful for those that spit blood. The roots boiled in vinegar helpeth the itch, scabs and breaking out of the skin, if it be bathed therewith. The distilled water of the herb and roots have the same virtue and cleanseth the skin from freckles. . . . All Docks being boiled with meat make it boil the sooner; besides Bloodwort is exceeding strengthening to the liver and procures good blood, being as wholesome a pot-herb as any growing in a garden.'

Another species of *Rumex* may also be termed of indirect medicinal use, for Turkey opium, as imported, comes in flattened masses enveloped in poppy leaves and covered with the reddish-brown, triangular winged fruit of a species of *Rumex*, to prevent the cakes adhering to one another.

See SORREL, RHUBARB.

DODDER

Cuscuta Europæa
N.O. Convolvulaceæ

Synonyms. Beggarweed. Hellweed. Strangle Tare. Scaldweed. Devil's Guts

Belonging to the same family as the Convolvulus is a small group of plants, the genus *Cuscuta*, that at first glance seem to have little in common with our common Bindweeds. All the members of this genus are parasites, with branched, climbing cord-like and thread-like stems, *no leaves* and globular heads of small wax-like flowers.

The seeds germinate in the ground in the

normal manner and throw up thready stems, which climb up adjoining plants and send out from their inner surfaces a number of small vesicles, which attach themselves to the bark of the plant on which they are twining. As soon as the young Dodder stems have firmly fixed themselves, the root from which they have at first drawn part of their nourishment withers away, and the Dodder, entirely losing its connection with the ground, lives completely on the sap of its 'host,' and participates of its nature.

One British species is very abundant on Furze, another on Flax, others on Thistles and Nettles, etc.

Cuscuta Epithymum, THE LESSER DODDER, is the species of Dodder that formerly was much used medicinally, and which is the commonest. It is parasitic on Thyme, Heath, Milk Vetch, Potentilla and other small plants, but most abundant on Furze, which it often entirely conceals with its tangled masses of red, thread-like stems. The flowers are in dense, round heads, each flower small, light flesh-coloured and wax-like, the corolla bell-shaped, four- to five-cleft. Soon after flowering, the stems turn dark brown and in winter disappear.

The Dodder which grows on Thyme, *C. Epithemum*, was often preferred to others.

The threads being boiled in water (preferably fresh gathered) with ginger and all-spice produced a decoction used in urinary complaints, kidney, spleen and liver diseases for its laxative and hepatic action. It was considered useful in jaundice, as well as in sciatica and scorbutic complaints.

The juice of two Brazilian species of Dodder is given for hoarseness and spitting of blood and their powder applied to wounds, to hasten healing.

Other species of Dodder which more or less resemble the Lesser Dodder are *C. Europæa*, THE GREATER OR COMMON DODDER, which is parasitical on Thistles and Nettles, and has stems as thick as twine, reddish or yellow, with pale orange-coloured flowers, $\frac{1}{2}$ to $\frac{3}{4}$ inch in diameter; *C. Epilinum*, FLAX DODDER, parasitical on Flax, to crops of which it is sometimes very destructive, and with seeds of which it is supposed to have been introduced; *C. Hassiaca*, parasitical on Lucerne, and *C. Trifolii*, CLOVER DODDER, parasitical on Clover.

Both the Greater Dodder and the Lesser Dodder have been employed medicinally.

Culpepper tells us:

'All Dodders are under Saturn. We confess Thyme is of the hottest herb it usually grows upon, and therefore that which grows upon thyme is hotter than that which grows upon colder herbs; for it draws nourishment from what it grows upon, as well as from the earth where its root is, and thus you see old Saturn is wise enough to have two strings to his bow. This is accounted the most effectual for melancholy diseases, and to purge black or burnt color, which is the cause of many diseases of the head and brain, as also for the trembling of the heart, faintings, and swoonings. It is helpful in all diseases and griefs of the spleen and melancholy that arises from the windiness of the hypochondria. It purges also the reins or kidneys by urine; it openeth obstructions of the gall, whereby it profiteth them that have the jaundice; as also the leaves, the spleen; purging the veins of choleric and phlegmatic humours and cures children in agues, a little wormseed being added.

'The other Dodders participate of the nature of those plants whereon they grow: as that which hath been found growing upon Nettles in the west country, hath by experience been found very effectual to procure plenty of urine, where it hath been stopped or hindered.'

Many of its popular and local names testify to the bad reputation it had among farmers, such as Beggarweed, Hellweed, Strangle Tare, and Scaldweed, the latter from the scalded appearance it gives to bean crops. The name 'Devil's Guts' shows how much its strangling threads were detested. An old writer comments:

'Hellweed grows upon tares more abundantly in some places, where it destroyeth the pulse, or at least maketh it much worse, and is called of the country people Hellweed, because they know not how to destroy it.'

It was not only considered useful in jaundice but also in sciatica and scorbutic complaints. Gathered fresh and applied externally after being bruised, the plant has been found efficacious in dispersing scrofulous tumours. The whole plant, of whatever species, is very bitter, and an infusion acts as a brisk purge.

DOG ROSE. *See* ROSE

DOG'S MERCURY. *See* MERCURY

DOGWOOD, JAMAICA
Part Used. Bark
Habitat. West Indies, Florida, Texas, Mexico, the northern part of South America

Piscidia erythrina (JACQ.)
N.O. Leguminosæ

¶ *Description.* A tree with very valuable wood and with the foliage and habit of Lonchocarpus. The pods bear four projecting longitudinal wings. The pounded leaves and young branches are used to poison fish; the method followed is to fill an open crate with the branches, drop it into the water, and swill it about till the water is impregnated with the liquid from the leaves, etc.; this quickly stupefies the fish and enables the fishers to catch them quickly. In commerce the bark is found in quilled pieces 1 or 2 inches long and ⅛ inch thick. The outer surface yellow or greyish brown, inner surface lighter coloured or white, and if damp a peculiar blue colour. Inside it is very fibrous and dark brown, taste very acrid and bitter, and produces burning sensation in mouth with a strong disagreeable smell like broken opium. In 1844 attention was called to its narcotic, analgesic and sudorific properties which are uncertain.

¶ *Constituents.* Resin, fat, a crystallizable substance called piscidin and in the aqueous extract of the bark piscidic acid, and a bitter glucoside.

¶ *Medicinal Action and Uses.* In some subjects it cures violent toothache, neuralgia and whooping-cough and promotes sleep, and acts as an antispasmodic in asthma. It also dilates the pupil and is useful in dysmenorrhœa and nervous debility. In other subjects it only causes gastric distress and nausea; over doses produce toxic effects.

¶ *Preparations and Dosages.* Fluid extract, 5 to 20 drops, which may be cautiously increased to 2 fluid drachms. Solid extract, 1 to 5 grains.

DRAGON'S BLOOD

Dæmomorops Draco (BLUME)
N.O. Palmaceæ

Synonyms. Calamus Draco. Draconis Resina. Sanguis draconis. Dragon's Blood Palm. Blume
Part Used. The resinous exudation of the fruits
Habitat. Sumatra

¶ *Description.* Dragon's Blood, as known in commerce, has several origins, the substance so named being contributed by widely differing species. Probably the best known is that from Sumatra. *Dæmomorops Draco*, formerly known as *Calamus Draco*, was transferred with many others of the species to *Dæmomorops*, the chief distinguishing mark being the placing of the flowers along the branches instead of their being gathered into catkins, as in those remaining under *Calamus*.

The long, slender stems of the genus are flexible, and the older trees develop climbing propensities. The leaves have prickly stalks which often grow into long tails, and the bark is provided with many hundreds of flattened spines. The berries are about the size of a cherry, and pointed. When ripe they are covered with a reddish, resinous substance which is separated in several ways, the most satisfactory being by steaming, or by shaking or rubbing in coarse, canvas bags. An inferior kind is obtained by boiling the fruits to obtain a decoction after they have undergone the second process. The product may come to market in beads, joined as if forming a necklace, and covered with leaves (Tear Dragon's Blood), or in small, round sticks about 18 inches long, packed in leaves and strips of cane. Other varieties are found in irregular lumps, or in a reddish powder. They are known as lump, stick, reed, tear, or saucer Dragon's Blood.

¶ *Uses.* It is used as a colouring matter for varnishes, tooth-pastes, tinctures, plasters, for dyeing horn to imitate tortoiseshell, etc. It is very brittle, and breaks with an irregular, resinous fracture, is bright red and glossy inside, and darker red, sometimes powdered with crimson, externally. Small, thin pieces are transparent.

¶ *Constituents.* Several analyses of Dragon's Blood have been made with the following results:

(1) 50 to 70 per cent. resinous compound of benzoic and benzoyl-acetic acid, with dracoresinotannol, and also dracon alban and dracoresene.

(2) 56·8 per cent. of red resin compounded of the first three mentioned above, 2·5 per cent. of the white, amorphous dracoalban, 13·58 of the yellow, resinous dracoresene, 18·4 vegetable debris, and 8·3 per cent. ash.

(3) 90·7 per cent. of red resin, draconin, 2·0 of fixed oil, 3·0 of benzoic acid, 1·6 of calcium oxalate, and 3·7 of calcium phosphate.

(4) 2·5 per cent. of draco-alban, 13·58 of draco resin, 56·86 of draco resin, benzoic dracoresinotannol ester and benzoylacetic-dracoresinotannol ester, with 18·4 of insoluble substances.

Dragon's Blood is not acted upon by water, but most of it is soluble in alcohol. It fuses by heat. The solution will stain marble a deep red, penetrating in proportion to the heat of the stone.

¶ *Medicinal Action and Uses.* Doses of 10 to 30 grains were formerly given as an astringent in diarrhœa, etc., but officially it is never at present used internally, being regarded as inert.

The following treatment is said to have

cured cases of severe syphilis. Mix 2 drachms of Dragon's Blood, 2 drachms of colocynth, $\frac{1}{2}$ oz. of gamboge in a mortar, and add 3 gills of boiling water. Stir for an hour, while keeping hot. Allow to cool, and add while stirring a mixture of 2 oz. each of sweet spirits of nitre and copaiba balsam.

¶ *Dosage.* $\frac{1}{2}$ oz. for catharsis, followed by 1 drachm two or three times a day.

¶ *Other Species.*

The Malay varieties are from *D. didynophyllos*, *D. micranthus* and *D. propinguus*.

The Borneo variety is from *D. draconcellus* and others. 'Zanzibar Drop' or Socotrine Dragon's Blood is imported from Bombay and Zanzibar, and is the product of *D. cinnabari*. It has no scales, and like other non-Sumatra varieties, is not soluble in benzene and carbon disulphide.

Dracæna Draco is a giant tree of the East Indies and Canary Islands, and shares with the baobab tree the distinction of being the oldest living representative of the vegetable kingdom, being much reverenced by the Guanches of the Canaries, who use its pro-duct for embalming in the fashion of the Egyptians.

The trunk cracks and emits a red resin used as 'tear' Dragon's Blood, now rarely seen in commerce.

Dracæna terminalis, or Chinese Colli, yields Chinese Dragon's Blood, used in China for its famous red varnish. In some countries a syrup, yielding sugar, is made from the roots (called Tii roots). An intoxicating drink can be made from it, and it has also been used in dysentery and diarrhœa, and as a diaphoretic.

Pterocarpus Draco, of the East Indies and South America, yields a resin found, as Guadaloupe Dragon's Blood, in small irregular lumps.

Croton Draco or Mexican Dragon's Blood, is called Sangre del Drago, and is used in Mexico as a vulnerary and astringent. Others used are from:

Croton hibiscifolius of New Granada.

Croton sanguifolius of New Andalusia, and *Calamus rotang* of the East Indies and Spanish America. *See* SEDGE (SWEET)

(POISON)
DROPWORT, HEMLOCK WATER

Œnanthe crocata (LINN.)
N.O. Umbelliferæ

Synonyms. Horsebane. Dead Tongue. Five-Fingered Root. Water Lovage. Yellow Water Dropwort

Part Used. Root

The name Water Hemlock is, though incorrectly, often popularly applied to several species of Œnanthe, the genus of the Water Dropworts, which of all the British umbelliferous plants are the most poisonous.

The species most commonly termed Water Hemlock is Œnanthe crocata, the Hemlock Water Dropwort, a common plant in England, especially in the southern counties, in ditches and watering places, but not occurring in Scandinavia, Holland, Germany, Russia, Turkey or Greece.

¶ *Description.* It is a large, stout plant, 3 to 5 feet high, the stems thick, erect, much branched above, furrowed, hollow, tough, dark green and smooth.

The roots are perennial and fleshy, of a pale yellow colour. They have a sweetish and not unpleasant taste, but are virulently poisonous. Being often exposed by the action of running water near which they grow, they are thus easily accessible to children and cattle, and the plant should not be allowed to grow in places where cattle are kept, as instances are numerous in which cows have been poisoned by eating these roots. They have also occasionally been eaten in mistake, either for wild celery or water parsnip, with very serious results, great agony, sickness, convulsions, or even death resulting. While the root of the Parsnip is single and conical in form, that of Œnanthe crocata consists of clusters of fleshy tubers similar to those of the Dahlia, hence, perhaps, one of its popular names: Dead Tongue.

The author of *Familiar Wild Flowers* states that the name 'Dead Tongue' was given from the paralysing effect of this plant on the organs of speech.

No British wild plant has been responsible for more fatal accidents than the one in question: a party of workmen repairing a breach in a towing-path dug up the plants and ate the roots, mistaking them for parsnips; another party, working in a field, thought that a few of the leaves with their bread and cheese would prove a tasty relish: in each case death occurred within three hours. On another occasion eight boys ate the roots, and five died – and the other three had violent convulsions and lost their reason for many hours.

The plant has been used to poison rats and moles.

Both stem and root, when cut, exude a yellowish juice, hence the specific name of the plant and one of the common names (Yellow Water Dropwort) by which it is known. The juice will stain the hands yellow. The generic name, *Œnanthe*, is derived from the Greek *ainos* (wine) and *anthos* (a flower), from the wine-like scent of the flowers.

The leaves are somewhat celery-like in form, and the flowers are in bloom in June and July, and are borne in large umbels. There is considerable variety in the form of the leaf-segments, the number of rays in the umbel, and of the involucre bracts. The lower leaves, with very short, sheathing footstalks, are large and spreading, reaching more than a foot in length, broadly triangular in outline and tri-pinnate. The leaflets are stalkless, 1 to 1½ inch long, roundish, with a wedge-shaped base, deeply and irregularly lobed, dark green, paler and shining beneath. The upper leaves are much smaller, nearly stalkless, the segments narrower and acute.

This most poisonous of our indigenous plants is not official and has never been used to any extent in medicine, though in some cases it has been taken with effect in eruptive diseases of the skin, being given at first in small doses, gradually increased.

Great caution must be exercised in the use of the tincture. The dose of the tincture is 1 to 5 drops. The roots have likewise been used in poultices to whitlows and to foul ulcers, both in man and horned cattle.

DROPWORT, WATER

Œnanthe phellandrium (LANK.)
N.O. Umbelliferæ

Synonyms. Water Fennel. Horsebane. Phellandrium aquaticum (Linn.)
Part Used. Fruit

Œnanthe phellandrium (syn. *Phellandrium aquaticum*), the Fine-leaved Water Dropwort, known popularly as Water Fennel, is a common British plant in ditches and by the sides of ponds.

It is a biennial, flowering from July to September in its second year of growth.

¶ *Description.* The stems are 2 to 3 feet high, very stout at the base, rising from fibrous roots. The leaves are divided into many fine segments, the lower ones submerged. The umbels are smaller than those of *Œ. crocata* and are on short stalks, springing either from the forks of the branches or from opposite the leaves.

The rootstock varies in appearance, according to the locality. If growing in deep or running water the rootstock and stem are long and slender; in other districts it is thicker and more erect. The variety that grows in deep running water is often considered a distinct species and is classed under *Œ. fluviatilis*.

Œ. phellandrium is less poisonous than *Œ. crocata*, but both produce ill-effects if eaten.

¶ *Constituents.* The fruits yield from 1 to 2½ per cent. of an ethereal oil, known as Water Fennel Oil, a yellow liquid of strong, pleasant, characteristic odour and burning taste, its specific gravity 0·85 to 0·89, containing as its chief constituent about 80 per cent. of the terpene Phellandrene.

¶ *Medicinal Action and Uses.* The fruits have been used in chronic pectoral affections such as bronchitis, pulmonary consumption and asthma, also in dyspepsia, intermittent fever, obstinate ulcers, etc. The dose when given in powdered form is 5 or 6 grains to commence with, so repeated as to amount to a drachm in four hours. An alcoholic extract and essence of the fruits has also been recommended as a very valuable and active remedy in the relief of consumption and bronchitis.

In overdoses, the fruits produce vertigo, intoxication and other narcotic effects.

Externally applied, the root has sometimes been used as a local remedy in piles. When eaten in mistake, like that of *Œ. crocata*, the results have sometimes proved fatal. The symptoms produced are those of irritation of the stomach, failure of circulation and great cerebral disturbance, indicated by giddiness, convulsions and coma.

The fresh leaves are injurious to cattle, producing a kind of paralysis when eaten. When dried, they lose their deleterious properties.

Œ. fistulosa, the Common Water Dropwort, is found in watery places. This has a mixture of slender and fleshy roots, and bears leaves with only a few narrow segments. It is also poisonous. A peculiar resinous principle, called œnanthin, has been found in this species.

Most of the other species of *Œnanthe* found both in Great Britain and in the United States are poisonous, although none appear to be as virulent as *Œ. crocata*. A few are, however, innocuous, and their roots, especially those of *Œ. pimpinelloides*, have been esteemed as food in certain districts. Burnett (*Medical Botany*) states 'they are replete with a bland farina and have something the flavour of a filbert.'

DYER'S GREENWEED. *See* GREENWEED

DYER'S MADDER. *See* MADDER

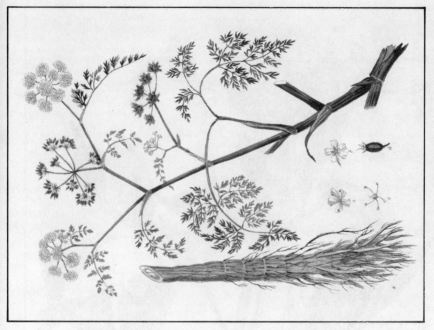

WATER DROPWORT
Œnanthe Phellandrium

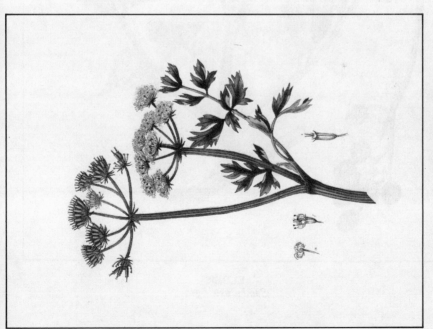

HEMLOCK WATER DROPWORT
Œnanthe Crocata

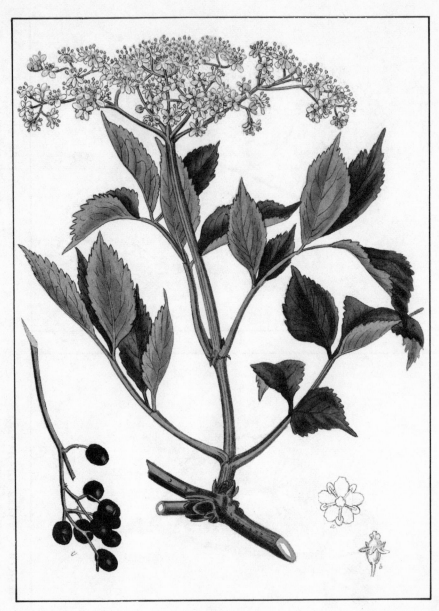

ELDER
Sambucus Nigra

ECHINACEA

Echinacea angustifolia (DE CANDOLLE)
N.O. Compositæ

Synonyms. Black Sampson. Coneflower. Niggerhead. Rudbeckia. *Brauneria pallida* (Nutt.)

Parts Used. Root, dried; also rhizome

Habitat. America, west of Ohio, and cultivated in Britain

¶ *Description.* Named *Echinacea* by Linnæus, and *Rudbeckia*, after Rudbeck, father and son, who were his predecessors at Upsala.

The flowers are a rich purple and the florets are seated round a high cone; seeds, four-sided achenes. Root tapering, cylindrical, entire, slightly spiral, longitudinally furrowed; fracture short, fibrous; bark thin; wood, thick, in alternate porous, yellowish and black transverse wedges, and the rhizome has a circular pith. It has a faint aromatic smell, with a sweetish taste, leaving a tingling sensation in the mouth not unlike *Aconitum napellus*, but without its lasting numbing effect.

¶ *Constituents.* Oil and resin both in wood and bark and masses of inulin, inuloid, sucrose, vulose, betaine, two phytosterols and fatty acids, oleic, cerotic, linolic and palmatic.

¶ *Medicinal Action and Uses.* Echinacea increases bodily resistance to infection and is used for boils, erysipelas, septicæmia, cancer, syphilis and other impurities of the blood, its action being antiseptic. It has also useful properties as a strong alterative and aphrodisiac. As an injection, the extract has been used for hæmorrhoids and a tincture of the *fresh* root has been found beneficial in diphtheria and putrid fevers.

¶ *Other Species.*

Echinacea purpurea has similar properties to *E. angustifolia*; the *fresh* root of this is the part used.

EGG PLANT. *See* NIGHTSHADE

ELATERIUM. *See* CUCUMBER (SQUIRTING).

ELDER

Sambucus nigra (LINN.)
N.O. Caprifoliaceæ

Synonyms. Black Elder. Common Elder. Pipe Tree. Bore Tree. Bour Tree. (*Fourteenth Century*) Hylder, Hylantree. (*Anglo-Saxon*) Eldrum. (*Low Saxon*) Ellhorn. (*German*) Hollunder. (*French*) Sureau

Parts Used. Bark, leaves, flowers, berries

The Elder, with its flat-topped masses of creamy-white, fragrant blossoms, followed by large drooping bunches of purplish-black, juicy berries, is a familiar object in English countryside and gardens. It has been said, with some truth, that our English summer is not here until the Elder is fully in flower, and that it ends when the berries are ripe.

The word 'Elder' comes from the Anglo-Saxon word *æld*. In Anglo-Saxon days we find the tree called Eldrun, which becomes Hyldor and Hyllantree in the fourteenth century. One of its names in modern German – Hollunder – is clearly derived from the same origin. In Low-Saxon, the name appears as Ellhorn. *Æld* meant 'fire,' the hollow stems of the young branches having been used for blowing up a fire: the soft pith pushes out easily and the tubes thus formed were used as pipes – hence it was often called Pipe-Tree, or Bore-tree and Bour-tree, the latter name remaining in Scotland and being traceable to the Anglo-Saxon form, Burtre.

The generic name *Sambucus* occurs in the writings of Pliny and other ancient writers and is evidently adapted from the Greek word *Sambuca*, the Sackbut, an ancient musical instrument in much use among the Romans, in the construction of which, it is surmised, the wood of this tree, on account of its hardness, was used. The difficulty, however, of accepting this is that the Sambuca was a stringed instrument, while anything made from the Elder would doubtless be a wind instrument, something of the nature of a Pan-pipe or flute. Pliny records the belief held by country folk that the shrillest pipes and the most sonorous horns were made of Elder trees which were grown out of reach of the sound of cock-crow. At the present day, Italian peasants construct a simple pipe, which they call *sampogna*, from the branches of this plant.

The popular pop-gun of small boys in the country has often been made of Elder stems, from which the pith has been removed, which moved Culpepper to declare: 'It is needless to write any description of this (Elder), since every boy that plays with a pop-gun will not mistake another tree for the Elder.' Pliny's writings also testify that pop-guns and whistles are manufactures many centuries old!

¶ *History.* A wealth of folk-lore, romance and superstition centre round this English tree. Shakespeare, in *Cymbeline*, referring to it as a symbol of grief, speaks slightingly of it as 'the stinking Elder,' yet, although many people profess a strong dislike to the scent of its blossom, the shrub is generally beloved by all who see it. In countrysides where the Elder flourishes it is certainly one of the most attractive features of the hedgerow, while its old-world associations have created for it a place in the hearts of English people.

In *Love's Labour Lost* reference is made to the common mediæval belief that 'Judas was hanged on an Elder.' We meet with this tradition as far back in English literature as Langland's *Vision of Piers Plowman* (middle of the fourteenth century, before Chaucer):

'Judas he japed with Jewen silver
And sithen an eller hanged hymselve.'

Why the Elder should have been selected as a gallows for the traitor Apostle is, considering the usual size of the tree, puzzling; but Sir John Mandeville in his travels, written about the same time, tells us that he was shown 'faste by' the Pool of Siloam, the identical 'Tree of Eldre that Judas henge himself upon, for despeyr that he hadde, when he solde and betrayed oure Lord.' Gerard scouts the tradition and says that the Judas-tree (*Cercis siliquastrum*) is 'the tree whereon Judas did hange himselfe.'

Another old tradition was that the Cross of Calvary was made of it, and an old couplet runs:

'Bour tree – Bour tree: crooked rong
Never straight and never strong;
Ever bush and never tree
Since our Lord was nailed on thee.'

In consequence of these old traditions, the Elder became the emblem of sorrow and death, and out of the legends which linger round the tree there grew up a host of superstitious fancies which still remain in the minds of simple country folk. Even in these prosaic days, one sometimes comes across a hedge-cutter who cannot bring himself to molest the rampant growth of its spreading branches for fear of being pursued by ill-luck. An old custom among gypsies forbade them using the wood to kindle their camp fires and gleaners of firewood formerly would look carefully through the faggots lest a stick of Elder should have found its way into the bundle, perhaps because the Holy Cross was believed to have been fashioned out of a giant elder tree, though probably the superstitious awe of harming the Elder descended from old heathen myths of northern Europe. In most countries, especially in Denmark, the Elder was intimately connected with magic. In its branches was supposed to dwell a dryad,

Hylde-Moer, the Elder-tree Mother, who lived in the tree and watched over it. Should the tree be cut down and furniture be made of the wood, Hylde-Moer was believed to follow her property and haunt the owners. Lady Northcote, in *The Book of Herbs*, relates:

'There is a tradition that once when a child was put in a cradle of Elder-wood, Hylde-Moer came and pulled it by the legs and would give it no peace till it was lifted out. Permission to cut Elder wood must always be asked first and not until Hylde-Moer has given consent by keeping silence, may the chopping begin.'

Arnkiel relates:

'Our forefathers also held the Ellhorn holy, wherefore whoever need to hew it down (or cut its branches) has first to make request, "Lady Ellhorn, give me some of thy wood, and I will give thee some of mine when it grows in the forest" – the which, with partly bended knees, bare head and folded arms was ordinarily done, as I myself have often seen and heard in my younger years.'

Mr. Jones (quoted in *The Treasury of Botany*), in his *Notes on Certain Superstitions in the Vale of Gloucester*, cites the following, said to be no unusual case:

'Some men were employed in removing an old hedgerow, partially formed of Elder-trees. They had bound up all the other wood into faggots for burning, but had set apart the elder and enquired of their master how it was to be disposed of. Upon his saying that he should of course burn it with the rest, one of the men said with an air of undisguised alarm, that he had never *heard* of such a thing as burning *Ellan Wood*, and in fact, so strongly did he feel upon the subject, that he refused to participate in the act of tying it up. The word Ellan (still common with us) indicates the origin of the superstition.'

In earlier days, the Elder Tree was supposed to ward off evil influence and give protection from witches, a popular belief held in widely-distant countries. Lady Northcote says:

'The Russians believe that Elder-trees drive away evil spirits, and the Bohemians go to it with a spell to take away fever. The Sicilians think that sticks of its wood will kill serpents and drive away robbers, and the Serbs introduce a stick of Elder into their wedding ceremonies to bring good luck. In England it was thought that the Elder was never struck by lightning, and a twig of it tied into three or four knots and carried in the pocket was a charm against rheumatism. A cross made of Elder and fastened to cow-houses and stables was supposed to keep all evil from the animals.'

In Cole's *Art of Simpling* (1656) we may read how in the later part of the seventeenth century:

'in order to prevent witches from entering their houses, the common people used to gather *Elder leaves* on the last day of April and affix them to their doors and windows,'

and the tree was formerly much cultivated near English cottages for protection against witches.

The use of the Elder for funeral purposes was an old English custom referred to by Spenser.

'The Muses that were wont green Baies to weave,
Now bringen bittre Eldre braunches seare.'
Shepheard's Calendar – November.

And Canon Ellacombe says that in the Tyrol:

'An Elder bush, trimmed into the form of a cross, is planted on a new-made grave, and if it blossoms, the soul of the person lying beneath it is happy.'

Green Elder branches were also buried in a grave to protect the dead from witches and evil spirits, and in some parts it was a custom for the driver of the hearse to carry a whip made of Elder wood.

In some of the rural Midlands, it is believed that if a child is chastised with an Elder switch, it will cease to grow, owing, in this instance, to some supposed malign influence of the tree. On the other hand, Lord Bacon commended the rubbing of warts with a green Elder stick and then burying the stick to rot in the mud, and for erysipelas, it was recommended to wear about the neck an amulet made of Elder 'on which the sun had never shined.'

In Denmark we come across the old belief that he who stood under an Elder tree on Midsummer Eve would see the King of Fairyland ride by, attended by all his retinue. Folkard, in *Plant-Lore, Legends and Lyrics*, relates:

'The pith of the branches when cut in round, flat shapes, is dipped in oil, lighted, and then put to float in a glass of water; its light on Christmas Eve is thought to reveal to the owner all the witches and sorcerers in the neighbourhood';

and again,

'On Bertha Night (6th January), the devil goes about with special virulence. As a safeguard, persons are recommended to make a magic circle, in the centre of which they should stand, with Elderberries gathered on St. John's night. By doing this, the mystic Fern-seed may be obtained, which possesses the strength of thirty or forty men.'

This is a Styrian tradition.

The whole tree has a narcotic smell, and it is not considered wise to sleep under its shade. Perhaps the visions of fairyland were the result of the drugged sleep! No plant will grow under the shadow of it, being affected by its exhalations.

Apart from all these traditions, the Elder has had from the earliest days a firm claim on the popular affection for its many sterling virtues.

¶ *Uses.* Its uses are manifold and important. The wood of old trees is white and of a fine, close grain, easily cut, and polishes well, hence it was used for making skewers for butchers, shoemakers' pegs, and various turned articles, such as tops for angling rods and needles for weaving nets, also for making combs, mathematical instruments and several different musical instruments, and the pith of the younger stems, which is exceedingly light, is cut into balls and is used for electrical experiments and for making small toys. It is also considerably used for holding small objects for sectioning for microscopical purposes.

In a cutting of Worlidge's *Mystery of Husbandry* (dated 1675) the Elder is included in the 'trees necessary and proper for fencing and enclosing of Lands.'

'A considerable Fence,' he writes, 'may be made of Elder, set of reasonable hasty Truncheons, like the Willow and may be laid with great curiosity: this makes a speedy shelter for a garden from Winds, Beasts and suchlike injuries,'

though he adds and emphasizes with italics, 'rather than from *rude Michers*.'

The word 'micher' is now obsolete, but it means a lurking thief, a skulking vagabond. By clipping two or three times a year, an Elder hedge may, however, be made close and compact in growth. There is an old tradition that an Elder stake will last in the ground longer than an iron bar of the same size, hence the old couplet:

'An eldern stake and a black thorn ether (hedge)
Will make a hedge to last for ever.'

The leaves have an unpleasant odour when bruised, which is supposed to be offensive to most insects, and a decoction of the young leaves is sometimes employed by gardeners to sprinkle over delicate plants and the buds of the flowers to keep off the attacks of aphis and minute caterpillars. Moths are fond of the blossoms, but it was stated by Christopher Gullet (*Phil. Trans.*, 1772, LXII) that if turnips, cabbages, fruit trees or corn be whipped with bunches of the green leaves, they gain immunity from blight. Though this does not sound a very practical procedure, there is evidently some foundation for this statement, as the following note which appeared in the *Chemist and Druggist*, January 6, 1923, would seem to prove:

'A liquid preparation for preventing, and also curing, blight in fruit trees, wherein the base is a liquid obtained by boiling the *young shoots of the Elder tree or bush*, mixed with suitable proportions of copper sulphate, iron sulphate, nicotine, soft soap, methylated spirit and slaked lime.'

The leaves, bruised, if worn in the hat or rubbed on the face, prevent flies settling on the person. In order to safeguard the skin from the attacks of mosquitoes, midges and other troublesome flies, an infusion of the leaves may be dabbed on with advantage. Gather a few fresh leaves from the elder, tear them from their stalks and place them in a jug, pouring boiling water on them and covering them at once, leaving for a few hours. When the infusion is cold, it is fit for use and should be at once poured off into a bottle and kept tightly corked. It is desirable to make a fresh infusion often. The leaves are said to be valued by the farmer for driving mice away from granaries and moles from their usual haunts.

The *bark* of the older branches has been used in the Scotch Highlands as an ingredient in dyeing black, also the *root*. The *leaves* yield, with alum, a green dye and the *berries* dye blue and purple, the juice yielding with alum, violet; with alum and salt, a lilac colour.

The botanist finds in this plant an object of considerable interest, for if a twig is partially cut, then cautiously broken and the divided portions are carefully drawn asunder, the spiral air-vessels, resembling a screw, may be distinctly seen.

Linnæus observed that sheep eat the leaves, also cows, but that horses and goats refuse it. If sheep that have the foot-rot can get at the bark and young shoots, they will cure themselves. Elderberries are eaten greedily by young birds and pigeons, but are said to have serious effects on chickens: the flowers are reported to be fatal to turkeys, and according to Linnæus, also to peacocks.

Elder Flowers and Elder Berries have long been used in the English countryside for making many home-made drinks and preserves that are almost as great favourites now as in the time of our great-grandmothers. The berries make an excellent home-made wine and winter cordial, which improves with age, and taken hot with sugar, just before going to bed, is an old-fashioned and well-established cure for a cold.

In Kent, there are entire orchards of Elder trees cultivated solely for the sake of their fruit, which is brought regularly to market and sold for the purpose of making wine. The berries are not only used legitimately for making Elderberry Wine, but largely in the manufacture of so-called British wines – they give a red colour to raisin wine – and in the adulteration of foreign wines. Judiciously flavoured with vinegar and sugar and small quantities of port wine, Elder is often the basis of spurious 'clarets' and 'Bordeaux.' 'Men of nice palates,' says Berkeley (*Querist*, 1735), 'have been imposed on by Elder Wine for French Claret.' Cheap port is often faked to resemble tawny port by the addition of Elderberry juice, which forms one of the least injurious ingredients of factitious port wines. Doctoring port wine with Elderberry juice seems to have assumed such dimensions that in 1747 this practice was forbidden in Portugal, even the cultivation of the Elder tree was forbidden on this account. The practice proving so lucrative, however, is by no means obsolete, but as the berries possess valuable medicinal properties, this adulteration has no harmful results. The circumstances under which this was proved are somewhat curious. In 1899 an American sailor informed a physician of Prague that getting drunk on genuine, old, dark-red port was a sure remedy for rheumatic pains. This unedifying observation started a long series of investigations ending in the discovery that while genuine port wine has practically no anti-neuralgic properties, the cheap stuff faked to resemble tawny port by the addition of elderberry juice often banishes the pain of sciatica and other forms of neuralgia, though of no avail in genuine neuritis. Cases of cure have been instanced, after many tests carried out by leading doctors in Prague and other centres abroad, the dose recommended being 30 grams of Elderberry juice mixed with 10 grams of port wine.

The Romans, as Pliny records, made use of it in medicine, as well as of the Dwarf Elder (*Sambucus Ebulus*). Both kinds were employed in Britain by the ancient English and Welsh leeches and in Italy in the medicine of the School of Salernum. Elder still keeps its place in the British Pharmacopœia, the cooling effects of Elder flowers being well known. In many parts of the country, Elder leaves and buds are used in drinks, poultices and ointments.

It has been termed 'the medicine chest of the country people' (Ettmueller) and 'a whole magazine of physic to rustic practitioners,' and it is said the great physician Boerhaave never passed an Elder without raising his hat, so great an opinion had he of its curative properties. How great was the popular estimation of it in Shakespeare's time may be gauged by the line in the *Merry Wives of Windsor*, Act II, Sc. 3:

'What says my Æsculapius? my Galen? my heart of Elder?'

John Evelyn, writing in praise of the Elder, says:

'If the medicinal properties of its leaves, bark and berries were fully known, I cannot tell what our countryman could ail for which he might not fetch a remedy from every hedge, either for sickness, or wounds.'

'The buds boiled in water gruel have effected wonders in a fever; the spring buds are excellently wholesome in pattages; and small ale in which Elder flowers have been infused is esteemed by many so salubrious that this is to be had in most of the eating-houses about our town.'

He also, as we have seen, recommends Elder flowers infused in vinegar as an ingredient of a salad, 'though the leaves are somewhat rank of smell and so not commendable in sallet they are of the most sovereign virtue,' and goes so far as to say, 'an extract composed of the berries greatly assists longevity. Indeed this is a catholicum against all infirmities whatever.'

Some twenty years before Evelyn's eulogy there had appeared in 1644 a book entirely devoted to its praise: *The Anatomie of the Elder*, translated from the Latin of Dr. Martin Blockwich by C. de Iryngio (who seems to have been an army doctor), a treatise of some 230 pages, that in Latin and English went through several editions. It deals very learnedly with the medicinal virtues of the tree – its flowers, berries, leaves, 'middle bark,' pith, roots and 'Jew's ears,' a large fungus often to be found on the Elder (*Hirneola auricula Judæ*), the name a corruption of 'Judas's ear,' from the tradition, referred to above, that Judas hanged himself on the Elder. It is of a purplish tint, resembling in shape and softness the human ear, and though it occurs also on the Elm, it grows almost exclusively on Elder trunks in damp, shady places. It is curious that on account of this connexion with Judas, the fungus should have (as Sir Thomas Browne says) 'become a famous medicine in quinses, sore-throats, and strangulation ever since.' Gerard says, 'the jelly of the Elder, otherwise called Jew's ear, taketh away inflammations of the mouth and throat if they be washed therewith and doth in like manner help the uvula,' and Salmon, writing in the early part of the eighteenth century, recommends an oil of Jew's ears for throat affections. The fungus is edible and allied species are eaten in China.

Evelyn refers to this work (or rather to the original by 'Blockwitzius,' as he calls him!) for the comprehensive statement in praise of the Elder quoted above. It sets forth that as every part of the tree was medicinal, so virtually every ailment of the body was curable by it, from toothache to the plague. It was used externally and internally, and in amulets (these were especially good for epilepsy, and in popular belief also for rheumatism), and in every kind of form – in rob and syrup, tincture, mixture, oil, spirit, water, liniment, extract, salt, conserve, vinegar, oxymel, sugar, decoction, bath, cataplasm and powder. Some of these were prepared from one part of the plant only, others from several or from all. Their properties are summed up as 'desiccating, conglutinating, and digesting,' but are extended to include everything necessary to a universal remedy. The book prescribes in more or less detail for some seventy or more distinct diseases or classes of diseases, and the writer is never at a loss for an authority – from Dioscorides to the Pharmacopœias of his own day – while the examples of cures he adduces are drawn from all classes of people, from Emylia, Countess of Isinburg, to the tradesmen of Heyna and their dependants.

The interest in the Elder evinced about this period is also demonstrated by a tract on 'Elder and Juniper Berries, showing how useful they may be in our Coffee Houses,' which was published with *The Natural History of Coffee*, in 1682.

¶ *Parts Used Medicinally*. The bark, leaves, flowers and berries.

¶ *Bark*. The Inner Bark should be collected in autumn, from young trees. It is best dried in a moderate sun-heat, being taken indoors at night. When ready for use, it is a light grey, soft and corky externally, with broad fissures; white and smooth on the inner surface. The taste of the bark is sweetish at first, then slightly bitter and nauseous. It is without odour.

¶ *Chemical Constituents.* The active princi-ple of the bark is a soft resin, and an acid, Viburnic acid, which has been proved identical with Valeric acid. Other constitu-ents are traces of a volatile oil, albumen, resin, fat, wax, chlorophyll, tannic acid, grape sugar, gum, extractive, starch, pectin and various alkaline and earthy salts. (*According to an analysis by Kramer in* 1881.)

¶ *Medicinal Action and Uses.* The bark is a strong purgative which may be employed with advantage, an infusion of 1 oz. in a pint of water being taken in wineglassful doses; in large doses it is an emetic. Its use as a purgative dates back to Hippocrates. It has been much employed as a diuretic, an aque-ous solution having been found very useful in cardiac and renal dropsies. It has also been successfully employed in epilepsy.

An emollient ointment is made of the green inner bark, and a homœopathic tincture, made from the fresh inner bark of the young branches, in diluted form, relieves asthmatic symptoms and spurious croup of children – dose, 4 or 5 drops in water.

Culpepper states :

'The first shoots of the common Elder, boiled like Asparagus, and the young leaves and stalks boiled in fat broth, doth mightily carry forth phlegm and choler. The middle or inward bark boiled in water and given in drink wortheth much more violently; and the berries, either green or dry, expel the same humour, and are often given with good success in dropsy; the bark of the root boiled in wine, or the juice thereof drunk, worketh the same effects, but more powerfully than either the leaves or fruit. The juice of the root taken, causes vomitings and purgeth the watery humours of the dropsy.'

Though the use of the root is now obsolete, its juice was used from very ancient times to promote both vomiting and purging, and taken, as another old writer recommends, in doses of 1 to 2 tablespoonsful, fasting, once in the week, was held to be 'the most excel-lent purge of water humours in the world and very singular against dropsy.' A tea was also made from the roots of Elder, which was con-sidered an effective preventative for incipient dropsy, in fact the very best remedy for such cases.

¶ *Leaves.* Elder leaves are used both fresh and dry.

Collect the leaves in June and July. Gather only in fine weather, in the morning, after the dew has been dried by the sun. Strip the leaves off singly, rejecting any that are stained or insect-eaten. Drying is then done in the usual manner.

¶ *Constituents.* Elder Leaves contain an alka-loid Sambucine, a purgative resin and the glucoside Sambunigrin, which crystallizes in white, felted needles. Fresh Elder leaves yield about 0·16 per cent. of hydrocyanic acid. They also contain cane sugar, in-vertin, a considerable quantity of potassium nitrate and a crystalline substance, Eldrin, which has also been found in other white flowering plants.

De Sanctis claims to have isolated the alka-loid Coniine from the branches and leaves of *Sambucus nigra.* Alpes (*Proc. Amer. Pharm. Assoc.*, 1900) found undoubted evidence of an alkaloid in the roots of the American Elder (*S. Canadensis*), its odour being somewhat similar to that of coniine and also suggesting nicotine. This alkaloid was evidently volatile. It appeared to be much less abundant in the dried roots after some months keeping. The fresh root of *S. Canadensis* has been found extremely poisonous, producing death in children within a short time after being eaten, with symptoms very similar to those of poisoning by Hemlock (*Conium*).

¶ *Uses.* Elder leaves are used in the prepara-tion of an ointment, *Unguentum Sambuci Viride*, Green Elder Ointment, which is a domestic remedy for bruises, sprains, chil-blains, for use as an emollient, and for apply-ing to wounds. It can be compounded as follows: Take 3 parts of fresh Elder leaves, 4 parts of lard and 2 of prepared suet; heat the Elder leaves with the melted lard and suet until the colour is extracted, then strain through a linen cloth with pressure and allow to cool.

Sir Thomas Browne (1655) stated: 'The common people keep as a good secret in cur-ing wounds the leaves of the Elder, which they have gathered the last day of April.' The leaves, boiled soft with a little linseed oil, were used as a healing application to piles. An ointment concocted from the green Elderberries, with camphor and lard, was formerly ordered by the London College of Surgeons to relieve the same complaint. The leaves are an ingredient of many cooling ointments: Here is another recipe, not made from Elder leaves alone, and very much re-commended by modern herbalists as being very cooling and softening and excellent for all kinds of tumours, swellings and wounds: Take the Elder leaves ½ lb., Plantain leaves ¼ lb., Ground Ivy 2 oz., Wormwood 4 oz. (all green); cut them small, and boil in 4 lb. of lard, in the oven, or over a slow fire; stir them continually until the leaves become crisp, then strain, and press out the ointment for use.

Oil of Elder Leaves (*Oleum Viride*), Green Oil, or Oil of Swallows, is prepared by digesting 1 part of bruised fresh Elder leaves in 3 parts of linseed oil. In commerce, it is said to be generally coloured with verdigris.

Like the bark, the leaves are also purgative, but more nauseous than the bark. Their action is likewise expectorant, diuretic and diaphoretic. They are said to be very efficacious in dropsy. The juice of Elder leaves is stated by the old herbalists to be good for inflammation of the eyes, and 'snuffed up the nostrils,' Culpepper declares, 'purgeth the brain.' Another old notion was that if the green leaves were warmed between two hot tiles and applied to the forehead, they would promptly relieve nervous headache.

The use of the leaves, bruised and in decoction, to drive away flies and kill aphides and other insect pests has already been referred to.

¶ *Flowers.* Elder Flowers are chiefly used in pharmacy in the fresh state for the distillation of Elder Flower Water, but as the flowering season only lasts for about three weeks in June, the flowers are often salted, so as to be available for distillation at a later season, 10 per cent. of common salt being added, the flowers being them termed 'pickled.' They are also dried, for making infusions.

The flowers are collected when just in full bloom and thrown into heaps, and after a few hours, during which they become slightly heated, the corollas become loosened and can then be removed by sifting. The Elder 'flowers' of pharmacy consist of the small, white wheel-shaped, five-lobed, monopetalous corollas only, in the short tube of which the five stamens with very short filaments and yellow anthers are inserted. When fresh, the flowers have a slightly bitter taste and an odour scarcely pleasant. The pickled flowers, however, gradually acquire an agreeable fragrance and are therefore generally used for the preparation of Elder Flower Water. A similar change also takes place in the water distilled from the fresh flowers.

In domestic herbal medicines, the *dried* flowers are largely used in country districts, and are sold by herbalists either in dried bunches of flowers, or sifted free from flower stalks. The flowers are not easily dried of good colour. If left too late exposed to the sun before gathering, the flowers assume a brownish colour when dried, and if the flower bunches are left too long in heaps, to cause the flowers to fall off, these heaps turn black. If the inflorescence is only partly open when gathered, the flower-heads have to be sifted more than once, as the flowers do not open all at the same time. The best and lightest-coloured flowers are obtained at the first

sifting, when the flowers that have matured and fallen naturally are free from stalks, and dried quickly in a heated atmosphere. They may be very quickly dried in a heated copper pan, being stirred about for a few minutes. They can also be dried almost as quickly in a cool oven, with the door open. Quickness in drying is essential.

The dried flowers, which are so shrivelled that their details are quite obscured, have a dingy, brownish-yellow colour and a faint, but characteristic odour and mucilaginous taste. As a rule, imported flowers have a duller yellow colour and inferior odour and are sold at a cheaper rate. When the microscope does not reveal tufts of short hairs in the sinuses of the calyx, the drug is not of this species. Most pharmacopœias specify that dark brown or blackish flowers should be rejected. This appearance may be due to their having been collected some time after opening, to carelessness in drying, or to having been preserved too long.

The flowers of the Dwarf Elder, a comparatively uncommon plant in this country, are distinguished from those of the Common Elder by having dark red anthers.

The flowers of the Yarrow (*Achillea millefolium*), and other composite plants, which have been used as adulterants of Elder flowers differ still more markedly in appearance and their presence in the drug is readily detected.

¶ *Constituents.* The most important constituent of Elder Flowers is a trace of semi-solid volatile oil, present to the extent only of 0.32, per cent. possessing the odour of the flowers in a high degree. It is obtained by distilling the fresh flowers with water, saturating the distillate with salt and shaking it with ether. On evaporating the ethereal solution, the oil is obtained as a yellowish, buttery mass. Without ether, fresh Elder flowers yield 0.037 per cent. of the volatile oil and the dried flowers 0.0027 per cent. only.

Elder Flower Water (*Aqua Sambuci*) is an official preparation of the British Pharmacopœia, which directs that it be made from 100 parts of Elder Flowers distilled with 500 parts of water (about 10 lb. to the gallon), and that if fresh Elder flowers are not obtainable, an equivalent quantity of the flowers preserved with common salt be used. The product has at first a distinctly unpleasant odour, but gradually acquires an agreeably aromatic odour, and it is preferable not to use it until this change has taken place.

Elder Flower Water is employed in mixing medicines and chiefly as a vehicle for eye and skin lotions. It is mildly astringent and a gentle stimulant. It is the *Eau de Sureau* of the Continent, *Sureau* being the French name of the Elder.

Here is a recipe that can be carried out at home: Fill a large jar with Elder blossoms, pressing them down, the stalks of course having been removed previously. Pour on them 2 quarts of boiling water and when slightly cooled, add 1½ oz .of rectified spirits. Cover with a folded cloth, and stand the jar in a warm place for some hours. Then allow it to get quite cold and strain through muslin. Put into bottles and cork securely.

Elderflower Water in our great-grand-mothers' days was a household word for clearing the complexion of freckles and sun-burn, and keeping it in a good condition. Every lady's toilet table possessed a bottle of the liquid, and she relied on this to keep her skin fair and white and free from blemishes, and it has not lost its reputation. Its use after sea-bathing has been recommended, and if any eruption should appear on the face as the effect of salt water, it is a good plan to use a mixture composed of Elder Flower Water with glycerine and borax, and apply it night and morning.

Elder Flowers, if placed in the water used for washing the hands and face, will both whiten and soften the skin – a convenient way being to place them in a small muslin bag. Such a bag steeped in the bathwater makes a most refreshing bath and a well-known French doctor has stated that he considers it a fine aid in the bath in cases of irritability of the skin and nerves.

The flowers were used by our forefathers in bronchial and pulmonary affections, and in scarlet fever, measles and other eruptive diseases. An infusion of the dried flowers, Elder Flower Tea, is said to promote expectoration in pleurisy; it is gently laxative and aperient and is considered excellent for inducing free perspiration. It is a good old-fashioned remedy for colds and throat trouble, taken hot on going to bed. An almost infallible cure for an attack of in-fluenza in its first stage is a strong infusion of dried Elder Blossoms and Peppermint. Put a handful of each in a jug, pour over them a pint and a half of boiling water, allow to steep, on the stove, for half an hour, then strain and sweeten and drink in bed as hot as possible. Heavy perspiration and refreshing sleep will follow, and the patient will wake up well on the way to recovery and the cold or influenza will probably be banished within thirty-six hours. Yarrow may also be added.

Elder Flower Tea, cold, was also con-sidered almost as good for inflammation of the eyes as the distilled Elder Flower Water.

Tea made from Elder Flowers has also been recommended as a splendid spring medicine, to be taken every morning before breakfast for some weeks, being considered an excellent blood purifier.

Externally, Elder Flowers are used in fomentations, to ease pain and abate inflam-mation. An old writer tells us:

'There be nothing more excellent to ease the pains of the hæmorrhoids than a fomen-tation made of the flowers of the Elder and *Verbusie*, or Honeysuckle in water or milk for a short time. It easeth the greatest pain.'

A lotion, too, can be made by pouring boiling water on the dried blossoms, which is healing, cooling and soothing. Add 2½ drachms of Elder Flowers to 1 quart of boiling water, infuse for an hour and then strain. The liquor can be applied as a lotion, by means of a linen rag, for tumours, boils, and affections of the skin, and is said to be effective put on the temples against head-ache and also for warding off the attacks of flies.

A salad of young Elder buds, macerated a little in hot water and dressed with oil, vine-gar and salt, has been used as a remedy against skin eruptions.

Elder Vinegar made from the flowers is an old remedy for sore throat.

A good ointment is also prepared from the flowers by infusion in warm lard, useful for dressing wounds, burns and scalds, which is used, also, as a basis for pomades and cos-metic ointments, Elder Flower Ointment (*Unguentum Sambuci*) was largely used for wounded horses in the War – the Blue Cross made a special appeal for supplies – but it is also good for human use and is an old remedy for chapped hands and chilblains. Equal quantities of the fresh flowers and of lard are taken; the flowers are heated with the lard until they become crisp, then strained through a linen cloth with pressure and allowed to cool. For use as a Face Cream,[1] the directions are a little more elaborate, but it is essentially the same: Melt lard in a pan, then add a small cup of cold water and stir well. Simmer with the lid on for about an hour and finally let the mixture boil with the lid off until all the water has evaporated; this will have happened when, on stirring, no steam arises. Place on one side to cool a little and then pass the liquid fat through a piece of muslin so that it may be well strained and free from impurities. Take a quantity

[1] This preparation is hardly suitable as a cosmetic, as lard induces the growth of hair. – EDITOR.

of Elder Flowers equal in weight to the lard and place these in the lard. Then boil up the mixture again, keeping it simmering for a good hour. At the end of that time, strain the whole through a coarse cloth and when cool, the ointment will be ready for use.

Elder Flowers, with their subtle sweet scent, entered into much delicate cookery, in olden days. Formerly the creamy blossoms were beaten up in the batter of flannel cakes and muffins, to which they gave a more delicate texture. They were also boiled in gruel as a fever-drink, and were added to the posset of the Christening feast.

¶ *Berries.* All the other parts of the Elder plant, except the wood and pith, are more active than either the flowers or the fruit. Fresh Elder Berries are found to contain sudorific properties similar to those of the flowers, but weaker. Chemically, the berries furnish Viburnic acid, with an odorous oil, combined with malates of potash and lime. The fresh, ripe fruits contain Tyrosin.

The blue colouring matter extracted from them has been considerably used as an indication for alkalis, with which it gives a green colour, being red with acids. (Alkalis redden some vegetable yellows and change some vegetable blues to green.) According to Cowie this colouring matter is best extracted in the form of a 20 per cent. tincture from the refuse remaining after the expression of the first juice. The colouring matter is precipitated blue by lead acetate. (*National Standard Dispensatory*, 1909.)

The Romans made use of Elderberry juice as a hair-dye, and Culpepper tells us that 'the hair of the head washed with the berries boiled in wine is made black.'

English Elder Berries, as we have seen, are extensively used for the preparation of Elder Wine. French and other Continental Elder berries, when dried, are not liked for this purpose, as they have a more unpleasant odour and flavour, and English berries are preferred. Possibly this may be due to the conditions of growth, or variety, or to the presence of the berries of the Dwarf Elder. Aubrey (1626–97) tells us that

'the apothecaries well know the use of the berries, and so do the vintners, who buy vast quantities of them in London, and some do make no inconsiderable profit by the sale of them.'

They were held by our forefathers to be efficacious in rheumatism and erysipelas. They have aperient, diuretic and emetic properties, and the inspissated juice of the berries has been used as an alterative in rheumatism and syphilis in doses of from one to two drachms, also as a laxative in doses of half an ounce or more. It promotes all fluid secretions and natural evacuations

For colic and diarrhœa, a tea made of the dried berries is said to be a good remedy.

In *The Anatomie of the Elder*, it is stated that the berries of the Elder and Herb Paris are useful in epilepsy. Green Elderberry Ointment has already been mentioned as curative of piles.

After enumerating many uses of the Elder, Gerard says:

'The seeds contained within the berries, dried, are good for such as have the dropsie, and such as are too fat, and would faine be leaner, if they be taken in a morning to the quantity of a dram with wine for a certain space. The green leaves, pounded with Deeres suet or Bulls tallow are good to be laid to hot swellings and tumors, and doth assuage the paine of the gout.'

Parkinson, physician to James I, also tells us of the same use of the seeds, which he recommends to be taken powdered, in vinegar.

Elderberry Wine has a curative power of established repute as a remedy, taken hot, at night, for promoting perspiration in the early stages of severe catarrh, accompanied by shivering, sore throat, etc. Like Elderflower Tea, it is one of the best preventives known against the advance of influenza and the ill effects of a chill. A little cinnamon may be added. It has also a reputation as an excellent remedy for asthma.

Almost from time immemorial, a 'Rob' (a vegetable juice thickened by heat) has been made from the juice of Elderberries simmered and thickened with sugar, forming an invaluable cordial for colds and coughs, but only of late years has science proved that Elderberries furnish Viburnic acid, which induces perspiration, and is especially useful in cases of bronchitis and similar troubles.

To make Elderberry Rob, 5 lb. of fresh, ripe, crushed berries are simmered with 1 lb. of loaf sugar and the juice evaporated to the thickness of honey. It is cordial, aperient and diuretic. One or two tablespoonsful mixed with a tumblerful of hot water, taken at night, promotes perspiration and is demulcent to the chest. The Rob when made can be bottled and stored for the winter. Herbalists sell it ready for use.

'Syrup of Elderberries' is made as follows: Pick the berries when throughly ripe from the stalks and stew with a little water in a jar in the oven or pan. After straining, allow $\frac{1}{2}$ oz. of whole ginger and 18 cloves to each gallon. Boil the ingredients an hour, strain again and bottle. The syrup is an excellent cure for a cold. To about a wineglassful of Elderberry syrup, add hot water, and if liked, sugar.

Both Syrup of Elderberries and the Rob were once official in this country (as they are still in Holland), the rob being the older of of the two, and the one that retained its place longer in our Pharmacopœia. In 1788, its name was changed to *Succus Sambuci spissatus*, and in 1809 it disappeared altogether. Brookes in 1773 strongly recommended it as a 'saponaceous Resolvent' promoting 'the natural secretions by stool, urine and sweat,' and, diluted with water, for common colds. John Wesley, in his *Primitive Physick*, directs it to be taken in broth, and in Germany it is used as an ingredient in soups.

There were six or seven robs in the old London Pharmacopœia, to most of which sugar was added. They were thicker than syrups, but did not differ materially from them; among them was a rob of Elderberries, and both Quincy and Bates had a syrup of Elder.

An old prescription for sciatica (called the Duke of Monmouth's recipe) was compounded of ripe haws and fennel roots, distilled in white wine and taken with syrup of Elder.

The use of the juicy berries, not as medicine, but as a pleasant article of food, in jam, jelly, chutney and ketchup has already been described.

¶ *Medicinal Preparations.* Fluid extract of bark, ½ to 1 drachm. Water, B.P.

SOME ELDER WINE RECIPES
An old recipe for Elder Wine

'To every quart of berries put 2 quarts of water; boil half an hour, run the liquor and break the fruit through a hair sieve; then to every quart of juice, put ¾ of a pound of Lisbon sugar, coarse, but not the very coarsest. Boil the whole a quarter of an hour with some Jamaica peppers, ginger, and a few cloves. Pour it into a tub, and when of a proper warmth, into the barrel, with toast and yeast to work, which there is more difficulty to make it do than most other liquors. When it ceases to hiss, put a quart of brandy to eight gallons and stop up. Bottle in the spring, or at Christmas. The liquor must be in a warm place to make it work.'

The following recipe for making Elder Wine is given by Mrs. Hewlett in a work entitled *Cottage Comforts*:

'If two gallons of wine are to be made, get one gallon of Elderberries, and a quart of damsons, or sloes; boil them together in six quarts of water, for half an hour, breaking the fruit with a stick, flat at one end; run off the liquor, and squeeze the pulp through a sieve, or straining cloth; boil the liquor up again with six pounds of coarse sugar, two ounces of ginger, two ounces of bruised allspice, and one ounce of hops; (the spice had better be loosely tied in a bit of muslin); let this boil above half an hour; then pour it off; when quite cool, stir in a teacupful of yeast, and cover it up to work. After two days, skim off the yeast, and put the wine into the barrel, and when it ceases to hiss, which will be in about a fortnight, paste a stiff brown paper over the bung-hole. After this, it will be fit for use in about 8 weeks, but will keep 8 years, if required. The bag of spice may be dropped in at the bung-hole, having a string fastened outside, which shall keep it from reaching the bottom of the barrel.'

Another Recipe

'Strip the berries, which must be quite ripe, into a dry pan and pour 2 gallons of boiling water over 3 gallons of berries. Cover and leave in a warm place for 24 hours; then strain, pressing the juice well out. Measure it and allow 3 pounds of sugar, half an ounce of ginger and ¼ ounce of cloves to each gallon. Boil for 20 minutes slowly, then strain it into a cask and ferment when lukewarm. Let it remain until still, before bunging, and bottle in six months.

'If a weaker wine is preferred, use 4 gallons of water to 3 gallons of berries and leave for two days before straining.

'If a cask be not available, large stone jars will answer: then the wine need not be bottled.'

Parkinson tells us that fresh Elder Flowers hung in a vessel of new wine and pressed every evening for seven nights together, 'giveth to the wine a very good relish and a smell like Muscadine.' Ale was also infused with Elder flowers.

The berries make good *pies*, if blended with spices, and formerly used to be preserved with spice and kept for winter use in pies when fruit was scarce. Quite a delicious *jam* can also be made of them, mixed with apples, which has much the flavour of Blackberry jam. They mix to very great advantage with Crab Apple, or with the hard Catillac cooking Pear, or with Vegetable Marrow, and also with Blackberries or Rhubarb.

The Fruit Preserving Section of the Food Ministry issued during the War the following recipe for *Elderberry and Apple Jam*: 6 lb. Elderberries, 6 lb. sliced apples, 12 lb. sugar.

Make a pulp of the apples by boiling in water till soft and passing through a coarse sieve to remove any seeds or cores. The Elderberries should also be stewed for half an hour to soften them. Combine the Apple pulp, berries and sugar and return to the fire to boil till thick.

Another Recipe

Equal quantities of Elderberries and Apples, ¾ lb. sugar and one lemon to each pound of fruit. Strip the berries from the stalks, peel, core and cut up the apples and weigh both fruits. Put the Elderberries into a pan over low heat and bruise them with a wooden spoon. When the juice begins to flow, add the Apples and one-third of the sugar and bring slowly to the boil. When quite soft, rub all through a hair sieve. Return the pulp to the pan, add the rest of the sugar, the grated lemon rind and juice and boil for half an hour, or until the jam sets when tested. Remove all scum, put into pots and cover.

Elderberry Jam without Apples.

To every pound of berries add ¼ pint of water, the juice of 2 lemons and 1 lb. of sugar. Boil from 30 to 45 minutes, until it sets when tested. Put into jars and tie down when cold.

The Elderberry will, of course, also make a *jelly*. As it is a juicy fruit, it will not need the addition of any more liquid than, perhaps, a squeeze of lemon. Equal quantities of Elderberry juice and apple juice, and apple juice from peeling, will require ¾ lb. of sugar to a pint. Elderberry Jelly is firm and flavorous, with a racy tang.

When the fruit is not quite ripe, it may be preserved in brine and used as a substitute for capers.

The juice from Elder Berries, too, was formerly distilled and mixed with vinegar for salad dressings and flavouring sauces. Vinegars used in former times frequently to be aromatized by steeping in them barberries, rosemary, rose leaves, gilliflowers, lavender, violets – in short, any scented flower or plant, though tarragon is now practically the only herb used in this manner to any large extent.

Elderflower Vinegar is made thus:

Take 2 lb. of dried flowers of Elder. If you use your own flowers, pluck carefully their stalks from them and dry them carefully and thoroughly. This done, place in a large vessel and pour over them 2 pints of good vinegar. Close the vessel hermetically, keep it in a very warm place and shake them from time to time. After 8 days, strain the vinegar through a paper filter. Keep in well-stoppered bottles.

This is an old-world simple, but rarely met with nowadays, but worth the slight trouble of making. It was well-known and appreciated in former days and often mentioned in old books; Steele, in *The Tatler*, says: 'They had dissented about the preference of Elder to Wine vinegar.'

One seldom has the chance of now tasting the old country pickle made from the tender young shoots and flowers. John Evelyn, writing in 1664, recommends Elder flowers infused in vinegar as an ingredient of a salad. The pickled blossoms are said by those who have tried them to be a welcome relish with boiled mutton, as a substitute for capers. Clusters of the flowers are gathered in their unripened green state, put into a stone jar and covered with boiling vinegar. Spices are unnecessary. The jar is tied down directly the pickle is cold. This pickle is very good and has the advantage of costing next to nothing.

The pickle made from the tender young *shoots* – sometimes known as 'English Bamboo' – is more elaborate. During May, in the middle of the Elder bushes in the hedges, large young green shoots may be observed. Cut these, selecting the greenest, peel off every vestige of the outer skin and lay them in salt and water overnight. Each individual length must be carefully chosen, for while they must not be too immature, if the shoots are at all woody, they will not be worth eating, The following morning, prepare the pickle for the Mock Bamboo. To a quart of vinegar, add an ounce of white pepper, an ounce of ginger, half a saltspoonful of mace and boil all well together. Remove the Elder shoots from the salt and water, dry in a cloth and slice up into suitable pieces, laying them in a stone jar. Pour the boiling mixture over them and either place them in an oven for 2 hours, or in a pan of boiling water on the stove. When cold, the pickle should be green in colour. If not, strain the liquor, boil it up again, pour over the shoots and repeat the process. The great art of obtaining and retaining the essence of the plant lies in excluding air from the tied-down jar as much as possible.

The young shoots can also be boiled in salted water with a pinch of soda to preserve the colour; they prove beautifully tender, resembling spinach, and form quite a welcome addition to the dinner table.

Good use can be made of the berries for *Ketchup* and *Chutney*, and the following recipes will be found excellent.

Elderberry Chutney

2 lb. Elderberries, 1 large Onion, 1 pint vinegar, 1 teaspoonful salt, 1 teaspoonful ground ginger, 2 tablespoonsful sugar, 1 saltspoonful cayenne and mixed spices, 1 teaspoonful mustard seed.

Stalk, weigh and wash the berries; put them into a pan and bruise with a wooden spoon; chop the onion and add with the rest of the ingredients and vinegar. Bring to the boil and simmer till it becomes thick. Stir well, being careful not to let it burn as it thickens. Put into jars and cover.

Another Recipe

Rub 1½ lb. of berries through a wire sieve, pound 1 onion, 6 cloves, ¼ oz. ground ginger, 2 oz. Demerara sugar, 3 oz. stoned raisins, a dust of cayenne and mace, 1 teaspoonful salt and ½ pint vinegar. Put all in an enamelled saucepan and boil with the pulp of the berries for 10 minutes. Take the pan from the fire and let it stand till cold. Put the chutney into jars and cork securely.

Elderberry Ketchup

1 pint Elderberries, 1 oz. shallots, 1 blade mace, ½ oz. peppercorns, 1½ oz. whole ginger, 1 pint vinegar.

Pick the berries (which must be ripe) from the stalks, weigh and wash them. Put them into an unglazed crock or jar, pour over the boiling vinegar and leave all night in a cool oven. Next day, strain the liquor from the berries through a cloth tied on to the legs of an inverted chair and put it into a pan, with the peeled and minced shallots, the ginger peeled and cut up small, the mace and peppercorns. Boil for 10 minutes, then put into bottles, dividing the spices among the bottles. Cork well.

All parts of the tree – bark, leaves, flowers and berries – have long enjoyed a high reputation in domestic medicine. From the days of Hippocrates, it has been famous for its medicinal properties.

ELDER, DWARF

Sambucus Ebulus (LINN.)
N.O. Caprifoliaceæ

Synonyms. Danewort. Walewort. Blood Hilder
  (*French*) Hièble
  (*German*) Attichwurzel
Part Used. Leaves
Habitat. This species is found less frequently in hedges, but inclines to waste places, not infrequently among rubbish and the ruined foundations of old buildings. Gerard speaks of the 'dwarf Elder' growing 'in untoiled places plentifully in the lane at Kilburne Abbey by London.' The celebrated natural historian of Selborne speaks of the Dwarf Elder as growing among the rubbish and ruined foundations of the Priory. Spots of equal interest with that of Selborne might be cited as favourite haunts of the Dwarf Elder. It grows profusely near Carisbrooke Castle, below the timeworn walls of Scarborough Castle, beside the old Roman Watling Street, where it is crossed by the footpath from Norton to Wilton, in Northamptonshire.

Its old names, Danewort and Walewort (wal-slaughter) are supposed to be traceable to an old belief that it sprang from the blood of slain Danes – it grows near Slaughterford in Wilts, that being the site of a great Danish battle. Another notion is that it was brought to England by the Danes and planted on the battlefields and graves of their slain countrymen. In Norfolk it still bears the name of Danewort and Blood Hilder (Blood Elder). In accounting for its English name, Sir J. E. Smith says: ' Our ancestors evinced a just hatred of their brutal enemies, the Danes, in supposing the nauseous, fetid and noxious plant before us to have sprung from their blood.'

The Dwarf Elder differs from the Common Elder in being a herbaceous plant, seldom exceeding 3 feet in height and dying back to the ground every year, spreading by underground shoots from the creeping root.

¶ *Description.* In leaf, flower and subsequent berry it bears a close resemblance to the Common Elder tree; the stem, however, is not woody and the leaves are distinguished by having a stipule, or small leaf, at the base of the finely-toothed leaflets, which are more numerous than those of the Common Elder, usually seven in number, larger and narrower and sometimes lobed. The flowers are whiter than those of the Common Elder, the corollas splashed with crimson on the outside and have dark red anthers. They are in bloom in July and August, have a less aromatic smell and do not always bring their fruit, a reddish-purple berry, to perfect ripeness in this country. The berries are, however, often present among imported Continental dried elderberries, the species being much more common there than here. In France it is called *Hièble*, in Germany *Attichwurzel*.

¶ *Medicinal Action and Uses.* Expectorant, diuretic, diaphoretic, purgative.

The Dwarf Elder has more drastic therapeutic action than the Common Elder, and it is only the leaves, or very occasionally the berries, that are used medicinally. The leaves are probably more used in herbal practice than those of *Sambucus nigra*, and are ingredients in medicines for inflammation of both kidney and liver. The drug is said to be very efficacious in dropsy. Dwarf Elder Tea, which has been considered one of the best remedies for dropsy, is prepared from the dried roots, cut up fine or ground to powder; the drug was much used by Kneipp.

The root, which is white and fleshy, has a nauseous, bitter taste and a decoction from it is a drastic purgative. Culpepper states that the decoction cures the bites of mad dogs and adders. The root-juice has been employed to dye hair black.

The leaves, bruised and laid on boils and scalds, have a healing effect, and boiled in wine and made into a poultice were employed in France to resolve swellings and relieve contusions.

A rob made from the berries is actively purgative.

An oil extracted from the seeds has been used as an application to painful joints.

Mice and moles are said not to come near the leaves, and in Silesia there is a belief that it prevents some of the diseases of swine, being strewn in sties.

In the United States, the name of Dwarf Elder is given to an entirely different plant, viz. *Aralia hispida* (N.O. Araliaceæ). In Homœopathy, it is the American Dwarf Elder which is employed. There it is also called Bristly Sarsaparilla and Wild Elder. It is found growing in rocky places in North America.

The homœopaths use a tincture from the fresh, root and a fluid extract is also prepared from it. It has sudorific, diuretic and alterative properties and is regarded as very valuable in dropsy, gravel and in suppression of urine. It is particularly recommended as a diuretic in dropsy, being more acceptable to the stomach than other remedies of the same class.

The 'Prickly Elder' of America is a closely related species, *A. spinosa*, also known as False Prickly Ash (the real Prickly Ash being *Xanthoxylum Americanum*), which contains a glucoside named Aralin. A decoction of the plant is used for the same purposes as Sarsaparilla.

The 'Poison Elder' of America is again no Elder, but a Sumach, its other name being Swamp Sumach, botanically *Rhus verni* (Linn.). It is a handsome shrub or small tree, 10 to 15 feet high, growing in swamps from Canada to California, with very small greenish flowers and small greenish-white berries and is extremely poisonous. It was confounded by the older botanists with *R. vernicifera* (D.C.) of Japan, the Japanese lacquer tree, which has similar poisonous properties. Its synonym is *R. venenata* (D.C.) *See* SUMACH.

There is a tree called the 'Box Elder,' mentioned by W. J. Bean in his *Trees and Shrubs hardy in the British Isles*; this is not a true Elder, however, but one of the American maples that yield sugar.

There are about half a dozen species of Elder hardy in Great Britain. The Common Elder (*S. nigra*), of which there are many varieties in cultivation, several of which are very ornamental, has leaves often very finely divided and jagged and variegated both with golden and silver blotches, a specially ornamental form being the 'golden cut-leaf Elder,' and another with yellow berries; the American Elder (*S. canadensis*) (the flowers of which, together with those of *S. nigra* are official in the United States Pharmacopœia) has berries smaller and deep purple rather than black, the leaves broader and the flowers more fragrant than our Common Elder, it never attains tree size, but is a shrub of from 6 to 10 feet in height; the Blue Elder (*S. glauca*), the intensely blue berries of which are used as a food, when cooked, in California; the Red-berried Elder (*S. racemosa*), a pretty species, native of Central and Southern Europe, cultivated in shrubberies, which flowers in March and towards the end of summer is highly ornamental, with large oval clusters of bright scarlet berries, is so attractive to birds that their beauty is rarely seen, except when cultivated close to a house; the Red-berried American Elder (*S. rubens* and *S. melanocarpa*).

¶ *Cultivation.* The Elders like moisture and a loamy soil; given these, they are not difficult to accommodate. The pruning of the sorts grown for their foliage should be done before growth recommences.

They can be easily propagated by cuttings or by seeds, but the former being the most expeditious method is generally followed. The season for planting the cuttings is any time from September to March, and no more care is needed than to thrust the cuttings 6 to 8 inches into the ground. They will take root very quickly, and can be afterwards transplanted where they are to remain. If their berries are allowed to fall upon the ground, they will produce abundance of plants in the following summer.

ELDER, DWARF, AMERICAN

Habitat. New England to Virginia

A perennial, stem 1 to 2 feet high, lower part woody and shrubby, beset with sharp bristles, upper part leafy and branching. Leaflets oblongovate, acute serrate, leaves bipinnate, many simple umbels, globose, axillary and terminal on long peduncles, has bunches of dark-coloured nauseous berries, flowers June to September. The whole plant smells unpleasantly. Fruit, black, round, one-celled, has three irregular-shaped seeds. The bark is used medicinally, but the root is the more active.

This plant must not be confused with the English Dwarf Elder (*Sambucus Ebulus*).
¶ *Medicinal Action and Uses.* Sudorific in warm infusion – bark diuretic and altera-

Herbaceous kinds like *S. Ebulus* may be increased by dividing the rootstocks in early autumn or spring.

Aralia hispida
N.O. Araliaceæ

tive and has a special action on kidneys. Most valuable in urinary diseases, dropsy, gravel, suppression of urine, etc. A decoction of the fresh roots and juice are efficacious in dropsy, being a good hydragogue and also an emetic. Dose, decoction, 2 to 4 oz. three times daily.

See ANGELICA TREE, BAMBOO BRIER, SARSAPARILLA, SPIKENARD (AMERICAN), SPIKENARD (CALIFORNIAN).

Aralia spinosa. The berries are used in an infusion of wine or spirits, relieving violent colic and rheumatic pains. It contains the glucoside Araliin.

See also GRUSENG, BAMBOO BRIER.

ELECAMPANE

Inula Helenium (LINN.)
N.O. Compositæ

Synonyms. Scabwort. Elf Dock. Wild Sunflower. Horseheal. Velvet Dock
(*French*) *Aunée*
(*German*) Alantwurzel
(*Welsh*) Marchalan
Part Used. Root
Habitat. Elecampane is one of our largest herbaceous plants. It is found widely distributed throughout England, though can scarcely be termed common, occurring only locally, in damp pastures and shady ground. It is probably a true native plant in southern England, but where found farther north may have originally only been an escape from cultivation, as it was cultivated for centuries as a medicinal plant, being a common remedy for sicknesses in the Middle Ages. When present in Scotland, it is considered to have been introduced. Culpepper says:

'It groweth in moist grounds and shadowy places oftener than in the dry and open borders of field and lanes and other waste places, almost in every county in this country, but it was probably more common in his days, cultivation of it being still general.'

It is found wild throughout continental Europe, from Gothland southwards, and extends eastwards in temperate Asia as far as Southern Siberia and North-West India. As a plant of cultivation, it has wandered to North America, where it has become thoroughly naturalized in the eastern United States, being found from Nova Scotia to Northern Carolina, and westward as far as Missouri, growing abundantly in pastures and along roadsides, preferring wet, rocky ground at or near the base of eastern and southern slopes

¶ *Description.* It is a striking and handsome plant. The erect stem grows from 4 to 5 feet high, is very stout and deeply furrowed, and near the top, branched. The whole plant is downy. It produces a radical rosette of enormous, ovate, pointed leaves, from 1 to 1½ feet long and 4 inches broad in the middle, velvety beneath, with toothed margins and borne on long foot-stalks; in general appearance the leaves are not unlike those of Mul-

lein. Those on the stem become shorter and relatively broader and are stem-clasping.

The plant is in bloom from June to August. The flowers are bright yellow, in very large, terminal heads, 3 to 4 inches in diameter, on long stalks, resembling a double sunflower. The broad bracts of the leafy involucre under the head are velvety. After the flowers have fallen, these involucral scales spread horizontally, and the removal of the fruit shows

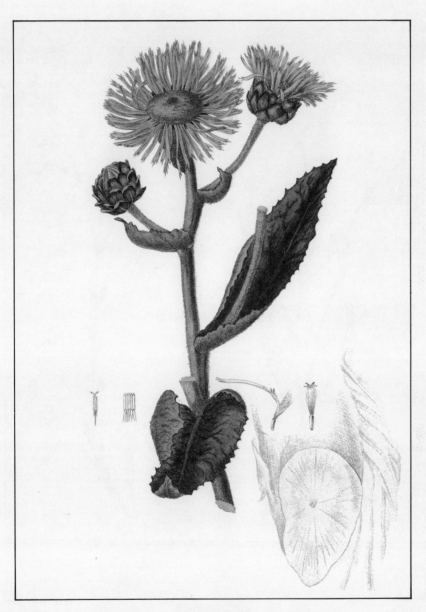

ELECAMPANE
Inula Helenium

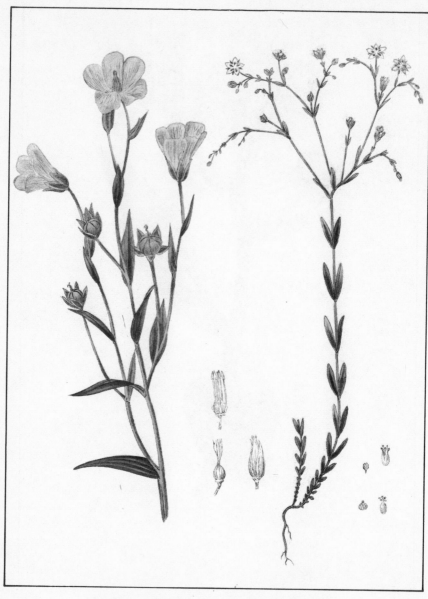

FLAX—LINSEED AND MOUNTAIN FLAX
Linum Usitatissimum and *Linum Catharticum*

the beautifully regular arrangement of the little pits on the receptacle, which form a pattern like the engine-turning of a watch. The fruit is quadrangular and crowned by a ring of pale-reddish hairs – the pappus.

The plant springs from a perennial rootstock, which is large and succulent, spindle-shaped and branching, brown and aromatic, with large, fleshy roots.

¶ *History*. Elecampane was known to the ancient writers on agriculture and natural history, and even the Roman poets were acquainted with it, and mention Inula as affording a root used both as a medicine and a condiment. Horace, in the Eighth Satire, relates how Fundanius first taught the making of a delicate sauce by boiling in it the bitter Inula, and how the Romans, after dining too richly, pined for turnips and the appetizing *Enulas acidas*:

> 'Quum rapula plenus
> Atque acidas mavult inulas.'

Inula, the Latin classical name for the plant, is considered to be a corruption of the Greek word *Helenion*, which in its Latinized form, *Helenium*, is also now applied to the same species. There are many fables about the origin of this name. Gerard tells us: 'It took the name Helenium of Helena, wife of Menelaus, who had her hands full of it when Paris stole her away into Phrygia.' Another legend states that it sprang from her tears: another that Helen first used it against venomous bites; a fourth, that it took the name from the island Helena, where the best plants grew.

Vegetius Renatus, about the beginning of the fifth century, calls it *Inula campana*, and St. Isidore, in the beginning of the seventh, names it *Inula*, adding 'quam Alam rustici vocant.' By the mediæval writers it was often written *Enula*. Elecampane is a corruption of the ante-Linnæan name *Enula campana*, so called from its growing wild in Campania.

The herb is of ancient medicinal repute, having been described by Dioscorides and Pliny. An old Latin distich celebrates its virtues: *Enula campana reddit præcordia sana* (Elecampane will the spirits sustain). 'Julia Augustus,' said Pliny, 'let no day pass without eating some of the roots of Enula, considered to help digestion and cause mirth.' The monks equally esteemed it as a cordial. Pliny affirmed that the root 'being chewed fasting, doth fasten the teeth,' and Galen that 'It is good for passions of the hucklebone called sciatica.'

Dioscorides, in speaking of Castus root, related that it is often mixed with that of Elecampane, from Kommagene (N.W. Syria) (Castus, derived from *Aplotaxis auriculata* (D.C.), is remarkably similar to Elecampane, both in external appearance and structure. It is an important spice, incense and medicine in the East.)

Elecampane is frequently mentioned in the Anglo-Saxon writings on medicine current in England prior to the Norman Conquest; it is also the 'Marchalan' of the Welsh physicians of the thirteenth century, and was generally known during the Middle Ages.

It was formally cultivated in all private herb-gardens, as a culinary and medicinal plant, and it is still to be found in old cottage gardens. Not only was its root much employed as a medicine, but it was also candied and eaten as a sweetmeat. Dr. Fernie tells us, in *Herbal Simples*:

'Some fifty years ago, the candy was sold commonly in London as flat, round cakes, being composed largely of sugar and coloured with cochineal. A piece was eaten each night and morning for asthmatical complaints, whilst it was customary when travelling by a river, to suck a bit of the root against poisonous exalations and bad air. The candy may still be had from our confectioners, but now containing no more of the plant Elecampane than there is of barley in Barley Sugar.'

In Denmark, Elecampane is sometimes called Elf-Doc. Here one sometimes comes across the name Elf-Dock locally, also Elf-wort.

¶ *Cultivation*. Although Elecampane is no longer grown to any extent in England, it is still cultivated for medicinal use on the Continent, mainly in Holland, Switzerland and Germany, most largely near the German town of Colleda, not far from Leipzig.

It grows well in moist, shady positions, in ordinary garden soil, though it flourishes best in a good, loamy soil, the ground being damp, but fairly well-drained.

It is easily cultivated. Seeds may be sown, either when ripe, in cold frames, or in spring in the open. It is best propagated, however, by off-sets, taken in the autumn from the old root, with a bud or eye to each. These will take root very readily, and should be planted in rows about a foot asunder, and 9 or 10 inches distant in the rows. In the following spring, the ground should be kept clean from weeds, and if slightly dug in autumn, it will greatly promote the growth of the roots, which will be fit for use after two years' growth.

By cutting the root into pieces about 2 inches long, covering with rich, light, sandy soil and keeping in gentle heat during the winter, a good stock of plants can also be obtained.

¶ *Part Used Medicinally.* The drug, Elecampane (*Radix Inulæ*), consists of both rhizome or rootstock and roots. It is official in most pharmacopœias.

For pharmaceutical use, the root is taken from plants two to three years old; when more advanced it becomes too woody. As a rule, it is dug in autumn.

Elecampane root has at first a somewhat glutinous taste, but by chewing, it becomes subsequently aromatic, and slightly bitter and pungent; it has an agreeably aromatic, somewhat camphoraceous orris-like odour.

The distinguishing characteristics of Elecampane root to be noted by a student are:

Its horny, not starchy nature.

The presence of oil-glands.

The absence of well-marked radiate structure in the wood.

Most roots of similar appearance to Elecampane root, such as Belladonna, Dandelion and Marsh Mallow, are devoid of oil-glands. Belladonna, moreover, is distinguished from it by its starchy fracture, Dandelion by its thick, ringed bark, and Marsh Mallow by its radiate structure and fibrous, easily separated bark. Pellitory root, which *has* oil-glands, is distinguished by its yellow, radiate wood, distinctive odour and taste.

¶ *Constituents.* The substance most abundantly contained in Elecampane root is Inulin, discovered by Valentine Rose, of Berlin, in 1804, who named it Alantin (the German name of the plant is *Alantwurzel*; French, *Aunée*), but the title, Inulin, proposed by Thompson, has been generally adopted. It has the same composition as starch, but stands to a certain extent in opposition to that substance, which it replaces in the root-system of *Compositæ*. In living plants, Inulin is dissolved in the watery juice, and on drying, is deposited within the cells in amorphous masses, which in polarized light are inactive. It resembles starch in appearance, but differs from it in giving a yellow instead of a blue colour with iodine, in being soluble in boiling water without forming a paste, and in being deposited unchanged from the hot aqueous solution when it cools. With nitric acid, Inula affords no explosive compound as starch does. By prolonged heat or the action of dilute acids, it is changed first to *inulin*, then to *levulin*, and finally to *levulose*. It is only slightly changed to sugar by ferments.

Sachs showed in 1864 that by immersing the roots of Elecampane or *Dahlia variabilis* in alcohol and glycerine, Inulin may be precipitated in globular aggregations of needle-shaped crystalline form.

Elecampane is the richest source of inulin.

The amount of Inulin varies according to the season, but is more abundant in the autumn. Dragendorff, who in 1870 made it the subject of a very exhaustive treatise, obtained from the root in October not less than 44 per cent., but in spring only 19 per cent., its place being taken by levulin, mucilage, sugar and several glucosides. Inulin is widely distributed in the perennial roots of *Compositæ*, and has been met with in the natural orders *Campanulacæ*, *Goodeniaceæ*, *Lobeliaceæ*, *Stylidiaceæ*, and in the root of the White Ipecacuanha of Brazil, belonging to the order *Violaceæ*.

Inulin is closely associated in Elecampane with *Inulenin*, obtainable in microscopical needles, slightly soluble in cold water and weak alcohol, and *pseudo-inulin*, which occurs in irregular granules, very soluble in hot water and weak, hot alcohol, but insoluble in cold alcohol.

It was observed by Le Febre as early as 1660 that when the root of Elecampane is subjected to distillation with water, a crystallizable substance collects in the head of the receiver, and similar crystals may be observed after carefully heating a thin slice of the root, and are often found as a natural efflorescence on the surface of roots that have been long kept. This was considered as a distinct body called *Helenin*, or Elecampane camphor, but the researches of Kallen in 1874 showed that it was resolvable into two crystallizable substances, which he named *Helenin*, a body without taste or colour, and *Alantcamphor*, with a peppermint odour and taste. As a result of further research, it is considered that the crystalline mass yielded by Elecampane root on distillation with water in the proportion of 1 to 2 per cent., and associated with about 1 per cent. volatile oil, consists of *Alantolactone, iso-alantolactone* and Alantolic acid, all of which are crystalline, nearly colourless, and have but slight odour and taste. The oily portion, *Alantol*, found in the distillate, a colourless liquid, has a peppermint-like odour.

¶ *Medicinal Action and Uses.* Diuretic, tonic, diaphoretic, expectorant, alterative, antiseptic, astringent and gently stimulant. It was employed by the ancients in certain diseases of women, also in phthisis, in dropsy and in skin affections. Its name 'Scabwort' arose from the fact that a decoction of it is said to cure sheep affected with the scab, and the name 'Horse-heal' was given it from its reputed virtues in curing the cutaneous diseases of horses.

In herbal medicine it is chiefly used for

coughs, consumption and other pulmonary complaints, being a favourite domestic remedy for bronchitis. It has been employed for many years with good results in chest affections, for which it is a valuable medicine, as it is in all chronic diseases of the lungs, asthma and bronchitis. It gives relief to the respiratory difficulties and assists expectoration. Its principal employment as a separate remedy is in acute catarrhal affections, and in dyspepsia attended with relaxation and debility, given in small, warm and frequently repeated doses. It is, however, seldom given alone, but most frequently preferred in combination with other medicines of a similar nature. It is best given in the form of decoction, the dose being a small teaspoonful, three times a day.

The root used not only to be candied and eaten as a sweetmeat, but lozenges were made of it. It has been employed in whooping-cough. It is sometimes employed in the form of a confection for piles, 1 oz. of powdered root being mixed with 2 oz. of honey.

In the United States, it has also been highly recommended, both for external use and internal administration in diseases of the skin, an old use of the root that has maintained its reputation for efficacy.

Externally applied, it is somewhat rubefacient, and has been employed as an embrocation in the treatment of sciatica, facial and other neuralgia.

Of late years, modern scientific research has proved that the claims of Elecampane to be a valuable remedy in pulmonary diseases has a solid basis. One authority, Korab, showed in 1885 that the active, bitter principle, Helenin, is such a powerful antiseptic and bactericide, that a few drops of a solution of 1 part in 10,000 immediately kills the ordinary bacterial organisms, being peculiarly destructive to the Tubercle bacillus. He gave it successfully in tubercular and catarrhal diarrhœas, and praised it also as an antiseptic in surgery. In Spain it has been made use of as a surgical dressing. Obiol, in 1886, stated it to be an efficient local remedy in the treatment of diphtheria, the false membrane being painted with a solution of Helenin in Oil of Almond.

¶ *Medicinal Preparations.* Powdered root ½ to 1 drachm. Fluid extract, ½ to 1 drachm. Inulin, 1 to 3 grains.

Gerard tells us: 'It is good for shortnesse of breathe and an old cough, and for such as cannot breathe unless they hold their neckes upright.' And further:

'The root of Elecampane is with good success mixed with counterpoisons; it is a remedy against the biting of serpents, it resisteth poison. It is good for them that are bursten and troubled with cramps and convulsions.'

And Culpepper says:

'The fresh roots of Elecampane preserved with sugar or made into a conserve, or a syrup, are very effectual to warm a cold windy stomach and stitches in the side, caused by spleen and to relieve cough, shortness of breath and wheezing in the lungs. The dried root made into powder and mixed with sugar, and taken, serveth the same purpose. . . . It cures putrid and pestilential fevers and even the plague. The roots and herbes beaten and put into new ale or beer and daily drunk, cleareth, strengtheneth and quickeneth the sight of the eyes. The decoction of the roots in wine or the juice taken therein, destroys worms in the stomach, and gargled in the mouth or the root chewed, fasteneth loose teeth and keeps them from putrefaction, and being drunk is good for spitting of blood, and it removes cramps or convulsions, gout, sciatica, pains in the joints, applied outwardly or inwardly, and is also good for those that are ruptured, or have any inward bruise. The root boiled well in vinegar, beaten afterwards and made into an ointment with hog's suet or oil of trotters is a most excellent remedy for scabs or itch in young or old; the places also bathed and washed with the decoction doth the same; it heals putrid sores or cankers. In the roots of this herb lieth the chief effect for the remedies aforesaid. The distilled water of the leaves and roots together is very good to cleanse the skin of the face or other parts from any morphew, spots or blemishes and make it clear.'

In Switzerland (Neufchâtel) Elecampane root is one of the substances used in the preparation of Absinthe, and it was also used for the same purpose in France. It furnishes the *Vin d'Aulnée* of the French.

A blue dye has been extracted from the root, bruised and macerated and mingled with ashes and whortleberries.

'The wine wherein the root of Elicampane hath steept,' says Markham (*Countrie Farme,* 1616), 'is singularly good against the colicke.' A cordial was made from the plant by infusing Elecampane roots with sugar and currants in white port.

See FLEABANE, (PLOUGHMAN'S) SPIKENARD, and (GOLDEN) SAMPHIRE.

ELM, COMMON
Ulmus campestris (LINN.)
N.O. Urticaceæ

Synonyms. Ulmi cortex. Broad-leaved Elm. Ulmus suberosa (var. Orme)
Part Used. The dried inner bark
Habitat. Britain (not indigenous), Europe, Asia, North Africa

¶ *Description.* The Elms belong to the natural order Ulmaceæ and to the genus *Ulmus,* which contains sixteen species, widely distributed throughout the north temperate zone, extending southwards as far as Mexico in the New World and the Sikkim Himalayas in the Old World.

The Common Elm (*U. campestris,* Linn.) is a doubtful native of England, found throughout the greater part of Europe, in North Africa, Asia Minor and eastwards to Japan.

It grows in woods and hedgerows, especially in the southern part of Britain and on almost all soils, thriving even in the smoky atmosphere of a city, but on a rich loam, in open, low-lying situations, attaining a height of 60 to 100 feet, even rising to 130 and 150 feet. In the first ten years of its growth the tree grows to 25 or 30 feet.

The branches are numerous and spreading, the bark rugged, the leaves alternate, ovate, rough, doubly toothed and unequal at the base. The flowers are small and numerous, appearing in March and April before the leaves, in purplish-brown tufts. If one of these tufts be examined, it will be found to be a short axis with a number of leaves, beginning two-ranked at the base, and going over to five-ranked above. There are no flowers in the axils of the lowest ten or twelve; in the axils of the upper leaves are flowers arranged in small cymes (in some species), but in *U. campestris* reduced to the one central flower. Each flower has a four-toothed, bell-shaped calyx, surrounding four stamens and a one-celled ovary bearing two spreading hairy styles.

The seed-vessels are green, membraneous, one-seeded and deeply cleft, but the tree seldom perfects its seed in England, being propagated by root-suckers from old trees, or by layers from stools.

In age and size, the Elm closely approaches the Oak, but is more varied, a large number of named varieties being grown.

¶ *Uses.* All parts of the tree, including sap-wood, are used in carpentry. The wood is close-grained, free from knots, hard and tough, and not subject to splitting, but it does not take a high polish. It does not crack when once seasoned and is remarkably durable under water, being specially adapted for any purpose which requires exposure to wet. To prevent shrinking and warping in drying,

it may be preserved in water or mud, but is best worked up soon after felling. In drying, the wood loses over 60 per cent. of its weight.

Elm wood is used for keels and bilge planks, the blocks and dead eyes of rigging and ship's pumps, for coffins, wheels, furniture, turned articles and general carpenter's work. Elm boards are largely used for lining the interior of carts, wagons and wheelbarrows on account of the extreme toughness of the wood, and it has been much employed in the past for making sheds, most of the existing farm buildings being covered with elm. Previous to the common employment of cast-iron, Elm was very much in use for waterpipes.

The inner bark is very tough and is made into mats and ropes. The leaves and young shoots have been found a suitable food for live stock.

¶ *Elm Tree Disease.* Investigations are at present being carried on as to the cause of a mysterious disease, known as the Dutch Elm disease, which is killing trees on many parts of the Continent. It first appeared in North Brabant in 1919, and spread until it is now all over Holland. By 1921, the disease was rampant in Belgium and in the same year it appeared in France, while in 1924 and 1925 it spread widely in Germany and it is also working havoc in Spain.

The first sign of the disease in trees up to thirty years old is a mass of dry twigs and leaves in the crown while the other parts are still green. Within a week, all the leaves of the tree may fall, or the leaves on one side of the tree may remain fresh, while on the other side they fall off. No cure has yet been discovered, and the tree eventually dies. Most investigators consider that the disease is caused by a fungus (*Graphium ulmus*), the infection being carried by spores blown from one tree to another.

To prevent the importation into Britain of this mysterious disease, the Ministry of Agriculture, early in 1927, prohibited live elms from the European mainland from being landed in England and Wales.

¶ *Constituents.* Analyses of Elm wood show 47·8 per cent. of lime, 21·9 of potash and 13·7 of soda.

A peculiar vegetable principle, called Ulmin or Ulmic Acid, was first discovered in the gummy substance which spontaneously exudes in summer from the bark of the Common Elm, becoming by the action of the air a dark-brown, almost black substance, without smell or taste, insoluble in cold, sparingly soluble in boiling water, which it colours yellowish-brown; soluble in alcohol and readily dissolved by alkaline solutions.

The *inner bark* is very mucilaginous, and contains a little tannic acid which gives it a somewhat bitter and slightly astringent taste; it also contains a great deal of starch.

¶ *Medicinal Action and Uses.* Tonic, demulcent, astringent and diuretic. Was formerly employed for the preparation of an antiscorbutic decoction recommended in cutaneous diseases of a leprous character, such as ringworm. It was applied both externally and internally. Under the title of Ulmus, the dried inner bark was official in the British Pharmacopœia of 1864 and 1867, directions for the preparation of *Decoc. Ulmi* being as follows: Elm Bark 1 part, water 8 parts; boil for 10 minutes, strain, make up to 8 parts.

A homœopathic tincture is made of the inner bark, and used as an astringent.

Fluid extract, dose 2 to 4 oz. three or four times daily.

A medicinal tea was also formerly made from the flowers.

In Persia, Italy and the south of France, galls, sometimes the size of a fist, are frequently produced on the leaves. They contain a clear water called *eau d'orme*, which is sweet and viscid, and has been recommended to wash wounds, contusions and sore eyes. Culpepper tells us:

'the water that is found in the bladders on the leaves of the elm-tree is very effectual to cleanse the skin and make it fair.'

Towards autumn, these galls dry, the insects in them die and there is found a residue in the form of a yellow or blackish balsam, called *beaume d'ormeau*, which has been recommended for diseases of the chest.

¶ *Other Species.*

A variety of the Common Elm, the CORK-BARKED ELM (*U. campestris*, var. *suberosa*), is

distinguished chiefly by its thick, deeply-fissured bark, the corky excrescences along the branchlets causing them to appear much thicker than they really are. A North American species with this feature most pronounced is *U. alata*, which well deserves its name of the WINGED ELM.

The SCOTCH ELM, or WYCH ELM (*U. montana*, With. – formerly called *U. glabra*, Huds.), is indigenous to Britain and is the common Elm of the northern part of the island.

It is a beautiful tree, both in form and foliage, usually attaining a height of about 50 feet, though tall-growing specimens have been known to attain 120 feet.

It has drooping branches and a smoother, thinner bark than *U. campestris*; its leaves, equally rough on the upper surface, though rather downy beneath, are longer, wider and more tapering and more deeply notched. A further distinction is that whereas the seeds of the Common Elm are placed near the end of their oblong envelope, those of the Wych Elm are set in the centre of their envelope. Moreover, the Common Elm has a profuse undergrowth of young shoots round the base of the trunk and few are to be seen round that of the Wych Elm. This is probably the 'French Elm' of Evelyn. An upright form of it is called the 'Cornish Elm.'

The wood, though more porous than that of the Common Elm, is tough and hardy when properly seasoned, and being very flexible when steamed, is well adapted for boat-building, though for the purposes of the wheelwright and millwright is inferior to that of the Common Elm. Branches of Wych Elm were formerly used for making bows and when forked were employed as divining rods. The bark of the young limbs is very tough and flexible, and is often stripped off in long ribands and used in Wales for securing thatch and other similar purposes.

On the leaves of *U. chenensis*, a number of galls are produced, which are used by the Chinese for tanning leather and dyeing.

ELM, SLIPPERY

Ulmus fulva (MICH.)
N.O. Urticaceæ

Synonyms. Red Elm. Moose Elm. Indian Elm
Part Used. The inner bark
Habitat. The United States, Canada

¶ *Description.* The Slippery Elm is a small tree abundant in various parts of North America.

The branches are very rough, the leaves long, unequally toothed, rough with hairs on both sides, the leaf-buds covered with a

dense yellow Wool. The flowers are stalkless.

The *inner bark* has important medicinal value and is an official drug of the United States Pharmacopœia.

The bark, which is the only part used, is

collected in spring from the bole and larger branches and dried. Large quantities are collected, especially in the lower part of the state of Michigan. As the wood has no commercial value, the tree is fully stripped and consequently dies.

The bark as it appears in commerce for use in medicine consists only of the inner bark or bast and is sold in flat pieces 2 to 3 feet long and several inches wide, but only about ⅛ to ¹⁄₁₆ of an inch in thickness. It is very tough and flexible, of a fine fibrous texture, finely striated longitudinally on both surfaces, the outer surface reddish-yellow, with patches of reddish brown, which are part of the outer bark adhering to the inner bast. It has an odour like Fenugreek and a very mucilaginous, insipid taste. The strips can be bent double without breaking: if broken, the rough fracture is mealy, strongly but finely fibrous. The clean transverse section shows numerous medullary rays and alternate bands of bast parenchyma, thus giving it a chequered appearance. A section moistened and left for a few minutes, and again examined, shows large swollen mucilage cells.

The *powdered* bark is sold in two forms: a coarse powder for use as poultices and a fine powder for making a mucilaginous drink. The disintegrated bark forms, when moistened, a flexible and spongy tissue, which is easily moulded into pessaries, teats, and suppositories.

It is recommended that ten-year-old bark should be used.

The powder should be greyish or fawn-coloured. If dark or reddish, good results will not be obtained. The powdered bark is said to be often adulterated with damaged flour and other starchy substances.

¶ *Constituents.* The principal constituent of the bark is the mucilage contained in large cells in the bast. This mucilage is very similar to that found in linseed. It is precipitated by solutions of acetate and sub-acetate of lead, although not by alcohol. The mucilage does not dissolve, but only swells in water and is so abundant that 10 grains of the powdered bark will make a thick jelly with an ounce of water.

Microscopic examination of the tissue of the bark shows round starch grains and very characteristic twin crystals of Calcium oxalate.

¶ *Medicinal Action and Uses.* Demulcent, emollient, expectorant, diuretic, nutritive. The bark of this American Elm, though not in this country as in the United States an official drug, is considered one of the most valuable remedies in herbal practice, the abundant mucilage it contains having wonderfully strengthening and healing qualities.

It not only has a most soothing and healing action on all the parts it comes in contact with, but in addition possesses as much nutrition as is contained in oatmeal, and when made into gruel forms a wholesome and sustaining food for infants and invalids. It forms the basis of many patent foods.

Slippery Elm Food is generally made by mixing a teaspoonful of the powder into a thin and perfectly smooth paste with cold water and then pouring on a pint of boiling water, steadily stirring meanwhile. It can, if desired, be flavoured with cinnamon, nutmeg or lemon rind.

This makes an excellent drink in cases of irritation of the mucous membrane of the stomach and intestines, and taken at night will induce sleep.

Another mode of preparation is to beat up an egg with a teaspoonful of the powdered bark, pouring boiling milk over it and sweetening it.

Taken unsweetened, three times a day, Elm Food gives excellent results in gastritis, gastric catarrh, mucous colitis and enteritis, being tolerated by the stomach when all other foods fail, and is of great value in bronchitis, bleeding from the lungs and consumption (being most healing to the lungs), soothing a cough and building up and preventing wasting.

A Slippery Elm compound excellent for coughs is made as follows: Cut obliquely one or more ounces of bark into pieces about the thickness of a match; add a pinch of Cayenne flavour with a slice of lemon and sweeten, infusing the whole in a pint of boiling water and letting it stand for 25 minutes. Take this frequently in small doses: for a consumptive patient, about a pint a day is recommended. It is considered one of the best remedies that can be given as it combines both demulcent and stimulating properties. Being mucilaginous, it rolls up the mucous material so troublesome to the patient and passes it down through the intestines.

In typhoid fever, the Slippery Elm drink, prepared as for coughs, is recommended, serving a threefold purpose, to cleanse, heal and strengthen, the patient being allowed to drink as much as desired until thirst has abated, and other remedies can be used. If the patient is not thirsty, a dose of 2 large tablespoonfuls every hour for an adult has been prescribed.

The bark is an ingredient in various lung medicines. A valuable remedy for *Bronchitis* and all diseases of the throat and lungs is compounded as follows: 1 teaspoonful Flax seed, 1 oz. Slippery Elm bark, 1 oz. Thoroughwort, 1 stick Liquorice, 1 quart water. Simmer slowly for 20 minutes. Strain and add 1 pint of the best vinegar and ½ pint of sugar. When cold, bottle. Dose: 1 tablespoonful two or three times a day.

In *Pleurisy*, the following is also recommended: Take 2 oz. each of Pleurisy root, Marsh Mallow root, Liquorice root and Slippery Elm bark. Boil in 3 pints of water down to 3 gills. Dose: ½ teaspoonful every half-hour, to be taken warm.

As a *heart* remedy, a pint of Slippery Elm drink has been prescribed alternately with Bugleweed compound.

Slippery Elm bark possesses also great influence upon diseases of the female organs.

It is particularly valuable both medicinally and as an *injection* in dysentery and other diseases of the bowels, cystitis and irritation of the urinary tract. The injection for inflammation of the bowels is made from an infusion of 1 oz. of the powder to 1 pint of boiling water, strained and used lukewarm. Other remedies should be given at the same time.

An injection for diarrhœa may also be made as follows: 1 drachm powdered Slippery Elm bark, 3 drachms powdered Bayberry, 1 drachm powdered Scullcap. Pour on ½ pint of boiling water, infuse for half an hour, strain, add a teaspoonful of tincture of myrrh and use lukewarm.

As an enema for *constipation*, 2 drachms of Slippery Elm bark are mixed well with 1 oz. of sugar, then ½ pint of warm milk and water and an ounce of Olive Oil are gently stirred in.

Injection for worms (*Ascarides*): ½ drachm Aloes powder, 1 drachm common salt, ½ drachm Slippery Elm powder (fine). When well mixed, add ½ pint warm water and sweeten with molasses, stirring well.

Slippery Elm mucilage is also prescribed to be mixed with Oil of Male Fern (2 oz. of the mucilage to 1 drachm of the oil) as a remedy for the expulsion of tapeworm.

The Red Indians have long used this viscous inner bark to prepare a healing salve, and in herbal medicine a Slippery Elm bark powder is considered one of the best possible poultices for wounds, boils, ulcers, burns and all inflamed surfaces, soothing, healing and reducing pain and inflammation.

It is made as follows: Mix the powder with hot water to form the required consistency, spread smoothly upon soft cotton cloth and apply over the parts affected. It is unfailing in cases of suppurations, abscesses, wounds of all kinds, congestion, eruptions, swollen glands, etc. In simple inflammation, it may be applied directly over the part affected; to abscesses and old wounds, it should be placed between cloths. If applied to parts of the body where there is hair, the face of the poultice should be smeared with olive oil before applying.

In old gangrenous wounds, an excellent antiseptic poultice is prepared by mixing with warm water or an infusion of Wormwood, equal parts of Slippery Elm powder and very fine charcoal and applying immediately over the part.

A very valuable poultice in cases where it is desirable to hasten suppuration or arrest the tendency to gangrene is made by mixing the Slippery Elm powder with brewer's yeast and new milk.

Compound Bran poultice is made by mixing with hot vinegar equal quantities of wheaten Bran with Slippery Elm powder. This is an excellent poultice for severe rheumatic and gouty affections, particularly of the joints, synovitis, etc.

Herbal poultices, generally made from the bruised, fresh leaves of special herbs, are frequently mixed with Slippery Elm and boiling water sufficient to give the mass consistency.

Marshmallow Ointment, one of the principal ointments used in herbal medicine, has a considerable proportion of Slippery Elm bark in its composition. It is made as follows: 3 oz. Marshmallow leaves, 2 oz. Slippery Elm bark powder, 2 oz. Beeswax, 16 oz. Lard. Boil the Marshmallow and Slippery Elm bark in 3 pints of water for 15 minutes. Express, strain and reduce the liquor to half a pint. Melt together the lard and wax by gentle heat, then add the extract while still warm, shake constantly till all are thoroughly incorporated and store in a cool place.

The bark of Slippery Elm is stated to preserve fatty substances from becoming rancid.

It has been asserted that a pinch of the Slippery Elm powder put into a hollow tooth stops the ache and greatly delays decay, if used as soon as there is any sign of decay.

Lozenges or troches containing 3 grains of Elm flavoured with methyl salicylate are used as a demulcent.

¶ *Preparations*. Mucilage, U.S.P., made by digesting 6 grams of bruised Slippery Elm in 100 c.c. and heated in a closed vessel in a water-bath for 1 hour and then strained.

¶ *Other Species*.

Fremontia Californica, or Californian Slippery Elm, has bark with similar properties, and is used in the same way, but is not botanically related.

EMBELIA
Embelia Ribes and robusta (BURM.)
N.O. Myrsinaceæ

Synonyms. Viranga. Birang-i-kabuli
Part Used. Dried fruits
Habitat. India, Indian Archipelago, Tropical Asia, Southern China, East Africa

¶ *Description.* A straggling shrub, almost a climber. The plant possesses petiolate leaves and has small, whity-pink flowers in racemes at ends of the branches. The berries (the drug) are minute, round, spherical fruits (not unlike peppercorns) and vary in colour from red to black – those of *E. Ribes* have ovate, lanceolate smooth leaves and warty fruits, and are often sold to traders to adulterate pepper, which they so much resemble as to render it almist impossible to distinguish them by sight, or by any other means, as they possess a considerable degree of the spice flavour. The fruits of *E. robusta*, however, are longitudinally finely striated. Both fruit have often a short stalk and calyx five-partite, removing this, a small hole is found in the fruit. The reddish seed, enclosed in a brittle pericarp, is covered by a thin membrane; when this is taken off, the seed is seen covered with light spots which disappear after immersion in water. The seed is horny, depressed at the base and has a ruminated endosperm. Taste, aromatic and astringent, with a slight pungency, owing to a resinous substance present in them.

¶ *Constituents.* Embelic acid, found in golden-yellow lamellar crystals (this acid is soluble in chloroform, alcohol and benzene, but not in water) and a quinone, Embelia.

¶ *Medicinal Action and Uses.* Anthelmintic, specially used to expel tapeworm, which are passed dead. In India and the Eastern Colonies the drug is given in the early morning, fasting, mixed with milk, and followed by a purgative. The dose is 1 to 4 drachms. The seeds are also made into an infusion, or ground to powder and taken in water or syrup, and being almost tasteless are not an unpleasant remedy.

Ammonium embelate is an effective tænicide for children: dose, 3 grains; adult dose, 6 or more grains.

The berries of *E. robusta* are considered cathartic.

¶ *Other Species.*
E. Basaal, an Indian variety, with larger elliptical leaves, more or less downy, is useful in various ways. The young leaves, in combination with ginger, are used as a gargle for sore throats, the dried bark of the root as a remedy for toothache, and the ground berries, mixed with butter or lard, made into an ointment and laid on the forehead for pleuritis.

EPHEDRA
Ephedra vulgaris (RICH.)
N.O. Gnetaceæ

Synonyms. Ephedrine. Epitonin. Ma Huang
Habitat. West Central China, Southern Siberia, Japan

¶ *Description.* It is found on sandy seashores and in temperate climates of both hemispheres. The plant has stamens and pistils on separate flowers – staminate flowers in catkins and a membraneous perianth, pistillate flowers terminal on axillary stalks, within a two-leaved involucre. Fruit has two carpels with a single seed in each and is a succulent cone, branches slender and erect, small leaves, scale-like, articulated and joined at the base into a sheath.

¶ *Constituents.* Ephedrine is salt of an alkaloid and is in shining white crystals very soluble in water.

¶ *Medicinal Action and Uses.* A sympathetic nerve stimulant resembling adrenaline, its effect on the unstriped muscular fibres is remarkable. It acts promptly in relieving swellings of the mucous membrane. It has valuable antispasmodic properties, acts on the air passages and is of benefit in asthma and hay fever; it is also employed for rheumatism; a 5 to 10 per cent. solution has mydriatic properties, prophylactically used for low blood pressure in influenza, pneumonia, etc. Used in tablet form for oral or hypodermic administration and in ampuls for hypodermic, intramuscular and intravenous use. It can advantageously be used in solution with liquid paraffin, either alone or in conjunction with methol camphor and oil of thyme. Dose, $\frac{1}{2}$ to 1 grain.

ERGOT. *See* FUNGI

ERYNGO. *See* (SEA) HOLLY

EUCALYPTUS

Eucalyptus globulus (LABILLE.)
N.O. Myrtaceæ

Synonyms. Blue Gum Tree. Stringy Bark Tree
Part Used. The oil of the leaves
Habitat. Australia. Now North and South Africa, India, and Southern Europe

The tree is indigenous with a few exceptions to Australia and Tasmania. The genus contains about 300 species and is one of the most characteristic genera of the Australian flora.

¶ *Description.* The leaves are leathery in texture, hang obliquely or vertically, and are studded with glands containing a fragrant volatile oil. The flowers in bud are covered with a cup-like membrane (whence the name of the genus, derived from the Greek *eucalyptos*, well-covered), which is thrown off as a lid when the flower expands. The fruit is surrounded by a woody, cup-shaped receptacle and contains numerous minute seeds.

Eucalyptus trees are quick growers and many species reach a great height. *Eucalyptus amygdalin* (Labille) is the tallest known tree, specimens attaining as much as 480 feet, exceeding in height even the Californian Big Tree (*Sequoia gigantea*). Many species yield valuable timber, others oils, kino, etc.

There are a great number of species of Eucalyptus trees yielding essential oils, the foliage of some being more odorous than that of others, and the oils from the various species differing widely in character. It necessarily follows that the term Eucalyptus oil is meaningless from a scientific point of view unless the species from which it is derived is stated.

The Eucalyptus industry is becoming of economic importance to Australia, especially in New South Wales and Victoria. Many of the old species which give the oil of commerce have given way to other species which have been found to gave larger yields or better oils. About twenty-five species are at the present time being utilized for their oil.

The oils may be roughly divided into three classes of commercial importance: (1) the *medicinal* oils, which contain substantial amounts of eucalyptol (also known as cineol); (2) the *industrial* oils, containing terpenes, which are used for flotation purposes in mining operations; (3) the *aromatic* oils, such as *E. citriodora*, which are characterized by their aroma.

The British Pharmacopœia describes Eucalyptus Oil as the oil distilled from the fresh leaves of *E. globulus* and other species.

E. globulus, the best-known variety (its name bestowed, it is said, by the French botanist De Labillardière, on account of the resemblance of its waxy fruit to a kind of button at that time worn in France), is the Blue Gum Tree of Victoria and Tasmania, where it attains a height of 375 feet, ranking as one of the largest trees in the world. It is also called the Fever Tree, being largely cultivated in unhealthy, low-lying or swampy districts for its antiseptic qualities.

The first leaves are broad, without stalks, of a shining whitish-green and are opposite and horizontal, but after four or five years these are succeeded by others of a more ensiform or sword-shaped form, 6 to 12 inches long, bluish-green in hue, which are alternate and vertical, i.e. with the edges turned towards the sky and earth, an arrangement more suited to the climate and productive of peculiar effects of light and shade. The flowers are single or in clusters, almost stalkless.

The Eucalyptus, especially *E. globulus*, has been successfully introduced into the south of Europe, Algeria, Egypt, Tahiti, South Africa and India, and has been extensively planted in California and also, with the object of lessening liability to droughts, along the line of the Central Pacific Railway.

It thrives in any situation, having a mean annual temperature not below 60° F., but will not endure a temperature of less than 27° F., and although many species of Eucalyptus will flourish out-of-doors in the south of England, they are generally grown, in this country, in pots as greenhouse plants.

It was Baron Ferdinand von Müller, the German botanist and explorer (from 1857 to 1873 Director of the Botanical Gardens in Melbourne), who made the qualities of this Eucalyptus known all over the world, and so led to its introduction into Europe, North and South Africa, California and the non-tropical districts of South America. He was the first to suggest that the perfume of the leaves resembling that of Cajaput oil, might be of use as a disinfectant in fever districts, a suggestion which has been justified by the results of the careful examination to which the Eucalyptus has been subjected since its employment in medicine. Some seeds, having been sent to France in 1857, were planted in Algiers and thrived exceedingly well. Trottoir, the botanical superintendent, found that the value of the fragrant antiseptic exhalations of the leaves in fever or marshy districts was far exceeded by the amazingly powerful drying action of the roots on the soil. Five years after planting the Eucalyptus, one of the most marshy and unhealthy districts of Algiers was converted into one of the healthiest and driest. As a result, the rapidly growing Eucalyptus trees are now largely cultivated in many temperate regions with the view of preventing malarial fevers. A noteworthy instance of this is the monastery of St. Paolo à la tre Fontana, situated in one of the most fever-stricken districts of the Roman Campagna. Since about 1870, when the tree was planted in its cloisters, it has become habitable throughout the year. To the remarkable drainage afforded by its roots is also ascribed the gradual disappearance of mosquitoes in the neighbourhood of plantations of this tree, as at Lake Fezara in Algeria.

In Sicily, also, it is being extensively planted to combat malaria, on account of its property of absorbing large quantities of water from the soil. Recent investigations have shown that Sicilian Eucalyptus oil obtained from leaves during the flowering period can compete favourably with the Australian oil in regard to its industrial and therapeutic applications. Oil has also been distilled in Spain from the leaves of *E. globulus*, grown there.

In India, considerable plantations of *E. globulus* were made in 1863 in the Nilgiris at Ootacamund, but though a certain amount of oil is distilled there locally, under simple conditions, little attempt has hitherto been made to develop the industry on a commercial scale, Australia remaining the source of supply.

A great increase in Eucalyptus cultivation has recently taken place in Brazil as a result of a decree published in 1919 awarding premiums and free grants of land to planters of Eucalyptus and other trees of recognized value for essence cultivation.

¶ *Constituents.* The essential Oil of Eucalyptus used in medicine is obtained by aqueous distillation of the fresh leaves. It is a colourless or straw-coloured fluid when properly prepared, with a characteristic odour and taste, soluble in its own weight of alcohol. The most important constituent is Eucalyptol, present in *E. globulus* up to 70 per cent. of its volume. It consists chiefly of a terpene and a cymene. Eucalyptus Oil contains also, after exposure to the air, a crystallizable resin, derived from Eucalyptol.

The British Pharmacopœia requires Eucalyptus Oil to contain not less than 55 per cent., by volume, of Eucalyptol, to have a specific gravity 0·910 to 0·930 and optical rotation – 10° to 10°. The official method for

the determination of the Eucalptol depends on the conversion of this body into a crystalline phosphate, but numerous other methods have been suggested (*see* Parry, *Essential Oils*, Vol. II).

A small amount of medicinal oil is still distilled from *E. globulus*, but its odour is less agreeable than those of many others. To-day, *E. polybractea* (Silver Malee Scrub – which is cultivated and the oil distilled near Bendigo in Victoria), containing 85 per cent. of Eucalyptol, and *E. Smithii* (Gully Ash) are favourites for distillation. Among others frequently employed, *E. Australiana* yields a valuable medicinal oil and also *E. Bakeri*, a large shrub or pendulous willow-like tree, about 30 to 50 feet high, with very narrow leaves, found from northern New South Wales to central Queensland, known locally as the 'Malee Box.' The oil from this species is of a bright reddish-yellow and contains 70 to 77 per cent. of Eucalyptol and other aromatic substances identical with those found in *E. polybractea*.

The oil used for flotation purposes in the extraction of ores is known as that of *E. amygdalina*, and is probably derived from this tree as well as from *E. dives*. It is an oil containing little Eucalyptol and having a specific gravity from 0·866 to 0·885, and an optical rotation −59° to −75°, its chief constituent is phellandrene, which forms a crystalline nitrate and is very irritating when inhaled. There is a considerable demand in New South Wales for the cheap phellandrene Eucalyptus oils for use in the mining industry in the separation of metallic sulphides from ores.

Of the perfume-bearing oils, that of *E. citriodora*, the CITRON-SCENTED GUM, whose leaves emit a delightful lemon scent, contains up to 98 per cent. of citronellol and is much used in perfumery, fetching four times as much as the medicinal oils. *E. Macarthurii* (' Paddy River Box ') contains up to 75 per cent. of geranyl acetate, and as a source of geraniol this tree would probably repay cultivation: it is now receiving special attention in Australia, as it is a very rapid grower. *E. odorata* yields also an odorous oil used by soapmakers in Australia. *E. Staigeriana*, the Lemon-scented Iron Bark, has also a very pleasing scent, and the fragrance of the leaves of *E. Sturtiana* is similar to that of ripe apples.

There are a number of Eucalypts which contain a ketone known as piperitone, such as *E. piperita*. This body can be used in the synthesis of menthol, but it remains to be seen whether the process can be made a commercial success. *E. dives* (Peppermint Gum) and *E. radiata* (White Top Peppermint) yield oils with a strong peppermint flavour.

Details of an enormous number of the oils of Eucalyptus can be found in *A Research on the Eucalypts*, by Baker and Smith.

¶ *Medicinal Action and Uses.* Stimulant, antiseptic, aromatic.

The medicinal Eucalyptus Oil is probably the most powerful antiseptic of its class, especially when it is old, as ozone is formed in it on exposure to the air. It has decided disinfectant action, destroying the lower forms of life. Internally, it has the typical actions of a volatile oil in a marked degree. Eucalyptus Oil is used as a stimulant and antiseptic gargle. Locally applied, it impairs sensibility. It increases cardiac action.

Its antiseptic properties confer some antimalarial action, though it cannot take the place of Cinchona.

An emulsion made by shaking up equal parts of the oil and powdered gum-arabic with water has been used as a urethral injection, and has also been given internally in drachm doses in pulmonary tuberculosis and other microbic diseases of the lungs and bronchitis.

In croup and spasmodic throat troubles, the oil may be freely applied externally.

The oil is an ingredient of 'catheder oil,' used for sterilizing and lubricating urethral catheters.

In large doses, it acts as an irritant to the kidneys, by which it is largely excreted, and as a marked nervous depressant ultimately arresting respiration by its action on the medullary centre.

For some years Eucalyptus-chloroform was employed as one of the remedies in the tropics for hookworm, but it has now been almost universally abandoned as an inefficient anthelmintic, Chenopodium Oil having become the recognized remedy.

In veterinary practice, Eucalyptus Oil is administered to horses in influenza, to dogs in distemper, to all animals in septicæmia. It is also used for parasitic skin affections.

¶ *Preparations.* The dose of the oil is ½ to 3 minims. Eucalyptol may be given in similar doses and is preferable for purposes of inhalation, for asthma, diphtheria, sore throat, etc.

As a local application for ulcers and sores, 1 oz. of the oil is added to 1 pint of lukewarm water. For local injections, ½ oz. to the pint is taken.

The Fluid Extract is used internally, the dose ½ to 1 drachm, in scarlet fever, typhoid and intermittent fever.

Eucalyptol, U.S.P.: dose, 5 drops. Ointment, B.P.

¶ *Other Species.*

EUCALYPTUS GUM or KINO

E. nostrata and some other species of Eucalyptus yield Eucalyptus or Red Gum, a ruby-coloured exudation from the bark (to be distinguished from Botany Bay Kino).

Red Gum is a very powerffl astringent and is given internally in doses 0 2 to 5 grains in cases of diarrhœa and pharyngeal inflammations. It is prepared in the form of tinctures, syrups, lozenges, etc.

Red Gum is official in Great Britain, being imported from Australia, though the Kino generally employed here as the official drug is derived from *Pterocarpus Marsupium*, a member of the order Leguminosæ, East Indian, or Malabar Kino, and is administered in doses of 5 to 20 grains powdered, or ½ to 1 drachm of the tincture.

In veterinary practice, Red Gum is occasionally prescribed for diarrhœa in dogs and is used for superficial wounds.

E. globulus, E. resinifera and other species yield what is known as Botany Bay Kino, an astringent, dark-reddish, amorphous resin, which is obtained in a semi-fluid state by making incisions in the trunk of the tree and is used for similar purposes.

J. H. Maiden (*Useful Native Plants of Australia*, 1889) enumerates more than thirty species as Kino-yielding.

MANNA

From the leaves and young bark of *E. mannifera, E. viminalis, E. Gunnii*, var. *rubida, E. pulverulenta*, etc., a hard, opaque sweet substance is procured, containing melitose. The Lerp Manna of Australia is, however, of animal origin. *See* KINOS.

TWO EUCALYPTUS OINTMENTS

Compound Resin Ointment, B.P.C. Resin, 20; Oil of Eucalyptus by weight, 15; Hard paraffin, 10; Soft paraffin, 55.

Eucalyptus Ointment (Benn's *Botanic Doctor's Adviser*). Elder Oil, 12 oz.; White Wax, 2 oz.; Spermaceti, 1½ oz.; Eucalyptus Oil, 2 drachms; Wintergreen Oil, 20 drops.

A good ointment for the skin, containing antiseptic and healing properties. It produces very satisfactory results in scurf, chapped hands, chafes, dandruff, tender feet, enlargements of the glands, spots on the chest, arms, back and legs, pains in the joints and muscles.

Apply a piece of clean cotton or lint to wounds after all dirt is washed away. For aches and pains rub the part affected well and then cover with lint. Repeat two or three times, taking a blood-purifying mixture at the same time.

EUONYMUS. *See* SPINDLE TREE.

EUPATORIUMS

N.O. Compositæ

The Eupatoriums are some of the most important plants used in herbal medicine.

Boneset, Hemp Agrimony and Gravel Root will be found described under their specific names.

The following species are not so well known in Great Britain, though they are familiar plants in different parts of America and Brazil. *Eupatorium teucrifolium*, or Wild Horehound (syn. *E. verbenæfolium*, Michx.), has small white flowerheads and abounds in the southern United States, and has similar though less powerful properties than *E. perfoliatum* (Boneset).

The whole herb is employed, and both this and the preceding species were formerly included in the Secondary List of the Materia Medica of the United States.

E. ageratoides, or White Snake-root, is also in use as an anti-spasmodic, diuretic and diaphoretic; it is this plant which has been supposed to cause the fatal disease called 'trembles' in cattle, and the equally fatal local disease of some of the western States called 'Milk Sickness' in the human subject. It has also been lately confirmed by experiment that another American species, *E. urticæfolium*, is poisonous to stock.

E. aromaticum (Linn.) and *E. incarnatum* (Walt.), the Texan 'Mata,' are also other American species, which have gained much reputation in diseases connected with inflammation and irritability of the bladder; they are said to contain a principle similar to, if not identical with, *coumarin*, which is obtained from the Tonka Bean. *E. incarnatum* is also used for flavouring tobacco.

E. Ayapana (Vent), a Brazilian species, is an aromatic bitter and febrifuge like *E. perfoliatum*, and is considered a sure remedy – if timely used – for antidoting the effects of the bites of poisonous reptiles and insects. It is regarded as the most powerful species of the genus, but has fallen into neglect, though still occasionally met with in European commerce. *E. fœniculem* (Willd.), *E. leucolepsis* (T. & G.) and *E. hyssopifolium* (Linn.) are also considered to be antidotes to the poisonous bites of reptiles and stings of insects.

E. nervosum, a Jamaican species commonly known as Bitter-Bush, is regarded as very efficacious in cholera, and also in typhus and typhoid fevers and in smallpox. Another Jamaican species, *E. villosum*, also known locally as Bitter-Bush, is used there in the preparation of beer as a tonic and a stimulant in low, zymotic diseases.

E. rotundifolium (Linn.), a native of New England and Virginia, has been considered a palliative in consumption, and *E. collinum* is included in the Mexican Pharmacopœia, for properties similar to those of *E. perfoliatum*.

The leaves of *E. glutinosum* (Larmarck) also constitute one of the substances known as 'Matico' in South America, the latter name, however, belonging by right to 'Herba Matico,' an infusion of which is a recognized styptic, used to staunch the bleeding of wounds and to cure internal hæmorrhage. The true Matico is *Piper Angustifolium* (Ruiz & P.), but other plants besides this species of Eupatorium are frequently brought into the market under the name of Matico. In Quito, *E. glutinosum* quite generally goes by the name of Matico or Chusalonga.

Attention has been drawn of late to another South American species, *E. rebaudiana*, a tiny shrub, native to the highlands of Paraguay, called by the Indians 'Sweet Herb,' a few leaves being said to be sufficient to sweeten a strong cup of tea or coffee, giving also a pleasant aromatic flavour. It would seem worth while to cultivate this species here for experiment, since it has been called the Sugar Plant of South America, and probably proving easy of cultivation might, as a paying crop, become a successful rival to the sugar beet. *See* BONESET, GRAVEL ROOT, AGRIMONY, HEMP.

EUPHORBIA, EUPHORBIUM. *See* SPURGES

EVENING PRIMROSE. *See* PRIMROSE

EVERLASTING FLOWERS. *See* BALSAM, CUDWEED, GNAPHALIUM, LIFE EVERLASTING

EYEBRIGHT

Euphrasia officinalis (LINN.)
N.O. Scrophulariaceæ

Synonyms. Euphrasia
(*French*) Casse-lunette
(*German*) Augentröst
Part Used. Herb

The Eyebright is the only British species of a genus containing twenty species distributed over Europe, Northern and Western Asia and North America.

¶ *Description*. It is an elegant little plant, 2 to 8 inches high, an annual, common on heaths and other dry pastures, especially on a chalky soil, and flowering from July to September, with deeply-cut leaves and numerous, small, white or purplish flowers variegated with yellow.

It varies much in size and in the colour of the corolla, which changes to quite white and yellow. On the mountains and near the sea, or in poor soil, it is often a tiny plant, only an inch or so high, with the stem scarcely branched, but in rich soil it assumes the habit of a minute shrub and forms a spreading tuft, 8 or 9 inches high. The leaves, also, are sometimes almost round, and at other times pointed and narrow, their margins, however, always deeply cut into teeth. The variability of the Eyebright has led to much discussion as to how many species of it are known: continental botanists define numerous species, but our botanists follow Bentham and Hooker, who considered that there is only *one* very variable species, with three principal varieties: *officinalis* proper, in which the corolla lip equals or exceeds the tube and the bracts of the 'flower-spike are broad at the base; *gracilis*, more slender, the corolla lip shorter than the tube, and the flower-spike bracts narrowed at the base, and *maritima*, found on the shores of the Shetland Islands, in which the capsule is much longer than the calyx.

The stem is erect and wiry, either unbranched in small specimens, or with many opposite branches. The leaves are $\frac{1}{8}$ to $\frac{1}{2}$ inch long and about $\frac{1}{4}$ inch broad, opposite to one another on the lower portion of the stem, alternate above, more often lance-shaped, though sometimes, as already stated, much broader, and with four to five teeth on each side.

The flowers, white, or lilac and purple-veined, are in terminal spikes, with leafy bracts interspersed. The structure of the flower places the plant in the family of the Foxglove and the Speedwell – Scrophulariaceæ. The corolla is two-lipped, its lower, tube-like portion being enclosed in a green calyx, tipped with four teeth. The upper lip is two-lobed and arches over the stamens, forming a shelter from the rain. The lower lip is spreading and three-lobed, each lobe being notched. A yellow patch emphasizes the central lobe and purple 'honey guides' on both upper and lower lips – marked streaks of colour – point the way down the throat. Four stamens, with brown, downy anthers, lie under the upper lip, in pairs, one behind the other; on the underside of each anther is a stiff spur, the two lowest spurs longer than the others and projecting over the throat of the flower. The upper spurs end in miniature brushes which are intended to prevent the pollen being scattered at the side and wasted.

When a bee visitor comes in search of the honey lying round the ovary at the bottom of the petal tube, it knocks against the projecting anther spurs, which sets free the pollen, so that it falls on the insect's head. On visiting the next flower, the bee will then rub its dusty head against the outstanding stigma which terminates the style, or long thread placed on the ovary and projects beyond the stamens, and thus cross-fertilization is effected. But though this is the normal arrangement, other and smaller flowers are sometimes found, which suggests that self-fertilization is aimed at. In these, the corolla elongates after opening, and as the stamens are attached to it, their heads are gradually brought almost up to the stigma and eventually their pollen will fertilize it.

The seeds in all kinds of the flowers are produced in tiny, flattened capsules, and are numerous and ribbed.

The Eyebright will not grow readily in a garden if transplanted, unless 'protected' apparently, by grass. The reason for this is that it is a semi-parasite, relying for part of its nourishment on the roots of other plants. Above ground, it appears to be a perfectly normal plant, with normal flowers and bright green leaves – the leaves of fully parasitic plants are almost devoid of green colouring matter – but below the surface, suckers from its roots spread round and lie on the rootlets of the grassplants among which it grows. Where they are in contact, tiny nodules form and send absorption cells into the grass rootlets. The grass preyed upon does not, however, suffer very much, as the cells penetrate but a slight distance, moreover the Eyebright being an annual, renewing itself from year to year, the suckers on the grass roots to which it is attached also wither in the autumn, so there is no permanent drain of strength from the grass.

¶ *History*. The name Euphrasia is of Greek origin, derived from *Euphrosyne* (gladness), the name of one of the three graces who was distinguished for her joy and mirth, and it is thought to have been given the plant from the valuable properties attributed to it as an eye medicine preserving eyesight and so bringing gladness into the life of the sufferer. The same Greek word is also given to the linnet, whence another old tradition says that it was the linnet who first made use of the leaf for clearing the sight of its young and who then passed on the knowledge to mankind, who named the plant in its honour.

Although always known under a name of Greek origin, the herb seems to have been unnoticed by the ancients and no mention of it is made by Dioscorides, Pliny, Galen or even by the Arabian physicians. In the fourteenth century, however, it was supposed to cure 'all evils of the eye' and is described as the source of 'a precious water to clear a man's sight.' Matthæus Sylvaticus, a physician of Mantua, who lived about the year 1329, recommended this plant in disorders of the eyes and Arnoldus Villanovanus, who died in 1313, was the author of a treatise on its virtues, *Vini Euphrasiati tantopere celebrati*. How long before Euphrasia was in repute for eye diseases it is impossible to say, but in Gordon's *Liticium Medicina*, 1305, among the medicines for the eyes, *Euphragia* is named 'and is recommended both outwardly in a compound distilled water and inwardly as a syrup.' *Euphragia* is not, however, mentioned in the *Schola Salernitana*, compiled about 1100.

Markham (*Countrie Farm*, 1616) says: 'Drinke everie morning a small draught of Eyebright wine.' In the eighteenth century Eyebright tea was used, and in Queen Elizabeth's time there was a kind of ale called 'Eyebright Ale.'

Eyebright, says Salmon (*Syn. Med.*, 1671), strengthens the head, eyes and memory and clears the sight.

Euphrasia was regarded as a specific in diseases of the eyes by the great herbalists of the sixteenth century, Tragus, Fuchsius, Dodoens, etc., and has been a popular remedy in most countries.

The French call it *Casse-lunette*, the Germans *Augentröst* (consolation of the eyes).

It was the Euphrasy of Spenser, Milton and other poets. Milton relates how the Archangel Michæl ministered to Adam after the Fall:

' . . . to nobler sights
Michael from Adam's eyes the film removed,
Then purged with euphrasine and rue
His visual orbs, for he had much to see.'

It is probable that the belief in its value as an eye medicine originated in the old Doctrine of Signatures, for as an old writer points out –

'the purple and yellow spots and stripes which are upon the flowers of the Eyebright doth very much resemble the diseases of the eye, as bloodshot, etc., by which signature it hath been found out that this herb is effectual for the curing of the same.'

¶ *Part Used*. A fluid extract is prepared from the plant in the fresh state, gathered when in flower, and cut off just above the root.

Euphrasia is best collected in July and August, when in full flower and the foliage in the best condition.

¶ *Constituents*. The precise chemical constituents of the herb have not yet been recorded; it is known to contain a peculiar tannin, termed Euphrasia-Tannin acid (which gives a dark-green precipitate with ferric salts and is only obtainable by combination with lead) and also Mannite and Glucose, but the volatile oil and acrid and bitter principle have not yet been chemically analysed.

¶ *Medicinal Action and Uses*. Slightly tonic and astringent.

Although neglected nowadays by the faculty, modern herbalists still retain faith in this herb and recommend its use in diseases of the sight, weakness of the eyes, ophthalmia, etc., combining it often with Golden Seal in a lotion stated to be excellent for general disorders of the eyes. The juice obtained by expression from the plant in the fresh state is sometimes employed, or an infusion in milk, but the simple infusion in water is the more usual form in which it is applied. An infusion of 1 oz. of the herb to a pint of boiling water should be used and the eyes bathed three or four times a day. When there is much pain, it is considered desirable to use a warm infusion rather more frequently for inflamed eyes till the pain is removed. In ordinary cases, the cold application is found sufficient.

In Iceland, the expressed juice is used for most ailments of the eye, and in Scotland the Highlanders make an infusion of the herb in milk and anoint weak or inflamed eyes with a feather dipped in it.

The dried herb is an ingredient in British Herbal Tobacco, which is smoked most usefully for chronic bronchial colds.

Homœopathists hold that Eyebright belongs to the order of scrofula-curing plants, and Dr. Fernie tells us that it has recently been found by experiment

'to possess a distinct sphere of curative operation, within which it manifests virtues which are as unvarying as they are potential. It acts specifically on the mucous lining of the eyes and nose and the upper part of the throat to the top of the windpipe, causing when given so largely as to be injurious, a profuse secretion from these parts; if given of reduced strength, it cures the troublesome symptoms due to catarrh. Hay Fever, and acute attacks of cold in the head may be checked by an immediate dose of the infusion repeated every two hours. A medicinal tincture is prepared from the whole plant with spirits of wine, of which a lotion is made with rose-water, for simple inflammation of the eyes. Thirty drops of the tincture should be mixed with a wineglassful of rose-water for making this lotion, which may be used several times a day.'

¶ *Preparation.* Fluid extract, ½ to 1 drachm.

'*A Marvelous Water to Preserve the Sight.*

'Take the leaves of red roses, mints, sage, maidenhaire (or leave out sage and mint and take eyebright and vervin), bittony, such of the mountain, and endive, of each 6 handfuls: steep them in Whitewine 24 hours: then distill them in A limpeck; the first water is like silver, the second like gold, the third like balme; keep it close in glasses.

'It helps all diseases of the eye.' (*A Plain Plantain.*)

Gerard said that the powder of the Eyebright herb, mixed with mace, 'comforteth the memorie,' and Culpepper says:

'If the herb was but as much used as it is neglected, it would half spoil the spectacle maker's trade and a man would think that reason should teach people to prefer the preservation of their natural before artificial spectacles, which that they may be instructed how to do, take the virtues of Eyebright as followeth: The juice or distilled water of the Eyebright taken inwardly in white wine, or broth, or dropped into the eyes for several days together helpeth all infirmities of the eye that cause dimness of sight. Some make conserve of the flowers to the same effect. Being used any of the ways, it strengthens the week brain or memory. This tunned with strong beer that it may work together and drunk, or the powder of the dried herb mixed with sugar, a little mace, fennel seed and drunk, or eaten in broth; or the said powder made into an electuary with sugar and taken, hath the same powerful effect to help and restore the sight decayed through age and Arnoldus de Villa Nova saith it hath restored sight to them that have been blind a long time.'

This is another eye lotion of Culpepper:

'*An Excellent Water to Clear the Sight.*

'Take of Fennel, Eyebright, Roses, white, Celandine, Vervain and Rue, of each a handful, the liver of a Goat chopt small, infuse them well in Eyebright Water, then distil them in an alembic, and you shall have a water will clear the sight beyond comparison.'

Hildamus also firmly believed that Eyebright would restore the sight of many persons at the age of seventy or eighty years! Many of the older herbalists describe a 'Red-flowered Eyebright,' which, however, is no longer considered another species of *Euphrasia*, but regarded as a very closely allied plant. Linnæus himself, though he afterwards made a new genus, *Bartsia*, for it, called it *Euphrasia*, both in his *Flora Suecia*, his monograph on the flora of Sweden, that appeared in 1755, and in his great work, *Systema Vegetabilium*, published in 1784. Later, however, he named it after his friend Dr. Johann Bartsch of Königsberg. *See* BARSTIA (RED)

FENNEL

Fœniculum vulgare (GÆRT.)
N.O. Umbelliferæ

Synonyms. Fenkel. Sweet Fennel. Wild Fennel
Parts Used. Seeds, leaves, roots
Habitat. Fennel, a hardy, perennial, umbelliferous herb, with yellow flowers and feathery leaves, grows wild in most parts of temperate Europe, but is generally considered indigenous to the shores of the Mediterranean, whence it spreads eastwards to India. It has followed civilization, especially where Italians have colonized, and may be found growing wild in many parts of the world, upon dry soils near the sea-coast and upon river-banks. It flourishes particularly on limestone soils and is now naturalized in some parts of this country, being found from North Wales southward and eastward to Kent, being most frequent in Devon and Cornwall and on chalk cliffs near the sea. It is often found in chalky districts inland in a semi-wild state.

For the medicinal use of its fruits, commonly called seeds, Fennel is largely cultivated in the south of France, Saxony, Galicia, and Russia, as well as in India and Persia.

This plant was attached by Linnæus to the genus *Anethum*, but was separated from it by De Candolle and placed with three or four others in a new genus styled *Fœniculum*, which has been generally adopted by botanists. (*Fœniculum* was the name given to this plant by the Romans, and is derived from the Latin word, *fœnum* = hay).

This was corrupted in the Middle Ages into *Fanculum*, and this gave birth to its alternative popular name, 'fenkel.'

The *Anethum Fœniculum* of Linnæus em-

293

braced two varieties, the Common or Wild Fennel and the Sweet Fennel. These are considered by De Candolle as distinct species named respectively *F. vulgare* (Gærtn.) – the garden form of which is often named *F. Capillaceum* (Gilibert) – and *F. dulce*.

¶ *History*. Fennel was well known to the Ancients and was cultivated by the ancient Romans for its aromatic fruits and succulent, edible shoots. Pliny had much faith in its medicinal properties, according no less than twenty-two remedies to it, observing also that serpents eat it 'when they cast their old skins, and they sharpen their sight with the juice by rubbing against the plant.' A very old English rhyming Herbal, preserved at Stockholm, gives the following description of the virtue of the plant:

'Whaune the heddere (adder) is hurt in eye
Ye red fenel is hys prey,
And yif he mowe it fynde
Wonderly he doth hys kynde.
He schall it chow wonderly,
And leyn it to hys eye kindlely,
Ye jows shall sang and hely ye eye
Yat beforn was sicke et feye.'

Many of the older herbalists uphold this theory of the peculiarly strengthening effect of this herb on the sight.

Longfellow alludes to this virtue in the plant:

'Above the lower plants it towers,
The Fennel with its yellow flowers;
And in an earlier age than ours
Was gifted with the wondrous powers
Lost vision to restore.'

In mediæval times, Fennel was employed, together with St. John's Wort and other herbs, as a preventative of witchcraft and other evil influences, being hung over doors on Midsummer's Eve to warn off evil spirits. It was likewise eaten as a condiment to the salt fish so much consumed by our forefathers during Lent. Like several other umbelliferæ, it is carminative.

Though the Romans valued the young shoots as a vegetable, it is not certain whether it was cultivated in northern Europe at that time, but it is frequently mentioned in Anglo-Saxon cookery and medical recipes prior to the Norman Conquest. Fennel shoots, Fennel water and Fennel seed are all mentioned in an ancient record of Spanish agriculture dating A.D. 961. The diffusion of the plant in Central Europe was stimulated by Charlemagne, who enjoined its cultivation on the imperial farms.

It is mentioned in Gerard (1597), and Parkinson (*Theatricum Botanicum*, 1640) tells us that its culinary use was derived from Italy, for he says:

'The leaves, seede and rootes are both for meate and medicine; the Italians especially doe much delight in the use thereof, and therefore transplant and whiten it, to make it more tender to please the taste, which being sweete and somewhat hot helpeth to digest the crude qualitie of fish and other viscous meats. We use it to lay upon fish or to boyle it therewith and with divers other things, as also the seeds in bread and other things.'

William Coles, in *Nature's Paradise* (1650) affirms that –

'both the seeds, leaves and root of our Garden Fennel are much used in drinks and broths for those that are grown fat, to abate their unwieldiness and cause them to grow more gaunt and lank.'

The ancient Greek name of the herb, *Marathron*, from *maraino*, to grow thin, probably refers to this property.

It was said to convey longevity, and to give strength and courage.

There are many references to Fennel in poetry. Milton, in *Paradise Lost* alludes to the aroma of the plant:

'A savoury odour blown,
Grateful to appetite, more pleased my sense
Than smell of sweetest Fennel.'

¶ *Description*. Fennel is a beautiful plant. It has a thick, perennial root-stock, stout stems, 4 to 5 feet or more in height, erect and cylindrical, bright green and so smooth as to seem polished, much branched bearing leaves cut into the very finest of segments. The bright golden flowers, produced in large, flat terminal umbels, with from thirteen to twenty rays, are in bloom in July and August.

In the kitchen garden this naturally ornamental, graceful plant, generally has its stems cut down to secure a constant crop of green leaves for flavouring and garnishing, so that the plant is seldom seen in the same perfection as in the wild state. In the original wild condition, it is variable as to size, habit, shape and colour of leaf, number of rays in the flower-head or umbel, and shape of fruit, but it has been under cultivation for so long that there are now several well-marked species. The Common Garden Fennel (*F. Capillaceum* or *officinale*) is distinguished from its wild relative (*F. vulgare*) by having much stouter, taller, tubular and larger stems, and less divided leaves, but the chief distinction is that the leaf-stalks form a curved sheath around the stem, often even as far as the base of the leaf above. The flower-stalks, or pedicels, of the umbels are also sturdier, and the fruits, $\frac{1}{4}$ to $\frac{1}{2}$ inch long, are double the size of the wild ones.

¶ *Cultivation.* Fennel will thrive anywhere, and a plantation will last for years. It is easily propagated by seeds, sown early in April in ordinary soil. It likes plenty of sun and is adapted to dry and sunny situations, not needing heavily manured ground, though it will yield more on rich stiff soil. From $4\frac{1}{2}$ to 5 lb. of seed are sown per acre, either in drills, 15 inches apart, lightly, just covered with soil, and the plants afterwards thinned to a similar distance, or sewn thinly in a bed and transplanted when large enough. The fruit is heavy and a crop of 15 cwt. per acre is an average yield.

The *roots* of Fennel were formerly employed in medicine, but are generally inferior in virtues to the fruit, which is now the only portion recognized by any of the Pharmacopœias.

The cessation of the supply of Fennel fruits from the Continent during the War led to its being grown more extensively here, any crop produced being almost certain to sell well.

There are several varieties of Fennel fruit known in commerce – sweet or Roman Fennel, German or Saxon Fennel, wild or bitter Fennel, Galician Russian and Roumanian Fennel, Indian, Persian and Japanese. The fruits vary very much in length, breadth, taste and other characters, and are of very different commercial value.

The most esteemed Fennel fruit vary from three to five lines in length, are elliptical, slightly curved, somewhat obtuse at the ends and pale greyish green in colour. *Wild* fruits are short, dark coloured and blunt at their ends, and have a less agreeable flavour and odour than those of sweet Fennel – they are not official.

Fennel fruits are frequently distinguished into 'shorts' and 'longs' in commerce, the latter being the most valued.

The odour of Fennel seed is fragrant, its taste, warm, sweet and agreeably aromatic. It yields its virtues to hot water, but more freely to alcohol. The essential oil may be separated by distillation with water.

For medicinal use, the fruits of the cultivated Fennel, especially those grown in Saxony, are alone official, as they yield the most volatile oil. Saxon fruits are greenish to yellowish-brown in colour, oblong, smaller and straighter than the French or Sweet Fennel (*F. dulce*). This French Fennel, known also as Roman Fennel, is distinguished by its greater length, more oblong form, yellowish-green colour and sweet taste; its anise-like odour is also stronger. It is cultivated in the neighbourhood of Nimes, in the south of France, but yields comparatively little oil, which has no value medicinally.

Indian Fennel is brownish, usually smaller, straighter and not quite so rounded at the ends with a sweet anise taste. Persian and Japanese fennel, pale greenish brown in colour, are the smallest and have a sweeter, still more strongly anise taste and an odour intermediate between that of French and Saxon.

The Saxon, Galician, Roumanian and Russian varieties all yield 4 to 5 per cent. of volatile oil, and these varieties are alone suitable for pharmaceutical use. In the ordinary way they furnish some of the best Fennel crops, and from their fruit a large portion of the oil of commerce is derived.

For family use, $\frac{1}{2}$ oz. of seed will produce an ample supply of plants and for several years, either from the established roots, or by re-seeding. Unless seed is needed for household or sowing purposes, the flower stems should be cut as soon as they appear.

¶ *Adulteration.* Commercial Fennel varies greatly in quality, this being either due to lack of care in harvesting, or deliberate adulteration. It may contain so much sand, dirt, stem tissues, weed seeds or other material, that it amounts to adulteration and is unfit for medicinal use, or it may have had some of its oil removed by distillation.

Fruits exhausted by water or steam are darker, contain less oil and sink at once in water, but those exhausted by alcohol still retain 1 to 2 per cent., and are but little altered in appearance; they acquire, however, a peculiar fusel oil odour.

Exhausted, or otherwise inferior fennel is occasionally improved in appearance by the use of a factitious colouring, but old exhausted fruits that have been re-coloured may be detected by rubbing the fruit between the hands, when the colour will come off.

¶ *Constituents.* As found in commerce, oil Fennel is not uniform.

The best varieties of Fennel yield from 4 to 5 per cent. of volatile oil (sp. gr. 0·960 to 0·930), the principal constituents of which are Anethol (50 to 60 per cent.) and Fenchone (18 to 22 per cent.). Anethol is also the chief constituent of Anise oil.

Fenchone is a colourless liquid possessing a pungent, camphoraceous odour and taste, and when present gives the disagreeable bitter taste to many of the commercial oils. It probably contributes materially to the medicinal properties of the oil, hence only such varieties of Fennel as contain a good proportion of fenchone are suitable for medicinal use.

There are also present in oil of Fennel, *d*-pinene, phellandrine, anisic acid and anisic aldehyde. Schimmel mentions limonene as also at times present as a constituent.

There is reason to believe that much of the commercial oil is adulterated with oil from which the anethol or crystalline constituent has been separated. Good oil will contain as much as 60 per cent.

Saxon Fennel yields 4·7 per cent. of volatile oil, containing 22 per cent. of fenchone.

Russian, Galician and Roumanian, which closely resembles one another, yield 4 to 5 per cent. of volatile oil, of which about 18 per cent. is fenchone. They have a camphoraceous taste.

French sweet or Roman Fennel yields only 2·1 per cent. of oil, containing much less anethol and with a milder and sweeter taste, probably due to the entire absence of the bitter fenchone.

French bitter Fennel oil differs considerably, anethol being only present in traces. The oil (*Essence de Fenouil amer*) is distilled from the entire herb, collected in the south of France, where the plant grows without cultivation.

Indian Fennel yields only 0·72 per cent. of oil, containing only 6·7 per cent. of fenchone.

Japanese Fennel yields 2·7 per cent. of oil, containing 10·2 of fenchone and 75 per cent. of anethol.

Sicilian Fennel oil is yielded from *F. piperitum*.

It was formerly the practice to boil Fennel with all fish, and it was mainly cultivated in kitchen gardens for this purpose. Its leaves are served nowadays with salmon, to correct its oily indigestibility, and are also put into sauce, in the same way as parsley, to be eaten with boiled mackerel.

The seeds are also used for flavouring and the carminative oil that is distilled from them, which has a sweetish aromatic odour and flavour, is employed in the making of cordials and liqueurs, and is also used in perfumery and for scenting soaps. A pound of oil is the usual yield of 500 lb. of the seed.

¶ *Medicinal Action and Uses.* On account of its aromatic and carminative properties, Fennel fruit is chiefly used *medicinally* with purgatives to allay their tendency to griping and for this purpose forms one of the ingredients of the well-known compound Liquorice Powder. Fennel water has properties similar to those of anise and dill water: mixed with sodium bicarbonate and syrup, these waters constitute the domestic 'Gripe Water,' used to correct the flatulence of infants. Volatile oil of Fennel has these properties in concentration.

Fennel tea, formerly also employed as a carminative, is made by pouring half a pint of boiling water on a teaspoonful of bruised Fennel seeds.

Syrup prepared from Fennel juice was formerly given for chronic coughs.

Fennel is also largely used for cattle condiments.

It is one of the plants which is said to be disliked by fleas, and powdered Fennel has the effect of driving away fleas from kennels and stables. The plant gives off ozone most readily.

Culpepper says:

'One good old custom is not yet left off, viz., to boil fennel with fish, for it consumes the phlegmatic humour which fish most plentifully afford and annoy the body with, though few that use it know wherefore they do it. It benefits this way, because it is a herb of Mercury, and under Virgo, and therefore bears antipathy to Pisces. Fennel expels wind, provokes urine, and eases the pains of the stone, and helps to break it. The leaves or seed boiled in barley water and drunk, are good for nurses, to increase their milk, and make it more wholesome for the child. The leaves, or rather the seeds, boiled in water, stayeth the hiccup and taketh away nausea or inclination to sickness. The seed and the roots much more help to open obstructions of the liver, spleen, and gall, and thereby relieve the painful and windy swellings of the spleen, and the yellow jaundice, as also the gout and cramp. The seed is of good use in medicines for shortness of breath and wheezing, by stoppings of the lungs. The roots are of most use in physic, drinks and broths, that are taken to cleanse the blood, to open obstructions of the liver, to provoke urine, and amend the ill colour of the face after sickness, and to cause a good habit through the body; both leaves, seeds, and roots thereof, are much used in drink, or broth, to make people more lean that are too fat. A decoction of the leaves and root is good for serpent bites, and to neutralize vegetable poison, as mushrooms, etc.'

'In warm climates,' says Mattiolus, 'the stems are cut and there exudes a resinous liquid, which is collected under the name of Fennel Gum.'

In Italy and France, the tender leaves are often used for garnishes and to add flavour to salads, and are also added, finely chopped, to sauces served with puddings. Roman bakers are said to put the herb under their loaves in the oven to make the bread taste agreeably.

The tender stems are employed in soups in Italy, though are more frequently eaten raw as a salad. John Evelyn, in his *Acetaria* (1680), held that the peeled stalks, soft and white, of the cultivated garden Fennel, when dressed like celery exercised a pleasant action conducive to sleep. The Italians eat these peeled stems, which they call 'Cartucci' as a salad, cutting them when the plant is about to bloom and serving with a dressing of vinegar and pepper.

Formerly poor people used to eat Fennel to satisfy the cravings of hunger on fast days and make unsavoury food palatable; it was also used in large quantities in the households of the rich, as may be seen by the record in the accounts of Edward I.'s household, 8½ lb. of Fennel were bought for one month's supply.

¶ *Preparations.* Fluid extract, 5 to 30 drops. Oil, 1 to 5 drops. Water, B.P. and U.S.P., 4 drachms.

FENNEL, DOG. *See* MAYWEED

FENNEL, FLORENCE

Fœniculum dulce
N.O. Umbelliferæ

Synonyms. Finnochio
Parts Used. Seeds, herb

Finnochio or Florence Fennel is a native of Italy, and bears a general resemblance to *Fœniculum vulgare*, but is an annual and a much smaller plant, being as a rule little more than a foot high. It is a very thick-set plant, the stem joints are very close together and their bases much swollen. The large, finely-cut leaves are borne on very broad, pale green, or almost whitish stalks, which overlap at their bases somewhat like celery, swelling at maturity to form a sort of head or irregular ball – often as big as a man's head and resembling a tuber. The flowers appear earlier than those of common Fennel, and the number of flowers in the umbel is only six to eight.

¶ *Cultivation.* The cultivation is much the same as for common Fennel, though it requires richer soil, and owing to the dwarf nature of the plant, the rows and the plants may be placed closer together, the seedlings only 6 to 8 inches apart. They are very thirsty and require watering frequently in dry weather. When the 'tubers' swell and attain the size of an egg, draw the soil slightly around them, half covering them. Cutting may begin about ten days later. The flower-heads should be removed as they appear.

Florence Fennel should be cooked in vegetarian or meat stock and served with either a rich butter sauce or cream dressing. It suggests celery in flavour, but is sweeter, and very pleasantly fragrant. In ordinary times, it can be bought from Italian green-grocers in London. In Italy it is one of the commonest and most popular of vegetables. It is grown in this country at Hitchin.

FENNEL FLOWER

Nigella sativa (LINN.)
N.O. Ranunculaceæ

Synonyms. Roman Coriander. Nutmeg Flower
(*French*) Faux cumin. Quatre épices. Toute épice
(*German*) Schwarzkummel
Parts Used. Seeds, herb

Fennel Flower, or Nutmeg Flower, is a small Asiatic annual, native to Syria, not in any way related to the Fennel, but belonging to the buttercup order of plants and grown to a limited extent in southern Europe and occasionally in other parts of the world.

Among the Romans it was esteemed in cooking, hence one of its common names, Roman Coriander.

French cooks employ the seeds of this plant under the name of *quatre épices* or *toute épice*. They were formerly used as a substitute for pepper.

¶ *Description.* The plant has a rather stiff, erect, branching stem, bears deeply-cut greyish-green leaves and terminal greyish-blue flowers, followed by odd, toothed seed-vessels, filled with small somewhat compressed seeds, usually three-cornered, with two sides flat and one convex, black or brown externally, white and oleaginous within, of a strong, agreeable aromatic odour, like that of nutmegs, and a spicy, pungent taste.

¶ *Cultivation.* The seed is sown in spring, after the ground gets warm. The drills may be 15 to 18 inches apart and the plants thinned to 10 to 12 inches asunder. No special attention is necessary until mid-summer when the seeds ripen. They are easily threshed and cleaned. After drying, they should be carefully stored in a cool, dry place.

¶ *Constituents.* The chief constituents of the seeds are a volatile oil and a fixed oil (1·3 per cent. of the former and 35 per cent. of the latter), and an amorphous, glucoside Melanthin, which is decomposed by diluted hydrochloric acid into Melanthigenin and sugar.

Rochebrune, *Toxicol Africaine*, has found a powerful paralysing alkaloid, to which he gives the name of Nigelline. Melanthin is stated to exhibit the typical physiological action of the most poisonous saponines.

¶ *Medicinal Action and Uses.* In India, the seeds are considered as stimulant, diaphoretic and emmenagogue, and are believed to increase the secretion of milk. They are also used as a condiment and as a corrigent or adjuvant of purgative and tonic medicines.

In Eastern countries they are commonly used for seasoning curries and other dishes, and the Egyptians spread them on bread or put them on cakes like comfits, believing them to be fattening. They are also used in India for putting among linen to keep away insects; and the native doctors employ them medicinally as a carminative in indigestion and bowel complaints.

FENNEL, HOG'S

Peucedanum palustre (LINN.)
Peucedanum officinale (LINN.)
N.O. Compositæ

Synonyms. Sow Fennel. Sulphurwort. Chucklusa. Hoar Strange. Hoar Strong. Brimstonewort. Milk Parsley. Marsh Parsley. Marsh Smallage
(*French*) Persil des Marais
(*German*) Sumpfsilge
Part Used. Herb

The Hog's Fennel, a native of Great Britain, though not commonly met with, is more closely allied to the dill than to the true Fennel, belonging to the same genus as the former.

The ordinary Hog's Fennel (*Peucedanum officinale*, Linn.) occurs, though somewhat rarely, in salt marshes on the eastern coast of England. It seems to have been less rare in the days of Culpepper, who states that it grows plentifully in the salt marshes near Faversham.

¶ *Description.* It grows to a height of 3 or 4 feet, and is remarkable for its large umbels of yellow flowers, which are in bloom from July to September. Its leaves are cut into long narrow segments, hence perhaps its popular name of Hog's Fennel.

The thick root has a strong odour of sulphur – hence one of the other popular names of the plant, Sulphurwort, and when wounded in the spring, yields a considerable quantity of a yellowish-green juice, which dries into a gummy resin and retains the strong scent of the root.

This plant is now naturalized in North America, where in addition to the name of Sulphurwort, it is called Chucklusa.

¶ *Constituents.* The active constituent of the root is Peucedanin, a very active crystalline principle, stated to be diuretic and emmenagogue.

¶ *Medicinal Action and Uses.* Culpepper gives Hog's Fennel the name of Hoar Strange, Hoar Strong, Brimstonewort and Sulphurwort, and tells us, on the authority of Dioscorides and Galen, that –

'the juice used with vinegar and rose-water, or with a little Euphorbium put to the nose benefits those that are troubled with the lethargy, frenzy or giddiness of the head, the falling sickness, long and inveterate headache, the palsy, sciatica and the cramp, and generally all the diseases of the sinews, used with oil and vinegar. The juice dissolved in wine and put into an egg is good for a cough or shortness of breath, and for those that are troubled with wind. It also purgeth gently and softens hardness of the spleen. . . . A little of the juice dissolved in wine and dropped into the ears or into a hollow tooth easeth the pains thereof. The root is less effectual to all the aforesaid disorders, yet the powder of the root cleanseth foul ulcers, and taketh out splinters of broken bones or other things in the flesh and healeth them perfectly; it is of admirable virtue in all green wounds and prevents gangrene.'

P. palustre, the Marsh Hog's Fennel, is also a rare plant, found in marshes in Yorks and Lincoln and a few other districts.

Its grooved stem grows 4 to 5 feet high,

bears white flowers and abounds in a milky juice which dries to a brown resin. The root is, when dried, of a brown colour externally, having a strong aromatic odour and an acrid, pungent, aromatic taste.

The resin in it has been found, by Peschier, to contain a volatile oil, a fixed oil and a peculiar acid which he named Selinic. It has

been used as a substitute for ginger in Russia and has been employed in that country as a remedy for epilepsy, having the same stimulating qualities as the former species, the dose given being from 20 to 30 grains thrice daily, rapidly increased to four times the amount.

See MASTERWORT.

(WATER) FENNEL. *See* (WATER) DROPWORT

FENUGREEK

Trigonella Fœnum-græcum (LINN.)
N.O. Leguminosæ

Synonyms. Bird's Foot. Greek Hay-seed
Part Used. Seeds
Habitat. Indigenous to the countries on the eastern shores of the Mediterranean. Cultivated in India, Africa, Egypt, Morocco, and occasionally in England

¶ *Description.* The name comes from *Fœnum-græcum,* meaning Greek Hay, the plant being used to scent inferior hay. The name of the genus, *Trigonella,* is derived from the old Greek name, denoting 'three-angled,' from the form of its corolla. The seeds of Fenugreek have been used medicinally all through the ages and were held in high repute among the Egyptians, Greeks and Romans for medicinal and culinary purposes.

Fenugreek is an erect annual herb, growing about 2 feet high, similar in habit to Lucerne. The seeds are brownish, about $\frac{1}{8}$ inch long, oblong, rhomboidal, with a deep furrow dividing them into two unequal lobes. They are contained, ten to twenty together, in long, narrow, sickle-like pods.

Taste, bitter and peculiar, not unlike lovage or celery. Odour, similar.

¶ *Constituents.* About 28 per cent. mucilage; 5 per cent. of a stronger-smelling, bitter fixed oil, which can be extracted by ether; 22 per cent. proteids; a volatile oil; two alkaloids, Trigonelline and Choline, and a yellow colouring substance. The chemical composition resembles that of cod-liver oil, as it is rich in phosphates, lecithin and nucleoalbumin, containing also considerable quantities of iron in an organic form, which can be readily absorbed. Reutter has noted the presence of trimethylamine, neurin and betain; like the alkaloids in cod-liver oil, these substances stimulate the appetite by their action on the nervous system, or produce a diuretic or ureo-poietic effect.

¶ *Medicinal Action and Uses.* In Cairo it is used under the name of *Helba.* This is an Egyptian preparation, made by soaking the seeds in water till they swell into a thick paste. Said to be equal to quinine in preventing fevers; is comforting to the stomach and has been utilized for diabetes. The seeds are

soaked in water, then allowed to sprout, and when grown about 2 or 3 inches high, the green eaten raw with the seeds.

The seeds yield the whole of their odour and taste to alcohol and are employed in the preparation of emollient cataplasms, ointments and plasters.

They give a strong mucilage, which is emollient and a decoction of 1 oz. seeds to 1 pint water is used internally in inflamed conditions of the stomach and intestines. Externally it is used as a poultice for abscesses, boils, carbuncles, etc. It can be employed as a substitute for cod-liver oil in scrofula, rickets, anæmia, debility following infectious diseases. For neurasthenia, gout and diabetes it can be combined with insulin. It possesses the advantage of being cheap and readily taken by children, if its bitter taste is disguised: 1 or 2 teaspoonful of the powder is taken daily in jam, etc.

The ground seeds are used also to give a maple-flavouring to confectionery and nearly all cattle like the flavour of Fenugreek in their forage. The powder is also employed as a spice in curry. At the present day, the ground seeds are utilized to an enormous extent in the manufactures of condition powders for horses and cattle; Funugreek is the principal ingredient in most of the quack nostrums which find so much favour among grooms and horsekeepers. It has a powerful odour of coumarin and is largely used for flavouring cattle foods and to make damaged hay palatable.

In India the fresh plant is employed as an esculent.

¶ *Other Species.*
Trigonella purpurascens, a British species, with small pinky-white flowers, one to three together, and straight, six- to eight-seeded pods, twice as long as the calyx.

FERNS

Ferns are herbs, with a perennial (rarely annual) short, tufted or creeping root-stock. The British genera comprise about forty-five species, only one of which, a small Jersey species, is annual.

The leaves of Ferns are mostly radical, partaking of the nature of branches and distinguished by the name of fronds. When divided laterally (as is generally the case) the leaflets are termed *pinnæ*, and their subdivisions *pinnules*.

The classification of the order *Filices* is according to fructification. The dust-like and almost invisible seeds or *spores* of Ferns are contained in little cases or *thecæ*, of a roundish shape, which are themselves encircled (except in some groups) by a jointed ring, the elasticity of which eventually bursts open the thecæ and scatters the spores when mature. These thecæ are in the majority of the genera arranged on the back of the pinnules in linear, oblong or circular clusters, called *sori*, mostly having above the mass a thin membrane called the *Indusium*, though in some genera the sori are naked. In some instances, as in the Maidenhairs, the sori are arranged on the margins of the fronds, the indusium being a continuation of the bleached, recurved margin of the pinnule itself. In a few genera, as in the Osmunda and Adder's Tongue, the plant is divided into barren and fertile fronds, either of a distinctly different or of the same form, the fructification rising at the top of the fertile fronds in spikes or panicles. The spores when sown develop minute green leafy expansions, called *Prothalli*. On each prothallus are produced tiny bodies which have been compared to stamens and pistils, from whence the young Fern is subsequently developed.

As regards culture, Ferns prefer a northern aspect, shade and shelter is not indispensable, but tends to their finer and most perfect con dition and growth. They flourish best in a soil that is a mixture of peat, earth and sand, pebbles being intermixed for the roots in many instances to cling to. The only manure needed is that from dried leaves or other vegetable matter. They should not be set too deep and are best kept rather moist. In all the wall species, the roots are best placed under the protection of the stones among which they are to grow. Attention should be paid in cultivation to the natural habits of the species. Ferns may be raised from the spores if carefully potted and looked after.

MALE FERN

Dryopteris Felix-mas (LINN.)
Aspidium Filix-mas (SCHWARZ)

Synonym. Male Shield Fern
Part Used. Root

The common Male Fern, often known as *Dryopteris Filix-mas* (Linn.), and assigned by other botanists to the genera *Lastrea*, *Nephrodium* and *Polypodium*, is one of the commonest and hardiest of British Ferns and, after the Bracken, the species most frequently met with, growing luxuriantly in woods and shady situations, and along moist banks and hedgerows. In sheltered spots it will sometimes remain green all the winter.

This Fern grows in all parts of Europe, temperate Asia, North India, North and South Africa, the temperate parts of the United States and the Andes of South America. It is very variable, some of its forms in this country markedly differing and described under the names of sub-species, the chief being *affine*, *Borreri*, *pumilum*, *abbreviatum*, and *elongatum*.

¶ *Description*. The root-stock or rhizome is short, stumpy and creeping, lying along the surface of the ground or just below it. From its under surface spring the slender, matted roots. The crown of the rhizome is a brown, tangled mass, with the hairy bases of the leaves, and in it is contained the mass of undeveloped fronds which, as they unroll, grow in a large circular tuft and attain a length of from 2 to 4 feet. Each frond is wide and spreading, stiff, erect, broadly lanceolate or lance-shaped, the stalk covered with brown scaly hairs. The pinnæ are arranged alternately on the mid-rib (which is also hairy), the lower ones decreasing in size, and each pinna divided again almost to its own mid-rib, the pinnules being oblong and rounded, with their edges slightly notched and their surface somewhat furrowed. The sori are on the upper half of the frond, at the back of the pinnules, in round masses towards the base of the segments, covered with a conspicuous, kidney-shaped indusium.

The name of this genus, *Aspidium*, is derived from *aspis* (a shield), because the spores are thus enclosed in bosses, resembling the shape of the round shields of ancient days.

¶ *Parts Used Medicinally*. An oil is extracted from the rhizome of this Fern, which, as far back as the times of Theophrastus and Dioscorides, was known as a valuable vermifuge, and its use has in modern times been widely revived.

Gerard writes:

'The roots of the Male Fern, being taken in the weight of half an ounce, driveth forth long flat worms, as Dioscorides writeth, being drunke in mede or honied water, and more effectually if it be given with two scruples, or two third parts of a dram of scammonie, or of black hellebore: they that will use it, must first eat garlicke.'

The famous remedy of Madame Nouffer, for expelling tapeworms, contained this plant as its basis.

Comparatively little Male Fern has so far been collected in this country, Germany until the War having supplied nearly all our requirements.

It may be collected in late autumn, winter or early spring, from the time the fronds die down, till February, late autumn being considered the best time. Only old rhizomes should be taken.

The rhizome varies in length and thickness according to its age. For medicinal purposes it should be from 3 to 6 inches or more long and from $1\frac{1}{2}$ to 2 inches or more broad. When removed from the ground, it is cylindrical and covered with the closely-arranged, overlapping remains of the leaf-stalks of the decayed fronds. These stalks are from 1 to 2 inches long, somewhat curved, angular, brown-coloured, and surrounded at the base with thin, silky scales, of a light brown colour. From between these remains of the leaf stalks, the black, wiry, branched roots may be seen. Internally in the fresh state, the rhizome is fleshy and of a light yellowish-green colour. It has very little odour, but a sweetish, astringent and subsequently nauseous and bitter taste.

Before drying, it is divested of its scales, roots and all dead portions, leaving the lower swollen portion attached to the rhizome, and is carefully cleansed from adhering soil. It is then sliced in half longitudinally. For pharmaceutical use, it is reduced to a coarse powder and at once exhausted with ether. Extract obtained in this way is more efficacious than that which has been obtained from rhizome that has been kept for some time. It should never be more than a year old.

There is also a market for Male Fern Fingers which are the bases of the fronds, collected in late summer, scraped when fresh (not peeled), cut up into pieces 2 to 3 inches long and then dried, when they present a wrinkled appearance externally and internally and should have the colour of pistachio nuts.

¶ *Substitutes.* English oil of Male Fern has always proved more reliable than that imported from the Continent, which is often extracted from an admixture of other species. The rhizomes of *Asplenium Filix-fœmina* (Bernh.), *Aspidium Oreopteris* (Sw.), and *A. spinulosum* (Sw.), resemble those of the Male Fern and have often been found mixed with it when imported. They are best distinguished by examining the transverse section of their leaf bases with a magnifying lens: in *Filix-mas*, the section exhibits eight wood bundles, forming an irregular circle, whilst in the three other ferns named only *two* are observed. The presence of secreting cells in the hard tissue, the number of bundles at the base of the leaf-stalk, and the absence of glandular hairs from the margin of the scales, readily distinguish Male Fern from the other species. The margin of the scales borne by the leaf-stalk has in the Male Fern merely hair-like projections, whereas in *A. spinulosum*, the hairs are glandular. *Filix-fœmina* has no glandular hairs, and has only two large bundles in the base of the leaf-stalk in distinction to the eight of *Filix-mas*. The United States Pharmacopœia includes the rhizome of a Canadian species, *A. marginale*, which in transverse section shows only six wood bundles.

This fern appears to have some qualities in common with the Bracken. The ashes of both have been used in soap and glassmaking, and the young curled fronds have been boiled and eaten like Asparagus. In times of great scarcity the Norwegians (over a century ago) used the fronds to mix with bread and also made them into beer. The leaves, cut green and dried, make an excellent bitter, and when infused in hot water make good fodder for sheep and goats.

The Scottish roots of Male Fern (according to an account published in the *Chemist and Druggist* of February 26, 1921) yield an oleoresin which contains 30 per cent. of filicin, whereas the British Pharmacopœia only requires 20 per cent.

¶ *Constituents.* By extraction with ether, Male Fern yields a dark green, oily liquid extract, Oil of Male Fern, containing the more important constituents of the drug. The chief constituents are about 5 per cent. of Filmaron – an amorphous acid, and from 5 to 8 per cent. of Filicic acid, which is also amorphous and tends to degenerate into its inactive crystalline anhydride, Filicin. The Filicic acid is regarded as the chief, though not the only active principle. Tannin, resin, colouring matter and sugar are also present in the rhizome. The drug has a disagreeable, bitter taste and an unpleasant odour.

¶ *Medicinal Action and Uses.* The liquid extract is one of the best anthelmintics against tapeworm, which it kills and expels. It is usual to administer this worm medicine last thing at night, after several hours of fasting, and to give a purgative, such as castor oil, first thing in the morning. A single sufficient dose will often cure at once. The powder, or the fluid extract, may be taken, but the ethereal extract, or oleoresin, if given in pill form, is the more pleasant way of taking it.

The drug is much employed for similar purposes by veterinary practitioners. In the powdered form, the dose varies from 60 to 180 grains, taken in honey or syrup, or infused in half a teacupful of boiling water.

The dose often given is too small, and failure is then due to the smallness of the dose. In too large doses, however, it is an irritant poison, causing muscular weakness and coma, and has been proved particularly injurious to the eyesight, even causing blindness.

The older herbalists considered that 'the roots, bruised and boiled in oil or lard, made a good ointment for healing wounds, and that the powdered roots cured rickets in children.'

¶ *Preparations and Dosages.* Powdered root, 1 to 4 drachms. Fluid extract, 1 to 4 drachms. Oleoresin, 5 to 20 drops. Ethereal extract, B.P., 45 to 90 drops.

SHIELD FERN, PRICKLY-TOOTHED

Aspidium spinulosum
N.O. Filices

Part Used. Root

The Prickly-toothed Shield Fern is allied to the Male Shield Fern, but is not so tall, about 8 to 14 inches, and has very much broader leaves. The rootstock is similar to Male Fern, but there are differences in the number of wood bundles in the stems, also in the hairs on the margins of the leaf-stalk scales. The fronds are more divided – twice or thrice pinnate – and are spinous, the pinnæ generally opposite and the lowest pair

much shorter than the others. The sori are circular, with kidney-shaped indusium, much smaller than in *Filix-mas*.

The Prickly-toothed Shield Fern is moderately erect and firm and grows in masses, being common in sheltered places on moist banks and in open woods.

The medicinal uses are as in Male Fern, with the rhizome of which, as imported from the Continent, it has always been much mixed.

LADY FERN

Asplenium Felix-fœmina (BERNH.)
N.O. Filices

Synonym. Athyrium Filix-fœmina

The Lady Fern is similar in size and general appearance to the Male Fern. It grows abundantly in Britain, in masses, in moist, sheltered woods, on hedgebanks and in ravines. The rootstock is short and woody; the fronds 2 to 3 feet high, grow in circular tufts and are light, feathery and succulent, generally drooping, and while young and tender, not infrequently soon shrivelling up after being gathered. The leaf base – as already stated – has only two large bundles, and the stalks are less scaly than in the Male Fern. The pinnæ are alternate, the lowest

decreasing much in size at the bottom, and are divided into numerous long, narrow, deeply-divided and toothed pinnules, with abundant sori on their undersides, the indusium attached along one side, in shape rather like an elongated and rather straightened kidney. The Lady Fern is very variable in form, tint and flexibility: it is more graceful and somewhat more delicate than the Male Fern, and is early cut down by autumn frosts. It is easy of cultivation.

The medicinal uses are as in Male Fern, but it is less powerful in action.

SPLEENWORT, COMMON

Asplenium ceterach (LINN.)
N.O. Filices

Synonyms. Scaly Fern. Finger Fern. Miltwaste. Ceterach (Arabian)

The Common Spleenwort grows on old walls and in the clefts of moist rocks. The fronds are 4 to 6 inches long, leathery, light green above, beneath densely covered with rusty, toothed scales, the sori hidden under the scales.

This Fern used also to be called 'Miltwaste,' because it was said to cure disorders of the milt or spleen, for which it was much recommended by the Ancients. Probably this

virtue has been attributed to the plant because the lobular milt-like shape of its leaf resembles the form of the spleen. The name of the genus, *Asplenium,* is derived from the Greek word for the spleen, for which the various species originally assigned to the genus were thought to have curative powers. This particular species was used to cure an enlarged spleen. It was also used as a pectoral and as an aperient in obstructions of the viscera, and an infusion of the leaves was prescribed for gravel. Meyrick considered that a decoction of the whole plant

SPLEENWORT, BLACK

Synonym. Black Maidenhair
Part Used. Herb

The Black Spleenwort is a small fern growing in rather circular masses, either on walls, where its fronds are only from 3 to 6 inches long, or on shady hedgebanks, where its oblong-triangular, evergreen fronds may attain as much as 20 inches in length. The pinnæ are alternate, slanting upwards; the pinnules thick, leathery, shiny, irregularly wedge-shaped. It is rather variable in form; when on exposed walls, it is more rigid and pointed and yellowish-green, instead of dark

WALL RUE

Synonyms. White Maidenhair. Tentwort
Part Used. Herb

The Wall Rue, named by some old writers *Salvis vitæ*, also White Maidenhair, is a small fern, only 2 to 3 inches high, growing in tufts and embedded in the crevices and joints of walls. It is much the colour of Garden Rue, its wedge-shaped pinnules being like those of the Rue, and also its slender stalks of a pale-green colour.

It was considered good for coughs and ruptures in children. One of its old names, 'Tentwort,' refers to its use as a specific for the cure of rickets, a disease once known as 'the taint.' It was also used to prevent hair from falling out.

Culpepper says:

'This is used in pectoral decoction. The

MAIDENHAIR, COMMON

A tea derived from our Common Maidenhair, a simple little fern, common on old walls, with long, simply pinnate fronds, their sori arranged on the back in oblique lines, has also demulcent effect. The fronds are sweet, mucilaginous, and expectorant, causing the tea to have been considered useful in pulmonary disorders. In Arran, the fronds have been dried and used as a substitute for tea; it acts as a laxative.

MAIDENHAIR, TRUE

Synonyms. Capillaire commun, or de Montpellier. Hair of Venus
Part Used. The herb
Habitat. Southern Europe. Southern and Central Britain

¶ *History.* Several varieties of Maidenhair Fern are used in medicine, the most common being the present species, when grown in France, and the Canadian *Adiantum pedatum.*

was efficacious, if persevered in, for removing all obstructions of the liver and spleen. Pliny considered that it caused barrenness.

Asplenium Adiantum nigrum (LINN.)
N.O. Filices

green. The sori are abundant, swelling over the edges of the pinnules. This is a very hardy and ornamental fern. Its stalks are polished and dark chestnut-brown in colour.

It is sometimes called Black Maidenhair, and has medicinal virtues similar to other Maidenhairs, a decoction of it relieving a troublesome cough and proving also a good hair wash.

¶ *Dosage of Infusion.* 3 tablespoonfuls.

Asplenium Ruta-muraria (LINN.)
N.O. Filices

decoction being drunk helps those that are troubled with coughs, shortness of breath, yellow jaundice, diseases of the spleen, stoppings of the urine, and helps to break the stone in the kidneys. . . . It cleanses the lungs, and by rectifying the blood causes a good colour to the whole body. The herb boiled in oil of camomile dissolves knots, allays swellings and drys up moist ulcers. The lye made thereof is singularly good to cleanse the head from scurf and from dry and running sores, stays the shedding or falling of the hair, and causes it to grow thick, fair and well-coloured, for which purpose boil it in wine, putting some smallage-seed thereto and afterwards some oil.'

Asplenium trichomanes (LINN.)
N.O. Filices

¶ *Other Species.*
The 'Golden Maidenhair,' which Culpepper also mentions, is not a Fern, but a Moss. He describes it as 'rarely used, but very good to prevent the falling off of the hair and to make it grow thick, being boiled in water or lye and the head washed with it.'

The above three species are the doradilles of France, sometimes used as rather unsatisfactory substitutes for the Maidenhair of Montpellier and Canada and Mexico.

Adiantum Capillus-veneris
N.O. Filices

¶ *Habitat. A. Capillus-veneris,* called the True Maidenhair, is a dainty little evergreen fern found in the milder parts of the West of England – in Dorset, Devon and

Cornwall – and in mild parts of the west of Ireland, growing in moist caves and on rocks near the sea, on damp walls and in wells.

¶ *Description.* The rootstock is tufted and creeping. The fern grows in masses, the fronds, however, separating and arching apart, giving the appearance of a perfect miniature tree. The stems are slender, of a shining, brownish black; the fronds themselves usually twice or three times pinnate, 6 inches to a foot long, the delicate pinnules fan-shaped, indented and notched. The sori are conspicuous, occupying the extremities of most of the lobes of the pinnules, in oval spots on the inner surface of the indusium, which is formed of the reflexed edge of the pinnule. The pinnules are very smooth: 'in vain,' said Pliny, 'do you plunge the Adiantum into water, it always remains dry.'

¶ *Constituents.* Tannin and mucilage. It has not been very fully investigated.

¶ *Medicinal Action and Uses.* Has been used from ancient times medicinally, being mentioned by Dioscorides. Its chief use has been as a remedy in pectoral complaints. A pleasant syrup is made in France from its fronds and rhizomes, called *Sirop de Capillaire*, which is given as a favourite medicine in pulmonary catarrhs. It is flavoured with orange flowers and acts as a demulcent with slightly stimulating effects. Narbonne Honey is generally added to the syrup.

Culpepper tells us:

'This and all other Maiden Hairs is a good remedy for coughs, asthmas, pleurisy, etc., and on account of its being a gentle diuretic also in jaundice, gravel and other impurities of the kidneys. All the Maidenhairs should be used green and in conjunction with other ingredients because their virtues are weak.'

Gerard writes of it:

'It consumeth and wasteth away the King's Evil and other hard swellings, and it maketh the haire of the head or beard to grow that is fallen and pulled off.'

It also enters into the composition of Elixir de Garus. It is employed on the Continent as an emmenagogue under the names of polytrichi, polytrichon, or kalliphyllon, administered as a sweetened infusion of 1 oz. to a pint of boiling water.

A. pedatum is a perennial fern of the United States and Canada, a little larger than the European variety, used in similar ways and more highly valued by many.

A. lunulatum of India is similarly employed.

A. trapeziforme of Mexico is more aromatic but less valuable medicinally.

A. radiatum and *A. fragile* of Jamaica and *A. Æthiopicum* of Ethiopia are both used in medicine.

HART'S TONGUE

Scolopendrium vulgare; Asplenium scolopendrium (LINN.)
N.O. Filices

Synonyms. Hind's Tongue. Buttonhole. Horse Tongue. God's-hair. Lingua cervina
Part Used. Fronds

The Hart's Tongue, a fern of common growth in England in shady copses and on moist banks and walls, is the *Lingua cervina* of the old apothecaries, and its name refers to the shape of its fronds.

¶ *Description.* Its broad, long, undivided dark-green fronds distinguish it from all other native ferns, and render it a conspicuous object in the situations where it abounds, as it grows in masses. It receives its name of *Scolopendrium* because its fructification is supposed to resemble the feet of *Scolopendra*, a genus of Mydrapods. The sori are in twin oblique lines, on each side of the midrib, covered by what looks like a single indusium, but really is *two*, one arranged partially over the other. In the early stages of its growth, the folding over of the indusium can be clearly seen through a lens. The fronds are stalked and the root, tufted, short and stout. This fern is evergreen and easy of cultivation.

¶ *Medicinal Action and Uses.* In common with Maidenhair, this fern was formerly considered one of the five great capillary herbs.

The older physicians esteemed it a very valuable medicine, and Galen gave it in infusion for diarrhœa and dysentery, for which its astringent quality made it a useful remedy. In country districts, especially in Wales and the Highlands, an ointment is made of its fronds for burns and scalds and for piles, and it has been taken internally for Bright's Disease, in a decoction made of 2 oz. to a pint of water, in wineglassful doses. In homœopathy, it is administered in combination with Golden Seal, for diabetes. It is specially recommended for removing obstructions from the liver and spleen, also for removing gravelly deposits in the bladder. Culpepper tells us:

'It is a good remedy for the liver, both to strengthen it when weak and ease it when afflicted. . . . It is commended for hardness and stoppings of the spleen and liver, and the heat of the stomach. The distilled water is very good against the passion of the heart, to stay hiccough, to help the falling of the palate and to stay bleeding of the gums by gargling with it.'

BRACKEN

Pteris aquilina (LINN.)
N.O. Filices

Synonyms. Brake Fern. Female Fern
Parts Used. Fronds, root

The Bracken or Brake Fern, often called by old writers the Female Fern, is found in almost every part of the globe, except the extreme north and south; it grows more freely than any other of the Fern tribe throughout Britain, flourishing luxuriantly on heaths and moors.

¶ *Description.* The rootstock is long and fibrous (creeping horizontally), very thick and succulent, throwing up solitary fronds at intervals, which soon cover large patches of ground. The stems are erect and tree-like, velvety at the base, very brittle at first, afterwards tough and wiry, ordinarily 2 to 3 feet high, though in favourable soil and situations attaining a height of 8 to 10 feet. They bear branched fronds, twice or thrice pinnate, the pinnæ more or less opposite, the pinnules long, narrow, smooth-edged, round-pointed and leathery. The sori on the back of the frond form a continuous line along the margin, being covered by an indusium attached to the slightly recurved edge of the pinnule.

The lower portion of the stem, when cut obliquely at the base, shows a pattern or figure formed of the wood bundles, which was supposed by Linnæus to represent a spread eagle, hence he gave the species the name of *Aquilina.* The name of the genus, *Pteris,* is derived from *pteron* (a feather), from the feathery appearance of the fronds, in the same way that the English name *Fern* is a contraction of the Anglo-Saxon *fepern* (a feather). In some parts of England it is called 'King Charles in the Oak Tree.' In Scotland, it is said to be an impression of the Devil's Foot, and yet witches were reputed to detest this fern, for the reason that it bears on its cut stem the Greek letter X, which is the initial of Christos. In Ireland, it is called the Fern of God, because if the stem is cut into three sections, on the first of these will be seen the letter G, on the second O, and on the third D.

The spores of this and other Ferns are too minute to be visible to the naked eye. Before the structure of Ferns was understood, their reproduction was thought to be due to unknown agencies – whence various superstitions arose.

'This kinde of Ferne,' writes Lyte in 1587, 'beareth neither flowers nor sede, except we shall take for sede the black spots growing on the backsides of the leaves, the whiche some do gather thinking to worke wonders, but to say the truth, it is nothing els but trumperi and superstition.'

The minute spores were reputed to confer invisibility on their possessor if gathered at the only time when they were said to be visible, i.e. on St. John's Eve, at the precise moment at which the saint was born. Shakespeare says, 1 *Henry IV*:

'We have the receipt of Fern seed – we walk
   invisible.'

and Ben Jonson:

'I had no medicine, Sir, to walk invisible
No fern seed in my pocket.'

The Fern was also said to confer perpetual youth.

¶ *Medicinal Action and Uses.* The Ancients used both the fronds and stems of the Bracken in diet-drinks and medicine for many disorders. Culpepper gives several uses for it:

'The roots being bruised and boiled in mead and honeyed water, and drunk kills both the broad and long worms in the body, and abates the swelling and hardness of the spleen. The leaves eaten, purge the belly and expel choleric and waterish humours that trouble the stomach. The roots bruised and boiled in oil or hog's grease make a very profitable ointment to heal the wounds or pricks gotten in the flesh. The powder of them used in foul ulcers causes their speedier healing.

'Fern, being burned, the smoke thereof drives away serpents, gnats, and other noisome creatures, which in fenny countries do, in the night-time, trouble and molest people lying in their beds with their faces uncovered.'

Gerard says that 'the root of Ferne cast into an hogshead of wine keepeth it from souring.' 'For thigh aches' (sciatica), says another old writer, 'smoke the legs thoroughly with Fern Bracken.'

¶ *Use as Food.* The rhizome is astringent and also contains much starch, and has been considered recently as a possible source of starch for food and industry. There seems, however, to be some doubt as to whether its astringent properties do not render the Bracken unsuitable for human food. Humboldt reported that the inhabitants of Palma and Gomera – islands of the Canary Group – use Bracken as food, grinding the rhizome to powder and mixing it with a small quantity of barley-meal, the composition being termed *goflo* – the use of such food being, however, a sign of the extreme poverty of the inhabitants. The rootstock of the Esculent Brake (*Pteris esculenta*) was much used by the aborigines of New Zealand as food, when the British first settled there, and is also eaten much by the natives of the Society Islands and Australia.

The young fronds used sometimes to be used as a vegetable, being sold in bundles like Asparagus, but although considered a delicacy in Japan, they are somewhat flavourless and insipid to our modern Western taste, though they are not indigestible, and in the absence of all other fresh vegetables might prove useful. In Japan, before cooking, the tender shoots are first washed carefully in fresh water, then plunged into boiling water for two minutes or so, and then immersed again in cold water for a couple of hours. After this preparation they may be used for cooking, either being prepared as a purée, like spinach, or like asparagus heads, being served with melted butter or some similar sauce.

In Siberia and in Norway, the uncoiled fronds have been employed with about two-thirds of their weight of malt for brewing a kind of beer.

¶ *Other Uses.* The astringent properties of the rhizome have caused a decoction to be recommended for the dressing and preparation of kid and chamois leather.

Before the introduction of soda from sea-salt and other sources, the large amount of alkali obtained from the ashes of Bracken was found serviceable for glassmaking, both in the northern parts of this Island and in other countries, and was used freely for the purpose. The ash contains enough potash to be used as a substitute for soap. The ashes are mixed with water and formed into balls; these made hot in the fire are used to make lye for the scouring of linen. In the East, tallow boiled with Bracken ash is made into soap.

The potash yield of Bracken ash is so considerable that in view of the present scarcity of fertilizers, this source of supply is well worth attention. Potash is a particularly valuable fertilizer for potato and sugar-beet land, especially for light loams and gravels and sandy soils. It should be borne in mind by persons having access to quantities of Bracken, that they have a usable supply of this almost indispensable manure at hand, either for cultivating flowers or crops, at the expense of a little trouble.

The best time for cutting Bracken for burning is from June to the end of October, but the ash from green Bracken is much more valuable than from the old and withered plant. In the month of June, the fronds and stems hold as much as 20 per cent. of potash, but in August that amount is reduced to 5 per cent., a large proportion having been given back to the rhizome or soil. Experiments have been contemplated by the Board of Agriculture to determine whether the cutting and incineration of Bracken in June, with a view to obtaining its potash content, would be economically feasible.

Where Bracken flourishes unchecked, it becomes injurious to sheep-farming by its encroachments on the grass on the runs, this being especially the case in the Lake District, and it would be of double advantage to cut it down and use it to supplement the reduced stocks of manures. Potash from Bracken is very soluble and should not be exposed to rain. The ashes as soon as cool should be collected and kept dry until required for use. It is stated that 50 tons of the dried fern produces 1 ton of potash. Instructions for dealing with Bracken are given by the Board of Agriculture for Scotland in Leaflets 18, 25, 39 and 42.

Formerly in both the green and the dried state, Bracken was used as fodder for cattle. When dry, it makes excellent litter for both horses and cattle, and forms also a very durable thatch. The young tops of the Fern are boiled in Hampshire for pigs' food, and the peculiar flavour of Hampshire bacon has sometimes been attributed to this custom. The fronds are much used as packing material for fruit, keeping it fresh and cool and imparting neither colour nor flavour. The dried fronds may be used in the garden for protecting tender plants.

In early spring, when dormant, large clumps may be lifted from moors or commons to serve as screens in the wilder parts of the garden, though the Fern is somewhat difficult to transplant and afterwards preserve with success, and is often destroyed by spring frosts. While growing in its natural habitats, Bracken is of value as cover and shelter for game.

In the seventeenth century it was customary to set growing Bracken on fire, believing that this would produce rain. A like custom of 'firing the Bracken' still prevails to-day on the Devonshire moors.

POLYPODY, COMMON

Polypodium vulgare (LINN.)
N.O. Filices

Synonyms. Polypody of the Oak. Wall Fern. Brake Root. Rock Brake. Rock of Polypody. Oak Fern
Parts Used. Root, leaves

The Common Polypody is a common Fern in sheltered places, on shady hedge-banks, and on roots and stumps of trees, moist rocks and old walls.

¶ *Description.* It has a creeping rhizome, which runs along the surface of the ground, or substance on which it grows, and is thick and woody, covered with yellowish scales. At intervals it throws up fronds, from a few inches to a foot in length, which hang down in tresses and have plain, long, narrow, smooth pinnæ, placed alternately on the stalk and joined together at the base. The stalk has no scales. The sori are rather large and prominent, white at first, ripening into a golden yellow, and in round masses, placed in two rows along the underside of the upper segments, equally distant from the centre and the margin. Unlike all the preceding species described, they are not covered with an indusium. The young fronds come out in May, but in sheltered places the plant is nearly evergreen.

The name is derived from *poly* (many) and *pous, podos* (a foot), from the many foot-like divisions of the caudex.

¶ *Part Used Medicinally.* The root, which is in perfection in October and November, though it may be collected until February. It is used both fresh and dried, and the leaves are also sometimes used.

This Fern was employed by the Ancients as a purgative: it is the Oak Fern of the older herbalists – not that of the modern botanists, *Polypodium dryopteris.* It was held that such Fern plants as grew upon the roots of an oak, which this Fern frequently does, owned special medicinal powers. In the same way the mistletoe that grew on the oak was esteemed by the Druids to have special powers of which that growing on other trees was devoid. The True Oak Fern is a much more delicate Fern and grows chiefly in mountainous districts, among the mossy roots of old oak-trees and sometimes in marshy places.

¶ *Medicinal Actions and Uses.* Alterative, tonic, pectoral and expectorant. Its principal use has been as a mild laxative. It serves as a tonic in dyspepsia and loss of appetite, and as an alterative in skin diseases is found perfectly safe and reliable. It is also used in hepatic complaints.

It proves useful in coughs and catarrhal affection, particularly in dry coughs: it promotes a free expectoration, and the infusion, prepared from ½ oz. of crushed root to a pint of boiling water and sweetened, is taken in teacupful doses frequently, proving valuable in the early stages of consumption. The powder is stated to have been used with success for some kinds of worms.

It sometimes produces a rash, but this disappears in a short time and causes no further inconvenience.

¶ *Preparation.* Fluid extract: dose, one drachm.

A mucilaginous decoction of the fronds was formerly, and probably still is, used in country places as a cure for whooping-cough in children; for this purpose the matured, fruitful fronds, gathered in the autumn, are dried, and when required for use are slowly boiled with coarse sugar. It is still used as a demulcent by the Italians.

The fresh root used to be employed in decoction, or powdered, for melancholia and also for rheumatic swelling of the joints. It is efficacious in jaundice, dropsy and scurvy, and combined with mallows removes hardness of the spleen, stitches in the side and colic. The distilled water of the roots and leaves was considered by the old herbalists good for ague, and the fresh or dried roots, mixed with honey and applied to the nose, were used in the cure of polypus.

Gerard tells us:

'Johannes Mesues reckoneth up Polypodie among those things that do especially dry and make thin: preadventure he had respect to a certain kind of arthritis or ache in the joints: in which not one part but many together most commonly are touched: for which it is very much commended by the Brabanders and other inhabitants about the river Rhene and the Maze. Furthermore Dioscorides saith that the root of Polypodie is very good for members out of joint and for chaps between the fingers.'

Culpepper considers Polypody

'a mild and useful purge, but being very slow, it is generally mixed by infusion or decoction with other ingredients, or in broths with beets, parsley, mallow, cummin, ginger, fennel or anise. The best form to take it for a complaint in the intestines is as follows: To an ounce of the fresh root bruised add an ounce and a half of the fresh roots of white beets and a quart of water, boiling hot and let it stand till next day, then drain it off.

A quarter of a pint of this liquor contains the infusion of 2 drams of this root. It should be sweetened with cane sugar or honey.'

The leaves of Polypody when burnt furnish a large proportion of carbonate of potash.

ROYAL FERN

Osmunda regalis (LINN.)
N.O. Filices

Synonyms. Osmund the Waterman. Heart of Osmund. Water Fern. Bog Onion
Part Used. Root

The Royal Fern grows abundantly in some parts of Great Britain, chiefly in the western counties of England and Scotland, and in Wales and the west of Ireland. It needs a soil of bog earth and is incorrectly styled the 'Flowering Fern,' from the handsome spikes of fructification. One of its old English names is Osmund the Waterman, and the white centres of its roots have been called the 'Heart of Osmund.'

There is a legend that the wife and daughter of Osmund, a waterman of Loch Tyne, took refuge among *Osmundes* during an invasion of the Danes.

Osmund is a Saxon word for domestic peace, from *os* (hoise) and *mund* (peace).

By some the name *Osmunda* is said to be derived from the god Thor (Osmunda). Others have traced its derivation from *os* (a bone) and *mundare* (to cleanse), in reference to the medicinal uses of the Fern.

The Fern is dedicated to St. Christopher.

¶ *Description.* The rootstock is tuberous, large and lobed, densely clothed with matted fibres, often forming a trunk rising perceptibly from the ground, sometimes to the height of a foot or more. It is many-headed and sends up tufts of fronds, the brown stems of which are cane-like, very tough and wiry, varying from 2 to 3 feet in drier situations, to from 8 to 10 feet in damp, sheltered places when very luxuriant. It is the tallest of our British ferns.

The fronds are twice pinnate, the pinnæ far apart, mostly opposite, the pinnules undivided, narrow and oblong, slightly tapering to their apex, smooth, very short-stalked. When young, they are of a very delicate texture and of a reddish colour, changing afterwards to a dull green. The fronds are divided into fertile and barren. The barren fronds are entirely leafy, the fertile fronds are terminated by long, branched spikes of fructification, composed of bunches of clustered thecæ or spore cases, green when young

and ripening into brown, not covered by an indusium. These fertile fronds are developed in April.

This handsome Fern is easy of cultivation and hardy, and is best transplanted when large.

¶ *Part Used Medicinally.* The root, or rhizome, which has a mucilaginous and slightly bitter taste. The actual curative virtues of this Fern have been said to be due to the salts of lime, potash and other earths which it derives in solution from the bog soil and from the water in which it grows.

¶ *Medicinal Action and Uses.* A decoction of the root is of good effect in the cure of jaundice, when taken in its early stages, and for removing obstructions of the viscera. The roots may also be made into an ointment for application to wounds, bruises and dislocations, the young fronds being likewise thought 'good to be put into balms, oyls and healing plasters.' A conserve of the root was used for rickets. Gerard says, drawing his information from Dodonæus and other older herbalists:

'The root and especially the heart or middle thereof, boiled or else stamped and taken with some kinde of liquor, is thought to be good for those that are wounded, dry-beaten and bruised; that have fallen from some high place.'

And Culpepper says:

'This has all the virtues mentioned in the former Ferns, and is much more effectual than they, both for inward and outward griefs: and is accounted singularly good in wounds, bruises or the like: the decoction to be drunk or boiled into an ointment of oil, as a balsam or balm, and so it is singularly good against bruises and bones broken or out of joint, and gives much ease to the colic and splenetic diseases: as also for ruptures and burstings.'

It has been recommended for lumbago.

ADDER'S TONGUE, ENGLISH

Ophioglossum vulgatum (LINN.)
N.O. Filices

Synonym. Christ's Spear
Parts Used. Root, leaves

The Adder's Tongue, known also in some parts of England as Christ's Spear, has no resemblance to any other Fern. The stems

which grow up solitarily from the small root – formed merely of a few stout, yellow fibres – are round, hollow and succulent, bearing on the upper part a simple spike, issuing from the sheath of a smooth, oblong-oval, tapering, concave, undivided, leafy frond. Embedded on each side of the stalk – at the top – is a single row of yellow thecæ, not covered by any indusium. The whole has much the appearance of the Arum flower.

The name is derived from *ophios* (a serpent) and *glossa* (a tongue).

This strange little Fern, growing only from 3 to 9 inches in height, is generally distributed over Great Britain, being not uncommon, buried in the grass in moist pastures and meadows. It is tolerably easy of cultivation.

¶ *Medicinal Action and Uses.* This Fern has long had a reputation as a vulnerary. A preparation of it, known as the 'Green Oil of Charity,' is still in request as a remedy for wounds.

The older herbalists called it 'a fine cooling herb.' The expressed juice of the leaves, drunk either alone, or with distilled water of Horse Tail, used much to be employed by country people for internal wounds and bruises, vomiting or bleeding at the mouth or nose. The distilled water was also considered good for sore eyes. An efficacious ointment for wounds was made as follows:

'Put 2 lb. of leaves chopped very fine into ½ pint of oil and 1½ lb. suet melted together. Boil the whole till the herb is crisp, then strain off from the leaves.'

This is a very ancient recipe for wounds.

MOONWORT

Botrychium lunaria (LINN.)
N.O. Filices

Part Used. Fronds

The Moonwort is said to possess similar vulnerary virtues to Adder's Tongue. The Ancients regarded it as a plant of magical power, if gathered by moonlight, and it was employed by witches and necromancers in their incantations.

Parkinson says that it was used by the alchemists, who thought it had power to condense or to convert quicksilver into pure silver.

Culpepper says: 'Moonwort (they absurdly say) will open locks and unshoe such horses as tread upon it; but some country people call it *unshoe the horse.*'

¶ *Description.* It is a very singular-looking plant, the stem hollow and succulent, throwing off a single, barren pinna, having on each side very peculiar stalked pinnules, occasionally deeply notched throughout to their base. The stem itself, continuing upwards, has near the top other very short, alternate, branched offshoots, on which, or on the spike itself, are arranged the thecæ in regular lines – like the *Osmunda* and *Ophioglossum*, uncovered by any indusium. This fructification appears in April.

The Moonwort is not uncommon on open heaths and pastures, where the soil is peaty, but not very wet.

This and *Ophioglossum*, alone among the Ferns, grow up straight, not with their fronds curled inward, crosier-fashion.

FEVER BUSH

Garrya fremonti (TORR.)
N.O. Cornaceæ

Synonyms. Skunk Bush. Californian Feverbush
Part Used. Leaves
Habitat. California, Oregon, Mexico, Cuba, Jamaica

¶ *Description.* This is a small evergreen bush. The leaves are broad, leathery, grey green on the upperside; on the underside mealy and lighter grey green. It has grown in the Author's garden, but needs care in the winter. The leaves are intensely bitter, and are largely used in California as an antiperiodic and tonic. A new alkaloid has been found in it called garryine. It is best administered as a fluid extract.

¶ *Dosages.* Powder, 10 to 30 grains – leaves. Fluid extract, 10 to 30 minims – leaves.

FEVERFEW

Chrysanthemum Parthenium (BERNH.)
N.O. Compositæ

Synonyms. Pyrethrum Parthenium (Sm.). Featherfew. Featherfoil. Flirtwort. Bachelor's Buttons
Part Used. Herb

¶ *Description.* Feverfew (a corruption of Febrifuge, from its tonic and fever-dispelling properties) is a composite plant growing in every hedgerow, with numerous, small, daisy-like heads of yellow flowers with outer white rays, the central yellow florets being arranged on a nearly *flat* receptacle, not conical as in the chamomiles. The stem is finely furrowed and hairy, about 2 feet high; the leaves alternate, downy with short hairs, or nearly smooth – about $4\frac{1}{2}$ inches long and 2 inches broad – bipinnatifid, with serrate margins, the leaf-stalk being flattened above and convex beneath. It is not to be confounded with other wild chamomile-like allied species, which mostly have more feathery leaves and somewhat large flowers; the stem also is upright, whereas that of the true garden Chamomile is procumbent. The delicate green leaves are conspicuous even in mild winter. The whole plant has a strong and bitter smell, and is particularly disliked by bees. A double variety is cultivated in gardens for ornamental purposes, and its flower-heads are sometimes substituted for the double Chamomile.

Country people have long been accustomed to make curative uses of this herb, which grows abundantly throughout England. Gerard tells us that it may be used both in drinks, and bound on the wrists is of singular virtue against the ague.

Pyrethrum is derived from the Greek *pur* (fire), in allusion to the hot taste of the root.

¶ *Cultivation.* Feverfew is a perennial, and herbaceous in habit. When once planted, it gives year after year an abundant supply of blossoms with only the merest degree of attention. Planting may be done in autumn, but the best time is about the end of April. Any ordinary good soil is suitable, but better results are obtained when well-drained, and of a stiff, loamy character, enriched with good manure. Weeding should be done by hand, the plants when first put out being small might be injured by hoeing.

There are three methods of propagation: by seed, by division of roots and by cuttings. If grown by *seed*, it should be sown in February or March, thinned out to 2 to 3 inches between the plants, and planted out early in June to permanent quarters, allowing a foot or more between the plants and 2 feet between the rows, selecting, if possible, a showery day for the operation. They will establish themselves quickly. To propagate by *division*, lift the plants in March, or whenever the roots are in an active condition, and with a sharp spade, divide them into three or five fairly large pieces. *Cuttings* should be made from the young shoots that start from the base of the plant, and should be taken with a heel of the old plant attached, which will greatly assist their rooting. They may be inserted at any time from October to May. The foliage must be shortened to about 3 inches, when the cuttings will be ready for insertion in a bed of light, sandy soil, in the open. Plant very firmly, surface the bed with sand, and water in well. Shade is necessary while the cuttings are rooting.

Keep a good watch at all times for snails, slugs and black fly. For the latter pest, try peppering the plants; for the others use soot, ashes or lime. Toads will keep a garden free of slugs.

'A few pots placed on their sides may be dotted about the garden, and it will be found that the toads will sit in these when they are not hunting around for their prey. The creatures are not at all likely to leave the garden, seeing that if the supply of slugs runs short they will turn their attention to all kinds of insects.' (S. L. B.)

¶ *Medicinal Action and Uses.* Aperient, carminative, bitter. As a stimulant it is useful as an emmenagogue. Is also employed in hysterical complaints, nervousness and lowness of spirits, and is a general tonic. The cold infusion is made from 1 oz. of the herb to a pint of boiling water, allowed to cool, and taken frequently in doses of half a teacupful.

A decoction with sugar or honey is said to be good for coughs, wheezing and difficult breathing. The herb, bruised and heated, or fried with a little wine and oil, has been employed as a warm external application for wind and colic.

A tincture made from Feverfew and applied locally immediately relieves the pain and swelling caused by bites of insects and vermin. It is said that if two teaspoonfuls of tincture are mixed with $\frac{1}{2}$ pint of cold water, and all parts of the body likely to be exposed to the bites of insects are freely sponged with it, they will remain unassailable. A tincture of the leaves of the true Chamomile and of the German Chamomile will have the same effect.

Planted round dwellings, it is said to purify the atmosphere and ward off disease.

An infusion of the flowers, made with boiling water and allowed to become cold, will allay any distressing sensitiveness to pain in a highly nervous subject, and will afford relief to the face-ache or earache of a dyspeptic or rheumatic person.

¶ *Preparations.* Fluid extract: dose, 1 to 2 drachms.

See CHAMOMILE, PELLITORY, PYRETHRUM.

¶ *Other Species.*

SWEET FEVERFEW (*Chrysanthemum Suaveolens*) and *C. maritima*, found by the seashore, especially in the north, with leaves broader, more fleshy, succulent and smaller flower-heads than the Common Feverfew.

(CORN) FEVERFEW. *See* MAYWEED

FIG, COMMON

Ficus Carica (LINN.)
N.O. Urticaceæ

Part Used. Fruit

Habitat. The *Common Fig-tree* provides the succulent fruit that in its fresh and dried state has been valued from the earliest days. It is indigenous to Persia, Asia Minor and Syria, but now is wild in most of the Mediterranean countries. It is cultivated in most warm and temperate climates and has been celebrated from the earliest times for the beauty of its foliage and for its 'sweetness and good fruit' (Judges ix. 2), there being frequent allusions to it in the Scriptures. The Greeks are said to have received it from Caria in Asia Minor – hence the specific name. Under Hellenic culture it was improved and Attic figs became celebrated in the East. It was one of the principal articles of sustenance among the Greeks, being largely used by the Spartans at their public table; and athletes fed almost entirely on figs, considering that they increased their strength and swiftness. To such an extent, indeed, were figs a part of the staple food of the people in ancient Greece that there was a law forbidding the exportation of the best fruit from their trees.

Figs were early introduced into Italy. Pliny gives details of no less than twenty-nine kinds known in his day, and specially praises those of Tarant and Caria and also those of Herculaneum. Dried Figs have been found in Pompeii in our days and in the wall-paintings of the buried city Figs are represented together with other fruits. Pliny states that homegrown Figs formed a large portion of the food of slaves, especially in the fresh state for agricultural workers.

The Fig plays an important part in Latin mythology. It was dedicated to Bacchus and employed in religious ceremonies. The wolf that suckled Romulus and Remus rested under a Fig tree, which was therefore held sacred by the Romans, and Ovid states that among the celebrations of the first day of the year by Romans, Figs were offered as presents. The inhabitants of Cyrene crowned themselves with wreaths of Figs when sacrificing to Saturn, holding him to be the discoverer of the fruit. Pliny speaks also of the Wild Fig, which is mentioned also in Homer, and further classical references to the Fig are to be found in Theophrastus, Dioscorides, Varro and Columella.

¶ *Description.* *Ficus Carica* is a bush or small tree, rarely more than 18 to 20 feet high, with broad, rough, deciduous, deeply-lobed leaves in the cultivated varieties, though in wild forms the leaves are often almost entire.

Considered botanically, the Fig, as we eat it, is a very remarkable form of fruit. It is actually neither fruit nor flower, though partaking of both, being really a hollow, fleshy receptacle, enclosing a multitude of flowers, which never see the light, yet come to full perfection and ripen their seeds – a contrary method from the strawberry, in which the minute pistils are scattered over the exterior of the enlarged succulent receptacle. In the Fig, the inflorescence, or position of the flowers, is concealed within the body of the 'fruit.' The Fig stands alone in this peculiar arrangement of its flowers. The edge of the pear-shaped receptacle curves inwards, so as to form a nearly-closed cavity, bearing the numerous fertile and sterile flowers mingled on its surface, the male flowers mostly in the upper part of the cavity and generally few in number. As it ripens, the receptacle enlarges greatly and the numerous one-seeded fruits become embedded in it. The fruit of the wild kind never attains the succulence of the cultivated kinds. The Figs are borne in the axils of the leaves, singly.

¶ *Cultivation.* The Fig is grown for its fresh fruit in all the milder parts of Europe, being cultivated in the Mediterranean countries, and in the United States of America. With protection in winter, it succeeds as far north as Pennsylvania. It is said to have been introduced into England by the Romans, but was probably introduced from Italy early in the sixteenth century, when the Fig tree still growing in Lambeth Palace garden is said to have been planted.

The trees live to a great age, and along the southern coast of England bear fruit abundantly as standard trees, though in Scotland and many parts of England a south wall is indispensable for their successful cultivation out of doors. Old quarries are good situations for them. The roots are free from stagnant water and they are sheltered from cold, while exposed to a hot sun, which ripens the fruit perfectly. The trees also succeed well planted in a paved court against a building with a south aspect.

The best soil for a Fig border is a friable loam, not too rich, but well-drained; a chalky subsoil is congenial to the tree. To correct the tendency to over-luxuriance of growth, the roots should be confined within spaces surrounded by a wall enclosing an area of about a square yard. Grown as a standard, the tree needs very little pruning. When against a wall, a single stem should be trained to a height of a foot and a shoot be trained to either side – one to the right and the other to the left.

The principal part needing protection in the winter is the main stem, which is more tender than the young wood.

Fig trees are *propagated* by cuttings, which should be put into pots and placed in a gentle hot-bed. They may be obtained more speedily from layers, and these when rooted will form plants ready to bear fruit the first or second year after planting.

There are numerous varieties of Fig in cultivation, bearing fruit of various colours, from deep purple to yellow or nearly white.

The Fig produces naturally two sets of shoots and two crops of fruit in the season. The first shoots generally show young Figs in July and August, but those in England rarely ripen and should therefore be rubbed off. The late midsummer shoots also put forth fruit buds which, however, do not develop till the following spring, ripening in late September and October, and these form the only crop of Figs on which the English gardener can depend.

There is sometimes a failure in the Fig crop, many immature receptacles dropping off in consequence of the pistils of the florets not having been duly fertilized by the pollen of the stamens. It is supposed that fertilization is caused naturally by the entry of insects through the very small orifice which remains open in the flowering Fig. Fig growers therefore adopt an artificial means of ensuring fertilization: a small feather is inserted and turned round in the internal cavity, the pollen thus being brushed against the pistils. This process is called 'Caprification,' from the Latin *caprificus* (a wild Fig), as the same result was originally obtained in the countries where the Fig grows wild, by placing branches of the Wild Fig in flower over the cultivated bushes, so that the pollen might be shaken out over the orifices of their receptacles, thus ensuring the development of the young fruit.

Most of our supplies of dried Figs come from Asia Minor, Spain, Malta and the South of France. When the fruits are ripe, they are collected and dried in the sun. 'Natural' Figs are those which are packed loose and retain to some extent their original shape. 'Pulled' Figs have been kneaded and pulled to make them supple; they are usually packed for exportation in small square or circular boxes – the latter being termed 'drums' – and are considered to be the best variety. A few bay leaves are put upon the top of each box, to keep the fruit from being injured by a gnat which feeds on it and is very destructive. 'Pressed' Figs have been closely packed into boxes so that they are compressed into discs. Maltese Figs are very good, but those from Smyrna, which are thin-skinned and soft (the best kind known as 'Elemi'), are most valued. Greek Figs are thicker skinned, tougher and have less pulp.

¶ *Constituents.* The chief constituent of Figs is dextrose, of which they contain about 50 per cent.

¶ *Uses.* Figs have long been employed for their nutritive value and in both their fresh and dried state form a large part of the food of the natives of both Western Asia and Southern Europe.

A sort of cake made by mashing up inferior Figs serves in parts of the Greek Archipelago as a substitute for bread.

Alcohol is obtained from fermented Figs in some southern countries, and a kind of wine, still made from the ripe fruit, was known to the Ancients and is mentioned by Pliny under the name of Sycites.

¶ *Medicinal Action and Uses.* Figs are used for their mild, laxative action, and are employed in the preparation of laxative confections and syrups, usually with senna and carminatives. It is considered that the laxative property resides in the saccharine juice of the fresh fruit and in the dried fruit is probably due to the indigestible seeds and skin. The three preparations of Fig of the British Pharmacopœia are *Syrup of Figs*, a mild laxative, suitable for administration to children; *Aromatic Syrup of Figs*, *Elixir of Figs*, or *Sweet Essence of Figs*, an excellent laxative for children and delicate persons, is compounded of compound tincture of rhubarb, liquid extract of senna, compound spirit of orange, liquid extract of cascara and Syrup of Figs. The *Compound Syrup of Figs* is a stronger preparation, composed of liquid extract of senna, syrup of rhubarb and Syrup of Figs, and is more suitable for adults.

Figs are demulcent as well as nutritive. Demulcent decoctions are prepared from them and employed in the treatment of catarrhal affections of the nose and throat.

Roasted and split into two portions, the soft pulpy interior of Figs may be applied as emollient poultices to gumboils, dental abscesses and other circumscribed maturating tumours. They were used by Hezekiah as a remedy for boils 2,400 years ago (Isaiah xxxviii. 21).

The milky juice of the freshly-broken stalk of a Fig has been found to remove warts on the body. When applied, a slightly inflamed area appears round the wart, which then shrivels and falls off. The milky juice of the stems and leaves is very acrid and has been used in some countries for raising blisters.

The wood of the tree is porous and of little value, though a piece, saturated with oil and spread with emery, is in France a common substitute for a hone.

Green Fig Jam is excellent. Choose very juicy Figs. Take off the stalks, but do not peel them. Make a syrup of ½ lb. of sugar and a glass of water (¼ pint) for each pound of fruit. Put the Figs into it and cook them till the syrup pearls. Boil a stick of cinnamon with them and remove it before pouring the jam into pots.

The Sycamore Fig (*Ficus Sycamorus*) is a tree of large size, with heart-shaped, somewhat mulberry-like leaves. It is a favourite tree in Egypt and Syria, being often planted along roads, deep shade being cast by its spreading branches. It bears a sweet, edible fruit, somewhat like that of the Common Fig, but produced in racemes, on the older branches. The Ancients, after soaking it in water, preserved it like the Common Fig. The porous wood is only fit for fuel.

Our northern Sycamore tree is in no way related to this Sycamore Fig, but has wrongly acquired its name, Prior says, through a mistake of the botanist Ruellius, who transferred the Greek name, *Sycamoros*, properly the name of the Wild Fig, to the great Maple.

'This mistake,' says Prior, 'arose perhaps from this tree, the great maple, being on account of the density of its foliage, used in the sacred dramas of the Middle Ages to represent the Fig tree into which Zaccheus climbed and that in which the Virgin Mary on her journey into Egypt had hidden herself and the infant Jesus to avoid the fury of Herod; a legend quoted by Stapel on Theophrastus and by Thevenot in his *Voyage de Levant*: "At Mathave is a large sycamore or Pharaoh's Fig, very old, but which bears fruit every year. They say that upon the Virgin passing that way with her son Jesus and being pursued by the people, this Fig tree opened to receive her and closed her in again, until the people had passed by and then opened again. The tree is still shown to travellers." ' (See Cowper's *Apocryphal Gospels*.)

See INDIARUBBER TREE

FIGWORT, KNOTTED

Scrophularia nodosa
N.O. Scrophulariaceæ

Synonyms. Throatwort. Carpenter's Square. Kernelwort.
(*Welsh*) Deilen Ddu
(*Irish*) Rose Noble
(*French*) Herbe du Siège
Part Used. Herb

The Knotted Figwort, common throughout England, is similar in general habit to the Water Figwort, but differs both in the form of its root and in having more acutely heart-shaped leaves. The stem, too, is without the projections or wings at its angles, and the lobes of the calyx have only a very narrow membraneous margin. The plant, also, though found in rather moist, bushy places, either in cultivated or waste ground, and in damp woods, is not distinctly an aquatic, like the Water Figwort.

The flowers, which resemble in appearance and character the Water Figwort, are in bloom during July and are specially visited by wasps.

During the thirteen months' siege of Rochelle by the army of Richelieu in 1628, the tuberous roots of this Figwort yielded support to the garrison for a considerable period, from which circumstance the French still call it *Herbe du siège*. The taste and smell of the tubers are unpleasant, and they would never be resorted to for food except in times of famine.

¶ *Medicinal Action and Uses.* It has been called the Scrofula Plant, on account of its value in all cutaneous eruptions, abscesses, wounds, etc., the name of the genus being derived from that of the disease for which it was formerly considered a specific.

It has diuretic and anodyne properties.

The whole herb is used, collected in June and July and dried. A decoction is made of it for external use, and the fresh leaves are also made into an ointment.

Of the different kinds of Figwort used, this species is most employed, principally as a fomentation for sprains, swellings, inflammations, wounds and diseased parts, especially in scrofulous sores and gangrene.

The leaves simply bruised are employed by the peasantry in some districts as an application to burns and swellings.

The Welsh so highly esteem the plant that they call it Deilen Ddu ('good leaf'). In Ireland, it is known as Rose Noble and as Kernelwort. Gerard tells us, referring to what he evidently considered an exaggerated estimate of its worth: 'Divers do rashly teach that if it be hanged about the necke or else carried about one, it keepeth a man in health.'

The herb was said to be curative of hydrophobia, by taking

'every morning while fasting a slice of bread and butter on which the powdered knots of the roots had been spread and eating it up with two tumblers of fresh spring water. Then let the patient be well clad in woollen garments and made to take a long, fast walk until in a profuse perspiration, the treatment being continued for seven days.'

A decoction of the herb has been successfully used as a cure for the scab in swine. Cattle, as a rule, will refuse to eat the leaves, as they are bitter, acrid and nauseating, producing purging and vomiting if chewed.

Preparation and Dosage. Fluid extract, ½ to 1 drachm.

Other Species.

BALM-LEAVED FIGWORT (*Scrophularia Scorodoma*), found only in Cornwall, and at Tralee, in Ireland; it is distinguished by its downy, wrinkled leaves.

YELLOW FIGWORT (*S. vernalis*) is a plant of local occurrence and is well distinguished by its remarkably bright green foliage and yellow flowers. It appears early in spring and is the only British species which can be called ornamental.

Gerard speaks of the 'yellow-flowered Figwort' as growing in his time 'in the moist medowes as you go from London to Hornsey.' He also speaks of the 'rare white-flowered Betony.'

FIGWORT, WATER

Scrophularia aquatica (LINN.)
N.O. Scrophulariaceæ

Synonyms. Water Betony. Fiddlewood. Fiddler. Crowdy Kit. Brownwort. Bishops' Leaves

Part Used. Leaves

The Water Figwort has obtained the name of Water Betony from a certain resemblance of its leaves to those of the Wood Betony, but it differs entirely from that plant in every other respect, not being even closely related to it, and nowadays is more generally called the Water Figwort, the name Figwort being derived from the form of the root in another member of the genus *Scrophularia*, the Knotted Figwort (*S. nodosa*), a fairly common plant.

Description. The root of the Water Figwort is perennial and throws out numerous large fibres. The plant is to be found only in damp ground, generally by the banks of rivers and ponds. It varies much in size, but on an average, the stems grow to a height of 5 feet. The general character of the stem is upright, though small lateral branches are thrown out from the rigid, straight, main stem, which is smooth and quadrangular, the angles being winged. The stems are often more or less reddish-purple in colour; though hollow and succulent, they become rigid when dead, and prove very troublesome to anglers owing to their lines becoming tangled in the withered capsules. The Figwort is named in Somersetshire, 'Crowdy Kit' (the word *kit* meaning a fiddle), or 'Fiddlewood,' because if two of the stalks are rubbed together, they make a noise like the scraping of the bow on violin strings, owing no doubt to the winged angles. In Devonshire, also, the plant is known as 'Fiddler.'

The leaves are placed in pairs on the stem, each pair at right angles to the pair below it;

all are on footstalks, the pairs generally rather distant from one another on the stem. The leaves are oblong and somewhat heart-shaped; smooth, with very conspicuous veining. The flowers grow at the top of the stems, arranged in loose panicles, under each little branch of which is a little floral leaf, or bract. They are in bloom during July and August. The calyx has five conspicuous lobes, fringed by a somewhat ragged-looking, brown, membranaceous border. The dark, greenish-purple, sometimes almost brown corolla is almost globular; the lobes at its mouth are very short and broad, the two upper ones stand boldly out from the flower, the two side ones taking the same direction, but are much shorter, and the fifth lobe turned sharply downward. The result is that the flowers look like so many little helmets. There are four anther-bearing stamens, and generally a fifth barren one beneath the upper lip of the corolla. The seed vessel when ripe is a roundish capsule, opening with two valves, the edges of which are turned in, and contains numerous small brown seeds.

Wasps and bees are very fond of the flowers, from which they collect much honey.

The leaves are used, collected in June and July, when in best condition, just coming into flower, and used both fresh and dried.

Medicinal Action and Uses. This plant has vulnerary and detergent properties, and has enjoyed some fame as a vulnerary, both when used externally and when taken in decoction.

In modern herbal medicine, the leaves are employed externally as a poultice, or boiled in lard as an ointment for ulcers, piles, scrofulous glands in the neck, sores and wounds. It is said to have been one of the ingredients in Count Matthei's noted remedy, 'Anti-Scrofuloso.'

In former days this herb was relied on for the cure of toothache and for expelling nightmare. It has also a reputation as a cosmetic, old herbalists telling us that

'the juice or distilled water of the leaves is good for bruises, whether inward or outward, as also to bathe the face and hands spotted or blemished or discoloured by sun burning.'

FIREWEED

Erechtites hieracifolia (LINN. and RAFIN.)
Cineraria Canadensis (WALTER.)
N.O. Compositæ

Synonyms. Senecio hieracifolius (Linn.)
Parts Used. Herb, oil
Habitat. Newfoundland and Canada, southward to South America

¶ *Description.* This coarse, homely American weed is an annual and derives its name from its habit of growing freely in moist open woods and clearings, and in greatest luxuriance on newly-burnt fallows. It has composite flowers, blooming from July to September.

Lactuca Canadensis, the wild Lettuce or Trumpet Weed, and *Hieracium Canadense*, are also given the designation of 'Fireweed' in America from their habit of growing on newly-burnt fallow, but *Erechtites hieracifolia* (Rafin.) may be called the true Fireweed, as it is the plant which commonly goes by that name.

Senecio is derived from *Senex* (an old man), in reference to the hoary pappus, which in this order represents the calyx; *Erechtites* comes from the ancient name of some troublesome Groundsel.

Fireweed is a rank, slightly hairy plant, growing from 1 to 7 feet high. The thick, somewhat fleshy stem is virgate, sulcate, leafy to the top, branching above, the branches erect. The leaves are alternate, delicate and thin, very variable in size and form, lance-ovate to linear, apex-pointed, margins irregular, sharply toothed, or divided right down to the midrib into leaflets, which are sometimes then bipinnatifid, the lower, very short-stalked and becoming sessile as they grow up the stem. The flowers are white or yellow, a corymbose panicle. The little fruits are oblong, slender, tapering at the end, striate and crowned with a very fine copious silky pappus, white or violet. The whole plant is succulent, the odour rank and slightly aromatic, with a bitterish and somewhat acrid and disagreeable taste.

In the United States Fireweed is a very troublesome weed; the fields often get infested with it, and when growing among Peppermint, it is definitely destructive, as it gets mingled with the plant in distilling and causes great deterioration of the oil.

¶ *Constituents.* A peculiar volatile oil – oil of Erechtites – transparent and yellow, obtained by distilling the plant with water, taste bitter and burning, odour fœtid, slightly aromatic, somewhat resembling oil of Erigeron, but not soluble as that is in an equal volume of alcohol. The specific gravity of the oil is variously given as 0·927 and 0·838–0·855, and its rotation 1 to 2. According to Bielstein and Wiegand, it consists almost wholly of terpenes boiling between 175° and 310° F.

¶ *Medicinal Action and Uses.* Astringent, alterative, tonic, cathartic, emetic. Much used among the aborigines of North America in various forms of eczema, muco-sanguineous diarrhœa, and hæmorrhages, also for relaxed throat and sore throat, and in the United States Eclectic Dispensatory in the form of oil and as an infusion, both herb and oil being beneficial for piles and dysentery. For its anti-spasmodic properties, it has been found useful for colic, spasms and hiccough. Applied externally, it gives great relief in the pains of gout, rheumatism and sciatica.

¶ *Dosage.* (Internally) 5 to 10 drops on sugar, in capsules or in emulsion.

The homœopathic tincture is made from the whole fresh flowering plant. It is chopped, pounded to a pulp and weighed. Then two parts by weight of alcohol are taken, the pulp mixed thoroughly with one-sixth part of it and the rest of the alcohol added. After having stirred the whole, it is poured into a well-stoppered bottle and allowed to stand for eight days in a dark, cool place.

The resulting tincture has a clear, beautiful, reddish-orange colour by transmitted light; a sourish odour, resembling that of claret, a taste at first sourish, then astringent and bitter, and an acid reaction.

FIRS. *See* PINES

FLEUR DE LUCE. *See* IRIS

FLUELLIN. *See* ROADFLAX

FOOL'S PARSLEY. *See* PARSLEY

FIVE-LEAF GRASS

Potentilla reptans (LINN.)
N.O. Rosaceæ

Synonyms. Cinquefoil. Five Fingers. Five-Finger Blossom. Sunkfield. Synkefoyle
Parts Used. Herb, root

Five-leaf Grass is a creeping plant with large yellow flowers like the Silverweed, each one growing on its own long stalk, which springs from the point at which the leaf joins the stem.

¶ *Description.* The rootstock branches at the top from several crowns, from which arise the long-stalked root-leaves and thread-like, creeping stems, which bear stalked leaves and solitary flowers. These stem-runners root at intervals and as they often attain a length of 5 feet, the plant is rapidly propagated, spreading over a wide area. It grows freely in meadows, pastures and by the wayside.

The name Five-leaved or Five Fingers refers to the leaves being divided into five leaflets. Each of these is about 1½ inch long, with scattered hairs on the veins and margin, the veins being prominent below. The margins of the leaflets are much serrated. In rich soils the leaflets are often six or seven. Out of a hundred blossoms once picked as a test, eighty had the parts of the corolla, calyx and epicalyx in fives, and the remaining twenty were in sixes.

Although the flowers much resemble those of the Silverweed, the two plants can readily be distinguished by the difference in their leaves. The flowers secrete honey on a ring-like ridge surrounding the base of the stamens. Insects alighting on the petals dust themselves with the pollen, but do not touch the stigmas, as the honey ring extends beyond. If they alight in the middle of the next flower, they dust the pollen against the stigma and cross-pollinate it. But the flower is often self-pollinated. The flowers close up in part in dull weather and completely at night, and it is then that the anthers touch the stigmas.

Bacon says that frogs have a predilection for sitting on this herb: 'The toad will be much under Sage, frogs will be in Cinquefoil.'

It was an ingredient in many spells in the Middle Ages, and was particularly used as a magic herb in love divinations. It was one of the ingredients of a special bait for fishing nets, which was held to ensure a heavy catch. This concoction consisted of corn boiled in thyme and marjoram water, mixed with nettles, cinquefoil and the juice of houseleek.

In an old recipe called 'Witches' Ointment' the juice of Five-leaf Grass, smallage and wolfsbane is mixed with the fat of children dug up from their graves and added to fine wheat flour.

¶ *Medicinal Action and Uses.* Astringent, febrifuge. The roots have a bitterish, styptic, slightly sweetish taste and have been employed medicinally since the time of Hippocrates and Dioscorides.

They were used to cure the intermittent fevers which prevailed in marshy, ill-drained lands, and especially ague.

Dioscorides stated that one leaf cured a quotidian, three a tertian, and four a quarten ague.

Culpepper says:

'It is an especial herb used in all inflammations and fevers, whether infectious or pestilential or, among other herbs, to cool and temper the blood and humours in the body; as also for all lotions, gargles and infections; for sore mouths, ulcers, cancers, fistulas and other foul or running sores.

'The juice drank, about four ounces at a time, for certain days together, cureth the quinsey and yellow jaundice, and taken for 30 days, cureth the falling sickness. The roots boiled in vinegar and the decoction held in the mouth easeth toothache.

'The juice or decoction taken with a little honey removes hoarseness and is very good for coughs.

'The root boiled in vinegar, being applied, heals inflammations, painful sores and the shingles. The same also, boiled in wine, and applied to any joint full of pain, ache or the gout in the hands, or feet or the hip-joint, called the sciatica, and the decoction thereof drank the while, doth cure them and easeth much pain in the bowels.

'The roots are also effectual to reduce ruptures, being used with other things available to that purpose, taken either inwardly or outwardly, or both; as also bruises or hurts by blows, falls or the like, and to stay the bleeding of wounds in any part, inward or outward.'

Robinson's *Herbal* directs that the roots are to be dug up in April and the outer bark taken off and dried, the rest not being used. To make the decoction, it is directed that 1½ oz. of the root be boiled in a quart of water down to a pint. This decoction is recommended not only as a remedy for diarrhœa, and of avail to stop bleeding of the lungs or bronchial tubes and bleeding at the nose, but as a good eyewash, as well as a gargle in relaxed sore throat.

The juice of the root, mixed with wheat bread, boiled first, is recommended as a good styptic.

(BLUE) FLAG. ⎫
 ⎬ *See* IRIS
(YELLOW) FLAG. ⎭

FLAX

Synonym. Linseed
Part Used. Seed

¶ *History.* Flax is one of the English-grown medicinal herbs, the products of which are included in the British Pharmacopœia, its seed known as Linseed, being much employed in medicine.

Its cultivation reaches back to the remotest periods of history, Flax seeds as well as the woven cloth having been found in Egyptian tombs. It has been cultivated in all temperate and tropical regions for so many centuries that its geographical origin cannot be identified, for it readily escapes from cultivation and is found in a semi-wild condition in all the countries where it is grown.

The 'fine linen' mentioned in the Bible has been satisfactorily proved to have been spun from Flax; it was the plant to which the plague of hail proved so disastrous (Exodus ix. 31). Joseph was arrayed in this product (Genesis xii. 42), and it also furnished the garments of the Jewish High-Priests (Exodus xxviii.) as well as the curtains of the Tabernacle (Exodus xxvi. 1). We learn that the knowledge of spinning this linen was known to the Canaanites (*see* Joshua ii. 6), and in New Testament times it formed the clothing of the Saviour in the tomb where Joseph of Arimathæa laid Him.

It was used for cord and sail-cloth ('white sails' are mentioned by Homer in the *Odyssey*), and it was used for lamp-wicks (Isaiah xlii. 3).

The seed-vessels with their five-celled capsules are referred to in the Bible as 'bolls,' and the expression 'the flax was *bolled*' (Exodus ix. 31) means that it had arrived at a state of

A scruple of the powder in wine is the dose prescribed to cure the ague.

In modern Herbal Medicine, the dried herb is more generally now employed, for its astringent and febrifuge properties.

An infusion of 1 oz. of the herb to a pint of boiling water is used in wineglassful doses for diarrhœa and looseness of the bowels, and for other complaints for which astringents are usually prescribed, and it is employed externally as an astringent lotion and as a gargle for sore throat.

¶ *Preparation and Dosage.* Fluid extract, ½ to 2 drachms.

See also AVENS, FIVE-LEAF GRASS (AMERICAN) SILVERWEED and TORMENTIL

Linum usitatissimum (LINN.)
N.O. Linaceæ

maturity. When the bolls are ripe, the Flax is pulled and tied in bundles, and in order to assist the separation of the fibre from the stalks, the bundles are placed in water for several weeks, and then spread out to dry. This custom is alluded to in Joshua ii. 6.

Pliny writes:

'What department is there to be found of active life in which flax is not employed? And in what production of the Earth are there greater marvels to us than in this? To think that here is a plant which brings Egypt to close proximity to Italy! – so much so, in fact, that Galerius and Balbillus, both of them prefects of Egypt, made the passage to Alexandria from the Straits of Sicily, the one in six days, the other in five! . . . What audacity in man! What criminal perverseness! Thus to sow a thing in the ground for the purpose of catching the winds and tempests; it being not enough for him, forsooth, to be borne upon the waves alone!'

Bartholomew, the mediæval herbalist, refers to the making of linen from the soaking of Flax in water till it is dried and turned in the sun and then bound in 'praty bundels' and afterwards 'knockyd, beten and brayd and carflyd, rodded and gnodded; ribbyd and heklyd, and at the last sponne'; of the bleaching, and finally of its many uses for making clothing, and for sails, and fish-nets, and thread and ropes, and strings ('for bows'), and measuring lines, and sheets ('to reste in'), and 'sackes and bagges, and purses (to put and to kepe thynges in').

317

Of the making of tow 'uneven and full of knobs' used for stuffing into the cracks in ships, and 'for bonds and byndynges and matches for candelles, for it is full drye and taketh sone fyre and brenneth.' 'And so,' he concludes somewhat breathlessly, 'none herbe is so needfull to so many dyurrse uses to mankynde as is the flexe.'

Darwin studied several species of *Linum*, and found that some like the primrose had flowers with two forms of stamens and pistil. His object was to test the relative degrees of fertility of the long and short-styled pistils. *L. perenne*, for instance, is dimorphic:

'Of the flowers on the long-styled plants he found that twelve were fertilized with their own form pollen, but from a different plant. A seed capsule was only set when pollinated from anthers of the same height as the stigmas.'

So Darwin concluded:

'We have the clearest evidence that the stigmas of each form require for full fertility that pollen from the stamens of a corresponding height, belonging to the opposite form, should be brought to them.' (*Forms of Flowers*, p. 92.)

This plant is visited by bees, who perform the function Darwin describes.

The Flax is a graceful little plant with turquoise blue blossoms, a tall, erect annual, 1 to 2 feet high, the stems usually solitary, quite smooth, with alternate, linear, sessile leaves, ¾ to 1 inch long.

Many traditions are associated with this useful plant. Flax flowers were believed in the Middle Ages to be a protection against sorcery. The Bohemians have a belief that if seven-year-old children dance among Flax, they will become beautiful, and the whole plant was supposed to be under the protection of the goddess Hulda, who, in Teuton mythology, was held to have first taught mortals the art of growing Flax, of spinning, and of weaving it.

¶ *Cultivation and Preparation for Market.* Linseed requires ground as rich as for wheat, and if cultivated for seed is not of much use for Flax.

Its cultivation in this country could only pay on a large scale. The very exhausting nature of the crop has prevented its extensive cultivation in England, and the area under cultivation has declined in consequence. This peculiarity was well known to the Ancients, and Pliny asserted that it scorched the ground. Its culture requires care and suitable soil to secure a good crop. It has been grown in large quantities in the alluvial soils of Lincolnshire and in the eastern counties, and flourishes well in Ireland. It succeeds best in deep, moist loams such as contain a large proportion of vegetable matter, in good condition, firm, not loose. Strong clays do not answer well, nor poor soils, nor such as are of a gravelly or sandy nature, nor should the soil be freshly manured.

It is best treated as a farm crop. Being quickly grown and quickly harvested, it can be grown after a winter root crop, being over and reaped in time to secure a catch crop for the following season. The seed, which must be kept dry, as damp injures it, is sown in March or April, in drills, 70 lb. to the acre, on land carefully prepared and freed from weeds by ploughing. The crop itself must be hand-weeded, or the roots, being surface rooted, will be injured. It should be reaped in August, before the seed is fully ripe. The fibres of the plant, when grown for Flax, are found to be softer and stronger when the blossom has just fallen and the stalk begins to turn yellow before the leaves fall, than if left standing till the seeds are quite mature. The seeds, however, will ripen after the plant is gathered, if they be allowed to remain on the plant for a time. The Dutch avail themselves of this fact with regard to their Flax crops. After pulling the plants they stack them. The seeds by this means ripen, while the fibres are collected at the most favourable period of their growth. They thus obtain both of the valuable products of the plant.

¶ *Parts Used Medicinally.* The fruit is a globular capsule, about the size of a small pea, containing in separate cells ten seeds, which are brown (white within), oval-oblong and flattened, pointed at one end, shining and polished on the surface, ⅛ to ¼ inch long. They are inodorous except when powdered, but the taste is mucilaginous and slightly unpleasant.

Linseed varies much in size and tint – a yellowish variety occurring in India. Holland, Russia, the United States, Canada, the Argentine and India furnish the principal supplies. The Russian seed or Dutch-grown of Russian origin, though small, is preferred for Flax-growing, as it is hardier than the large southern seed from the Mediterranean and India. For medicinal purposes, English and Dutch seeds are preferred, on account of their freedom from weed-seeds and dirt. If containing more than 4 per cent. of weed-seeds, linseed may be said to be adulterated. Of English and Dutch seeds about twelve weigh 1 grain, but some of the Indian and Mediterranean varieties are twice as large and heavy.

¶ *Constituents.* The envelope or testa of the seed contains about 15 per cent. of mucilage. The seeds themselves contain in the cotyledons and endosperm from 30 to 40 per cent. of a fixed oil, of a light yellow colour, and about 25 per cent. proteids, together with wax, resin, sugar, phosphates, acetic acid, and a small quantity of the glucoside Linamarin. On incineration, linseed should not yield more than 5 per cent. of ash.

The oil is obtained by expression, with little or no heat. The cake which remains after expressing the oil, and which contains the farinaceous and mucilaginous part of the seed, is familiarly known as oil-cake, and is largely used as a fattening food for cattle. It is also used as a manure. When ground up, it is known as linseed meal, which is employed for making poultices. The meal is sold in two forms, crushed linseed and linseed meal. Formerly linseed meal was always obtained by grinding English oil-cake to powder and contained little oil, but now the crushed seeds, containing all the oil, are official. Crushed linseed of good quality usually contains from 30 to 35 per cent. of oil.

Linseed oil rapidly absorbs oxygen from the air and forms, when laid on in thin layers, a hard, transparent varnish. It is largely used in the arts for its properties as a drying oil. It is a viscid, yellow liquid, its chief constituent being Linolein. It also contains palmitin, stearin and myristin, with glyceride of linoleic acid. *Boiled oil,* produced by heating raw linseed oil to a temperature of 150° C., together with a small proportion of a metallic drier, possesses the drying properties of linseed oil to an enhanced degree. It becomes of a brown colour and dries much more rapidly, and in this state is used in the manufacture of printer's ink.

¶ *Medicinal Action and Uses.* Emollient, demulcent, pectoral. The crushed seeds or linseed meal make a very useful poultice, either alone or with mustard. In ulceration and superficial or deep-seated inflammation a linseed poultice allays irritation and pain and promotes suppuration. The addition of a little lobelia seed makes it of greater value in cases of boils. It is commonly used for abscesses and other local affections.

Linseed is largely employed as an addition to cough medicines. As a domestic remedy for colds, coughs and irritation of the urinary organs, linseed tea is most valuable. A little honey and lemon juice makes it very agreeable and more efficacious. This demulcent infusion contains a large quantity of mucilage, and is made from 1 oz. of the ground or entire seeds to 1 pint of boiling water. It is taken in wineglassful doses, which may be repeated *ad libitum.*

Linseed oil, mixed with an equal quantity of lime water, known then as Carron Oil, is an excellent application for burns and scalds.

Internally, the oil is sometimes given as a laxative; in cases of gravel and stone it is excellent, and has been administered in pleurisy with great success. It may also be used as an injection in constipation. Mixed with honey, linseed oil has been used as a cosmetic for removing spots from the face.

The oil enters into veterinary pharmacy as a purgative for sheep and horses, and a jelly formed by boiling the seeds is often given to calves.

Linseed is often employed, with other seeds, as food for small birds.

Plantain seeds, also a favourite food of small birds, can, it is said, be used instead of linseed in making poultices, as they contain much mucilage, though not so much oil.

Linseed has occasionally been employed as human food – we hear of the seeds being mixed with corn by the ancient Greeks and Romans for making bread – but it affords little actual nourishment and is apparently unwholesome, being difficult of digestion and provoking flatulence.

The meal has sometimes been used fraudulently for adulterating pepper.

FLAX, MOUNTAIN

Linum catharticum (LINN.)
N.O. Linaceæ

Synonyms. Purging Flax. Dwarf Flax. Fairy Flax. Mill Mountain
Part Used. Whole herb

Mountain Flax is a pretty little herb, which grows profusely in hilly pastures.

¶ *Description.* It is an annual, with a small, thready root, which sends up several slender, smooth, straight stems, which rise to a height of 6 to 8 inches, and are sometimes branched towards the upper part. The leaves are small, linear-oblong and obtuse, the lower ones opposite, and the upper alternate. The flowers, $\frac{1}{8}$ to $\frac{1}{4}$ of an inch in diameter, are white. The plant at first glance much resembles chickweed, being glaucous and glabrous.

¶ *Part Used.* The whole herb is used medicinally, both fresh and dried, collected in July, when in flower, in the wild state.

¶ *Constituents.* A green, bitter resin and a neutral, colourless, crystalline principle of a persistently bitter taste, called Linin, to which the herb owes its activity.

¶ *Medicinal Action and Uses*. This herb was highly extolled by Gerard as a purgative. It operates chiefly as a gentle cathartic, and is useful in all cases where a brisk purgative is required. As a laxative, it is preferred to senna, though the action is very similar. It

is generally taken combined with a carminative, such as peppermint.

The dried herb has been found very useful in muscular rheumatism and catarrhal affections, the infusion of 1 oz. in a pint of boiling water being taken in wineglassful doses. In liver complaints and jaundice, it has been employed with benefit.

FLAX, PERENNIAL

Linum perenne
N.O. Linaceæ

Part Used. Seeds

¶ *Preparations and Dosage*. Fluid extract, 10 to 30 drops.

A tincture is also made from the entire fresh plant, 2 or 3 drops in water being given every hour or two for diarrhœa.

Country people boil the fresh herb and take it for rheumatic pains, colds, coughs and dropsy.

The Perennial Flax is a native plant not uncommon in some parts of the country upon calcareous soils. It grows about 2 feet in height and is readily distinguished from the annual kind by its paler flowers and narrower leaves. The rootstock usually throws up many stems. It flowers in July.

This species has been recommended for cultivation as a fibre plant, but it has been little adopted, the fibre being coarser and the seeds smaller than those of the Common Flax.

As the plant will last several years and yields an abundant crop of stems, it

might be advantageously grown for paper making.

The seeds contain the same kind of oil as the ordinary species.

The All-Seed or Flax-Seed (*Radiola linoides*) belongs to the Flax family also; it is a minute annual with very fine, repeatedly forked branches. The leaves are opposite. Flowers in clusters very small, and seeding abundantly. It occurs inland on gravelly and sandy places, but is not common, from the Orkneys to Cornwall, e.g., near St. Ives, on the hills, and in the New Forest, near Lyndhurst.

Culpepper mentions remedies which include 'Lin-seed,' more than once – usually in the form of 'mussilage of Lin-seed'; in one he mentions 'the seeds of Flax' and (later in the same prescription) 'Linseed.' He says it 'heats and moistens, helps pains of the breast, coming cold and pleurises, old aches, and stitches, and softens hard swellings.'

FLEABANE, CANADIAN

Erigeron Canadense (LINN.)
N.O. Compositæ

Synonyms. Fleawort. Coltstail. Prideweed
Parts Used. Herb, seeds
Habitat. This species of Fleabane is an American annual, common in Northern and Middle States, as well as in Canada, growing in fields and meadows and by roadsides, and closely allied to the Common Fleabane

¶ *History*. It was introduced into Europe in the seventeenth century. Parkinson, in his *Theatrum Botanicum* (1640), mentions it as having been brought to Europe, but describes it as an American species, not yet growing in England. In 1653 we hear of it growing in the Botanic Gardens of Paris, and soon after it had become a weed about Paris. We first hear of it in England in 1669, and since its introduction it has often been found in the neighbourhood of London and in the Thames Valley, where it appears to have naturalized itself here and there, though it is very rare in the rest of England. Green (*Universal Herbal*, 1832) stated that it was to be found on cultivated ground in Glamorganshire and also on rubbish heaps.

The name *Erigeron* denotes 'soon becom-

ing old,' and is most appropriate, for in many of the species the plant, even when in flower, has a worn-out appearance, giving the idea of a weed which has passed its prime.

Parkinson says Fleabane 'bound to the forehead is a great helpe to cure one of the frensie.'

Culpepper says 'Flea-wort' (Fleabane) obtained its name 'because the seeds are so like Fleas'!

¶ *Description*. It has an unbranched stem, with lance-shaped leaves, the lower ones with short stalks and with five teeth, the upper ones with uncut edges and narrower, 1 to 2 inches long. The stem is bristly and grows several feet high, bearing composite heads of flowers, small, white and very numerous, blossoming from June to September.

¶ *Part Used.* The whole herb is gathered when in bloom and dried in bunches. The seeds are also used.

¶ *Constituents.* The herb contains a bitter extractive, tannic and gallic acids and a volatile oil, to which its virtues are due.

¶ *Medicinal Action and Uses.* Astringent, diuretic, tonic. It is considered useful in gravel, diabetes, dropsy and many kidney diseases, and is employed in diarrhœa and dysentery.

Oil of Erigeron resembles in its action Oil of Turpentine, but is less irritating. It has been used to arrest hæmorrhage from the lungs or alimentary tract, but this property is not assigned to it in modern medicine.

It is said to be a valuable remedy for inflamed tonsils and ulceration and inflammation of the throat generally.

The drug has a feeble odour and an astringent, aromatic and bitter taste. It is given in infusion (dose, wineglassful to a teacupful), oil (dose, 2 to 5 drops) on sugar. Fluid extract, ½ to 1 drachm.

FLEABANE, COMMON

Inula dysenterica (LINN.)
N.O. Compositæ

Synonyms. Pulicaria dysenterica (Gærtn.). Middle Fleabane
(*Arabian*) Rarajeub
Parts Used. Herb, root
Habitat. This species is a native of most parts of Europe, in moist meadows, watery places, by the sides of ditches, brooks and rivers, growing in masses and frequently overrunning large tracts of land on account of its creeping underground stems. In Scotland, however, it is rare, though common in Ireland

The Common Fleabane is nearly related to elecampane and other species of *Inula*, and by Linnæus, whom Hooker follows, is assigned to the same genus, although placed, with a smaller variety, in a separate genus, *Pulicaria*, by the botanist Gærtner.

This plant has medicinal properties, and though in England it has never had much reputation as a curative agent, it has ranked high in the estimation of herbalists abroad. It was formerly used in dysentery, and on this account received its specific name from Linnæus, who in his *Flora Suecia* says that he had been informed by General Keit, of the Russian Army, that his soldiers, in one of their expeditions against Persia, were cured of dysentery by means of this plant. Our old authors call it 'Middle Fleabane' – Ploughman's Spikenard being the Great Fleabane; both names being derived from the fact that, if burnt, the smoke from them drives away fleas and other insects. The generic name, *Pulicaria*, refers to this property, the Latin name for the flea being Pulex.

By the Arabians, it is called *Rarajeub*, or Job's Tears, from a tradition that Job used a decoction of this herb to cure his ulcers. It was formerly recommended for the itch and other cutaneous disorders.

¶ *Description.* It is a rough-looking plant, well marked by its soft, hoary foliage, and large terminal flat heads of bright yellow flowers, single, or one or two together, about an inch across, large in proportion to the size of the plant, the ray florets very numerous, long and narrow, somewhat paler than the florets in the centre or disk.

The creeping rootstock is perennial, and sends up at intervals stems reaching a height of 1 to 2 feet. These stems are woolly, branched above and very leafy, the leaves oblong, 1½ to 2½ inches long, heart or arrow-shaped at the base, embracing the stem, irregularly waved and toothed. Like the stem, the leaves are more or less covered with a woolly substance, varying a good deal in different plants. The under surface is ordinarily more woolly than the upper, and though the general effect of the foliage varies according to its degree of woolliness, it is at best a somewhat dull and greyish green.

The plant is in bloom from the latter part of July to September. The fruit is silky and crowned by a few short, unequal hairs of a dirty-white, with an outer ring of very short bristles or scales, a characteristic which distinguishes it from Elecampane and other members of the genus *Inula*, whose pappus consists of a *single* row of hairs this being the differing point which has led to its being assigned to a distinct genus, *Pulicaria*.

Another English plant bears the name of Fleabane (*Erigeron acris*), a member of the same order. For the sake of distinction, it is commonly known as the Blue Fleabane, its flowerheads having a yellow centre, and being surrounded by purplish rays. It is a smaller, far less striking plant, growing in dry situations.

¶ *Medicinal Action and Uses.* The leaves when bruised have a somewhat soap-like smell. The sap that lies in the tissues is bitter, astringent and saltish, so that animals will not eat the plant, and this astringent character, to which no doubt the medicinal properties are to be ascribed, is imparted to decoctions and infusions of the dried herb.

The following is taken from Miss E. S.

Rohde's *Old English Herbals*: 'Fleabane bound to the forehead is a great helpe to cure one of the frensie.'

'*Fleabane* on the lintel of the door I have hung,
S. John's wort, caper and wheatears
With a halter as a roving ass

Thy body I restrain.
O evil spirit, get thee hence!
Depart, O evil Demon.'
(Trans. of Utukke Limnûte Tablet 'B.' R. C. Thompson, *Devils and Evil Spirits of Babylonians*).

See ELECAMPANE

FLEABANE, GREAT. *See* SPIKENARD (PLOUGHMAN'S)

FORGET-ME-NOT

Myosotis symphytifolia
N.O. Boraginaceæ

Part Used. Herb

This plant has a strong affinity for the respiratory organs, especially the left lower lung. On the Continent it is sometimes made into a syrup and given for pulmonary affections. There is a tradition that a decoction or juice of the plant hardens steel.

(POISON)
FOXGLOVE

Digitalis purpurea (LINN.)
N.O. Scrophulariaceæ

Synonyms. Witches' Gloves. Dead Men's Bells. Fairy's Glove. Gloves of Our Lady. Bloody Fingers. Virgin's Glove. Fairy Caps. Folk's Glove. Fairy Thimbles
(*Norwegian*) Revbielde
(*German*) Fingerhut
Part Used. Leaves
Habitat. The Common Foxglove of the woods (*Digitalis purpurea*), perhaps the handsomest of our indigenous plants, is widely distributed throughout Europe and is common as a wild-flower in Great Britain, growing freely in woods and lanes, particularly in South Devon, ranging from Cornwall and Kent to Orkney, but not occurring in Shetland, or in some of the eastern counties of England. It flourishes best in siliceous soil and grows well in loam, but is entirely absent from some calcareous districts, such as the chain of the Jura, and is also not found in the Swiss Alps. It occurs in Madeira and the Azores, but is, perhaps, introduced there. The genus contains only this one indigenous species, though several are found on the Continent.

Needing little soil, it is found often in the crevices of granite walls, as well as in dry hilly pastures, rocky places and by roadsides. Seedling Foxgloves spring up rapidly from recently-turned earth. Turner (1548), says that it grows round rabbit-holes freely

¶ *Description*. The normal life of a Foxglove plant is two seasons, but sometimes the roots, which are formed of numerous, long, thick fibres, persist and throw up flowers for several seasons.

In the first year a rosette of leaves, but no stem, is sent up. In the second year, one or more flowering stems are thrown up, which are from 3 to 4 feet high, though even sometimes more, and bear long spikes of drooping flowers, which bloom in the early summer, though the time of flowering differs much, according to the locality. As a rule, the flowers are in perfection in July. As the blossoms on the main stem gradually fall away, smaller lateral shoots are often thrown out from its lower parts, which remain in flower after the principal stem has shed its blossoms. These are also promptly developed if by mischance the central stem sustains any serious injury.

The radical leaves are often a foot or more long, contracted at the base into a long, winged footstalk, the wings formed by the lower veins running down into it some distance. They have slightly indented margins and sloping lateral veins, which are a very prominent feature. The flowering stems give off a few leaves, that gradually diminish in size from below upwards. All the leaves are covered with small, simple, unbranched hairs.

The flowers are bell-shaped and tubular, 1½ to 2½ inches long, flattened above, inflated beneath, crimson outside above and paler beneath, the lower lip furnished with long hairs inside and marked with numerous dark crimson spots, each surrounded with a white border. The shade of the flowers varies much, especially under cultivation, sometimes the corollas being found perfectly white.

In cultivated plants there frequently occurs a malformation, whereby one or two of the uppermost flowers become united, and form an erect, regular, cup-shaped flower, through the centre of which the upper extremity of the stem is more or less prolonged.

The Foxglove is a favourite flower of the honey-bee, and is entirely developed by the visits of this insect. For that reason, its tall and stately spikes of flowers are at their best in those sunny, midsummer days when the bees are busiest. The projecting lower lip of the corolla forms an alighting platform for the bee, and as he pushes his way up the bell, to get at the honey which lies in a ring round the seed vessel at the top of the flower, the anthers of the stamens which lie flat on the corolla above him, are rubbed against his back. Going from flower to flower up the spike, he rubs pollen thus from one blossom on to the cleft stigma of another blossom, and thus the flower is fertilized and seeds are able to be produced. The life of each flower, from the time the bud opens till the time it slips off its corolla, is about six days. An almost incredible number of seeds are produced, a single Foxglove plant providing from one to two million seeds to ensure its propagation.

It is noteworthy that although the flower is such a favourite with bees and is much visited by other smaller insects, who may be seen taking refuge from cold and wet in its drooping blossoms on chilly evenings, yet no animals will browse upon the plant, perhaps instinctively recognizing its poisonous character.

The Foxglove derives its common name from the shape of the flowers resembling the finger of a glove. It was originally Folksglove – the glove of the 'good folk' or fairies, whose favourite haunts were supposed to be in the deep hollows and woody dells, where the Foxglove delights to grow. Folksglove is one of its oldest names, and is mentioned in a list of plants in the time of Edward III. Its Norwegian name, *Revbielde* (Foxbell), is the only foreign one that alludes to the Fox, though there is a northern legend that bad fairies gave these blossoms to the fox that he might put them on his toes to soften his tread when he prowled among the roosts.

The earliest known form of the word is the Anglo-Saxon *foxes glofa* (the glove of the fox).

The mottlings of the blossoms of the Foxglove and the Cowslip, like the spots on butterfly wings and on the tails of peacocks and pheasants, were said to mark where the elves had placed their fingers, and one legend ran that the marks on the Foxglove were a warning sign of the baneful juices secreted by the plant, which in Ireland gain it the popular name of 'Dead Man's Thimbles.'

In Scotland, it forms the badge of the Farquharsons, as the Thistle does of the Stuarts. The German name *Fingerhut* (thimble) suggested to Leonhard Fuchs (the well-known German herbalist of the sixteenth century, after whom the Fuchsia has been named) the employment of the Latin adjective *Digitalis* (from *Digitabulum*, a thimble) as a designation for the plant, which, as he remarked, up to the time when he thus named it, in 1542, had had no name in either Greek or Latin.

The Foxglove was employed by the old herbalists for various purposes in medicine, most of them wholly without reference to those valuable properties which render it useful as a remedy in the hands of modern physicians. Gerard recommends it to those 'who have fallen from high places,' and Parkinson speaks highly of the bruised herb or of its expressed juice for scrofulous swellings, when applied outwardly in the form of an ointment, and the bruised leaves for cleansing for old sores and ulcers. Dodoens (1554) prescribed it boiled in wine as an expectorant, and it seems to have been in frequent use in cases in which the practitioners of the present day would consider it highly dangerous.

Culpepper says it is of

'a gentle, cleansing nature and withal very friendly to nature. The Herb is familiarly and frequently used by the Italians to heal any fresh or green wound, the leaves being but bruised and bound thereon; and the juice thereof is also used in old sores, to cleanse, dry and heal them. It has been found by experience to be available for the King's evil, the herb bruised and applied, or an ointment made with the juice thereof, and so used. . . . I am confident that an ointment of it is one of the best remedies for a scabby head that is.'

Strangely enough, the Foxglove, so handsome and striking in our landscape, is not mentioned by Shakespeare, or by any of the old English poets. The earliest known descriptions of it are those given about the middle of the sixteenth century by Fuchs and Tragus in their Herbals. According to an old manuscript, the Welsh physicians of the thirteenth century appear to have frequently made use of it in the preparation of external medicines. Gerard and Parkinson advocate its use for a number of complaints, and later Salmon, in the *New London Dispensatory*, praised the plant. It was introduced into the London Pharmacopœia in 1650, though it did not come into frequent use until a century later, and was first brought prominently under the notice of the medical profession by Dr. W. Withering, who in his *Account of the Foxglove*, 1785, gave details of upwards of 200 cases, chiefly dropsical, in which it was used.

A domestic use of the Foxglove was general throughout North Wales at one time, when the leaves were used to darken the lines engraved on the stone floors which were fashionable then. This gave them a mosaic-like appearance.

The plant is both cultivated and collected in quantities for commercial purposes in the Harz Mountains and the Thuringian Forest. ¶ *Cultivation.* The Foxglove is cultivated by a few growers in this country in order to provide a drug of uniform activity from a true type of *Digitalis purpurea.* It is absolutely necessary to have the true medicinal seeds to supply the drug market: crops must be obtained from carefully selected wild seed and all variations from the new type struck out.

The plant will flourish best in well-drained loose soil, preferably of siliceous origin, with some slight shade. The plants growing in sunny situations possess the active qualities of the herb in a much greater degree than those shaded by trees, and it has been proved that those grown on a hot, sunny bank, protected by a wood, give the best results.

It grows best when allowed to seed itself, but if it is desired to raise it by sown seed, 2 lb. of seed to the acre are required. As the seeds are so small and light, they should be mixed with fine sand in order to ensure even distribution. They should be thinly covered with soil. The seeds are uncertain in germination, but the seedlings may be readily and safely transplanted in damp weather, and should be pricked out to 6 to 9 inches apart. Sown in spring, the plant will not blossom till the following year. Seeds must be gathered as soon as ripe. The flowers of the true medicinal type must be pure, dull pink or magenta, not pale-coloured, white or spotted externally.

It is estimated that one acre of good soil will grow at least two tons of the Foxglove foliage, producing about ½ ton of the dried leaves. ¶ *Preparation for Market.* The leaves alone are now used for the extraction of the drug, although formerly the seeds were also official.

No leaves are to be used for medicinal purposes that are not taken from the two-year-old plants, picked when the bloom spike has run up and about two-thirds of the flowers are expanded, because at this time, before the ripening of the seeds, the leaves are in the most active state. They may be collected as long as they are in good condition: only green, perfect leaves being picked, all those that are insect-eaten or diseased, or tinged with purple or otherwise discoloured, must be discarded. Leaves from seedlings are valueless, and they must also not be collected in the spring, before the plant flowers, or in the autumn, when it has seeded, as the activity of the alkaloids is in each case too low.

If the *fresh* leaves are sent to the manufacturing druggists for Extract-making, they should be in ½ cwt. bundles, packed in air-covered railway cattle-trucks, or if in an open truck, must be covered with tarpaulin. The fresh crop should, if possible, be delivered to the wholesale buyer the same day as cut, but if this is impossible, on account of distance, they should be picked before the dew falls in the late afternoon and despatched the same evening, packed loosely in wicker baskets, lined with an open kind of muslin. Consignments by rail should be labelled: 'Urgent, Medicinal Herbs,' to ensure quick delivery. The weather for picking must be absolutely dry – no damp or rain in the air – and the leaves must be kept out of the sun and not packed too closely, or they may heat and turn yellow.

The odour of the fresh leaves is unpleasant, and the taste of both fresh and dried leaves is disagreeably bitter.

Foxglove leaves have in some places been recklessly gathered by over-zealous and thoughtless collectors without due regard to the future supply of the plants. The plant should not be roughly treated and never cut off just above the root, but the bottom leaves should in all cases be left to nourish the flower-spikes, in order that the seed may be ripened. In patches where Foxgloves grow thickly, the collection and redistribution of seed in likely places is much to be recommended.

The dried leaves as imported have occasionally been found adulterated with the leaves of various other plants. The chief of these are *Inula Conyza* (Ploughman's Spikenard), which may be distinguished by their greater roughness, the less-divided margins, the teeth of which have horny points, and odour when rubbed; *I. Helenium* (Elecampane), the leaves of which resemble Foxglove leaves, though they are less pointed, and the lower lateral veins do not form a 'wing' as in the Foxglove; the leaves of *Symphytum officinale* (Comfrey), which, however, may be recognized by the isolated stiff hairs they bear, and *Verbascum Thapsus*

(Great Mullein), the leaves of which, unlike those of the Foxglove, have woolly upper and under surfaces, and the hairs of which, examined under a lens, are seen to be branched. Primrose leaves are also sometimes mingled with the drug, though they are much smaller than the average Foxglove leaf, and may be readily distinguished by the *straight*, lateral veins, which divide near the margins of the leaves. Foxglove leaves are easy to distinguish by their veins running *down* the leaf.

There is no reason why Foxglove leaves, properly prepared, should not become a national export.

Digitalis has lately been grown in Government Cinchona plantations in the Nilgiris, Madras, India. The leaves are coarser and rather darker in colour than British or German-grown leaves, wild or cultivated, but tests show that the tincture prepared from them contains glucosides of more than average value.

¶ *Constituents.* Digitalis contains four important glucosides of which three are cardiac stimulants. The most powerful is Digitoxin, an extremely poisonous and cumulative drug, insoluble in water; Digitalin, which is crystalline and also insoluble in water; Digitalein, amorphous, but readily soluble in water, rendering it, therefore, capable of being administered subcutaneously, in doses so minute as rarely to exceed $\frac{1}{100}$ of a grain; Digitonin, which is a cardiac depressant, containing none of the physiological action peculiar to Digitalis, and is identical with Saponin, the chief constituent of Senega root. Other constituents are volatile oil, fatty matter, starch, gum, sugar, etc.

The amount and character of the active constituents vary according to season and soil: 100 parts of dried leaves yield about 1·25 of Digitalin, which is generally found in a larger proportion in the wild than in the cultivated plants.

The active constituents of Digitalis are not yet sufficiently explored to render a chemical assay effective in standardizing for therapeutic activity. The different glucosides contained varying from each other in their physiological action, it is impossible to assay the leaves by determining one only of these, such as Digitoxin. No method of determining Digitalin is known. Hence the chemical means of assay fail, and the drug is usually standardized by a physiological test. One of our oldest firms of manufacturing druggists standardizes preparations of this extremely powerful and important drug by testing their action upon frogs.

¶ *Preparations.* The preparations of Foxglove on the market vary considerably in composition and strength. Powdered Digitalis leaf is administered in pill form. The pharmacopœial tincture, which is the preparation in commonest use, is given in doses of 5·15 minims, and the infusion is the unusually small dose of 2 to 4 drachms, the dose of other infusions being an ounce or more. The tincture contains a fair proportion of both Digitalin and Digitoxin.

The following note from the *Chemist and Druggist* (December 30, 1922) is of interest here:

'Cultivation of Digitalis

'As is well known, for many years prior to the War digitalis was successfully cultivated on a large scale in various parts of the former Austro-Hungarian monarchy, and indeed the Government actively promoted the cultivation of this as well as of other medicinal plants. B. Pater, of Klausenburg, gives a résumé of his experiences in this direction (*Pharmazeutische Monatshefte*, 7, 1922), dealing not only with the best methods for cultivating digitalis from the seeds of this plant, but also with his investigations into certain differences and abnormalities peculiar to *Digitalis purpurea*. Apart from the fact that, occasionally, some plants bear flowers already in the first year of growth, the observation was made that the colour of the flowers showed a wide scale of variation, ranging from the well-known distinctive purple shade through dark rose, light rose, to white. These variations in colour of the flowers of cultivated digitalis plants induced the author to undertake a study of the activity of the several varieties, based on the digitoxin content of the stem leaves collected from flowering plants. In the case of *Digitalis purpurea* with normal purple flowers, the content of purified digitoxin, ascertained by Keller's method, averaged 0·17 per cent., while the leaves of plants bearing white flowers showed a slightly lower content, i.e. an average of 0·155 per cent. of purified digitoxin. On the other hand, the plants with rose-coloured flowers were found to possess a very low content of digitoxin, averaging only 0·059 per cent. In the course of these investigations the fact was confirmed that the upper stem leaves are more active than the lower leaves.'

¶ *Medicinal Action and Uses.* Digitalis has been used from early times in heart cases. It increases the activity of all forms of muscle tissue, but more especially that of the heart and arterioles, the all-important property of the drug being its action on the circulation. The first consequence of its absorption is a

contraction of the heart and arteries, causing
a very high rise in the blood pressure.

After the taking of a moderate dose, the
pulse is markedly slowed. Digitalis also
causes an irregular pulse to become regular.
Added to the greater force of cardiac contraction is a permanent tonic contraction of
the organ, so that its internal capacity is reduced, which is a beneficial effect in cases of
cardiac dilatation, and it improves the nutrition of the heart by increasing the amount of
blood.

In ordinary conditions it takes about twelve
hours or more before its effects on the heart
muscle is appreciated, and it must thus always
be combined with other remedies to tide the
patient over this period and never prescribed
in large doses at first, as some patients are
unable to take it, the drug being apt to cause
considerable digestive disturbances, varying
in different cases. This action is probably
due to the Digitonin, an undesirable constituent.

The action of the drug on the kidneys is of
importance only second to its action on the
circulation. In small or moderate doses, it is
a powerful diuretic and a valuable remedy in
dropsy, especially when this is connected
with affections of the heart.

It has also been employed in the treatment
of internal hæmorrhage, in inflammatory
diseases, in delirium tremens, in epilepsy,
in acute mania and various other diseases,
with real or supposed benefits.

The action of Digitalis in all the forms in
which it is administered should be carefully
watched, and when given over a prolonged
period it should be employed with caution,
as it is liable to accumulate in the system and
to manifest its presence all at once by its
poisonous action, indicated by the pulse becoming irregular, the blood-pressure low and
gastro-intestinal irritation setting in. The
constant use of Digitalis, also, by increasing
the activity of the heart, leads to hypertrophy
of that organ.

Digitalis is an excellent antidote in
Aconite poisoning, given as a hypodermic
injection.

When Digitalis fails to act on the heart as
desired, Lily-of-the-Valley may be substituted and will often be found of service.

FRANKINCENSE
  Synonym. Olibanum.
  Part Used. The gum resin
  Habitat. Arabia, Somaliland

¶ *Description.* Obtained from the leafy forest
tree *Boswellia Thurifera*, with leaves deciduous, alternate towards the tops of
branches, unequally pinnated; leaflets in

In large doses, the action of Digitalis on
the circulation will cause various cerebral
symptoms, such as seeing all objects blue, and
various other disturbances of the special
senses. In cases of poisoning by Digitalis,
with a very slow and irregular pulse, the
administration of Atropine is generally all
that is necessary. In the more severe cases,
with the very rapid heart-beat, the stomach
pump must be used, and drugs may be used
which depress and diminish the irritability of
the heart, such as chloral and chloroform.

Preparations of Digitalis come under
Table II of the Poison Schedule.

¶ *Preparations and Dosages.* Tincture, B.P.,
5 to 15 drops. Infusion, B.P., 2 to 4
drachms. Powdered leaves, ½ to 2 grains.
Fluid extract, 1 to 3 drops. Solid extract,
U.S.P., ⅛ grain.

A method of preparing the drug in a non-
injurious manner is given in the *Chemist and
Druggist* (December 30, 1922):

'*Digitalis Maceration*

'On preparing an infusion of digitalis
leaves in the usual manner, one of the active
principles, gitalin, is destroyed by the action
of the boiling water. To obviate the possibility of destroying any of the active principles in the leaves, Th. Koch (*Süddeutsche
Apotheker-Zeitung*, 63, 1922) has for some
years past adopted the following procedure:
20 gm. powdered standardized digitalis
leaves, 1000 gm. chloroform water (7·1000)
and 40 drops of 10 per cent. Solution of
Sodium Carbonate are shaken for four hours.
The liquid is then passed through a flannel
cloth, and, after standing for some time,
filtered in the ordinary way, taking the precaution to cover the filter with a glass plate.
The use of chloroform water as the solvent
serves a threefold purpose: It promotes the
solution of the gitalin present in the leaves,
ensures the stability and keeping properties
of the maceration, and prevents the occurrence of gastric troubles. The presence of
Sodium Carbonate prevents the plant acid
from reacting with the chloroform to produce
hydrochloric acid. In this maceration no
digitoxin is present, the principle which is
assumed to exert a deleterious action on the
heart as well as a cumulative effect.'

Boswellia Thurifera
N.O. Burseraceæ

about ten pairs with an odd one opposite,
oblong, obtuse, serrated, pubescent, sometimes alternate; petioles short. Flowers, white
or pale rose on short pedicels in single

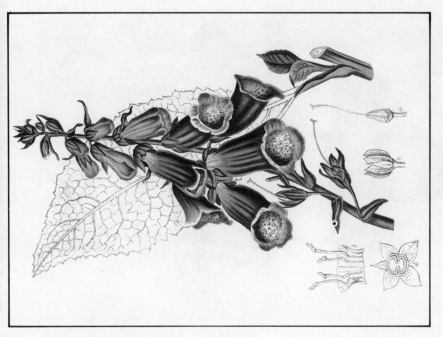

FOXGLOVE
Digitalis Purpurea

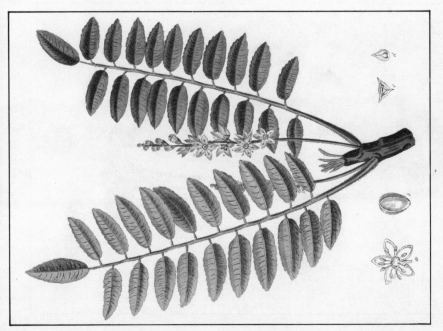

FRANKINCENSE
Boswellia Thurifera

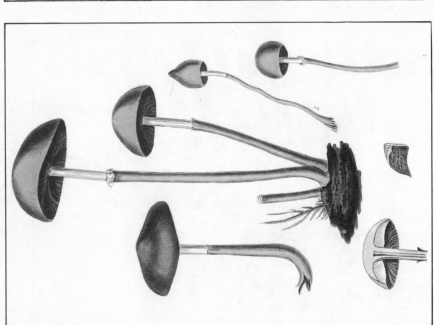

FUNGI
Agaricus Bulbosus

FUNGI
Agaricus Semiglobatus

axillary racemes shorter than the leaves. Calyx, small five-toothed, persistent; corolla with five obovate-oblong, very patent petals, acute at the base, inserted under the margin of the disk; æstivation slightly imbricative. Stamens, ten, inserted under the disk, alternately shorter; filaments subulate, persistent. Anthers, caducous, oblong. Torus a cup-shaped disk, fleshy, larger than calyx, crenulated margin. Ovary, oblong, sessile. Style, one caducous, the length of the stamens; stigma capitate, three-lobed. Fruit capsular, three-angled, three-celled, three-valved, septicidal, valves hard. Seeds, solitary in each cell surrounded by a broad membranaceous wing. Cotyledons intricately folded multifid.

The trees on the Somali coast grow, without soil, out of polished marble rocks, to which they are attached by a thick oval mass of substances resembling a mixture of lime and mortar. The young trees furnish the most valuable gum, the older yielding merely a clear, glutinous fluid, resembling copal varnish.

To obtain the Frankincense, a deep, longitudinal incision is made in the trunk of the tree and below it a narrow strip of bark 5 inches in length is peeled off. When the milk-like juice which exudes has hardened by exposure to the air, the incision is deepened. In about three months the resin has attained the required degree of consistency, hardening into yellowish 'tears.' The large, clear globules are scraped off into baskets and the inferior quality that has run down the tree is collected separately. The season for gathering lasts from May till the middle of September, when the first shower of rain puts a close to the gathering for that year.

The coast of Southern Arabia is yearly visited by parties of Somalis, who pay the Arabs for the privilege of collecting Frankincense, and in the interior of the country, about the plain of Dhofar, during the southwest Monsoon, Frankincense and other gums are gathered by the Bedouins. (The incense of Dhofar is alluded to by the Portuguese poet, Camoens.)

¶ *Constituents*. Resins 65 per cent., volatile oil 6 per cent., water-soluble gum 20 per cent., bassorin 6 to 8 per cent., plant residue 2 to 4 per cent.; the resins are composed of boswellic acid and alibanoresin.

¶ *Medicinal Action and Uses*. It is stimulant, but seldom used now internally, though formerly was in great repute. Pliny mentions it as an antidote to hemlock. Avicenna (tenth century) recommends it for tumours, ulcers, vomiting, dysentery and fevers. In China it is used for leprosy.

Its principal use now is in the manufacture of incense and pastilles. It is also used in plasters and might be substituted for Balsam of Peru or Balsam or Tolu. The inhalation of steam laden with the volatile portion of the drug is said to relieve bronchitis and laryngitis.

The ceremonial incense of the Jews was compounded of four 'sweet scents,' of which pure Frankincense was one, pounded together in equal proportion. It is frequently mentioned in the Pentateuch. Pure Frankincense formed part of the meet offering and was also presented with the shew-bread every Sabbath day. With other spices, it was stored in a great chamber of the House of God at Jerusalem.

According to Herodotus, Frankincense to the amount of 1,000 talents weight was offered every year, during the feast of Bel, on the great altar of his temple in Babylon. The religious use of incense was as common in ancient Persia as in Babylon and Assyria. Herodotus states that the Arabs brought every year to Darius as tribute 1,000 talents of Frankincense, and the modern Parsis of Western India still preserve the ritual of incense.

Frankincense, though the most common, never became the only kind of incense offered to the gods among the Greeks. According to Pliny, it was not sacrificially employed in Trojan times. Among the Romans, the use of Frankincense (alluded to as *mascula thura* by Virgil in the *Eclogues*) was not confined to religious ceremonials. It was also used on state occasions, and in domestic life.

The *kohl*, or black powder with which the Egyptian women paint their eyelids, is made of charred Frankincense, or other odoriferous resin mixed with Frankincense. Frankincense is also melted to make a depilatory, and it is made into a paste with other ingredients to perfume the hands. A similar practice is described by Herodotus as having been practised by the women of Scythia and is alluded to in Judith x. 3 and 4. In cold weather, the Egyptians warm their rooms with a brazier whereon incense is burnt, Frankincense, Benzoin and Aloe wood being chiefly used for the purpose.

The word 'incense,' meaning originally the aroma given off with the smoke of any odoriferous substance when burnt, has been gradually restricted almost exclusively to Frankincense, which has always been obtainable in Europe in greater quantity than any other of the aromatics imported from the East.

There is no fixed formula for the incense now used in the Christian churches of Europe, but it is recommended that Frankincense should enter as largely as possible into its composition. In Rome, Olibanum alone is employed: in the Russian church, Benzoin is chiefly employed.

The following is a formula for an incense used in the Roman Church: Olibanum, 10 oz. Benzoin, 4 oz. Storax, 1 oz. Break into small pieces and mix.

FRINGE TREE

Chionanthus virginica (LINN.)
N.O. Oleaceæ

Synonyms. Old Man's Beard. Fringe Tree Bark. Chionathus. Snowdrop Tree. Poison Ash
Part Used. The dried bark of the root
Habitat. The United States, from Pennsylvania to Tennessee

¶ *Description.* A small tree, bearing in June white flowers like snowdrops, and with large leaves like those of Magnolia, it presents a charming appearance. The root-bark is found in single, transversely-curved pieces, often heavy enough (though small) to sink in water. The outside is reddish or greyish-brown, with root scars and whiter patches. The inner surface is a yellowish-brown. The fracture is short, coarsely granular, and yellowish-white. It is almost odourless, but very bitter in taste. The powder is light brown in colour.

¶ *Constituents.* It is said that both saponin and a glucoside have been found, but neither appears to have been officially confirmed.
¶ *Medicinal Action and Uses.* Aperient, diuretic. Some authorities regard it as tonic and slightly narcotic. It is used in typhoid, intermittent, or bilious fevers, and externally, as a poultice, for inflammations or wounds. Is useful in liver complaints.
¶ *Dosage.* Of fluid extract, ½ to 1 fluid drachm two or three times a day. Of infusion, ½ to 2 fluid ounces two or three times a day. Chiomanthin, 1 to 3 grains.

FRITILLARY, COMMON

Fritillaria Meleagris (LINN.)
N.O. Liliaceæ

Synonyms. Lilium variegatum. Chequered Daffodil. Narcissus Caparonius. Turkey Hen. Ginny Flower

Fritillaria Meleagris (Linn.), the Snake's Head Fritillary, is a native of Great Britain, found in meadows and pastures in the southern and eastern counties of England, chiefly in Oxfordshire. It is not common and does not occur farther north than Norfolk, or farther west than Somerset.

It has a tiny, solid bulb, not larger than a good-sized black currant, with two or three long, narrow leaves, on a stem about a foot high, which bears a single, drooping flower of a dull red colour, marked curiously with pink and dark purple, in quaint squares and blotches. The petals are only overlapping and not joined together in any way, although the flowers look bell-like. Though the open flower is pendulous, the bud stands erect, and so does the capsule. The plant is in bloom in April and May, in mild seasons in March.

The botanical name, *meleagris*, is derived from a Greek term applied to a guinea-hen,

and many of the popular English names have a similar allusion to the markings of the flower, viz. Guinea-hen flower, Turkey-hen flower, Pheasant Lily, Leopards Lily, Chequered Lily, Chequered Daffodil and Lazarus Bell.

Bees visit the flower for the nectar secreted largely at the base of the perianth.

Many garden varieties are now cultivated. The best mode of propagation is by offsets, but also by seed, which ripens readily. Rabbits are very fond of this plant and will destroy it wholesale.

The bulb is poisonous and very distasteful to the palate and is said to have no medicinal value, though from its presence on the elaborate allegorical frontispiece of the old Herbal of Clusius, *Rariorum Plantarum Historia*, published in 1601, it bore at that time a reputation as a herb of healing.

See LILY (CROWN IMPERIAL).

FROSTWORT

Helianthemum Canadense (MISCH.)
N.O. Cistaceæ

Synonyms. Cistus. Frostweed. Frostplant. Rock Rose. Canadisches Sonnenroschen. Helianthemum Ramultoflorum. Helianthemum Rosmarinifolium. Helianthemum michauxii. Helianthemum Corymbosum. Cistus Canadensis. Lechea Major. Heterameris Canadensis
Part Used. The dried herb
Habitat. Eastern United States

¶ *Description.* The official name comes from the Greek *helios* (the sun) and *anthemon* (a flower). The genus differs from the *Cistus*

in having imperfectly three-celled instead of five or ten-celled capsules. Two distinct varieties of the species are known, the early and late flowering forms. They grow in sandy soil, from 6 to 12 inches high, with upright stems, branching or almost without branches, leaves light or dark green, small and lanceolate, and flat, yellow flowers, solitary or in terminal clusters. The popular names spring from the peculiarity of thin, curved, ice-crystals projecting in early winter from fissures in the bark near the root. The taste is astringent, slightly aromatic and bitter. It has no odour.

¶ *Constituents.* A volatile oil, wax, tannin, fatty oil, and a glucoside that will crystallize into white needles. Chlorophyll, gum and inorganic salts were also found in *Helianthemum Corymbosum.*

¶ *Medicinal Action and Uses.* Antiscrofulous, astringent, alterative and tonic. It has for long been used in secondary syphilis, diarrhœa, ulcerations, ophthalmia, and any conditions arising from a scrofulous constitution. Locally it is useful as a wash in prurigo and as a gargle in scarlatina, and in poultice form for scrofulous tumours and ulcers.

It is said that an oil helpful in cancer has been obtained from it.

It may be combined with Corydalis Formosa and Stillingia, in secondary syphilis, and the infusion may be used in chronic diarrhœa and dysentery.

FUCHSIA. *See* WILLOW HERBS

An overdose may produce nausea and vomiting.

¶ *Dosage.* Of extract, 2 grains. Of fluid extract, 1 fluid drachm as an alternative and astringent.

¶ *Other Species.*
H. Corymbosum may be used indiscriminately as officinal.

Cistus Creticus, or European Rock Rose, the only other plant of the order used in medicine, yields the gum resin Ladanum or Labdanum, a natural exudation valued as a stimulant expectorant and emmenagogue. It has been used in plasters, and formerly in catarrh and dysentery. An oil with the odour of ambergris has been obtained from the resin.

Labdanum is found in masses weighing up to several pounds, enclosed in bladders. It softens in the hand when broken, becoming adhesive and balsamic. It burns with a clear flame. An adulterated kind is in contorted, hard pieces, mixed with sand and earth.

C. Landaniferous, C. Ledon and *C. Laurifolius* are said to yield the same substance, most of which comes from the Grecian Islands.

All these Cistus and Helianthenums grow in the author's garden at Chalfont St. Peters.

FUMITORY

Fumaria officinalis (LINN.)
N.O. Fumariaceæ

Synonyms. Earth Smoke. Beggary. Fumus. Vapor. Nidor. Fumus Terræ. Fumiterry, Scheiteregi. Taubenkropp. Kaphnos. Wax Dolls
Part Used. Herb
Habitat. Europe and America. Parts of Asia, Australia and South Africa

¶ *Description.* A small annual plant, a common weed in many parts of Europe, including Britain, and naturalized in the United States.

The Fumitories, of which *Corydalis* and *Fumaria* are the only two fully British genera, are distinguished in the Order of Fumariaceæ by having one of the petals swollen or spurred at the base, and a one-seeded capsule which does not open. The name is said to be derived either from the fact that its whitish, blue-green colour gives it the appearance of smoke rising from the ground, or, according to Pliny, because the juice of the plant brings on such a flow of tears that the sight becomes dim as with smoke, and hence its reputed use in affections of the eye. According to the ancient exorcists, when the plant is burned, its smoke has the power of expelling evil spirits, it having been used for this purpose in the famous geometrical gardens of St. Gall.

There is a legend that the plant was produced, not from seed, but from vapours arising out of the earth.

The herb is small and slender, with weak, straggling, or climbing stems, decompound leaves, and clusters or spikes of small flowers of a pinkish hue, topped with purple, or more rarely, white. The leaves have no odour, but taste bitter and saline. The plant flowers almost throughout the summer in fields, gardens, and on banks, and in ditches, spreading with great rapidity. At Mudgee, in New South Wales, it was reported to have smothered a wheat crop. Shakespeare makes several references to the herb. An interesting peculiarity is that it is very seldom visited by insects. It is self-fertile, and sets every seed.

The flowers are used to make a yellow dye for wool.

¶ *Constituents.* The leaves yield by expression a juice which has medicinal properties. An extract, prepared by evaporating

329

the expressed juice, or a decoction of the leaves, throws out upon its surface a copious saline efflorescence. Fumaric acid was early identified as present, and its isomerism with maleic acid was established later. The alkaloid Fumarine has been believed to be identical with corydaline, but it differs both in formula and in its reaction to sulphuric and nitric acids. It occurs in colourless, tasteless crystals, freely soluble in chloroform, less so in benzine, still less so in alcohol and ether, sparingly soluble in water.

¶ *Medicinal Action and Uses.* A weak tonic, slightly diaphoretic, diuretic, and aperient; valuable in all visceral obstructions, particularly those of the liver, in scorbutic affections, and in troublesome eruptive diseases, even those of the leprous order. A decoction makes a curative lotion for milk-crust on the scalp of an infant. Physicians and writers from Dioscorides to Chaucer, and from the fourteenth century to Cullen and to modern times value its purifying power. The Japanese make a tonic from it. Cows and sheep eat it, and the latter are said to derive great benefit from it. The leaves, in decoction or extract, may be used in almost any doses. The inspissated juice has also been employed, also a syrup, powder, cataplasm, distilled water, and several tinctures.

French and German physicians still prefer it to most other medicines as a purifier of the blood; while sometimes the dried leaves are smoked in the manner of tobacco, for disorders of the head. Dr. Cullen, among its good effects in cutaneous disorders, mentions the following:

'There is a disorder of the skin, which, though not attended with any alarming symptoms of danger to the life of the patient, is thought to place the empire of beauty in great jeopardy; the complaint is frequently brought on by neglecting to use a parasol, and may be known by sandy spots, vulgarly known as freckles, scattered over the face. Now, be it known to all whom it may concern, that the infusion of the leaves of the above-described plant is said to be an excellent specific for removing these freckles and clearing the skin; and ought, we think, to be chiefly employed by those who have previously removed those moral blemishes which deform the mind, or degrade the dignity of a reasonable and an immortal being.'

¶ *Dosage.* Of Fumarine, $\frac{1}{8}$ or $\frac{1}{4}$ of a grain is moderately excitant; 3 grains are first irritant, then sedative. Of the expressed juice, 2 fluid ounces or more, twice a day. Of fluid extract, $\frac{1}{2}$ to 1 drachm.

For dyspepsia, 2 oz. of the flowers and tops may be macerated in 3 pints of Madeira wine, and taken twice a day in doses of 2 to 4 fluid ounces.

Fluid extract, $\frac{1}{2}$ to 1 drachm.

¶ *Old Recipes and Prescriptions.*

The Liquid Juice four or five spoonfuls in the morning, fasting, with a glass of white Port wine. It purges a little downwards, but more especially if mixed with an infusion of Senna in wine. It purifies the blood from salt, choleric, or viscous humours, and strengthens all the Viscera, not leaving any evil quality behind it.

The Essence has all the virtues of the former, but is more efficacious. A safe remedy also against adult choler and melancholy or obstructions which are the cause of choleric and putrid fevers, jaundice, Strangury of Urine through Gravel, Sand, or Viscous Matter, all of which it expels in abundance.

Dose, 5 or 6 spoonfuls in white wine or clarified whey.

The Syrup. Whether made of the juice or greenherb, has all the virtue, but is weaker in operation, and therefore ought to be given mixed with the Syrup of Damask Roses or Peach Blossoms, or Tincture of Senna. Very effectual against Jaundice, Dropsy, and Gout; and is a most singular thing against hypochondriack melancholy in any person whatsoever.

The Decoction in Water or Wine. Weaker than the above, and 6 to 8 oz. may be given in the morning, fasting.

The Power of the Dried Herb. A drachm, with half a drachm of Powder of Esula Root, and given in 5 or 6 spoonsful of the essence of juice, causes vomiting and cleanses the stomach and bowels, effectual against Dropsy, Scurvy, Jaundice, Gout and Rheumatism; but because it stirs up much wind, should be corrected with a few drops of oil of Anise or Fennel Seed, or with the Powder of the same.

The Collurium. 3 ounces of Juice or Essence of Fumitory, mixed with one ounce each of distilled Water of Fumitory, and honey. An excellent thing against sores, inflamed, running and watery Eyes. Also a healing Gargle. Drops in the Eyes clear the sight and take away redness. If the Juice be mixed with equal parts of Juice of Sharp-pointed Docks and Wine Vinegar, and a contaminated Skin be washed therewith, it cures it of Scabs, Itch, Wheals, Pimples, Scurf, etc.

The Distilled Water has the virtues of the

Juice, but is much weaker, and may be used as a Vehicle for any of the other Preparations. Taken with good Venice Treacle, it is good against Plague, driving forth the Malignity by sweat.

The Spirituous Tincture is good against Plague, Fevers, Colic, and Griping of the Guts, whether in Young or Old.

Dose, 2 to 3 drachms in Canary or other fit vehicle.

The Acid Tincture is an excellent Antiscorbutick, good against Vapors and Tumors which cause fiery Eruptions. Causes a good Appetite and a strong Digestion. To be given in all the patient drinks, so many drops as may give the Liquor a grateful or pleasant acidity, and to be continued for some time.

The Saline Tincture cures Scabs, Pimples, Leprosy, etc., by bathing or well washing the parts affected therewith, as hot as can be endured, and continuing for some considerable time.

The Powder of the Seed. Stronger than the Powder of the Herb, prevalent against the Dropsy, being given daily with 10 to 12 grains of Scammony. A drachm of the simple powder, morning and night, especially in an infusion of Senna, may do wonders in Melancholy.

¶ *Other Fumitories.*

American Fumitory (*Fumaria Indica,* or *Codder Indian*) of Virginia and Canada has the virtues of Common Fumitory, but is more bitter and more powerful. The tuberous American or Indian Fumitory is much weaker.

Bulbous Fumitory, so-called, is *Adoxa Meschatellina,* and belongs to the *Octandria* class.

The Lyre Flower of Japan and Siberia (*Dicentra* or *F. spectabilis*) belongs to the Fumitory Order.

F. cucullaria (Naked- talked Fumitory) is a native of Canada.

F. fungosa (Spongy-flowered Fumitory) is a native of North America.

F. mobilis (Great-flowered Fumitory) is a native of Siberia.

F. sempervirens (Glaucous Fumitory) is a native of North America.

F. lutea (Yellow Fumitory) is a native of Barbary.

F. Sibirica (Siberian Fumitory) is a native of Siberia.

F. capnoides (White-flowered Fumitory) is a native of South Europe.

F. enneaphylla (White-flowered Fumitory) is a native of Spain and Italy.

F. capreolata (Ramping Fumitory) is a native of Provence, Silesia and Britain.

F. spicula (Narrow-leaved Fumitory) is a native of Spain, Portugal, Italy, and France.

F. claviculata (Climbing Fumitory) is a native of Southern Europe and Britain.

F. vesicaria (Bladdered Fumitory) is a native of the Cape of Good Hope.

F. parviflora (Small-flowered Fumitory) is a native of hot countries. Rare in Britain.

F. densiflora is a native of Southern Europe and Britain.

Some of these differences may merely be due to situation.

In ancient history they are all included among medicinal species.

FUNGI

Fungi are those plants which are colourless; they have no green chlorophyll within them, and it is this green substance which enables the higher plants to build up, under the influence of sunlight, the starches and sugars which ultimately form our food. Having no chlorophyll, fungi cannot use the energy of the sun and must therefore adopt another method of life. They either live as parasites on other living plants or animals, or they live on decaying matter. In either case they derive their energy by breaking up highly complex substances and, when these are broken up in the living plant, the living plant suffers. Many Fungi, such as the bacteria, are microscopic; others form visible growths; from moulds and mildews to the familiar mushroom and toadstools they increase in size and conspicuousness.

Fungi differ from flowering plants in their chemical influence upon the air. They absorb oxygen and exhale carbonic acid, performing the same office in this respect as animals, which they most resemble in chemical composition. The odours they emit in decay are more like putrescent animal than vegetable matter. Some species, e.g., the Stinkhorns, emit a most intolerably offensive stench; others, on the contrary, are very agreeable to the smell and some 'toadstools' acquire in drying a fine aroma. They are quite as variable to the taste.

Numerically, Fungi rank next to flowering plants and in many portions of the globe far exceed them. In Great Britain, indeed, we have just over 5,000 species of Fungi, which number exceeds that of our flowering plants, ferns, mosses, lichens and algæ all added together.

¶ *Uses of Fungi.* The uses of Fungi are various. Their office in the organized world is to check exuberance of growth, to facilitate decomposition, to regulate the balance of the component elements of the atmosphere, to promote fertility and to nourish myriads of the smaller members of the animal kingdom. As disease producers, both in plants and animals, not excluding man himself, they are responsible for much damage; nor do they leave alone the works of man. The subject of Mycology (Fungology) is of growing importance and is attracting the attention of scientific research, especially in America, as to the action of Fungi in human diseases. The fact is recognized in medical science that more than 20 per cent. of tropical diseases, in the strict sense, are caused by Fungi and that the diseases due to Fungi are also not at all rare in temperate climates.

Certain of the species represent a danger to our existing food supply; the parasites on wheat and on potato plants have of recent years been the object of study by scientific agriculturists. The Imperial Bureau of Entomology, which grapples with injurious insects, has its counterpart in the Imperial Bureau of Mycology, which was inaugurated in 1920, and is equally effective in helping to control the fungus pests of our Colonies.

Yet all members of this great division of flowerless and chlorophyll-free plants are not harmful. Many of them perform useful and even beneficent functions, playing an important part in the welfare of humanity. Yeast, for instance, converts sugary solution into alcohol. Yeasts are everywhere and the various vintage wines are to some extent due to the particular yeast which is found amongst the grapes. Other Fungi (bacteria) help one to digest. As food plants, Fungi deserve more attention than they have received, at least in this country, although it has been estimated that we possess at least 200 edible forms. In ancient times the eating of Fungi was a common practice. The Romans especially favoured the *Boleti*, while Celsus makes allusion to the use of certain of the edible varieties. Throughout Europe and the East, Fungi are much more widely used as food than in Great Britain. In France, Germany, Italy and Japan the mushroom trade is officially recognized: in France, the *prefecture de police* has established a centre of inspection for mushrooms at the 'Halles' of Paris. Not only are all consignments of mushrooms entering this market inspected and passed before being put up for sale, but all amateur gatherers of Fungi may also have their spoil classified by the inspector free of charge, whereas a most useful addition to our food resources in this country is almost entirely neglected.

Formerly it was stated by enthusiastic fungus-eaters that Fungi contained more nitrogenous material than beef, but recent chemical analysis proves that the amount of nitrogenous matter that can be assimilated or used as food is actually but small and that Fungi practically contain no more flesh-forming material than does a cabbage. Notwithstanding this, Fungi have their special flavours, often combined with a very pleasant aroma, and in this way serve a purpose, like condiments, rendering more palatable other essential foods and often aiding their digestion and assimilation.

A considerable number of Fungi have been employed in *medicine*, and although Ergot alone represents these plants in the Pharmacopœia, yet the medicinal properties attributed by tradition to certain species of Fungi (as a writer in the *Lancet* pointed out, September 26, 1925) may possibly represent an untapped source of therapeutic value.

Up to the present time, no less than 64,000 species of Fungi have been described. They are divided into two great classes, the *Sporifera*, or spore-bearing, in which the spores are naked or exposed, and the *Sporidifera*, in which the spores are contained in bags or sacs called *asci*. The sporiferous division is by far the larger: in its family Hymenomycetes, which includes all the mushrooms and toadstools, the hymenium, or spore-bearing surface, is distributed over gills, tubes, pores or fissures. It is the most important group, both from the view of the toxicologist and the epicure, and comprises about 14,000 species.

The Agaricaceæ order of gill-bearing Fungi comprises about 4,600 species. Some members are poisonous, as the *Amanitas* (Fly and Deadly Agarics), whereas others, as *Agaricus*, *Cantharellus*, etc., are among the best edible varieties.

The name *Agaricum* (as it stands in Pliny) was applied by Dioscorides to a peculiar drug supplied by the *Polyporus* of the Larch, which was obtained principally, if not solely, from Agraria, a region in Sarmatia and which was formerly of considerable repute and is still to be had from herbalists. Other *Polypori* were often substituted for that of the larch, and the name *Agaricus* became to a certain extent generic for *Polyporus*, but was applied by Linnæus erroneously to the Toadstool class of Fungi bearing gills, and from that time adopted, though the earlier herbalists applied the name rightly to the corky tree Fungi, as Agaric of the Oak, etc.

¶ *Discrimination between Edible and Poisonous Fungi*. Of the 1,100 species of gill-bearing Fungi of the Mushroom type which are native to Great Britain, less than one hundred are known to be poisonous, though unfortunately these are mostly very virulent; and so it is essential, before attempting to enjoy the novelty of a dish of Fungi, to well study descriptions and figures of both edible and poisonous species, and not attempt to experiment on any unknown kind, as some of the really good and edible Fungi unfortunately *superficially* resemble extremely poisonous species.

There are no absolute *general* rules by which good or harmless Fungi can be distinguished, but there should be no difficulty in recognizing all the best kinds by means of ordinary care. In the Mushrooms and Toadstools, the gill-bearing Fungi, the colour of the gills and spores they contain are, for instance, of considerable importance and must be taken into account in determining a fungus. Hairs, scales, wool and gluten are found on the stem and cap of some species and present important data for identification. It must be noted, also, whether the stem is hollow or solid.

Many of the old statements as to the methods of distinguishing between edible and poisonous Fungi are quite valueless. It is quite an erroneous notion that only those Fungi are good to eat which grow in open places, and also that if the skin of the cap cannot be peeled off, as in the common Mushroom, a fungus is unfit for food, for many good species grow in woods (though comparatively few of these actually grow on trees), and in many excellent species which are constantly eaten there is no separable cuticle, whereas in numerous deadly species, it is as readily peeled off as in the Mushroom. Equally without foundation is the statement that if a silver spoon placed among Fungi that are cooking turns black, it is a proof that such Fungi are poisonous.

Good Fungi have usually a pleasant mushroomy odour, some have a smell of new meal, others a faint anise-like scent, or no particular odour at all. Evil-smelling Fungi are always to be regarded with distrust. It is a suspicious sign of dangerous qualities, if a fungus on being cut or bruised quickly turns deep blue or greenish, also if it is noticed that a small piece broken from a freshly-gathered fungus when tasted leaves, instead of an agreeable, nutty flavour, a sharp tingling on the tongue, or is in any way bitter. All such should be avoided. It is as well, also, not to eat any Fungi which contain a milky juice which exudes freely on being cut, without carefully identifying the species first, as some of these, belonging to the genus *Lactarius*, are dangerous, though one of them, dis-

tinguished by a reddish juice, ranks as one of the best.

The majority are acrid and dangerous, producing severe or even fatal gastric enteritis, due to the presence of an irritant resin. As, however, most species are used, when pickled, in considerable quantities almost indiscriminately by the Russians, it would seem that the dangerous properties are neutralized by the acid.

The *Amanita* genus of the large order Agaricaceæ was formerly included in the genus *Agaricus*, but is now generally recognized to be quite distinct. It is remarkable for including two closely-allied species which are respectively one of the best of our edible species, *Amanita rubescens*, the Blusher Toadstool, and certainly our most poisonous species: *A. phalloides*, the Deadly Agaric or Death Cap.

Species of *Amanita* are usually of large size, grown on the ground and speedily decay after maturity. In the most highly evolved species, the entire plant when young is enclosed in a universal veil, which remains intact until the stem, cap and gills are completely differentiated, when by increase in length of the stem and the expansion of the cap, it is ruptured, leaving a more or less loose sheath round the base of the stem called the *volva*. The upper part of the universal veil remains on the surface of the cap, where by the gradual expansion of the same, it is broken up into irregular patches, which in most cases remain throughout the life of the fungus, hence one of the popular names – Wart Caps. After the universal veil has been ruptured and the cap has commenced to expand, the secondary veil, or *velum*, may be seen as a firm, felted or interwoven membrane stretched between the upper part of the stem and the edge or margin of the cap. This secondary veil serves to protect the gills until the spores are formed, when by the gradual growth and straightening out of the edge of the cap, it breaks away from the edge of the cap and remains as a ring or collar round the stem. After these phases of development have passed, the cap expands to its full size, the stem attains its full length, the spores mature and are dispersed and the entire fungus rapidly decays. No other Agarics have a complete volva and ring present. Although one species of *Amanita* and various other Fungi possessing a volva are edible, yet the safest plan for those not familiar to them is to avoid all species possessing this organ.

The Amanitas may also be distinguished from the mushrooms by their white *lamellæ* or gills and the relatively thin edge of the cap.

The poisonous Amanitas should not be very liable to be mistaken for the mushroom, since the top of the cap is usually coloured, from yellow through shades of orange to red or occasionally olive brown. *A. phalloides*, though generally of a pale primrose yellow, is, however, frequently white, in which case its other characters must be depended on for recognition. The species, the Death Cap, is the most fatally poisonous of all Fungi, though it has a pleasant taste and smell and looks perfectly harmless. Its volva is partly a ragged, edged, basal cup, partly in scales upon the top of the cap, one or the other position predominating in different cases. It has a well-developed, partly drooping, white veil. It is one of the commonest found in our woods, liking damp spots.

A. muscaria, the 'Fly Agaric,' is one of our most handsome toadstools. The cap is large (4 to 6 inches) and spreads out quite horizontally. It is a brilliant scarlet, studded with scattered white scales, fragments of the volva in which it was wrapped when young. The white stem is thick and provided with a prominent ring. The skin of the cap is viscid, so that débris, such as pine-needles, stick to it. The gills underneath the cap are white, It is intensely poisonous and should be handled with great care. Poison extracted from it was once used for the destruction of flies and other insects – hence its name. Throughout the autumn, it may frequently be found, solitary and in groups, in birch and pine woods, in damp parts. Although justly considered injurious, it is used as a means of intoxication by the natives of Kamschatka. *A. pantherina* is used in Japan for like purposes.

This fungus is used in Homœopathy as *Agaricus* or *Aga*. Hahnemann, naming it 'Bug Agaric,' described it as 'surmounted with a scarlet-coloured top with white excrescences and white leaflets.'

Hahnemann's and his students' proving was published in Stapf's *Archives* in 1830, with some toxic symptoms, and *Aga* was included in Hahnemann's second edition of his *Chronic Diseases* as one of the antipsorics, and present-day homœopaths assert that its powers over such chronic affections as chorea and chilblains proves its right to the title. C. T. Allen (*Hom. Rec.*, March, 1913) has recorded the power of *Aga* to clear up certain cataracts. In this he used sometimes the ordinary preparations of *Aga* at other times *Agaricin*, or Agaric Acid.

A. Cæsarea (Cæsar's Mushroom), largely consumed in Southern Europe, is closely allied to the poisonous species and shares their general appearance, and it is in seeking for this that most of the recorded fatal mistakes are made. Its stem, veil and gills are yellow, and it has a white volva in the form of a cup.

The nature of Amanita toxin from *A. phalloides* is not yet determined, but poisons of a similar nature appear to be widespread throughout the whole genus.

Poisonous principles in Fungi.

The poisonous principles in Fungi may be divided into:

(1) Those acting purely upon the nerves, as *muscarine* and *fungus-atropine*.
(2) Those that produce local irritation, as various species of *Lactarius* and *Russula*.
(3) Those acting primarily upon the blood, as *helvellic acid* and *phallin*.

The most important constituents are the alkaloid Muscarine, especially in *A. muscaria* and the albuminoid Phallin, especially in *A. phalloides*, which appears to be related to serpent venom, though differing in its greater activity when absorbed through the stomach. The action of *A. muscaria* depends principally upon the alkaloid Muscarine, which prolongs the diastolic action of the heart and acts as a decided depressant upon the vaso-motor system and the respiratory centre. Muscarine has been employed as a remedy for epilepsy, but is probably of little value. It has also been used in the treatment of the nightsweats of phthisis: the reports as to its effect vary. When poisonous doses are taken, large doses of atropine should be injected by hypodermic syringe, external heat applied and the stomach pump or emetics promptly employed. Purgatives such as castor oil should be freely given as early as possible.

The symptoms produced by poisoning from eating *A. phalloides* are usually delayed for nearly twenty-four hours – they consist of great respiratory and circulatory depression; a cold heavy sweat breaks out, accompanied by severe headache and delirium often sets in. Jaundice may occur and a high temperature is frequent. Sometimes convulsions precede collapse. If Fly Agaric (*A. muscaria*) has been eaten, Muscarine poisoning is added to these symptoms, viz. profuse salivation, contracted pupils and slowing of pulse. Treatment consists in the administration of stimulants and the emptying of the alimentary canal by means of promptly-acting emetics and purges to prevent absorption. Atropine is to be freely used as an antidote.

The Polyporaceæ order of Tube-bearing Fungi includes about 2,000 species, many of which are parasites on trees and destructive to timber. Some are edible, as *Boletus*

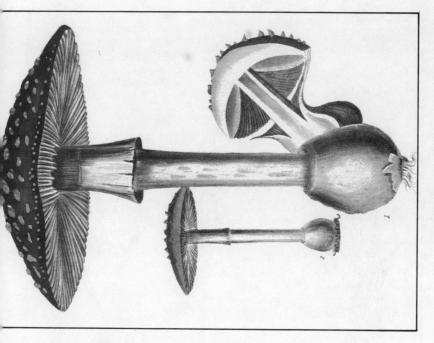

FUNGI (FLY AGARIC)
Amanita Muscaria

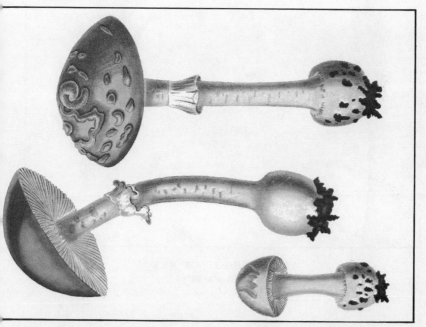

FUNGI
Amanita Muscaria (Var)

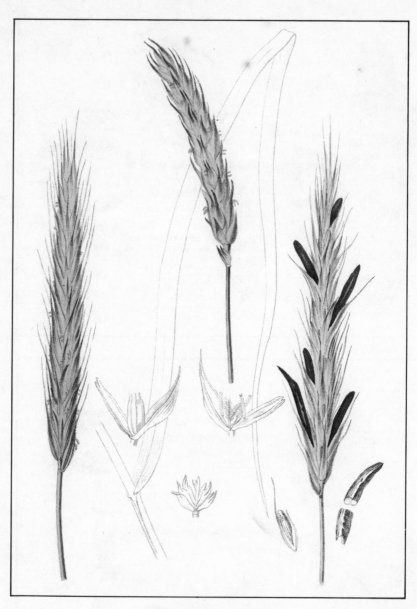

FUNGI—ERGOT OF RYE
Claviceps Purpurea

edulis, whereas others are poisonous, as *B. satanus.*

The genus *Polyporus*, which has its pores so closely packed and united together that they are not easily separable, is a very large one, containing very varied forms, some succulent, others very hard and dense, form and colour being as varied as the texture. In most cases there is no stem, and when present it is often lateral.

P. officinalis was once a celebrated drug, known as White Agaric, or Larch Agaric, but it is now little used, though it is still to be obtained in the herbalists' shops. The term 'Agaric' is, of course, more properly applied to the Fungi of the genus *Agaricus* (see above), but in medicine it has long been applied to this species of fungus, *P. officinalis* (Fries), syn. *B. laricis* (Jacqui.), *B. purgans* (Person), which is found upon the old trunks of the European Larch, and *Larix siberica* (Ledebour) of Asia. The same species is found upon various coniferous trees in some of the western United States and in British Columbia. It is stemless, of various sizes, from that of the fist to that of a child's head or even larger, hard and spongy, externally brown or reddish, but as found in commerce, deprived of its outer coat, it consists of a light, white, spongy somewhat farinaceous mass, which though capable of being rubbed into powder upon a sieve, is not easily pulverized in the ordinary way, as it flattens under the pestle. The best is considered to be that from Siberia, but it is probably produced wherever the European Larch grows. It is collected in the autumn, chiefly in the larch forests of Archangel, then dried, deprived of its firm, upper rind, and exported to Hamburg.

The powdered drug has a faint odour and a sweetish taste, which is afterwards bitter. It yields to boiling alcohol not less than 50 per cent. of a resinous extract, and when burnt yields not more than 2 per cent. of a white ash, rich in phosphates. White Agaric owes its medicinal virtues to Agaric acid, which is also called Laricic and Agaricinic acid. It contains a small amount of soft resin and from 4 to 6 per cent. of a fatty body. Sodium, Lithium and Bismuth Agaricinates have been prepared and introduced into medicine.

In moderate doses, Agaric acid is stated to have no effect upon the system except to paralyse the nerves of the sweat glands. Large doses act as an irritant to the stomach and intestines. The most important use of Agaric is in the treatment of sweats in wasting conditions such as phthisis. Its value in checking these profuse sweats has been confirmed by clinical experience. It is used in the preparation of *Tincture antiperiodica.* When Agaric acid is applied to abraded surfaces or mucous membrane, it acts as a distinct counter-irritant.

An Agaric growing on the *L. leptolepsis*, used in Japan as a sacred medicine, under the name of *Toboshi* or *Eburiko*, has been found to contain Agaric acid.

Under the name of Agaricin are marketed preparations containing the active Agaric acid with larger or smaller amount of impurities. The dose of the pure principle is from $\frac{1}{6}$ to $\frac{1}{2}$ of a grain.

P. suaveolens (on willows), *P. annosus* (on birches), *P. squamosus* and other species have apparently a similar composition and similar properties. *P. anthelminticus* (*Chu-tau* of the Chinese) is used as a worm-dispeller. *P. hirsutus*, or 'Pugak,' and *P. tinctorius* yield dye-stuffs.

B. chirurgorum (SURGEON'S AGARIC, OAK AGARIC, PUNK, TOUCHWOOD) is the product of *P. fomentarius*, which is found upon the oak and beech trees of Europe and is a very different substance, its uses being mechanical, as tinder, and to staunch bleeding.

It is shaped somewhat like the horse's foot, with a diameter of from 6 to 10 inches. It is soft like velvet when young, but afterwards becomes hard and ligneous. It usually rests immediately upon the bark of the tree, without any supporting foot-stalk. On the upper surface, it is smooth, but marked with circular ridges of different colours, more or less brown or blackish. On the under surface, it is whitish or yellowish and full of small pores; internally, it is fibrous, tough and of a tawny brown colour. It is composed of short, tubular fibres, compactly arranged in layers, one of which is added every year.

It is collected in Central and Southern Europe, in August and September, chiefly from oak and beech, the best being from oak and prepared for use by removing the exterior rind and cutting the inner part into thin slices, which are washed first in weak alkali, then in water and then beaten with a hammer and worked until they become soft, pliable and easily torn by the fingers. In this state, it was formerly much used by surgeons for arresting hæmorrhage, being applied with pressure. When it is steeped in a solution of nitre and afterwards dried, it constitutes 'Spunk,' 'punk' or tinder, the *Amadou* of the French, which occurs in flat pieces, of a consistence somewhat like that of very soft, rotten buckskin leather, of a brownish-yellow colour, capable of absorbing liquids and inflammable by the slightest spark. Though as a styptic, it has now gone out of use, as tinder it is still an article of commerce and in Northern Europe has been much used by smokers, manufactured also into fusees, and used to be found here in tobacconists' shops under the name of Amadou or German tinder.

Among its constituents are extractive, resin (in very similar proportion), nitrogenous matter, also in small quantity, potassium chloride and calcium sulphate, and in its ashes are found iron and calcium and magnesium phosphate.

Similar but harder products are yielded by *P. igniarius* and *P. marginatus*, the former internally rust-brown, or dark cinnamon-brown, the latter yellowish, but *P. fomentarius* is considered to supply the best Amadou.

P. squamosus, one of the large fan-shaped species with a lateral stem, that grows mostly on decayed oak trees and becomes very tough, has often, when carefully dried and cut, been used as a razor strop, *P. betulina*, a stemless variety found on birch trees, serving a like purpose. When quite young, they have been recommended as esculents, but cannot be said to be excellent.

Many trees, especially beeches, often bear a number of overlapping sulphur-coloured fungus tufts of the consistency of mellow cheese. This is *P. sulphureus*. When wounded, quantities of yellow juice exude, which has been used for dyeing. When dry, the fungus becomes covered with beautiful crystals of oxalate of potash and during decomposition, it is luminous. It is absolutely unfit for food.

The STRIPED STUMP FLAP (*Polystictus versicolor*), one of our commonest and most beautiful Fungi, is also poisonous. It has no stalk, but grows out horizontally in a bracket-like way, layer upon layer, from trunks and tree-stumps and branches.

The TINDER BRACKET (*Fomes fomentarius*) is one of the large Fungi which cause much destruction in beech forests. This species causes the condition of timber known as white rot. After doing serious damage to the interior wood, a dark, hoof-shaped knob bursts through the bark and spreads horizontally into an inverted bracket, a foot across, with a white layer of spore-bearing tubes on its flat underside.

A much larger beech fungus is the GIANT POLYPORE (*P. giganteus*), the largest of our Bracket Fungi, which attacks the roots and base of the trunks, demoralizing the foundations, so that a huge beech that appears to have the solidity of a lighthouse, is snapped across in the first severe gale. The external manifestation of the fungus is made in autumn, when about twenty handsome, overlapping, fleshy fans, a foot across, and of a pale brown tint, with darker zones, make their appearance at the base of the trunk. The pallid underside of the flaps becomes dark at once when bruised. Its esculent qualities are appreciated on the Continent.

The JEW'S EAR (*Hirneola auricula-Judæ*) has never been regarded here as an edible fungus, but in some parts of the world has that reputation. It is a somewhat gelatinous, flabby, thin, expanded saucer-like fungus of a brownish colour when fresh, more or less folded, the fructifying surface uppermost, spread all over the inequalities of the fungus. It is smooth in the inside and veined or plaited, having some resemblance to the human ear; minutely velvety outside and greyish olive in colour. It is thin and elastic when moist, rigid when dry. It varies in size from 1 to 3 inches across and is attached to the tree-bark by a point at the back, rather on one side.

Our native species had at one time a reputation for medicinal qualities and was on that account included in most of the old Herbals; for its astringent properties it was considered a cure for sore throats, and because of its faculty of absorbing and holding water like a sponge, was also used as a medium for applying eye-water and for similar purposes, but its virtues are no longer recognized, nor is it here regarded as an article of food, though it is in all probability edible, but a very closely allied species, *H. polytricha*, not uncommon in tropical and sub-tropical countries, is esteemed as a dainty by the Chinese, under the name of *Mu-esh*, and is one of the species of Fungi cultivated in China, where it grows wild on the bark of the wild cherry, but is cultivated on rotten poles of the China oak. It is of great commercial importance, the quantity annually produced being very large. It is largely used by the Chinese in soups with farinaceous seeds and also as a medicine, being highly valued. The demand for it is so large that much is imported into China from the small Pacific islands and especially from New Zealand, and its collection and exportation to China adds to the revenue of this part of the British Empire.

A fungus growing on the Elder, *Fungus sambuci*, has been used as a local application in conjunctivitis: according to Steckel, it is capable of taking up from nine to twelve times its weight of water. (*N.R. Pharm.*, XIII, 476, 1864.)

In the PUFF-BALLS (*Lycoperdon, Bovista*, etc.), belonging to the family Gasteromycetes, the hymenium remains completely enclosed in a continuous wall of *peridium* (Gr. *perideo*,

I wrap round) until the spores are fully formed, when the peridium is ruptured and the spore-producing portion of the fungus is enabled to liberate its spores. In the Puff-balls there is a specialized opening or mouth in the wall of the peridium through which the spores can escape into the air. There are also present, mixed with the dry mass of spores, certain very fine, elongated threads or *hyphæ*. This mass of thread is termed the *capillitium*, and is considered to assist in the expulsion of the spores.

The Puff-balls are distinctive enough to be readily recognized. Although generally wantonly kicked to pieces when found, they can be used as food, being excellent eating when young. Two species of *Bovista* are very common in pastures, resembling small balls, white when young, which when ripe discharge their dust-like spores from openings in the top of the peridium. In the GIANT PUFF-BALL (*L. gigantea*), instead of there being a well-defined opening at the apex, the upper part of the wall breaks away in irregular patches. This giant Puff-ball is often not larger than a moderately-sized turnip, but the size is very variable, ranging from 4 inches to a foot in diameter, and specimens are said to have been met with a yard in diameter. It is usually found singly, or only two or three together, among grass in pastures, meadows, etc. It forms a globose, white mass, depressed a little at the top, often puckered at the base, the wall thick, somewhat downy, becoming smooth and fragile, breaking away above and leaving a wide, irregular opening. The base is spongy. The mass of spores is yellow, then olive, finally brownish olive, the interspersed threads or *capillitium*, dark coloured, long and inter-twining.

Young Puff-balls in nearly all European countries but our own are used as food. Cut in slices, about $\frac{1}{2}$ inch thick, the outer skin peeled off, and dipped in egg and bread-crumbs and fried in butter, with salt and pepper, they are quite palatable and digestible. But it is only in the immature condition, whilst the interior remains fleshy and perfectly white, that they are edible, and on no account should any Puff-ball be cooked after the flesh has commenced discoloration, as poisonous properties are apt to be developed when old, even before decomposition sets in, so that it is essential they should be eaten only before the development of the spores. Gradually the flesh assumes a faint yellow tinge, deepening to canary yellow and in the dry, powdery condition to a brownish-olive colour. It is juicy and good about the end of July or in August, reaching the powdery state in September. The Giant Puff-ball is said to have been an article of diet among the North American Indians.

The smaller Puff-balls are not made use of, probably only on account of their small size, as they are not considered to be harmful, but the Giant Puff-balls, besides being edible, have been employed also in other ways.

The Puff-ball has a reputation in country districts for arresting hæmorrhage. In former times, it was not unusual among cottagers to find the woolly interior mass, with its profusion of minute, snuff-coloured spores, considered an excellent remedy to apply for the staunching of blood in wounds, pieces of Puff-ball being kept year after year for use in case of emergency, being bound over the wound and allowed to remain until healed. The smoke from the burning plant has been employed for the purpose of stupefying bees in order that their honey may be collected without difficulty. It was formerly thought to contain a narcotic principle, but it has been determined that the stupefying effect of the smoke is due to the presence of carbon dioxide. If inhaled in large amount, it causes anæsthesia and excessive quantities cause death by respiratory failure. A 25 per cent. tincture has been recommended in 1 drachm doses as a sedative in the treatment of nervous affections, but the drug is now considered of little importance in internal medicine. There is a tradition that in the days of flint and steel, housewives employed the dried substance of Puff-balls as tinder, Gerard remarking that 'In divers parts of England, where people dwell farre from neighbours, they carry them kindled with fire, which lasteth long.'

The spores prove very irritating to the nose and eyes if blown into the face when dry and powdery.

In the family Ascomycetes the spores are produced inside special cells or *asci*. The great majority of the species are minute and come under the definition of microscopic Fungi, and many of these are parasitic, and in many instances prove very destructive to cultivated plants: among such are the species causing Apple Scab, Potato Disease, American Gooseberry Mildew. Though none are known to be distinctly poisonous, except the fungus called ERGOT and a few others, very few are edible, those best known in this country being the large, fleshy MORELS and the subterranean TRUFFLES.

Under the name of *Lycoperdon Nuts*, HART'S TRUFFLE, or Deer Balls, a species closely allied to the Truffles, *Elophomyces granulatus*, had formerly some medicinal reputation, the drug being termed in old

Herbals *B. cervinus*, though it has nothing to do with the modern genus *Boletus*, belonging to the tube-bearing order Polyporaceæ. This old-fashioned drug was a few years ago offered in the London market, but it met with no sale. In the time of Dr. Pereira (middle of last century) it was stated by him that it was no longer used in medicine officially, but that he met with it in the stock of a London herbalist, and it was sold in Covent Garden as *Lycoperdon* nuts, so it could not long have gone out of use. It was formerly used by apothecaries for the preparation of *Balsamus apoplecticus*, and great power was ascribed to it in promoting parturition and the secretion of milk. Parkinson (*Theatrum Botanicum*, 1640) says the dose of it is 1½ drachms in powder, taken in sweet wine. An analysis by Biltz is given by Pereira, from which it appears to contain a bitter substance in the coat; sugar, inuline, and various salts of lime and ammonia, and some proteid substances. An excellent illustration is given of the drug in Pereira's *Materia Medica*, Vol. II, Part 1, 1850. According to Volg, *Pharmacognisie*, 1892, it is still used in Central Europe in veterinary medicine, and Ludwig and Busse (1869) found it to contain mannite, mycose, pectin, mycogum, mycodextrin and mycoinulin. The fungus is found in woods under pine-trees from June to October, and it may usually be detected by the presence of orange-yellow branched threads or hyphæ in the decayed leaf-mould where it occurs. It is brown and warty, about as large as a walnut, and purplish-brown internally.

Claviceps, or ERGOT, is one of the few species of Fungi that has sustained its reputation as a medicine, its value having been proved to be so considerable that it is official in all Pharmacopœias. It is the winter resting stage of *Claviceps purpurea*, parasitic on wheat, rye and various other grasses. The stigmas of the flower of a grass becomes infected by the spores of the fungus brought by some insect visiting the flower. The spore germinates on the stigma and the mycelium grows down into the ovary, where it appropriates the food intended to nourish the grain or seed that should normally develop there. Instead of this, the fungus grows out as a long, black, slightly curved body, the *sclerotium* (a mass of cells compacted into a solid body), which bears minute conidia on its surface. These conidia are carried by insects to other grasses which in turn become infected. When the grass is ripe, the black sclerotia fall to the ground, where they remain in an unaltered condition until the following spring, when they give origin to one or more sub-globose ascophores, or heads supported on slender stems. Spores produced by these ascophores escape and are carried by wind, etc., on to the stigmas of grasses and cereals, and the course of development commences anew.

The firm dark-coloured sclerotium, which when mature stands out conspicuously from the glumes of the ears of rye, constitutes the drug known as Ergot. It has attained its full development when the ears of rye have ripened, and is then collected by hand or separated from the grain, after it has been threshed, by specially designed machinery. After collection, it is carefully dried, and is then ready for use.

The drying of Ergot has to be carefully performed. Its quality is injuriously affected by too great drying, wherefore the official requirement that it be 'only moderately dried,' whereas incomplete drying subjects it to danger of mouldiness. Its oil is subject to rancidity, and insects are very liable to destroy it. The Pharmacopœia therefore directs it to be preserved in a close vessel and a few drops of chloroform added from time to time, and that it be not used after being kept longer than a year. It is very prone to chemical change if kept in a damp place.

The chief commercial varieties of the drug are the Russian, Spanish and German; but Austrian, Swiss, Norwegian and Swedish Ergots also come into the market occasionally. The Spanish drug is generally largest and of the finest appearance, but it contains much starch and is less active than Russian Ergot. The drug is dark violet-black, tapering towards both ends, longitudinally furrowed, especially on the concave side, breaks with a short fracture and is whitish within. The odour and taste are characteristic and disagreeable.

¶ *Constituents.* According to the most recent investigations, Ergot owes its activity to specific complex alkaloids, Ergotoxine and Ergotamine; in good Ergots the alkaloidal content may be 0·02. A large number of other substances have been isolated from Ergot, the most important (quantitatively) is a fatty oil, which occurs to the extent of 30 to 35 per cent. A red colouring matter, Sclererythrin, is extracted by alcohol and by alkalis and serves for the recognition of Ergot in flour. The drug also contains mannitol, partly combined as a glucoside, and the sugar trehalose. About 3 per cent. of ash is yielded.

¶ *Uses.* Ergot stimulates plain muscle, directly and indirectly throughout the body; its action on the uterus is like that on other plain muscle, and it is employed almost entirely to excite uterine contraction in the final stages of parturition. It is also employed, though rarely, to arrest internal hæmorrhage, but its use should be restricted to cases of uterine hæmorrhage, as it has been found to raise blood pressure in pulmonary and cerebral hæmorrhage.

It has a strongly sedative action on the central nervous system and has proved a useful remedy in delirium tremens and spinal congestion and has been employed in certain forms of asthma, hysteria, amenorrhœa and in menstrual disorders. It increases the secretion of milk and is used to check the night-sweats of phthisis.

It is usually administered in the form of extract (Ergotin), liquid extract, infusion or ammoniated tincture.

Ergot is scheduled under Part I of the Poisons Act. Its long-continued use is dangerous, resulting sometimes in gangrene, and it should only be used in the hands of fully qualified practitioners.

Sometimes a fatal gangrenous disease, known as Ergotism, has spread over large districts on the Continent, as if it were a visitation of the plague, as the result of eating bread made with grain which has been contaminated by Ergot.

Ergot was in olden times written *argot* in French, and there is little doubt that this is the origin of our name, the old French signification being 'a cock's spur,' to which Ergot has a marked similarity of form.

The earliest reference to Ergot is found in Loneer's 1582 edition of Rhodion's *Kreutterbuch*, where the occurrence of Ergot on rye and its obstetric virtues are mentioned. Camerarius about the same time stated that it was a popular remedy for accelerating parturition, and in France and Italy it was in quite general use for the same purpose for many years before it was employed by professional physicians. A Dutch physician used it for obstetric work in 1747; but the first to give it extended trials and to bring it under the notice of the profession in France was Dr. J. B. Desgranges of Lyons, in 1777. But it was not until Dr. J. Stearns, of New York, published his *Account of the 'Pulvis Parturiens (Secale cornutum),'* a remedy for quickening childbirth in 1805 that the knowledge of its value became general among English-speaking practitioners, and it was not until 1836 that it appeared in the London Pharmacopœia, as Ergota: *Acinula Clavus* (Fries).

In regard to the botanical history of Ergot, it was for a long time regarded merely as a malformation of the rye, due to luxuriance of sap or to insect bite. Its fungoid nature was first recognized by Baron Otto von Munchhausen in a work on *Rural Economy*, dated 1764. He placed it between the genera *Clavaria* and *Lycoperdon*. De Candolle definitely classified it as a fungus under the name of *Sclerotium clavus*, and Tulasne worked out its life-history and named it *Claviceps purpurea*.

Chemical investigations of Ergot go back to the eighteenth century, but the first of any importance was due to Vauquelin (*Ann. Chim. Phys.* 1816), and was doubtless suggested by the introduction of Ergot into scientific medicine.

Its purely vegetable origin was, however, still disputed, for Rennie, in the fourth edition (1837) of his *New Supplement*, after referring to De Candolle and Fries, adds that he has himself 'ascertained beyond doubt' that it is 'an exudation caused by the puncture of an insect – namely, *Aphis graminis*.'

Ergot can also be obtained from wheat and grasses, but that on Rye is alone official and is distinguished by its size, attaining a length often double that on other cereals, in which the sclerotium may not project at all.

¶ *Ustilago.* Innumerable 'smuts' of this and related genera are known and various specimens have been noted as poisonous, but the only other that has found a place in medicine is *Ustilago maydis* (Corn Smut or Corn Ergot), a very well-known substance wherever Indian Corn is grown, deforming the young ears into huge, misshapen, irregularly lobed, or branched bluish-black masses, covered by a delicate, transparent, shining, sometimes whitish skin, which encloses a brownish-black powder, consisting of innumerable spores.

Corn Smut is employed as an emmenagogue and parturient and has been used also in hæmorrhages of lungs and bowels.

GALANGAL

Alpinia officinarum (HANCE.)
N.O. Zingaberaceæ or Scilaminæ

Synonyms. Galanga. China Root. India Root. East India Catarrh Root. Lesser Galangal. Rhizoma Galangæ. Gargaut. Colic Root. Kæmpferia Galanga

Part Used. Dried rhizome

Habitat. China (Hainan Island), Java

¶ *Description.* The genus *Alpinia* was named by Plumier after Prospero Alpino, a famous Italian botanist of the early seventeenth century. The name Galangal is derived from the Arabic *Khalanjan*, perhaps a perversion of a Chinese word meaning 'mild ginger.'

The drug has been known in Europe for seven centuries longer than its botanical origin, for it was only recognized in 1870, when specimens were examined that had been found near Tung-sai, in the extreme south of China, and later, on the island of Hainan, just opposite. The name of *Alpinia officinarum* was given to the herb, as the source of Lesser Galangal. The Greater Galangal is a native of Java (*A. Galanga* or *Maranta Galanga*), and is much larger, of an orange-brown colour, with a feebler taste and odour. It is occasionally seen at London drug sales, but is scarcely ever used. There is also a resemblance to *A. calcarata*. The herb grows to a height of about 5 feet, the leaves being long, rather narrow blades, and the flowers, of curious formation, growing in a simple, terminal spike, the petals white, with deep-red veining distinguishing the lip-petal.

The branched pieces of rhizome are from $1\frac{1}{2}$ to 3 inches in length, and seldom more than $\frac{3}{4}$ inch thick. They are cut while fresh, and the pieces are usually cylindrical, marked at short intervals by narrow, whitish, somewhat raised rings, which are the scars left by former leaves. They are dark reddish-brown externally, and the section shows a dark centre surrounded by a wider, paler layer which becomes darker in drying. Their odour is aromatic, and their taste pungent and spicy. They are tough and difficult to break, the fracture being granular, with small, ligneous fibres interspersed throughout one side. The drug is exported, chiefly from Shanghai, in bales made of split cane, plaited,

and bound round with cane. The root has been used in Europe as a spice for over a thousand years, having probably been introduced by Arabian or Greek physicians, but it has now largely gone out of use except in Russia and India. Closely resembling ginger, it is used in Russia for flavouring vinegar and the liqueur 'nastoika': it is a favourite spice and medicine in Lithuania and Esthonia. Tartars prepare a kind of tea that contains it, and it is used by brewers. The reddish-brown powder is used as snuff, and in India the oil is valued in perfumery.

¶ *Constituents.* The root contains a volatile oil, resin, galangol, kæmpferid, galangin and alpinin, starch, etc. The active principles are the volatile oil and acrid resin. Galangin is dioxyflavanol, and has been obtained synthetically. Alcohol freely extracts all the properties, and for the fluid extract there should be no admixture of water or glycerin.

¶ *Medicinal Action and Uses.* Stimulant and carminative. It is especially useful in flatulence, dyspepsia, vomiting and sickness at stomach, being recommended as a remedy for sea-sickness. It tones up the tissues and is sometimes prescribed in fever. Homœopaths use it as a stimulant. Galangal is used in cattle medicine, and the Arabs use it to make their horses fiery. It is included in several compound preparations, but is not now often employed alone.

The powder is used as a snuff for catarrh.

¶ *Dosage.* From 15 to 30 grains in substance, and double in infusion. Fluid extract, 30 to 60 minims.

GALBANUM

Part Used. Gum resin
Habitat. Persia; also Cape of Good Hope

Ferula Galbaniflua (BOISS. ET BUHSE)
N.O. Umbelliferæ

¶ *Description.* There are two kinds of Galbanum in commerce, viz. Levant Galbanum and the Persian Galbanum. The latter is softer than the Levant, has a more terebinthic odour, has the smell and consistency of Venice turpentine, and contains fruit and fragments of stalks in place of bits of sliced roots. Several species of *Ferula* are used as a source for commercial Galbanum, but the official plant is *Ferula galbaniflua*, a perennial, with smooth stem, and shining leaflets, ovate, wedge-shaped, acute and finely serrated on the edges. The umbels of flowers are few, the seeds shiny.

The whole plant abounds with a milky juice, which oozes from the joints of old plants, and exudes and hardens from the base of the stem after it has been cut down, then

is finally obtained by incisions made in the root. The juice from the root soon hardens and forms the tears of the Galbanum of Commerce. The best tears are palish externally and about the size of a hazel nut and when broken open are composed of clear white tears. The taste is unpleasant, bitterish, acrid, with a strong, peculiar, somewhat aromatic smell. The common kind is an agglutinated mass, showing reddish and white tears, this is of the consistency of firm wax, and can easily be torn to pieces and softened by heat; when cold it is brittle, and mixed with seeds and leaves, when imported in lumps it is often considered preferable to the tears as it contains more volatile oil. Distilled with water it yields a quantity of essential oil, about 6 drachms, to 1 lb. of gum. It was well known to the ancients and Pliny called it 'bubonion.' Galbanum under dry distillation yields a thick oil of a bluish colour, which after purification becomes the blue colour of the oil obtained from the flowers of *Matricaria Chamomilla*.

¶ *Constituents.* Gum resin, mineral constituents, volatile oil, umbelliferine, galbaresino-tannol.

¶ *Medicinal Action and Uses.* Stimulant, expectorant in chronic bronchitis. Anti-spasmodic and considered an intermediate between ammoniac and asafœtida for relieving the air passages, in pill form it is specially good, in some forms of hysteria, and used externally as a plaster for inflammatory swellings.

¶ *Preparations and Dosage.* In pill form 10 to 20 grains, or as an emulsion, mixed with gum, sugar and water.

¶ *Other Species.* In Beyrout the people use the root of *F. Hermonic*, commonly known as Zalou root, as an aphrodisiac.

GALE, SWEET

Myrica Gale (LINN.)
N.O. Myricaceæ

Synonyms. Bayberry. English Bog Myrtle. Dutch Myrtle. Herba Myrti Rabanitini. Gale palustris (Chevalier)
Parts Used. Leaves, branches
Habitat. Higher latitudes of Northern Hemisphere; Great Britain, especially in the north; abundant on the Scottish moors and bogs

¶ *Description.* The badge of the Campbells. A deciduous, bushy shrub, growing to 4 feet high. The wood and leaves fragrant when bruised. The leaves, not unlike a willow or myrtle, are oblanceolate, tapering entire at the base, toothed and broadest at the apex, the upper side dark glossy green, the underside paler and slightly downy, under which are a few shining glands. The male plant produces flowers in May and June in crowded, stalkless catkins. The fruit catkins about the same size, but thicker, are closely-set, resinous nutlets, the flowers being borne on the bare wood of one year's growth. The sexes are on different plants. The leaves are often dried to perfume linen, etc., their odour being very fragrant, but the taste bitter and astringent. The branches have been used as a substitute for hops in Yorkshire and put into a beer called there 'Gale Beer.' It is extremely good to allay thirst. The catkins, or cones, boiled in water, give a scum beeswax, which is utilized to make candles. The bark is used to tan calfskins; if gathered in autumn, it will dye wool a good yellow colour and is used for this purpose both in Sweden and Wales. The Swedes use it in strong decoction to kill insects, vermin and to cure the itch. The dried berries are put into broth and used as spice. In China, the leaves are infused like tea, and used as a stomachic and cordial.

¶ *Constituents.* Said to contain a poisonous volatile oil and to have properties similar to those of *Myrica cerifera*.

¶ *Medicinal Action and Uses.* The leaves have been used in France as an emmenagogue and abortifacient.

¶ *Other Species.*
M. Gale, var. *tomentosa*. The young wood and leaves on both sides are very downy and specially so on the underside.
See BAYBERRY.

GALLS. *See* OAK GALLS, SUMACHS

GAMBOGE

Garcinia Hanburyii (HOOK)
N.O. Guttiferæ

Synonyms. Gutta gamba. Gummigutta. Tom Rong. Gambodia. Garcinia Morella
Part Used. Gum resin
Habitat. Siam, Southern Cochin-China, Cambodia, Ceylon

¶ *Description.* The commercial Gamboge is obtained from several varieties, though *Garcinia Hanburyii* is the official plant; an almost similar gum is obtained from Hypericum (St. Johnswort). The Gamboge tree grows to a height of 50 feet, with a diameter of 12 inches, and the gum resin is extracted by incisions or by breaking off the leaves and shoots of the trees; the juice, which is a milky yellow resinous gum, re-sides in the ducts of the bark and is gathered in vessels, and left to thicken and become hardened. Pipe Gamboge is obtained by letting the juice run into hollowed bamboos, and when congealed the bamboo is broken away from it. The trees must be ten years old before they are tapped, and the gum is collected in the rainy season from June to October. The term 'Gummi Gutta,' by which Gamboge is generally known, is de-

341

rived from the method of extracting it in drops. Gamboge was first introduced into England by the Dutch about the middle of the seventeenth century; it is highly esteemed as a pigment, owing to the brilliancy of its orange colour. It has no odour, and little taste, but if held in the mouth a short time it gives an acrid sensation. The medicinal properties of Gamboge are thought to be contained in the resin. It is official in the United States Pharmacopœia.

¶ *Constituents*. Resin gum, vegetable waste, garonolic acids; the gum is analogous to gum acacia.

¶ *Medicinal Action and Uses*. A very powerful drastic hydragogue, cathartic, very useful in dropsical conditions and to lower blood pressure, where there is cerebral congestion. A full dose is rarely given alone, as it causes vomiting, nausea and griping, and a dose of 1 drachm has been known to cause death. It is usually combined with other purgatives which it strengthens. A safe dose is from 2 to 6 grains, but in the treatment of tapeworm the dose is often as much as 10 grains. It provides copious watery evacuations with little pain, but must be used with caution. Dose, 2 to 5 grains in an emulsion or in an alkaline solution.

¶ *Other Species*.

The tree *G. Morella* is the Indian Gamboge; a gum resin is obtained from it; it has a similar action to Gamboge and is used as its equivalent in India and Eastern Colonies. Dose, $\frac{1}{2}$ to 2 grains.

GARLIC

Allium sativum (LINN.)
N.O. Liliaceæ

Synonym. Poor Man's Treacle
Part Used. Bulb

The Common Garlic, a member of the same group of plants as the Onion, is of such antiquity as a cultivated plant, that it is difficult with any certainty to trace the country of its origin. De Candolle, in his treatise on the *Origin of Cultivated Plants*, considered that it was apparently indigenous to the southwest of Siberia, whence it spread to southern Europe, where it has become naturalized, and is said to be found wild in Sicily. It is widely cultivated in the Latin countries bordering on the Mediterranean. Dumas has described the air of Provence as being 'particularly perfumed by the refined essence of this mystically attractive bulb.'

¶ *Description*. The leaves are long, narrow and flat like grass. The bulb (the only part eaten) is of a compound nature, consisting of numerous bulblets, known technically as 'cloves,' grouped together between the membraneous scales and enclosed within a whitish skin, which holds them as in a sac.

The flowers are placed at the end of a stalk rising direct from the bulb and are whitish, grouped together in a globular head, or umbel, with an enclosing kind of leaf or spathæ, and among them are small bulbils.

To prevent the plant running to leaf, Pliny (*Natural History*, XIX, 34) advised bending the stalk downward and covering it with earth; seeding, he observed, may be prevented by twisting the stalk.

In England, Garlic, apart from medicinal purposes, is seldom used except as a seasoning, but in the southern counties of Europe it is a common ingredient in dishes, and is largely consumed by the agricultural population. From the earliest times, indeed, Garlic has been used as an article of diet.

¶ *History*. Garlic was placed by the ancient Greeks (Theophrastus relates) on the piles of stones at cross-roads as a supper for Hecate, and according to Pliny garlic and onion were invocated as deities by the Egyptians at the taking of oaths.

It was largely consumed by the ancient Greeks and Romans, as we may read in Virgil's *Eclogues*. Horace, however, records his detestation of Garlic, the smell of which, even in his days (as much later in Shakespeare's time), was accounted a sign of vulgarity. He calls it 'more poisonous than hemlock,' and relates how he was made ill by eating it at the table of Mæcenas. Among the ancient Greeks, persons who partook of it were not allowed to enter the temples of Cybele. Homer, however, tells us that it was to the virtues of the 'Yellow Garlic' that Ulysses owed his escape from being changed by Circe into a pig, like each of his companions.

Homer also makes Garlic part of the entertainment which Nestor served up to his guest Machaon.

There is a Mohammedan legend that

'when Satan stepped out from the Garden of Eden after the fall of man, Garlick sprang up from the spot where he placed his left foot, and Onion from that where his right foot touched.'

There is a curious superstition in some parts of Europe, that if a morsel of the bulb be chewed by a man running a race it will prevent his competitors from getting ahead of

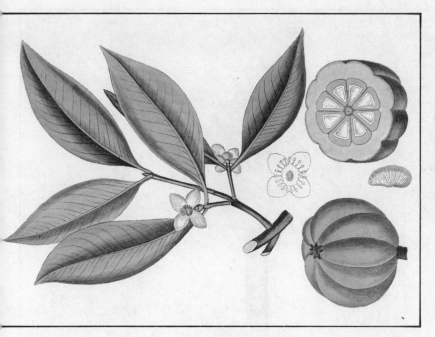

GAMBOGE
Garcinia Hanburyii

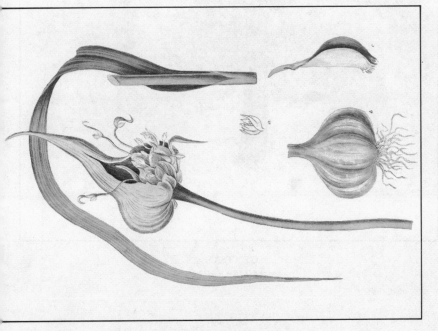

GARLIC
Allium Sativum

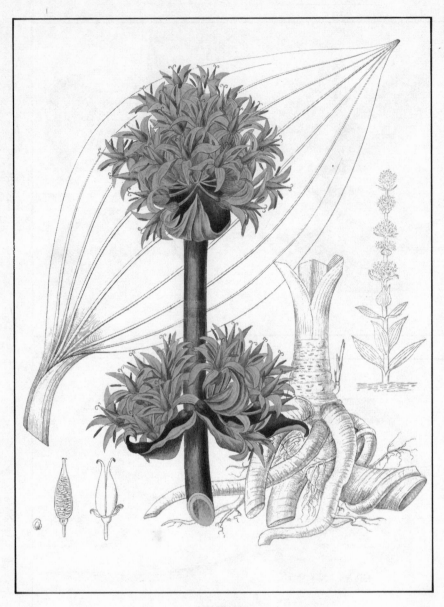

GENTIAN
Gentiana Lutea

him, and Hungarian jockeys will sometimes fasten a clove of Garlic to the bits of their horses in the belief that any other racers running close to those thus baited, will fall back the instant they smell the offensive odour.

Many of the old writers praise Garlic as a medicine, though others, including Gerard, are sceptical as to its powers. Pliny gives an exceedingly long list of complaints, in which it was considered beneficial, and Galen eulogizes it as the rustics' *Theriac*, or Heal-All. One of its older popular names in this country was 'Poor Man's Treacle,' meaning *theriac*, in which sense we find it in Chaucer and many old writers.

A writer in the twelfth century – Alexander Neckam – recommends it as a palliative for the heat of the sun in field labour, and in a book of travel, written by Mountstuart Elphinstone about 100 years ago, he says that

'the people in places where the Simoon is frequent, eat Garlic and rub their lips and noses with it when they go out in the heat of the summer to prevent their suffering from the Simoon.'

Garlic is mentioned in several Old English vocabularies of plants from the tenth to the fifteenth centuries, and is described by the herbalists of the sixteenth century from Turner (1548) onwards. It is stated to have been grown in England before the year 1540. In Cole's *Art of Simpling* we are told that cocks which have been fed on Garlic are 'most stout to fight, and so are Horses': and that if a garden is infested with moles, Garlic or leeks will make them 'leap out of the ground presently.'

The name is of Anglo-Saxon origin, being derived from *gar* (a spear) and *lac* (a plant), in reference to the shape of its leaves.

¶ *Cultivation.* The ground should be prepared in a similar manner as for the closely-allied onion.

The soil may be sandy, loam or clay, though Garlic flourishes best in a rich, moist, sandy soil. Dig over well, freeing the ground from all lumps and dig some lime into it. Tread firmly. Divide the bulbs into their component 'cloves' – each fair-sized bulb will divide into ten or twelve cloves – and with a dibber put in the cloves separately, about 2 inches deep and about 6 inches apart, leaving about 1 foot between the rows. It is well to give a dressing of soot.

Garlic beds should be in a sunny spot. They must be kept thoroughly free from weeds and the soil gathered up round the roots with a Dutch hoe from time to time.

When planted early in the spring, in February or March, the bulbs should be ready for lifting in August, when the leaves will be beginning to wither. Should the summer have been wet and cold, they may probably not be ready till nearly the middle of September.

The use of Garlic as an antiseptic was in great demand during the past war. In 1916 the Government asked for tons of the bulbs, offering 1s. per lb. for as much as could be produced. Each pound generally represents about 20 bulbs, and 5 lb. divided up into cloves and planted, will yield about 38 lb. at the end of the growing season, so it will prove a remunerative crop.

The following appeared in the *Morning Post* of December 12, 1922:

'A Dog's Recovery

'Mr. W. H. Butlin, Tiptree, records the following experience: A fox-terrier, aged 14 years, appeared to be developing rapidly a pitiable condition, with a swollen neck and an ugly intractable sore at the root of the tail, and dull, coarse coat shedding abundantly. I administered "Yadil Antiseptic" in his drinking water and in less than a month the dog became perfectly sound and well, a *mirabile dictu*, his coat became firm, soft, and glossy.' (Yadil is a patent medicine said to contain Garlic.)

'In cases of arterial tension, MM. Chailley-Bert, Cooper, and Debrey, at the Society of Biology, recommended about 30 drops of alcoholic extract as a remedy. To be administered by the mouth or intravenously.'

Although only the cultivated Garlic is utilized medicinally, all of the other species have similar properties in a greater or less degree. Several of the species of Allium are natives of this country.

The CROW GARLIC (*A. vineale*) is widely distributed and fairly common in many districts, but the bulbs are very small and the labour of digging them would be great. It is frequent in pastures and communicates its rank taste to mik and butter, when eaten by cows.

NOTE.—Professor Henslow calls *A. vineale* the Field Garlic, and *A. oleraceum* the Crow Garlic.

RAMSONS (*A. ursinum*) grows in woods and has a very acrid taste and smell, but it also has very small bulbs, which would hardly render it of practical use.

Ransoms is also very generally known as 'Broad-leaved Garlic.'

The FIELD GARLIC (*A. oleraceum*) is rather a rare plant. Both this and the Crow Garlic have, however, occasionally been employed as potherbs or for flavouring. It is an old country notion that if crows eat Crow Garlic, it stupefies them.

Ramsons, the wild Wood Garlic, but for its evil smell would rank among the most beautiful of our British plants. Its broad leaves are very similar to those of the Lily-of-the-Valley, and its star-like flowers are a dazzling white, but its odour is too strong to admit of it being picked for its beauty, and many woods, especially in the Cotswold Hills, are spots to be avoided when it is in flower, being so closely carpeted with the plants that every step taken brings out the offensive odour.

There are many species of Allium grown in the garden, the flowers of some of which are even sweet-smelling (as *A. odorum* and *A. fragrans*), but they are the exceptions, and even these have the Garlic scent in their leaves and roots.

¶ *Constituents.* The active properties of Garlic depend on a pungent, volatile, essential oil, which may readily be obtained by distillation with water. It is a sulphide of the radical Allyl, present in all the onion family. This oil is rich in sulphur, but contains no oxygen. The pecular penetrating odour of Garlic is due to this intensely smelling sulphuret of allyl, and is so diffusive that even when the bulb is applied to the soles of the feet, its odour is exhaled by the lungs.

¶ *Medicinal Action and Uses.* Diaphoretic, diuretic, expectorant, stimulant. Many marvellous effects and healing powers have been ascribed to Garlic. It possesses stimulant and stomachic properties in addition to its other virtues.

As an antiseptic, its use has long been recognized. In the late war it was widely employed in the control of suppuration in wounds. The raw juice is expressed, diluted with water, and put on swabs of sterilized Sphagnum moss, which are applied to the wound. Where this treatment has been given, it has been proved that there have been no septic results, and the lives of thousands of men have been saved by its use.

It is sometimes externally applied in ointments and lotions, and as an antiseptic, to disperse hard swellings, also pounded and employed as a poultice for scrofulous sores. It is said to prevent anthrax in cattle, being largely used for the purpose.

In olden days, Garlic was employed as a specific for leprosy. It was also believed that it had most beneficial results in cases of smallpox, if cut small and applied to the soles of the feet in a linen cloth, renewed daily.

It formed the principal ingredient in the 'Four Thieves' Vinegar,' which was adapted so successfully at Marseilles for protection against the plague when it prevailed there in 1722. This originated, it is said, with four thieves who confessed, that whilst protected by the liberal use of aromatic vinegar during the plague, they plundered the dead bodies of its victims with complete security.

It is stated that during an outbreak of infectious fever in certain poor quarters of London, early last century, the French priests who constantly used Garlic in all their dishes, visited the worst cases with impunity, whilst the English clergy caught the infection, and in many instances fell victims to the disease.

Syrup of Garlic is an invaluable medicine for asthma, hoarseness, coughs, difficulty of breathing, and most other disorders of the lungs, being of particular virtue in chronic bronchitis, on account of its powers of promoting expectoration. It is made by pouring a quart of water, boiled hot, upon a pound of the fresh root, cut into slices, and allowed to stand in a closed vessel for twelve hours, sugar then being added to make it of the consistency of syrup. Vinegar and honey greatly improve this syrup as a medicine. A little caraway and sweet fennel seed bruised and boiled for a short time in the vinegar before it is added to the Garlic, will cover the pungent smell of the latter.

A remedy for asthma, that was formerly most popular, is a syrup of Garlic, made by boiling the bulbs till soft and adding an equal quantity of vinegar to the water in which they have been boiled, and then sugared and boiled down to a syrup. The syrup is then poured over the boiled bulbs, which have been allowed to dry meanwhile, and kept in a jar. Each morning a bulb or two is to be taken, with a spoonful of the syrup.

Syrup made by melting 1½ oz. of lump sugar in 1 oz. of the raw expressed juice may be given to children in cases of coughs without inflammation.

The successful treatment of tubercular consumption by Garlic has been recorded, the freshly expressed juice, diluted with equal quantities of water, or dilute spirit of wine, being inhaled antiseptically.

Bruised and mixed with lard, it has been proved to relieve whooping-cough if rubbed on the chest and between the shoulder-blades.

An infusion of the bruised bulbs, given before and after every meal, has been considered of good effect in epilepsy.

A clove or two of Garlic, pounded with honey and taken two or three nights successively, is good in rheumatism.

Garlic has also been employed with advantage in dropsy, removing the water which may already have collected and preventing its future accumulation. It is stated that some dropsies have been cured by it alone.

If sniffed into the nostrils, it will revive a hysterical sufferer. Amongst physiological results, it is reported that Garlic makes the eye retina more sensitive and less able to bear strong light.

The juice of Garlic, and milk of Garlic – made by boiling the bruised bulbs in milk – is used as a vermifuge.

¶ *Preparations.* Juice, 10 to 30 drops. Syrup, 1 drachm. Tincture, ½ to 1 drachm.

Wine of Garlic – made by macerating three or four bulbs in a quart of proof spirit – is a good stimulant lotion for baldness of the head.

Used in cookery it is a great aid to digestion, and keeps the coats of the stomach healthy. For this reason, essential oil is made from it and is used in the form of pills.

If a very small piece is chopped fine and put into chicken's food daily, it is a sure preventative of the gapes. Pullets will lay finer eggs by having garlic in their food *before* they start laying, but when they commence to lay it must be stopped, otherwise it will flavour the eggs.

See ONION, ASAFETIDA.

Mrs. Beeton (in an old edition of her *Household Management*, 1866) gives the following recipe for making 'Bengal Mango Chutney,' which she states was given by a native to an English lady who had long been a resident in India, and who since her return to England had become quite celebrated amongst her friends for the excellence of this Eastern relish.

Ingredients. 1½ lb. moist sugar, ¾ lb. salt, ¼ lb. Garlic, ¼ lb. onions, ¾ lb. powdered ginger, ¼ lb. dried chillies, ¾ lb. dried mustard-seed, ¾ lb. stoned raisins, 2 bottles of best vinegar, 30 large, unripe, sour apples.

Mode. The sugar must be made into syrup; the Garlic, onions and ginger be finely pounded in a mortar; the mustard-seed be washed in cold vinegar and dried in the sun; the apples be peeled, cored and sliced, and boiled in a bottle and a half of the vinegar. When all this is done, and the apples are quite cold, put them into a large pan and gradually mix the whole of the rest of the ingredients, including the remaining half-bottle of vinegar. It must be well stirred until the whole is thoroughly blended, and then put into bottles for use. Tie a piece of wet bladder over the mouths of the bottles, after which they are well corked. This chutney is very superior to any which can be bought, and one trial will prove it to be delicious.

(*POISON*)
GELSEMIUM

Gelsemium nitidum (MICH.)
N.O. Loganiaceæ

Synonyms. Yellow Jasmine. Gelsemium Sempervirens (Pers.). False Jasmine. Wild Woodbine. Carolina Jasmine

Part Used. Root

Habitat. Gelsemium is one of the most beautiful native plants of North America, occurring in rich, moist soils, by the sides of streams, along the seacoast from Virginia to the south of Florida, extending into Mexico

The important drug *Gelsemium*, official in the principal Pharmacopœias, is composed of the dried rhizome and root of *Gelsemium nitidum* (Michaux), a climbing plant growing in the southern States of North America and there known as Yellow Jasmine, though it is in no way related to the Jasmines, and is best distinguished as Caroline Jasmine, as it belongs to the Loganiaceæ, an order that forms a connecting link between the orders Gentianaceæ, Apocynaceæ, Scrophulariaceæ and Rubiaceæ. The plant is not to be confounded with the true Yellow Jasmine (*Jasminum odoratissimum*), of Madeira, which is often planted in the southern States for the sake of its fragrant flowers and has also been known there under the name of Gelseminum; this has only two stamens, while Gelsemium has five.

¶ *Description.* Its woody, twining stem often attains great height, its growth depending upon its chosen support, ascending lofty trees and forming festoons from one tree to another. It contains a milky juice and bears opposite, shining and evergreen lanceolate leaves and axillary clusters of from one to five large, funnel-shaped, very fragrant yellow flowers, which during its flowering season, in early spring, scent the atmosphere with their delicious odour. The fruit is composed of two separable, jointed pods containing numerous, flat-winged seeds.

The stem often runs underground for a considerable distance, and these portions (the rhizome) are used indiscriminately with the roots in medicine, and exported from the United States in bales.

The plant was first described in 1640 by John Parkinson, who grew it in his garden from seed sent by Tradescant from Virginia; at the present time it is but rarely seen, even in botanic gardens, in Great Britain, and specimens grown at Kew have not flowered.

¶ *Description of the Drug.* The drug in commerce mostly consists of the underground stem or rhizome, with occasional pieces of the root. The rhizome is easily distinguished by occurring in nearly straight pieces, about 6 to 8 inches long, and $\frac{1}{4}$ to $\frac{3}{4}$ inch in diameter, having a small dark pith and a purplish-brown, longitudinally fissured bark. The root is smaller, tortuous, and of a uniform yellowish-brown colour, finely wrinkled on the surface.

Both rhizome and root in transverse section exhibit a distinctly radiate appearance, the thin cortex or bark enclosing a large, pale, yellowish-white wood, which consists of narrow bundles with small pores, alternating with straight, whitish, medullary rays about six or eight cells in thickness. In the case of the rhizome, a small pith, frequently divided into four nearly equal parts, is also present, particularly in smaller and younger pieces.

The drug is hard and woody, breaking with an irregular splintery fracture, and frequently exhibits silky fibres in the bast, which are isolated, or occur in groups of two or three and form an interrupted ring, whereas in the aerial stem, they are grouped in bundles.

The drug has a bitter taste, due to the presence of alkaloids, which occur chiefly in the bark. The slight aromatic odour is probably due to the resin in the drug.

¶ *Collection. Adulterations.* The drug is commonly collected in the autumn and dried. Though consisting usually of the dried rhizomes with only the larger roots attached, sometimes smaller roots are present, and it is often adulterated with the aerial portions of the stem, which can be easily detected by the thinness and dark-purplish colour of the latter. It is stated to be destitute of alkaloid and therefore of no medicinal value.

Similar roots of Jasmine, especially those of *Jasminum fruticans*, are sometimes intermixed, and can be distinguished by the absence of indurated pith cells, which occur in Gelsemium, by the abundance of thin-walled starch cells in the pith and in the medullary ray cells (those of Gelsemium being thick-walled and destitute of starch), and by the bast fibres round the sieve tubes.

¶ *Constituents.* Gelsemium contains two potent alkaloids, Gelseminine and Gelsemine.

Gelseminine is a yellowish, bitter and poisonous amorphous alkaloid, readily soluble in ether and alcohol, forming amorphous salts.

The alkaloid Gelsemine is colourless, odourless, intensely bitter and forms crystalline salts. It is only sparingly soluble in water, but readily forms a hydrochloride, which is completely so. This alkaloid is not to be confounded with the resinoid known as 'Gelsemin,' an eclectic remedy, a mixture of substances obtained by evaporating an alcoholic extract of Gelsemium to dryness.

The rhizome also contains Gelsemic acid, a crystalline substance which exhibits an intense bluish-green fluorescence in alkaline solution; it is probably identical with methyl-æsculatin or chrysatropic acid found in Belladonna root.

There are also present in the root 6 per cent. of a volatile oil, 4 per cent. of resin and starch.

¶ *Poisoning by Gelsemium.* The drug is a powerful spinal depressant; its most marked action being on the anterior cornus of grey matter in the spinal cord.

The drug kills by its action on the respiratory centre of the medulla oblongata. Shortly after the administration of even a moderate dose, the respiration is slowed and is ultimately arrested, this being the cause of death.

Poisonous doses of Gelsemium produce a sensation of languor, relaxation and muscular weakness, which may be followed by paralysis if the dose is sufficiently large. The face becomes anxious, the temperature subnormal, the skin cold and clammy and the pulse rapid and feeble. Dropping of the upper eyelid and lower jaw, internal squint, double vision and dilatation of the pupil are prominent symptoms. The respiration becomes slow and feeble, shallow and irregular, and death occurs from centric respiratory failure, the heart stopping almost simultaneously. Consciousness is usually preserved until late in the poisoning, but may be lost soon after the ingestion of a fatal dose. The effects usually begin in half an hour, but sometimes almost immediately. Death has occurred at periods varying from 1 to $7\frac{1}{2}$ hours.

The treatment of Gelsemium poisoning consists in the prompt evacuation of the stomach by an emetic, if the patient's condition permits; and secondly, and equally important, artificial respiration, aided by the early administration, subcutaneously, of ammonia, strychnine, atropine or digitalis.

An allied species, *G. elegans* (Benth.) of Upper Burma, is used in China as a criminal poison; its effects are very rapid.

¶ *Medicinal Action and Uses.* Antispasmodic, sedative, febrifuge, diaphoretic.

The medical history of the plant is quite modern. It is stated to have been brought into notice by a Mississippi planter, for whom, in his illness, the root was gathered in mistake for that of another plant. After partaking of an infusion, serious symptoms arose, but when, contrary to expectations, he recovered, it was clear that the attack of bilious fever from which he had been suffering had disappeared. This accidental error led to the preparation from the plant of a proprietary nostrum called the 'Electric Febrifuge.' Later, in 1849, Dr. Porcher, of South Carolina, brought Gelsemium to the notice of the American Medical Association. Dr. Henry, in 1852, and after him many others, made provings of it, the chief being that of Dr. E. M. Hale, whose *Monograph on Gelsemium* was an efficient help to the true knowledge of the new American drug.

In America, it was formerly extensively used as an arterial sedative and febrifuge in various fevers, more especially those of an intermittent character, but now it is considered probably of little use for this purpose, for it has no action on the skin and no marked action on the alimentary or circulatory system.

It has been recommended and found useful in the treatment of spasmodic disorders, such as asthma and whooping cough, spasmodic croup and other conditions depending upon localized muscular spasm. In convulsions, its effects have been very satisfactory.

It is, at present, mainly used in the treatment of neuralgic pains, especially those involving the facial nerves, particularly when arising from decaying teeth.

It is said it will suspend and hold in check muscular irritability and nervous excitement with more force and power than any known remedy. While it relaxes all the muscles, it relieves, by its action on the general system, all sense of pain.

The drug is also said to be most useful in the headache and sleeplessness of the drunkard and in sick headache.

It has been used in dysmenorrhœa, hysteria, chorea and epilepsy, and the tincture has been found efficacious in cases of retention of urine.

Some recommend its use in acute rheumatism and pleurisy, in pneumonia and in bronchitis, and it has been advocated, though not accepted by all authorities, as of avail in the early stages of typhoid fever.

GENTIANS

The Gentians are an extensive group of plants, numbering about 180 species, distributed throughout all climates, though mostly in temperate regions and high mountains, being rare in the Arctic. In South America and New Zealand, the prevailing colour of the flower is red, in Europe blue (yellow and white being of rarer occurrence).

N.O. Gentianaceæ

The name of the genus is derived from Gentius, an ancient King of Illyria (180–167 B.C.), who, according to Pliny and Dioscorides, discovered the medicinal value of these plants. During the Middle Ages, Gentian was commonly employed as an antidote to poison. Tragus, in 1552, mentions it as a means of diluting wounds.

GENTIAN, YELLOW

Gentiana lutea (LINN.)

Part Used. Root

Habitat. The Yellow Gentian is a native of the Alpine and sub-alpine pastures of central and southern Europe, frequent in the mountains of Spain and Portugal, the Pyrenees, Sardinia and Corsica, the Apennines, the Mountains of Auvergne, the Jura, the lower slopes of the Vosges, the Black Forest and throughout the chain of the Alps as far as Bosnia and the Balkan States. It does not reach the northern countries of the Continent, nor the British Isles. At an elevation of from 3,000 to 4,500 feet, it is a characteristic species of many parts of France and Switzerland, where, even when not in flower, the numerous barren shoots form conspicuous objects: the leaves are at first sight very similar to *Veratrum album*, the White Hellebore, which is its frequent companion. Out of Europe, the plant occurs in the mountains of Lydia. In some parts it occupies large tracts of country, being untouched by any kind of cattle.

All the known species are remarkable for the intensely bitter properties residing in the root and every part of the herbage, hence they are valuable tonic medicines. That most commonly used in Europe is *Gentiana lutea*, the Yellow Gentian. The root of this species is the principal vegetable bitter employed in medicine, though the roots of several other species, including our native ones, are said to be equally efficacious. Before the introduction of hops, Gentian, with many other bitter herbs, was used occasionally in brewing.

Gentian roots are collected and dried in central and southern Europe, much of the supply for this country having formerly come from Germany, though it is also imported from Switzerland, France and Spain, and French Gentian is considered of special excellence.

Yellow Gentian is one of the many herbs

347

so far not cultivated in England for medicinal use, though preparations of the root are in constant use in every dispensary, and it is much prescribed also by veterinary surgeons. Though the plant is indigenous in central Europe, it can readily be grown from seed in England, and could quite easily be cultivated as a garden or field crop in this country. Though not often met with, it has been grown in gardens since the time of Gerard, who tells us that a learned French physician sent him from Burgundy plants of this species for his garden on Holborn Hill. It is a highly ornamental plant, forming one of the most stately hardy herbaceous perennials for the garden border, and when successfully treated will grow luxuriantly, even if in the neighbourhood of London.

¶ *Description.* The root is long and thick, generally about a foot long and an inch in diameter, but sometimes even a yard or more long and 2 inches in diameter, of a yellowish-brown colour and a very bitter taste. The stem grows 3 or 4 feet high or more, with a pair of leaves opposite to one another, at each joint. The lowest leaves have short foot-stalks, but the upper ones are stalkless, their bases almost embracing the stem. They are yellowish-green in colour, oblong in shape and pointed, rather stiff, with five prominent veins on the underside, and diminish gradually in size as they grow up the stem. The large flowers are in whorls in the axils of the uppermost few pairs of leaves, forming big orange-yellow clusters. The corollas are wheel-shaped, usually five-cleft, 2 inches across, sometimes marked with rows of small brown spots, giving a red tinge to the otherwise deep yellow. Seeds in abundance are produced by strong plants, and stock is easily raised from them.

¶ *Cultivation.* For the successful cultivation of *G. lutea*, a strong, loamy soil is most suitable, the deeper the better, as the stout roots descend a long way down into the soil. Plenty of moisture is also desirable and a position where there is shelter from cold winds and exposure to sunshine. Old plants have large crowns, which may be divided for the purpose of propagation, but growing it on a large scale, seeds would be the best method. They could be sown in a frame, or in a nursery bed in a sheltered part of the garden and the young seedlings transplanted. They take about three years to grow to flowering size. It is, however, likely that the roots are richest in medicinal properties before the plants have flowered. A big clump of *G. lutea* is worthy of a conspicuous position in any large flower garden, quite apart from its medicinal value.

¶ *Part Used.* The rhizome and roots collected in autumn and dried. When fresh, they are yellowish-white externally, but gradually become darker by slow drying. Slow drying is employed to prevent deterioration in colour and to improve the aroma. Occasionally the roots are longitudinally sliced and quickly dried, the drug being then pale in colour and unusually bitter in taste, but this variety is not official.

The dried root as it occurs in commerce is brown and cylindrical, 1 foot or more in length, or broken up into shorter pieces, usually $\frac{1}{2}$ inch to 1 inch in diameter, rather soft and spongy, with a thick reddish bark, tough and flexible, and of an orange-brown colour internally. The upper portion is marked with numerous rings, the lower longitudinally wrinkled. The root has a strong, disagreeable odour, and the taste is slightly sweet at first, but afterwards very bitter.

¶ *Substitutes. G. purpurea, G. pannonica, G. punctata* and *G. acaulis* are European gentians having similar medicinal properties to *G. lutea* and are used indiscriminately with each other and the official root, from which they differ but little in appearance, though are somewhat smaller.

American Gentian root is derived from *G. puberula, G. saponaria* and *G. Andrewsii.* This drug is said to have properties practically identical with those of European varieties.

Belladonna and Aconite roots, and the rhizomes of Orris and White Hellebore have been found mixed with the genuine root, and the powdered root of commerce is frequently adulterated, ground almond shells and olive stones having been used for this purpose.

¶ *Constituents.* The dried Gentian root of commerce contains Gentiin and Gentiamarin, bitter glucosides, together with Gentianic acid (gentisin), the latter being physiologically inactive. Gentiopicrin, another bitter glucoside, a pale yellow crystalline substance, occurs in the fresh root, and may be isolated from it by treatment with boiling alcohol. The saccharine constituents of Gentian are dextrose, lævulose, sucrose and gentianose, a crystallizable, fermentable sugar. It is free from starch and yields from 3 to 4 per cent. ash.

¶ *Medicinal Action and Uses.* Gentian is one of the most useful of our bitter vegetable tonics. It is specially useful in states of exhaustion from chronic disease and in all cases of general debility, weakness of the digestive organs and want of appetite. It is one of the best strengtheners of the human system, and is an excellent tonic to combine with a purgative to prevent its debilitating effects. Many dyspeptic complaints are more effectually relieved by Gentian bitters than by Peruvian Bark. It is of extreme value in jaundice and is prescribed extensively.

Besides being unrivalled as a stomachic tonic, Gentian possesses febrifuge, emmenagogue, anthelmintic and antiseptic properties, and is also useful in hysteria, female weakness, etc. Gentian with equal parts of Tormentil or galls has been used with success for curing intermittent fever.

As a simple bitter, Gentian is considered more palatable combined with an aromatic, and for this purpose orange peel is frequently used. A tincture made with 2 oz. of the root, 1 oz. of dried orange peel, and ½ oz. bruised cardamom seeds in a quart of brandy is an excellent stomachic tonic, and is efficacious in restoring appetite and promoting digestion. A favourite form in which Gentian has been administered in country remedies is as an ingredient in the so-called Stockton bitters, in which Gentian and the root of Sweet Flag play the principal part.

The dose of the fluid extract is ½ to 1 teaspoonful in water, three times daily.

Fresh Gentian root is largely used in Germany and Switzerland for the production of an alcoholic beverage. The roots are cut, macerated with water, fermented and distilled; the distillate contains alcohol and a trace of volatile oil, which imparts to it a characteristic odour and taste.

¶ *Preparations and Dosages.* Fluid extract, ½ to 1 drachm. Compound infusion, B.P., ½ to 1 oz. Compound tincture, B.P. and U.S.P., ½ to 1 drachm. Solid extract, B.P., 2 to 8 grains.

Culpepper states that our native Gentians 'have been proved by the experience of divers physicians not to be a whit inferior in virtue to that which comes from beyond sea.'

Gentian

'comforts the heart and preserves it against faintings and swoonings: The powder of the dry roots helps the biting of mad dogs and venomous beasts. . . . The herb steeped in wine, and the wine drank, refreshes such as be over-weary with traveling, and grow lame in their joints, either by cold or evil lodgings: it helps stitches, and griping pains in the sides: is an excellent remedy for such as are bruised by falls . . . when Kine are bitten on the udder by any venomous beast, do but stroke the place with the decoction of any of these and it will instantly heal them.'

In the eighteenth century Gentian wine was drunk as an aperitif before dinner.

Gentiana scabræ

GENTIAN, JAPANESE
    Synonym. Ryntem Root
    Part Used. Root

¶ *Description.* The rhizome is dark greyish brown, attaining about 10 cm. in length and 5 mm. in diameter. It is irregularly annulate, and bears on the top stem-bases occasionally stem-remnants, and on the lateral and lower sides numerous roots. The cross-section of the rhizome is dark brown, and shows in the wood fibro-vascular bundles, running irregularly. The roots are brownish-yellow, attaining about 20 cm. in length and 3 mm. in diameter, and longitudinally wrinkled. The cross-section of the root is brown, having a darker coloured wood, which shows radially arranged trachea at the periphery. It does not contain sclerenchymatous cells; the parenchymatous cells contain many oxalate crystals, but no starch grains. It has a very bitter taste. It may be used as a substitute for radix gentianæ. (From *The Chemist and Druggist* of August 19, 1922.)

GENTIAN, AUTUMN
    Synonyms. Bitterwort. Felwort. Baldmoney
    Part Used. Root

The Autumn Gentian (*Gentiana amarella*, Linn.) is not uncommon in calcareous soils and in dry pastures, in most parts of Europe,

¶ *Other Species.*
    The two most frequently found native Gentians are *Gentiana amarella*, the Autumn Gentian, and *G. campestris*, the Field Gentian, which were formerly pronounced by both Linnæus and Scopoli to be merely variations of the same species, but are now universally described as separate species.

Both have been used for their bitterness instead of hops, and also as a medicine, in common with others of the same genus, and the dried root and dried herb of the Field Gentian are still sold by herbalists for use as a bitter tonic, having the same properties as the foreign Gentian. The old English names for these Gentians – Bitterwort and Felwort (Fel being an old word for the gall) – testify to their bitter qualities being popularly known.

Gentiana amarella (LINN.)

flowering from July to September. It has an annual root, twisted and yellowish, somewhat thready. The stem is square, erect, bearing several pairs of stalkless, dark green leaves, each with three prominent veins, and clothed from top to bottom with flowers on short stalks in the axils of the leaves, one flower terminating the stem. The calyx is pale, with green ribs, divided half-way down into five lance-shaped, nearly equal segments. The corolla is salver-shaped, blue-purple in

colour, the tube quite as long as the calyx, and five-cleft, the lobes being nearly equal; the mouth of the tube is provided with a purple, upright fringe, which conceals the stamens. In sunshine, the lobes of the corolla are spread wide horizontally, forming conspicuous blue stars.

GENTIAN, FIELD

Synonyms. Bitterroot. Felwort
Part Used. Root

Gentiana campestris (LINN.)

The Field Gentian (*Gentiana campestris*, Linn.) resembles the Autumn Gentian in general character, though the plant is as a rule smaller, 4 to 12 inches high. Its stems are erect and much branched, the branches long, with leaves and flowers scattered the whole length, whereas *G. amarella*, when branched, has the branches short, even the lower ones not exceeding the length of the leaves from which they spring, and the upper ones mostly much shorter. The flowers are fewer in number than those of *amarella*, though larger and on longer flower-stalks. The essential difference between the species, however, is that both calyx and corolla are

four-cleft in *G. campestris*, the two outer, oval lobes of the calyx being also much larger, completely enfolding and concealing the two smaller ones, which are not a fifth part as broad. The salver-shaped corolla is of a dull purplish colour, fringed in the throat, as in *G. amarella*. The roots are small, but penetrate some distance into the soil. This species grows in pastures, particularly near the sea, but is not so much confined to a calcareous soil as *G. amarella*. It is an annual, and flowers in August and September. This is the principal species used by the peasantry in Sweden in lieu of hops in brewing beer.

GENTIAN, MARSH

Part Used. Root

Gentiana Pneumonanthe (LINN.)

The Marsh Gentian (*Gentiana Pneumonanthe*, Linn.), though occasionally found on moist, boggy heaths, is a plant of much more local occurrence in Great Britain than the two previous species. Its stems are 3 to 18 inches high, the leaves 1 to 2 inches long. The flowers, 1½ to 2 inches long, are rather few in number, pale blue externally, with five paler stripes and dark, vivid blue within, variegated with white in the throat. Gerard

tells us of this pretty little plant, which is quite worthy of cultivation, that 'the gallant flowers hereof bee in their bravery about the end of August,' and goes on to say that 'the later physicians hold it to be effectual against pestilent diseases and the bitings and stingings of venomous beasts.' It has the bitterness and other qualities of the preceding species.

This variety grows in moist places on heaths near Swanage, Dorset.

GENTIAN, SPRING

Part Used. Root

Gentiana Verna

The flowers are of such a startling blue that A. C. Benson has described it as 'the pure radiance of the untroubled heaven.'

The flowers grow singly on exceedingly short stalks, and only open if the sun is shining, when they stretch their blue petals wide and face the blue above them. There is a narrow, green calyx-cup and a blue tube issuing therefrom which opens out into five lobes star-wise. The leaves grow in pairs, stalkless, clasping the stem. They are not very numerous on the short flower-stalks, but form close rosettes of foliage near the soil. The flower-stems are rigidly erect, about 4 to

12 inches being their usual height. It flowers in April and May and is to be found in Westmorland, but is not so much at home in England as it is on Irish soil; it grows in profusion, too, on the Isle of Arran. It likes limestone and chalky ground.

We have only six varieties of Gentians in Great Britain, one of which (*G. nivalis*) is found on the Breadalbane and Clora Mountains. Another species (*G. acaulis*) most nearly resembles our *G. Pneumonanthe*. The flowers are bright blue and rather elongated, 1 to 2 inches in length.

GENTIAN, CROSS-LEAVED   Gentiana cruciata
   Part Used. Root

Gentiana cruciata (Cross-leaved Gentian), so called because its leaves grow in the form of a cross, has been recommended in hydro-phobia. In homœopathic medicine a tincture of the root is used in hoarseness and sore throat.

GENTIAN, FIVE-FLOWERED   Gen tiana quinqueflora
   Part Used. Root

A tincture is also made from the fresh flowering plant of *Gentiana quinqueflora* (Five-flowered Gentian) and used in homœo-pathy as a tonic and stomachic, and in intermittent fevers.

See also CENTAURY.

GERANIUM. *See* CRANESBILL

GERMANDER, SAGE-LEAVED   Teucrium scorodonia (LINN.)
                                         N.O. Labiatæ

Synonyms. Wood Sage. Large-leaved Germander. Hind Heal. Ambroise. Garlic Sage
Part Used. Herb
Habitat. Sage-leaved Germander (*Teucrium scorodonia*) is a common woodland plant in healthy districts. It is a native of Europe and Morocco, found in woody and hilly situations among bushes and under hedges, where the soil is dry and stony. It is frequent in such places in most parts of Great Britain, flowering from July to September

¶ *Description.* The roots are perennial and creeping, the stems square, a foot or two in height, of a shrubby character, with opposite greyish-green, sage-like leaves, in form somewhat oblong heart-shaped, the edges coarsely toothed, very much wrinkled in texture like those of the Sage, hence its familiar names, Wood Sage and Sage Germander.

The whole plant is softly hairy or pubescent. The small labiate flowers are in one-sided spike-like clusters, the corollas greenish-yellow in colour, with four stamens, which have yellow anthers, and very noticeable purple and hairy filaments. The terminal flowering spike is about as long again as those that spring laterally below it from the axils of the uppermost pair of leaves.

The generic name of *Teucrium* was bestowed by Linnæus, it has been suggested, from a belief that this plant is identical with the plant that Dioscorides says was first used medicinally by an ancient king of Troy, named Teucer, but it is also said that Linnæus named the genus after a Dr. Teucer, a medical botanist.

The specific name, *scorodonia*, is derived from the Greek word for Garlic, and does not appear to be particularly appropriate to this species.

It has been popularly called ' Hind Heal,' from a theory that the hind made use of it when sick or wounded, and was probably the same herb as *Elaphoboscum*, the Dittany taken by harts in Crete.

In taste and smell, the species resembles Hops. It is called 'Ambroise' in Jersey, and used there and in some other districts as a substitute for hops. It is said that when this herb is boiled in wort the beer becomes clear sooner than when hops are made use of, but that it is apt to give the liquor too much colour.

The bitter taste is due to the presence of a peculiar tonic principle found in all the species of this genus.

There are about 100 species of *Teucrium* widely dispersed throughout the world, but chiefly abounding in the northern temperate and subtropical regions of the Eastern Hemisphere. Of the three other British species besides the Wood Sage, two have been used medicinally, *T. Chamædrys* (Wall Germander), a famous old gout medicine, and *T. Scordium* (Water Germander).

¶ *Cultivation.* Wood Sage is generally collected in the wild state, but will thrive in any moderately good soil, and in almost any situation.

It may be increased by seeds, by cuttings, inserted in sandy soil, under a glass, in spring and summer; or by division of roots in the autumn.

¶ *Part Used.* The whole herb, collected in July.

¶ *Constituents.* A volatile oil, some tannin and a bitter principle.

¶ *Medicinal Action and Uses.* Alterative and diuretic, astringent tonic, emmenagogue. Much used in domestic herbal practice for skin affections and diseases of the blood, also in fevers, colds, inflammations, and as an emmenagogue.

Fluid extract, ½ to 1 drachm.

It is useful for quinsy, sore throat, and in kidney and bladder trouble.

In chronic rheumatism it has been used with benefit, and is considered a valuable tonic and restorer of the system after an attack of rheumatism, gout, etc.

The infusion (freshly prepared) is the proper mode of administration, made from 1 oz. of the dried herb to 1 pint of boiling water, taken warm in wineglassful doses, three or four times a day.

Wood Sage is an appetizer of the first order, and as a tonic will be found equal to Gentian. It forms an excellent bitter combined with Comfrey and Ragwort, which freely influences the bladder.

It is also good to cleanse old sores. If used in the green state with Comfrey and Ragwort, the combination makes an excellent poultice

GERMANDER, WALL

Synonyms. Petit Chêne. Chasse fièvre
Part Used. Whole herb

The Common or Wall Germander (*Teucrium Chamædrys*) is a native of many parts of Europe, the Greek Islands and also of Syria, being found near Jerusalem, but in England is scarce and hardly indigenous, being chiefly found on the ruins of old buildings and in other places where it has escaped from cultivation. It was formerly much cultivated in this country for medicinal purposes.

¶ *Description*.—The roots are perennial and creeping, the square stem, 6 to 18 inches high, erect, much branched, leafy. The opposite, dark green leaves are ½ to 1½ inch long and indented, somewhat like an oak leaf, hence the name Chamædrys, from *chamai* (ground) and *drus* (oak). The name Germander is considered also to be a corruption of Chamædrys. The French term this plant *Petit Chêne*, from the shape of the leaves, as well as *Chasse fièvre*, from its use in medicine.

The rose-coloured, labiate flowers, which bloom in June and July, are in three to six flowered whorls, in the axils of leafy bracts, and in leafy, terminal spikes. The whole plant is almost roughly hairy.

The fresh leaves are bitter and pungent to the taste and when rubbed, emit a strong odour somewhat resembling garlic.

¶ *Cultivation*. Germander will grow in almost any soil and is propagated by seeds, by cuttings taken in spring or summer, and by division of roots, in the autumn. Plant about a foot apart each way.

¶ *Part Used*. The whole herb, collected in July and dried in the same manner as Wood Sage.

¶ *Medicinal Action and Uses*. Stimulant, tonic, diaphoretic, diuretic. Germander acts as a slight aperient, as well as a tonic.

for old wounds and inflammations in any part of the body. Culpepper tells us:

'The decoction of the green herb with wine is a safe and sure remedy for those who by falls, bruises or blows suspect some vein to be inwardly broken, to disperse and void the congealed blood and consolidate the veins. The drink used inwardly and the herb outwardly is good for such as are inwardly or outwardly bursten, and is found to be a sure remedy for the palsy. The juice of the herb or the powder dried is good for moist ulcers and sores. It is no less effectual also in green wounds to be used upon any occasion.'

A snuff has been made from its powdered leaves to cure nasal polypi.

Teucrium Chamædrys (LINN.)
N.O. Labiatæ

The reputation of Germander as a specific for gout is of very old date, the Emperor Charles V having been cured by a decoction of this herb taken for sixty days in succession.

It has been employed in various forms and combinations, of which the once celebrated Portland Powder is one of the chief instances.

It was also used as a tonic in intermittent fevers, and is recommended for uterine obstructions.

The expressed juice of the leaves, with the addition of white wine, is held to be good in obstruction of the viscera.

Possessing qualities nearly allied to those of Horehound, a decoction of the green herb, taken with honey, has been found useful in asthmatic affections and coughs, being recommended for this purpose by Dioscorides. The decoction has also been given to relieve dropsy in its early stages.

Culpepper tells us that it is

'most effectual against the poison of all serpents, being drunk in wine and the bruised herb outwardly applied. . . . Used with honey it cleanseth ulcers and made into an oil and the eyes anointed therewith, taketh away dimness and moisture. It is also good for pains in the side and cramp. . . . The decoction taken for four days driveth away and cureth tertian and quartan agues. It is also good against diseases of the brain, as continual headache, falling sickness, melancholy, drowsiness and dulness of spirits, convulsions and palsies.'

He further states that the powdered *seeds* are good against jaundice. The tops, when in flower, steeped twenty-four hours in white wine will destroy worms.

GERMANDER, WATER

Teucrium Scordium (LINN.)
N.O. Labiatæ

Part Used. Herb

The Water Germander (*Teucrium Scordium*) is a creeping plant growing in marshy places in various parts of Europe, but very rare in Great Britain except in the Isle of Ely. It was formerly cultivated in gardens for medicinal uses.

¶ *Description.* The square, hairy stalks, are of a dirty green colour and very weak. The leaves are short, broad, woolly and soft, and indented at the edges. The flowers are small, of a purplish-rose colour, in whorls, in the axils of the leaves. It flowers in July and August.

The whole plant is bitter and slightly aromatic.

The fresh leaves, when rubbed, have a penetrating odour, like Garlic, and it is said that when cows eat it through hunger, it gives the flavour of Garlic to their milk.

¶ *Medicinal Action and Uses.* It was once esteemed as an antidote for poisons and as an antiseptic and anthelmintic, but is now scarcely used, though its tonic and aromatic bitter qualities and diaphoretic action make a decoction of it an excellent remedy in all inflammatory diseases, and it may be used with advantage in weak, relaxed constitutions.

The tincture in small doses is considered a good remedy for exhilarating and rousing torpid faculties.

For intermittent fever and scrofulous complaints the infusion of 1 oz. of the dried herb to 1 pint of boiling water, taken in wineglassful doses, is recommended.

The dried leaves have been employed as a vermifuge, and decoction is said to be a good fomentation in gangrenous cases.

¶ *Preparation.* Fluid extract, $\frac{1}{2}$ to 1 drachm.

GINGER

Zingiber officinale (ROSC.)
N.O. Zingiberaceæ

Part Used. Root
Habitat. Said to be a native of Asia. Cultivated in West Indies, Jamaica, Africa

¶ *Description.* Naturalized in America after the discovery of that country by the Spaniards. Francisco de Mendosa transplanted it from the East Indies into Spain, where Spanish-Americans cultivated it vigorously, so that in 1547 they exported 22,053 cwt. into Europe.

It is now cultivated in great quantities in Jamaica and comes into this country dried and preserved. The root from the West Indies is considered the best. Also imported from Africa, there are several varieties known in commerce. Jamaica or White African is a light-brown colour with short rhizome, very pungent. Cochin has a very short rhizome, coated red-grey colour. 'Coated or Uncoated' is the trade term for peel on or skinned. Green Ginger is the immature undried rhizome. Preserved Ginger is made by steeping the root in hot syrup. Ratoon is uncultivated Ginger. Ginger is a perennial root which creeps and increases underground, in tuberous joints; in the spring it sends up from its roots a green reed, like a stalk, 2 feet high, with narrow lanceolate leaves; these die down annually. The flowering stalk rises directly from the root, ending in an oblong scallop spike; from each spike a white or yellow bloom grows. Commercial Ginger is called black or white, according to whether it is peeled or unpeeled; for both kinds the ripened roots are used, after the plant has died down. The black are scalded in boiling water, then dried in the sun. The white (best) are scraped clean and dried, without being scalded. For preserve young green roots are used; they are scalded and are washed in cold water and then peeled. The water is changed several times, so that the process takes three or four days. The tubers are then put into jars and covered with a weak syrup; this is changed after a few days' soaking for a stronger syrup, which is again changed for a still stronger one. The discarded syrups are fermented and made into a liquor called 'cool drink'; a few drops of chloroform or chloride are generally added to the preserve to prevent insects breeding in it. Ginger flowers have an aromatic smell and the bruised stem a characteristic fragrance, but the root is considered the most useful part of the plant, and must not be used under a year's growth. The peeling has to be done very thinly or the richest part of the resin and volatile oil is lost. It is sometimes soaked in lime-juice instead of plain water, and the colour is improved by a final coating of chalk. The Chinese fresh Ginger is grated into powder. African and Cochin Ginger yield the most resin and volatile oil. The root must be kept in a dry place, or it will start growing and is then spoilt. The odour of Ginger is penetrating and aromatic, its taste spicy, hot and biting; these properties are lost by exposure. The most common adulterants are flour, curcuma, linseed, rapeseed, the hulls of cayenne pepper and waste ginger.

¶ *Constituents.* Volatile oil, acrid soft resin, resin insoluble in ether and oil, gum, starch, lignin, vegeto matter, asmazone, acetic acid, acetate of potassa, sulphur.

¶ *Medicinal Action and Uses.* Stimulant, carminative, given in dyspepsia and flatulent colic, excellent to add to bitter infusions; specially valuable in alcoholic gastritis; of use for diarrhœa from relaxed bowel where there is no inflammation. Ginger Tea is a hot in-fusion very useful for stoppage of the menses due to cold, externally it is a rubefacient. Essence of Ginger should be avoided, as it is often adulterated with harmful ingredients.

¶ *Dosage. Infusion:* ½ oz. bruised or powdered root to 1 pint boiling water is taken in 1 fluid ounce. Dose, 10 to 20 grains.

¶ *Preparation:* Fluid extract, 10 to 20 drops. Tincture, B.P., ½ to 1 drachm. Syrup, B.P. and U.S.P., ½ to 1 drachm. Oleoresin, U.S.P., ½ grain.

GINGER, WILD

Asarum Canadense (LINN.)
N.O. Aristolochiaceæ

Synonyms. Canada Snakeroot. Indian Ginger. Coltsfoot
Parts Used. Rhizome dried and roots
Habitat. North America, North Carolina, Kansas

¶ *Description.* An inconspicuous but fragrant little plant, not over 12 inches high, found growing in rich soil on roadsides and in woods. A stemless perennial, much resembling the European Asarum, but with larger leaves, provided with a short spine, leaves usually only two, kidney-shaped, borne on thin fine hairy stems, dark above and paler green under-surface, 4 to 8 inches broad, strongly veined. A solitary bell-shaped flower, dull brown or brownish purple, drooping between the two leaf stems, woolly, the inside darker than the outside and of a satiny texture, the fruit a leathery six-celled capsule. It has a yellowish creeping rootstock, slightly jointed, with thin rootlets from the joints. In commerce the rootstock is found in pieces 4 to 5 inches long, ⅛ inch thick, irregular quadrangular, brownish end wrinkled outside, whitish inside, showing a large centre pith hard and brittle, breaking with a short fracture. Odour fragrant, taste aromatic, spicy and slightly bitter—it is collected in the autumn.

¶ *Constituents.* A volatile oil once largely used in perfumery, also resin, a bitter principle called asarin, mucilage, alkaloid, sugar and a substance like camphor.

The plant yields its properties to alcohol and to hot water.

¶ *Medicinal Action and Uses.* Stimulant, carminative, diuretic, diaphoretic. Used in chronic chest complaints, dropsy with albuminaria, painful spasms of bowels and stomach.

¶ *Dosage.* ½ oz. of the powdered root in 1 pint of boiling water, taken hot, produces copious perspiration.

Dry powder, 20 to 30 grains.

As an adjuvant to tonic mixtures or infusions, ½ to 1 drachm.

¶ *Other Species.*

ASARUM EUROPÆUM (*Syn.* Hazlewort; Wild Nard, very similar in properties to above).

¶ *Part Used.* Root and leaves dried.

¶ *Description.* A European plant growing in most hilly woods, flowering from May till August. The root smells like pepper, with a spicy taste and gives an ash-coloured powder. The leaves give a green powder and have the same properties as the root.

¶ *Medicinal Action and Uses.* Emetic, cathartic and errhine, for which latter purpose it is principally used in affections of the brain, eyes, throat, toothache and paralysis of the mouth. In France drunkards use it as an emetic, and it promotes sneezing and is therefore helpful for colds in the head.

¶ *Dosage.* Powder, 10 to 12 grains. As an emetic, ½ to 1 drachm.

A. ARIFOLIUM yields an oil with the odour of sassafras.

See ASARABACCA.

GINSENG

Panax quinquefolium (LINN.)
N.O. Araliaceæ

Synonyms. Aralia quinquefolia. Five Fingers. Tartar Root. Red Berry. Man's Health
Part Used. Root
Habitat. Ginseng is distinguished as Asiatic or Chinese Ginseng. It is a native of Manchuria, Chinese Tartary and other parts of eastern Asia, and is largely cultivated there as well as in Korea and Japan

Panax, the generic name, is derived from the Greek *Panakos* (a panacea), in reference to the miraculous virtue ascribed to it by the Chinese, who consider it a sovereign remedy in almost all diseases.

It was formerly supposed to be confined to

Chinese Tartary, but now is known to be also a native of North America, from whence Sarrasin transmitted specimens to Paris in 1704.

The word ginseng is said to mean 'the wonder of the world.'

¶ *Description*. The plant grows in rich woods throughout eastern and central North America, especially along the mountains from Quebec and Ontario, south to Georgia. It was used by the North American Indians. It is a smooth perennial herb, with a large, fleshy, very slow-growing root, 2 to 3 inches in length (occasionally twice this size) and from ½ to 1 inch in thickness. Its main portion is spindle-shaped and heavily annulated (ringed growth), with a roundish summit, often with a slight terminal, projecting point. At the lower end of this straight portion, there is a narrower continuation, turned obliquely outward in the opposite direction and a very small branch is occasionally borne in the fork between the two. Some small rootlets exist upon the lower portion. The colour ranges from a pale yellow to a brownish colour. It has a mucilaginous sweetness, approaching that of liquorice, accompanied with some degree of bitterness and a slight aromatic warmth, with little or no smell. The stem is simple and erect, about a foot high, bearing three leaves, each divided into five finely-toothed leaflets, and a single, terminal umbel, with a few small, yellowish flowers. The fruit is a cluster of bright red berries.

The plant was first introduced into England in 1740 by the botanist Collinson.

Chinese Ginseng is a larger plant, but presents practically the same appearance and habits of growth. Its culture in the United States has never been attempted, though it would appear to be a promising field for experiment.

Father Jartoux, who had special privileges accorded him in the study of this plant, says that it is held in such esteem by the natives of China, that the physicians deem it a necessity in all their best prescriptions, and regard it as a remediable agency in fatigue and the infirmities of old age. Only the Emperor has the right to collect the roots. The prepared root is chewed by the sick to recover health, and by the healthy to increase their vitality; it is said to remove both mental and bodily fatigue, to cure pulmonary complaints, dissolves tumours and prolongs life to a ripe old age.

Father Jartoux was satisfied that its praise was justified, and he adds his own testimony to its efficacy in relieving fatigue and increasing vitality. The roots are called, by the natives of China, *Jin-chen*, meaning 'like a man,' in reference to their resemblance to the human form. The American Indian name for the plant, *garantoquen*, has the same meaning.

Owing to the enormous demand for the root in China recourse was had to the American species, *Panax quinquefolium* (Linn.), and in 1718 the Jesuits of Canada began shipping the roots to China, and the first shipment from North America to Canton yielded enormous profits. In 1748 the roots sold at a dollar a pound in America and nearly five in China. Afterwards, the price fluctuated, but the root is still eagerly purchased by Chinese traders for export to China, and at the present time commands a yet higher price in the American markets, though it is not an official medicine and has only a place in the eclectic Materia Medica. The American Consul at Amoy stated a few years ago that it is possible to market twenty million dollars worth of American Ginseng annually to China, if it could be produced; but since its collection for exportation, it has been so eagerly sought that it has become exterminated in many districts where it was formerly abundant.

This has led to its cultivation and to various devices for preserving the natural supply. In Canada a fine is imposed for collecting between January and the 1st of September. Among the Indians, it is customary to collect the root only after the maturity of the fruit and to bend down the stem before digging the root, thus providing for its propagation. Indian collectors assert that a large number of such seeds will germinate, and that they have been able to increase their area of collection by this method.

In 1876, 550,624 lb. were exported at an average price of 1 dollar 17 cents; the amount available for export since then has steadily decreased and the price has gone up in proportion, till in 1912 the export was only 155,308 lb., at an average price of 7 dollars 20 cents per pound.

¶ *Cultivation*. On account of the growing scarcity of the American Ginseng plant, experiments have been made by the State of Pennsylvania to determine whether it can be grown profitably, resulting in the conclusion that in five years, starting with seeds and one year plants (or sooner if a start were made with older plants), an acre of ground would yield a profit of 1,500 dollars, without allowance for rental, but many precautions are necessary for success. The cultivated plants produced larger roots than those of the wild plant.

In 1912 it was estimated that the acreage of cultivated Ginseng in the United States was about 150 acres, and it is calculated that to supply China with twenty million dollars' worth of dry root would require the American growers to plant 1,000 acres annually for five years, before this estimated annual supply could be sold. The cultivation of Ginseng would therefore appear to offer a rich field to American agriculture. It presents, however, considerable difficulty, owing to the great care and special methods required and to the fact that it is a very slow-growing crop, so that rapid returns can hardly be anticipated, and it is doubtful if its cultivation can be carried on profitably except by specialists in the crop. None the less, the percentage returns for the industrious, patient and painstaking farmer are large, and the demand for a fine article for export is not at all likely to be exceeded by the supply.

For successful cultivation of Ginseng in America, it is stated that a loose, rich soil, with a heavy mulch of leaves and about 80 per cent. shade – generally provided artificially – is necessary.

It is difficult to cultivate it here with success. A rich compost is necessary. Most of the species of this genus need greenhouse treatment in this country. Propagation by cuttings of the roots is the most successful method, the cuttings being placed in sand, under a handglass. Seeds, generally obtained from abroad, are sown in pots in the early spring and require gentle heat. When the plants are a few inches high, they must be transplanted into beds or sheltered borders. They require a good, warm soil, but much shade. To grow on a commercial basis is not considered feasible in this country.

¶ *Harvesting, Preparation for Market*. The root should be collected only in the autumn, in which case it retains its plump and handsome appearance after drying. It is much more highly prized when of a fine light colour, which it is more apt to assume when grown in deep, black, fresh mould.

The best root is said to be that collected by the Sioux Indian women, who impart this white appearance by rotating it with water in a partly-filled barrel, through which rods are run in a longitudinal direction. In no other way, it is said, can the surface be so thoroughly and safely cleansed.

The structure of the root is fleshy and somewhat elastic and flexible, and it is of a firm, solid consistence if collected at the proper time and properly cured. The bark is very thick, yellowish-white, radially striate in old roots and contains brownish-red resin cells. The wood is strongly and coarsely radiate, with yellowish wood wedges and whitish rays.

The best roots for the Chinese market are sometimes submitted before being dried to a process of clarification, which renders them yellow, semi-transparent and of a horny appearance and enhances their value. This condition is gained by first plunging them in hot water, brushing until thoroughly scoured and steaming over boiling seed. Its commercial value is determined in a high degree by its appearance. The roots are valued in accordance with their large size and light colour, their plumpness and fine consistence, their unbroken and natural form, and above all by the perfectly developed condition of the branches.

¶ *Constituents*. A large amount of starch and gum, some resin, a very small amount of volatile oil and the peculiar sweetish body, *Panaquilon*. This occurs as a yellow powder, precipitating with water a white, amorphous substance, which has been called *Panacon*.

¶ *Medicinal Action and Uses*. *Panax* is not official in the British Pharmacopœia, and it was dismissed from the United States Pharmacopœia at a late revision. It is cultivated almost entirely for export to China.

In China, both varieties are used particularly for dyspepsia, vomiting and nervous disorders. A decoction of $\frac{1}{2}$ oz. of the root, boiled in tea or soup and taken every morning, is commonly held a remedy for consumption and other diseases.

In Western medicine, it is considered a mild stomachic tonic and stimulant, useful in loss of appetite and in digestive affections that arise from mental and nervous exhaustion.

A tincture has been prepared from the genuine Chinese or American root, dried and coarsely powdered, covered with five times its weight of alcohol and allowed to stand, well-stoppered, in a dark, cool place, being shaken twice a day. The tincture, poured off and filtered, has a clear, light-lemon colour, an odour like the root and a taste at first bitter, then dulcamarous and an acid reaction.

¶ *Substitutes*. A substitute for Ginseng, somewhat employed in China, is the root of *Codonopsis Tangshen*, a bell-flowered plant, used by the poor as a substitute for the costly Ginseng.

Ginseng is sometimes accidentally collected with Senega Root (*Polygala Senega*, Linn.) and with Virginian Snake Root (*Aristolochia Serpentaria*, Linn.), but is easily detected, being less wrinkled and twisted and yellower in colour. It is occasionally found with the collected root of *Cypripedium parviflorum* (Salis) and *Stylophorum diphyllum* (Nuttall).

Blue Cohosh (*Caulophyllum thalictroides*, Linn.) is often called locally in the United States 'Blue' or 'Yellow Ginseng,' and Fever Root (*Triosteum perfoliatum*, Linn.) also is sometimes given the name of Ginseng.

GIPSYWEED, COMMON

Lycopus Europæus
N.O. Labiatæ

Synonyms. Water Horehound. Gipsy-wort. Egyptian's Herb
Part Used. Herb

Common Gipsyweed (*Lycopus Europæus*), frequent throughout Europe, yields a black dye, stated to give a permanent colour to wool and silk. As its name implies, it was formerly used by gipsies to stain their skins darker. It is common by the banks of streams, flowers from July to September, and is an erect plant with scarcely branched stems, about 2 feet high, with deeply-cut, pointed leaves and small, pale flesh-coloured flowers, growing in crowded whorls in the axils of the upper leaves.

Anne Pratt says it received its old name of Egyptian's Herb 'because of the rogues and runnegates which call themselves Egyptians, and doe colour themselves black with this herbe.'

¶ *Medicinal Action and Uses*. Astringent, sedative.

See BUGLE.

GLADWYN, STINKING

Iris fœtidissima (LINN.)
N.O. Iridaceæ

Synonyms. Gladwin. Spurge Plant. Roast Beef Plant
Part Used. Root

Stinking Gladwyn is found only locally in England, but is common in all the south-western counties, growing in woods and shady places, on hedgebanks and sloping grounds.

¶ *Description*. The creeping rhizomes are thick, tufted and fibrous. The leaves are firm, deep green, sword-shaped, shorter, narrower and less rigid and of a darker green than those of the Yellow Flag, and are ever-green in winter. When bruised or crushed, they emit a strong odour, at a distance not unlike that of hot, roast beef, hence its country name of 'Roast Beef Plant.' On closer acquaintance, the scent becomes dis-agreeable, hence the more usual common name 'Stinking Gladwyn,' and the Latin specific name.

It flowers from June to August, but sparingly, and the corollas, of a dull, livid purple colour, rarely bluish or yellowish, are smaller than those of the other flags and not fragrant at night.

The flowers are followed by triangular seed-vessels, which, when ripe, open, dis-closing beautiful orange-red coloured seeds.

¶ *Cultivation*. Stinking Gladwyn flourishes in moist and partially-shaded places, in ordinary garden soil. Seeds scattered in semi-wild places soon make good plants and plants may also be increased by division of the rhizomes. The brilliant seeds in their gaping capsules make it an effective garden plant in autumn.

¶ *Medicinal Action and Uses*. Antispasmodic, cathartic, anodyne. *Iris fœtidissima* has been employed for the same medicinal pur-poses as the Yellow Flag and is equally violent in its action. A decoction of the roots acts as a strong purge. It has also been used as an emmenagogue and for cleansing erup-tions. The dried root, in powder or as an infusion, is good in hysterical disorders, fainting, nervous complaints and to relieve pains and cramps.

Taken inwardly and applied outwardly to the affected part, it is an excellent remedy for scrofula.

The use of this Iris was well known to the Ancients and is referred to by Theophrastus, in the fourth century before Christ.

See IRIS.

GLASSWORTS

N.O. Chenopodiaceæ
Salicornia herbacea (LINN.)

GLASSWORT, JOINTED
Synonym. Marsh Samphire

Many species of the genera *Salsola*, *Suæda* and *Salicornia* belonging to Chenopodiaceæ are rich in soda and were formerly much em-ployed in making both soap and glass, hence the name Glasswort. Large quantities of the ashes of these plants were formerly imported from southern Europe and northern Africa under the name of *Barilla*, the chief sources being *Salsola Kali* (Linn.) and *Salsola Soda* (Linn.), the Spanish *Salsola sativa* (Loft) and *S. tragus* (Linn.). On the introduction of Le Blanc's process of obtaining soda from common salt, the importance of Barilla as an article of commerce ceased.

Our native plant, the Jointed Glasswort (*Salicornia herbacea*, Linn.), was, as its name implies, also regarded as of value in the manufacture of glass.

¶ *Description.* It is a low-growing, annual herb, common in salt marshes and on muddy seashores all round the British Islands and was much used for this purpose. It has no leaves, but is formed of cylindrical, jointed branches of a light green colour, smooth, very succulent and full of a salt, bitterish juice, its minute flowers produced in threes in little pits in the axils of the branches.

The whole plant is greedily devoured by cattle for its saltish taste. Steeped in malted vinegar, the tender shoots make a good pickle and were often used as a substitute for Samphire in those parts of the coast where the latter did not abound, on which account the plant is also called Marsh Samphire. Sir Thomas More, enumerating the useful native plants that would improve 'many a poor knave's pottage' if he were skilled in their properties, says that 'Glasswort might afford him a pickle for his mouthful of salt meat.'

Parkinson relates a theory in connexion with Glasswort in his days:

'If the soap that is made of the lye of the ashes be spread upon a piece of thicke coarse brown paper cut into the forme of their shooe sole that are casually taken speechless and bound to the soles of their feete, it will bring again the speech and that within a little time after the applying thereof if there be any hope of being restored while they live: this hath been tried to be effectuall upon diverse persons.'

There are references in the Bible to the uses of Glasswort for soap and for glass.

GLASSWORT, PRICKLY
Salsola Kali (LINN.)

The Prickly Glasswort (*Salsola Kali*, Linn.) has a thick, round, brittle stem, with few, rigid leaves of a bluish-green colour and small, yellow flowers.

¶ *Medicinal Action and Uses.* The juice of the fresh plant was said to be an excellent diuretic, the twisted seed-vessels having the same virtue and being given in infusion.

The whole plant was likewise burnt for its fixed salt used in making glass.

See ARRACH, BLITES, BEETROOTS, CHENO-PODIUM, GOOSEFOOTS, SPINACH, WORMSEED.

GLEDITSCHIA
Gleditschia triacanthos (LINN.)
N.O. Leguminosæ

Synonyms. Gleditschine. Honey Locust. Gleditschia Ferox. Three-(t)horned Acacia
Parts Used. The twigs and leaves
Habitat. Eastern and Central United States

¶ *Description.* A small, thorny tree, with pinnated leaves and greenish flowers growing in dense spikes. The younger and smaller branches have strong, triple tapering thorns. In the autumn they bear thin, flat pods resembling apple-parings. They contain seeds surrounded by a sweetish pulp from which it is stated that sugar has been extracted. The wood is chiefly used for fencing.

¶ *Constituents.* An alkaloid, Gleditschine, has been abstracted, and another called Stenocarpine. It also contains cocaine, and probably atropine.

¶ *Medicinal Action and Uses.* Stenocarpine was introduced as a local anæsthetic in 1887. Gleditschine was found to produce stupor and loss of reflex activity in a frog.

¶ *Other Species.*
G. Macracantha possesses similar properties, and is indigenous to China.

GLOBE FLOWER
Trollius Europæus
N.O. Ranunculaceæ

Synonyms. Globe Trollius. Boule d'Or. European Globe Flower. Globe Ranunculus. Globe Crowfoot. Lucken-Gowans
Part Used. The whole plant, fresh
Habitat. Northern and Central Europe, from the Caucasus and Siberia to Wales and sometimes Ireland. Found wild in northern counties of England and in Scotland

¶ *Description.* The plant grows usually in moist woods and mountain pastures, and is about 2 feet high, the stalk being hollow, smooth, and branching towards the top, each branch bearing one yellow flower without a calix, shaped like that of Crowfoot. The leaves are beautifully cut into five, indented sections. It is a favourite bloom for rustic festivals, and early in June collections of it are made by youths and maidens to decorate cottage doors.

It is often cultivated as a border flower, as are the other two species of the genus.

¶ *Constituents*. The Swedish naturalist Peter Kalm affirms that these plants have medicinal properties, but lose the greater part of their active principles in drying. The irritant, acrid principle is not well defined, and appears to be destroyed by the action of heat.

¶ *Medicinal Action and Uses*. It is stated that Trollius is used in Russia in certain ob-

scure maladies, while another authority claims that it has cured a scorbutic case declared incurable by doctors. It is a plant to be investigated.

¶ *Other Species*.
T. Asiaticus, or Asiatic Globe Flower. The leaves of this species are larger than in the European plant, resembling those of Yellow Monk's Hood, although the stature of *T. Asiaticus* is less. The flowers are an orange-tinged yellow. It is a native of Siberia, but can be grown in any garden with shade and a moist soil.

T. Laxus is yellow, and grows in shady, wet places on the mountains of New York and Pennsylvania.

See CROWFOOT.

GNAPHALIUMS

N.O. Compositæ

The Gnaphaliums are a group of plants, individual species of which are known as Life Everlasting, Eternal Flowers, etc. They are used by the aborigines of America, who taught the white settlers their medical properties.

The *Antennaria Dioica*, known under the name of Life Everlasting or Catsfoot, is the only British species and must not be confused with *Antennaria Plantaginifolia*, or White Plantain, which is also sometimes called Life Everlasting.

GNAPHALIUM ARENARIUM
Habitat. Scania, Denmark, Germany, Japan

¶ *Medicinal Action and Uses*. Formerly much recommended for dysentery. Said to preserve woollen cloths from moth. In Japan it is used for moxas and as tobacco.

¶ *Description*. Leaves lanceolate, lower ones obtuse, flowers compound corymb, stalks simple. An annual hoary plant, stem upright, white, downy, about 1 foot high, with shiny yellow heads of flowers – the calicine scales ovate, blunt, lemon-coloured; also the corollets. Found in dry sandy pastures and

hills. Blooming in Germany, Denmark and Scania July to December, in Japan December to April.

¶ *Other Species*.
Gnaphalium Cymosum, or Branching Everlasting. The leaves when rubbed emit an odour like Southern Wood.

G. Plantaginifolia. For a small fee the American Indians allow themselves to be bitten by a rattlesnake and immediately cure themselves with this herb.

GNAPHALIUM STŒCHAS[1]

Helichrysum Stœchas
N.O. Compositæ

Synonyms. Eternal Flower. Goldilocks. Stœchas Citrina. Gnaphalium citrinum. Common Shrubby Everlasting
Parts Used. Tops and the flowers
Habitat. Germany, France, Spain, Italy

¶ *Medicinal Action and Uses*. Expectorant, deobstruent, used for colds, flowers formerly used as attenuants, discutients, diaphoretics.

¶ *Description*. Leaves linear; compound corymb; branches wand-like; stem 3 feet high, with long slender irregular branches, lower ones have blunt leaves, 2½ inches

long ⅛ inch broad at end; those on flower stalks very narrow, ending in acute points. Whole plant very woolly, calyces at first silvery, then turn a sulphur yellow. Taste warm, pungent, bitter, agreeable odour when rubbed.

See also CUDWEED, LIFE EVERLASTING, WHITE BALSAM, CATSFOOT.

GOA. *See* ARAROBA.

[1] In homœopathic medicine, a tincture is made from *Gnaphalium polycephalum* which has proved very useful in sciatica, lumbago and some forms of arthritis. – EDITOR.

GOAT'S BEARD

Tragopogon pratensis (LINN.)
N.O. Compositæ

Synonyms. Noon Flower. Jack-go-to-bed-at-noon

Habitat. Goat's Beard (*Tragopogon pratensis*), a rather close relation of the Hawkweeds, is a handsome plant fairly common throughout Britain in meadows and on the broad green strips that often border country roads, being very common in the north of England

¶ *Description.* It has an erect, slightly branching stem, rising to a height of 1 to 2 feet, from a perennial tap-root. The leaves are long, narrow and grass-like in character, without any indentations, broadening at the base and sheathing the stem, bluish-green in colour, the lower ones 8 or 9 inches long, the upper ones much shorter.

The plant is in bloom during June and July. Each flower-stem has at its summit a single, large flower-head, the stem being slightly thickened just below it. The involucre or cup at the base of the flower-head is composed of a ring of about eight narrow lance-shaped, leaf-like bracts, which, when the flower is expanded, spread out in rays beyond the florets, which are golden-yellow in colour, and all of the 'ligulate' or strap-shaped type. After flowering, the green rays of the involucre elongate and the lower portion becomes thicker, till finally a big, round head of winged, long seeds – like the familiar clock of the Dandelion – develops, which becomes broken up by the wind. The pappus, or feathery down crowning each seed, is very beautiful, being raised on a long stalk and interlaced, so as to form a kind of shallow cup. By means of the pappus, the seeds are wafted by the wind and freely scattered.

The Goat's Beard opens its blossoms at daybreak and closes them before noon, except in cloudy weather, hence its old country name of 'Noon-flower' and 'Jack-go-to-bed-at-noon,' a peculiarity noticed more than once by the poets and referred to in Cowley's lines:

'The goat's beard, which each morn abroad doth peep
But shuts its flowers at noon and goes to sleep.'

The name of the genus, *Tragopogon*, is formed from two Greek words, having the same signification as the popular English name, Goat's Beard, which is thought to have been suggested by the fluffy character of the seed-ball.

Gerard says:

'it shutteth itselfe at twelve of the clocke, and sheweth not his face open untill the next dayes Sun doth make it flower anew. Whereupon it was called go-to-bed-at-noone; when these flowers be come to their full maturitie and ripenesse they grow into a downy Blowball like those of Dandelion, which is carried away by the winde.'

¶ *Medicinal Action and Uses.* In mediæval times, the Goat's Beard had some reputation as a medicinal plant, though it has fallen out of use.

The tapering roots were formerly eaten as we now eat parsnips, and the young stalks, taken before the flowers appear, were cut up into lengths and boiled like asparagus, of which they have somewhat the flavour, and are said to be nearly as nutritious. The roots were dug up in the autumn and kept in dry sand for winter use.

The fresh juice of the young plant has been recommended as 'the best dissolvent of the bile, relieving the stomach without danger and without introducing into the blood an acrid, corrosive stimulant, as is frequently done by salts when employed for this purpose.'

Culpepper tells us:

'A large double handful of the entire plant, roots, flowers and all, bruised and boiled and then strained with a little sweet oil, is an excellent clyster in most desperate cases of strangury or suppression of urine. A decoction of the roots is very good for the heartburn, loss of appetite, disorders of the breast and liver; expels sand and gravel, and even small stone. The roots dressed like parsnips with butter are good for cold, watery stomachs, boiled or cold, or eaten as a raw salad; they are grateful to the stomach strengthen the lean and consumptive, or the weak after long sickness. The distilled water gives relief to pleurisy, stitches or pains in the side.'

Another close relation of the above is the Bristly Ox-Tongue (*Helmintha Echioides*), a stout, much-branched plant, 2 to 3 feet high, well distinguished by its numerous prickles, each of which springs from a raised white spot, and by the large heart-shaped bracts at the base of the yellow flowers. The fruit, which is beaked and singularly corrugated, bears some resemblance to 'a little worm,' which is the meaning of the systematic name. The English name 'Ox-Tongue' has reference to the shape and roughness of the leaves. Not uncommon.

See SALSAFY.

GOAT'S RUE. *See* RUE (GOAT'S)

GOLD THREAD

Coptis trifolia (SALIS.)
N.O. Ranunculaceæ

Synonyms. Helleborus triflius or trilobus. Helleborus pumilus. Coptis. Anemone grœn-
landica. Coptide. Mouthroot. Vegetable Gold. Chrusa borealis
Parts Used. The dried rhizome, with roots, stems, and leaves
Habitat. Northern America and Asia. Greenland and Iceland

¶ *Description.* The name of the genus *Coptis* is suggested by the form of the leaflets, and means 'to cut.' The popular name is derived from the thin, creeping, gold-coloured rhizome, which yields a yellow dye. The solitary, yellowish flowers, and obovate, evergreen leaves grow in tufts with yellow scales surrounding the base. The herb is a small perennial, usually found creeping in swamps or damp, sandy places. In commerce, the dried herb is found in loose masses, odourless, and with a pure, bitter taste. The powder is yellowish-green. It resembles gentian and quassia in its properties.

The *Coptis* family is closely linked to that of the Hellebores.

¶ *Constituents.* Its bitterness is imparted to both water and alcohol, but more readily to the latter. As there is neither tannic nor gallic acid, the activity is due to berberia or berberine, which is associated with another alkaloid called Coptine or Coptina, resembling hydrastia. It also contains albumen, fixed oil, colouring matter, lignin, extractive, and sugar. Authorities differ as to the presence of resin.

¶ *Medicinal Action and Uses.* It may be used as other pure bitters. In New England it is valued as a local application in thrush, for children.

It is stated to be good for dyspepsia, and combined with other drugs is regarded as helpful in combating the drink habit.

¶ *Dosage.* Of powder, 10 to 30 grains. Of tincture of 1 oz. of root to a pint of diluted alcohol, 1 fluid drachm. Of fluid extract, 30 minims.

¶ *Other Species and Substitutes.*
Statice monopetala, used as an astringent in the United States, sometimes used to adulterate *C. trifolia.*

Coptis Teeta, or Coptidis Rhizoma, Coptidis Radix, Mahmira, Tita, Mishmi Bitter, Mishmi Tita, Hwang-lien, Honglane, Chuen-lien, Chonlin, Mu-lien, is official in the Pharmacopœia of India. It grows in the Mishmi Mountains, East Assam, is imported into Bengal in little rattan bags, and is thus sold in the Indian bazaars. Large quantities have been sold in London. It contains a higher percentage of berberia than any other drug, and is much used as a tonic in India and China, especially for the stomach, and in Scind for inflammation of the eyes.

The Chinese and Japanese variations (var. *chinensis* and *C. anemonæfolia*) imported into Bombay are thinner and duller than the Assam rhizomes. In Japan, the last variety is used for intestinal catarrh.

GOLDEN ROD

Solidago virgaurea (LINN.)
N.O. Compositæ

Synonyms. Verge d'Or. Solidago. Goldruthe. Woundwort. Aaron's Rod
Part Used. Leaves
Habitat. Europe, including Britain. Central Asia. North America

¶ *Description.* The generic name comes from *solidare*, for the plant is known as a vulnerary, or one that 'makes whole.' It grows from 2 to 3 feet in height, with alternate leaves, of a clear green, and terminal panicles of golden flowers, both ray and disk. It is the only one (of over eighty species) native to Great Britain.

The leaves and flowers yield a yellow dye. When bruised, the herb smells like Wild Carrot.

¶ *Constituents.* The plant contains tannin, with some bitter and astringent principles.

¶ *Medicinal Action and Uses.* Aromatic, stimulant, carminative. Golden Rod is

an ingredient in the Swiss Vulnerary, *faltrank.* It is astringent and diuretic and efficacious for stone in the bladder. It is recorded that in 1788 a boy of ten, after taking the infusion for some months, passed quantities of gravel, fifteen large stones weighing up to 1¼ oz., and fifty over the size of a pea. It allays sickness due to weak digestion.

In powder it is used for cicatrization of old ulcers. It has been recommended in many maladies, as it is a good diaphoretic in warm infusion, and is in this form also helpful in dysmenorrhœa and amenorrhœa. As a spray and given internally, it is of great value in diphtheria.

¶ *Dosage.* ½ to 1 drachm of the fluid extract.

¶ *Other Species.*
S. *Rigida*, Hardleaf Goldenrod, and *S. Gigantea*, Smooth Three-Ribbed Golden Rod, have leaves and blossoms which are valuable for all forms of hæmorrhage, being astringent and styptic. The oil is diuretic.

S. *Odora*, or Sweet-scented, or Fragrant-leaved Goldenrod, also of the United States, is used as an astringent in dysentery and ulceration of the intestines. The essence has been used as a diuretic for infants, as a local application in headache, and for flatulence and vomiting. The flowers are aperient, tonic, and astringent, and their infusion is beneficial in gravel, urinary obstructions, and simple dropsy.

S. *Canadensis*, or Gerbe d'Or, of Canada, and *S. sempervirens* of North America, are used as vulneraries.

RAYLESS GOLDEN ROD is an American name for Bigelovia.

GOLDEN ROD TREE is *Bosea Yervamora*.

GOLDEN ROD is also the common name of *Leontice Chrysogonum*.

GOLDEN SEAL

Hydrastis Canadensis (LINN.)
N.O. Ranunculaceæ

Synonyms. Yellow Root. Orange Root. Yellow Puccoon. Ground Raspberry. Wild Curcuma. Turmeric Root. Indian Dye. Eye Root. Eye Balm. Indian Paint. Jaundice Root. Warnera

Part Used. Root

Habitat. The plant is a native of Canada and the eastern United States, the chief States producing it being Ohio, Kentucky, West Virginia, Indiana, New York and in Canada, Ontario. Most of the commercial supplies are obtained from the Ohio Valley, the chief market being Cincinnati. It is scarce east of the Alleghany Mountains, having become quite rare in New York State, where it has been almost exterminated by collectors. It is found in the rich soil of shady woods and moist places at the edge of wooded lands

The North American plant Golden Seal produces a drug which is considered of great value in modern medicine. The generic name of the plant, *Hydrastis*, is derived from two Greek words, signifying water and to accomplish, probably given it from its effect on the mucous membrane.

Golden Seal belongs to the Buttercup family, Ranunculaceæ, though its leaves and fruit somewhat resemble those of the Raspberry and the *Rubus* genus generally.

¶ *Description.* It is a small perennial herb, with a horizontal, irregularly knotted, bright yellow root-stock, from ¼ inch to ¾ inch thick, giving off slender roots below and marked with scars of the flower-stems of previous years. The flowering stem, which is pushed up early in the spring, is from 6 to 12 inches high, erect, cylindrical, hairy, with downward-pointing hairs, especially above, surrounded at the base with a few short, brown scales. It bears two prominently-veined and wrinkled, dark green, hairy leaves, placed high up, the lower one stalked, the upper stalkless, roundish in outline, but palmately cut into 5 to 7 lobes, the margins irregularly and finely toothed. There is one solitary radical leaf on a long foot-stalk, similar in form to the stem leaves, but larger, when full-grown being about 9 inches across.

The flower, which is produced in April, is solitary, terminal, erect, small, with three small greenish-white sepals, falling away immediately after expansion, no petals and numerous stamens. The fruit is a head of small, fleshy, oblong, crimson berries, tipped with the persistent styles and containing one or two hard black, shining seeds. It is ripe in July and has much the appearance of a Raspberry (whence the name 'Ground Raspberry'), but is not edible.

Hydrastis Canadensis was first introduced into England by Miller in 1760, under the name of *Warnera*, after Richard Warner of Woodford, and later was grown at Kew, Edinburgh and Dublin. Having no claims to horticultural attractiveness, its cultivation has not been attempted in this country except in botanical gardens – and on a slight experimental scale – nor has it been cultivated on any scale in any other country until quite recently, when owing to its growing scarcity in the woods of Ohio, where it used to be abundant, plantations were started in a few parts of America, but the amount under cultivation there is still very small.

In 1905 the United States Department of Agriculture called attention to the increasing demand for Golden Seal for medicinal purposes in a Bulletin (No. 51). There it is stated that the early settlers learnt of the virtues of Golden Seal from the American Indians, who used the root as a medicine and its yellow juice as a stain for their faces and a dye for their clothing. It was not until

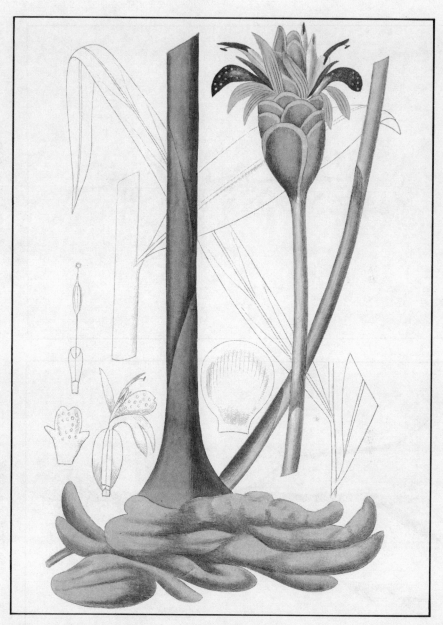

GINGER
Zingiber Officinale

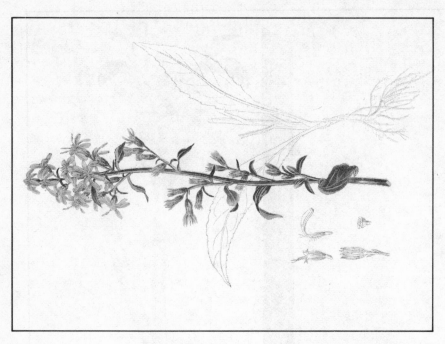

GOLDEN ROD
Solidago Virgaurea

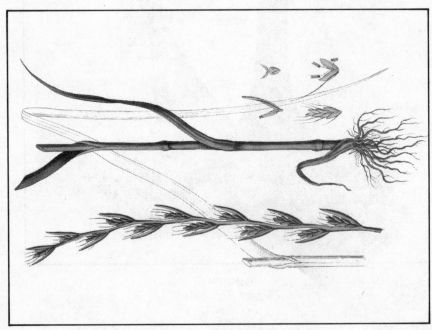

DARNEL GRASS
Lolium Temulentum

about 1850 that the root became an article of commerce, and in 1905 the annual supply of it was estimated at from 200,000 lb. to 300,000 lb., about one-tenth of which was exported, with an ever-increasing demand. Thirty years ago it was plentiful in its wild haunts and sold for 8 cents per lb., but as its supply diminished, not only from over-collection, but from the forests in the central States being cut away, the price rose in proportion and is now almost prohibitive.

¶ *Cultivation.* Experimental growing of the drug here has not been attended with much success, as it is of somewhat difficult culture.

The best conditions for the cultivation of Golden Seal are said to be a well-drained soil, rich in humus, in a partially shaded situation. Lath blinds (placed overhead on wires and light runners) are used by American cultivators – as with Ginseng – and these are considered to be preferable to the shade of trees, the roots of which interfere with operations. The plant requires from 60 to 75 per cent. shade. The root-stocks are divided into small pieces and then planted about 8 inches apart in rows. Seeds are not considered reliable. Fresh plantations are made in autumn, after the plants have died down, or earlier, if they are lifted for a supply of marketable rhizomes. The strong fibrous roots sometimes develop buds which can be used as stock. Plantations thus formed take two or three years to grow to marketable size, the rhizomes deteriorating in their fourth year. According to an American grower, 32 sturdy plants set to each square yard, in three years' growth will produce 2 lb. of dry root. Experiments conducted by the United States Department of Agriculture recommend growing it only two years and marketing. It is stated that the plant may be transplanted at any time of the year with safety.

It has proved difficult to obtain a supply of living roots with which to start plantations in this country. The market is in the hands of American growers, collectors and dealers, and it may be that they are unwilling to spoil their monopoly by aiding other countries to grow their own Golden Seal, but the drug is growing in favour with medical practitioners, therefore its production on a commercial scale in this country would appear to be desirable, if it could be carried out with success.

The fresh rhizome is juicy and loses much of its weight in drying. When fresh, it has a well-marked, narcotic odour, which is lost in a great measure by age, when it acquires a peculiar sweetish smell, somewhat resembling liquorice root. It has a very bitter, feebly opiate taste, more especially when freshly dried.

The rhizome is irregular and tortuous, much knotted, with a yellowish-brown, thin bark and bright yellow interior, $\frac{1}{2}$ inch to $1\frac{1}{2}$ inch long, and from $\frac{1}{8}$ to $\frac{1}{4}$ inch thick. The upper surface bears short ascending branches, which are usually terminated by cup-like scars, left by the aerial stems of previous years. From the lower surface and sides, numerous thin, wiry, brittle roots are given off, many of them breaking off, leaving small protuberances on the root.

The colour of the rhizome, though yellow in the fresh root, becomes a dark, yellowish-brown by age; that of the rootlets and the interior of the root is yellow and that of the powder still more so.

When dry, the rhizome is hard and breaks with a clean, resinous fracture; the smooth, fractured surface is of a brownish-yellow, or greenish-yellow colour, and exhibits a ring of bright yellow, somewhat distant, narrow wood bundles surrounding a large pith.

¶ *Constituents.* The chief constituents of Hydrastis rhizome are the alkaloids Berberine (3·5 to 4 per cent.), which constitutes the yellow colouring matter of the drug, Hydrastine (2 to 4 per cent.), a peculiar crystallizable substance and a third alkaloid, Canadine; resin, albumin, starch, fatty matter, sugar, lignin and a small quantity of volatile oil, to which its odour is due, are also present. The rhizome is stated to be much richer in alkaloid than the roots.

Hydrastis owes its virtues almost entirely to Hydrastine, the alkaloid Berberine, apart from some effect as a bitter being practically inert. The United States Pharmacopœia requires Hydrastis to yield not less than 2·5 per cent. of Hydrastine.

For many years the alkaloids and the powdered root were the chief forms administered, but now the fluid extract is the form most used. The tincture is also official in both the British and the United States Pharmacopœias.

¶ *Medicinal Action and Uses.* The American aborigines valued the root highly as a tonic, stomachic and application for sore eyes and general ulceration, as well as a yellow dye for their clothing and weapons.

It is official in most Pharmacopœias, several of which refer to its yellowing the saliva when masticated.

The action is tonic, laxative, alterative and detergent. It is a valuable remedy in the disordered conditions of the digestion and has a special action on the mucous membrane, making it of value as a local remedy in various forms of catarrh. In chronic inflammation of the colon and rectum, injections of Hydrastine are often of great service, and it has been used in hæmorrhoids with excellent results, the alkaloid Hydrastine having an astringent action. The powder has proved useful as a snuff for nasal catarrh.

It is employed in dyspepsia, gastric catarrh, loss of appetite and liver troubles. As a tonic, it is of extreme value in cases of habitual constipation, given as a powder, combined with any aromatic. It is an efficient remedy for sickness and vomiting.

¶ *Preparations.* Powdered root, 10 grains. Fluid extract, ¼ to 1 drachm. Tincture, B.P. and U.S.P., ½ to 1 drachm. Solid extract, 5 to 8 grains.

As an infusion, it has great influence in preventing and curing night-sweats. It is sometimes used as a wash for ulcerated mouth.

Externally, it is used as a lotion in treatment of eye affections and as a general cleansing application.

It is said to be a specific to prevent pitting by smallpox.

In large amounts the drug proves very poisonous.

The employment of Hydrastis as a dye by the Indians has led to investigations as to its possible commercial employment in this direction. Durand (*Amer. Journ. Pharm.,* Vol. XXIII) states that 'it imparts to linen a rich and durable light yellow colour, of great brilliancy, which might probably by proper mordants give all the shades of that colour, from the pale yellow to the orange. The lake produced by the bichloride of tin might also prove a useful pigment in oil and water-colour painting.' With indigo, it is said to impart a fine green to wool, silk and cotton.

¶ *Substitutes.* Owing to the high price of Hydrastis, the quality of the commercial article has steadily deteriorated, and in recent years, about every drug native to the soil which resembles this rhizome, either in fibre or in colour, has been known to be mixed with it. The yellow colour of Hydrastis rhizome, the appearance of a transverse section and the characteristic odour of the drug distinguish it readily from Blood Root, obtained from *Sanguinaria Canadensis,* which is usually of a dark reddish-brown colour, while a transverse section exhibits a more or less pronounced red colour and no evident wood bundles.

None of the substitutes can be reasonably mistaken for the drug in the entire condition.

GOOD KING HENRY. *See* GOOSEFOOT

GOOSEBERRY

Ribes Grossularia
N.O. Grossulariaceæ

Synonyms. Fea. Feverberry. Feabes. Carberry. Groseille. Grozet. Groser. Krusbaar. Deberries. Goosegogs. Honeyblobs. Feaberry

Parts Used. Fruit, leaves

Habitat. Central and Northern Europe, especially Britain. *Ribes Uva Crispa*, also, as far east as Nepal and south to Morocco

¶ *Description.* The well-known fruit grows on shrubs 3 to 4 feet high, with many branches, spreading prickles, and small, three- or five-lobed, hairy leaves. The flowers are green and hang singly or in pairs from little tufts of young leaves. The berries may be red, green, yellow, or white, hairy (*Ribes Grossularia*) or smooth (*R. Uva Crispa*), over 200 varieties being recognized. It is especially cultivated in Lancashire and in the Lothians, in Scotland, the former district aiming at size, and the latter at flavour. The shrub may attain great age and size. In 1821, at Duffield, near Derby, a bush had been planted for at least forty-six years, and was 12 yards in circumference, while two, trained against a wall near Chesterfield, reached upwards of 50 feet in growth from end to end.

The yellow gooseberries have usually the richest flavour for dessert, and the best wine made from them very closely resembles champagne. The red are generally the most acid, supporting the fact that acids change vegetable blues to red.

The fruit does not appear to be highly valued in the South of Europe, but further North is very popular for tarts, pies, sauces, chutneys, jams, and dessert, also for preserving in bottles for winter use. The young and tender leaves are eaten in salads.

¶ *Constituents.* Citric acid, pectuse, sugar, and mineral matters, the pectuse causing the fruit to be excellent for jellies.

¶ *Medicinal Action and Uses.* The juice was formerly said to 'cure all inflammations.' In the green berries it is sub-acid and is corrective of putrescent foods, such as mackerel or goose. The light jelly made from the red berries is valuable for sedentary, plethoric, and bilious subjects.

As a spring medicine, gooseberry is more

valuable than rhubarb. In one of the many books on the Plague, published in the sixteenth century, the patient is recommended to eat 'Goseberries.' Gerard, describing it under the name of 'Feaberry,' says:

'the fruit is much used in diners, sawces for meates and used in brothe instead of Verjuyce, which maketh the brothe not only pleasant to taste, but is greatly profitable to such as are troubled with a hot, burning ague.'

The leaves were formerly considered very wholesome and a corrective of gravel. An infusion taken before the monthly period will be found a useful tonic for growing girls.

¶ *Dosage.* Of an infusion of 1 oz. of dried leaves to 1 pint of water, 1 teacupful three times a day.

GOOSEFOOTS

N.O. Chenopodiaceæ

GOOD KING HENRY

Chenopodium Bonus Henricus

Synonyms. English Mercury. Mercury Goosefoot. Allgood. Tola Bona. Smearwort. Fat Hen
(*German*) Fette Henne
Part Used. Herb
Habitat. Good King Henry grows abundantly in waste places near villages, having formerly been cultivated as a garden pot-herb

¶ *Description.* It is a dark-green, succulent plant, about 2 feet, high, rising from a stout, fleshy, branching root-stock, with large, thickish, arrow-shaped leaves and tiny yellowish-green flowers in numerous close spikes, 1 to 2 inches long, both terminal and arising from the axils of the leaves. The fruit is bladder-like, containing a single seed.

The leaves used to be boiled in broth, but were principally gathered, when young and tender, and cooked as a pot-herb. In Lincolnshire, they are still eaten in place of spinach. Thirty years ago, this Goosefoot was regularly grown as a vegetable in Suffolk, Lincolnshire, and other eastern counties, and was preferred to the Garden Spinach, its flavour being somewhat similar, but less pronounced. In common with several other closely allied plants, it was sometimes called 'Blite' (from the Greek, *bliton*, insipid), Evelyn says in his *Acetaria*, 'it is well-named being insipid enough.' Nevertheless, it is a very wholesome vegetable. If grown on rich soil, the young shoots, when as thick as a lead pencil, may be cut when 5 inches in height, peeled and boiled and eaten as Asparagus. They are gently laxative.

¶ *Cultivation.* Good King Henry is well worth cultivating. Being a perennial, it will continue to produce for a number of years, being best grown on a deep loamy soil. The ground should be rich, well drained, and deeply dug. Plants should be put in about April, 1 foot apart each way, or seeds may be sown in drills at the same distance. During the first year, the plants should be allowed to establish themselves, but after that, both shoots and leaves may be cut or picked, always leaving enough to maintain the plant in health. Manure water is of great assistance in dry weather, or a dressing of 1 oz. of nitrate of soda, or sulphate of ammonia may be given.

As with many of the wild plants, it does not always adapt itself to a change of soil when transplanted from its usual habitat and success is more often ensured when grown from seed.

Dodoens says the name, Good King Henry, was given it to distinguish the plant from another, and poisonous one, called *Malus Henricus* ('Bad Henry'). The name *Henricus* in this case was stated by Grimm to refer to elves and kobolds ('Heinz' and 'Heinrich'), indicating magical powers of a malicious nature. The name has no connexion with our King Hal.

The plant is also known as Mercury Goosefoot, English Mercury and Marquery (to distinguish it from the French Mercury), because of its excellent remedial qualities in indigestion, hence the proverb: 'Be thou sick or whole, put Mercury in thy Koole.'

The name 'Smear-wort' refers to its use in ointment. Poultices made of the leaves were used to cleanse and heal chronic sores, which, Gerard states, 'they do scour and mundify.'

The roots were given to sheep as a remedy for cough and the seeds have found employment in the manufacture of shagreen.

The plant is said to have been used in Germany for fattening poultry and was called there *Fette Henne*, of which one of its popular names, Fat Hen, is the translation.

GOOSEFOOT, WHITE   Chenopodium album (LINN.)

Synonyms. Frost Blite. Mutton Tops. Dirtweed. Lamb's Quarters. Dirty Dick. Midden Myles. Pigweed (Canada). Baconweed. Fat Hen

Part Used. Herb

The White Goosefoot (*Chenopodium album*, Linn.), so called from its mealy leaves, rejoices in old manure heaps, and if the manure is stacked up on a farm ready for use at a later season, it is soon overrun by this weed, which has thus gained the popular names of 'Midden Myles,' 'Dirtweed' and 'Dirty Dick.'

It shares with its near relative Good King Henry the names of Allgood and Fat Hen from its usefulness as a pot-herb and its reputed value in feeding poultry. 'Boil Myles in water and chop them in butter and you will have a good dish,' is an old English saying. It is a very wholesome medicine, as well as a pleasant vegetable, and an excellent substitute for spinach.

¶ *Description.* The stem is erect, from 1 to 3 feet high, the leaves oval, wedge-shaped, with wavy teeth, the flowers in dense spikes. The mealiness is most apparent in the flowers and undersides of the leaves, but has not the objectionable odour of that of the Stinking Goosefoot.

This nutritious plant is grown as food for pigs and sheep in Canada, where it is called 'Pigweed.'

The young and tender plants are collected by the Indians of New Mexico and Arizona, and boiled as herbs, alone or with other food; large quantities also are eaten in the raw state. The seeds of this species are gathered by many tribes, ground into flour after drying and made into bread. The flour resembles that of Buckwheat in colour and taste and is regarded as equally nutritious. The small grey seeds are not unpleasant when eaten raw.

GOOSEFOOT, RED   Chenopodium rubrum (LINN.)

Synonyms. Sowbane. Pigweed

The seeds of the Red Goosefoot (*Chenopodium rubrum*, Linn.) are a favourite food of birds and are also good for poultry. This species has a reddish stem, 1 to 3 feet high, usually upright, its leaves triangular to oval, with large blunt lobes and notches, but very variable in size and shape. It is very common about manure heaps. Its erect flower-spikes, intermixed with leaves, distantly resemble those of Dock.

¶ *Other Species.*

The leaves of another Goosefoot, *C. hybridum*, are sometimes found as an adulterant of Stramonium leaves, when these are imported in a broken condition, but they can be detected by their small epidermal cells, with nearly straight walls, and hairs terminated by a large, bladdery, water-storing cell.

See ARRACHS, BEETS, BLITES, GLASSWORTS, QUINOA, SPINACH, WORMSEEDS.

GORSE, GOLDEN

Ulex Europæus (LINN.)

N.O. Leguminosæ

Synonyms. Furze. Broom. Whin. Prickly Broom. Ruffet. Frey. Goss

Parts Used. Flowers, seed

Habitat. It is found from Denmark to Italy, the Canaries and Azores, and in every part of Great Britain, though it is rarer in the north. There is probably hardly a heath in the country which lacks a patch, however small, of the dry-soil-loving Furze

The Golden Gorse (*Ulex Europæus*, Linn.) is conspicuous in waste places and on commons throughout Great Britain, from its spiny branches and bright yellow flowers, situated on the spines, either solitary or in pairs. It is thought to be the *Scorpius* of Theophrastus and the *Ulex* of Pliny. By botanists before Linnæus, it was known as a Broom and called *Genista spinosa*. Linnæus restored to it the name of *Ulex*, by which it has ever since been recognized.

Although it looks so sturdy, it is not very hardy. Severe frosts are liable to injure it, and during some exceptionally severe winters whole tracts of it on open commons have perished. Linnæus, we are told in Johnson's *Useful Plants of Great Britain*:

'lamented that he could not keep Furze alive in Sweden, even in a greenhouse. It was one of his favourite plants, though the well-known story of his falling on his knees when first seeing it in this country and thanking Heaven for having created a flower so beautiful is of rather doubtful authenticity as it is likewise related of Dillenius.'

¶ *Description.* The plant is a dense, much-branched, stunted shrub, rarely attaining a height of more than 6 feet. It is evergreen, but the leaves are very minute and fall off early, not being present in the older stages, when they take the form of long, thread-like spines, which are straight and furrowed, or branching. The stem is hairy and spreading.

The golden-yellow, papilionaceous flowers have a powerful scent, perfuming the air. They open from early spring right up to August, or even later, but the bushes are to be found in blossom, here and there, practically all the year round, hence the old saying:

'When Gorse is out of bloom, Kissing's out of season,'

and an old custom in some parts of the country of inserting a spray of Gorse in the bridal bouquet, is an allusion to this.

The following reference to its continuous flowering appeared in the *Chemist and Druggist* of January 15, 1921. The writer says:

'Sir, The impression that is prevalent concerning the perennial flowering of the common Furze is a very natural, although a mistaken one.

'The ordinary furze, *U. Europæus*, begins to flower in December, is in full bloom in March and April, and continues sometimes in a desultory manner as late as June. Then the Dwarf Furze begins to flower, and is in full bloom in August. When mixed with the heather – then in blossom – it forms gorgeous purple and gold carpets wherever, as in Jersey, it is abundant. *U. Gallii* then takes up the tale, and from August to November blossoms freely. *U. Europæus* is rarely less than 2 ft. high when it begins to flower: the *U. Nanus* has a decumbent habit, and is rarely more than 1½ ft. high, and the flowers are paler and do not expand the wings widely. *U. Gallii* is easily recognized by the larger lateral spines of the branches being decurved, and the flowers more of an orange tint. But an ordinary observer would discount these differences, if noticed at all, and merely regard the other species as more or less dwarf plants. *U. Gallii* is sometimes as short as *U. nanus*, and sometimes as tall as *U. Europæus*, but may always be recognized by the stout spines curved backwards.

'Yours truly,
'SEMPERVIRENS.'

Its elastic seed-vessels, like those of the Broom, burst with a crackling noise in hot weather and scatter the seeds on all sides.

The Gorse has not as many uses as the Broom, nor is it of such importance medicinally.

'In France,' to quote Syme and Sowerby, *British Botany*, 1864, 'it is used for burning, being cut down every few years, in places where it grows naturally. In Surrey and other counties, it is used largely as fuel, especially by bakers in their ovens and is cultivated for that purpose and cut down every three years. When burned, it yields a quantity of ashes rich in alkali, which are sometimes used for washing, either in the form of a solution or lye, or mixed with clay and made into balls, as a substitute for soap. The ashes form an excellent manure and it is not uncommon where the ground is covered with Furze bushes to burn them down to improve the land and to secure a crop of young shoots, which are readily eaten by cattle. In some parts of England, it is usual to put the Furze bushes into a mill to crush the thorns and then to feed horses and cows with the branches. When finely cut or crushed, sheep will readily eat it.'

The bruised shoots form a very nutritious fodder and when well bruised are eaten with much relish by horses, and cows are said to give good milk upon this food alone. When crushed, it is necessary to use it quickly, as the mass soon ferments. The variety of Furze found in the west of England and in Ireland, called *U. strictus*, is the best for this purpose, its shoots being softer and more succulent. It has terminal bunches of flowers.

Professor Henslow (*Uses of British Plants*, 1905) states that Furze 'has also been used chopped up into small pieces and sown in drills with Peas, proving a good defence against the attack of birds and mice.'

The leaf-buds have been used as a substitute for tea and the flowers yield a beautiful yellow dye.

The seeds are said to be nutritious, but do not appear to have been used for cattle feeding, though in earlier days they were sometimes employed medicinally.

Goldsmith calls the Furze 'unprofitably gay,' but Furze is not 'unprofitable.' It is usually cut once in three years, and its ashes, after burning, yield a serviceable dressing for the land.

Gorse is frequently sown as a shelter to very young trees in plantations and as a cover for game and makes excellent hedges when kept closely cut, but is only to be recommended for this purpose in mild climates or sheltered situations, as it is always liable to be cut off by hard frost. Wherever sown, it requires to be kept free from weeds during the first year or two. Like Broom, it grows well near the sea.

The name *Ulex* was given it by Pliny, but

its signification is unknown. He states that the plant was used in the collection of gold, being laid down in water to catch any gold-dust brought down by the water.

The word Furze is derived from the Anglo-Saxon name *fyrs*, while Gorse is also from the A.-S. *gorst* (a waste), a reference to the open moorlands on which it is found.

¶ *Medicinal Action and Uses.* The plant has never played an important part in herbal medicine.

Parkinson tells us that 'some have used the flowers against the jaundice.' An infusion of the blossoms used to be given to children to drink in scarlet-fever.

Gerard states: 'the seeds are employed in medicines against the stone and staying of the laske' (laxness of the bowels). They have some astringent property, containing tannin.

Old writers also tell us that 'sodden with honey, it clears the mouth' and that it 'is good against snake-bite.'

It had an old reputation as an insecticide: 'Against fleas, take this same wort, with its seed, sodden; sprinkle it into the house; it killeth the fleas.'

In 1886 A. W. Gerrard discovered an alkaloid in the seeds, more powerful as a purgative than the Sparteine obtained from *Cytisus scoparius* (Link) (*Pharm. Journal*, Aug. 7, 1886). This was named Ulexine. In 1890 the German scientist Kobert, as the result of much investigation, came to the conclusion that Ulexine and Cytisine are identical. He also found indication of a second alkaloid. The suggestion gave rise to a considerable chemico-physiological discussion (see *Pharm. Journal*, Feb. 1891). Ulexine has been used in cardiac dropsy, the dose being from $\frac{1}{15}$ to $\frac{1}{25}$ of a grain.

See BROOM, MELILOT, LABURNUM.

GOUTWEED

Ægopodium podagraria (LINN.)
N.O. Umbelliferæ

Synonyms. Jack-jump-about. Goatweed. Herb Gerard. Ashweed. Achweed. English Masterwort. Wild Masterwort. Pigweed. Eltroot. Ground Elder. Bishop's Elder. Weyl Ash. White Ash. Bishopsweed. Bishopswort. Ground Ash

Parts Used. Herb, root

Habitat. Europe (except Spain) and Russian Asia. Not really indigenous to England

¶ *Description.* The generic name is a corruption of the Greek *aix, aigos* (a goat) and *pous, podos* (a foot), from some fancied resemblance in the shape of the leaves to the foot of a goat. The specific name is derived from the Latin word for gout, *podagra*, because it was at one time a specific for gout.

It is a stout, erect plant, coarse and glabrous, a perennial; in height, $1\frac{1}{2}$ to 2 feet, sometimes more, the stem round, furrowed and hollow. It has a creeping root-stock and by this means it spreads rapidly and soon establishes itself, smothering all vegetation less rampant than its own. It is a common pest of orchards, shrubberies and ill-kept gardens, and is found on the outskirts of almost every village or town, being indeed rarely absent from a building of some description. It is possible that Buckwheat might drive it out if planted where Goutweed has gained a hold.

It was called Bishopsweed and Bishopswort, because so frequently found near old ecclesiastical ruins. It is said to have been introduced by the monks of the Middle Ages, who cultivated it as a herb of healing. It was called Herb Gerard, because it was dedicated to St. Gerard, who was formerly invoked to cure the gout, against which the herb was chiefly employed.

Its large leaves are alternate, the lobes ovate and sharply-toothed, 2 to 3 inches long. The radical leaves are on long stalks, bi- and tri-ternate. There are fewer stem-leaves; they are less divided, with smaller segments.

The umbels of flowers are rather large, with numerous, small white flowers, which are in bloom from June to August and are followed by flattened seed-vessels which when ripe are detached and jerked to a distance by the wind, hence its local name, 'Jack-jump-about.'

Gerard says:

'Herbe Gerard groweth of itself in gardens without setting or sowing and is so fruitful in its increase that when it hath once taken root, it will hardly be gotten out againe, spoiling and getting every yeare more ground, to the annoying of better herbe.'

An Alpine species, which appears to possess all the bad properties of its congener, is found in Asia.

The plant is eaten by pigs, hence one of its names. The following charm is from an Anglo-Saxon Herbal:

'To preserve swine from sudden death take the worts lupin, *bishopwort* and others, drive the swine to the fold, hang the worts upon the four sides and upon the door' (Lacnunga, 82).

John Parkinson recommends cummin seed and bishopsweed 'for those who like to look pale.'

The white root-stock is pungent and aromatic, but the flavour of the leaves is strong and disagreeable.

Culpepper gives 'Bishop-weed' a separate description, and states it is also called 'Æthiopian Cummin-Seed,' and 'Cummin-Royal,' also 'Herb William' and 'Bull-Wort.' He also (like Parkinson) says that 'being drank or outwardly applied, it abates an high colour, and makes pale.'

Linnæus recommends the young leaves boiled and eaten as a green vegetable, as in Sweden and Switzerland, and it used also to be eaten as a spring salad.

¶ *Medicinal Action and Uses.* Diuretic and sedative. Can be successfully employed *internally* for aches in the joints, gouty and sciatic pains, and *externally* as a fomentation for inflamed parts.

The roots and leaves boiled together, applied to the hip, and occasionally renewed, have a wonderful effect in some cases of sciatica.

Culpepper says:

'It is not to be supposed Goutwort hath its name for nothing, but upon experiment to heal the gout and sciatica; as also joint-aches and other cold griefs. The very bearing of it about one eases the pains of the gout and defends him that bears it from the disease.'

Gerard tells us that –

'with his roots stamped and laid upon members that are troubled or vexed with gout, swageth the paine, and taketh away the swelling and inflammation thereof, which occasioned the Germans to give it the name of Podagraria, because of his virtues in curing the gout.'

¶ *Other Species.* Bishopsweed is also the common name of *Ammi majus.*

GRAPE, MOUNTAIN

Berberis aquifolium (PURSH.)
N.O. Berberidaceæ

Synonyms. Mahonia aquifolia. Holly-leaved Barberry. Oregon Grape Root
Part Used. Root
Habitat. Western United States

¶ *Description.* Several varieties of the subgenus *Mahonia* contribute to the drug of commerce under the name of *Berberis aquifolium.* It is a quickly-growing shrub about 6 feet high: the oddly compound leaves have no spine at the base; they are evergreen and shining. The flowers grow in terminal racemes, are small and yellowish-green in colour, and the purple berries are three- to nine-seeded. The bark is brown on the surface and yellow beneath. The root is from ½ inch in diameter to 3 inches at the base of the stem, odourless, and with a bitter taste. The shrub was introduced into England from North America in 1823. It was formerly known as *Mahonia aquifolia* and is very hardy.

¶ *Constituents.* The principal constituent is a high proportion of berberin, and there is also oxycanthin.

¶ *Medicinal Action and Uses.* Tonic and alterative, recommended in psoriasis, syphilis and impure blood-conditions. It may be used like colombo, berberis, etc., in dyspepsia and chronic mucous complaints. In constipation it is combined with Cascara Sagrada. It improves digestion and absorption.

¶ *Preparation.* Fluid extract, 10 to 30 drops.

¶ *Other Species.*
B. nervosa and *B. repens* are frequently found in the drug.

GRASSES

N.O. Graminaceæ

The family of Grasses is, perhaps, of all groups in the plant world, the most important to mankind. The seeds of the valuable cereals, wheat, barley, oats, rye, etc., furnish us with indispensable farinaceous food and their stems with straw – the coarser kinds are useful for litter and fodder, also for thatching and other purposes, such as the making of mats, etc. – the finer varieties are widely employed in the making of hats, and our native Grasses furnish nutritious herbage, either as green pasture, or as hay, and some of them with mucilaginous roots possess distinctive medicinal virtues.

COUCH-GRASS   Agropyrum repens (BEAUV.)

Synonyms. Twitch-grass. Scotch Quelch. Quick-grass. Dog-grass. Triticum repens (Linn.)

Part Used. Rhizome

Habitat. Couch-grass is widely diffused, being not only abundant in fields and waste places in Britain and on the Continent of Europe, but also in Northern Asia, Australia and North and South America. It was formerly known as *Triticum repens*, though now assigned to the genus *Agropyrum*

Among these the Couch-grass (*Agropyrum repens*) is pre-eminent, though anything but a favourite with the farmer, for it has a slender, creeping rhizome, or underground stem, which extends for a considerable distance just beneath the surface of the ground, giving off lateral branches occasionally, and marked at intervals of about an inch by nodes, from which leaf-buds and slender branching roots are produced. These long, creeping, subterranean stems increase with great rapidity, and the smallest piece left in the ground will vegetate and quickly extend itself, so that it is almost impossible to extirpate it when once established in the soil, while its exhaustive powers render it very injurious to the crops. Its very name, *Couch*, is supposed to be derived from the Anglo-Saxon, *civice* (vivacious), on account of its tenacity of life. It is said that the only way to extirpate it, is to lay the ground down in pasture for some years, when the Couch will soon be destroyed by the close-growing Grasses, for it flourishes only in loose soil.

The name *Agropyron* is from the Greek *agros* (field), and *puros* (wheat).

On sandy seashores, the grass is often very abundant and assists in binding the sand and preventing the dunes from shifting, its long rhizome answering the purpose nearly as well as those of the Mat and Lyme Grasses.

Though commonly regarded in this country as a worthless and troublesome weed, its roots are, however, considered on the Continent to be wholesome food for cattle and horses. In Italy, especially, they are carefully gathered by the peasants and sold in the markets. The roots have a sweet taste, somewhat resembling liquorice, and Withering relates that, dried and ground into meal, bread has been made with them in time of scarcity.

¶ *Description.* From its long creeping, pointed root-stock, it produces in July several round, hollow flower stems, 2 to 3 feet high, thickened at the joints, bearing five to seven leaves and terminated by long, densely-flowered, two-rowed spikes of flowers, somewhat resembling those of rye or beardless wheat, composed of eight or more oval spikelets on alternate sides of the spike, each containing four to eight florets, the awns, when present, being not more than half the length of the flower. The leaves are flat, with a long, cleft sheath, and are rough on the upper surface, having a row of hairs on each principal vein.

One of the names of this grass is Dog's-grass, from its efficacy in relieving dogs when ill. They are often to be seen searching for its rough leaves, which they chew in order to procure vomiting. Culpepper closes his description of the grass by saying: 'If you know it not by this description, watch the dogs when they are sick and they will quickly lead you to it,' and concludes his account of its medicinal virtues with: 'and although a gardener be of another opinion, yet a physician holds half an acre of them to be worth five acres of carrots twice told over.'

Gerard wrote:

'Although that Couch-grasse be an unwelcome guest to fields and gardens, yet his physicke virtues do recompense those hurts; for it openeth the stoppings of the liver and reins without any manifest heat.' He says concerning a variety of Couch-grass that –

'the roots of this grass and tuberous in early spring, but in summer-time these bulbs lose all shape or form. . . . The learned Societie of London and the Physitions of the Colledge do hold this bulbous Couch grass in temperature agreeing with the common Couch Grass, but in vertues more effectual,' and mentions it as 'growing in the fields next to St. James' Wall, as ye go to Chelsea, and in the fields as ye go from the Tower Hill of London to Radcliffe.'

Culpepper greatly praises its virtues for diseases of the kidneys.

The juice of the roots drank freely is recommended by Boerhaave in obstruction of the viscera, particularly in cases of scirrhous liver and jaundice, and it is noteworthy that cattle having scirrhous livers in winter soon get cured when turned out to grass in spring. Sheep and goats eat the leaves as well as cows; horses eat them when young, but leave them untouched when fully grown.

The ancients were familiar with a grass – under the names of *Agrostis* and *Gramen* – having a creeping root-stock like the Couch-grass. Dioscorides asserts that its root, taken in the form of decoction is a useful remedy in suppression of urine and stone in the bladder. The same statements are made by Pliny, and are found in the writings of Oribasius and Marcellus Empiricus in the fourth century and of Ætius in the sixth century, and figures of the plant may be found in Dodoens's herbal. The drug is also met with in the German pharmaceutical tariffs of the sixteenth century.

Formerly the decoction of Couch-grass roots was a popular drink taken to purify the blood in spring. The drug is still a domestic remedy in great repute in France, being taken as a demulcent and sudorific in the form of a *tisane*. Readers of *Trilby* will remember Little Billee being dosed with this, as most Parisians have been. The French also use the Cocksfoot-grass (*Cynodon Dactylon*), which they term *Pied-de-poule*, in a similar way and for a similar purpose.

¶ *Part Used.* The rhizome, or underground stem, collected in the spring and freed from leaves and roots.

Couch-grass rhizome is long, stiff, pale yellow and smooth, about $\frac{1}{15}$ inch in diameter, hollow except at the nodes and strongly furrowed longitudinally, with five or six longitudinal ridges. Where the nodes occur, traces of rootlets may be found on the under surfaces and the fibrous remains of sheathing leaf-bases on the upper surfaces, but all traces of rootlets and leaves must be removed before use.

As found in commerce, the rhizome is always free from rootlets, cut into short lengths of $\frac{1}{8}$ to $\frac{1}{4}$ inch and dried, being thus in the form of little shining, straw-coloured, many-edged tubular pieces, which are without odour, but have a sweet taste.

¶ *Constituents.* Couch-grass rhizome contains about 7 to 8 per cent. of Triticin (a carbohydrate resembling Inulin) and yielding levulose on hydrolysis. It appears to occur in the rhizome of other grasses, and possibly is widely diffused in the vegetable kingdom. Sugar, Inosite, Mucilage and acid malates are also constituents of the drug. Lactic acid and mannite may occur in an extract of the rhizome, but are understood to be fermentation products. Starch is not present and no definite active constituent has yet been discovered. The rhizome leaves about $4\frac{1}{2}$ per cent. ash on incineration.

¶ *Medicinal Action and Uses.* Diuretic, demulcent. Much used in cystitis and the treatment of catarrhal diseases of the bladder. It palliates irritation of the urinary passages and gives relief in cases of gravel.

It is also recommended in gout and rheumatism. It is supposed to owe its diuretic effect to its sugar, and is best given in the form of an infusion, made from 1 oz. to a pint of boiling water, which may be freely used, taken in wineglassful doses. A decoction is also made by putting 2 to 4 oz. in a quart of water and reducing down to a pint by boiling. Of the liquid extract $\frac{1}{2}$ to 2 teaspoonful are given in water.

Couch-grass is official in the Indian and Colonial Addendum of the British Pharmacopœia for use in the Australasian, Eastern and North American Colonies, where it is much employed.

¶ *Substitutes. Agropyrum acutum* (R. et S.) *A. pungens* (R. et S.) and *A. junceum* (Beauv.), by some botanists regarded as mere maritime varieties of *A. repens*, have root-stocks similar to the latter.

Other Species.

COUCH-GRASS, DOG'S TOOTH   Cynodon dactylon (PERS.)

Synonyms. (French) Chien-dent. Pied-de-poule
Part Used. Rhizome

Cynodon dactylon (Pers.), a grass very common in the south of Europe and the warmer parts of Western Europe, also indigenous to Northern Africa as far as Abyssinia, affords the *Gros Chien-dent* or *Chiendent* and *Pied-de-poule* of the French. It is a rhizome differing from that of Couch-grass, in being a little stouter and in containing much starch, of which there is no trace in Couch-grass. Under the microscope it displays an entirely different structure, inasmuch as it contains a large number of much stronger fibrovascular bundles and a cellular tissue loaded

with starch, and is, therefore, in appearance much more woody. It thus approximates to the rhizome of *Carex arenaria* (Linn.) which is as much used in Germany as that of *Cynodon* in France and Southern Europe. The latter appears to contain Asparagin, or a substance similar in composition to it.

The herb of *Hygrophila spinosa* (Linn.) has been used for the same purpose as Couch-grass rhizome, and was formerly included in the Indian and Colonial Addendum to the British Pharmacopœia. It contains much mucilage.

DARNEL, BEARDED · Lolium temulentum (LINN.)

Synonyms. Ray-grass. Drake. Cheat
  (*Old English*) Cokil
  (*French*) Ivraie
  (*Arabic*) Zirwan
Part Used. Seeds

The Bearded Darnel, a common grass weed in English cornfields, is easily distinguished by its long glumes or awns and turgid, fruiting pales, containing the large grains, from the common Ray or Rye-grass (*Lolium perenne*), which is one of the best of the cultivated grasses, peculiarly adapted for both hay and pasture, especially in wet or uncertain climates. Both are often indiscriminately called Darnel or Ray-grass.

The seeds or grains of the Bearded Darnel were used medicinally by the ancient Greeks and Romans, but were never official in our Pharmacopœia.

The admixture of the grain with those of the nutritious cereals amongst which it is often found growing should be guarded against, as its properties are generally regarded as deleterious. Gerard tells us: 'the new bread wherein Darnel is eaten hot causeth drunkenness.' When Darnel has been given medicinally in a harmful quantity, it is recorded to have produced all the symptoms of drunkenness: a general trembling, followed by inability to walk, hindered speech and vomiting. For this reason the French call Darnel: '*Ivraie*,' from *Ivre* (drunkenness); the word Darnel is itself of French origin and testifies to its intoxicating qualities, being derived from an old French word *Darne*, signifying stupefied. The ancients supposed it to cause blindness, hence with the Romans, *lolio victitare*, to live on Darnel, was a phrase applied to a dim-sighted person.

The alleged poisonous properties of Darnel are now generally believed to be due to a fungus.

Darnel is in some provincial districts known as Cheat, and there is reason to suspect that the old custom of using Darnel to adulterate malt and distilled liquors has not been entirely abandoned.

Culpepper terms it 'a pestilent enemy among the corn,' and in olden days its name was so commonly used as a synonym for a pernicious weed that it has been said that the expression in Matthew xiii. 25, would have been better translated *Darnel* than *tares*.

The Arabs still give the name *zirwan* to a noxious grass (which is only too common in the cornfields of Palestine) simulating the wheat when undeveloped, though easily distinguishable at 'harvest' time.

In connection with this similarity, it may be of interest to relate an experiment made by a friend of the writer. She procured some ears of Palestine wheat and also some of Palestine 'Darnel' ('tares'), for the purpose of illustrating the truth of the Parable of the Tares to her Bible-class. After sowing both kinds in a patch of ground she asked her scholars to watch the appearance of the respective 'blades' as they appeared. They attached small strands of wool to distinguish each. In many cases wheat grew from the tare seeds, and tares from the wheat.

It is said that the country people of Cheshire believed Darnel to be 'degenerated wheat.'

In the East it is a more serious enemy to the farmer; and in the low-lying districts of the Lebanon and other parts of Palestine it becomes alarmingly plentiful. If inadvertently eaten it produces sickness, dizziness, and diarrhœa. It would seem that the 'malice aforethought' of sowing this wild grass deliberately (as in our Lord's parable), was a not unusual practice. The following is a quotation from an old newspaper:

'*The Country of Ill-Will* is the by-name of a district hard by St. Arnaud, in the north of France. There tenants, when ejected by a landlord, or when they have ended their tenancy on uncomfortable terms, have been in the habit of spoiling the crop to come by vindictively sowing *tares*, and other coarse strangling weeds, among the wheat, whence has been derived the sinister name of the district. The practice has been made penal, and any man proved to have tampered with any other man's harvest will be dealt with as a criminal.'

Virgil speaks of 'unlucky darnel' (*Georg.*, lib. i. 151–4) and groups it with thistles, thorns, and burs, among the enemies of the husbandman, and Shakespeare says:

'Darnel and all the idle weeds that grow
In our sustaining corn.'

In the Middle Ages it was sometimes called Cokil, as well as Ray, and in the fourteenth century we hear of it being used against 'festour and morsowe,' and of Cokkilmeal being thought good for freckles and to make the face white and soft. Culpepper, after calling it 'a malicious part of sullen Saturn,' adds: 'as it is not without some vices, so

hath it also many virtues . . . the meal of darnel is very good to stay gangrenes; it also
cleanseth the skin of all scurvy, morphews,
ringworms, if it be used with salt and reddish
(Radish) roots.' Also: 'a decoction thereof
made with water and honey, and the places
bathed therewith cures the sciatica,' and
finally: 'Darnel meal applied in a poultice
draweth forth splinters and broken bones in
the flesh.'

¶ *Medicinal Action and Uses.* Darnel is
usually regarded as possessing sedative and
anodyne properties. It was not only employed medicinally by the Greeks and Romans and in the Middle Ages, but in more
modern practice in the form of a powder or
pill in headache, rheumatic meningitis, sciatica and other cases. Cases are on record of
serious effects having resulted from the use
of bread, containing by accidental admixture
the flour of Darnel seeds. Chemically the

seeds contain an acrid fixed oil and a yellow
glucoside, but as far as microscopical appear-
ances indicate, the Darnel contains nothing
that is not contained in wheat, and analysis
has not yet revealed its poisonous elements.

Of late years, it has been questioned
whether the ill-effects of Darnel are inherent
in the grain themselves, or whether they may
not be ascribed to their having been ergotized. Lindley in his *Vegetable Kingdom* takes
the latter view, stating moreover, 'this is the
only authentic instance of unwholesome
qualities in the order of grasses,' and Professor Henslow considers too that as the use
of Darnel in the sixteenth century was similar
to that of Ergot – a diseased condition of the
grain of Rye – it is more probable that the
injurious nature of Darnel has been due to
an ergotized condition, especially as experiments have shown that perfectly healthy
Darnel seeds have no injurious effects.

VERNAL GRASS, SWEET SCENTED
Anthoxanthum odoratum (LINN.)

Part Used. Flowers

The Sweet-scented Vernal Grass – with
yellow anthers, not purple, as so many other
grasses – gives its characteristic odour to
newly-mown meadow hay, and has a pleasant
aroma of Woodruff. It is, however, specially
provocative of hay fever and hay asthma.
The flowers contain Coumarin, the same substance that is present in the Melilot flowers,
and the volatile pollen impregnates the atmosphere in early summer, causing much distress to hay-fever subjects. The sweet perfume is due chiefly to benzoic acid.

A medicinal tincture is made from this
grass with spirit of wine, and it said that if
poured into the open hand and sniffed well
into the nose, almost immediate relief is
afforded during an attack of hay fever. It is
recommended that 3 or 4 drops of the tincture be at the same time taken as a dose with
water, repeated if required, at intervals of
twenty to thirty minutes.

The name *Anthoxanthum* is from the Greek
anthos (flower) and *xanthos* (yellow).

¶ *Other Species.*

A. Puelii is a smaller species than *A.
odoratum*, with many slender much-branched
stems; lax panicles; long, slender awns, and
a fainter perfume. It occurs occasionally as
a modern introduction in sandy fields.
Flowers from July to September.

The following British grasses have varying
degrees of utility, though are not all medicinally valuable.

COMMON CORD-GRASS (*Spartina stricta*).
The generic name is from the Greek *spartiné*
(a cord) from the use to which the leaves

have been put. It grows on muddy salt-
marshes in the south. It is cut at Southampton by the poorer classes for thatching.
Another variety grows on the mud-flats at
Southampton, and is known as MANY-SPIKED
CORD-GRASS (*S. Towsendi*) with shorter leaves;
broader, larger spikelets, more lanceolate
downy glumes, and a flexuous tip to the
rachis; it also occurs on Southampton Water
and in the Isle of Wight.

CANARY - GRASS (*Phalaris canariensis*).
Though probably an escape in England, it is
much cultivated as 'canary-seed' in Central
and Southern Europe for caged 'song birds.'

SOFT-GRASS (*Holcus*). Name said to be from
the Greek *holkos*, connected with *helko* (I
draw), referring to a supposed power of
drawing thorns out of the flesh. There are
two British species, *H. Mollis* (Creeping Soft-
grass), abundant on light soil, and *H. lanatus*
(Yorkshire Fog, Meadow Soft-grass) larger
than the preceding.

DOG'S-TOOTH GRASS (*Fibichia*), of which the
only British species is *F. umbellata*, a low
prostrate grass, with long tough runners and
short fat glaucous leaves, distinguished from
all other British grasses (except *Panicum
sanguinale* and *P. glabrum*) by the digitate
arrangement of the three to five slender
purplish spikes in the panicle, each of which
is 1 to 1½ inches long; and from those two
species by having its awnless spikelets arranged singly, instead of in pairs, along the
spikes. It is found in sandy pastures by the
sea in the south-western counties, but is very
rare. It is a good sand-binder, and one of
the best pasture grasses of many dry climates.

In India it is called *Doorba* or *Doab-grass*, and in Bermuda, *Bermuda-grass*. It was named after J. Fibich, a German botanist.

REED (*Phragmites*), of which *P. communis* (Common Reed) is the only species, is a stout grass, 5 to 10 feet high, with a long creeping root-stock. It is common all over the world, is very serviceable on river banks for binding the soil, and is used also for thatch (especially in Norfolk).

The runners are nutritious, containing much sugar, and might be used as fodder.

Name said to be from the Greek, *phragma* (a hedge).

CRESTED DOG'S-TAIL (*Cynosurus cristatus*). Is a most useful grass, but the wiry stalks, when not eaten by sheep, remain in a dry state and are known as 'bents' or 'bennets.'

PURPLE MOLINIA (*Molinia varia*). The only species, and a rather coarse, stiff plant, sometimes 3 feet high, with one node near the base of the stem. It grows in tussocks in company with *Scabiosa succisa* (Premorse, or Devil's-bit Scabious). The stems of this grass are sold in bundles by tobacconists for cleaning pipes. It was named after G. F. Molina, a Chilian botanist.

WATER WHORL-GRASS (*Catabrosa aquatica*). The only species is a soft smooth pale-green plant, creeping or floating; sometimes much-branched, 1 to 2 feet high. It grows in ditches and by the margins of ponds. Rather scarce, though distributed over the whole island. One of the sweet grasses; water-fowl and cattle are fond of it; but it is unsuitable for cultivation from the character of its habitat. Its name is derived from the Greek *Katabrosis*, an 'eating out,' alluding to the torn ends of the glumes.

REED MANNA-GRASS (*Glyceria aquatica*). A conspicuous and imposing grass, 4 to 6 feet high, frequent in England and Ireland but rare in Scotland.

It is a fine covert for waterfowl.

SCENTED GRASSES

Among the Grasses may be included the SCENTED GRASSES, growing in tropical climates, largely cultivated in India, Ceylon and the Straits Settlements. They furnish very important essential oils for perfumery.

LEMONGRASS OIL is prepared from *Cymbopogon citratus*, formerly known as *Andropogon Schoenanthus*, a species growing abundantly in India and cultivated in Ceylon and Seychelles. It owes its scent almost entirely to its chief constituent, citral, and is one of the chief sources of the citral used in the manufacture of Tonone or artificial violet perfume. It is sometimes called Oil of Verbena from its similarity to the odour of the true Verbena Oil which is rarely found in commerce. It is frequently used to adulterate Lemon Oil. Samples of the oil produced experimentally in the West Indies, Uganda, and new districts of India were examined in the laboratories of the Imperial Institute in 1911, and as a result of the recommendations made, the production of Lemongrass has been taken up on a considerable scale in Uganda.

CITRONELLA OIL is derived from *C. nardus*, grown in Ceylon, Java and Burmah. The oil is distilled on an enormous scale and used for perfuming the cheapest household soaps and in the manufacture of coarse scents, and is also added as an adulterant to more expensive oils. Its scent is chiefly due to two substances, Geraniol and Citronellel.

PALMAROSA, Rosha or Indian Geranium Oil, is derived from *C. martine*. It is grown in India and was formerly known as 'Turkish Geranium Oil,' because it was imported into Europe *via* Turkey and Bulgaria as an adulterant to Otto of Roses. It has a strong geranium-like odour and is used in the commercial preparation of pure Geraniol, its chief constituent. The distillation of this oil was started in the eighteenth century.

GINGERGRASS OIL is also the product of the last-named grass, an oil of poorer quality, which is only suitable for cheap perfumes.

See SEDGES

GRAVELROOT

Eupatorium purpureum (LINN.)
N.O. Compositæ

Synonyms. Trumpet-weed. Gravelweed. Joe-pye Weed. Jopi Weed. Queen-of-the-Meadow Root. Purple Boneset. Eupatorium purpureum, trifoliatum, and maculatum. Eupatorium verticillatum. Eupatorium ternifolium. Hempweed

Part Used. Fresh root

Habitat. Is indigenous to North America, and common from Canada to Florida, growing in swampy and rich low grounds, where it blossoms throughout the summer months

¶ *Description.* This species varies greatly in form and foliage, the type being very tall and graceful.

The stem is rigidly erect, usually about 5 or 6 feet high, though sometimes even reaching a height of 12 feet, and is stout, unbranched and either hollow, or furnished with an incomplete pith. It is purple above the joints and often covered with elongated spots and lines (this variety having been called *maculata* by Linnæus). The leaves, oblong and pointed, rough above, but downy beneath, are placed in whorls of four or five on the stem (mostly in fives) and are nearly destitute of resinous dots. The margins are coarsely and unequally toothed, the leaf-stalks either short or merely represented by the contracted bases of the leaves. The flowers are purple, in a dense terminal inflorescence, the heads very numerous, five to ten flowered, contained in an eight-leaved, fresh-coloured involucre.

It grows in low, swampy ground. There are over forty species of the genus, many of which are used medicinally. The name is derived from a king of Pontus, Mithridates Eupator, who first used the plant as a remedy, and the popular name of Jopi or Joe-pye is taken from an American Indian who cured the typhus with it.

The taste is aromatic, astringent, and bitter. The roots should be collected in the autumn.

¶ *Constituents.* The chief constituent is Euparin. It is yellow, neutral, and crystalline, and received the formula $C_{12} = H_{11} = O_3$.

Eupurpurin, a so-called oleoresin, has been precipitated from a tincture of the drug.

A tincture and a fluid extract are prepared.

¶ *Medicinal Action and Uses.* Diuretic, nervine. Formerly the use of this purple-flowered Boneset was very similar to that of the ordinary Boneset. It is especially valuable as a diuretic and stimulant as well as an astringent tonic, and is considered a valuable remedy in dropsy, strangury, gravel, hematuria, gout and rheumatism, exerting a special influence upon chronic renal and cystic troubles.

¶ *Preparations.* Fluid extract, ½ to 1 drachm. Eupatorin, 3 to 5 grains.

See BONESET, HEMP AGRIMONY.

GREENWEED (DYERS')

Genista tinctoria (LINN.)
N.O. Leguminosæ

Synonyms. Greenweed. Greenwood. Woad or Wood-waxen, formerly Wede-wixen or Woud-wix. Base-broom. Genet des Teinturiers. Färberginster. Dyers' Broom
Part Used. Whole plant
Habitat. Mediterranean countries. Canary Islands. Western Asia. Britain. Established in the United States

¶ *Description.* The name of the genus is derived from the Celtic *Gen* (a small bush). *Genista tinctoria* is a small, tufted shrub, bearing short racemes of yellow flowers. The bright, luxuriant growth of the latter has led to its cultivation in greenhouses in the United States.

The bright green, smooth stems, 1 to 2 feet high, are much branched, the branches erect, rather stiff, smooth or only slightly hairy and free from spines. The leaves are spear-shaped, placed alternately on the stem, smooth, with uncut margins, ½ to 1 inch in length, very smoothly stalked, the margins fringed with hairs.

The shoots terminate in spikes of bright-yellow, pea-like flowers, opening in July. They are ½ to ¾ inch long, on foot-stalks shorter than the calyx. Like those of the Broom, they 'explode' when visited by an insect. The 'claws' of the four lower petals are straight at first, but in a high state of tension, so that the moment they are touched, they curl downwards with a sudden action and the flower bursts open. The flowers are followed by smooth pods, 1 to 1¼ inch long, much compressed laterally, brown when ripe, containing five to ten seeds.

A dwarf kind grows in tufts in meadows in the greater part of England and is said to enrich poor soil.

Cows will sometimes eat the plant, and it communicates an unpleasant bitterness to their milk and even to the cheese and butter made from it.

All parts of the plant, but especially the flowering tops, yield a good yellow dye, and from the earliest times have been used by dyers for producing this colour, especially for wool: combined with woad, an excellent green is yielded, the colour being fixed with alum, cream of tartar and sulphate of lime. In some parts of England, the plant used to be collected in large quantities by the poor and sold to the dyers.

Tournefort (1708) describes the process of dyeing linen, woollen, cloth or leather by the use of this plant, which he saw in the island of Samos. It is still applied to the same purpose in some of the Grecian islands. The Romans employed if for dyeing and it is described by several of their writers.

In some countries the buds are prepared and served as seasoning. As a dye the plant has largely been superseded by *Reseda luteola.*

The seeds have been suggested as a substitute for coffee.

In Spain and Italy strong cloths that take dyes well are woven from the fibres.

¶ *Constituents.* The active principle, *Scopnarine*, is found as starry, yellow crystals, and is soluble in boiling water and in alcohol. From the liquid which remains another principle, *Spartéine*, is extracted, an organic base, liquid and volatile, with strong narcotic properties.

¶ *Medicinal Action and Uses.* Diuretic, cathartic, emetic. Both flower tops and seeds have been used medicinally.

The powdered seeds operate as a mild purgative, and a decoction of the plant has been used medicinally as a remedy in dropsy and is also stated to have proved effective in gout and rheumatism, being taken in wineglassful doses three or four times a day.

The ashes form an alkaline salt, which has also been used as a remedy in dropsy and other diseases.

In the fourteenth century it was used, as well as Broom, to make an ointment called *Unguentum geneste*, 'goud for alle could goutes,' etc. The seed was used in a plaister for broken limbs.

A decoction of the plant was regarded in the Ukraine as a remedy for hydrophobia, but its virtues in this respect do not seem to rest on very good evidence.

Dioscorides and Pliny speak of the purgative properties of the seeds and flowers, and the latter also regarded them as diuretic and good for sciatica. Cullen used a decoction of the young shoots for the same purpose. An infusion of the flowers has been found useful for albuminuria, and a combination of the tips with mustard, in dropsy. A poultice has benefited cold abscesses and scrofulous tumours. The infusion can be taken in wineglassful doses three or four times a day.

It has been stated that scoparine can replace all preparations, while one drop of spartéine dissolved in alcohol is a strong narcotic.

¶ *Other Species.*

G. scoparia, *G. purgans*, and *G. griot* have similar properties. The last two are employed by the peasants as purgatives.

The flowers of *G. Hispanica* have been used in dropsy combined with albuminaric.

Dyers' Wood or Dyers' Weed is also the common name of *Isatis tinctoria*, and *Reseda Luteola*, or Yellow Weed or Weld, used in dyeing and painting.

See BROOM

GRINDELIA

Grindelia camporum (GREENE)
Grindelia cuneifolia
Grindelia squarrosa
N.O. Compositæ

Synonyms. Hardy Grindelia. Gum Plant. California Gum Plant. Scaly Grindelia. Rosin Weed. Grindelia robusta (Nutt.)

Parts Used. Dried leaves and flowering tops

Habitat. The western United States

¶ *Description.* Until the work of Perredes in 1906 the drug was supposed to be derived from *Grindelia robusta*, and the species now regarded as official were thought to be merely varieties. *G. robusta*, however, is rarely used.

There are about twenty-five species of the genus, seven or eight being found in South America. The early growth of most of them is covered with a glutinous varnish. They are perennial or biennial herbs or small shrubs, with stems up to half-a-yard long, round, yellow, and smooth, with alternate, light-green, coarsely-toothed leaves having a clasping base. They are easily broken off when dried, so are often found loose in packages. The solitary, terminal flower-heads are large and yellow, both disk and radiate. Taste and odour are slightly aromatic, the former bitter.

The distinctive mark of the genus is the limb of the calyx, consisting of two to eight rigid, narrow awns, which fall early.

The plant was only made widely known to the medical profession in the latter part of the nineteenth century, by Dr. C. A. Canfield, and Mr. J. G. Steele of San Francisco.

¶ *Constituents.* Grindelia may contain as much as 21 per cent. of amorphous resins. Two are dark-coloured, one being soluble in ether, and one soft and greenish, soluble in petroleum spirit. There is also found tannin, lævoglucose, and a little volatile oil. The presence of glucosides has not been confirmed.

¶ *Medicinal Action and Uses.* Expectorant and sedative, with an action resembling atropine. It has been recommended in cystitis and catarrh of the bladder, but its principal use is in bronchial catarrh, especially when there is any asthmatic tendency. It relieves dyspnœa due to heart disease, has been successfully employed in whooping cough, and as a local application in rhus poisoning, burns, genito-urinary catarrh, etc. As its active principle is excreted from the kidneys, it sometimes produces signs of renal irritation; in chronic catarrh of the bladder it stimulates the mucous membrane.

A homœopathic tincture is prepared.

¶ *Dosage.* Of fluid extract, ½ to 1 fluid drachm. Of Grindelia, 30 to 40 grains.

The Fluid extract is sometimes continued with liquorice in the proportion of ½ drachm of Grindelia to 1 drachm of the Fluid extract of Liquorice, mucilage to 1 oz.[1]

¶ *Other Species.*
G. cuneifolia is a marsh plant, darker green and less glutinous than *G. camporum*. It has a variety called *paludosa*.

G. squarrosa grows on prairies and dry banks. The bracts of the involucre are linear-lanceolate and spreading.

G. robusta var. *latifolia* is large, hardy, and a native of California.

These are all official varieties.

GROUND IVY. *See* IVY

(AMERICAN) GROUND PINE. *See* PINE

(EUROPEAN) GROUND PINE. *See* (YELLOW) BUGLE

GROUNDSEL, COMMON
Senecio vulgaris (LINN.)
N.O. Compositæ

Synonyms. (*Scotch*) Grundy Swallow, Ground Glutton. (*Norfolk*) Simson, Sention
Part Used. Whole herb
Habitat. A very common weed throughout Europe and Russian Asia, not extending to the tropics. It is abundant in Britain, being found up to the height of 1,600 feet in Northumberland. It grows almost everywhere, and is to be found as frequently on the tops of walls as among all kinds of rubbish and waste ground, but especially in gardens. Groundsel is one of those plants which follows civilized man wherever he settles, for there is hardly a European colony in the world in which it does not spring up upon the newly tilled land, the seeds probably having mingled with the grain which the European takes with him to the foreign country. Other home weeds, such as the thistle, have made their way across the seas in the same manner

Groundsel, so well known as a troublesome weed, is connected in the minds of most of us with caged birds, and probably few people are aware that it has any other use except as a favourite food for the canary. And yet in former days, Groundsel was a popular herbal remedy, is still employed in some country districts, and still forms an item in the stock of the modern herbalist, though it is not given a place in the British Pharmacopœia.

The name Groundsel is of old origin, being derived from the Anglo-Saxon *groundeswelge*, meaning literally, 'ground swallower,' referring to the rapid way the weed spreads. In Scotland and the north of England it is still in some localities called Grundy Swallow – only a slight corruption of the old form of the word – and is also there called Ground Glutton. In Norfolk it is often called Simson or Sention, which has by some been considered an abbreviation of 'Ascension Plant.' It seems more probable that 'Sention' is a corruption of the Latin, *Senecio*, derived from *Senex* (an old man), in reference to its downy head of seeds; 'the flower of this herb hath white hair and when the wind bloweth it away, then it appeareth like a bald-headed man.'

The genus *Senecio*, belonging to the large family *Compositæ*, includes about 900 species, which are spread over all parts of the globe, but are found in greatest profusion in temperate regions. Nine are natives of this country. The essential character of the genus is an involucre (the enveloping outer leaves of the composite heads of flowers) consisting of a single series of scales of equal length. The florets of the flower-heads are either all tubular, or more commonly, the central tubular and the marginal strap-shaped. The prevailing colour of the flowers in this genus is yellow purple (white or blue being comparatively rare).

¶ *Description.* It is an annual, the root consisting of numerous white fibres and the round or slightly angular stem, erect, 6 inches to nearly 1 foot in height, often branching at the top, is frequently purple in colour. It is juicy, not woody, and generally smooth, though sometimes bears a little loose, cottony wool. The leaves are oblong, wider and clasping at the base, a dull, deep green colour, much cut into (pinnatifid), with irregular, blunt-toothed or jagged lobes, not unlike the shape of oak leaves. The cylindrical flower-heads, each about ¼ inch long and ⅛ inch across, are in close terminal clusters or corymbs, the florets yellow and all tubular; the scales surrounding the head

---

[1] It combines well with yerba santa in equal proportions. – EDITOR.

and forming the involucre are narrow and black-tipped, with a few small scales at their base. The flowers are succeeded by downy heads of seeds, each seed being crowned by little tufts of hairs, by means of which they are freely dispersed by the winds. Groundsel is in flower all the year round and scatters an enormous amount of seed in its one season of growth, one plant if allowed to seed producing one million others in one year.

A variety of *Senecio vulgaris*, named *S. radiata* (Koch), with minute rays to the outer florets, is found in the Channel Islands.

According to Linnæus, goats and swine eat this common plant freely, cows being not partial to it and horses and sheep declining to touch it, but not only are caged birds fond of it, but its leaves and seeds afford food for many of our wild species. Groundsel, in common with many other common garden weeds, such as Chickweed, Dandelion, Bindweed, Plantain, etc., may be freely given to rabbits. It is said that Groundsel will at times entice a rabbit to eat when all other food has been refused. Rabbit-keeping is a very practical way of reducing the butcher's bill, and no means of feeding the rabbits economically should be neglected. Stores of both Groundsel and Chickweed might well be dried in the summer for giving to the rabbits in winter time with their hay.

¶ *Parts Used Medicinally.* The whole herb, collected in May, when the leaves are in the best condition and dried. The fresh plant is also used for the expression of the juice.

¶ *Constituents.* Chemically, Groundsel contains senecin and seniocine. The juice is slightly acrid, but emollient.

¶ *Medicinal Action and Uses.* Diaphoretic, antiscorbutic, purgative, diuretic, anthelmintic.

It was formerly much used for poultices and reckoned good for sickness of the stomach. A weak infusion of the plant is now sometimes given as a simple and easy purgative, and a strong infusion as an emetic: it causes no irritation or pain, removes bilious trouble and is a great cooler, or as Culpepper puts it:

'This herb is Venus's mistress piece and is as gallant and universal a medicine for all diseases coming of heat, in what part of the body soever they be, as the sun shines upon: it is very safe and friendly to the body of man, yet causes vomiting if the stomach be afflicted, if not, purging. It doth it with more gentleness than can be expected: it is moist and something cold withal, thereby causing expulsion and repressing the heat caused by the motion of the internal parts in purges and vomits. The herb preserved in a syrup, in a distilled water, or in an ointment, is a remedy in all hot diseases, and will do it: first, safely; secondly, speedily.'

'The decoction of the herb, saith Dioscorides, made with wine and drunk, helpeth the pains in the stomach proceeding from choler (bile). The juice thereof taken in drink, or the decoction of it in ale gently performeth the same. It is good against the jaundice and falling sickness (epilepsy), and taken in wine expelleth the gravel from the reins and kindeys. It also helpeth the sciatica, colic, and pains of the belly. The people in Lincolnshire use this externally against pains and swelling, and as they affirm with great success. The juice of the herb, or as Dioscorides saith, the leaves and flowers, with some Frankinsense in powder, used in wounds of the body, nerves or sinews, help to heal them. The distilled water of the herb performeth well all the aforesaid cures, but especially for inflammation or watering of the eye, by reason of rheum into them.'

Gerard says that 'the down of the flower mixed with vinegar' will also prove a good dressing for wounds, and recommends that when the juice is boiled in ale for the purpose of a purge, a little honey and vinegar be added, and that the efficacy is improved by the further addition of 'a few roots of Assarbace.' He states also that 'it helpeth the King's Evil, and the leaves stamped and strained into milk and drunk helpeth the red gums and frets in children.'

Another old herbalist tells us that the fresh roots smelled when first taken out of the ground are an immediate cure for many forms of headache. But the root must not be dug up with a tool that has any iron in its composition.

Some of the old authorities claimed that Groundsel was especially good for such wounds as had been caused by being struck by iron.

Groundsel in an old-fashioned remedy for chapped hands. If boiling water be poured on the fresh plant, the liquid forms a pleasant swab for the skin and will remove roughness.

For gout, it was recommended to 'pound it with lard, lay it to the feet and it will alleviate the disorder.'

A poultice of the leaves, applied to the pit of the stomach, is said to cause the same emetic effect as a dose of the strong infusion. A poultice made with salt is said to 'disperse knots and kernels in the flesh.'

In this country, farriers give Groundsel to horses as a cure for bot-worms, and in Germany it is said to be employed as a popular vermifuge for children.

A drachm of the juice is sufficient to take, internally.

See CHICKWEED, RAGWORT

GROUNDSEL, GOLDEN
Senecio aureus (LINN.)

Synonyms. Life Root. Squaw Weed. Golden Senecio
Part Used. Herb

Senecio aureus, Golden Groundsel, an American species, native of Virginia and Canada, is considered a most useful plant, deserving of attention. The root and whole herb are employed medicinally for their emmenagogue, diuretic, pectoral, and astringent qualities. It has often been used in the first stage of consumption for the beneficial effects of its tonic properties, combined with its pectoral qualities, 1 teaspoonful of the fluid extract prepared from it being taken in water or combined with other pectorals. It is also of value in gravel, stone, diarrhœa, etc. The plant has slender, fluted, unbranched and cottony stems, 1 to 2 feet high. The rhizome is perennial, 1 to 2 inches long, the bark of the roots hard and blackish. The root-leaves are roundish and kidney-shaped, up to 6 inches long, on long leaf-stalks. The stem leaves decrease in size as they grow up the stem, and are cut into as far as the midrib, the upper ones being stalkless. The flower-heads are few in number, loosely arranged at the summit of the stem, the flowers two-thirds to nearly an inch broad, of a golden yellow, with the outer ray florets slightly reflexed. The plant has only a slight odour, but a bitter, astringent, slightly acrid taste.

¶ *Preparations.* Senecin, 1 to 3 grains. Powdered root, ½ to 1 drachm. Fluid extract, ½ to 1 drachm. Solid extract, 5 to 10 grains.

GROUNDSEL, HOARY
Senecio erucifolius (LINN.)

Senecio erucifolius, the Hoary Groundsel, which has similar properties to *S. vulgaris*, has been employed in poultices, ointments and plasters. It is a perennial, distributed over Europe and Siberia, growing not infrequently here on dry banks and by roadsides in limestone or chalky districts from Berwick southwards, but rarely in Ireland. It is a tall plant, in growth similar to *S. Jacobœ*, but sending up several stems from its shortly creeping root. The whole plant is cottony, or softly hairy, with curled hairs, especially on the upper surfaces of the leaves, which have much narrower, regularly-divided segments, slightly rolled back at the edges. The flower-heads are larger. It flowers from July to August.

All forms of this genus are not of such beneficial use, and one at least has lately been found to be distinctly harmful, for Molteno disease, a cattle and horse disease prevalent in certain parts of South Africa, has been definitely traced to the presence of a poisonous alkaloid in a plant eaten by the animals, this plant being *Senecio latifolius*, a near relative of the Common Groundsel of this country.

SENECIO MARITIMA
Cineraria maritima (LINN.)

Senecio maritima, sometimes looked on as a variety of *S. campestris* (D.C.), and known by Linnæus as *Cineraria maritima*, is found on maritime rocks at Holyhead. It is a shrubby plant, divided into many branches, which have a white, downy covering of hairs. The flowers bloom from June to August, and are about ⅜ inches across, arranged in a similar manner to Ragwort. The leaves are 5 to 8 inches long and about 2 to 2¼ inches wide, the segments broadly-toothed, about three-lobed and with soft hairs, which form a dense white covering. One or two drops of the fresh juice of the plant dropped into the eye is said to be of use in removing cataract.

GROUNDSEL, MOUNTAIN
Senecio sylvaticus

Senecio sylvatica, Mountain Groundsel, is distinguished from Common Groundsel by its larger size, being 1 to 2 feet high, and by its having conical, rather than cylindrical heads of dull yellow flowers, with a few rays rolled back and often wanting. The stems are branched and the leaves pinnatifid, with narrower lobes, toothed. It is an annual, grows common on gravelly soil, on dry heaths and commons, growing in the Highlands up to 1,000 feet above sea-level and

flowers from July to September. It has a somewhat unpleasant odour, and detergent and antiscorbutic properties.

GROUNDSEL, VISCID

Senecio viscosus

Synonym. Stinking Groundsel

Senecio viscosus, Viscid Groundsel, is near the last-named species in habit, though its erect stem is not so tall, and it is distinguished by being clothed with viscid down, causing the leaves, which are finely cut into, to be thick and clammy to the touch and lighter in colour. The flower heads are less numerous, with the outer bracts of the involucre about half as long as the inner, and the flowers pale. It grows in similar situa-

tions, mostly on dry ditch banks and waste dry ground, from Forfar downwards, but is more local than *S. sylvaticus,* and is rare in Ireland. It, also, is an annual, flowering from July to September, and has a fœtid odour, obtaining for it the popular name of Stinking Groundsel. The leaves are carminative: its emetic properties are slightly less than those of *S. vulgaris.*

GUAIACUM

Guaiacum officinale (LINN.)
N.O. Zygophyllaceæ

Synonym. Lignum Vitæ
Parts Used. Resin, bark, wood
Habitat. West Indian Islands. North Coast of South America

¶ *Description.* An ornamental evergreen tree with pretty rich blue flowers, the trunk is a greenish-brown colour, the wood of slow growth but attains a height of 40 to 60 feet, stem almost always crooked, bark furrowed; the wood is extraordinarily heavy, solid and dense, fibres cross-grained; pinnate leaves, oval obtuse; fruit obcordate capsule; seeds solitary, hard, oblong. The old heart wood is dark green, the sap wood little in quantity and of a much lighter yellowish colour; the wood is largely used by turners, where weight is not an obstacle; it is very hard and durable, suitable for making black sheaves, pestles, pulleys, rulers, skittle boards, etc.; it has a slight acrid taste and is odourless, unless heated, when it emits an agreeable scent. The bark yields 1 per cent. volatile oil of delicious fragrance.

Guaiacum sanctum. Habitat, Bahamas and South Florida) is also used for the same purposes as *G. officinale;* it is easily distinguished from the latter, by its five-celled fruit, and its oblong leaflets, six to eight to each leaf. The leaves are sometimes used as a substitute for soap.

Guaiacum Resin. This is obtained from both the above trees and is procured by raising one end of the log and firing it; this melts the resin, which runs out of a hole cut in the other end, and is then caught into vessels. The resin is found in round or ovoid tears; some are imported the size of walnuts, but usually it is in large blocks; these break easily; the fracture is clean and glassy, in thin pieces, colour yellow-reddish brown. The powder is grey, and must be kept in

dark-coloured bottles, as exposure to the light and air soon turns it green.

¶ *Medicinal Action and Uses.* The wood is very little used in medicine; it obtained a great reputation about the sixteenth century, when it was brought into notice as a cure for syphilis and other diseases; later on the resin obtained from the wood was introduced and now is greatly preferred, for medicinal use, to the wood. The wood is sometimes sold by chemists in the form of fine shavings, and as such called Lignum Vitæ, which are turned green by exposure to the air, and bluish green by the action of nitric fumes. This test proves its genuiness.

It is a mild laxative and diuretic. For tonsilitis it is given in powdered form. Specially useful for rheumatoid arthritis, also in chronic rheumatism and gout, relieving the pain and inflammation between the attacks, and lessening their recurrence if doses are continued. It acts as an acrid stimulant, increasing heat of body and circulation; when the decoction is taken hot and the body is kept warm, it acts as a diaphoretic, and if cool as a diuretic. Also largely used for secondary syphilis, skin diseases and scrofula.

¶ *Dosage.* Of the wood 30 to 60 grains, Decoction, 2 oz. to 4 oz. in a pint of water. Fluid extract, ½ to 1 drachm. Guaiacum tincture, B.P. and U.S.P., ½ to 1 drachm. Ammoniated tincture Guaiacum, B.P. and U.S.P., ½ to 1 drachm. Resin, 5 to 15 grains. Guaiacum mixture, B.P., ½ to 1 fluid ounce. Guaiacum Resin Lozenges, B.P., 1 to 6 may be taken.

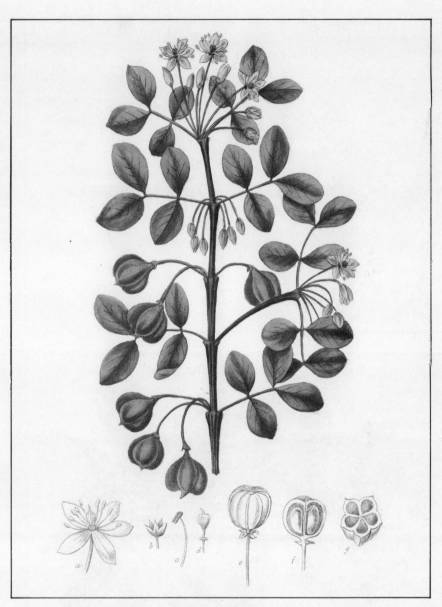

GUAIACUM
Guaiacum Officinale

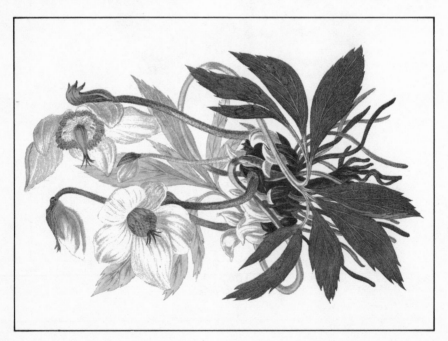

WHITE HELLEBORE
Veratrum Album

BLACK HELLEBORE
Helleborus Niger

GUARANA
Paullinia Cupana, Kunth. (H. B. and K.)
N.O. Sapindaceæ

Synonyms. Paullinia. Guarana Bread. Brazilian Cocoa. Uabano. Uaranzeiro. Paullinia Sorbilis
Part Used. Prepared seeds, crushed
Habitat. Brazil, Uruguay

¶ *Description*. This climbing shrub took the name of its genus from C. F. Paullini, a German medical botanist who died 1712. It has divided compound leaves, flowers yellow panicles, fruit pear shaped, three sided, three-celled capsules, with thin partitions, in each a seed like a small horse-chestnut half enclosed in an aril, flesh coloured and easily separated when dried. The seeds of *Paullinia Sorbilis* are often used or mixed with those of *P. Cupana*. Guarana is only made by the Guaramis, a tribe of South American Indians.

After the seeds are shelled and washed they are roasted for six hours, then put into sacks and shaken till their outside shell comes off; they are then pounded into a fine powder and made into a dough with water, and rolled into cylindrical pieces 8 inches long; these are then dried in the sun or over a slow fire, till they became very hard and are then a rough and reddish-brown colour, marbled with the seeds and testa in the mass. They break with an irregular fracture, have little smell, taste astringent, and bitter like chocolate without its oiliness, and in colour like chocolate powder; it swells up and partially dissolves in water.

¶ *Constituents*. A crystallizable principle, called guaranine, identical with caffeine, which exists in the seeds, united with tannic acid, catechutannic acid starch, and a greenish fixed oil.

¶ *Medicinal Action and Uses*. Nervine, tonic, slightly narcotic stimulant, aphrodisiac, febrifuge. A beverage is made from the guaran sticks, by grating half a tablespoonful into sugar and water and drinking it like tea. The Brazilian miners drink this constantly and believe it to be a preventive of many diseases, as well as a most refreshing beverage. Their habit in travelling is to carry the stick or a lump of it in their pockets, with a palate bone or scale of a large fish with which to grate it. *P. Cupana* is also a favourite national diet drink, the seeds are mixed with Cassava and water, and left to ferment until almost putrid, and in this state it is the favourite drink of the Orinoco Indians. From the tannin it contains it is useful for mild forms of leucorrhœa, diarrhœa, etc., but its chief use in Europe and America is for headache, especially if of a rheumatic nature. It is a gentle excitant and serviceable where the brain is irritated or depressed by mental exertion, or where there is fatigue or exhaustion from hot weather. It has the same chemical composition as caffeine, theine and cocaine, and the same physiological action. Its benefit is for nervous headache or the distress that accompanies menstruation, or exhaustion following dissipation. It is not recommended for chronic headache or in cases where it is not desirable to increase the temperature, or excite the heart or increase arterial tension. Dysuria often follows its administration. It is used by the Indians for bowel complaints, but is not indicated in cases of constipation or blood pressure.

¶ *Dosage*. Powder, 10 grains to $\frac{1}{2}$ drachm. Fluid extract of Guarana, U.S.P., 30 minims sweetened with one teaspoonful of syrup in water three times a day.

As a strong diuretic $7\frac{1}{2}$ grains can be taken daily and in 24 hours it has been known to increase urine from 27 oz. to 107 oz.

Tincture of Guarana, B.P.C., for sick headaches, 1 to 2 fluid drachms in water.

GUELDER ROSE
Viburnum opulus (LINN.)
N.O. Caprifoliaceæ

Synonyms. Cramp Bark. Snowball Tree. King's Crown. High Cranberry. Red Elder. Rose Elder. Water Elder. May Rose. Whitsun Rose. Dog Rowan Tree. Silver Bells. Whitsun Bosses. Gaitre Berries. Black Haw
Part Used. Bark
Habitat. The 'Gaitre-Beries' of which Chaucer makes mention among the plants that 'shal be for your hele' to 'picke hem right as they grow and ete hem in,' are the deep red clusters of berries of the Wild Guelder Rose (*Viburnum Opulus*, Linn.), a shrub growing 5 to 10 feet high, belonging to the same family as the Elder, found in copses and hedgerows throughout England, though rare in Scotland, and also indigenous to North America, where it is to be found in low grounds in the eastern United States

¶ *Description*. It resembles the Common Elder in habits of growth, hence in some districts we find it called Red Elder or Rose Elder. The conspicuous, large, nearly flat-topped heads of snow-white flowers are 3 to 5 inches across, the inner ones very small, but with an outer ring of large, showy, sterile blossoms, containing undeveloped stamens with no pollen and an ovary without ovules. Only the inner, complete flowers provide the nectar for the attraction of insects who are to fertilize them. The resulting fruits, which ripen very quickly, form a drooping cluster of bright red berries, shining and translucent, perhaps the most ornamental of our wild fruits, the tree presenting a very beautiful appearance in August, when they are ripe, especially as the leaves assume a rich purple hue before falling. But although edible, the berries, in spite of Chaucer's recommendation, are too bitter to be palatable eaten fresh off the trees, and when crushed, smell somewhat disagreeable, though birds appreciate them and in Siberia the berries used to be, and probably still are, fermented with flour and a spirit distilled from them. They have been used in Norway and Sweden to flavour a paste of honey and flour.

In Canada, they are employed to a considerable extent as a substitute for Cranberries and are much used for making a piquant jelly, their sourness gaining for them there the name of High Bush Cranberry, though the tree is, of course, quite unrelated to the true Cranberry.

The name Guelder comes from Gueldersland, a Dutch province, where the tree was first cultivated. It was introduced into England under the name of 'Gueldres Rose.' The garden variety, Viburnum sterile, with snowball flowers, does not produce the showy fruit of the wild species.

The berries have anti-scorbutic properties. They turn black in drying and have been used for making ink.

The wood, like that of the Spindle Tree and Dogwood, is used for making skewers.

¶ *Medicinal Action and Uses.* The bark, known as Cramp Bark, is employed in herbal medicine. It used formerly to be included in the United States Pharmacopœia, but is now omitted though it has been introduced into the National Formulary in the form of a Fluid Extract, Compound Tincture and Compound Elixir, for use as a nerve sedative and anti-spasmodic in asthma and hysteria.

In herbal practice in this country, its administration in decoction and infusion, as well as the fluid extract and compound tincture is recommended. It has been employed with benefit in all nervous complaints and debility and used with success in cramps and spasms of all kinds, in convulsions, fits and lock-jaw, and also in palpitation, heart disease and rheumatism.

The decoction ($\frac{1}{2}$ oz. to a pint of water) is given in tablespoon doses.

The bark is collected chiefly in northern Europe and appears in commerce in thin strips, sometimes in quills, $\frac{1}{20}$ to $\frac{1}{12}$ inch thick, greyish-brown externally, with scattered brownish warts, faintly cracked longitudinally. It has a strong, characteristic odour and its taste is mildly astringent and decidedly bitter.

¶ *Constituents.* The active principle of Cramp Bark is the bitter glucoside Viburnine; it also contains tannin, resin and valerianic acid.

¶ *Preparations and Dosages.* Fluid extract, $\frac{1}{2}$ to 2 drachms. Viburnin, 1 to 3 grains.

Its constituents are identical with the species of *Viburnum* that is more widely used and is an official drug in the United States, viz. *Viburnum Prunifolium* or Black Haw, though Cramp Bark contains $\frac{1}{8}$ the resin contained in Black Haw and its similar properties are considered much weaker.

Fluid Extract of Cramp Bark has a reddish-brown colour and the slight odour and somewhat astringent taste of the bark.

HAIR CAP MOSS. *See* MOSS

HARDHACK

Spiræa tomentosa (LINN.)
N.O. Rosaceæ

Synonyms. Steeple Bush. White Cap. White Leaf. Silver Leaf

Parts Used. Leaves, root, flowers

Habitat. Canada, New Brunswick, Nova Scotia to the mountains of Georgia westward

¶ *Description.* Indigenous shrub, with leaves ovate, lanceolate, serrate, greenish-white and downy. The rose-coloured flowers are in panicles underneath.

¶ *Constituents.* The root is said to contain gallic and tannic acid, and, when freshly dug, some volatile oils.

¶ *Medicinal Action and Uses.* The flowers give feebly the medicinal action of salicylic acid and are used in decoction for their diuretic and tonic effect.

The root and leaves are astringent and useful in diarrhœa when there are no inflammatory symptoms.

Dose for diarrhœa, 30 to 60 minims of the fluid extract.

HART'S TONGUE. *See* FERNS

HAWKBIT, AUTUMNAL

HAWKBIT, ROUGH

Leontodon autumnalis (LINN.)

Leontodon hispidus (LINN.)
N.O. Compositæ

Part Used. Herb

Assigned also at one time to the genus *Hieracium*, but now placed by most botanists in the genus *Leontodon*, and sometimes in the genus *Apargia*, are the Hawkbits, of which there are two British species, the Autumnal Hawkbit and the Rough Hawkbit, both abundantly distributed throughout Britain, in meadowland, and on commons and waste ground.

The Rough Hawkbit has been used medicinally in the same manner as the Hawkweeds and the Dandelion, for its action on the kidneys, and as a remedy for jaundice and dropsy, and is still used for its diuretic qualities in country districts in Ireland.

It is a plant somewhat resembling the Dandelion in appearance, the leaves all springing from the root, 3 to 4 inches long, jaggedly cut into, with the lobes pointing backwards, but instead of being smooth like the Dandelion, they are rough with forked bristles. The few flowers which the plant bears are borne singly on slender stems, 6 inches to a foot or more high, swollen at the top beneath the heads, which are 1½ inches in diameter when expanded; when in bud, they droop.

The name of the genus, *Leontodon*, is formed from two Greek words, meaning Lion's tooth, referring to the toothed leaves. *Apargia* is derived from the name bestowed by the Greeks on this or some similar plant, and is taken from two Greek words, meaning 'From idleness,' the implication being that where these weeds are allowed to abound, the farmer has his own idleness to thank. The name of the genus, *Hieracium*, derived from the Greek, *hieras* (a hawk), refers to an ancient belief that hawks ate these plants to sharpen their sight, a belief also indicated in the popular English names, Hawkweed and Hawkbit.

All the Hawkweeds abound in honey and have a sweet honey-like smell when expanded in the full sunshine.

¶ *Other Species.*

Hieracium Aurantiacum, called also 'Grim-the-Collier,' from the black hairs which clothe the flower-stalk and involucre, is an ornamental plant with orange flowers.

HAWKWEED, WALL

Hieracium murorum (LINN.)
N.O. Compositæ

Part Used. Herb

HAWKWEED, WOOD

Hieracium sylvaticum (LINN.)
N.O. Compositæ

Part Used. Herb

The Hawkweeds, together with the Hawkbits, Goat's Beard and Salsify, belong to the Chicory group of the great order Compositæ, which includes also the Dandelion and Sowthistles. All the plants of this group have milky juice, and the flowers – mostly yellow – have not *two* kinds of florets, like the daisy, but consist only of strap-shaped florets, each one of which is a complete flower in itself, not lacking stamens, as do the outer similarly shaped ray florets of the Daisy.

It is often a perplexing matter to distinguish the different members of the Hawkweed family. Some botanical authorities have recognized no less than thirty different species, but many of these are considered by other authorities to be merely variations or sub-species, and, as a rule, about ten species are regarded as distinct, of which the commonest among the taller species are the Wall Hawkweed (*Hieracium murorum*), and the Wood Hawkweed (*H. sylvaticum*), and the little Mouse-ear Hawkweed.

The older writers have often grouped together, as far as their medicinal qualities are concerned, the Hawkweeds, the Hawkbits and the Hawkbeards, all of which have yellow, dandelion-like flowers, and are much alike in appearance. Culpepper says:

'Saturn owns it. Hawkweed, saith Dioscorides, is cooling, somewhat drying and binding, and good for the heat of the stomach and gnawings therein, for inflammation and the bad fits of ague. The juice of it in wine helps digestion, dispels wind, hinders crudities abiding in the stomach; it is good against the biting of venomous serpents, if the herb be applied to the place, and is good against all other poisons. A scruple of the dried root given in wine and vinegar is profitable for dropsy. The decoction of the herb taken in honey digesteth the phlegm in the chest or lungs, and with hyssop helps the cough. The decoction of the herb and of wild succory made with wine, cures windy colic and hardness of the spleen, it procures rest and sleep, cools heat, purges the stomach, increases blood and helps diseases of the reins and bladder. Outwardly applied it is good for all the defects and diseases of the eyes, used with new milk; it is used with good success for healing spreading ulcers, especially in the beginning. The green leaves, bruised and with a little salt, applied to any place burnt with fire before blisters arise, help them: as also St. Anthony's fire(erysipelas)and all eruptions. Applied with meal and water as a poultice, it eases and helps cramps and convulsions. The distilled water cleanseth the skin and taketh away freckles, spots, or wrinkles in the face.'

The Wall Hawkweed, probably the commonest of the genus, grows freely in Great Britain in woods and on heaths, walls and rocks. It is a very variable plant, 1 to 2 feet high; the leaves, which are more or less hairy, mostly rise directly from the root and lie in a rosette on the ground. They are egg-shaped and toothed at the base and have slender footstalks. The stem is many-flowered and rarely bears more than one large leaf, sometimes none. The yellow flowers, which are in bloom in July and August, are from ¾ to 1 inch in diameter, their stalks below the heads being covered with scattered, simple and gland-tipped black hairs.

The Wood Hawkweed is found on banks and in copses, flowering in August and September. It is also very variable, but is best distinguished from *H. murorum* by its more robust habit, rather larger heads of flowers and by the narrower leaves, less crowded in a rosette, the stem being as a rule more leafy, but some varieties of *murorum* would rank with this in form of foliage. The leaves are sometimes very slightly toothed, the teeth pointing upwards, at other times deeply so, and are often spotted with purple. The stems are 1 to 3 feet high and many flowered, the involucres of the heads being hoary with down.

HAWKWEED, MOUSE-EAR

Hieracium Pilosella (LINN.)
N.O. Compositæ

Synonyms. Hawkweed. Pilosella. Mouse Ear
Part Used. Herb

None of the Hawkweeds are now much used in herbal treatment, though in many parts of Europe they were formerly employed as a constant medicine in diseases of the lungs, asthma and incipient consumption, but the small Mouse-ear Hawkweed, known commonly as Mouse-ear, is still collected and used by herbalists for its medicinal properties. It is very common on sunny banks and walls, and in dry pastures, and is well distinguished from all other British plants of the order, by its creeping scions or runners, which are thrown out in the same manner as in the strawberry, by its small rosettes of hairy, undivided leaves, greyish green above and hoary beneath, with a dense white coat of stellately branched hairs, and by its bright lemon-coloured flowers, which are borne singly on the almost leafless stems, which are only a few inches high. The flower-heads, which are about an inch in diameter, are composed of about fifty florets, the outer having a broad, purple stripe on the under side. They open daily at 8 a.m. and close about 2 p.m. The plant is in bloom from May to September.

The Mouse-ear differs from all other milky plants of this class, in its juice being less bitter and more astringent, and on account of this astringency, it was much employed as a medicine in the Middle Ages under the name of *Auricula muris*, from which the popular name is taken. It has sudorific, tonic and expectorant properties, and is considered a good remedy for whooping cough (for which, indeed, it has been regarded as a specific) and all affections of the lungs.

The infusion of the whole herb is employed, made by pouring 1 pint of boiling water on 1 oz. of the dried herb. This is well sweetened with honey and taken in wineglassful doses. A fluid extract is also prepared, the dose being ½ to 1 drachm. The powdered leaves prove an excellent astringent in hæmorrhage, both external and internal, a strong decoction being good for hæmorrhoids, and the leaves boiled in milk are a good external application for the same purpose.

Drayton has written:

'To him that hath a flux, of Shepherd's Purse he gives,
And *Mouse-ear* unto him whom some sharp rupture grieves.'

The name 'Mouse-ear' is also applied to 'Mouse-ear Chickweed,' a plant of the genus *Cerastium*, to a plant of the genus *Myosotis*, valued for its medicinal properties, and to various kinds of Woundworts.

Culpepper gives many uses for Mouse-ear Hawkweed. He tells us that

'The juice taken in wine, or the decoction drunk, cures the jaundice, though of long continuance, to drink thereof morning and evening, and abstain from other drink two or three hours after. It is a special remedy for the stone and the tormenting pains thereof; and griping pains in the bowels. The decoction with Succory and Centaury is very effectual in dropsy and the diseases of the spleen. It stayeth fluxes of blood at the mouth or nose, and inward bleeding also, for it is a singular wound herb for wounds both inward and outward. . . . There is a syrup made of the juice and sugar by the apothecaries of Italy, which is highly esteemed and given to those that have a cough, and in phthisis, and for ruptures and burstings.

The green herb bruised and bound to any cut or wound doth quickly close the lips thereof, and the decoction or powder of the dried herb wonderfully stays spreading and fretting cankers in the mouth and other parts. The distilled water of the plant is applicable for the diseases aforesaid and apply tents of cloths wet therein.'

The herb is collected in May and June, when in flower and is dried.

Parkinson states that if 'Mouseare' be given to any horse it 'will cause that he shall not be hurt by the smith that shooeth him.' Also that skilful shepherds are careful not to let their flocks feed in pastures where mouseare abounds 'lest they grow sicke and leane and die quickly after.'

See DANDELION, HAWKBITS, GOATSBEARD

HAWTHORN

Cratægus oxyacantha (LINN.)
N.O. Rosaceæ

Synonyms. May. Mayblossom. Quick. Thorn. Whitethorn. Haw. Hazels. Gazels. Halves. Hagthorn. Ladies' Meat. Bread and Cheese Tree
(*French*) L'épine noble
(*German*) Hagedorn
Part Used. Dried haws or fruits
Habitat. Europe, North Africa, Western Asia

¶ *Description.* The Hawthorn is the badge of the Ogilvies and gets one of its commonest popular names from blooming in May. Many country villagers believe that Hawthorn flowers still bear the smell of the Great Plague of London. The tree was formerly regarded as sacred, probably from a tradition that it furnished the Crown of Thorns. The device of a Hawthorn bush was chosen by Henry VII because a small crown from the helmet of Richard III was discovered hanging on it after the battle of Bosworth, hence the saying, 'Cleve to thy Crown though it hangs on a bush.' The Hawthorn is called *Cratægus Oxyacantha* from the Greek *kratos*, meaning hardness (of the wood), *oxus* (sharp), and *akantha* (a thorn). The German name of *Hagedorn*, meaning Hedgethorn, shows that from a very early period the Germans divided their land into plots by hedges; the word *haw* is also an old word for hedge. The name Whitethorn arises from the whiteness of its bark and Quickset from its growing as a quick or living hedge, in contrast to a paling of dead wood.

This familiar tree will attain a height of 30 feet and lives to a great age. It possesses a single seed-vessel to each blossom, producing a separate fruit, which when ripe is a brilliant red and this is in miniature a stony apple. In some districts these mealy red fruits are called Pixie Pears, Cuckoo's Beads and Chucky Cheese. The flowers are mostly fertilized by carrion insects, the suggestion of decomposition in the perfume attracts those insects that lay their eggs and hatch out their larvæ in decaying animal matter.

¶ *Constituents.* In common with other members of the Prunus and Pyrus groups of the order Rosaceæ, the Hawthorn contains Amyddalin. The bark contains the alkaloid Cratægin, isolated in greyish-white crystals, bitter in taste, soluble in water, with difficulty in alcohol and not at all in ether.

¶ *Medicinal Action and Uses.* Cardiac, diuretic, astringent, tonic. Mainly used as a cardiac tonic in organic and functional heart troubles. Both flowers and berries are astringent and useful in decoction to cure sore throats. A useful diuretic in dropsy and kidney troubles.

¶ *Preparation and dosage.* Fluid Extract of Berries, 10 to 15 drops.

The leaves have been used as an adulterant for tea. An excellent liquer is made from Hawthorn berries with brandy.

Formerly the timber, when of sufficient size, was used for making small articles. The root-wood was also used for making boxes and combs; the wood has a fine grain and takes a beautiful polish. It makes excellent fuel, making the hottest wood-fire known and used to be considered more desirable than

Oak for oven-heating. Charcoal made from it has been said to melt pig-iron without the aid of a blast.

The stock is employed not only for grafting varieties of its own species, but also for several of the garden fruits closely allied to it, such as the medlar and pear.

¶ *Other Species.*

C. Aronia is a bushy species giving larger fleshy fruit than *C. Oxyacantha*. It is indigenous to Southern Europe and Western Asia and is common about Jerusalem and the Mount of Olives, where its fruit is used for preserves.

C. odoratissima is very agreeable also as a fruit.

C. Azarole. Its fruit in the same way is highly esteemed in Southern Europe.

HEARTSEASE

Viola tricolor (LINN.)
N.O. Violaceæ

Synonyms. Wild Pansy. Love-Lies-Bleeding. Love-in-Idleness. Live-in-Idleness. Loving Idol. Love Idol. Cull Me. Cuddle Me. Call-me-to-you. Jack-jump-up-and-kiss-me. Meet-me-in-the-Entry. Kiss-her-in-the-Buttery. Three-Faces-under-a-Hood. Kit-run-in-the-Fields. Pink-o'-the-Eye. Kit-run-about. Godfathers and God-mothers. Stepmother. Herb Trinitatis. Herb Constancy. Pink-eyed-John. Bouncing Bet. Flower o' luce. Bird's Eye. Bullweed

(*Anglo-Saxon*) Banwort, Banewort.

(*French*) Pensée

Part Used. Herb

Habitat. The Heartsease, or Wild Pansy, very different in habit from any other kind of *Viola*, is abundantly met with almost throughout Britain. Though found on hedgebanks and waste ground, it seems in an especial degree a weed of cultivation, found most freely in cornfields and garden ground. It blossoms almost throughout the entire floral season, expanding its attractive little flowers in the early days of summer and keeping up a succession of blossom until late in autumn

¶ *Description.* The Heartsease is as variable as any of the other members of the genus, but whatever modifications of form it may present, it may always be readily distinguished from the other Violets by the general form of its foliage, which is much more cut up than in any of the other species and by the very large leafy stipules at the base of the true leaves. The stem, too, branches more than is commonly found in the other members of the genus. Besides the free branching of the stem, which is mostly 4 to 8 inches in height, it is generally very angular. The leaves are deeply cut into rounded lobes, the terminal one being considerably the largest. In the other species of *Viola* the foliage is ordinarily very simple in outline, heart-shaped, or kidney-shaped, having its edge finely toothed.

The flowers ($\frac{1}{4}$ to $1\frac{1}{4}$ inch across) vary a great deal in colour and size, but are either purple, yellow or white, and most commonly there is a combination of all these colours in each blossom. The upper petals are generally most showy in colour and purple in tint, while the lowest and broadest petal is usually a more or less deep tint of yellow. The base of the lowest petal is elongated into a spur, as in the Violet.

The flowers are in due course succeeded by the little capsules of seeds, which when ripe, open by three valves. Though a near relative of the Violet, it does not produce any of the curious bud-like flowers – cleisto-gamous flowers – characteristic of the Violet, as its ordinary showy flowers manage to come to fruition so that there is no necessity for any others. Darwin found that the humble bee was the commonest insect visitor of the Heartsease, though the moth *Pluvia* visited it largely – another observer mentions *Thrips* – small wingless insects – as frequent visitors to the flowers. Darwin considered that the cultivated Pansy rarely set seed if there were no insect visitors, but that the little Field Pansy can certainly fertilize itself if necessary.

The flower protects itself from rain and dew by drooping its head both at night and in wet weather, and thus the back of the flower and not its face receives the moisture.

The wild species is an annual, but from it the countless varieties of the perennial garden pansies, with blossoms of large size and singular beauty, are supposed to have originated. It is a very widely distributed plant, found not only throughout Britain, but in such diverse places as Arctic Europe, North Africa, Siberia and N.W. India. Several of the varieties have been distinguished as sub-species: the most marked of these are *V. arvensis*, most common in cornfields, with white or yellowish flowers, with spreading petals; and *lutea*, which has a branched rootstock, short stems, with underground runners, and blue, purple or yellow flowers with spreading petals much longer than the sepals.

Miss Martineau tells us that many kinds are common in meadows in America, and says that as early as February the fields about Washington are quite gay with their flowers.

The Pansy is one of the oldest favourites in the English garden and the affection for it is shown in the many names that were given it. The Anglo-Saxon name was Banwort or Bonewort.

Miss Rohde is of opinion that Banwort was the old name for the daisy.

She says: 'It would be interesting to know if the *daisy* is still called banwurt in the north,' and she quotes from Turner's *Herbal* in support of this, 'The Northern men call thys herbe banwurt because it helpeth bones to knyt againe. . . .'

Its common name of Pansy (older form 'Pawnce,' as in Spenser) is derived from the French *pensées*, the name which is still used in France.

'Love in Idleness' is still in use in Warwickshire. In ancient days the plant was much used for its potency in love charms, hence perhaps its name of Heartsease. It is this flower that plays such an important part as a love-charm in the *Midsummer Night's Dream*.

The celebrated Quesnay, founder of the 'Economists,' physician to Louis XV, was called by the king his 'thinker,' and given, as an armorial bearing, three pansy flowers.

In many old Herbals the plant is called Herba Trinitatis, being dedicated by old writers to the Trinity, because it has in each flower three colours.

Stepmother is a familiar name for it in both France and Germany, from a fanciful reference to the different-shaped petals, supposed to represent a stepmother, her own daughters and her stepchildren.

¶ *Part Used Medicinally and Preparation for Market.* The whole herb, collected in the wild state and dried.

The Wild Pansy may be collected any time from June to August, when the foliage is in the best condition.

¶ *Constituents.* The herb contains an active chemical principle, Violine (a substance similar to Emetin, having an emeto-cathartic action), mucilage, resin, sugar, salicylic acid and a bitter principle. When bruised, the plant, and especially the root, smells like peach kernels or prussic acid. The seeds are considered to have the same therapeutic activity as the leaves and flowers.

¶ *Medicinal Action and Uses.* The Pansy has very similar properties to the Violet.

It was formerly in much repute as a remedy for epilepsy, asthma and numerous other complaints, and the flowers were considered cordial and good in diseases of the heart, from which may have arisen its popular name of Heartsease as much as from belief in it as a love potion.

Gerard states:

'It is good as the later physicians write for such as are sick of ague, especially children and infants, whose convulsions and fits of the falling sickness it is thought to cure. It is commended against inflammation of the lungs and chest, and against scabs and itchings of the whole body and healeth ulcers.'

A strong decoction of syrup of the herb and flowers was recommended by the older herbalists for skin diseases and a homœopathic medicinal tincture is still made from it with spirits of wine, using the entire plant, and given in small diluted doses for the cure of cutaneous eruptions.

It was formerly official in the United States Pharmacopœia, and is still employed in America in the form of an ointment and poultice in eczema and other skin troubles, and internally for bronchitis.

Some years ago attention was called to this herb by a writer in the *Medical Journal* as a valuable remedy for the cutaneous disorder called *crusta lactes,* or Scald head, in children. For this purpose, ½ drachm of dried leaves, or a handful of the fresh herb boiled in milk, was recommended to be given every morning and evening: poultices formed of the leaves were likewise applied with success. By several medical writers its use is said to have proved very efficacious in this complaint.

On the Continent, the herbaceous parts of the plant have been employed for their mucilaginous, demulcent and expectorant properties. The root and seeds are also emetic and purgative, which properties as well as the expectorant action of the plant are doubtless due to the presence of the violine.

Pansy leaves are used on the Continent in place of litmus in acid and alkali tests.

HEDGE-HYSSOP. *See* HYSSOP

HEDGE MUSTARD. *See* MUSTARD

HELIOTROPE

Synonyms. Turnsole. Cherry Pie

Heliotropium Peruviana
N.O. Heliotropeæ

A sweet-scented plant which is called Heliotrope because it follows the course of the sun. After opening it gradually turns from the east to the west and during the night turns again to the east to meet the rising sun. The Ancients recognized this characteristic of the plant and applied it to mythology.

(*POISON*)
HELLEBORE, BLACK

Helleborus niger (LINN.)
N.O. Ranunculaceæ

Synonyms. Christe Herbe. Christmas Rose. Melampode
Parts Used. Rhizome, root
Habitat. It is a native of the mountainous regions of Central and Southern Europe, Greece and Asia Minor, and is cultivated largely in this country as a garden plant. Supplies of the dried rhizome, from which the drug is prepared, have hitherto come principally from Germany.
Two allied species are natives of this country, but this particular kind does not grow wild here

The Black Hellebore – once known as Melampode – is a perennial, low-growing plant, with dark, shining, smooth leaves and flower-stalks rising directly from the root, its pure white blossoms appearing in the depth of winter and thereby earning for it the favourite name of Christmas Rose.

The generic name of this plant is derived from the Greek *elein* (to injure) and *bora* (food), and indicates its poisonous nature. The specific name refers to the dark-coloured rootstock.

The Black Hellebore used by the Greeks has been identified by Dr. Sibthorp as *Helleborus officinalis*, a handsome plant, with a branching stem, bearing numerous serrated bracts, and three to five whitish flowers. It is a native of Greece, Asia Minor, etc.

The two species found wild in many parts of England, especially on a limestone soil, are *H. Fœtidus*, the Bearsfoot, and *H. Viridis*, the Green Hellebore; the latter has injurious effects on cattle if eaten by them.

Both these British species possess powerful medicinal effects and are at times substituted for the true *H. niger*.

¶ *History.* According to Pliny, Black Hellebore was used as a purgative in mania by Melampus, a soothsayer and physician, 1,400 years before Christ, hence the name Melampodium applied to Hellebores. Spenser in the *Shepheard's Calendar*, 1579, alludes to the medicinal use of Melampode for animals. Parkinson, writing in 1641, tells us

'a piece of the root being drawne through a hole made in the eare of a beast troubled with cough or having taken any poisonous thing cureth it, if it be taken out the next day at the same houre.'

Parkinson believed that White Hellebore would be equally efficacious in such a case, but Gerard recommends the Black Horehound only, as being good for beasts. He says the old farriers used to 'cut a slit in the

¶ *Medicinal Action and Uses.* In homœopathic medicine a tincture of the whole fresh plant is used for clergyman's sore throat and uterine displacement.

dewlap, and put in a bit of Beare-foot, and leave it there for daies together.'

Gerard describes the plant in these words:

'It floureth about Christmas, if the winter be mild and warm . . . called Christ herbe. This plant hath thick and fat leaves of a deep green colour, the upper part whereof is somewhat bluntly nicked or toothed, having sundry diversions or cuts, in some leaves many, in others fewer, like unto a female Peony. It beareth rose-coloured flowers upon slender stems, growing immediately out of the ground, an handbreadth high, sometimes very white, and ofttimes mixed with a little shew of purple, which being faded, there succeed small husks full of black seeds; the roots are many; with long, black strings coming from one end.'

Once, people blessed their cattle with this plant to keep them from evil spells, and for this purpose, it was dug up with certain mystic rites. In an old French romance, the sorcerer, to make himself invisible when passing through the enemy's camp, scatters powdered Hellebore in the air, as he goes.

The following is from Burton's *Anatomy of Melancholy*:

'Borage and hellebore fill two scenes,
Sovereign plants to purge the veins
Of melancholy, and cheer the heart
Of those black fumes which make it smart.'

¶ *Cultivation.* All kinds of Hellebore will thrive in ordinary garden soil, but for some kinds prepared soil is preferable, consisting of equal parts of good fibry loam and well-decomposed manure, half fibry peat and half coarse sand. Thorough drainage is necessary, as stagnant moisture is very injurious. It prefers a moist, sheltered situation, with partial shade, such as the margins of shrubberies. If the soil is well trenched and manured, Hellebore will not require replanting for at least seven years, if grown for flowering, but a top dressing of well-decayed manure and a little liquid manure might be given during the growing season, when plants are making their foliage. Propagation is by seeds, or division of roots. Seedlings should be pricked off thickly into a shady border, in a light, rich soil. The second year they should be transplanted to permanent quarters, and will bloom in the third year. For division of roots, the plant is strongest in July, and the clumps to be divided must be well established, with rootstocks large enough to cut. The plants will be good flowering plants in two years, but four years are required to bring them to perfection.

¶ *Part Used.* The rhizome, collected in autumn and dried.

The root has a slight odour, when cut or broken, somewhat resembling Senega root. The dry powder causes violent sneezing. It has a somewhat bitter-sweet and acrid taste.

¶ *Constituents.* Two crystalline glucosides, Helleborin and helleborcin, both powerful poisons. Helleborin has a burning, acrid taste and is narcotic, helleborcin has a sweetish taste and is a highly active cardiac poison, similar in its effects to digitalis and a drastic purgative. Other constituents are resin, fat and starch. No tannin is present.

¶ *Medicinal Action and Uses.* The drug possesses drastic purgative, emmenagogue and anthelmintic properties, but is violently narcotic. It was formerly much used in dropsy and amenorrhœa, and has proved of value in nervous disorders and hysteria. It is used in the form of a tincture, and must be administered with great care.

Applied locally, the fresh root is violently irritant.

¶ *Preparations and Dosages.* Fluid extract, 2 to 10 drops. Solid extract, 1 to 2 grains. Powdered root, 10 to 20 grains as a drastic purge, 2 to 3 grains as an alterative. Decoction, 2 drachms to the pint, a fluid ounce every four hours till effective.

A tincture of the fresh root of *H. fœtidus* is used in homœopathy.

HELLEBORE, FALSE (*POISON*)

Adonis autumnalis
Adonis vernalis
N.O. Ranunculaceæ

Synonyms. Red Chamomile. Pheasant's Eye. Adonis. Red Morocco. Rose-a-rubie. Red Mathes. Sweet Vernal

Part Used. Herb

The Pheasant's Eye (*Adonis autumnalis*), a plant very nearly allied to the Anemone, is sometimes found wild in England, mostly in cornfields in Kent, but is often regarded as a mere garden escape. Though generally only a cultivated species in this country, it is common enough on the Continent.

It is a graceful plant, growing about a foot high, with finely cut leaves and terminal flowers like small scarlet buttercups.

¶ *History.* Its Latin name is derived from the ill-fated Adonis, from whose blood it sprang, according to the Greek legends. 'Red Morocco' was a somewhat strange old English name for this plant, also 'Rose-a-rubie' and 'Red Mathes,' 'by which name,' says Gerard, 'it is called of them that dwell where it groweth naturally and generally red camomill' – the latter on account of the finely-cut leaves. It is now aptly called Pheasant's Eye, on account of its brilliant little scarlet and black blossoms.

Although named *A. autumnalis*, it blossoms throughout the summer, commencing to flower in June, and the seeds ripen in August and September. It is an annual, propagated by its seeds, which may be sown at almost any season, but should always be sown where the plant is to grow, because it does not bear transplanting. Any soil will suit it: it blos-soms more freely in the sunshine, but will also flourish in shade.

In olden days it was considered to have some medicinal value, but is no longer used. Its near relative, *A. vernalis* (or 'Ox-eye'), though not official, is still regarded of medicinal value, and is a perennial species, not a native of this country, but common in central Europe, where its root is often used in the place of Black Hellebore.

'*A. vernalis* is one of the brightest and most effective of spring plants, known in many places as Sweet Vernal. It might be said of this, as of the Daffodil, that it "takes the winds of March with beauty," for often before the month is out it opens its rich, golden Anemone-like cups to the sun, and when planted in profusion, presents a glowing mass of colour. The plant is only about 9 inches high, and its foliage is one of its beauties. It makes a good addition to the rockery. Another species, *A. amurensis*, which is among the earliest of all the flowers, for it comes into bloom in February and March, is rather taller, and the foliage is more finely cut. There is a double variety, *flore pleno*, with large, yellow flowers. These plants will grow in any good garden soil, well drained and not too heavy. They should have a sunny position, but should not be allowed to suffer from drought during summer. They are quite hardy, and if left undisturbed improve from year to year.'

¶ *Constituents.* *A. vernalis* contains a glucoside Adonidin and has an action almost exactly like that of digitalin, but is much stronger and is said not to be cumulative. It appears to be about ten times as powerful as digitoxin. It has been prescribed instead of digitalis, and sometimes succeeds where digitalis fails, especially where there is kidney disease. It is, however, less certainly beneficial in valvular disease than digitalis, and should be used only where digitalis fails. It produces vomiting and diarrhœa more readily than digitalis. It is given in the form of an infusion.

¶ *Preparations and Dosages.* Fluid extract, 1 to 2 drops. Glucoside adonidin, ¼ to ½ grain.

The infusion is made with ¼ oz. of the herb to a pint of boiling water and given in tablespoonful doses every three hours.

(POISON)
HELLEBORE, GREEN

Veratrum viride
N.O. Melanthaceæ or Liliaceæ

Synonyms. American Hellebore. Swamp Hellebore. Indian Poke. Itch-weed
Parts Used. Dried rhizome and roots
Habitat. Swamps, low grounds, and moist meadows of the United States

¶ *Description.* For commercial convenience, the roots are usually broken into small pieces or fragments, but are sometimes sliced, the cut surface being of a dingy white colour, or whole, the outside dark brown, with characteristic markings. Often, portions of the dried stem or leafstalks remain attached, and these, being inert, should be rejected.

American Hellebore closely resembles the German *Veratrum album*, or White Hellebore, and the Mexican *V. officinale*, or Sabadilla (Cevadilla), N.O. Liliaceæ. The name Veratrine is given to the mixture of bases obtained from Sabadilla by extracting with alcohol, distilling off the alcohol, and precipitating the mixed bases with ammonia. Official in the Pharmacopœia of 1898. The British Pharmacopœia Codex preparation is *Oleinatum Veratrinæ*.

¶ *Constituents.* It has been found that the alkaloids contained in *V. viride* are not the same as the veratrine contained in *V. album* and the seeds of Sabadilla. The principal alkaloids are Pseudojervine, Rubijervine, Jervine, Cevadine, Protoveratrine, and Protoveratridine. The last is probably a decomposition product, it is highly poisonous, and sternutatory. Starch and resin are also present.

¶ *Medicinal Action and Uses.* Emetic, diaphoretic, sedative, highly poisonous. The German White Hellebore, resembling the American, but without its cevadine, is rarely given internally, but the powder has been used in preparing an ointment for itch.

Veratrine, a pale grey amorphous powder, is used externally as an analgesic, and also as a parasiticide. It is not known to affect the living blood, but when the latter is drawn, veratrine kills the white corpuscles. Violent pain and irritation are caused if it is given internally or subcutaneously. It prolongs the ontractions of heart and muscles. Its only justifiable use is as an anodyne counter-irritant, especially for neuralgia. It was emphatically decided a few years ago that *V. viride* should *whenever possible* be used instead of the European *V. album*, which is more likely to upset the intestines. The various alkaloids present act in very different manners, and none in exactly the same way as the whole drug – jervine, for example, is less poisonous than the drug itself, while protoveratrine, although present in small quantity, is extremely toxic.

A moderate dose of veratrum produces a reduction in the rate of the pulse, with a fall in the arterial pressure. There may be slowing of respiration. It has been used in the treatment of pneumonia, peritonitis, and other sthenic fevers, but is chiefly useful in chronic diseases, such as arterio-sclerosis and interstitial nephritis. It differs from digitalis in that it diminishes cardiac tone, and has been used for threatened apoplexy and 'irritable heart'; also for puerperal eclampsia.

Sabadilla is the principal ingredient of the *pulvis capocinorum*, sometimes used in Europe for the destruction of vermin in the hair.

¶ *Dosages.* *V. viride*, from 1 to 3 minims of the fluid extract every two or three hours until pulse rate is reduced. 1 to 2 grains. Of U.S. tincture, 10 to 30 minims.

V. album, 1 to 2 grains in powder. Rarely given internally.

Veratrine, $\frac{1}{30}$ grain.

¶ *Poisons, if any, and Antidotes.* Causes vomiting, with much nausea and retching. Pulse slow, later, rapid and irregular. Prostration, perspiration, pallor, with shallow and sometimes stertorous breathing.

If there is vomiting, two glasses of water should be given and 20 grains of tannic acid as an imperfect chemical antidote. Should vomiting not occur, it must be provoked, or a stomach pump employed. The patient

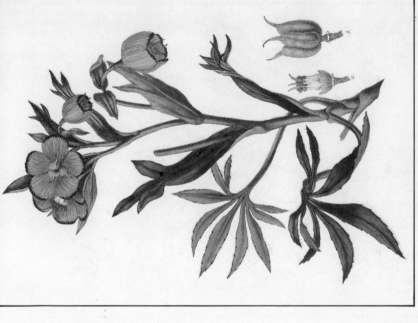

XLIX

(BLACK) STINKING HELLEBORE (ENGLISH BEARSFOOT)
Helleborus Fœtidus

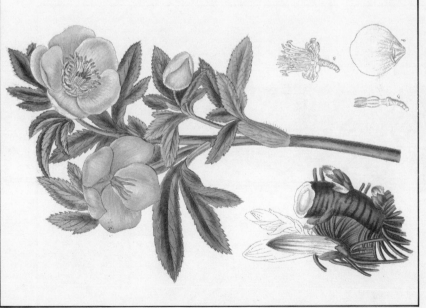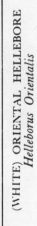

(WHITE) ORIENTAL HELLEBORE
Helleborus Orientalis

L

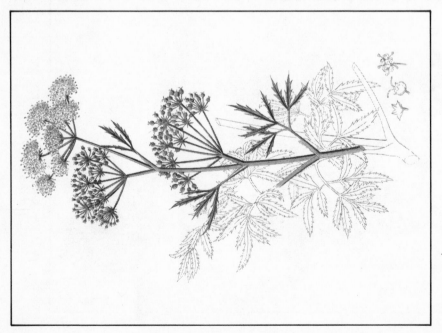

HEMLOCK
Conium Maculat

WATER HEMLOCK (COWBANE)
Cicuta Vir

must be kept in a horizontal position, not even being allowed to sit up to vomit. To stop the vomiting a counter-irritant must be used over the epigastrium and morphine employed *very cautiously*. In the early stages, when the pulse is low, atropine is very valuable, or active respiratory stimulants, such as hypodermic injections of ammonia and strychnine. If the bodily temperature is low, heat can be applied externally.

See BEARSFOOT (STINKING HELLEBORE), SABADILLA and HELLEBORE, WHITE

(POISON)
HELLEBORE, WHITE

Veratrum album
N.O. Lilaceæ

Synonyms. Veratrum Lobelianium. Veratrum Californicum. Weiszer Germer. Weisze Nieszwurzel

Parts Used. Rhizome, root

Habitat. Europe, from Lapland to Italy. Does not occur in the British Isles

¶ *Description. Veratrum album* closely resembles the American species, but is distinguished by its yellowish-white flower.

The fresh rhizome has an alliaceous odour, but when dried it has no marked smell. Its taste is first sweet, then bitter and acrid, leaving the tongue tingling and numb. Its powder is ash-coloured. White Hellebore deteriorates by keeping. It is *scarcely ever used internally* owing to the severity of its action. It is stated to have been one of the principal poisons used in Europe for arrows, daggers, etc.

¶ *Constituents.* Authorities differ as to the presence or absence of the *veratria* of cevadilla. It contains jervine, pseudo-jervine, rubijervine, veratralbine and veratrine. Cevadine is stated to be absent. There is fatty matter, composed of olein, stearin and a volatile acid, supergallate of Veratia, yellow colouring matter, starch ligneous matter, and gum; the ashes contain much phosphate and carbonate of lime, carbonate of potassa and some traces of silica, and sulphate of lime. There has been found in it a white, crystalline, fusible and inflammable substance called barytin, of which the properties have not been thoroughly investigated.

¶ *Medicinal Action and Uses.* A violent, irritant poison. When snuffed up the nose it occasions profuse running of the nose; when swallowed, severe vomiting and profuse diarrhœa. It was formerly used in cerebral affections, such as mania, epilepsy, etc., and for gout, as a substitute for colchicum or the Eau Mediciale of Husson, when 3 parts of the wine of White Hellebore added to 1 part of laudanum was given in doses of from ½ fluid drachm to 2 fluid drachms.

It is occasionally used in the form of an ointment or decoction in obstinate skin diseases such as scabies, or to kill lice, but even this use is not free from danger. It is also occasionally used as an errhine or sternutatory, diluted with starch or other mild powder, in cases of amaurosis and chronic affections of the brain.

The principal use of the plant is in veterinary medicine.

¶ *Dosages.* Of the powder, 1 to 8 grains, gradually and cautiously increased, commencing with 1 grain. Of the vinous tincture, from 20 to 60 minims.

¶ *Poisons, if any, and Antidotes.* Narcotic symptoms, such as stupor and convulsions, appear in addition to vomiting and diarrhœa, when the dose is fatal. The poison may be treated by drinks and injections of coffee, stimulants to overcome the depressed condition of the heart and arteries, and opiates and demulcents to relieve internal inflammation.

¶ *Other Species.*

Helleborus orientalis (Lam.). A tincture of the root is used in homœopathy for indigestion and diarrhœa.

See also BEARSFOOT (HELLEBORE, STINKING), SABADILLA.

(POISON)
HEMLOCK

Conium maculatum (LINN.)
N.O. Umbelliferæ

Synonyms. Herb Bennet. Spotted Corobane. Musquash Root. Beaver Poison. Poison Hemlock. Poison Parsley. Spotted Hemlock. Kex. Kecksies

Parts Used. Leaves, fruit, seeds

Habitat. It is by no means an uncommon plant in this country, found on hedgebanks, in neglected meadows, on waste ground and by the borders of streams in most parts of England, occurring in similar places throughout Europe (except the extreme north) and also in temperate Asia and North Africa. It has been introduced into North and South America

The Hemlock is a member of the great order Umbelliferæ, the same family of plants to which the parsley, fennel, parsnip and carrot belong.

391

Many of the umbelliferous plants abound in an acrid, watery juice, which is more or less narcotic in its effects on the animal frame, and which, therefore, when properly administered in minute doses, is a valuable medicine. Among these the most important is *Conium*, or Hemlock. Every part of this plant, especially the fresh leaves and fruit, contains a volatile, oily alkaloid, which is so poisonous that a few drops prove fatal to a small animal.

¶ *History.* The Ancients were familiar with the plant, which is mentioned in early Greek literature, and fully recognized its poisonous nature. The juice of hemlock was frequently administered to criminals, and this was the fatal poison which Socrates was condemned to drink.

The old Roman name of *Conium* was *Cicuta*, which prevails in the mediæval Latin literature, but was applied about 1541 by Gesner and others to another umbelliferous plant, *Cicuta virosa*, the Water Hemlock, which does not grow in Greece and southern Europe. To avoid the confusion arising from the same name for these quite dissimilar plants, Linnæus, in 1737, restored the classical Greek name and called the Hemlock (*Conium maculatum*), the generic name being derived from the Greek word *Konas*, meaning to whirl about, because the plant, when eaten, causes vertigo and death. The specific name is the Latin word, meaning 'spotted,' and refers to the stem-markings. According to an old English legend, these purple streaks on the stem represent the brand put on Cain's brow after he had committed murder.

Hemlock was used in Anglo-Saxon medicine, and is mentioned as early as the tenth century. The name Hemlock is derived from the Anglo-Saxon words *hem* (border, shore) and *leác* (leek or plant). Another authority derives the British name 'hemlock' from the Anglo-Saxon word *healm* (straw), from which the word 'haulm' is derived.

The use of Hemlock in modern medicine is due chiefly to the recommendation of Storch, of Vienna, since when (1760) the plant has been much employed, though it has lost some of its reputation owing to the uncertain action of the preparations made from it.

¶ *Description.* Hemlock is a tall, much-branched and gracefully growing plant, with elegantly-cut foliage and white flowers. Country people very generally call by the name of Hemlock many species of umbelliferous plants, but the real Hemlock may be distinguished by its slender growth, perfectly smooth stem which is marked with red, and its finely-divided leaves which are also smooth.

It is a biennial plant, usually growing from 2 to 4 feet high, but in sheltered situations sometimes attaining nearly double that height. The *root* is long, forked, pale yellow and $\frac{1}{2}$ to $\frac{3}{4}$ inch in diameter. The erect, smooth *stem*, stout below, much branched above and hollow, is bright green, but (as already stated) is distinctively mottled with small irregular stains or spots of a port-wine colour and also covered with a white ' bloom' which is very easily rubbed off.

The *leaves* are numerous, those of the first year and the lower ones very large, even reaching 2 feet in length, alternate, long-stalked, tripinnate (divided along the midrib into opposite pairs of leaflets and these again divided and subdivided in similar manner). The upper leaves are much smaller, nearly stalkless, with the short footstalk dilated and stem-clasping, often opposite or three together, more oblong in outline, dipinnate or pinnate, quite smooth, uniform dull green, segments toothed, each tooth being tipped with a minute, sharp white point.

The *umbels* are rather small, $1\frac{1}{4}$ to 2 inches broad, numerous, terminal, on rather short flower stalks, with 12 to 16 rays to the umbel. At the base of the main umbel there are 4 to 8 lance-shaped, deflexed bracts; at the base of the small umbels there are three or four spreading bractlets. The flowers are small, their petals white with an inflexed point, the stamens a little longer than the petals, with white anthers.

The *fruit* is small, about $\frac{1}{8}$ inch long, broad, ridged, compressed laterally and smooth. Both flowers and fruit bear a resemblance to caraway, but the prominent crenate (wavy) ridges and absence of *vittæ* (oil cells between the ridges) are important characters for distinguishing this fruit from others of the same natural order of plants.

The entire plant has a bitter taste and possesses a disagreeable mousy odour, which is especially noticeable when bruised. When dry, the odour is still disagreeable, but not so pronounced as in the fresh plant. The seeds or fruits have very marked odour or taste, but when rubbed with a solution of potassium bi-oxide, the same disagreeable mouse-like odour is produced.

The poisonous property occurs in all parts of the plant, though it is stated to be less strong in the root. Poisoning has occurred from eating the leaves for parsley, the roots for parsnips and the seeds in mistake for anise seeds. Many children, too, have suffered by using whistles made from the hollow stems of the Hemlock, which should be extirpated from meadows and pastures since many domestic animals have been killed by eating it, though goats are said to eat it with impunity.

¶ *Parts Used, Harvesting and Drying.* The leaves and fruit. The fresh green Hemlock is employed in the preparation of Juice of Conium, Conium Ointment, and the green Extract of Conium.

The British Pharmacopœia directs that the leaves and young branches should be gathered from wild British plants when the flowers are fully matured, and the fruits are just beginning to form, as they then possess their greatest medicinal activity. This is about the end of June. The smaller leaves are selected and the larger stalks picked out and discarded.

The leaves separated from the branches and *dried* are also official.

The dried ripe fruit is official in the British Pharmacopœia, and the Pharmacopœia of India, but in the Pharmacopœia of the United States the full-grown fruit, gathered before it turns from green to yellow and carefully dried, is directed to be used.

Hemlock fruits were introduced into British medicine in 1864 as a substitute for the dried leaf in making the tincture, but it has been shown that a tincture, whether of leaf or fruit, is far inferior to the preserved juice of the herb.

¶ *Constituents.* By far the most important constituent of hemlock leaves is the alkaloid Coniine, of which they may contain, when collected at the proper time, as much as 2·77 per cent. the average being 1·65 per cent. When pure, Coniine is a volatile. colourless, oily liquid, strongly alkaline, with poisonous properties and having a bitter taste and a disagreeable, penetrating, mouse-like odour.

There are also present the alkaloids, Methyl-coniine, Conhydrine, Pseudoconhydrine, Ethyl piperidine, mucilage, a fixed oil and 12 per cent. of ash.

Hemlock fruits have essentially the same active constituents, but yield a greater portion of Coniine than the leaves.

¶ *Medicinal Action and Uses.* As a medicine, Conium is sedative and antispasmodic, and in sufficient doses acts as a paralyser to the centres of motion. In its action it is, therefore, directly antagonistic to that of Strychnine, and hence it has been recommended as an antidote to Strychnine poisoning, and in other poisons of the same class, and in tetanus, hydrophobia, etc. (In mediæval days, Hemlock mixed with betony and fennel seed was considered a cure for the bite of a mad dog.)

On account of its peculiar sedative action on the motor centres, Hemlock juice (*Succus*

conii) is prescribed as a remedy in cases of undue nervous motor excitability, such as teething in children, epilepsy from dentition. cramp, in the early stages of paralysis agitans, in spasms of the larynx and gullet, in acute mania, etc. As an inhalation it is said to relieve cough in bronchitis, whooping-cough, asthma, etc.

The drug has to be administered with care, as narcotic poisoning may result from internal use, and overdoses produce paralysis. In poisonous doses it produces complete paralysis with loss of speech, the respiratory function is at first depressed and ultimately ceases altogether and death results from asphyxia. The mind remains unaffected to the last. In the account of the death of Socrates, reference is made to loss of sensation as one of the prominent symptoms of his poisoning, but the dominant action is on the motor system. It is placed in Table II of the Poison Schedule.

Hemlock was formerly believed to exercise an alterative effect in scrofulous disorders. Both the Greek and Arabian physicians were in the practice of using it for the cure of indolent tumours, swellings and pains of the joints, as well as for affections of the skin. Among the moderns Baron Storch was the first to call the attention of medical men to its use, both externally and internally, for the cure of cancerous and other ulcers, and in the form of a poultice or ointment it has been found a very valuable application to relieve pain in these cases.

In the case of poisoning by Hemlock, the antidotes are tannic acid, stimulants and coffee, emetics of zinc, or mustard and castor oil, and, if necessary, artificial respiration. It is essential to keep up the temperature of the body.

Like many other poisonous plants, when cut and dried, Hemlock loses much of its poisonous properties, which are volatile and easily dissipated. Cooking destroys it.

Its disagreeable odour has prevented its fatal use as a vegetable in the raw state.

Larks and quails are said to eat Hemlock with impunity, but their flesh becomes so impregnated with the poison that they are poisonous as food. Thrushes eat the fruits with impunity, but ducks have been poisoned by them.

Coles' *Art of Simpling*:

'If Asses chance to feed much upon Hemlock, they will fall so fast asleep that they will seeme to be dead, in so much that some thinking them to be dead indeed have flayed off their skins, yet after the Hemlock had done operating they have stirred and wakened out of their sleep, to the griefe and amazement of the owners.'

¶ *Adulteration.* Commercial Conium occasionally contains the leaves of other umbelliferous plants somewhat like it in appearance, or it may even be almost wholly composed of such plants. Anise has been used as an adulterant of the fruit.

Among umbelliferous plants most frequently mistaken for the true Hemlock, *Anthriscus sylvestris* (Wild Chervil) and *Æthusa Cynapium* (Fool's Parsley) have similar general characteristics, but are readily distinguished. *A. sylvestris* has *hairy*, not smooth leaves, its fruit is *elongated*, not broad, and the bracts of the partial involucre (or involucels) are not directed outwards, as in the Hemlock. The stem also is *unspotted.*

¶ *Preparations and Dosages.* Powdered leaves, 1 to 3 grains. Fluid extract of leaves, 5 to 10 drops. Fluid extract of seeds, 2 to 5 drops. Tincture seeds, B.P., ½ to 1 drachm. Juice of leaves, B.P., 1 to 2 drachms. Solid extract, 2 to 6 grains. Ointment, B.P.

See FOOL'S PARSLEY, WATER DROPWORT, WATER FENNEL, WATER PARSNIP, SKIRRET.

(*POISON*)
HEMLOCK, WATER

Cicuta virosa
N.O. Umbelliferæ

Synonym. Cowbane
Part Used. Root

The leaves of the Water Hemlock are sometimes found admixed with those of Conium. This is a semi-aquatic plant growing in ditches and on the banks of pools and rivers, though not very common in England. It has similar properties to the true Hemlock.

¶ *Description.* Water Hemlock is a perennial, with a short, thick, vertical, hollow rootstock, in shape somewhat like a parsnip, giving off whorls of slender, fibrous roots. The erect, very stout, hollow stem, rising 2 to 4 feet high or more, is smooth, branched and slightly furrowed. The lower leaves are large, 1 to 2 feet long and long-stalked; they are tripinnate, like the Hemlock. The upper leaves are divided into three leaflets, and each again into three (twice ternate). The flowers are pure white, arranged in rather large, long-stalked umbels of 12 to 16 long, slender, curved rays. There is no general involucre.

The Water Hemlock may be distinguished from the true Hemlock as follows: (i) The pinnæ of the leaves are larger and lance-shaped; (ii) the umbel of the flowers is denser and more compact; (iii) the stem is not spotted like the true Hemlock; (iv) the odour of the plant resembles that of smallage or parsley.

Both plants are poisonous; but while the *root* of the Water Hemlock is acrid and powerfully poisonous in its fresh state, though it loses its virulent qualities when dried, that of the true Hemlock possesses little or no active power.

The Water Hemlock produces tetanic convulsions, and is fatal to cattle. In April, 1857, two farmer's sons were found lying paralysed and speechless close to a ditch where they had been working. Assistance was soon rendered, but they shortly expired. A quantity of the Water Hemlock grew in the ditch, where they had been employed. A piece of the root was subsequently found with the marks of teeth in it, near to where the men lay, and another piece of the same root was discovered in the pocket of one of them.

¶ *Constituents.* A resinous body has been obtained from *Cicuta virosa* named Cicutoxin, an amorphous substance of acid reaction, of slight odour, but disagreeable taste; the dry root yields 3 to 5 per cent. The presence of a volatile alkaloid termed Cicutine has also been traced.

Other Species.
AMERICAN COWBEAN (*POISON*)

Circuta maculata
N.O. Umbelliferæ

The American Cowbane is closely analogous to the European species, and also possesses very poisonous properties. In several instances, children have been fatally poisoned by eating its roots. It is said to be the most poisonous plant native to the United States.

Although it has been recommended as a remedy in nervous and sick headaches, it is very rarely used.

No complete analysis of the plant has been published, but the alkaloid termed Cicutine, present in the European species, is said to exist in it. The seed is stated to contain an alkaloid identical with Coniine.

The root of this American variety is even more virulent than the English one.

See HEMLOCK, WATER DROPWORT, WILD CHERVIL, WATER FENNEL, WATER PARSNIP, FOOL'S PARSLEY.

HEMP, AGRIMONY. *See* AGRIMONY

HEMP, CANADIAN

Apocynum Cannabinum (LINN.)
Apocynum Androsæmum
N.O. Apocynaceæ

Synonyms. Black Indian Hemp. Dogsbane
Parts Used. Dried rhizome, roots
Habitat. United States of America, Canada

¶ *Description*. This plant must not be confused with Indian Hemp (*Cannabis Indica*). Both species have a milky juice and a tough fibrous bark, which when macerated affords a substitute for hemp, hence its common name. It is used in California for making twine, bags, cordage, fishing-nets, lines, and a coarse kind of linen. When the milky juice is properly dried it exhibits the properties of india-rubber. The corolla of this plant secretes a sweet liquid, which attracts flies and other insects to settle on them; the scales in the throat of the corolla are very sensitive, and as soon as the insects settle on them, they bend inwards and make them prisoners. None of these plants possess any great beauty, all are more or less poisonous and acrid. In *Apocynum Cannabinum*, a perennial herb, the stems and branches are upright, headed by erect, many-flowered stems, leaves nearly sessile; it grows in gravelly or sandy soil, mostly near streams. While *A. Androsæmifolium*, or Dogsbane, has spreading forked branches, leaves slender petioled cymes, loose and spreading, grows in dry thickets and open woods, and is distinguished from *A. Cannabinum* by the root, thick-walled stone cells which are arranged in a broken circle, near middle of the bark, short fracture, with some pith occurring in pieces of the rhizome, very slight odour, taste starchy, afterwards bitter and acrid.

¶ *Constituents*. The activity of the plants is due to a very bitter principle of a glucose nature, to which is applied the name of Symarin. Apocynum belongs to the digitalis group of heart tonics, and acts very much in the same way, differing only from foxglove in the relative degree of its different effects. It is the most powerful of the group, often causing sickness and diarrhœa; it acts more irritantly on the mucous membrane than either strophanthus, or digitalis, and it may be this stimulating effect which is the cause of its violent diuretic action, though some authorities consider that this is caused by dilatation of the renal arteries. *A. Docymum* is the crystalline lactone cynotoxin, the crystalline substance. Apocynin is identical with acetovanillone. *A. Androsæmifolium* contains apocyanamarin, identical with cynotoxin, also apocynin and its glucoside, androsin ipuranil; the two phytosterols androsterol and homo-androsterol, and other fatty acids.

¶ *Medicinal Action and Uses*. Diuretic, diaphoretic, expectorant. Should only be prescribed with the greatest caution. It is a very valuable heart tonic of great service in dropsy resulting from heart failure; it is also to be highly recommended in the ascites of hepatic cirrhosis, but care must be taken that it does not accumulate in the system. It causes violent vomiting.·

¶ *Dosage*. 1 to 5 grains.

¶ *Preparations*. Fluid extract of Apocynum, U.S.P., 15 minims. Tincture of Apocynum, 5 to 10 minims.

¶ *Other Species*.

HEMP, AFRICAN, or Bowstring (*Sansev01era guineenesis*, N.O. Liliaceae), native of tropical Africa, also *S. Roxburghiana*, a native of India, and *S. Angolensis*, native of western tropical Africa. The leaves contain much fibre for making ropes, the latter producing the best kind of fibre for deep-sea soundings and dredging lines.

HEMP, KENTUCKY (*Urtica Canadensis* and *Cannabina*, N. O. Urticaceae), natives of Canada and Northern U.S. These also contain a strong fibre and are known by the name given above.

HEMP, MANILLA, the fibre of *Musitextilis* (N.O. Musaceae), native of the Philippines, cultivated in India, and other countries, for its fibre, of which there are two qualities, the finer made into shawls and the coarser into ropes.

HEMP, SUNN, the Indian name for the fibre of *Crotalaria Juncea* (N.O. Leguminosæ), native of India; it gives a very strong fibre, useful for ropes, canvas, etc.

HEMP, JUBBULPORE (*Crotalaria tenuifolia*), The plant closely resembles Sunn Hemp (*C. Juncea*).

(*POISON*)
HEMP, INDIAN

Cannabis sativa (LINN.)
N.O. Urticaceæ

Synonyms. Cannabis Indica. Cannabis Chinense. Ganeb. Ganja. Kif. Hanf. Tekrouri. Chanvre

Part Used. The dried, flowering tops of the female, or pistillate plants

Habitat. India

Habitat. In Britain, and formerly else-where, only Hemp grown in India was recognized as official, but the heavy tax has resulted in the admission by the United States of any active *Cannabis sativa*, whether grown in the States or in Africa, Turkey, Turkestan, Asia Minor, Italy, or Spain.

¶ *Description*. The plant is an annual, the erect stems growing from 3 to 10 feet or more high, very slightly branched, having greyish-green hairs. The leaves are palmate, with five to seven leaflets (three on the upper leaves), numerous, on long thin petioles with acute stipules at the base, linear-lanceolate, tapering at both ends, the margins sharply serrate, smooth and dark green on the upper surface, lighter and downy on the under one. The small flowers are unisexual, the male having five almost separate, downy, pale yellowish segments, and the female a single, hairy, glandular, five-veined leaf enclosing the ovary in a sheath. The ovary is smooth, one-celled, with one hanging ovule and two long, hairy thread-like stigmas extending beyond the flower for more than its own length. The fruit is small, smooth, light brownish-grey in colour, and completely filled by the seed.

Hemp grows naturally in Persia, Northern India and Southern Siberia, and probably in China. It is largely cultivated in Central and Southern Russia. It is sometimes found as a weed in England, probably due to seeds from birdcages, as they are much used in feeding tame birds. The drug that is official in Europe comes from Bogra and Rajshabi, north of Calcutta, or sometimes from Guzerat and Madras. It is called *Guaza* by London merchants.

It is imported in parcels of small masses, with flowers, smaller leaves and a few ripe fruits pressed together by sticky, resinous matter. It is rough, brittle, dull-green in colour and almost tasteless, with a peculiar, slightly narcotic odour. It should be freed from resin by macerating in spirit and then soaking in water. The leaves are said to be picked off to form *bhang*, and the little shoots which follow these are used as above, and called *ganja*. It is exported from Bombay in wooden cases. Two-year-old ganja is almost inert, and the law requires it to be burnt in the presence of excise officers. In the Calcutta areas the short tops are rolled under foot instead of being trodden, the weight of the

workers being supported by a horizontal bamboo pole. This variety is very active, and is usually re-exported from England to the West Indies.

Hemp is prepared in various forms. *Ganja* is smoked like tobacco. *Bhang, sidhee*, or *subjee* is the dried, larger leaves, broken or mixed with a few fruits. It is pounded with water to make a drink, and is the chief ingredient of the sweetmeat *majun*. *Churrus* or *charas* is the resin which exudes spontaneously from the leaves, tops and stems. A usual way of collecting it is for men in leathern garments to rush through the bushes, the resin being afterwards scraped off the clothes. In Nepal the plant is squeezed between the palms of the hands, and in Baluchistan the resin is separated by rubbing the dried plant carefully between carpets. This is the *hashish, haschisch*, or *hashash* of the Arabians, the word 'assassin' being said to be derived from it, owing to the wild, fanatical courage given by its use. In Persia the woollen carpets, after scraping, are washed with water, and the evaporated extract is sold cheaply. Another way is to collect the dust after stirring dry bhang, this impure form of resin being only used for smoking.

Flat cakes called *hashish* by the Russians are a preparation made from Hemp in Central Asia, and also called *nasha*.

In Thibet *momea* or *mimea* is said to be made with Hemp and human fat.

Many electuaries and pastes are made with butter or other oily foundation, such as *majun* of Calcutta, *mapouchari* of Cairo, and the *dawames* of the Arabs.

The *madjound* of the Algerians is a mixture of honey and hashish powder.

Hemp Fibre is best produced by the plants in cooler latitudes, the best being obtained from Italy, but much from Russia. About one and a half million hundredweight are imported annually for cordage, sacking, and sail-cloths.

A *varnish* is made from the pressed *seeds*.

Two or three green twigs collected in spring and placed in beds will drive bedbugs from the room.

¶ *Constituents*. Cannabinone or Hemp resin is soluble in alcohol and ether. Cannabinol is separated from it. It is fawn-coloured, in thin layers, and burns with a clear, white flame, leaving no ash. This is the active principle. There is a small amount of amber-coloured volatile oil, one of the linseed-oil group. It has been resolved into a colourless liquid called *cannabene*, and a solid hydride of this.

It is said that a volatile alkaloid has been found in the tops, resembling nicotine. It also contains alcoholic extract, ash, and the alkaloid Choline.

¶ *Medicinal Action and Uses.* The principal use of Hemp in medicine is for easing pain and inducing sleep, and for a soothing influence in nervous disorders. It does not cause constipation nor affect the appetite like opium. It is useful in neuralgia, gout, rheumatism, delirium tremens, insanity, infantile convulsions, insomnia, etc.

The tincture helps parturition, and is used in senile catarrh, gonorrhœa, menorrhagia, chronic cystitis and all painful urinary affections. An infusion of the seed is useful in after pains and prolapsus uteri. The resin may be combined with ointments, oils or chloroform in inflammatory and neuralgic complaints.

The drug deteriorates rapidly and hence is very variable, so that it is best given in ascending quantities to produce its effect. The deterioration is due to the oxidation of cannabinol and it should be kept in hermetically-sealed containers.

The action is almost entirely on the higher nerve centres. It can produce an exhilarating intoxication, with hallucinations, and is widely used in Eastern countries as an intoxicant, hence its names 'leaf of delusion,' 'increaser of pleasure,' 'cementer of friendship,' etc. The nature of its effect depends much on the nationality and temperament of the individual. It is regarded as dangerous to sleep in a field of hemp owing to the aroma of the plants.

¶ *Dosage.* Tincture, B.P. and U.S.P., 5 to 15 drops. Solid extract, B.P., ¼ to 1 grain. Fluid extract, 1 to 3 drops. Of cannabis, 1 to 3 grains. Of best hashish, for smoking, ¼ to 1 grain. Of tincture, 10 to 30 minims. Of tincture for menorrhagia, 5 to 10 minims. three to four times a day (i.e. 24 grains of resinous extract in a fluid ounce of rectified spirit).

Of extract, from ½ to 20 grains, according to quality.

The following is stated to be a certain cure for gonorrhœa. Take equal parts of tops of male and female hemp in blossom. Bruise in a mortar, express the juice, and add an equal portion of alcohol. Take 1 to 3 drops every two to three hours.

HENBANE (*POISON*)

Hyoscyamus niger (LINN.)
N.O. Solaneæ

Synonyms. Common Henbane. Hyoscyamus. Hog's-bean. Jupiter's-bean. Symphonica. Cassilata. Cassilago. Deus Caballinus

(*Anglo-Saxon*) Henbell

(*French*) Jusquiame

Parts Used. Fresh leaves, flowering tops and branches, seeds

Habitat. It is found throughout Central and Southern Europe and in Western Asia, extending to India and Siberia. As a weed of cultivation it now grows also in North America and Brazil. It had become naturalized in North America prior to 1672, as we find it mentioned in a work published in that year among the plants 'sprung up since the English planted and kept cattle in New England.'

It is not considered truly indigenous to Great Britain, but occurs fairly frequently in parts of Scotland, England and Wales, and also in Ireland, and has been found wild in sixty British counties, chiefly in waste, sandy places, by road-sides, on rubbish heaps and near old buildings, having probably first escaped from the old herb gardens. It is frequently found on chalky ground and particularly near the sea. It appears to have been more common in Gerard's time (Queen Elizabeth's reign) than it is now.

Henbane (*Hyoscyamus niger*, Linn.) is a member of the important order Solaneæ, to which belong the Potato, Tobacco and Tomato, and also the valuable Belladonna.

There are about eleven species of the genus *Hyoscyamus*, distributed from the Canary Islands over Europe and Northern Africa to Asia. All those which have been investigated contain similar principles and possess similar properties.

The medicinal uses of Henbane date from remote ages; it was well known to the Ancients, being particularly commended by Dioscorides (first century A.D.), who used it to procure sleep and allay pains, and Celsus (same period) and others made use of it for the same purpose, internally and externally, though Pliny declared it to be 'of the nature of wine and therefore offensive to the understanding.' There is mention of it in a work by Benedictus Crispus (A.D. 681) under the names of Hyoscyamus and Symphonica. In the tenth century, we again find its virtues recorded under the name of Jusquiasmus (the modern French name is *Jusquiame*). There is frequent mention made of it in Anglo-Saxon works on medicine of the eleventh century, in which it is named 'Henbell,' and in the old glossaries of those days it also appears as Caniculata, Cassilago and Deus Caballinus.

Later it fell into disuse. It was omitted from the London Pharmacopœia of 1746 and 1788, and only restored in 1809, its re-introduction being chiefly due to experiments and recommendations by Baron Storch, who gave it in the form of an extract, in cases of epilepsy and other nervous and convulsive diseases.

It is supposed that this is the noxious herb referred to by Shakespeare in *Hamlet*:

'Sleeping within mine orchard,
My custom always of the afternoon
Upon my secure hour thy uncle stole,
With juice of cursed *hebenon* in a vial,
And in the porches of mine ear did pour
The leprous distillment.'

Other authorities argue that the name used here is a varied form of that by which the Yew is known in at least five of the Gothic languages, and which appears in Marlowe and other Elizabethan writers as 'hebon.' There can be little doubt that Shakespeare took both the name and the use of this plant from Marlowe, who mentions 'juice of hebon' as a deadly poison. Hebenus, according to Gower, is a 'sleepy tree.' Spenser, too, makes 'heben' a tree, and speaks of 'the deadly heben bow,' a weapon that could hardly be made of Henbane. 'This tree,' wrote Lyte in his *Herball*, 1578, 'is altogether venomous and against man's nature; such as do only sleepe under the shadow thereof become sicke and sometimes they die,' whereas he *recommends* the juice of Henbane as an application for earache.

Speaking of Henbane, Gerard says:

'The leaves, the seeds and the juice, when taken internally cause an unquiet sleep, like unto the sleep of drunkenness, which continueth long and is deadly to the patient. To wash the feet in a decoction of Henbane, as also the often smelling of the flowers causeth sleep.'

Culpepper says:

'I wonder how astrologers could take on them to make this an herb of Jupiter: and yet Mizaldus, a man of penetrating brain, was of that opinion as well as the rest: the herb is indeed under the dominion of Saturn and I prove it by this argument: All the herbs which delight most to grow in saturnine places are saturnine herbs. Both Henbane delights most to grow in saturnine places, and whole cart loads of it may be found near the places where they empty the common Jakes, and scarce a ditch to be found without it growing by it. Ergo, it is a herb of Saturn. The leaves of Henbane do cool all hot inflammations in the eyes. . . . It also assuages the pain of the gout, the sciatica, and other pains in the joints which arise from a hot cause. And applied with vinegar to the forehead and temples, helps the headache and want of sleep in hot fevers. . . . The oil of the seed is helpful for deafness, noise and worms in the ears, being dropped therein; the juice of the herb or root doth the same. The decoction of the herb or seed, or both, kills lice in man or beast. The fume of the dried herb, stalks and seeds, burned, quickly heals swellings, chilblains or kibes in the hands or feet, by holding them in the fume thereof. The remedy to help those that have taken Henbane is to drink goat's milk, honeyed water, or pine kernels, with sweet wine; or, in the absence of these, Fennel seed, Nettle seed, the seed of Cresses, Mustard or Radish; as also Onions or Garlic taken in wine, do all help to free them from danger and restore them to their due temper again. Take notice, that this herb must never be taken inwardly; outwardly, an oil, ointment, or plaister of it is most admirable for the gout . . . to stop the toothache, applied to the aching side. . . .'

The leaves or roots eaten produce maniacal delirium, if nothing worse. Another old writer says:

'If it be used either in sallet or in pottage, then doth it bring frenzie, and whoso useth more than four leaves shall be in danger to sleepe without waking.'

It is poisonous in all its parts, and neither drying nor boiling destroys the toxic principle. The leaves are the most powerful portion, even the odour of them when fresh will produce giddiness and stupor. Accidental cases of poisoning by Henbane are, however, not very common, as the plant has too unpleasant a taste and smell to be readily mistaken for any esculent vegetable, but its roots, which are thick and somewhat like those of salsafy, have sometimes been gathered and eaten. In one case recorded, a woman pulled up a quantity of Henbane roots which she found in a field, supposing them to be parsnips. She boiled them in soup, which was eaten by the family. The whole of the nine persons who had partaken of them suffered severely, being soon seized with indistinctness of vision, giddiness and sleepiness, followed by delirium and convulsions.

It is also recorded that the whole of the inmates of a monastery were once poisoned by using the roots instead of chicory. The monks partaking of the roots for supper were all more or less affected during the night and following day, being attacked with a sort of delirious frenzy, accompanied in many cases by such hallucinations that the establishment resembled a lunatic asylum.

The herb was used in magic and diabolism, for its power of throwing its victims into convulsions. It was employed by witches in their midnight brews, and from the leaves was prepared a famous sorcerer's ointment.

Anodyne necklaces were made from the root and were hung about the necks of children as charms to prevent fits and to cause easy teething.

In mythology, we read that the dead in Hades were crowned with it as they wandered hopelessly beside the Styx.

The herb is also called Hog's-bean, and both its botanical name *Hyoscyamus* and the tenth-century *Jusquiasmus* are derived from the Greek words *hyos* and *cyamos*, signifying 'the bean of the hog,' which animal is supposed to eat it with impunity. An old Anglo-Saxon name for it was 'Belene,' probably from the bell-shaped flowers; then it became known as 'Hen-bell,' and from the time that its poisonous properties were recognized this name was changed to 'Henbane,' because the seeds were thought to be fatal to poultry. Dr. Prior is inclined to think that the name Henbane is derived from the Spanish *hinna* (a mule), e.g. 'henna bell,' referring to the similarity of its seed-vessel to the bell hung upon the neck of the mules.

Although swine are said to feed upon the leaves and suffer no ill effects, this plant should not be allowed to grow in places to which cattle have access, though they seldom touch it, and its effects seem less violent on most of the larger domestic animals than on man; sheep will sometimes eat it when young, and it has occasionally been noticed that no bad effects have followed. Cows, however, have been poisoned by having Henbane mixed with their forage, it is said for the purpose of fattening them. A small quantity of the seeds of the Stramonium or Thornapple, as well as those of Henbane, are also sometimes added; the idea appears to be that the tendency to stupor and repose caused by these plants is conducive to fattening. In some districts, horse-dealers mix the seeds of Henbane with their oats, in order to fatten their animals.

¶ *Description. H. niger* is susceptible of considerable diversity of character, causing varieties which have by some been considered as distinct species. Thus the plant is sometimes *annual*, the stem almost unbranched, smaller and less downy than in the *biennial* form, the leaves shorter and less hairy and the flowers often yellow, without any purple markings. The annual plant also flowers in July or August, the biennial in May and June.

The annual and biennial form spring indifferently from the same crop of seed, the former growing during summer to a height of from 1 to 2 feet, and flowering and perfecting seed, the latter producing the first season only a tuft of radical leaves, which disappear in winter, leaving underground a thick, fleshy root, from the crown of which arises in spring a branched, flowering stem, usually much taller and more vigorous than the flowering stems of the annual plants. The annual form is apparently produced by the weaker and later developed seeds formed in the fruit at the ends of the shoots; it is considered to be less active than the typical species and differs in being of dwarfed growth and having rather paler flowers. The British drug of commerce consists of dense flowering shoots only, and of larger size.

Both varieties are used in medicine, but the biennial form is the one considered official. The leaves of this biennial plant spread out flat on all sides from the crown of the root like a rosette; they are oblong and egg-shaped, with acute points, stalked and more or less sharply toothed, often more than a foot in length, of a greyish-green colour and covered with sticky hairs. These leaves perish at the appearance of winter. The flowering stem pushes up from the root-crown in the following spring, ultimately reaching from 3 to 4 feet in height, and as it grows, becoming branched and furnished with alternate, oblong, unequally lobed, stalkless leaves, which are stem-clasping and vary considerably in size, but seldom exceed 9 or 10 inches in length. These leaves are pale green in colour, with a broad conspicuous mid-rib, and are furnished on both sides (but particularly on the veins on the under surface) with soft, glandular hairs, which secrete a resinous substance that causes the fresh leaves to feel unpleasantly clammy and sticky. Similar hairs occur on the sub-cylindrical branches. The flowers are shortly stalked, the lower ones growing in the fork of the branches, the upper ones stalkless, crowded together in one-sided, leafy spikes, which are rolled back at the top before flowering, the hairy, leafy, coarsely-toothed bracts becoming smaller upwards. The flowers have a hairy, pitcher-shaped calyx, which remains round the fruit and is strongly veined, with five stiff, broad, almost prickly lobes. The corollas are obliquely funnel-shaped, upwards of an inch across, of a dingy yellow or buff, marked with a close network of lurid purple veins. A variety sometimes occurs in which the corolla is not marked with these purple veins. The seed-capsule opens transversely by a convex lid and contains numerous small seeds. Perhaps the most striking feature of the plant are these curious seed-vessels, a very detailed description of which is given in the works of Flavius Josephus, as it was upon this capsule that one of the ornaments of the Jewish High Priests' head-dress was modelled. The whole plant has a powerful, oppressive, nauseous odour.

¶ *Cultivation.* Henbane is in such demand for medicinal purposes that it is necessary to cultivate it, the wild plants not yielding a sufficient supply. Both varieties were formerly cultivated in England, but at present the biennial is almost solely grown. English-grown Henbane has always been nearly sufficient to provide enough fresh leaves for the preparation of the juice, or green extract, but large quantities, chiefly of the annual kind, were imported before the War from Germany, Austria and Russia, in the form of dry leaves.

Henbane will grow on most soils, in sandy spots near the sea, on chalky slopes, and in cultivation flourishing in a good loam.

It is, however, very capricious in its growth, the seeds being prone to lie dormant for a season or more, refusing to germinate at all in some places, and the crop varying without any apparent reason, sometimes dying in patches. In some maritime localities it can be grown without any trouble. It requires a light, moderately rich and well-drained soil for successful growth and an open, sunny situation, but does not want much attention beyond keeping the ground free from weeds.

The seed should be sown in the open early in May or as soon as the ground is warm, as thinly as possible, in rows 2 to 2½ feet apart, the seedlings thinned out to 2 feet apart in the rows, as they do not stand transplanting well. Only the larger seedlings should be reserved, especially those of a bluish tint. The soil where the crop is to be, must have been well manured, and must be kept moist until the seeds have germinated, and also during May and June of the first year. It is also recommended to sow seeds of biennial Henbane at their natural ripening time, August, in porous soil.

The ground must never be water-logged, especially in the first winter; it runs to stalk in a wet season. Drought and late frosts stunt the growth and cause it to blossom too early, and if the climatic conditions are unsuitable, especially in a dry spring and summer, the biennial Henbane will flower in its first year, while the growth is quite low, but well-manured soil may prevent this.

Care must be taken in selecting the seed: commercial Henbane seed is often kiln-dried and useless for sowing. In order to more readily ensure germination, it is advisable to soak the seeds in water for twenty-four hours before planting: the unfertile seeds will then float on the top of the water and may thus be distinguished. Ripe seed should be grey, and yellowish or brown seeds should be rejected, as they are immature. Let the seeds dry and then sift out the smallest, keeping only the larger seeds.

Henbane seed being very small and light should be well mixed with fine dry soil as it is sown.

As seedlings often die off, a reserve should be kept in a box or bed to fill gaps, even though they do not always transplant successfully.

If it is desired to raise a crop of the annual variety the plants, being smaller and not branching so freely, may be grown at a distance of 18 inches apart each way, but the annual is very little cultivated in this country.

If any annuals come up among the biennials sown, the flowers should be cut off until the leaves get larger and the stem branches.

There is usually some difficulty in growing Henbane owing to its destruction by insects: sometimes the whole of the foliage is destroyed by the larvæ of a leaf-mining fly, *Pegomyia Hyoscyami*, and the crop is rendered worthless in a week. And when the large autumnal leaves of the first-year plants of the biennial variety decay, the large terminal bud is often destroyed by one of the various species of macro-lepidopterous caterpillars which hide themselves in the ground. The crown or bud should be covered as soon as the leaves have rotted away with soil mixed with soot or naphthaline, to prevent the depredations of these and other insects.

Floods may also rot the plants in winter, if grown on level ground. Potato pests are fond of the prickly leaves and will leave a potato patch to feed on the Henbane plant.

If mildew develops on the foliage in summer, dust the plants with powdered sulphur or spray with ½ oz. of liver of sulphur in 2 gallons of water.

When it is desired to preserve seed for propagation, it is well to cut off the top flowering shoots at an early stage of flowering (these may be dried and sold as flowering tops), and allow only about six seed-capsules to ripen. This will ensure strong seed to the capsules left, and this seed will probably produce biennial Henbane, weaker seeds being apt to produce the less robust and less valuable annual Henbane.

Seeds sown as soon as ripe in August may germinate in autumn, and thus constitute a biennial by growing on all through the winter and flowering the next summer.

Although the cultivation of Henbane in sandy ground near the sea, especially on the rich soil of estuaries, would probably pay well, it is hardly a profitable plant to grow in small gardens, more especially as the yield of dried leaf is very small. It is estimated that about 15 cwt. of dry herb are obtained from an acre of ground.

¶ *Parts Used. – Preparation for Market.* Henbane leaves are official in all pharmacopœias. Some require that it be collected from uncultivated plants, others that it be not used after keeping for more than a year.

The official drug, according to the British Pharmacopœia, consists of the *fresh* leaves, flowering tops and branches of the biennial variety of *H. niger*, and the same parts of the plant carefully dried.

The drug is preferably given in the form of the fluid extract or tincture. The smaller branches and leaves of the plant, with the leaves and flowers, is the drug from which the green extract and juice of Henbane are prepared, whilst the leaves and flowering tops are separated from the branches and dried and used for making tincture. The inspissated juice of the fresh leaves is considered exceedingly variable in its operation, and is not so much recommended.

The commercial drug presents three varieties, distinguished by the trade names 'Annual,' 'First Biennial' (the leaves from the biennial plant in its first year), and 'Biennial,' or 'Second Biennial,' the official drug, which is scarce and high-priced, the first two kinds commanding lower prices.

When grown in this country, the official Henbane plant, as already mentioned, is usually biennial. The leaves of the first year's growth are collected and sold under the name of 'First Biennial Henbane.' This variety consists of large, stalked leaves, attaining 10 inches or more in length, and is of course free from flower.

Under certain conditions the biennial plant will flower in the first year: this is also collected and sold as 'Annual (English) Henbane.' It closely resembles the biennial, but the flowering tops are usually less dense, and the drug often contains portions of the stem.

Such plants are much stronger than the foreign imported annual, and being more carefully dried are richer in alkaloids.

Formerly the second year's growth of the biennial plant was thought to contain a considerably larger percentage of alkaloid than either the first year's growth of the same plant, or the annual plant, and only the actual flowering tops of such plants were official, but it is now held that leaves from the *English-grown* species of all the above are practically of equal alkaloidal value, though the imported drug is of much less value.

Much Henbane is imported from Germany and Russia; this is probably collected mostly from annual plants, and often arrives in very poor condition, sometimes mixed with other species of Henbane. In consequence, English Henbane has always commanded a much higher price. Foreign annual Henbane is usually a much more slender plant than the English, and as imported its alkaloidal value is lower than that of the English-grown varieties. This may be due to the large proportion of stem, sand, etc., that the drug contains, the whole plant being cut and dried. It is probable that the well-dried *leaves* alone of all the varieties are of approximately equal alkaloidal strength.

¶ *Harvesting.* Much of the efficacy of Henbane depends upon the time at which it is gathered. The leaves should be collected when the plant is in full flower. In the biennial plant, those of the second year are preferred to those of the first; the latter are less clammy and fœtid, yield less extractive, and are medicinally considered less efficient. Sometimes, however, the plant is destroyed by a severe winter in England, and then no leaves of the second year's growth are obtainable, and it has been suggested that this is, perhaps, one of the causes of the great uncertainty of the medicine as found in commerce.

The leaves of the biennial variety are collected in June or the first week of July and those of the annual in August.

The leaves and flowering tops which constitute the 'Second Biennial Henbane' are collected either with or without the smaller branches to which they are attached and carefully dried, unless they are required for the preparation of the juice or green extract, when they should be sent to the distillery at once on cutting.

The herb when required in the fresh state should be cut the first week in June, because in the second week the leaf-mining insect attacks the leaves, leaving only patches of white epidermis.

The herb requires very careful drying, as

its properties are liable to be in great measure destroyed if kept too long in a damp state.

The fresh herb loses 80 to 86 per cent. of its weight on drying, 100 lb. yielding 14 to 20 lb. of dry herb.

The fresh leaves have, when bruised, a strong, disagreeable narcotic odour, somewhat like that of tobacco: their taste is mucilaginous and very slightly acrid. The characteristic odour disappears to a large extent on drying, but the bitter taste then becomes more pronounced.

When the dried leaves are thrown upon the fire they burn with a crackling noise from the nitrate they contain, and at the same time they emit a strong odour.

The dried drug consists principally of the flowering tops. In commerce, it is commonly found in irregular rounded or flattened masses, in which the coarsely-toothed hairy bracts, the yellowish corolla with deep purple lines and two-celled ovary, with numerous ovules, can easily be identified.

The *root* is not employed in medicine, but experiments have shown that the *seeds* not only possess all the properties of the plant, but have ten times the strength of the leaves. They are also employed in pharmacy, having been much used in the Middle Ages. At the present time, they are much prescribed by the Mohammedan doctors of India.

The seed should be gathered in August; it may be kiln-dried for medicinal purposes, but the treatment renders it useless for culture, and if required for propagation seeds should be sun-dried. The capsules should be harvested before the lids split off, the seeds then being shaken out and dried in the sun.

¶ *Constituents.* The chief constituent of Henbane leaves is the alkaloid Hyoscyamine, together with smaller quantities of Atropine and Hyoscine, also known as Scopolamine.

The proportion of alkaloid in the British Pharmacopœia dried drug varies from 0·045 to 0·14 per cent. Higher yields are exceptional. The amount of Hyoscyamine is many times greater than that of Hyoscine.

Other constituents of Henbane are a glucosidal bitter principle called hyoscytricin, choline, mucilage, albumin, calcium oxalate and potassium nitrate. On incineration, the leaves yield about 12 per cent. of ash. By destructive distillation, the leaves yield a very poisonous empyreumatic oil.

The chief constituent of the seeds is about 0·5 to 0·6 per cent. of alkaloid, consisting of Hyoscyamine, with a small proportion of Hyoscine. The seeds also contain about 20 per cent. of fixed oil.

¶ *Medicinal Action and Uses.* Antispasmodic, hypnotic, mild diuretic. The leaves

have long been employed as a narcotic medicine. It is similar in action to belladonna and stramonium, though milder in its effects.

The drug combines the therapeutic actions of its two alkaloids, Hyoscyamine and Hyoscine. Because of the presence of the former, it tends to check secretion and to relax spasms of the involuntary muscles, while through the narcotic effects of its hyoscine it lessens pain and exercises a slight somnifacient action.

Its most important use is in relief of painful spasmodic affections of the unstriped muscles, as in lead colic and irritable bladder. It will also relieve pain in cystitis.

It is much employed to allay nervous irritation, in various forms of hysteria or irritable cough, the tincture or juice prepared from the bruised, fresh leaves and tops being given in mixtures as an antispasmodic in asthma.

Combined with silver nitrate, it is especially useful in the treatment of gastric ulcer and chronic gastric catarrh.

It is used to relieve the griping caused by drastic purgatives, and is a common ingredient of aperient pills, especially those containing aloes and colocynth.

In small repeated doses, Henbane has been found to have a tranquillizing effect upon persons affected by severe nervous irritability, producing a tendency to sleep, not followed by the disorder of the digestive organs and headache, which too frequently result from the administration of repeated doses of opium, to which Henbane is often preferred when an anodyne or sedative is required. The comparatively small amount of atropine present does not give rise to the excitation and delirium occasioned by belladonna. It is, therefore, used in insomnia, especially when opium cannot be given. Except for this, it acts like atropine.

A watery solution of the extract applied to the eye has a similar effect to that of atropine, in dilating the pupil and thus preparing the eye for an operation, or assisting the cure of its internal inflammation. This dilution leaves no injurious effect afterwards.

In the form of extract or tincture, it is a valuable remedy, either as an anodyne, a hypnotic or a sedative, and will take effect when other drugs fail. When used for such a purpose, it is the active principle, Hyoscine, that is employed. This is very powerful – only a very small amount is used, from $\frac{1}{200}$ to $\frac{1}{70}$ of a grain of the Hydrobromate of Hyoscine. This drug comes under Table I of the Poisons Schedule. In poisonous doses Henbane in any form causes dimness of sight, faintness, delirium, and sometimes death.

Hyoscine, in combination with other drugs,

has of late come into use in the treatment known as Twilight Sleep. This is on account of its sedative action on brain and spine, causing loss of recollection and insensibility. Hyoscine is also used to a considerable extent in asylum practice, for the treatment of acute mania and delirium tremens.

A sedative application for external use is prepared by macerating Henbane leaves in alcohol, mixing the strong tincture with olive oil and heating in a water-bath, until the alcohol is dissipated. A compound liniment of Henbane, when applied to the skin, is of great service for relieving obstinate rheumatic pains.

The fresh leaves, crushed and applied as a poultice, or fomentation, will similarly relieve local pains of gout or neuralgia. They have been employed also to allay pain in cancerous ulcers, irritable sores and swellings, but their use for this purpose is of doubtful real advantage, and seems only a palliative. The extract, in form of suppositories, is also frequently used to alleviate the pain of hæmorrhoids.

¶ *Preparations and Dosages.* Powdered leaves, 2 to 10 grains. Fluid extract, 2 to 10 drops. Tincture, B.P. and U.S.P., $\frac{1}{2}$ to 1 drachm. Juice, B.P., $\frac{1}{2}$ to 1 drachm. Solid extract, 2 to 8 grains. Hyoscyamine, $\frac{1}{8}$ to 1 grain.

The *seeds* possess all the properties of the plant. Their expressed oil was formerly used externally.

Henbane seeds are used in some parts of the country as a domestic remedy for toothache; the smoke obtained by heating the seeds on a hot plate is applied to the mouth by means of a funnel, or a poultice is sometimes made from the crushed drug. The seeds were a favourite remedy for toothache in the Middle Ages, but their use is dangerous, having caused convulsions and even insanity in some instances. Both leaves and seeds have also been smoked in a pipe as a remedy for neuralgia and rheumatism, but with equal risk, being too uncertain and violent in their effect to be safe.

Children have been known to eat the seeds with serious results.

Sir Hans Sloane records the case of four children who, having eaten some of the capsules in mistake for filberts, exhibited all the symptoms of narcotic poisoning, continuing for two days and nights in a profound sleep.

In the case of adults, twenty seeds have been proved insufficient to prove fatal, though they induced grave results, the effects being the same as in poisoning by atropine or belladonna, the remedies to be employed being an emetic of mustard, followed by large draughts of warm water, strong tea or coffee, with powdered charcoal; stimulants (whisky, etc.), if necessary; the patient to be roused if drowsy; heat and friction to be applied to the extremities and finally, in acute cases, artificial respiration.

Gerard writes with regard to the use of the seed of Henbane by mountebanks for obstinate toothache:

'Drawers of teeth who run about the country and pretend they cause worms to come forth from the teeth by burning the seed in a chafing dish of coals, the party holding his mouth over the fume thereof, do have some crafty companions who convey small lute strings into the water, persuading the patient that these little creepers came out of his mouth, or other parts which it was intended to ease.'

Another old writer says: 'These pretended worms are no more than an appearance of worms which is always seen in the smoak of Henbane seed.' As a matter of fact, the small white, cylindrical embryos of the seed are forced out of some of them by the heat (especially if the seed be put into a basin with boiling water), and these were mistaken by ignorant sufferers for 'worms' coming out of their teeth.

¶ *Other Species of Hyoscyamus.*
Henbane, except for the use of the unofficial forms, is scarcely subject to adulteration in the entire condition. It, however, frequently contains an excessive amount of stem, which reduces its alkaloidal percentage and value.

In the south of Europe, RUSSIAN HEN-BANE (*H. albus*) – a native of the region of the Mediterranean, and so called from the pale colour of its flowers – is used as the official Henbane, and is regarded as equal in medicinal value. In France it is used indiscriminately with *H. niger*, though here it is not recognized as having identical properties. It is easily distinguished by the bracts, as well as the leaves being all stalked, and by the pale-yellow colour of the flower. According to *Pharmacographia*, the Hyoscyamus of the Ancients was probably *H. albus*, and the white variety was preferred for internal use in the practice of more modern times. Both the black and the white occur in our first Pharmacopœia, but the use of the former was confined to external applications, such as *unguentum populeum*, while the latter was an ingredient of the famous electuary, *Philonium Romanum*, the original of the Confection of Opium. In France, too, White Henbane had the preference, though it was held to be milder in operation: only the seeds were official, whereas in the black variety only the leaves were official.

The alkaloidal contents of *H. muticus*, EGYPTIAN HENBANE, from Egypt and the East Indies, often exceeds 1·25 per cent. This is mostly pure Hyoscyamine: its medicinal action is thus different, and its use as a substitute is dangerous.

The drug is readily distinguished, consisting chiefly of very light and light-coloured stems, often as thick as the finger, and capsules which are equally light-coloured and far more elongated than those of *H. niger*. The calyx limb is also further prolonged beyond the capsule. The leaves are much narrower; they are coarsely toothed or lobed at the summit, but lack the very large and sharp lateral lobe of the European Henbane.

The presence of *H. muticus*, as an admixture of the official imported drug, may be detected by the presence of characteristic branching non-glandular hairs, which are found on both the stems and leaves.

H. muticus is one of the most important medicinal herbs produced in Egypt, and is a valuable source of the alkaloids, Hyoscyamine, Hyoscine and Atropine, Hyoscyamine, practically pure, occurring in the drug in considerably greater proportion than in the European herb, the Egyptian-grown plant being much richer than the Indian, and being chiefly imported into this country for the manufacture of Hyoscyamine.

The drug occurs in three forms, as a mixture of broken stem, leaf and fruit, in which stem predominates – as leaves with little stem, and as seeds; the first named is the variety usually met with.

Although *H. muticus* is grown in Egypt, a British Protectorate before the War, the Ger-

mans had a monopoly of the supply. The Imperial Institute, during the War, investigated *H. muticus* as a source of atropine, and reported that if a sufficient supply of the drug could be imported, it would be an additional inducement to British manufacturers to take up the preparation of atropine. As a result, pressed bales have reached this country in fair supply, and the manufacture of atropine is now carried on here in increased quantities.

It has been grown in this country, but not to any great extent. In 1916 it was reported that it was proposed to experiment with the seed of this plant in certain districts in the West Indian islands.

In Egypt the drug is called *Sakran*, meaning 'the drunken.' In India it is considerably used as a narcotic.

Scopola carniolica, a common plant in Austria and Hungary, Bavaria and southwest Russia, which appears in our trade lists of plants recommended for our pleasure gardens, also yields the alkaloid Hyoscine (Scopolamine) and is worth attention. By selective cultivation, its yield of alkaloid might be raised.

In 1916 (reported in the *Chemist and Druggist*, Feb. 17, 1924) Wild Hyoscyamus was discovered growing in Montana, U.S.A., the plant growing to the height of about 6 feet near Bearmouth, also Big Timber and other nearby places. It is assumed that it was introduced by some foreigners who were working on a building at Big Timber, Montana. From here it spread and became such a pest that every property-owner was ordered to rid his place of it. The climate and soil seem to suit it and the plants yield the normal quantity of alkaloid.

HENNA

Lawsonia alba (LANK.)
Lawsonia inermis
N.O. Lythraceæ

Synonyms. Henne. Al-Khanna. Al-henna. Jamaica Mignonette. Mehndi. Mendee. Egyptian Privet. Smooth Lawsonia

Parts Used. Flowers, powdered leaves, fruit

Habitat. Egypt, India, Kurdistan, Levant, Persia, Syria

¶ *Description*. The small, white and yellow, heavy, sweet-smelling flowers are borne on dwarf shrubs 8 to 10 feet high. A distilled water prepared from them is used as a cosmetic, and the powdered leaves have been in use from the most ancient times in Eastern countries for dyeing the hair and the nails a reddish-yellow.

Since 1890 it has been widely used in Europe for tinting the hair, usually in the form of a shampoo, many shades being obtainable by mixing with the leaves of other

plants, such as indigo. As a dye for the skin or nails the powder may be mixed with catechu or lucerne, made into a paste with hot water, and spread on the part to be dyed, being allowed to remain for one night.

¶ *Constituents*. There has been found in it a brown substance of a resinoid fracture, having the chemical properties which characterize the tannins, and therefore named *hennotannic acid*.

¶ *Medicinal Action and Uses*. It has been employed both internally and locally in jaundice, leprosy, smallpox, and affections of the skin. The fruit is thought to have emmenagogue properties.

HEPATICA. *See* LIVERWORT (AMERICAN)

HERB PARIS. *See* PARIS

HOG'S FENNEL. *See* FENNEL

HOLLY

The Egyptians are said to have prepared both an oil and an ointment from the flowers for making the limbs supple.

Ilex aquifolium (LINN.)
N.O. Aquifoliaceæ

Synonyms. Hulver Bush. Holm. Hulm. Holme Chase. Holy Tree. Christ's Thorn
Parts Used. Leaves, berries, bark
Habitat. The Holly is a native of most of the central and southern parts of Europe. It grows very slowly: when planted among trees which are not more rapid in growth than itself, it is sometimes drawn up to a height of 50 feet, but more frequently its greatest height in this country is 30 to 40 feet, and it rarely exceeds 2 feet in diameter. In Italy and in the woods of France, especially in Brittany, it attains a much larger size than is common in these islands

Holly, the most important of the English evergreens, forming one of the most striking objects in the wintry woodland, with its glossy leaves and clusters of brilliant scarlet berries, is in the general mind closely connected with the festivities of Christmas, having been from very early days in the history of these islands gathered in great quantities for Yuletide decorations, both of the Church and of the home. The old Christmas Carols are full of allusions to Holly:

'Christmastide
Comes in like a bride,
With Holly and Ivy clad.'

¶ *History.* Christmas decorations are said to be derived from a custom observed by the Romans of sending boughs, accompanied by other gifts, to their friends during the festival of the Saturnalia, a custom the early Christians adopted. In confirmation of this opinion, a subsequent edict of the Church of Bracara has been quoted, forbidding Christians to decorate their houses at Christmas with green boughs at the same time as the pagans, the Saturnalia commencing about a week before Christmas. The origin has also been traced to the Druids, who decorated their huts with evergreens during winter as an abode for the sylvan spirits. In old church calendars we find Christmas Eve marked *templa exornantur* (churches are decked), and the custom is as deeply rooted in modern times as in either pagan or early Christian days.

An old legend declares that the Holly first sprang up under the footsteps of Christ, when He trod the earth, and its thorny leaves and scarlet berries, like drops of blood, have been thought symbolical of the Saviour's sufferings, for which reason the tree is called

'Christ's Thorn' in the languages of the northern countries of Europe. It is, perhaps, in connexion with these legends that the tree was called the Holy Tree, as it is generally named by our older writers. Turner, for instance, refers to it by this name in his *Herbal* published in 1568. Other popular names for it are Hulver and Holme, and it is still called Hulver in Norfolk, and Holme in Devon, and Holme Chase in one part of Dartmoor.

Pliny describes the Holly under the name of *Aquifolius*, needle leaf, and adds that it was the same tree called by Theophrastus *Cratægus*, but later commentators deny this. Pliny tells us that Holly, if planted near a house or farm, repelled poison, and defended it from lightning and witchcraft, that the flowers cause water to freeze, and that the wood, if thrown at any animal, even without touching it, had the property of compelling the animal to return and lie down by it.

¶ *Description.* It sometimes sends up a clean stem furnished with a bushy head, or it may form a perfect pyramid, leafy to the base. The trunk, like that of the Beech, frequently has small wood knots attached to it: these are composed of a smooth nodule of solid wood embedded in bark, and may be readily separated from the tree by a smart blow. The bark is of a remarkably light hue, smooth and grey, often touched with faint crimson, and is very liable to be infected with an exceedingly thin lichen, the fructification of which consists of numerous curved black lines, closely resembling Oriental writing.

The leaves are thick and glossy, about 2 inches long and 1¼ inch broad, and edged with stout prickles, whose direction is alternately upwards and downwards, and of which the terminal one alone is invariably in the same plane as the leaf. The upper leaves have mostly only a single prickle. The leaves have neither taste nor odour. They remain attached to the tree for several years, and when they fall, defy for a long time the action of air and moisture, owing to their leathery texture and durable fibres, which take a long time to decay.

Professor Henslow says:

'It has been gravely asserted that holly leaves are only prickly on trees as high as a beast can reach, but at the top it has no spines; that spiny processes of all sorts are a provision of Nature against browsing animals. The truth is that they are the result of drought. A vigorous shoot of Holly may have small leaves without spines at the base, when vigour was beginning; normal, large leaves in the middle when growth was most active; and later on small spineless leaves again appear as the annual energy is declining. Moreover, hollies of ten grow to twenty feet in height, with spiny leaves throughout, and if spineless ones *do* occur at the top, it is only the result of lessened energy. A cow has been known to be partial to some holly bushes within reach, which had to be protected, just as another would eat stinging-nettles: and the camel lives upon the "Camel-thorn." This animal has a hardened pad to the roof of its mouth, so feels no inconvenience in eating it.'

In May, the Holly bears in the axils of the leaves, crowded, small, whitish flowers, male and female flowers being usually borne on different trees. The fertile flowers are succeeded by the familiar, brilliant, coral-red berries. The same tree rarely produces abundant crops of flowers in consecutive seasons, and Hollies sometimes produce abundance of flowers, but never mature berries, this barrenness being caused by the *male* flowers alone being properly developed. Berries are rarely produced abundantly when the tree is much clipped, and are usually found in the greatest number on the upper part of the tree, where the leaves are less spiny.

The berries, though eaten by birds, are injurious to human beings, and children should be warned against them. Deer will eat the leaves in winter, and sheep thrive on them. They are infested with few insects.

The ease with which Holly can be-kept trimmed renders it valuable as a hedge plant: it forms hedges of great thickness that are quite impenetrable.

It has been stated by M. J. Pierre, that the young stems are gathered in Morbihan by the peasants, and made use of as a cattle-food from the end of November until April, with great success. The stems are dried, and having been bruised are given as food to cows three times daily. They are found to be very wholesome and productive of good milk, and the butter made from it is excellent.

It is also well known to rabbit-breeders that a Holly-stick placed in a hutch for the rabbits to gnaw, will act as a tonic, and restore their appetite.

The wood of Holly is hard, compact and of a remarkable even substance throughout. Except towards the centre of very old trees, it is beautifully white, and being susceptible of a very high polish, is much prized for ornamental ware, being extensively used for inlaying, as in the so-called Tunbridge ware. The evenness of its grain makes it very valuable to the turner. When freshly cut, it is of a slightly greenish hue, but soon becomes perfectly white, and its hardness makes it superior to any other white wood. As it is very retentive of its sap and warps in consequence, it requires to be well dried and seasoned before being used. It is often stained blue, green, red or black; when of the latter colour, its principal use is as a substitute for ebony, as in the handles of metal teapots. Mathematical instruments are made of it, also the blocks for calico printing, and it has been employed in wood engraving as a substitute for boxwood, to which, however, it is inferior. The wood of the silver-striped variety is said to be whiter than that of the common kind.

A straight Holly-stick is much prized for the stocks of light driving whips, also for walking-sticks.

The common Holly is the badge of the Drummonds.

¶ *Cultivation.* The Holly will grow in almost any soil, provided it is not too wet, but attains the largest size in rich, sandy or gravelly loam, where there is good drainage, and a moderate amount of moisture at the roots, for in very dry localities it is usually stunted in its growth, but it will live in almost any earth not saturated with stagnant water. The most favourable situation seems to be a thin scattered wood of Oaks, in the intervals of which it grows up at once. It is rarely injured by even the most severe winters.

Holly is raised from seeds, which do not germinate until the second year, hence the berries are generally buried in a heap of earth for a year previously to being sown. The young plants are transplanted when about a foot or 18 inches high, autumn being the best time for the process. If intended for a hedge, the soil around should be previously well trenched and moderately manured if necessary. Holly exhausts the soil around it to a greater extent than most deciduous trees. At least two years will be needed to recover the check given by transplanting.

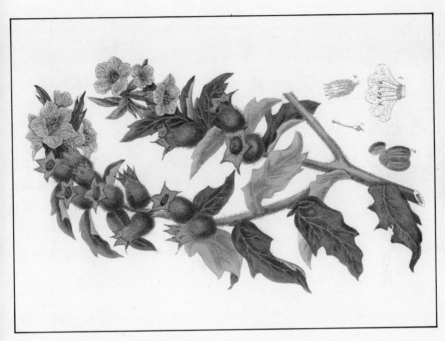

LI

.HENBANE
Hyoscyamus Niger

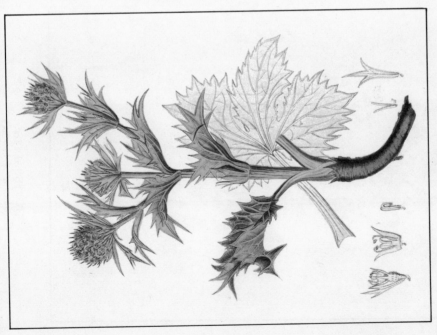

SEA HOLLY
Eryngium Campestre

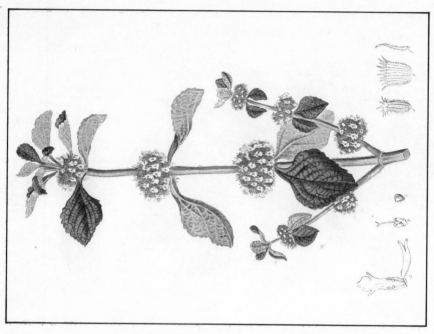

WHITE HOREHOUND
Marrubium Vulgare

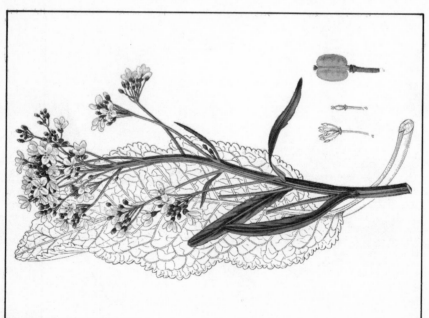

HORSERADISH
Cochlearia Armoracia

Although always a slow grower, Holly grows more quickly after the first four or five years.

The cultivated varieties of Holly are very numerous: of these one is distinguished by the unusual colour of its berries, which are yellow. Other forms are characterized by the variegated foliage, or by the presence of a larger or smaller number of prickles than ordinary.

In winter the garden and shrubbery are much indebted to the more showy varieties for the double contrast afforded by their leaves and berries. They are propagated by grafting on four- or five-year-old plants of the common sort and by cuttings.

The best time to cut down Holly is early in the spring, before the sap rises. A sloping cut is preferable to a straight one, as moisture is thus prevented from remaining on the cut portion, and as an additional precaution the wound should be covered with a coating of tar. The side growths should be left, as they will help to draw up the sap.

¶ *Part Used.* The leaves and berries, also the bark. The leaves are used both fresh and dried, but usually in the dried condition, for which they are collected in May and June. They should be stripped off the tree on a dry day, the best time being about noon, when there is no longer any trace of dew on them. All stained or insect-eaten leaves must be rejected.

¶ *Medicinal Action and Uses.* Holly leaves were formerly used as a diaphoretic and an infusion of them was given in catarrh, pleurisy and smallpox. They have also been used in intermittent fevers and rheumatism for their febrifugal and tonic properties, and powdered, or taken in infusion or decoction, have been employed with success where Cinchona has failed, their virtue being said to depend on a bitter principle, an alkaloid named Ilicin. The juice of the fresh leaves has been employed with advantage in jaundice.

The berries possess totally different qualities to the leaves, being violently emetic and purgative, a very few occasioning excessive vomiting soon after they are swallowed, though thrushes and blackbirds eat them with impunity. They have been employed in dropsy; also, in powder, as an astringent to check bleeding.

Culpepper says 'the bark and leaves are good used as fomentations for broken bones and such members as are out of joint.' He considered the berries to be curative of colic.

From the bark, stripped from the young shoots and suffered to ferment, birdlime is made. The bark is stripped off about midsummer and steeped in clean water; then boiled till it separates into layers, when the inner green portion is laid up in small heaps till fermentation ensues. After about a fortnight has elapsed, it becomes converted into a sticky, mucilaginous substance, and is pounded into a paste, washed and laid by again to ferment. It is then mixed with some oily matter, goosefat being preferred, and is ready for use. Very little, however, is now made in this country. In the north of England, Holly was formerly so abundant in the Lake District, that birdlime was made from it in large quantities and shipped to the East Indies for destroying insects.

The leaves of Holly have been employed in the Black Forest as a substitute for tea. Paraguay Tea, so extensively used in Brazil, is made from the dried leaves and young shoots of another species of Holly (*Ilex Paraguayensis*), growing in South America, an instance of the fact that similar properties are often found in more than one species of the same genus.

I. Gongonha and *I. Theezans*, also used in Brazil as tea, and like *I. Paraguayensis* are valuable diuretics and diaphoretics. The leaves of *I. Paraguayensis* and several others are used by dyers; the unripe fruits of *I. Macoucoua* abound in tannin, and bruised in a ferruginous mud, are used in dyeing cotton, acting something like galls.

See PARAGUAY.

HOLLY, SEA

Eryngium maritimum
Eryngium campestre
N.O. Umbelliferæ

Synonyms. Eryngo. Sea Hulver. Sea Holme
(*French*) Panicaut
(*German*) Krausdistel
Part Used. Root
Habitat. It abounds on most of our sandy seashores and is very plentiful on the East Coast, also on the sands of Mounts Bay, Cornwall, but is rare in Scotland

Closely allied to the Wood Sanicle, not only belonging to the same order, Umbelliferæ, but placed by Hooker in the same

Tribe or subdivision of the order, *Saniculæ,* is the Sea Holly (*Eryngium maritinum*).

This spiny plant, which at first sight might

be taken rather for a thistle than a member of the umbelliferous order, is sometimes called by old English writers Sea Hulver and Sea Holme.

¶ *Description.* The roots are perennial, large, fleshy and brittle, penetrating far into the sand, often reaching several feet in length.

The stems, 6 to 12 inches high, thick and solid, are branched at the summit. The radical leaves are on stalks, 2 to 7 inches long, the blades cut into three broad divisions at the apex, coarsely toothed, the teeth ending in spines and undulated. The margin of the leaf is thickened and cartilaginous. The lower stem-leaves are shortly stalked, resembling the radical ones, but the upper ones are sessile and half embracing the stem, which terminates in a shortly-stalked head, below which it gives off two or three spreading branches, all from one point, which is surrounded by a whorl of three leaves, spreading like the rays of the sun.

The heads of flowers appear in July and are at first round, afterwards egg-shaped, ¾ to 1 inch across, the flowers stalkless, whitish-blue, ⅛ inch across. The calyx tube is thickly covered with soft, cartilaginous bristles; the calyx teeth end in a spine.

The plant is intensely glaucous tinged with blue towards the top, especially on the flower-heads and the leaves immediately below them.

The name of this genus has reference to its supposed efficacy in flatulent disorders, coming from the Greek word *eruggarein* (to eructate). Dioscorides recommended the roots for this purpose.

Another derivation is from the diminutive of *eerungos* (the beard of a goat), possibly from its appearance. Plutarch relates a curious story about the plant, saying:

'They report of the Sea Holly, if one goat taketh it into her mouth, it causeth her first to stand still and afterwards the whole flock, until such time as the shepherd takes it from her.'

According to Linnæus, the young flowering-shoots, when boiled and eaten like asparagus, are palatable and nourishing. The leaves are sweetish, with a slight aromatic, warm pungency. The roots, boiled or roasted, resemble chestnuts in taste, and are palatable and nutritious.

The roots are supposed to have the same aphrodisiac virtues as those of the Orchis tribe, and are still regarded by the Arabs as an excellent restorative. They are sold in some places in a candied form, and used to be obtainable in London shops as a sweetmeat. They are said to have been prepared in this manner by Robert Burton, an apothe-

cary of Colchester, in the seventeenth century, who established a manufactory for the purpose, but the roots were in use long before, being considered both antiscorbutic and excellent for health, and we are told that the 'kissing comfits,' alluded to by Falstaff, were made of them. We read that once the town of Colchester presented royalty with a sample of their candied Sea Holly roots, whereon the sale of the article increased greatly, and many wonderful cures were supposed to be effected by the confection.

Gerard says:

'The roots if eaten are good for those that be liver sick; and they ease cramps, convulsions and the falling sickness. If condited, or preserved with sugar, they are exceeding good to be given to old and aged people that are consumed and withered with age, and who want natural moisture.'

He gives an elaborate recipe for 'conditing' the roots of Sea Holly or Eringos.

He also cultivated in his garden the Field Eryngo (*E. campestre*), a native of most parts of Europe, but not common in Britain, though a troublesome weed in the few spots where it does appear, as the roots run deep into the ground, and are not easily destroyed by the plough and spread greatly. The whole plant is very stiff and of a pale-green colour, less glaucous and more branched than the Sea Holly; the corolla are blue, sometimes white or yellow. It is taller and more slender, also, than the Sea Holly. By many authorities it is considered a doubtful native of these islands.

¶ *Cultivation.* The Sea Holly, in common with the ornamental varieties, Eryngo, now cultivated, will grow in a garden, if planted in a warm, well-drained and preferably a gravel soil, but the roots will not grow as large or as fleshy as those which are found upon the seashore within reach of salt water. Plenty of sun is essential for all varieties.

The best time to transplant the roots is in autumn, when the leaves decay; the young roots are much better to transplant than the old, because, being furnished with fibres, they will readily take root. They will require no further culture than to be kept free from weeds.

If propagated by seeds, they are more likely to succeed if the seeds are sown in the autumn, as the germination is very slow. They may be sown where intended to grow and thinned out to about a foot or more apart, to avoid transplanting, as the long roots may break in the process. The seedlings are, in any case, not ready for transplanting for a year, so that the mode of propagation generally preferred is by division of roots in spring. Cuttings of the roots will succeed in light soil, if planted about 2 inches deep.

¶ *Part Used.* The root, dug in autumn, from plants at least two years old.

Culpepper says:

'The distilled water of the whole herb' (Sea Holly) 'when the leaves and stalks are young is profitably drank for all the purposes aforesaid, and helps the melancholy of the heart, and is available in quartan and quotidian agues; as also for them that have their necks drawn awry, and cannot turn them without turning their whole body.'

Eryngo roots when dry are in pieces from 2 to 4 inches long, or more, transversely wrinkled, blackish-brown, crowned with the bristly remains of leaf-stalks. The fracture is spongy and coarsely fibrous, with a small radiate, yellow centre.

The taste is sweetish and mucilaginous, but the root has no odour.

The roots of both the Common Sea Holly and of the Field Eryngo are both sold under the name of Eryngo Root.

¶ *Medicinal Action and Uses.* Diaphoretic, diuretic, aromatic, stimulant, expectorant. Eryngo promotes a free expectoration and possessing an aromatic principle is very serviceable in debility attendant upon coughs of chronic standing in the advanced stages of pulmonary consumption, in which it has been used in the candied form with great benefit.

It is useful in paralysis and chronic nervous diseases, alike in simple nervousness and in delirium produced by diseases.

Boerhaave, the celebrated Danish physician, much recommended Eryngo, considering that a decoction of the roots, drunk freely, acted on the kidneys and is serviceable in scorbutic complaints. It is used with good results in cases of bladder disease.

The roots are also considered good in obstructions of the liver and in jaundice, operating as a diuretic and a good restorative.

They have been pronounced balsamic, as well as diuretic, old writers telling us that bruised and applied outwardly, they are good for King's Evil, and that when bruised and boiled in hog's fat and applied to broken bones, thorns in the flesh, etc., they draw the latter out and heal up the place again, 'gathering new flesh where it was consumed.'

¶ *Other Species.*

E. campestre was formerly abundant about Watling Street.

Of the foreign species, which are numerous, the most worthy of notice is *E. amethystinum*, so called from the brilliant blue tint not of its flowers only, but of the bracts and upper part of the stem; it is a native of Dalmatia and Croatia, but is frequently cultivated in English gardens; while *E. Alpinum*, a smaller plant of a still more brilliant colour, is a native of the Swiss Alps.

E. aquaticum (Button Snake-root), a North American plant, is used in Homœopathy, a tincture being made from the root both fresh and dried.

HOLLYHOCK

Althæa Rosea (LINN.)
N.O. Malvaceæ

Synonym. Garden Hollyhock
Part Used. Flowers

The Hollyhock, first brought to this country from China, was once eaten as a pot-herb, though it is not particularly palatable.

Its flowers are employed medicinally for their emollient, demulcent and diuretic properties, which make them useful in chest complaints. Their action is similar to Marshmallow.

The flowers are also used for colouring purposes. They are sold freed from the calyx and should be gathered in July and early August, when in full bloom, and dried in trays, in thin layers, in a current of warm air immediately after picking. When dry, they are a deep, purplish-black, about 2½ inches in diameter, united with the stamens, which form a tube, the one-celled, reniform anthers remaining free.

See MALLOWS.

HONEYSUCKLES

Lonicera caprifolium (LINN.)
Lonicera Periclymenum (LINN.)
N.O. Caprifoliaceæ

Synonyms. Dutch Honeysuckle. Goats' Leaf
(*French*) Chèvre-feuille
(*German*) Geisblatt
(*Italian*) Capri-foglio
Parts Used. Flowers, seeds, leaves

Caprifoliaceæ, the order to which the Honeysuckles belong, includes about 300 species, chiefly shrubs, growing in the north temperate zone or extending into the higher cool tropical regions. Besides the *Viburnums* and *Sambucus*, a number have found more or less important uses in medicine, but they exhibit but little uniformity in composition or properties.

¶ *Medicinal Action and Uses.* A dozen or more of the 100 species of *Lonicera* or Honeysuckle are used medicinally, the fruits generally having emiticocathartic properties. Several of these drugs have more than a local repute.

The herbage of *L. caprifolium* (Linn.), the smaller, or ITALIAN HONEYSUCKLE, of Mid- and Southern Europe, is used as a cutaneous and mucous tonic and vulnerary and the seeds as a diuretic.

L. Periclymenum (Linn.), our common ENGLISH WILD HONEYSUCKLE, is used similarly and the stems as a substitute or adulterant for *Solanum Dulcamara*, the Bittersweet.

Waller says: 'The leaves and flowers of Honeysuckle are possessed of diuretic and sudorific properties,' and adds:

'a decoction of the flowers has been celebrated as an excellent antispasmodic and recommended in asthma of the nervous kind. An elegant water may be distilled from these flowers, which has been recommended for nervous headache.'

Gerard says: 'The Honeysuckle is "neither cold nor binding, but hot and attenuating or making thin."' He quotes Dioscorides as saying that—

'the ripe seed gathered and dried in the shadow and drunk for four days together, doth waste and consume away the hardness of the spleen and removeth wearisomeness, helpeth the shortness and difficulty of breathing, cureth the hicket (hiccough), etc. A syrup made of the flowers is good to be drunk against diseases of the lungs and spleen.'

He also recommends it for sores in various parts of the alimentary canal.

Salmon in his *Herbal* (1710) speaks only of the Meadow Honeysuckle, 'which was the name given by the agriculturists of his day to the Meadow Trefoil (*Trifolium pratense*).'

The herbage of the true Honeysuckles is a favourite food of goats, hence the Latin name *Caprifolium* (Goats' Leaf), the French *Chèvre-feuille*, German *Geisblatt* and Italian *Capri-foglio*, all signifying the same. The berries have been used as food for chickens. The name of the genus, *Lonicera*, was given by Linnæus in honour of Adam Lonicer, a physician and naturalist, born at Marburg in 1528, who wrote, among other works, the *Naturalis Historiæ Opus novum*, which contains much curious information about plants. Our native Honeysuckle has expectorant and laxative properties. The flowers in the form of syrup have been used for diseases of the respiratory organs and in asthma and the leaves as decoction in diseases of the liver and spleen. It was also considered a good ingredient in gargles.

L. tartarica, a native of Siberia, an upright species, a shrub, not a climber, has berries which are nauseously bitter and purgative. The wood of *L. Xylosteum*, native of Eastern Europe and Asia, but found naturalized in Sussex, also of shrub-like nature, is used by the Russians to prepare an empyrheumatic oil for 'cold tumours and chronic pains.' It is sold in China as *Jin-tung*. Animals seldom touch the leaves of this species and birds eat its berries only in hard weather – they are reputed to be purgative and emetic.

L. brachypoda repens is used in Japan as a drastic purgative, and *L. Japonica* (Thunb.) is sold in China as *Kin-yin-keva*.

Diervilla, the Bush Honeysuckle, especially *Diervilla Diervilla* (*L. Diervilla*, Linn.), has a similar repute, especially as a diuretic and as an application to relieve itching.

Various species of *Symphoricarpus*, Snowberry, Wax-berry, Coral-berry, Indian Currant, Turkey-berry, Wolf-berry, to give a few of its names, of North America, are similarly employed. *S. racemosa* (Mich.) is often planted in hedges.

Culpepper says:

'Honeysuckles are cleansing, consuming and digesting, and therefore no way fit for inflammations. Take a leaf and chew it in your mouth and you will quickly find it likelier to cause a sore mouth and throat than cure it. If it be not good for this, what is it good for? It is good for something, for God and nature make nothing in vain. It is a herb of Mercury, and appropriated to the lungs; the celestial Crab claims dominion over it, neither is it a foe to the Lion; if the lungs be afflicted by Jupiter, this is your cure. It is fitting a conserve made of the flowers should be kept in every gentlewoman's house; I know no better cure for the asthma than this besides it takes away the evil of the spleen: provokes urine, procures speedy delivery of women in travail, relieves cramps, convulsions, and palsies, and whatsoever griefs come of cold or obstructed perspiration; if you make use of it as an ointment, it will clear the skin of morphew, freckles, and sunburnings, or whatever else discolours it, and then the maids will love it. Authors say, the flowers are of more effect than the leaves, and that is true: but they say the seeds are the least effectual of all. But there is a vital spirit in every seed to beget its like; there is a greater heat in the seed than any other part of the plant; and heat is the mother of action.'

HOPS

Part Used. Flowers

The Hop (*Humulus Lupulus*, Linn.) is a native British plant, having affinities, botanically speaking, with the group of plants to which the Stinging Nettles belong. The sole representative of its genus in these islands, it is found wild in hedges and copses from York southwards, being only considered an introduced species in Scotland, and rare and not indigenous in Ireland. It is found in most countries of the North temperate zone.

The root is stout and perennial. The stem that arises from it every year is of a twining nature, reaching a great length, flexible and very tough, angled and prickly, with a tenacious fibre, which has enabled it to be employed to some extent in Sweden in the manufacture of a coarse kind of cloth, white and durable, though the fibres are so difficult of separation, that the stems require to be steeped in water a whole winter. Paper has also been made from the stem, or *bine*, as it is termed.

The leaves are heart-shaped and lobed, on foot-stalks, and as a rule placed opposite one another on the stem, though sometimes the upper leaves are arranged singly on the stem, springing from alternate sides. They are of a dark-green colour with their edges finely toothed.

The flowers spring from the axils of the leaves. The Hop is diœcious, i.e. male and female flowers are on separate plants. The male flowers are in loose bunches or panicles, 3 to 5 inches long. The female flowers are in leafy cone-like catkins, called *strobiles*. When fully developed, the strobiles are about 1¼ inch long, oblong in shape and rounded, consisting of a number of overlapping, yellowish-green bracts, attached to a separate axis. If these leafy organs are removed, the axis will be seen to be hairy and to have a little zigzag course. Each of the bracts enfolds at the base a small fruit (achene), both fruit and bract being sprinkled with yellow translucent glands, which appear as a granular substance. Much of the value of Hops depends on the abundance of this powdery substance, which contains 10 per cent. of Lupulin, the bitter principle to which Hops owe much of their tonic properties.

As it is, these ripened cones of the female Hop plant that are used in brewing, female plants only are cultivated, since from these alone can the fruits be obtained. Those with undeveloped seeds are preferred, to ensure which the staminate plants are excluded, only a few male plants being found scattered over a plantation of hops.

We find the Hop first mentioned by Pliny, who speaks of it as a garden plant among the Romans, who ate the young shoots in spring, in the same way as we do asparagus, and as country people frequently do in England at the present day. The young tops of Hop used formerly to be brought to market tied up in small bundles for table use. The tender first foliage, blanched, is a good pot-herb.

The leaves and flower-heads have been used also to produce a fine brown dye.

The origin of the name of the Hop genus, *Humulus*, is considered doubtful, though it has been assumed by some writers that it is derived from *humus*, the rich moist ground in which the plant grows. The specific name, *Lupulus*, is derived from the Latin, *lupus* (a wolf), because, as Pliny explains, when produced among osiers, it strangles them by its light, climbing embraces, as the wolf does a sheep. The English name *Hop* comes from the Anglo-Saxon *hoppan* (to climb).

Hops appear to have been used in the breweries of the Netherlands in the beginning of the fourteenth century. In England they were not used in the composition of beer till nearly two centuries afterwards. The liquor prepared from fermented malt formed the favourite drink of our Saxon and Danish forefathers. The beverage went by the name of Ale (the word derived from the Scandinavian *öl* – the Viking's drink) and was brewed either from malt alone, or from a mixture of the latter with Honey and flavoured with Heath tops, Ground Ivy, and various other bitter and aromatic herbs, such as Marjoram, Buckbean, Wormwood, Yarrow, Woodsage or Germander and Broom. They knew not, however, the ale to which Hops give both flavour and preservation. For long after the introduction of Hops, the liquor flavoured in the old manner retained the name of *Ale*, while the word of German and Dutch origin, *Bier* or *Beer*, was given only to that made with the newly-introduced bitter catkins.

It has been stated that the planting of Hops in this country was forbidden in the reign of Henry VI, but half a century later the cultivation was introduced from Flanders, though only to a limited extent, and it did not become sufficient for the needs of the kingdom till the end of the seventeenth century. The prejudice against the use of Hops was at first great. Henry VIII forbade brewers to put hops and sulphur into ale, Parliament having been petitioned against the Hop as 'a wicked weed that would spoil the taste of the drink and endanger the people.' In the fifth year of Edward VI, however, privileges were granted to Hop growers, though in the reign of James I the plant was still not sufficiently cultivated to supply the consumption, as we find a statute of 1608 against the importation of spoiled Hops.

Hops were at first thought to engender melancholy.

'Hops,' says John Evelyn, in his *Pomona* (1670), 'transmuted our wholesome ale into beer, which doubtless much alters its constitution. This one ingredient, by some suspected not unworthily, preserves the drink indeed, but repays the pleasure in tormenting diseases and a shorter life.'

¶ *Cultivation.* It has been estimated that in pre-war times 70 per cent. of the Hops used in brewing was home produce and 30 per cent. imported, chiefly from the United States and Germany.

Hops are also grown in France, South Russia, Australia and New Zealand.

The cultivation of Hops in the British Islands is restricted to England, where it is practically confined to half a dozen counties: four in the south-east (Kent, Surrey, Hants and Sussex) and two in the western Midland counties (Worcester and Hereford). As a rule, over 60 per cent. of home-grown Hops are grown in Kent.

In the years 1898–1907, the average annual acreage of Hops under cultivation in this country was 48,841 acres (being 51,127 acres in 1901 and 33,763 acres in 1907). The average annual yield per acre for these ten years was 8·84 cwt., and the average annual home produce 434,567 cwt. In 1907 Kent had under cultivation 28,169 acres; Hereford, 6,143; Sussex, 4,243; Worcester, 3,622; Hants; 1,842, and Surrey, 744.

Hops require deep, rich soil, on dry bottom, with south or south-west aspect – free circulation of air is necessary. The ground is generally well pulverized and manured to considerable depth by plough or spade before planting. Hops in Kent are usually planted in October or November, the plants being placed 6 feet apart each way, thus giving 1,210 plant centres to the acre. The plants are usually set in 'stools' of from three to five, a few inches apart. They are obtained from cuttings or suckers taken from the healthiest old shoots, which are usually planted out closely in nursery lines a year before being planted permanently.

Very little growth takes place the first year. Some planters still grow potatoes or mangels between the rows of the first year, as the plants do not bear much till the second

year, but this is considered a mistake, as it exhausts the ground.

As a rule, the plants are not full bearing till the third year, when four to six poles from 14 to 18 feet long are required for each stool. The most used timber for Hop poles is Spanish Chestnut, which is largely grown for this special purpose in coppices in hop-growing districts. Ash is also used. The poles are set to the plants in spring, before growth commences, and removed when the latter are cut away in autumn. The plants are then dressed with manure, and the soil between the stools stirred lightly. Much of the Hop-land is ploughed between the rows, but it is better to dig Hop-land if possible, the tool used being the Kent spud.

Experiments in Hop manuring have been conducted in connexion with the South-East Agricultural College, Wye. The main results have been to demonstrate the necessity of a liberal supply of phosphates, if the full benefit is to be reaped from application of nitrogenous manures. Manuring is applied in the winter and dug or ploughed in. London manure from stables is used to an enormous extent. Rags, fur waste, sprats, wood waste and shoddy, are also put on in the winter. In the summer, rape dust, guano, nitrate of soda and various patent Hop-manures are chopped in with the Canterbury hoe. Fish guano, or desiccated fish, is largely used; it is very stimulating and more lasting than some of the forcing manures.

Hop-land is ploughed or dug between November and March. After this, the plants are trimmed or 'dressed,' i.e. all the old bine ends are cut off with a sharp curved Hop-knife and the plant centres kept level with the ground. Much attention is required to keep the bines in their places on the poles, strings or wire during the summer.

The Hop cones – or strobiles – are fit to gather when a brown-amber colour and of a firm consistence. The stalks are then cut at the base and removed with the poles and laid horizontally on frames of wood, to each of which is attached a large sack into which the Hops fall as they are picked. When picked, the Hops are at once taken to the kiln or oast-house, and dried, as they are liable to become spoiled in a few hours, especially when picked moist. During the process of drying which is carried out in a similar manner to the drying of malt, great care is required to prevent overheating, by which the essential oil would become volatilized. The Hops are spread 8 to 12 inches deep, on hair-cloth, also being sometimes exposed to fumes of burning sulphur. When the ends of the stalks shrivel, they are removed from the kiln and laid on a wooden floor till quite cool, when they are packed in bales, known as 'pockets.'

The difficulties attendant upon the cultivation of Hops have been aggravated and the expenses increased in recent years by the regularly recurring attacks of aphis blight, due to the insect *Aphis humuli*, which make it necessary to spray or syringe every Hop plant, every branch and leaf with insecticidal solutions three or four times and sometimes more often in each season. Quassia and soft soap solutions are usually employed: the soft soap serves as a vehicle to retain the bitterness of the quassia upon the bines and leaves, making them repulsive to the Aphides, which are thus starved out. The solution is made from 4 to 8 lb. of quassia chips to 100 gallons of water.

Another pest, the Red Spider (*Tetranychus telarius*) is most destructive in very hot summers. Congregating on the under surfaces of the leaves, the red spiders exhaust the sap and cause the leaves to fall. The Quassia and Soft Soap Hopwash is of little avail in the case of Red Spider. Some success has attended the use of a solution consisting of 8 to 10 lb. of soft soap to 100 gallons of water, with 3 pints of paraffin added. It must be applied with great force, to break through the webs with which the spiders protect themselves.

Hop washing is done by means of large garden engines worked by hand or by horse-engines: even steam-engines have sometimes been employed.

Among fungoid parasites, Mould or Mildew is frequently the cause of loss to Hop planters. It is due to the action of the fungus *Podosphæra castagnei*, and the mischief is more especially that done to the cones. The remedy is sulphur, employed usually in the form of flowers of sulphur, from 40 to 60 lb. per acre being applied at each sulphuring, distributed by means of a blast pipe. The first sulphuring takes place when the plants are fairly up the poles and is repeated three or four weeks later, and even again if indications of mildew are present. Sulphur is also successfully employed in the form of an alkaline sulphur, such as a solution of liver of sulphur, a variety of potassium sulphide.

¶ *Parts Used Medicinally*. (*a*) The strobiles, collected and dried as described. (*b*) The Lupulin, separated from the strobiles by sifting.

¶ *Chemical Constituents*. The aromatic odour of the Hop strobiles is due to a volatile oil, of which they yield about 0·3 to 1·0 per cent. It appears to consist chiefly of the sesquiterpene Humulene. Petroleum spirit extracts 7 to 14 per cent. of a powerfully antiseptic soft resin, and ether extracts a hard resin. The petroleum spirit extract contains the two crystalline bitter principles (*a*) Lupamaric acid (Humulone), (*b*) Lupamaric acid (Lupulinic acid). These bodies are chiefly contained in the glands at the base of the bracts. The leafy organs contain about 5 per cent. of tannin which is not a constituent of the glands. Hops yield about 7 per cent. Ash.

The oil and the bitter principle combine to make Hops more useful than Chamomile, Gentian or any other bitter in the manufacture of beer: hence the medicinal value of *extra-hopped* or *bitter* beer. The tannic acid contained in the strobiles adds to the value of Hops by causing precipitation of vegetable mucilage and consequently the cleansing of beer.

Fresh Hops possess a bitter aromatic taste and a strong characteristic odour. The latter, however, changes and becomes distinctly unpleasant as the Hops are kept. This change is ascribed to oxidation of the soft resin with production of Valerianic acid. On account of the rapid change in the odour of Hops, the recently dried fruits should alone be used: these may be recognized by the characteristic odour and distinctly green colour. Those which have been subjected to the treatment of *sulphuring* are not to be used in pharmacy. This process is conducted with a view of improving the colour and odour of the Hops, since sulphuric acid is found to retard the production of the Valerianic odour and to both preserve and improve the colour of the Hops.

Lupulin, which consists of the glandular powder present on the seeds and surface of the scales, may be separated by shaking the strobiles. The drug occurs in a granular, brownish-yellow powder, with the strong odour and bitter aromatic taste characteristic of Hops. The glands readily burst on the application of slight pressure and discharge their granular oleo-resinous contents. Commercial Lupulin is often of a very inferior quality, and consists of the sifted sweepings from the floors of hop-kilns. It should contain not more than 40 per cent. of matter insoluble in ether and not yield more than 12 per cent. of ash on incineration. A dark colour and disagreeable odour indicates an old drug.

The chief constituent of Lupulin is about 3 per cent. of volatile oil, which consists chiefly of Humulene, together with various oxygenated bodies to which the oil owes its peculiar odour. Other constituents are the two Lupamaric acids, cholene and resin.

Lupulin is official both in the British Pharmacopœia and the United States Pharmaco-pœia.

¶ *Medicinal Action and Uses.* Hops have tonic, nervine, diuretic and anodyne properties. Their volatile oil produces sedative and soporific effects, and the Lupamaric acid or bitter principle is stomachic and tonic. For this reason Hops improve the appetite and promote sleep.

The official preparations are an infusion and a tincture. The infusion is employed as a vehicle, especially for bitters and tonics: the tincture is stomachic and is used to improve the appetite and digestion. Both preparations have been considered to be sedative, were formerly much given in nervousness and hysteria and at bedtime to induce sleep; in cases of nervousness, delirium and inflammation being considered to produce a most soothing effect, frequently procuring for the patient sleep after long periods of sleeplessness in overwrought conditions of the brain.

The bitter principle in the Hop proves one of the most efficacious vegetable bitters obtainable. An infusion of ½ oz. Hops to 1 pint of water will be found the proper quantity for ordinary use. It has proved of great service also in heart disease, fits, neuralgia and nervous disorders, besides being a useful tonic in indigestion, jaundice, and stomach and liver affections generally. It gives prompt ease to an irritable bladder, and is said to be an excellent drink in cases of delirium tremens. Sherry in which some Hops have been steeped makes a capital stomachic cordial.

A pillow of warm Hops will often relieve toothache and earache and allay nervous irritation.

An infusion of the leaves, strobiles and stalks, as Hop Tea, taken by the wineglassful two or three times daily in the early spring, is good for sluggish livers. Hop Tea in the leaf, as frequently sold by grocers, consists of Kentish Hop leaves, dried, crushed under rollers and then mixed with ordinary Ceylon or Indian Tea. The infusion combines the refreshment of the one herb with the sleep-inducing virtues of the other.

Hop juice cleanses the blood, and for calculus trouble nothing better can be found than the bitter principle of the Hop. A decoction of the root has been esteemed as of equal benefit with Sarsaparilla.

As an external remedy, an infusion of Hops is much in demand in combination with chamomile flowers or poppy heads as a fomentation for swelling of a painful nature, inflammation, neuralgic and rheumatic pains, bruises, boils and gatherings. It removes pain and allays inflammation in a very short time. The Hops may also be applied as a poultice.

The drug Lupulin is an aromatic bitter and is reputed to be midly sedative, inducing sleep without causing headache.

It is occasionally administered as a hypnotic, either in pills with alcohol, or enclosed in a cachet.

Preparations of Lupulin are not much used in this country, although official, but in the United States they are considered preferable for internal use.

RECIPES FOR HERB BEERS

Formerly every farmhouse inn had a brewing plant and brewhouse attached to the buildings, and all brewed their own beer till the large breweries were established and supplanted home-brewed beers. Many of these farmhouses then began to brew their own 'stingo' from wayside herbs, employing old rustic recipes that had been carried down from generation to generation. The true value of vegetable bitters and of herb beers have yet to be recognized by all sections of the community. Workmen in puddling furnaces and potteries in the Midland and Northern counties find, however, that a tea made of tonic herbs is cheaper and less intoxicating than ordinary beer and patronize the herb beers freely, *Dandelion Stout* ranking as one of the favourites. It is also made in Canada.

Dandelion is a good ingredient in many digestive or diet drinks. A dinner drink may be made as follows: Take 2 oz. each of dried Dandelion and Nettle herbs and 1 oz. of Yellow Dock. Boil in 1 gallon of water for 15 minutes and then strain the liquor while hot on to 2 lb. of sugar, on the top of which is sprinkled 2 tablespoonsful of powdered Ginger. Leave till milk-warm, then add boiled water gone cold to bring the quantity up to 2 gallons. The temperature must then not be above 75° F. Now dissolve ½ oz. solid yeast in a little of the liquid and stir into the bulk. Allow to ferment 24 hours, skim and bottle, and it will be ready for use in a day or two.

A good, pleasant-tasting botanic beer is also made of the *Nettle* alone. Quantities of the young fresh tops are boiled in a gallon of water, with the juice of two lemons, a teaspoonful of crushed ginger and 1 lb. of brown sugar. Fresh yeast is floated on toast in the liquor, when cold, to ferment it, and when it is bottled the result is a specially wholesome sort of ginger beer.

Meadow Sweet was also formerly much in favour. The mash when worked with barm made a pleasant drink, either in the harvest field or at the table. It required little sugar, some even made it without any sugar at all.

Another favourite brew was that of arms-ful of Meadowsweet, Yarrow, Dandelion and Nettles, and the mash when 'sweetened with old honey' and well worked with barm, and then bottled in big stoneware bottles, made a drink strong enough to turn even an old toper's head.

Old honeycomb from the thatch of an ancient cottage, filled with rich and nearly black honey, when boiled into syrup and then strained, was used in the making of herb beer, while the wax was put at the mouths of the hives for the bees.

Dandelion, Meadowsweet and Agrimony, equal quantities of each, would also be boiled together for 20 minutes (about 2 oz. each of the dried herbs to 2 gallons of water), then strained and 2 lb. of sugar and ½ pint of barm or yeast added. This was bottled after standing in a warm place for 12 hours. This recipe is still in use.

A Herb Beer that needs no yeast is made from equal quantities of Meadowsweet, Betony, Agrimony and Raspberry leaves (2 oz. of each) boiled in 2 gallons of water for 15 minutes, strained, then 2 lb. of white sugar added and bottled when nearly cool.

In some outlying islands of the Hebrides there is still brewed a drinkable beer by mak-ing two-thirds Heath tops with one-third of malt.

HOP BITTERS, as an appetiser, to be taken in tablespoonful doses three times in the day before eating, may be made as follows: Take 2 oz. of Buchu leaves and ½ lb. of Hops. Boil these in 5 quarts of water in an iron vessel for an hour. When lukewarm add essence of Winter green (Pyrola) 2 oz. and 1 pint alcohol.

Another way of making Hop Bitters is to take ½ oz. Hops, 1 oz. Angelica Herb and 1 oz. Holy Thistle. Pour 3 pints of boiling water on them and strain when cold. A wineglassful may be taken four times a day.

To make a good HOP BEER, put 2 oz. Hops in 2 quarts of water for 15 minutes. Then strain and dissolve 1 lb. of sugar in the liquor. To this add 4 quarts of cold water and 2 tablespoonsful of fresh barm. Allow to stand for 12 hours in a warm place and it will then be ready for bottling.

HOREHOUND, WHITE

Marrubium vulgare (LINN.)
N.O. Labiatæ

Synonym. Hoarhound
Part Used. Herb
Habitat. White Horehound is a perennial herbaceous plant, found all over Europe and indigenous to Britain. Like many other plants of the Labiate tribe, it flourishes in waste places and by roadsides, particularly in the counties of Norfolk and Suffolk, where it is also cultivated in the corners of cottage gardens for making tea and candy for use in coughs and colds. It is also brewed and made into Horehound Ale, an appetizing and healthful beverage, much drunk in Norfolk and other country districts

¶ *Description.* The plant is bushy, produc-ing numerous annual, quadrangular and branching stems, a foot or more in height, on which the whitish flowers are borne in crowded, axillary, woolly whorls. The leaves are much wrinkled, opposite, petiolate, about 1 inch long, covered with white, felted hairs, which give them a woolly appearance. They have a curious, musky smell, which is dimin-ished by drying and lost on keeping. Hore-hound flowers from June to September.

The Romans esteemed Horehound for its medicinal properties, and its Latin name of *Marrubium* is said to be derived from *Maria urbs*, an ancient town of Italy. Other authors derive its name from the Hebrew *marrob* (a bitter juice), and state that it was one of the bitter herbs which the Jews were ordered to take for the Feast of Passover.

The Egyptian Priests called this plant the 'Seed of Horus,' or the 'Bull's Blood,' and the 'Eye of the Star.' It was a principal in-gredient in the negro Cæsar's antidote for vegetable poisons.

Gerard recommends it, in addition to its uses in coughs and colds, to 'those that have drunk poyson or have been bitten of ser-pents,' and it was also administered for 'mad dogge's biting.'

It was once regarded as an anti-magical herb.

According to Columella, Horehound is a serviceable remedy against Cankerworm in trees, and it is stated that if it be put into new milk and set in a place pestered with flies, it will speedily kill them all.
¶ *Cultivation.* White Horehound is a hardy plant, easily grown, and flourishes best in a dry, poor soil. It can be propagated from seeds sown in spring, cuttings, or by dividing the roots (the most usual method). If raised from seed, the seedlings should be planted out in the spring, in rows, with a space of about 9 inches or more between each plant. No further culture will be needed than weed-ing. It does not blossom until it is two years old.

Until recently, it was chiefly collected in

Southern France, where it is much cultivated. It is in steady demand, and it would
probably pay to cultivate it more in this
country.

White Horehound is distinguished from
other species by its woolly stem, the densely
felted hairs on the leaves, and the ten-
toothed teeth of the calyx.

¶ *Constituents.* The chief constituent is a
bitter principle known as Marrubium, with
a little volatile oil, resin, tannin, wax, fat,
sugar, etc.

¶ *Medicinal Action and Uses.* White Horehound has long been noted for its efficacy
in lung troubles and coughs. Gerard says of
this plant:

'Syrup made of the greene fresh leaves and
sugar is a most singular remedie against the
cough and wheezing of the lungs . . . and
doth wonderfully and above credit ease such
as have been long sicke of any consumption
of the lungs, as hath beene often proved
by the learned physitions of our London
College.'

And Culpepper says:

'It helpeth to expectorate tough phlegm
from the chest, being taken with the roots of
Irris or Orris. . . . There is a syrup made of
this plant which I would recommend as an
excellent help to evacuate tough phlegm and
cold rheum from the lungs of aged persons,
especially those who are asthmatic and short
winded.'

Preparations of Horehound are still largely
used as expectorants and tonics. It may, indeed, be considered one of the most popular
pectoral remedies, being given with benefit
for chronic cough, asthma, and some cases of
consumption.

Horehound is sometimes combined with
Hyssop, Rue, Liquorice root and Marshmallow root, ½ oz. of each boiled in 2 pints of
water, to 1½ pint, strained and given in ½
teacupful doses, every two to three hours.

For children's coughs and croup, it is given
to advantage in the form of syrup, and is a
most useful medicine for children, not only
for the complaints mentioned, but as a tonic
and a corrective of the stomach. It has quite
a pleasant taste.

Taken in large doses, it acts as a gentle
purgative.

The powdered leaves have also been employed as a vermifuge and the green leaves,
bruised and boiled in lard, are made into an
ointment which is good for wounds.

For ordinary cold, a simple infusion of
Horehound (Horehound Tea) is generally
sufficient in itself. The tea may be made by
pouring boiling water on the fresh or dried
leaves, 1 oz. of the herb to the pint. A wineglassful may be taken three or four times a
day.

Candied Horehound is best made from the
fresh plant by boiling it down until the juice
is extracted, then adding sugar before boiling
this again, until it has become thick enough
in consistence to pour into a paper case and
be cut into squares when cool.

Two or three teaspoonsful of the expressed
juice of the herb may also be given as a dose
in severe colds.

¶ *Preparations and Dosages.* Fluid extract,
½ to 1 drachm. Syrup, 2 to 4 drachms.
Solid extract, 5 to 15 grains.

HOREHOUND, BLACK

Ballota nigra (LINN.)
N.O. Labiatæ

Synonyms. Marrubium nigrum. Black Stinking Horehound
Part Used. Herb

¶ *Description.* Black Horehound is distinguished by its disagreeable odour. It also
belongs to the Labiatæ order, among which
it is distinguished by the strongly ten-ribbed
salver-shaped calyx. The *Ballota* are natives
of the temperate regions of the Eastern
Hemisphere, and are remarkable for their
strong offensive odour, on account of which
they are for the most part rejected by cattle;
hence the name from the Greek *ballo* (to reject). This plant (*Ballota nigra*) is sometimes
given the opprobrious name of 'Black Stinking Horehound.' It is a common wayside
perennial, has stout-branched stems, egg-
shaped wrinkled leaves, and whorls of
numerous dull purple flowers.

The whole plant is as offensive in odour as
it is unattractive in appearance. It is mostly
found growing near towns and villages, and
has accompanied our colonists to many
remote countries.

It has a perennial root of a woody and
fibrous nature. The leaves are arranged in
pairs on the stem, each pair being at right
angles to the pair it succeeds. They are
stalked, with margins coarsely serrate, dull
green in colour, their surfaces clothed with
soft grey hairs, and with rather conspicuous
veining.

The flowers are arranged in more or less
dense whorls at the axils of the leaves; their
colour occasionally varies to white.

The corolla of the Horehound has its
upper lip erect and slightly concave, and the
lower lip cleft into three, the lateral lobes
being considerably smaller than the central

ones. The calyx is tubular, its mouth having five short spreading teeth terminating in a stiff bristly point. The body of the calyx is sharply ridged and furrowed.

It is found in flower from June to October. The name *ballote* was given to this plant as early as the time of Dioscorides.

It has been suggested that the name Horehound came from two Anglo-Saxon words signifying the hoary honey-yielding plant; but other authorities find other derivations.

Dioscorides (like Gerard) declared that the *Ballota* was an antidote for the bite of a mad dog.

Beaumont and Fletcher's *Faithful Shepherdess* has a reference to this property of the plant:

'This is the clote bearing a yellow flower,
And this *black horehound*: both are very good
For sheep or shepherd bitten by a wood-Dog's venom'd tooth.'

¶ *Medicinal Action and Uses.* Antispasmodic, stimulant and vermifuge.

¶ *Preparation.* Liquid extract.

HORSE CHESTNUT. *See* CHESTNUT

HORSEMINT. *See* MINTS

HORSENETTLE

Solanum carolinense (LINN.)
N.O. Solanaceæ

Synonyms. Bull Nettle. Treadfoot. Sand Brier. Apple of Sodom. Poisonous Potato
Parts Used. Air-dried ripe berries, root
Habitat. United States of America. This weed is a hardy, coarse perennial, found growing in waste sandy ground as far west as Iowa and south to Florida

¶ *Description.* Bears orange yellow berries which is the most active part of the plant, they are glabrous and fleshy, with an odour like pepper; taste, bitter and acrid.

¶ *Constituents.* Probably Solanine and Solanidine and an organic acid.

¶ *Medicinal Action and Uses.* Sedative, antispasmodic; has long been used by the Southern negroes in the treatment of epilepsy; is a useful remedy in infantile convulsions and menstrual hysteria, has no unpleasant effects, but its usefulness is said to be limited, unless given with bromides.

¶ *Preparations and Dosages.* Fluid drachm three times a day. Berries are given in doses of 5 to 60 grains. Root, 10 grains.

HORSERADISH

Cochlearia Armoracia (LINN.)
N.O. Cruciferæ

Synonyms. Mountain Radish. Great Raifort. Red Cole
(*French*) Moutarde des Allemands
Part Used. Root
Habitat. This plant has been in cultivation from the earliest times, but its exact place of origin seems to be obscure. Hooker considers that it is possibly a cultivated form of *Cochlearia macrocarpa*, a native of Hungary; other authorities consider it indigenous to the eastern parts of Europe, from the Caspian and through Russia and Poland to Finland. In Britain and other parts of Europe from Sicily northwards, it occurs cultivated, or semi-wild as a garden escape. It is probably the plant mentioned by Pliny under the name of *Amoracia*, and recommended by him for its medicinal qualities, being then apparently employed exclusively in physic, not as food or condiment. It is possible that the Wild Radish, or *Raphanos agrios* of the Greeks was this plant. It is said to be one of the five bitter herbs, with Coriander, Horehound, Lettuce and Nettle, which the Jews were made to eat during the Feast of Passover

Both the root and leaves of Horseradish were universally used as a medicine during the Middle Ages, and as a condiment in Denmark and Germany. It was known in England as 'Red Cole' in the time of Turner (1548), but is not mentioned by him as a condiment. Gerard (1597), who describes it under the name of *Raphanus rusticanus*, states that it occurs wild in several parts of England, and after referring to its medicinal uses, goes on to say:

'the Horse Radish stamped with a little vinegar put thereto, is commonly used among the Germans for sauce to eate fish with and such like meates as we do mustarde,'

showing that the custom was unfamiliar to his countrymen, with whom the root had not yet passed from a drug to a condiment. He mentions this plant as an illustration of the old idea of 'Antipathies,' saying:

'Divers thinke that this Horse Radish is an

enimie to Vines, and that the hatred between them is so great, that if the rootes heerof be planted neere to the vine, it bendeth backward from it as not willing to have fellowship with it.'

Nearly half a century later, the taste for Horseradish as a condiment had spread to England, for Parkinson, writing in 1640, describes its use as a sauce 'with country people and strong labouring men in some countries of Germany,' and adds 'and in our owne land also, but, as I said, it is too strong for tender and gentle stomaches,' and a few years later, in 1657, Coles states as a commonly-known fact, 'that the root, sliced thin and mixed with vinegar is eaten as a sauce with meat, as among the Germans.' That the use of Horseradish in France was in like manner a custom adopted from their neighbours, is proved by its old French name, *Moutarde des Allemands*.

The root was included in the *Materia Medica* of the London Pharmacopœias of the eighteenth century, under the name of *R. rusticanus*, the same name Gerard gave it. Its present botanical name, *Cochlearia Armoracia*, was given it by Linnæus, *Cochleare* being the name of an old-fashioned spoon to which its long leaves are supposed to bear a resemblance. The popular English name, Horseradish, means a coarse radish, to distinguish it from the edible radish (*R. sativus*), the prefix 'Horse' being often used thus, comp. Horse-Mint, Horse Chestnut. It was formerly also known as the Mountain Radish and Great Raifort.

The common Scurvy-grass (*C. officinalis*) is of the same genus, as are also the English Scurvy-grass (*C. Anglica*) and the Danish Scurvy-grass (*C. Danica*).

¶ *Cultivation*. To grow fine Horseradish roots a plot of tilled ground must be chosen, manure being placed 18 to 24 inches deep; the ground in which they are planted ought to be very rich, or they will not thrive.

In order to obtain good sticks for winter an early start must be made, and some time in January the ground should be deeply dug. Planting is carried out in February by means of root cuttings, straight, young roots, 8 or 9 inches long, and about ½ inch wide being chosen, each having a crown or growing point. Make deep holes with the dibber, 12 to 15 inches deep and 12 to 18 inches apart each way; carefully divest the sets of all side roots and drop each in a hole, trickling a little fine soil round them before filling up the holes firmly. Beyond hoeing to keep the soil clear of weeds, no further care is needed.

During winter, the crop may either be lifted or stored like Beetroot, or the roots be lifted as required. In the latter case, the ground must be protected in frosty weather. The roots may be preserved for some time in their juicy state by putting them in dry sand.

It is necessary every few years to replant the bed, otherwise the crop deteriorates. The plants will stand through two seasons without deterioration. They may either be replanted elsewhere or another bed made on the same site, just as may be expedient. When it is desired to destroy plantations of Horseradish, it is absolutely necessary to rid the soil of even the smallest particle of root: if this is not done, much annoyance will be caused the following summer.

¶ *Part Used*. The root is the only part now used, and in the fresh state only. It is nearly cylindrical, except at the crown, where it is somewhat enlarged.

¶ *Constituents*. When unbroken, it is inodorous, but exhales a characteristic pungent odour when scraped or bruised, and has a hot, biting taste, combined with a certain sweetness. It has properties very similar to Black Mustard seeds, containing Sinigrin, a crystalline glucoside, which is decomposed in the presence of water by Myrosin, an enzyme found also in the root, the chief produce being the volatile oil Allyl, isothiocyanate, which is identical with that of Black Mustard seed. This volatile oil, which is easily developed by scraping the root when in a fresh state, does not pre-exist in the root, the reaction not taking place in the root under normal conditions, because the Sinigrin and Myrosin exist in separate cells, and it is only the bruising of the cells that brings their contents together.

The oil is highly diffusible and pungent on account of the Myrosin contained, 1 drop being sufficient to odorize the atmosphere of a whole room. On exposure to the air, the root quickly turns colour and loses its volatile strength. It likewise becomes vapid and inert by being boiled. It contains also a bitter resin, sugar, starch, gum, albumin and acetates.

¶ *Medicinal Action and Uses*. Stimulant, aperient, rubefacient, diuretic and antiseptic. It is a powerful stimulant, whether applied internally or externally as a rubefacient, and has aperient and antiseptic properties. Taken with oily fish or rich meat, either by itself or steeped in vinegar, or in a plain sauce, it acts as an excellent stimulant to the digestive organs, and as a spur to complete digestion.

It is a very strong diuretic, and was employed by old herbalists in calculus and like affections. It is useful in the treatment of dropsy. Boerhaave recommended it to be given in scurvy when there was not much fever, and administered it for various other complaints.

An infusion for dropsy is prepared by pouring 1 pint of boiling water on 1 oz. of Horseradish and ½ oz. of Mustard seed, crushed. The dose is 2 to 3 tablespoonsful three times a day.

The chief official preparation of Horseradish in the British Pharmacopœia is Comp. Sp. Horseradish; a fluid extract is also prepared. A compound spirit of Horseradish may be prepared with slices of the fresh root, orange peel, nutmeg and spirit of wine, which proves effective in languid digestion, as well as for chronic rheumatism, 1 or 2 teaspoonsful being taken two or three times daily after meals with half a wineglassful of water.

The root is expectorant, antiscorbutic, and if taken too freely, emetic. It contains so much sulphur that it is serviceable used externally as a rubefacient in chronic rheumatism and in paralytic complaints. Culpepper says: 'If bruised and laid to a part grieved with the sciatica, gout, joint-ache or hard swellings of the spleen and liver, it doth wonderfully help them all.' A poultice of the scraped root serves instead of a mustard plaister. Scraped horseradish if applied to chilblains, secured with a light bandage, will help to cure them. For facial neuralgia, some of the fresh scrapings, if held in the hand of the affected side, will give relief – the hand in some cases within a short time becoming bloodlessly white and benumbed.

When infused in wine, Horseradish root will stimulate the whole nervous system and promote perspiration.

An infusion of sliced Horseradish in milk, by its stimulating pungency and the sulphur it contains, makes an excellent cosmetic for the skin when lacking clearness and freshness of colour. Horseradish juice mixed with white vinegar will also, applied externally, help to remove freckles. The same mixture, well diluted with water and sweetened with glycerine, gives marked relief to children in whooping-cough, 1 or 2 desertspoonsful being taken at a time. Horseradish syrup is very effectual in hoarseness: 1 drachm of the root, fresh scraped, with 4 oz. of water, is infused two hours in a close vessel and made into a syrup with double its weight in sugar. The dose is a teaspoonful or two, occasionally repeated.

If eaten at frequent intervals during the day and at meals, Horseradish is said to be most efficacious in getting rid of the persistent cough following influenza.

Horseradish was formerly much employed as a remedy for worms in children. Coles says: 'Of all things given to children for worms, horseradish is not the least, for it soon killeth and expelleth them.'

¶ *Preparations and Dosages.* Fluid extract, ½ to 1 drachm. Comp. Spirit of Horseradish, B.P., 1 to 2 drachms.

HORSETAILS

Equisetum arvense
Equisetum hyemale
Equisetum maximum
Equisetum sylvaticum
N.O. Equisetaceæ

Synonyms. Shave-grass. Bottle-brush. Paddock-pipes. Dutch Rushes. Pewterwort
Part Used. Herb
Habitat. They are chiefly distributed in the temperate northern regions: seven of the twenty-five known species are British, the most frequent being *Equisetum arvense*, *E. sylvaticum*, *E. maximum* and *E. hyemale*. *E. arvense*, the CORN HORSETAIL, is a very troublesome weed, most difficult to extirpate from cultivated land. Many of the species are very variable

The Horsetails belong to a class of plants, the Equisetaceæ, that has no direct affinity with any other group of British plants. They are nearest allied to the Ferns. The class includes only a single genus, *Equisetum*, the name derived from the Latin words *equus* (a horse) and *seta* (a bristle), from the peculiar bristly appearance of the jointed stems of the plants, which have also earned them their popular names of Horsetail, Bottle-brush and Paddock-pipes.

Large plants of this order probably formed a great proportion of the vegetation during the carboniferous period, the well-known fossils Calamites being the stems of gigantic fossil Equisetaceæ, which in this period attained their maximum development – those now existing being mere dwarfish representatives.

The Equisetaceæ have an external resemblance in habit to *Casuarina* or *Ephedra*, and as regards the heads of fructification to *Zamia* (a genus of Cycadaceæ). The *Casuarina* have very much the appearance of gigantic Horsetails, being trees with thread-like, jointed, furrowed, pendent branches without leaves, but with small toothed sheaths at the joints. They are met with most abundantly in tropical Australia, less frequently in the Indian Islands, New Caledonia, etc. In Australia they are said by Dr. Bennett to be called Oaks. The wood is used for fires, as it burns readily and the ashes retain the heat for a long time. The wood is much valued for steam-engines, ovens, etc., and the timber furnished by these trees is appreciated for its extreme hardness. From its colour it is called in the Colonies 'Beefwood.'

Though mostly inhabitants of watery places, flourishing where they can lodge their perennial roots in water or string clay which holds the wet, the Equisetums will grow in a garden near water, under a wall, or in the shade and will spread rapidly.

¶ *Description.* The stems spring from a creeping rhizome, or root-stock, which produces at its joints a number of roots. Two kinds of stems are produced, fertile and barren: they are erect, jointed, brittle and grooved, hollow except at the joints and with air-cells in their walls under the grooves. There are no leaves, the joints terminating in toothed sheathes, the teeth corresponding with the ridges and representing leaves. Branches, if present, arise from the sheath-bases and are solid. In most cases, the fertile or fruiting stem is unbranched and withers in spring, almost before the barren fronds appear. It bears a terminal cone-like catkin, consisting of numerous closely-packed peltæ, upon the under margins of which are the *sporanges*, containing microscopic spores, attached to elastic threads, which are coiled round the spore when moist and uncoil when dry.

The development of young Horsetails from the spores is similar to that of Ferns, germination and impregnation being effected in the same manner. The Equisitaceæ are also propagated in a vegetative non-sexual manner by means of subterranean stolons and by tubers.

The barren summer fronds give off numerous, slender, jointed branches in whorls of about a dozen; in some British species, the fruiting and barren stems are often both unbranched.

A quantity of silica is deposited in the stems, especially in the epidermis or outer skin. In one species, *E. hyemale* (Linn.), the epidermis contains so much silica that bunches of the stem have been sold for polishing metal and used to be imported from Holland for the purpose, hence the popular name of Dutch Rushes. It is also called Scouring Rush, and by old writers Shave-grass, and was formerly much used by white-smiths and cabinet-makers. Gerard tells us that in his time it was employed for scouring pewter and wooden kitchen utensils, and thence called Pewterwort, and that fletchers and combmakers rubbed and polished their work with it, and long after his day, the dairy-maids of the northern counties of England used it for scouring their milk-pails. Linnæus tells us that this species, among others, forms excellent food for horses in some parts of Sweden, but that cows are apt to lose their teeth by feeding on it and to be afflicted with diarrhœa. As a matter of fact, cattle, in this country, usually instinctively avoid these plants and would probably only eat them in the absence of better fodder.

The young shoots of the larger species of Horsetail, especially *E. maximum* (Lamk.) – the *E. fluviatile* of Linnæus – were formerly said to be eaten, dressed like asparagus, or fried with flour and butter. It is recorded that the poorer classes among the Romans occasionally ate them as a vegetable, but they are neither palatable nor very nutritious. Linnæus stated that the reindeer, who refuses ordinary hay, will eat this kind of Horsetail, which is about 3 feet high and juicy, and that it is cut as fodder in the north of Sweden for cows, with a view to increasing their milk, but that horses will not touch it.

Several of the species have been used medicinally, and the older herbalists considered them useful vulneraries, and recommended them for consumption and dysentery. The FIELD HORSETAIL (*E. arvense*), the species of British Horsetail most commonly met with, is the one now generally collected and sold for medicinal purposes. It is common in cornfields and wet meadows, its presence being supposed to indicate subterranean, flowing waters or springs. In this species, the fruiting stems are simple, very rarely branched, appearing early in spring and soon decaying. The barren stems which appear later are branched, six to nineteen grooved, the angles rough and sharp, and terminate generally in a long, naked point; the joints are about 1 inch long and $\frac{1}{24}$ to $\frac{1}{16}$ inch in diameter, the teeth of the sheaths long and acute. The shoots have neither colour nor taste. The fertile stems are yellowish, shorter and stouter, somewhat succulent, with only two to five joints.

In warmer climates, and even in Lisbon, as *E. debile* and *elongatum*, they require the support of bushes to which they cling. They sometimes attain a great size as does *E. giganteum*, though they never reach the dimensions of the fossil Equisetaceæ.

The rhizomes contain a considerable quantity of starch-cells.

E. sylvaticum, the WOOD HORSETAIL, which grows in copses and on hedgebanks, has slender, angular stems, 1 to 2 feet high, nearly smooth, ten to eighteen grooved. It is readily recognized by the elegant appearance of the whorls of recurved branches, generally twelve or more branches to a whorl, which are very slender, about 5 inches long, quadrangular and beset by several secondary whorls so that the plant resembles a miniature pine tree. The cones of the fertile stems are ¾ to 1 inch long.

It is this species that Linnæus informs us is a principal food for horses in some parts of Sweden. It is used medicinally in the same manner as the preceding species.

E. maximum, the GREAT or RIVER HORSETAIL, already mentioned, is found in bogs, ditches, and on the banks of rivers and ponds. It is the largest of the European species, the barren stems attaining a height of from 3 to 6 feet, sometimes nearly an inch in diameter. They are twenty to forty grooved, with numerous joints, pale in colour and smooth, the branchlets quadrangular. The fertile stems are quite short, only 8 to 10 inches high, but thicker; their cones, 2 to 3 inches long.

¶ *Part Used Medicinally.* The barren stems only are used medicinally, appearing after the fruiting stems have died down, and are used in their entirety, cut off just above the root. The herb is used either fresh or dried, but is said to be most efficacious when fresh. A fluid extract is prepared from it. The ashes of the plant are also employed.

¶ *Medicinal Action and Uses.* Diuretic and astringent. Horsetail has been found beneficial in dropsy, gravel and kidney affections generally, and a drachm of the dried herb, powdered, taken three or four times a day, has proved very effectual in spitting of blood.

The ashes of the plant are considered very valuable in acidity of the stomach, dyspepsia, etc., administered in doses of 3 to 10 grains.

Besides being useful in kidney and bladder trouble, a strong decoction acts as an emmenagogue; being cooling and astringent, it is of efficacy for hæmorrhage, cystic ulceration and ulcers in the urinary passages.

The decoction applied externally will stop the bleeding of wounds and quickly heal them, and will also reduce the swelling of eyelids.

¶ *Preparation and Dosage.* Fluid extract, 10 to 60 drops.

Horsetail was formerly official under the name of *Cauda equina* and was much esteemed as an astringent. Culpepper quotes Galen in saying that it will heal sinews, 'though they be cut in sunder,' and speaks of it highly for bleeding of the nose, a use to which it is still put by country people.

Culpepper says:

'It is very powerful to stop bleeding, either inward or outward, the juice or the decoction being drunk, or the juice, decoction or distilled water applied outwardly . . . It also heals inward ulcers. . . . It solders together the tops of green wounds and cures all ruptures in children. The decoction taken in wine helps stone and strangury; the distilled water drunk two or three times a day eases and strengthens the intestines and is effectual in a cough that comes by distillation from the head. The juice or distilled water used as a warm fomentation is of service in inflammations and breakings-out in the skin.'

HOUND'S TONGUE

Cynoglossum officinale (LINN.)
N.O. Boraginaceæ

Synonyms. Lindefolia spectabilis. Dog's Tongue
Part Used. Herb

Hound's Tongue is a rough, bristly perennial, belonging to the Borage tribe. Its scientific name of *Cynoglossum* is derived from the Greek, and signifies 'Dog's Tongue,' from the shape and texture of the leaves, under which name, and still more frequently as Hound's Tongue, it is properly known.

It is a stout, herbaceous plant, found occasionally in this country on waste ground, though more frequently on the Continent, especially in Switzerland and Germany.

The stem, hairy and leafy, 1 to 2 feet high, branched above, arises from amidst large, narrow, radical, stalked leaves.

In Culpepper's days, the root was also used in decoction and as pills for coughs, colds in the head and shortness of breath, and the leaves were boiled in wine as a cure for dysentery. He also tells us:

'Bruising the leaves or the juice of them boiled in hog's lard and applied helpeth to preserve the hair from falling and easeth the pain of a scald or burn. A bruised leaf laid to a green wound speedily heals the same. The baked roots are good for piles, also the distilled water of the herb and root is used with good effect for all the aforesaid purposes, taken inwardly or applied outwardly, especially as a wash for wounds or punctures.'

Gerard says of this plant: 'It will tye the tongues of Houndes so that they shall not bark at you, if it be laid under the bottom of your feet,' and in his days the ointment and decoction were very generally reputed to be a cure for the bites of mad dogs.

HOUSELEEK

Synonyms. Jupiter's Eye. Thor's Beard. Ayron. Ayegreen
(*French*) Joubarbe des toits
(*German*) Donnersbart
Part Used. Fresh leaves

The Houseleek was dedicated of old to Jupiter or Thor, and bore also the names of Jupiter's Eye, Thor's Beard, Jupiter's Beard, Barba Jovis (in France, Joubarbe des toits), from its massive clusters of flowers, which were supposed to resemble the beard of Jupiter. The German name of *Donnersbart* and the English *Thunderbeard* have the same meaning, being derived from Jupiter the Thunderer.

It was in high esteem among the Romans, who grew it in vases before their houses.

It is not really indigenous to this country, being a native of the mountain ranges of Central and Southern Europe and of the Greek islands, but it was introduced into Great Britain many centuries ago and is now found abundantly throughout the country, its large rosettes of fleshy leaves being a familiar sight on many an old cottage roof.

The word Leek is from the Anglo-Saxon *leac*, a plant, so that Houseleek means literally the House Plant. It was also called, in the fourteenth century, Ayron, Ayegreen and Sengreen, i.e. Evergreen.

The generic name *Sempervivum*, from the Latin *semper* (always) and *vivo* (I live), refers to its retention of vitality under almost all conditions, and the specific name *tectorum* bears witness to its usual place of growth – a roof.

It was supposed to guard what it grows upon against fire and lightning, and we read that Charlemagne ordered it to be planted upon the roof of every house, probably with this view. Whatever the origin of the custom, it prevails in many other parts of Europe, as well as in England and France. Welsh peasants believe it protects their houses from storms, and ensures the prosperity of their inmates. Superstitious country-folk in Wiltshire are often found to have a strong objection to the removal of a plant of Houseleek from their roof, or even to the plucking of the flowers by a stranger, believing it will bring death to the dwellers; it was formerly believed to be an efficient guard against sorcery as well as against lightning.

The root is perennial and is fibrous. The thick succulent leaves enable the plant to

In modern medicine it is often used internally and externally to relieve piles. It is soothing to the digestive organs.

Sempervivum tectorum (LINN.)
N.O. Crassulaceæ
Jupiter's Beard. Bullock's Eye. Sengreen.

retain vitality even in the driest weather, acting as reservoirs of moisture. The leaves, arising directly from the root, grow in compact, rose-like tufts, 2 to 4 inches in diameter. They are extremely fleshy and juicy, flat, 1 to 2 inches long, sessile, oblong, though broader towards the middle of the rosette, sharply pointed, and the edges fringed with hairs and of a purple colour.

The flowers are produced in July, but generally very sparingly. The flower-stems do not arise from the rosettes of leaves, but are on separate, upright shoots, which are from 9 inches to a foot or more in height, round, fleshy and stout, slightly downy, with the leaves scattered thickly on them. The flowers are clustered together on only one side of the stem and are numerous, $\frac{2}{3}$ to 1 inch in diameter, of a dull, pale red-purple. Like other flowers in this genus they are absolutely regular and symmetrical throughout, the sepals, petals and pistils being all of the same number – twelve in this species – and the stamens just twice as many, twenty-four in this case, twelve of which are arranged alternately with the petals and are imperfect, frequently bearing in their anthers instead of pollen dust, embryo seeds, which never attain maturity. The flowers are quite scentless.

This is a most useful as well as effective plant for an old wall, or to cover the high part of a rock-garden; it can be absolutely relied upon to withstand drought.

¶ *Cultivation.* This species will grow on rock-work, as well as on a roof, flourishing better than on ordinary ground. When once fixed, it will spread fast by means of its offsets. It may easily be made to cover the whole roof of a building, whether of tiles, thatch or wood, by sticking the offsets on with a little earth. Linnæus stated that the plant was used in this manner as a preservative to the coverings of houses in certain parts of Sweden, and it is certain that it tends to preserve thatched roofs.

The flowering-heads die soon after they have blossomed, but the offsets soon supply their places.

¶ *Part Used Medicinally.* The fresh leaves and the expressed juice from them. The leaves have a saline, astringent and acid taste, but no odour.

¶ *Constituents.* The leaves contain malic acid in combination with lime.

¶ *Medicinal Action and Uses.* Refrigerant, astringent, diuretic. In rural districts, the bruised leaves of the fresh plant, or its juice, are often applied as a poultice to burns, scalds, contusions, scrofulous ulcers, and in inflammatory conditions of the skin generally, giving immediate relief. If the juice be mixed with clarified lard and applied to an inflamed surface, the inflammation is quickly reduced.

It can be used in many skin diseases. Some old authorities recommend mixing the juice with cream.

With honey, the juice has been used to assuage the soreness and ulcerated condition of the mouth in thrush, the mixture being used with a hair pencil.

Boerhaave, the famous Dutch physician, found 10 oz. of the juice beneficial in dysentery, but it is not admitted into modern practice.

In large doses, Houseleek juice is emetic and purgative.

Dose, 2 to 10 drops.

It is said to remove warts and corns. Parkinson tells us:

'The juice takes away corns from the toes and feet if they be bathed therewith every day, and at night emplastered as it were with the skin of the same House Leek.'

The leaves sliced in two and the inner surface applied to warts, act as a positive cure for them.

Culpepper informs us that

'Our ordinary Houseleek is good for all inward heats, as well as outward, and in the eyes or other parts of the body: a posset made of the juice is singularly good in all hot agues, for it cooleth and tempereth the blood and spirits and quencheth the thirst; and is also good to stay all defluction or sharp and salt rheums in the eyes, the juice being dropped into them. If the juice be dropped into the ears, it easeth pain. . . . It cooleth and restraineth all hot inflammations, St. Anthony's fire (Erysipelas), scaldings and burnings, the shingles, fretting ulcers, ringworms and the like; and much easeth the pain and the gout.'

After describing the use of the leaves in the cure of corns, he goes on to say:

'it easeth also the headache, and the distempered heat of the brain in frenzies, or through want of sleep, being applied to the temples and forehead. The leaves bruised and laid upon the crown or seam of the head, stayeth bleeding at the nose very quickly. The distilled water of the herb is profitable for all the purposes aforesaid. The leaves being gently rubbed on any place stung with nettles or bees, doth quickly take away the pain.'

Gerard tells us the

'iuice of Houseleeke, Garden Nightshade, and the buds of Poplar, boiled in hog's grease, maketh the most singular Populeon that ever was used in Chirugerie.'

Galen recommends Houseleek for erysipelas and shingles, and Dioscorides as a remedy for weak and inflamed eyes. Pliny says it never fails to produce sleep.

In the fourteenth century it was used as an ingredient of a preparation for neuralgia, called hemygreyne, i.e. megrim, and an ointment used at that time for scalds and burns.

Culpepper speaks of the Small Houseleek, the Stonecrop Houseleek, the Common Stonecrop or Wallpepper, the Orpine, the Kidneywort and the Water Houseleek, some of which are known now under different names, the name Houseleek nowadays being reserved exclusively for the above-described species, *Sempervivum tectorum.*

See STONECROPS.

HYACINTH, GRAPE

Muscari racemosum (MILL.)
N.O. Liliaceæ

Synonym. Starch Hyacinth

The Grape Hyacinth, very much cultivated in England as a garden plant and occasionally met with in sandy soils in the eastern and southern counties, has, like the Wild Hyacinth, a poisonous bulb. The leaves are narrow and rather thick, 6 inches to a foot long, the flower-stem usually shorter, with a close, terminal raceme, or head of small, dark blue flowers, looking almost like little berries and having a sweet scent. A few of the uppermost are of a pale blue, erect, much narrower and without stamens or pistils. As the flowers of the various species of *Muscari* secrete much nectar, they are – like the garden *Scillas* – to be reckoned among the useful bee plants of the spring.

The Grape Hyacinth has sometimes been called Starch Hyacinth, as the flowers have been supposed to smell of wet starch. The name of the genus, *Muscari*, comes from the Greek word for musk, a smell yielded by some species.

¶ *Medicinal Action and Uses.* The American species, *Muscari comosum* (Mill.) (Feather Hyacinth), or Purse Tassel, has been used, as well as other species of *Muscari*, for its diuretic and stimulant properties. Comisic acid has been extracted from the bulb, and apparently acts like Saponin.

The innumerable varieties of Garden Hyacinth are derived from an Eastern plant, *Hyacinthus orientalis.*

HYACINTH, WILD

Hyacinthus nonscriptus
N.O. Rosaceæ

Synonyms. Bluebell. Scilla nutans. Nodding Squill. Scilla nonscriptus. Agraphis nutans

Part Used. Roots

Habitat. Woods of Britain

¶ *History.* The Wild Hyacinth is in flower from early in April till the end of May, and being a perennial, and spreading rapidly, is found year after year in the same spot, forming a mass of rich colour in the woods where it grows. The long leaves remain above ground until late in the autumn. From the midst of very long, narrow leaves, rising from the small bulb and overtopping them, rises the flower-stem, bearing the pendulous 'bluebells' arranged in a long, curving line. Each flower has two small bracts at the base of the short flower-stalk of pedicel. The perianth (the term applied when the parts of the calyx and corolla are so similar in form and colour that no difference is perceptible) is bluish-purple and composed of six leaflets. The flowers have a slight, starch-like scent.

This is the 'fair-hair'd hyacinth' of Ben Jonson, a name alluding to the old myth, for tradition associates the flower with the Hyacinth of the Ancients, the flower of grief and mourning, so Linnæus first called it Hyacinthus. Hyacinthus was a charming and handsome Spartan youth, loved by both Apollo and Zephyrus. Hyacinthus preferred the Sun-God to the God of the West, who sought to be revenged. One day, when Apollo was playing quoits with the youth, a quoit that he threw was blown by Zephyrus out of its proper course and it struck and killed Hyacinthus. Apollo, stricken with grief, raised from his blood a purple flower on which the letters 'ai, ai,' were traced, so that the cry of woe might for evermore have existence on the earth. As our English variety of Hyacinth had no trace of these mystic letters, our older botanists called it *Hyacinthus nonscriptus*, or 'not written on.' A later generic name, *Agraphis*, is of similar meaning, being a compound of two Greek words, meaning 'not to mark.'

The bulbs are poisonous in the fresh state. The viscid juice so abundantly contained in them and existing in every part of the plant has been used as a substitute for starch and in the days when stiff ruffs were worn was much in request, being thought second only to Wake-robin roots. It was also used for fixing feathers on arrows, instead of glue and as bookbinders' gum for the covers of books.

The roots, dried and powdered, are balsamic, having some styptic properties which have not been fully investigated.

It has been found to be one of the best remedies for leucorrhœa. The decoction of the juice of the root operates by urine.

¶ *Dosage.* From 1 to 3 grains.

HYDNOCARPUS. *See* CHAULMOOGRA

HYDRANGEA

Hydrangea arborescens (LINN.)
N.O. Saxifragaceæ

Synonyms. Wild Hydrangea. Seven Barks. Hydrangea vulgaris. Common Hydrangea

Parts Used. Dried rhizome, roots

Habitat. The United States

¶ *History.* The Hydrangeas are marsh or aquatic plants, and hence the name is derived from a Greek compound signifying water-vessel. Four of the known species are natives of America; one, the garden Hydrangea (*Hydrangea hortensis*), is widely cultivated in the gardens of China and Japan. Many methods are employed in this country for imparting the blue tinge to its petals. The oak-leaved Hydrangea (*H. quercifolia*), a native of Florida, is also cultivated for its beauty.

The bark of *H. arborescens* is rough, with a tendency to peel, each layer being of a different colour, from which it has probably derived its name 'Seven Barks.' The roots are of variable length and thickness, having numerous radicles, reaching a diameter of more than half an inch. They are externally pale grey, tough, with splintery fracture; white inside, without odour, having a sweetish, rather pungent taste. When fresh, the root and stalks are very succulent, containing much water, and can easily be cut. When dry, they are tough and resistant, so that they should be bruised or cut into short, transverse sections while fresh. The taste of the bark of the dried root resembles that of cascarilla. The stalks contain a pith which is easily removed, and they are used in some parts of the country for pipe-stems.

¶ *Constituents.* The root has been found to contain two resins, gum, sugar, starch, albumen, soda, lime potassa, magnesia, sulphuric and phosphoric acids, a protosalt of iron, and a glucoside, Hydrangin. No tannin has been found, but a fixed oil and a volatile oil have been obtained. From the alcoholic extract of the flowers of *H. hortensia*, two crystalline substances were isolated, Hydragenol and Hydrangeaic acid.

¶ *Medicinal Action and Uses.* Diuretic, cathartic, tonic. The decoction is said to have been used with great advantage by the

Cherokee Indians, and later, by the settlers, for calculous diseases. It does not cure stone in the bladder, but, as demonstrated to the medical profession by Dr. S. W. Butler, of Burlington, N.J., it removes gravelly deposits and relieves the pain consequent on their emission. As many as 120 calculi have been known to come from one person under its use.

The fluid extract is principally used for earthy deposits, alkaline urine, chronic gleet, and mucous irritations of the bladder in aged persons. A concentrated syrup with sugar or honey, or a simple decoction of the root, may also be used. In overdoses, it will cause vertigo, oppressions of the chest, etc. The leaves are said by Dr. Eoff to be tonic, silagogue, cathartic and diuretic.

¶ *Dosage.* 30 grains. Of fluid extract, 30 to 100 minims. Of syrup, 1 teaspoonful, three times a day.

HYDROCOTYLE

Hydrocotyle Asiatica (LINN.)
N.O. Umbelliferæ

Synonyms. Indian Pennywort. Marsh Penny. White Rot. Thick-leaved Pennywort
Part Used. Leaves
Habitat. Asia and Africa

¶ *Description.* A small umbelliferous plant growing in Southern Africa and India, indigenous to the Southern United States. The special characteristics of the leaflets are petiolate, reniform, crenate, seven nerved and nearly glabrous.

¶ *Constituents.* An oily volatile liquid called vellarin (which has a strong smell reminiscent of the plant, and a bitter, pungent, persistent taste) and tannic acid.

¶ *Medicinal Action and Uses.* A valuable medicine for its diuretic properties; has long been used in India as an aperient or alterative tonic, useful in fever and bowel complaints and a noted remedy for leprosy, rheumatism and ichthyosis; employed as a

poultice for syphilitic ulcers. In small doses it acts as a stimulant, in large doses as a narcotic, causing stupor and headache and with some people vertigo and coma.

¶ *Other Species.*
The native species is not unlike the Indian variety, but there is a slight difference in the leaves.

European hydrocotyle vulgaris (syn. Common Pennywort). Leaves orbicular and peltate. The plant appears to have no noxious qualities; it grows freely in boggy places on the edges of lakes and rivers.

The plant has come into disfavour because it is said to cause footrot in sheep.

HYDROPHILIA

Hydrophilia spinosa
N.O. Acanthaceæ

Synonym. Asteracantha Longifolia
Parts Used. Root, seeds, dried herb
Habitat. India, widely distributed in the sub-tropical regions of the world

¶ *Description.* The name is derived from the Greek, and refers to the medical doctrine of fluids in the body. It has tapering roots, a number of rootlets, and upright square stems; leaves and branches opposite, nodes swollen near them; the stem and leaves have three- to five-celled stiff hairs. Flowers, four pairs awl-shaped and like leaves in shape. Corolla glabrous on lower lip. Fruit has four to eight flattened brownish seeds, which contain a quantity of strong mucilage. The drug has no special odour or taste.

¶ *Constituents.* Chiefly mucilage, fixed oil, phytosterol, and a trace of an alkaloidal

substance, properties similar to Couchgrass.

¶ *Medicinal Action and Uses:* Demulcent and a diuretic for catarrh of the urinary organs; the dried herb and root, or rhizome, has long been used in India for dropsy, especially when accompanied by hepatic obstruction. It is a popular aphrodisiac. In Southern India the root is the commercial part, but in Bombay the seeds are mostly used.

¶ *Preparation.* Decoction, 2 oz. of root to 3 pints of water boiled down to 1 pint. Dose, ½ to 2 fluid ounces. Official in India and the Eastern Colonies.

HYSSOP

Part Used. Herb

Hyssopus officinalis (LINN.)
N.O. Labiatæ

Hyssop is a name of Greek origin. The Hyssopos of Dioscorides was named from *azob* (a holy herb), because it was used for cleaning sacred places. It is alluded to in the Scriptures: 'Purge me with Hyssop, and I shall be clean.'

¶ *Cultivation.* It is an evergreen, bushy herb, growing 1 to 2 feet high, with square stem, linear leaves and flowers in whorls, six- to fifteen-flowered. Is a native of Southern Europe not indigenous to Britain, though stated to be naturalized on the ruins of Beaulieu Abbey in the New Forest.

Hyssop is cultivated for the use of its flower-tops, which are steeped in water to make an infusion, which is sometimes employed as an expectorant. There are three varieties, known respectively by their blue, red and white flowers, which are in bloom from June to October, and are sometimes employed as edging plants. Grown with cat-mint, it makes a lovely border, backed with Lavender and Rosemary. As a kitchen herb, it is mostly used for broths and decoctions, occasionally for salad. For medicinal use the flower-tops should be cut in August.

It may be propagated by seeds, sown in April, or by dividing the plants in spring and autumn, or by cuttings, made in spring and inserted in a shady situation. Plants raised from seeds or cuttings, should, when large enough, be planted out about 1 foot apart each way, and kept watered till established. They succeed best in a warm aspect and in a light, rather dry soil. The plants require cutting in, occasionally, but do not need much further attention.

¶ *Medicinal Action and Uses.* Expectorant, diaphoretic, stimulant, pectoral, carminative. The healing virtues of the plant are due to a particular volatile oil, which is stimulative, carminative and sudorific. It admirably promotes expectoration, and in chronic catarrh its diaphoretic and stimulant properties combine to render it of especial value. It is usually given as a warm infusion, taken frequently and mixed with Horehound. Hyssop Tea is also a grateful drink, well adapted to improve the tone of a feeble stomach, being brewed with the green tops of the herb, which are sometimes boiled in soup to be given for asthma. In America, an infusion of the leaves is used externally for the relief of muscular rheumatism, and also for bruises and discoloured contusions, and the green herb, bruised and applied, will heal cuts promptly.

The infusion has an agreeable flavour and is used by herbalists in pulmonary diseases.

It was once much employed as a carminative in flatulence and hysterical complaints, but is now seldom employed.

A tea made with the fresh green tops, and drunk several times daily, is one of the old-fashioned country remedies for rheumatism that is still employed. Hyssop baths have also been recommended as part of the cure, but the quantity used would need to be considerable.

¶ *Preparation.* Fluid extract, 30 to 60 drops.

The Hyssop of commerce (*Hyssopus officinalis*) occurs in Palestine, but is not conspicuous among the numerous Labiatæ of the Syrian hillsides, which include thyme and marjoram, mint, rosemary and lavender. Tradition identifies the Hyssop of Scripture with the familiar herb, *Marjoram* (*origanum*), of which six species are found in the Holy Land. The common kind, so well known in cottage gardens (*O. vulgare*), grows only in the north, but an allied species (*O. maru*) abounds through the central hills, and a variety is common in the southern desert.

Dr. J. F. Royle disagrees, and identifies the Hyssop of the Bible with the Caper-plant (*Capparis spinosa*) which grows in the Jordan Valley, in Egypt, and the Desert, in the gorges of Lebanon, and in the Kedron Valley. It 'springs out of the walls' of the old Temple area. This view is supported by Canon Tristram and others. The Arabs call it *azaf*.

The leaves, stems and flowers of *H. officinalis* possess a highly aromatic odour and yield by distillation an essential oil of exceedingly fine odour, much appreciated by perfumers, its value being even greater than Oil of Lavender. It is also much employed in the manufacture of liqueurs, forming an important constituent in Chartreuse. Bees feed freely on the plant and the odour of the honey obtained from this source is remarkably good. The leaves are used locally as a medicinal tea. As a kitchen herb it has gone out of use because of its strong flavour, but on account of its aroma it was formerly employed as a strewing herb.

RECIPE FOR HYSSOP TEA

'Infuse a quarter of an ounce of dried hyssop flowers in a pint of boiling water for ten minutes; sweeten with honey, and take a wineglassful three times a day, for debility of the chest. It is also considered a powerful vermifuge.' (Old Cookery Book.)

HYSSOP, HEDGE

Gratiola officinalis (LINN.)
N.O. Scrophulariaceæ

Parts Used. Root, herb

¶ *Description.* Hedge-Hyssop was formerly an official drug. The root and herb are still used in herbal medicine.

The plant, a perennial, is a native of the south of Europe, growing in meadows and moist grounds. The square stem rises from a creeping, scaly rhizome to the height of 6 to 12 inches, and has opposite stalkless, lance-shaped, finely serrate, smooth, pale-green leaves, and whitish, or reddish flowers, placed singly in the axils of the upper pairs of leaves, the corollas two-lipped, with yellow hairs in the tube.

The plant is inodorous, but has a bitter, nauseous, somewhat acrid taste, which earns it the name of Hedge Hyssop.

¶ *Constituents.* Its active constituent is the bitter crystalline glucoside Gratiolin and a reddish, amorphous, bitter principle, Gratiosolin, likewise a glucoside.

¶ *Medicinal Action and Uses.* A drastic cathartic and emetic, possessing also diuretic properties. Has been used for the relief of dropsy, and is recommended in scrofula, chronic affections of the liver, jaundice, and enlargement of the spleen, and as a worm dispeller.

¶ *Preparations.* The infusion of ½ oz. of powdered root is taken in tablespoonful doses. Powdered root, 15 to 30 grains.

Gratiola officinalis was in former times called *Gratia Dei*, on account of its active medicinal properties. In large doses it is said to be poisonous. Haller says that the abundance of this plant in some of the Swiss meadows renders it dangerous to allow cattle to feed in them. *G. peruviane* has similar properties.' (*Treasury of Botany*.)

The tropical American herb *Vandellia diffusa* (Linn.) is used like Gratiola. The dried plant has a strong odour of tobacco.

A decoction of *V. diffusa* is employed medicinally in Guiana in fevers and disorders of the liver. The species are natives of the East Indies, China, Burma, and South America. Some of them are grown in this country. The generic name commemorates a Professor of Botany at Lisbon.

Curanga amara (Juss.), known as *Herpestis amara* (Benth.) and *Gratiola amara* (Roxb.), yields the important East Indian tonic and febrifuge Curanja or *Kœn-tao-tjao*. It contains the bitter alcohol-soluble glucoside curanjiin.

Bonnaya rotundifolia (Benth.) is the East Indian *Tsjanga-puspam* used as an antispasmodic.

Scoparia dulcis (Linn.), a common weed of tropical America, is used as an astringent and antispasmodic under the name *Vacourinha*.

Many other species, native to different parts of the world, belonging to this family, are in medicinal use in a lesser degree. Nearly all of them contain bitter substances, and many possess anthelmintic properties.

HYSTERONICA

Hysteronica Baylahuen
N.O. Compositæ

Synonym. Haplopappus Baylahuen
Habitat. Western United States of America, Chile

¶ *Description.* Belongs to the same group as *Solidago* (Golden Rod) and is closely allied to *Grindelia* botanically and as a drug.

¶ *Constituents.* Volatile oil, fatty oil which has the same odour as the plant, acid resin which is a mixture of four other resines, and tannin.

¶ *Medicinal Action and Uses.* Stimulant, expectorant. The medicinal properties lie principally in its resin and volatile oil, the resin acting chiefly on the bowels and urinary passages, and the volatile oil on the lungs. It does not cause disorder to the stomach and bowels, it is a valuable remedy in dysentery, chronic diarrhœa specially of tuberculous nature and in chronic cystitis.

The tincture, by its stimulating and protective action (like tinc. benzoin), has served as a dressing for wounds and ulcers.

¶ *Preparations.* Infusion (1 : 150) has been advised, also a tincture (100 : 500) in a dose of 15 to 25 drops.

See GRINDELIA.

A
MODERN HERBAL

VOLUME II

ICELAND MOSS. *See* MOSS

IGNATIUS BEANS (*POISON*)

Strychnos Ignatii (BERG.)
N.O. Loganiaceæ

Synonyms. Faba Ignatic. Ignatia amara (Linn.)
Part Used. Ripe dried seeds
Habitat. Philippine Islands

¶ *Description.* A large woody climbing shrub, introduced into Cochin China, and highly esteemed there as a medicine. It attracted the attention of the Jesuits, hence its name. In commerce the beans are about one full inch long; ovate, a dull blacky brown colour, very hard and horny, covered in patches with silvery adpressed hairs; endosperm translucent, enclosing an irregular cavity with an oblong embryo; no odour; taste extremely bitter. Each fruit contains about twelve to twenty seeds embedded in the pulp from which they have to be separated.

¶ *Constituents.* The beans have the same properties as Nux Vomica, but contain more strychnine, also brucine, a volatile principle extractive, gum, resin, colouring matter, a fixed oil, and bassorin; they contain no albumen or starch.

¶ *Medicinal Action and Uses.* Tonic and stimulant in action like Nux Vomica, which, being cheaper, is nearly always used as a substitute. Old writers lauded these beans as a remedy against cholera. They are useful in certain forms of heart trouble, but must be used with the greatest caution, as they are a very active and powerful poison.

¶ *Antidotes.* Same as for strychnine, chloroform, belladonna, aconite, tobacco, chloral hydrate 1 drachm doses, morphia.

¶ *Preparations and Dosages.* Tincture of Ignatia, 5 to 20 minims. Alkaline Tincture of Ignatia (*syn.* Goute Ameres de Beaume), 5 to 20 minims.

INDIAN HEMP. *See* HEMP

INDIAN PHYSIC

Gillenia trifoliata (MŒNCH.)
N.O. Rosaceæ

Synonyms. Bowman's Root. American Ipecacuanha. Gillenia. Indian Hippo. Spiræa trifoliata. Spiræa stipulata
Part Used. Root-bark
Habitat. Eastern United States

¶ *Description.* A perennial herb, indigenous to the United States, its irregular, brownish root gives rise to several stems 2 or 3 feet in height, and has depending from it many long, thin fibres. The leaves and leaflets are of various shapes, and the white, reddish-tinged flowers grow in a few loose, terminal panicles.

The dried root is reddish brown, the bark being easily removed and pulverized. Within, it is light, ligneous, and comparatively inert. The bitterness of the bark is extracted by alcohol, or by water at 212° F., to which a red colour is given.

It grows well in the author's garden, in slightly moist, rich soil, not in the full blaze of the mid-day sun.

¶ *Constituents.* The roots have been found to contain gum, starch, gallotannic acid, fatty matter, wax, resin, lignin, albumen, salts and colouring matter.

Gillenin was obtained by W. B. Stanhope by exhausting coarsely powdered bark with alcohol, evaporating the resulting red tincture to the consistency of an extract, dissolving this in cold water, filtering, evaporating, and finally drying on glass.

Half a grain caused nausea and retching.

Two glucosides were found, Gillein, from the ethereal extract, and Gilleenin, from the aqueous infusion.

¶ *Medicinal Action and Uses.* Tonic, emetic, slightly diaphoretic, cathartic, and expectorant. The American Indians and early colonists knew the uses of the roots, the action of which resembles Ipecacuanha.

Recommended in dyspepsia, dropsy, rheumatism, chronic costiveness, and whenever an emetic is required. It is safe and reliable.

¶ *Dosages.* Of powdered root, as an emetic, 20 to 30 grains. In dyspepsia, as a tonic, 2 to 4 grains. As a sudorific, in cold water, 6 grains at intervals of two or three hours. It may be combined with opium. Frequent large doses of the infusion cause vomiting and purging.

¶ *Other Species.*
Gillenia stipulata, taller and more bushy, with fewer flowers and roots more like those of Ipecac; grows as far west as Kansas.

It is, equally with *G. trifoliata*, the source of Gillenia.

See MEADOWSWEET, HARDHACK.

INDIGO

Indigofera tinctoria
N.O. Leguminosæ

Synonyms. Pigmentum Indicum
Part Used. The plant
Habitat. India; cultivated in sub-tropical countries

¶ *Description*. A blue dyestuff is obtained from the various species of Indigofera. It does not exist ready formed, but is produced during fermentation from another agent existing in the plant. This is called Indocan, and is yellow, amorphous, of a nauseous bitter taste with an acid reaction; readily soluble in water, alcohol and ether.

¶ *Medicinal Action and Uses*. Indigo was at one time much used in medicine, but now is rarely employed. It is said to produce nausea and vomiting.

It is a very well-known and highly important dye, millions of pounds being exported from India annually.

An artificial product, Indigotine, is manufactured chemically and used as a substitute.

INDIGO (WILD)

Baptisia tinctoria (R. BR.)
N.O. Leguminosæ

Synonyms. Baptisia. Horse-fly Weed. Rattlebush. Indigo-weed. Sophora tinctoria (Linn.). Podalyria tinctoria (Michx.)
Parts Used. Root, bark, leaves
Habitat. Dry hilly woods from Canada to Carolina

¶ *Description*. An herbaceous perennial which takes its name from the Greek *Bapto* (to dye); has a black woody root, yellowish internally with many rootlets; stem about 3 feet high, smooth, glabrous, round, and branched; leaves, small, subsessile, alternate and palmately trifoliate; leaflets rounded at end; calyx four-cleft; flowers, yellow, blooming August and September, in small loose terminal racemes. Legume short, bluish-black seeds, subreniform.

¶ *Constituents*. The root is non-odorous and of a nauseous acrid taste, containing gum, albumen, starch, a yellowish resin and a crystalline substance.

¶ *Medicinal Action and Uses*. Used internally in form of decoction or syrup in scarlatina, typhus, and in all cases where there is a tendency to putrescency; it is purgative, emetic, stimulant, astringent, and antiseptic; principally used for its antiseptic qualities.

¶ *Dosage*. Of the decoction, 1 tablespoonful. Fluid extract, $\frac{1}{4}$ to $\frac{1}{2}$ drachm. Baptisin, 1 to 3 grains.

IPECACUANHA

Psychotria Ipecacuanha (STOKES)
N.O. Rubiaceæ

Synonym. Cephælis Ipecacuanha
Part Used. Root
Habitat. The root used in medicine under this name is that of a small, shrubby plant about a foot high, belonging to the order Rubiaceæ, which is found in most parts of Brazil, growing in clumps or patches, in moist, shady woods.

    The drug is chiefly collected in the interior, in the province of Matto Grosso and near the German colony of Philadelphia, north of Rio de Janeiro. It is also found in New Granada and in Bolivia.

¶ *Description*. The plant has a slender stem, which grows partly underground and is often procumbent at the base, the lower portion being knotted.

Fibrous rootlets are given off from the knots, and some of them develop an abnormally thick bark, in which much starch is deposited.

The thickened rootlets alone are collected and dried for medicinal use, since the active constituents of the drug are found chiefly in the bark.

Ipecacuanha roots are collected, chiefly by the Indians, during the months of January and February, when the plant is in flower and are prepared by separation from the stem, cleaning and hanging in bundles to dry in the sun.

The drug is known in commerce as Brazilian or Rio Ipecacuanha.

¶ *History*. The name of the plant is the Portuguese form of the native word, *i-pe-kaa-guéne*, which is said to mean 'road-side sick-making plant.'

In an account of Brazil, written by a Portuguese friar who had resided in that country from about 1570 to 1600, mention is made of three remedies for the bloody flux, one of which is called Igpecaya, or Pigaya, which is probably this root.

Although in common use in Brazil, Ipecacuanha was not employed in Europe prior to the year 1672, when a traveller named Legros brought a quantity of the root to Paris from South America. In 1680, a merchant of Paris named Garnier became possessed of 150 lb. of Ipecacuanha, and informed his assistant and the physician Helvetius of its usefulness in treating dysentery.

Helvetius prescribed the new drug, and it formed the basis of a patent medicine for dysentery. Trials were made of the composition, and Helvetius was granted by Louis XIV the sole right of vending the remedy. A few years after, the secret was bought from him by the French Government for 1,000 louis d'or and the formula was made public in 1688.

The botanical source of Ipecacuanha was the subject of much dispute, until it was finally settled by Gomez, a physician of the Portuguese Navy, who brought authentic specimens from Brazil to Lisbon in 1800.

Ipecacuanha occurs in commerce as slender and somewhat tortuous closely annulated pieces, which seldom exceed 6 inches in length and $\frac{1}{4}$ inch in thickness. It varies in colour from very dark brown to dark red, the latter colour being partly due to adhering particles of earth. Difference in colour may also be due to difference of age or mode of drying. The bark is constricted at short intervals, so as to give the root the appearance of a number of discs somewhat irregularly strung together. The constrictions are sometimes quite shallow in Brazilian or Rio Ipecacuanha, though they may penetrate nearly to the wood. The root is hard and breaks with a very short fracture, the fractured surface exhibiting a thick, dark grey bark or cortex, with a horny, resinous or starchy appearance and a hard, wiry centre – small dense wood, in which no distinct pores or pith can be discerned; when examined with a lens though it is radiate.

The drug has a bitter taste, but only a slight, rather musty odour.

It is generally mixed with more or less of the slender subterranean stem, which has only a very thin bark, surrounding a ring of wood which encloses a distinct pith, and is thus easily distinguished from the root. The activity of the drug resides chiefly in the cortical portion, hence the presence of the stem diminishes its value.

The variety imported from Colombia and known as Cartagena Ipecacuanha, the product of *Psychotria acuminata*, differs only in its larger size and in being less conspicuously annulated, the constrictions of the bark assuming the form of narrow merging ridges.

¶ *Substitutes*. In addition to the Cartagena Ipecacuanha, various other roots have been offered as substitutes, but all differ considerably.

East Indian Ipecacuanha, from *Cryptocarpus spiralis*, exhibits a typically monocotyledonous structure in transverse section, scattered bundles running the pith, and a white starchy bark.

The name *poaya* is applied in Brazil to emetic roots of several genera belonging to the natural orders Rubiaceæ, Violaceæ and Polygalaceæ, and hence several roots have from time to time been sent over to England as Ipecacuanha, but none of them possess the ringed or annulated appearance of the true drug. Of these, the root of *Ionidium Ipecacuanha*, *Richardsonia scabra* and *P. emetica* are those which have most frequently been exported from Brazil or Colombia.

Undulated Ipecacuanha, from *R. scabra*, is only lightly annulated, the wood is porous and the starchy bark often has a violet colour.

Lesser Striated Ipecacuanha from another species of *Richardsonia* is dark purplish brown in colour, longitudinally wrinkled, not annulated, and has porous wood.

Greater Striated Ipecacuanha from *P. emetica*, known as *Black or Peruvian Ipecacuanha*, closely resembles the preceding, but contains no starch and has dense wood. It grows in Peru and New Grenada, and in earlier days was for a long time considered as the source of the new drug, but is much less active.

White Ipecacuanha, from *I. Ipecacuanha* is greyish-white, or yellowish in colour and is also free from starch. This likewise was for long believed to be the plant which produces the genuine drug. It is a member of the order Violaceæ. The root is almost insipid and inodorous and is used in Brazil as an emetic, though it has been considered doubtful whether it possesses any well-defined properties.

The roots of several species of *Borreria*, as *B. ferruginia* and *B. Poaya*, are also used in Brazil as substitutes for Ipecacuanha.

¶ *Constituents*. The chief constituents of Ipecacuanha root are the alkaloids Emetine, Cephaelin and Psychotrine, of which the bark may contain from 1·5 to 2 per cent., of which about 72 per cent. consists of Emetine and 26 per cent. of Cephaelin, while only 2 per cent. consists of Psychotrine.

Emetine, to which Ipecacuanha owes its properties and which, with the exception of traces, occurs only in the cortical portion of the root, is an amorphous white powder, but it forms crystalline salts. It has a bitter taste, no odour and turns yellow when exposed to air and light.

Other constituents are a crystalline saponin-like glucoside, an amorphous, bitter gluco-side, which is a modification of tannin, and is known as Ipecacuanhic acid, choline, resin, pectin, starch, sugar, calcium oxalate, odorous, fatty matter and a disagreeable-smelling volatile oil.

Cartagena Ipecacuanha contains 2 to 3 per cent. more alkaloidal matter than the Brazilian drug, but a smaller proportion of Emetine, Cephaelin being the alkaloid present in largest quantities.

East Indian Ipecacuanha and White Ipeca-cuanha contain minute quantities of emetic principles, which differ from the alkaloids of true Ipecacuanha, but the Undulated and Striated Ipecacuanha contain Emetine.

¶ *Medicinal Action and Uses.* In large doses, Ipecacuanha root is emetic; in smaller doses, diaphoretic and expectorant, and in still smaller, stimulating to the stomach, intestines and liver, exciting appetite and facilitating digestion.

The dose of the powdered root is ¼ to 2 grains when an expectorant action is desired (it is frequently used in the treatment of bronchitis and laryngitis, combined with other drugs, aiding in the expulsion of the morbid product), and from 15 to 30 grains when given as an emetic, which is one of its most valuable functions.

The Pharmacopœias contain a very large number of preparations of Ipecacuanha, most of which are standardized.

Ipecacuanha has been known for more than a century to benefit amœbic (or tropical) dysentery, and is regarded as the specific treatment, but the administration of the drug by mouth was limited by its action as an emetic. Sir Leonard Rogers showed in 1912 that subcutaneous injections of the alkaloid Emetine, the chief active principle present in Ipecacuanha usually produced a rapid cure in cases of amœbic dysentery. The toxic action of Emetine on the heart must be watched. A preparation from which the Emetine has been removed, known as de-emetized Ipecacu-anha, is also in use for cases of dysentery.

IRISES

The Iris belongs to a family of plants that is justly popular in this country for its many varieties of handsome garden blooms, beautifying the borders in spring and early summer.

The plant is named after the rainbow god-dess, 'Iris,' from the beauty and variety of colours in the flowers of the genus.

From ancient times the stately Iris stood as a symbol of power and majesty – it was dedi-

The great value of the drug in dysentery and its rapid increase in price from an average of 2s. 9½d. per lb. in 1850 to about 8s. 9d. per lb. in 1870, led to attempts to acclimatize the plant in India, but without much commercial success, owing to the difficulty of finding suitable places for its cultivation and to its slowness of growth. It is grown to a limited extent in the Malay States, at Johore, near Singapore. In December, 1915, the Brazil root was valued at 24s. per lb. and the Johore root at 20s. per lb. At the same time, Cartagena root sold for 16s. per lb. It would probably pay to grow this plant more extensively in the British Colonies.

The diaphoretic properties are employed in the *Pulvis Ipecacuanhæa compositus*, or Dover's Powder, which contains 1 part of Ipecacuanha powder and 1 part of Opium in 10.

When applied to the skin, Ipecacuanha powder acts as a powerful irritant, even to the extent of causing pustulations.

When inhaled, it causes sneezing and a mild inflammation of the nasal mucous membrane.

Toxic doses cause gastro-enteritis, cardiac failure, dilation of the blood-vessels, severe bronchitis and pulmonary inflammation.

¶ *Preparations and Dosages.* Powdered root, 5 to 30 grains. Fluid extract, B.P., 2 to 20 drops. Comp. Tinct. (Dover's), U.S.P., 8 drops. Wine, B.P., 10 drops to 6 drachms. Syrup, U.S.P., ¼ to 4 drachms. Dover's Powder, B.P., 5 to 15 grains.

Other plants possessing emetic properties to a greater or less degree, to which the name of Ipecacuanha has been popularly applied are: American Ipec., *Gillenia stipulacea*; Wild Ipec., *Euphorbia Ipecacuanha*; Guinea Ipec., *Bœrhavia decumbens*; Venezuela Ipec., *Sarcostemma glaucum*; Ipecacuanha des Alle-mands, *Vincetoxicum officinale*, and the Bastard Ipecacuanha, *Asclepias cuirassavica*, of the West Indies. This plant is used by the negroes as an emetic and the root is purgative; the juice of the plant, made into a syrup, is said to be a powerful anthelmintic, and as such is given to children in the West Indies.

N.O. Iridaceæ

cated to Juno and was the origin of the sceptre, the Egyptians placing it on the brow of the Sphinx and on the sceptre of their kings, the three leaves of its blossoms typifying faith, wisdom and valour.

Cultivation has produced a great number of varieties, both among the bulbous or Spanish Iris (*Iris xiphium*) and the herbaceous, or Flag Irises, which have fleshy, creeping root-stocks or rhizomes. Among the latter, many have a considerable reputation for their medicinal virtues; in all the species belonging to this genus, the roots being more or less acrid, are possessed of cathartic and emetic properties. The chief economic use of the Iris at the present time is for the production of Orris Root (*Rhizoma Iridis*), which is derived from *I. Germanica*, *I. pallida* and *I. Florentina*, collected indiscriminately in Italy from these three species, well-known and very beautiful ornamental plants, natives of the eastern Mediterranean region, extending into Northern India and Northern Africa, and largely cultivated for their rhizomes in Southern Europe, mostly on the mountain slopes.

I. pseudacorus, *I. fœtidissima* and *I. tuberosa* are the European species that have been employed in medicine, though their use has much declined, but the American species, *I. versicolor*, produces a drug official in the United States Pharmacopœia.

Only two of these Irises are naturally wild plants in this country, *I. pseudacorus* (the Yellow Flag) and *I. fœtidissima* (the Stinking Iris). *I. tuberosa* (the Snakeshead Iris), which has cathartic properties, is occasionally but very rarely found in Cornwall and South Devon, but it is not native, and where it occurs it is considered a garden escape.

I. Germanica and other Flag Irises are cultivated in this country for their beautiful flowers, but no attempts have been made to supply the market with the rhizomes.

In ancient Greece and Rome, Orris Root was largely used in perfumery, and Macedonia, Elis and Corinth were famous for their unguents of Iris.

Theophrastus and Dioscorides were well acquainted with Orris Root; Dioscorides and Pliny remark that the best comes from Illyricum (the modern Dalmatia). Probably *I. Germanica* is the Illyrian Iris of the ancients, as it is plentiful there and *I. Florentina* and *I. pallida* do not occur. The latter were probably introduced into Northern Italy in the early Middle Ages. The ancient arms of Florence – a white Lily or Iris on a red shield – seem to indicate that the city was famed for the growth of these plants. A writer of the thirteenth century, Petrus de Crescentiro of Bologna, mentions the cultivation of the White, as well as of the Purple Iris, and states at what season the root should be collected for medicinal use.

IRIS GERMANICA (Linn.), Blue Flower de Luce, German Iris, is a handsome plant with sword-like leaves of a bluish-green colour, narrow and flat, the largest of all the species. The flower-stems are 2 to 3 feet high, the flowers, which bloom in May and June, are large and deep blue, or purplish-blue in colour. The three bending petals, or falls, are of a faint purple, inclining to blue, with purple veins running lengthwise; the beard on them is yellow and the three erect petals or standards are bright blue, with faint purple stripes. The flowers have an agreeable scent, reminiscent of orange blossoms. The creeping root-stocks are thick and fleshy, spreading over the surface of the ground and of a brownish colour.

¶ *Habitat*. The plant is a native of Southern Europe, very frequent in Italy, apart from its cultivation there, and is also cultivated in Morocco. In England, this German Flag or Flag Iris is by far the commonest of the family in gardens and justly deserves its popularity, for it will grow and flower well in the most unpromising situations and will bear with apparent equanimity hardships that few other plants would endure without loss of vitality. It is not moisture-loving – ordinary border soil, well cultivated, suits it well and the heavy clay soils are more or less inimical to its growth. If the best results are to be obtained, deep and rich beds should be prepared for these Irises, for they will well repay liberal treatment by the production of larger and more numerous flowers. Although they may be moved at any time of the year, April is the best month. They will not flower the same year, but they will during the summer, if attended to, become sufficiently strong to bloom freely the succeeding year. Winter is the worst time to move them, as in heavy soil, the plants often remain dormant without forming a single root-fibre until the spring. But they are easily increased in spring by dividing the root-stocks and replanting and watering into rich soil.

The German Iris, or Flag Iris of the nurseryman as it now exists, is a compound of many species and more varieties, as hybridization has been extensively carried on for many years.

¶ *Medicinal Action and Uses*. The juice of the fresh roots of this Iris, bruised with wine, has been employed as a strong purge of great efficiency in dropsy, old physic writers stating that if the dropsy can be cured by the hand of man, this root will effect it. The juice is also sometimes used as a cosmetic and for the removal of freckles from the skin.

IRIS PALLIDA (Lamarck) has sweet-scented flowers of a delicate, pale blue. It is a native of the Eastern Mediterranean countries and grows very freely in Italy. It yields, with *I. Germanica*, the bulk of the drug.

IRIS FLORENTINA (Linn.), called by our old writers White Flower de Luce, or Flower de Luce of Florence, has large, white flowers tinged with pale lavender and a bright yellow beard on the falls. Less commonly, a purple form occurs, of smaller growth.

¶ *Medicinal Action and Uses*. The fresh root, like that of *I. Germanica*, is a powerful cathartic, and for this reason its juice has been employed in dropsy.

It is chiefly used in the dry state, being said to be good for complaints of the lungs, for coughs and hoarseness, but is now more valued for the pleasantness of its violet-like perfume than for any other use.

Fresh roots have an earthy smell, the characteristic violet odour is gradually developed during the drying process and does not attain its maximum for at least two years, and even intensifies after that time. The essential oil may, therefore, be included in the class of so-called 'ferment-oils.'

The rhizomes of *I. Germanica*, *I. pallida* and *I. Florentina* so closely resemble one another that they are not easily distinguished. Contractions occur at intervals of about two inches, indicating the limit of a year's growth in each case.

When fresh, the rhizomes are extremely acrid and when chewed excite a pungent taste in the mouth, which continues some hours. This acridity is almost entirely dissipated when dried, the taste then being slightly bitter and the smell agreeable, closely approaching that of violets, though in the fresh state the rhizomes are practically odourless. The loss of acridity appears to be due to the disappearance of a volatile acrid principle on drying the rhizome.

All three species of Iris from which Orris root is derived were already cultivated in England in the time of Gerard, though not on a commercial scale.

¶ *Collection*. In Tuscany and other parts of Italy, large districts are given over to the cultivation of these three Irises. They are also cultivated, but only to a slight degree, in other parts of Europe, in Morocco and in India.

The planting of the Orris root in Tuscany – locally known as 'giaggiolo' – is a matter of great importance. When the Iris begins to grow, the ground is carefully and systematically weeded, this being chiefly done by women, who traverse the rows of the plants barefoot, hoeing up the weeds; whole families of peasants work together at this, and in the subsequent collection, trimming and drying of the roots. The Orris plant takes two or even three years to arrive at maturity, only a somewhat sparse growth being attained during the second year: the flowers are very fine, but the roots are as yet immature. In the third year of its growth, the plant attains almost the height of a man. The full beauty of the flowers lasts during May and June, in July they fade and wither and the glory of the plantation is over.

The product of a good harvest at a large Orris plantation at San Polo, in the hilly region midway between Florence and Siena in Tuscany, is about a million kilogrammes of fresh roots (about 1,000 tons), yielding after peeling and drying, roughly 300 tons of dry root.

Orris root, in the decorticated, dried condition, is imported into England in large casks, mainly from Leghorn, Trieste and Mogador.

There are several varieties of Orris in commerce, differing chiefly in colour and the care with which they have been peeled. The finest is Florentine Orris, from *I. Florentina*, which is carefully peeled, nearly white, plump and very fragrant, irregular in shape, bearing small marks where the rootlets have been removed. Veronese Orris, from *I. Germanica*, is usually somewhat compressed and elongated, less suddenly tapering than the Florentine root, less carefully peeled, yellowish in colour, and somewhat wrinkled and has not the fine fragrance of the Florentine Orris.

Morocco or Mogadore Orris, also obtained from *I. Germanica*, bears particles of reddish-brown cork, is darker in colour generally and less fragrant; the pieces are also smaller, flatter, more shrunken and often bear the shrivelled remains of leaves at the apex. This variety is sometimes bleached with sulphur dioxide. It is altogether inferior to both the foregoing varieties. Bombay Orris is also of small size, dark-coloured and of inferior fragrance.

¶ *Constituents*. The chief constituent of Orris root is the oil of Orris (0·1 to 0·2 per cent.), a yellowish-white to yellow mass, containing about 85 per cent. of odourless myristic acid, which appears to be liberated from a fat present in the rhizome during the process of steam distillation. Oil of Orris is known commercially as Orris Butter.

Other constituents are fat, resin, a large quantity of starch, mucilage, bitter extractive and a glucoside named Iridin, which is not to be confused with the powdered extracti Iridin or Irisin, prepared from the rhizome of the American plant *I. versicolor*, by precipitating a tincture of the drug with water and mixing the precipitate with an equal weight of powdered liquorice root, or other absorbent powder.

The odorous constituent of oil of Orris is a liquid ketone named Irone, to which the violet-like odour is due (though it is not absolutely identical with oil of Violets obtained from the natural flower), and it is the presence of this principle in the rhizome that has long led to the employment of powdered Orris root in the preparation of Violet pow-

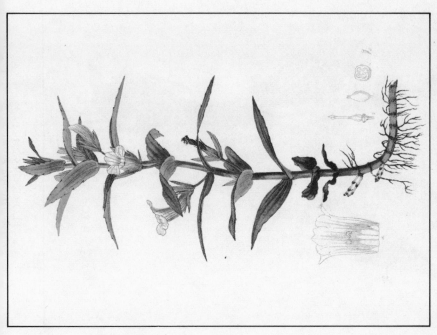

HEDGE HYSSOP
Gratiola Officinalis

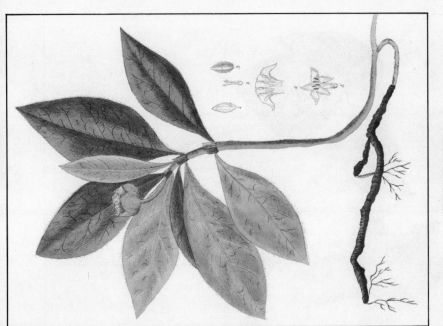

IPECACUANHA
Psychotria Ipecacuanha

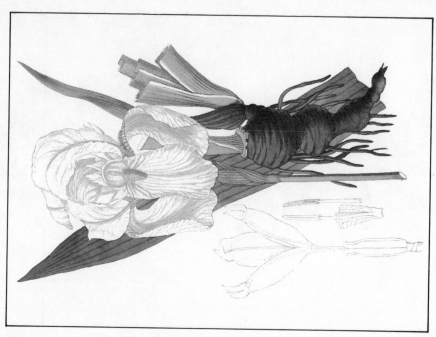

FLORENTINE IRIS
Iris Florentina

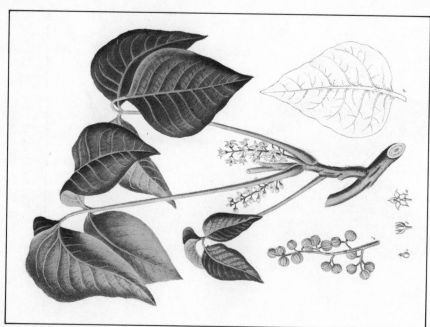

POISON IVY
Rhus Toxicodendron

ders, which owe very little of their scent to the real Violet perfume. It was first isolated by the eminent chemist Tiemann and formed the basis of his researches on artificial Violet perfume, and in 1893 he succeeded in preparing an allied body, which was termed Ionone and which had an odour even more like that of Violets than had Irone, and is now largely manufactured for the perfumery trade in making toilet waters and handkerchief extracts. The discovery of Ionone, which costs about one-eighth of the natural oil of Violets, has popularized Violet perfume to an enormous extent: most of the cheaper Violet perfumes on the market contain no trace of true Violet, but are made entirely with the artificial Ionone.

Otto of Orris is a golden-yellow oily liquid, which contains the odorous principles of the concrete oil of the rhizome without the solid, fatty inodorous constituents.

The important industry of Orris root still requires the light of scientific research to be thrown upon the life history of the plant to determine the conditions under which the largest percentage of the volatile oil can be developed.

¶ *Medicinal Action and Uses*. Orris Root is rarely employed in *medicine* at the present time.

The fresh root possesses diuretic, emetic and cathartic properties. If given in large doses, it will occasion nausea, vomiting, purging and colic.

The drug was formerly employed in the treatment of bronchitis and chronic diarrhœa, and was considered a useful remedy in dropsy. The internal dose is stated to be from 5 to 15 grains.

The starch of the rhizome was formerly reckoned medicinal.

The dried powder is said to act as a good snuff, useful to excite sneezing to relieve cases of congested headache.

Pieces of the dried root are occasionally chewed for the purpose of overcoming a disagreeable breath.

The principal use of the dried root is, however, in *perfumery*, in sachet powders and to flavour dentifrices, toothpowders and cachous.

Oil of Orris, obtained by distilling powdered Orris root with steam, has an intense and extremely delicate odour of the fresh Violet and commands a high price. It is used commercially in the preparation of the finest scents and is also blended with artificial Violet perfumes, the odour of which it renders more subtle. Orris has the power of strengthening the odour of other fragrant bodies and is used as a fixative in perfumery.

Powdered Orris root is sometimes put into rinsing water in laundries and imparts a refreshing and fragrant scent to the linen.

Orris root, mixed with Anise, was used in England as a perfume for linen as early as 1480, under which date it is mentioned in the Wardrobe accounts of Edward IV.

One of the most interesting of the MS. still-room books of the later seventeenth century is *Mary Doggett: Her Book of Receipts*, 1682. In it we find 'A perfume for a sweet bagg,' as follows:

'Take half a pound of Cypress Roots, a pound of *Orris*, 3 quarter of a pound of Calamus, 3 Orange stick with Cloves, 2 ounces of Benjamin, 3 quarters of a pound of Rhodium, a pound of Coriander seed, and an ounce of Storax and 4 pecks of Damask Rose leaves, a peck of dryed sweet Marjerum, a pretty stick of Juniper shaved very thin, some lemon pele dryed and a stick of Brasill; let all these be powdered very grosely for ye first year and immediately put into your baggs; the next year pound and work it and it will be very good again.'

Dr. Rhind (*History of the Vegetable Kingdom*, 1868) states that Orris gives the peculiar flavour to artificial brandies made in this country, and the root is much used in Russia to flavour a drink made of honey and ginger which is sold in the streets.

The larger and finer roots are often turned into pretty forms to be used for ornamental purposes, rosary beads, etc., and long pieces of Verona Orris are often shaped for infants' use when teething. The less handsome rhizomes, as well as the chips, are distilled.

Lyte says 'the Iris is knowen of the clothworkers and drapers, for with these rootes they use to trimme their clothes to make them sweete and pleasant.' This was probably the 'swete clothe' so celebrated in the reign of Elizabeth.

IRIS PSEUDACORUS (LINN.)

N.O. Iridaceæ

Synonyms. Iris Aquatica. Iris lutia. Yellow Flag. Yellow Iris. Fleur de Luce. Dragon Flower. Myrtle Flower. Fliggers. Flaggon. Segg. Sheggs. Daggers. Jacob's Sword. Gladyne. Meklin. Levers. Livers. Shalder

Part Used. Root

Of all British wild plants, none can rival in stately beauty this native representative of the Irises, one of the most distinguished plants in the marginal vegetation of watery places, not only in this country, being universally distributed in Great Britain and growing also in

Ireland, but also throughout Europe, North Africa and Siberia.

It is found on river-banks, by the side of lakes, ponds, etc., in ditches and hedges, but any moist, shady place will suit it, and it is quite worthy of a place in our gardens.

Propagation is effected in autumn or spring, by division of the root-stocks. It should not, however, be allowed to grow where cattle feed.

¶ *Description*. From the thick, creeping rhizome, brownish on the outside, reddish and spongy within, which pushes through the moist ground parallel to the surface, many rootlets pass downwards. From above it, rise the broad, flat, sword-shaped, stalkless leaves, bound several together into a sheath at the base. The lower, radical leaves are 2 to 3 feet tall, the upper leaves much shorter, embracing the flower-stalk, which is round and seldom rises as high as the outer leaves. On the top of the stem are the beautiful, very conspicuous, deep yellow flowers, two or three together, the buds being very large and pointed. The mature flowers consist of three large, drooping, yellow petal-like sepals (the falls) with brownish mottled markings on their upper surfaces, inside which are the three petalloid stigmas, also yellow, which arch gracefully over the stamens, forming a rain-protecting roof for the pollen, as in all the Irises. The honey is contained in canals on the inner side, towards the base of the small, erect petals and out of these it exudes and lies round the ovary in the heart of the flower. The Yellow Iris is adapted to receive two kinds of insect visitors, the Bumble Bee (*Bombus*), and the Honey Bee (*Apis mellifica*), and also the long-tongued Hover-Fly (*Rhingia rostrata*), which in seeking the honey, push through the outer perianth segments and the style, the anther being between, dusting its back with the pollen.

After fertilization, the floral leaves fade and drop away from the top of the capsule, which increases in size. When ripe, the capsule opens above and allows the smooth, flattened seeds, when blown by the wind, to fall some distance away.

This Iris is in bloom from May to July.

Locally, the plant is often called 'Segg,' 'Skeggs' or 'Cegg,' all of which names come down from Anglo-Saxon days, 'Segg' being the Anglo-Saxon for a small sword, an obvious allusion to the shape of its leaves. The names 'Daggers' and 'Jacob's Sword ' have a similar allusion, and 'Yellow Saggen,' 'Seag,' 'Seggin' are variations of Seg. In the days of Chaucer, it was called Gladyne. To the popular mind in early days, the fluttering segment of the perianth suggested the waving

of a flag, hence the origin of the names 'Yellow Flag,' 'Water Flag' and 'Sword Flag,' and corruptions of the name such as 'Flaggon,' 'Flaggon's' and perhaps 'Fliggers,' the latter stated to be applied to it from the motion of its leaves by the slightest breeze. The strange name 'Cheiper' is explained 'because children make a shrill noise with its leaves,' and 'Cucumbers' refers to the seed-vessels, which when green resemble young cucumbers.

Culpepper calls it 'Myrtle Flag or Myrtle Grass.'

It is also called the Flower de Luce, or Fleur de Lys, being the origin of the heraldic emblem of the Kings of France. The legend is that early in the sixth century, the Frankish King Clovis, faced with defeat in battle, was induced to pray for victory to the god of his Christian wife, Clothilde. He conquered and became a Christian and thereupon replaced the three toads on his banner by three Irises, the Iris being the Virgin's flower. Six hundred years later, it was adopted by Louis VII of France as his heraldic bearings in his Crusade against the Saracens, and it is said that it then became known as Fleur de Louis, corrupted into Fleur de Luce and then into Fleur de Lys or Lis, though another theory for the name is that it was not named Fleur de Lys from Louis, but from the river Lys, on the borders of Flanders, where it was peculiarly abundant.

Its specific name, *Pseudacorus*, refers to its similarity to another plant, *pseudo* being the Greek for false, while *acorus* is the generic name of the Sweet Sedge (*Acorus calamus*), with which it is supposed to have been confused, the plants when not in flower resembling it and growing in the same situations. The Sweet Sedge, however, has an aromatic scent, while *Iris Pseudacorus* is odourless.

The Romans called the plant *consecratix*, from its being used in purifications, and Pliny mentions certain ceremonies used in digging up the plant.

¶ *Medicinal Action and Uses*. The Yellow Flag rhizome was formerly much employed as a medicine, acting as a very powerful cathartic, but from its extremely acrid nature is now seldom used. An infusion of it has been found to be effective in checking diarrhœa, and it is reputed of value in dysmenorrhœa and leucorrhœa.

It was formerly held in the highest esteem, the juice of the root being considered a cure for obstinate coughs, 'evil spleens,' convulsions, dropsies and serpents' bites, and as Gerard also says, 'doth mightilie and vehementlie draw forth choler.' Gerard recommended it as a cosmetic, saying:

'The root, boiled soft, with a few drops of rosewater upon it, laid plaisterwise upon the face of man or woman, doth in two daies at the most take away the blacknesse and blewnesse of any stroke or bruise,'

though he adds as a warning that if the skin

'be very tender and delicate, it shall be needful that ye lay a piece of silke, sindall or a piece of fine lawne betweene the plaister and the skinne for otherwise in such tender bodies it often causeth heat and inflammation.'

He recommends

'an oil made of the roots and flowers of the Iris, made in the same way as oil of roses and lilies. It is used to rub in the sinews and joints to strengthen them, and is good for cramp.'

Parkinson, of all the varieties, most esteems 'for his excellent beautie and raretie the great Turkie Flower de luce.'

'And for a sweet powder to lay among linnen and garments and to make sweet waters to wash hand-gloves or other things to perfume them' the roots of the sweet-smelling Flag.

The acrid juice snuffed up the nostrils excites violent sneezing, and on the authority of Dr. Thornton, 'in this way it has cured complaints of the head of long standing in a marvellous way.' The root powdered was also used as snuff.

The old authorities praised it as a cure for toothache, a slice of the rhizome rubbed against the aching tooth or held in the mouth between the teeth, being supposed to cause the pain to disappear at once.

The root was also an ingredient in an antidote to poison. Withering (*Arrangement of Plants*) mentions it as having cured swine bitten by a mad dog.

Culpepper (1652) says that the distilled water of the whole herb is a sovereign remedy for weak eyes, either applied on a wet bandage, or dropped into the eye, and that an ointment made of the flowers is very good for ulcers or swellings.

A French chemist, early last century, discovered that the seeds, when ripe, freed from the friable skin which envelops them, produces a beverage similar to coffee and even much superior to it in flavour, but they must be well roasted before using.

The flowers afford a beautiful yellow dye, and the root, with sulphate of iron, a good black dye.

The acrid properties are entirely dissipated by drying, after which it acts only as an astringent, so powerful from the amount of tannin contained, that it has been used in the place of Galls in the making of ink.

IRIS LENAX

N.O. Iridaceæ

Synonym. Iris Minor
Habitat. The hillsides of Oregon

A tincture of the whole plant, or of the bulbous stems, is given in bilious vomiting, and is recommended for depression.

The Indians use the fibres of this plant for making ropes.

IRIS VERSICOLOR (LINN.)

N.O. Iridaceæ

Synonyms. Blue Flag. Poison Flag. Flag Lily. Liver Lily. Snake Lily. Dragon Flower. Dagger Flower. Water Flag
Part Used. Root

Iris Versicolor (Linn.) is a perennial herb, found abundantly in swamps and low grounds throughout eastern and central North America, common in Canada, as well as in the United States, liking a loamy or peaty soil. It is not a native of Europe.

It grows 2 to 3 feet high, with narrow, sword-shaped leaves, and from May to July produces large, handsome flowers, blue, except for the yellow and whitish markings at the base of the sepals.

¶ *Description.* Blue Flag Rhizome has annual joints, 2 or more inches long, about ¾ inch in diameter, cylindrical in the lower half, becoming compressed towards the crown, where the cup-shaped stem-scar is seen, when dry, and numerous rings, formed of leaf scars are apparent above and scars of rootlets below. It is dark brown externally and longitudinally wrinkled. The fracture is short, purplish, the vascular bundles scattered through the central column. The rootlets are long, slender and simple. The rhizome has a very slight but peculiar odour, and a pungent, acrid and nauseous taste.

Owing to the similarity of name, and the appearance before blooming, this flag is sometimes mistaken by American children for Sweet Flag or Calamus, which grows in the same localities, often with disastrous results.

Of the 100 species of true Iris, twenty-two inhabit the United States, but only one, *Iris*

Missouriensis, much resembles this species (the rhizome of which yields an official American drug), or has a rhizome likely to be mistaken for it.

When *cultivated*, the American Blue Flag succeeds best in heavy, rich, moist soil. If planted in August or September, it can be harvested at the end of October the following year. The yield per acre is 3 to 4 tons of the rhizome.

¶ *Constituents.* The rhizome contains starch, gum, tannin, volatile oil, 25 per cent. of acrid, resinous matter, isophthalic acid, traces of salicylic acid and possibly an alkaloid, though a number of substances contained are still unidentified. It owes its medicinal virtues to an oleoresin.

Distilled with water, the fresh rhizome yields an opalescent distillate, from which is separated a white, camphoraceous substance with a faint odour. The oil possesses the taste and smell, but only partly the medicinal activity of the drug.

¶ *Medicinal Action and Uses.* The root is an official drug of the United States Pharmacopœia and is the source of the Iridin or Irisin of commerce, a powdered extractive, bitter, nauseous and acrid, with diuretic and aperient properties.

Iridin acts powerfully on the liver, but, from its milder action on the bowels, is preferable to podophyllin.

The fresh Iris is quite acrid and if employed internally produces nausea, vomiting, purging and colicky pains. The dried root is less acrid and is employed as an emetic, diuretic and cathartic. The oleoresin in the root is purgative to the liver, and useful in bilious sickness in small doses.

It is chiefly used for its alterative properties, being a useful purgative in disorders of the liver and duodenum, and is an ingredient of many compounds for purifying the blood. It acts as a stimulant to the liver and intestinal glands and is used in constipation and biliousness, and is believed by some to be a hepatic stimulant second only to podophyllin, but if given in full doses it may occasion considerable nausea and severe prostration.

Its chief use is for syphilis and some forms of low-grade scrofula and skin affection. It is also valuable in dropsy.

It is said to have been used by the southern North American Indians as a cathartic and emetic.

The flowers afford a fine blue infusion, which serves as a test for acids and alkalies.

¶ *Preparations and Dosages.* Powdered root, as a cathartic, 20 grains. Irisin, 1 to 3 grains. Solid extract, 10 to 15 grains. Fluid extract, ½ to 1 drachm. Tincture, 1 to 3 drachms.

IRISH MOSS. *See* MOSS

ISPAGHUL. *See* PLANTAIN

IVY, AMERICAN. *See* VIRGINIA CREEPER

IVY, COMMON   Hedera Helix (LINN.)
                                    N.O. Araliaceæ

Parts Used. Leaves, berries

Habitat. The plant is found over the greater part of Europe and Northern and Central Asia, and is said to have been particularly abundant at Nyssa, the fabled home of Bacchus in his youth. There are many varieties, but only two accepted species, i.e. *Hedera Helix* and the Australian species, which is confined to the southern Continent

This well-known evergreen climber, with its dark-green, glossy, angular leaves is too familiar to need detailed description. It climbs by means of curious fibres resembling roots, which shoot out from every part of the stem, and are furnished with small disks at the end, which adapt themselves to the roughness of the bark or wall against which the plant grows and to which it clings firmly. These fibres on meeting with soil or deep crevices become true roots, obtaining nourishment for the plant, but when dilated at the extremity, they merely serve to attach the stems and do not absorb nourishment from the substance to which they adhere. The Ivy is therefore liable to injure the trees around which it twines by abstracting the juices of the stem.

When it attains the summit of a tree or wall, it grows out in a bushy form, and the leaves instead of being five-lobed and angular, as they are below, become ovate, with entire margins. Ivy only produces flowers when the branches get above their support, the flowering branches being bushy and projecting a foot or two from the climbing stems, with flowers at the end of every shoot.

440

Professor Henslow has an interesting note on the Ivy and its shoots, in his *Floral Rambles in Highways and Byways*:

'The shoots turn to the darker side, as may be seen when Ivy reaches the top of a wall, from *both* sides; wherever the sun may be the shoots lie flat upon the top. The roots themselves only come out from the darker side of the shoots, so that both of these acquired habits have their purposes. When the Ivy is going to flower, the shoots *now* turn to the light and stand out freely into the air; moreover the form of the leaf changes from a fine-pointed one to a much smaller oval type. As the shoot now has to support itself, if a section be made and compared with one of the same diameter which is supported by the adhesive roots, it will be found that it has put on more wood with less pith, than in that of the supported stem. It at once, so to speak, *feels* the strain and makes wood sufficient to meet it.'

The form of Ivy which creeps over the ground on banks and in woods, etc., never blossoms. The branches root into the soil, but they are of the ordinary kind deriving nourishment from it. On endeavouring to train this kind on a wall, it was found to have practically lost the power of climbing; for it kept continually falling away from the wall instead of adhering to it; just as cucumbers refuse to climb by their tendrils, if the stem and branches are supported artificially.

The flowers of Common Ivy are small, in clusters of nearly globular umbels and of a yellowish-green, with five broad and short petals and five stamens. They seldom open before the latter end of October, and often continue to expand till late in December. Though they have little or no scent, they yield abundance of nectar and afford food to bees late in the autumn, when they can get no other.

The berries, which do not become ripe till the following spring, provide many birds, especially wood pigeons, thrushes and blackbirds with food during severe winters. When ripe, they are about the size of a pea, black or deep purple, smooth and succulent, and contain two to five seeds. They have a bitter and nauseous taste, and when rubbed, an aromatic and slightly resinous odour.

¶ *History.* Ivy was in high esteem among the ancients. Its leaves formed the poet's crown, as well as the wreath of Bacchus, to whom the plant was dedicated, probably because of the practice of binding the brow with Ivy leaves to prevent intoxication, a quality formerly attributed to the plant. We are told by old writers that the effects of intoxication by wine are removed if a handful of Ivy leaves are bruised and gently boiled in wine and drunk.

It is the Common Ivy that is alluded to in the Idylls of Theocritus, but the Golden Ivy of Virgil is supposed to be the yellow-berried variety (*Hedera Chrysocarpa*), now so rare.

The Greek priests presented a wreath of Ivy to newly-married persons, and the Ivy has throughout the ages been regarded as the emblem of fidelity. The custom of decorating houses and churches with Ivy at Christmas was forbidden by one of the early Councils of the Church, on account of its pagan associations, but the custom still remains.

An Ivy leaf is the badge of the Gordons.

The Roman agricultural writers much recommended Ivy leaves as cattle food, but they are not relished by cows, though sheep and deer will sometimes eat them in the winter. The broad leaves being evergreen afford shelter to birds in the winter, and many prefer Ivy to other shrubs, in which to build their nests.

The wood when it attains a sufficient size is employed by turners in Southern Europe, but being very soft is seldom used in England except for whetting the knives of leather-dressers. It is very porous, and the ancients thought it had the property of separating wine from water by filtration, an error arising from the fact that wood absorbs the colour of the liquid in its passage through the pores. On the Continent it has sometimes been used in thin slices as a filter.

In former days, English taverns bore over their doors the sign of an Ivy bush, to indicate the excellence of the liquor supplied within: hence the saying 'Good wine needs no bush.'

The medicinal virtues of Ivy are little regarded nowadays. Its great value is as an ornamental covering for unsightly buildings, and it is said to be the only plant which does not make walls damp. It acts as a curtain, the leaves from the way they fall, forming a sort of armour and holding and absorbing the rain and moisture.

Ivy is very hardy; not only are the leaves seldom injured by frost, but they suffer little from smoke, or from the vitiated air of manufacturing towns. The plant lives to a great age, its stems become woody and often attain a considerable size – Ivy trunks of a foot in diameter are often to be seen where the plant has for many years climbed undisturbed over rocks and ruins.

The spring months are the best times for planting.

¶ *Medicinal Action and Uses.* Robinson tells us that a drachm of the flowers decocted in wine restrains dysentery, and that the yellow berries are good for those who spit blood and against the jaundice.

Culpepper says of the Ivy: 'It is an enemy to the nerves and sinews taken *inwardly*, but most excellent *outwardly*.'

To remove sunburn it is recommended to smear the face with tender Ivy twigs boiled in butter; according to the old English *Leechbook of Bald.*

IVY, GROUND

Glechoma Hederacea (LINN.)
N.O. Labiatæ

Synonyms. Nepeta Glechoma (Benth.). Alehoof. Gill-go-over-the-Ground. Haymaids. Tun-hoof. Hedgemaids. Lizzy-run-up-the-Hedge. Gill-go-by-the-Hedge. Cats-foot. Robin-run-in-the-Hedge
Part Used. Herb

¶ *Description.* Ground Ivy is one of the commonest plants, flourishing upon sunny hedge banks and waste ground in all parts of Great Britain. The root is perennial, throwing out long, trailing, unbranched square stems, which root at intervals and bear numerous, kidney-shaped leaves of a dark green tint, somewhat downy with many-celled hairs, and having regular, rounded indentations on the margins. The leaves are stalked and opposite to one another, the undersides paler and dotted with glands.

The flowers are placed three or four together in the axils of the upper leaves, which often have a purplish tint and are two-lipped, of a bright purplish blue, with small white spots on the lower lip, or more rarely white or pink and open early in April. The plant continues in blossom through the greater part of the summer and autumn.

Its popular name is attributed to the resemblance borne by its foliage to that of the true Ivy.

It varies in size, as well as the degree of colour in the flower, according to its situation and remains green not only in summer, but, like the true Ivy, at all times of the year, even throughout winter, unless the frost is very severe.

Green (*Universal Herbal*, 1832) tells us that Ground Ivy expels the plants which grow near it, and in consequence impoverishes pastures. Cattle seem in general to avoid it, though Linnæus says that sheep eat it; horses are not fond of it, and goats and swine refuse it. It is thought to be injurious to those horses that eat much of it, though the expressed juice, mixed with a little wine and applied morning and evening, has been said to destroy the white specks which frequently form on their eyes.

The whole plant possesses a balsamic odour and an aromatic, bitter taste, due to its particular volatile oil, contained in the glands on the under surface of the leaves. It was one of the principal plants used by the early Saxons to clarify their beers, before hops had been introduced, the leaves being steeped in the hot liquor. Hence the names it has also borne: Alehoof and Tunhoof. It not only improved the flavour and keeping qualities of the beer, but rendered it clearer. Until the reign of Henry VIII it was in general use for this purpose.

The plant also acquired the name of Gill from the French *guiller* (to ferment beer), but as Gill also meant 'a girl,' it came also to be called 'Hedgemaids.'

Some hairy tumours may often be seen in the autumn on the leaves of Ground Ivy, caused by the puncture of the *Cynips glechomæ*, from which these galls spring. They have a strong flavour of the plant and are sometimes eaten by the peasantry of France.

¶ *Part Used Medicinally.* The whole herb, gathered early in May, when most of the flowers are still quite fresh.

¶ *Medicinal Action and Uses.* Diuretic, astringent, tonic and gently stimulant. Useful in kidney diseases and for indigestion.

From early days, Ground Ivy has been endowed with singular curative virtues, and is one of the most popular remedies for coughs and nervous headaches. It has even been extolled before all other vegetable medicines for the cure of consumption.

An excellent cooling beverage, known in the country as Gill Tea, is made from this plant, 1 oz. of the herb being infused with a pint of boiling water, sweetened with honey, sugar or liquorice, and drunk when cool in wineglassful doses, three or four times a day. This used to be a favourite remedy with the poor for coughs of long standing, being much used in consumption. Ground Ivy was at one time one of the cries of London for making a tea to purify the blood. It is a wholesome drink and is still considered serviceable in pectoral complaints and in cases of weakness of the digestive organs, being stimulating and tonic, though it has long been discarded from the *Materia Medica* as an official plant, in favour of others of greater certainty of action. As a medicine useful in pulmonary complaints, where a tonic for the kidneys is required, it would appear to possess peculiar suitability, and is well adapted to all kidney complaints.

A fluid extract is also prepared, the dose being from $\frac{1}{2}$ to 1 drachm. It has a bitter and acrid taste and a strong and aromatic odour.

The expressed juice of the fresh herb is diaphoretic, diuretic and somewhat astringent; snuffed up the nose, it has been considered curative of headache when all other remedies have failed. A snuff made from the dried leaves of Ground Ivy will render marked relief against a dull, congestive headache of the passive kind.

The expressed juice may also be advantageously used for bruises and 'black eyes.' It is also employed as an antiscorbutic, for which it has a long-standing reputation. Combined with Yarrow or Chamomile Flowers it is said to make an excellent poultice for abscesses, gatherings and tumours.

In America, painters used the Ground Ivy as a preventive of, and remedy for lead colic, a wineglassful of the freshly-made infusion being taken frequently.

The infusion is also used with advantage as a wash for sore and weak eyes.

Gerard says:

'it is commended against the humming noise and ringing sound of the ears, being put into them, and for them that are hard of hearing. Matthiolus writeth that the juice being tempered with Verdergrease is good against fistulas and hollow ulcers. Dioscorides teacheth that "half a dram of the leaves being drunk in foure ounces and a half of faire water for 40 or 50 days together is a remedy against sciatica or ache in the huckle-bone."

Galen hath attributed all the virtues to the flowers. Ground Ivy, Celandine and Daisies, of each a like quantity, stamped, strained and a little sugar and rose-water put thereto, and dropt into the eyes, takes away all manner of inflammation, etc., yea, although the sight were well-nigh gone. It is proved to be the best medicine in the world. The women of our Northern parts, especially Wales and Cheshire, do turn Herbe-Ale-hoof into their ale – but the reason I know not. It also purgeth the head from rheumatic humours flowing from the brain.'

Culpepper, repeating much that Gerard has already related of the virtues of Ground Ivy, adds that it is

'a singular herb for all inward wounds, ulcerated lungs and other parts, either by itself or boiled with other like herbs; and being drank, in a short time it easeth all griping pains, windy and choleric humours in the stomach, spleen, etc., helps the yellow jaundice by opening the stoppings of the gall and liver, and melancholy by opening the stoppings of the spleen; the decoction of it in wine drank for some time together procureth ease in sciatica or hip gout; as also the gout in the hands, knees or feet; if you put to the decoction some honey and a little burnt alum, it is excellent to gargle any sore mouth or throat, and to wash sores and ulcers; it speedily heals green wounds, being bruised and bound thereto.'

He concludes his account of the herb by saying:

'It is good to tun up with new drink, for it will clarify it in a night that it will be the fitter to be drank the next morning; or if any drink be thick with removing or any other accident, it will do the like in a few hours.'

(*POISON*)
IVY, POISON

Rhus Toxicodendron (LINN.)
N.O. Anacardiaceæ

Synonyms. Poison Oak. Poison Vine
Part Used. Leaves
Habitat. The American Poison Ivy is one of the species of Sumachs, an attractive group of plants widely distributed in Europe, Asia and North America, varying much in habit from low bushes to moderately-sized trees, and many of them familiar denizens of our gardens, for the sake of their ornamental foliage, which mostly assume beautiful tints in autumn, some of the varieties also bearing showy fruits. It grows in thickets and low grounds in North America, where it is quite common

Its sap is of an extremely poisonous character, and in many persons the slightest contact with the leaves causes a rash of a most distressing character, the hands and arms and sometimes the whole body becoming greatly swollen from simply touching or carrying a branch of the plant, the swelling being accompanied with intolerable pain and inflammation,

ending in ulceration. Some persons, however, are able to handle the plant with impunity. It has been sometimes known as *Ampelopsis Hoggii,* and under this name has occasionally been introduced with other climbers, but it has nothing to do with the group of Vines known under the name of *Ampelopsis,* and its presence in our gardens should be avoided.

443

¶ *Description.* The root is reddish and branching; the leaves rather large, three-parted (which will readily distinguish it from the five-parted *Ampelopsis*). The central leaflet has a longer stalk, the lateral ones are almost stalkless. The leaflets are entire when young, but when full-grown they are variously indented, downy beneath, thin and about 4 inches long. They abound with an acrid juice, which darkens when exposed to air, and when applied to the skin produces the inflammation and swelling referred to. When dry, the leaves are papery and brittle, sometimes with black spots of exuded juice turned black on drying. The flowers are in loose, slender clusters or panicles, in the axils of the leaves and are small, some perfect, others unisexual, and are greenish or yellowish-white in colour. They blossom in June, and are followed by clusters of small, globular, dun-coloured, berry-like fruit.

There are almost as many antidotes for the inflammation caused by Poison Ivy as for the bites of the rattlesnake. Alkaline lotions, especially carbonate of soda, alum and hyposulphite of soda, are all recommended, and the patient is advised to moisten the skin constantly with the agent in solution. A hot solution of potassium permanganate applied locally is also recommended as a cure, also solutions of lead and ammonia. *Rhus venenata* has similar poisonous qualities.

¶ *Part Used Medicinally.* The fresh leaves, from which a fluid extract is prepared.

¶ *Constituents.* The activity of the drug was formerly ascribed to a fixed oil, Toxicodendrol, but has been attributed more recently to a yellow resin, to which the name Toxicodendrin is applied.

¶ *Medicinal Action and Uses.* Irritant, rubefacient, stimulant, narcotic.

R. Toxicodendron was introduced into England first in 1640, but not used as a medicine till 1798, when Du Fressoy, a physician at Valenciennes, had brought to his notice a young man, who had been cured of a herpetic eruption on his wrist of six years' standing, on being accidentally poisoned by this plant. He thereupon commenced the use of the plant in the treatment of obstinate herpetic eruptions and in palsy, many cases yielding well to the drug. Since then it has rapidly gained a place in general practice, meeting with some success in the treatment of paralysis, acute rheumatism and articular stiffness, and in various forms of chronic and obstinate eruptive diseases.

It is not official in the British Pharmacopœia, but was formerly official in the United States Pharmacopœia. It is in extensive use by homœopathists for rheumatism, ringworm and other skin disorders, and is considered by them one of the most useful remedies in a great majority of cases of Nettlerash, especially if caused by some natural predisposition of constitution, in which the eruption is due to the use of some particular food.

The fluid extract, prepared from the fresh leaves, is mostly given in the form of a tincture, in doses of 5 to 30 drops. In small doses it is an excellent sedative to the nervous system, but must be given with care, as internally it may cause gastric intestinal irritation, drowsiness, stupor and delirium.

It has been recommended in cases of incontinence of urine. For this, the bark of the root of *R. aromatica* is also employed very successfully, an infusion of 1 oz. to a pint of boiling water being taken in wineglassful doses.

The fluid extract of *R. Toxicodendron* can be used as a vesicant or blister producer, like cantharides, mezeron, and oil of Mustard.

The best preparation is a concentrated alcoholic tincture made from the green plant in the strength of 1 in 4. The dose of 25 per cent. tincture is given in 1 to 5 drops three times a day. A solid extract is not used owing to the extreme volatility of the active principles of the crude drug.

Its milky juice is also used as an indelible ink for marking linen, and as an ingredient of liquid dressings or varnishes for finishing boots or shoes, though *R. venenata* is more extensively used for the latter purpose.

See SUMACHS.

JABORANDI

Pilocarpus Jaborandi (HOLMES.)
N.O. Rutaceæ

Synonyms. Arruda do Mato. Arruda brava. Jamguarandi. Juarandi
Part Used. Dried leaflets
Habitat. Brazil

¶ *Description.* There is divergence of opinion among recognized authorities as to the origin of the drug known as Jaborandi. Not only is the name applied to plants of quite different species in South America, but various shrubs are recognized as official in some countries that are classed as inferior substitutes in others.

Until 1914 *Pilocarpus Jaborandi* only was regarded as official in the British Pharmacopœia, but in the edition of that year it was omitted. In the United States *P. Jaborandi* is

JABORANDI

recognized as Pernambuco Jaborandi, and *P. microphyllus* as Maranham Jaborandi. Pernambuco Jaborandi was at first referred to *P. pennatifolius*, the leaves of which are now rarely found in commerce, and some writers describe this as being probably the true source of the drug. The uncertainty appears to be due to the fact that the fruit of the different species is not known to botanists, the drug being only introduced into Europe in 1847.

The names of Jaborandi, Iaborandi, and Jamborandi are applied to sundry pungent plants of the Rutaceæ and Piperaceæ orders, and especially to *Piper Jaborandi*.

The shrub grows from 4 to 5 feet high; the bark is smooth and greyish; the flowers are thick, small, and reddish-purple in colour, springing from rather thick, separate stalks about ¼ inch long. The leaves are large, compound, pinnate with an odd terminal leaflet, with two to four pairs of leaflets.

They are chiefly exported from Ceara and Pernambuco, and only the leaflets are officinal, though they arrive mixed with petioles and small fruits. The colour is brownish-green, the margin entire, with a notch cut out at the blunt tip of the leaf, which except in the case of the terminal leaflet, is unequal at the base. They are hairless, leathery, with large oil-glands, from 2½ to 4 inches long, and when crushed have a slightly aromatic odour. The taste is bitter and aromatic, becoming pungent. The powder is dark green or greenish brown.

¶ *Constituents.* A volatile oil, containing dipentene and other hydrocarbons, tannic acid, a peculiar volatile acid, and potassium chloride. The principal constituents are the three alkaloids, Pilocarpine (not found in all species), Isopilocarpine and Pilocarpidine.

Pilocarpine, only in the proportion of 0·5 per cent., is found as a soft, viscous mass yielding crystalline salts, freely soluble in alcohol, ether, and chloroform, and only slightly soluble in water. The nitrate should melt at 1·78° C. It is a white, crystalline powder, soluble in 95 per cent. alcohol, and giving a yellowish solution with strong sulphuric acid.

Various hypodermic solutions are prepared from it.

Hydrochlorate of Pilocarpine is official in the United States, and in some European Pharmacopœias.

¶ *Medicinal Action and Uses.* The crude drug is rarely used, its virtues being due to the alkaloid, Pilocarpine. It is antagonistic to atropine, stimulating the nerve-endings paralysed by that drug, and contracting the pupil of the eye. Its principal use is as a powerful and rapid diaphoretic, the quantity of sweat brought out by a single dose being as much as 9 to 15 oz. It induces also free salivation and excites most gland secretions, some regarding it as a galactagogue.

Jaborine, of which there is a small quantity in the leaves, resembles atropine, and is antagonistic to pilocarpine, so that an impure pilocarpine may vary largely in effect.

Jaborandi may irritate the stomach and cause vomiting and nausea, as may pilocarpine, even when given as a subcutaneous injection, but these symptoms yield to morphine.

It is useful in psoriasis, prurigo, deafness depending on syphilitic disease of the labyrinth, baldness, chronic catarrh, catarrhal jaundice, tonsillitis, and particularly dropsy. Probably it is most popularly known in preparations for the hair. In small doses it quenches thirst in fever or chronic renal diseases.

It is contra-indicated in fatty heart or pleurisy.

¶ *Dosages.* Of Powdered leaves, 5 to 60 grains. Of Pilocarpine, $\frac{1}{20}$ to ¼ grain. Of Pilocarpine Nitrate, $\frac{1}{20}$ to ¼ grain. Of Fluid extract, B.P., 10 to 30 drops. Of Tincture, B.P., ½ to 1 drachm.

¶ *Poisons with Antidotes.* An overdose may cause flushing, profuse sweating and salivation, nausea, rapid pulse, contracted pupils, diarrhœa, and even fatal pulmonary œdema. The stomach should be emptied and a full dose of atropine given.

¶ *Other Species.*

P. microphyllus, with smaller and more yellowish leaves, is regarded as identical in constituents in the United States.

P. pennatifolius, or *P. pinnatus* or *P. simplex*, inhabits Southern Brazil and Paraguay. The leaves are paler than the official ones, and contain little alkaloid. They are sometimes known as 'Paraguay Jaborandi.'

P. Selloamus, a variety of the above, with fleshier leaflets, yields Rio Janeiro Jaborandi. It was formerly official in the United States.

P. trachylophus, with smaller leaves, gives Ceara Jaborandi. It grows in Northern Brazil.

P. spicatus, giving Aracati Jaborandi, has simple lanceolate leaves said to have a high percentage of alkaloid.

P. racemosus of the West Indies, including a good percentage of alkaloids, yields Guadeloupe Jaborandi.

¶ *Substitutes.* Logwood leaves have been substitutes for Paraquay Jaborandi under the name of 'Feuilles de Bois d'inde.'

Leaves of *Tunatea decipiens*, or *Swartzia decipiens* are often mixed in parcels of *P. microphyllus*.

445

JACOB'S LADDER

Polemonium cœruleum (LINN.)
N.O. Polemoniaceæ

Synonyms. Greek Valerian. Charity
Part Used. Herb

Habitat. This species is found wild in bushy places and by the side of streams, apparently indigenous, from Stafford and Derby northwards to the Cheviots, but doubtedly indigenous elsewhere, and when found in Scotland and Ireland, only an escape from gardens

The Greek Valerian (*Polemonium cœruleum*, Linn.) is not a Valerian at all, but belongs to the natural order Polemoniaceæ, the family of the Phloxes. Cats are, however, nearly as fond of the smell of this plant as of the true Valerian, and will frequently roll on it and injure it, and hence, perhaps, it has been popularly termed Valerian. It does not possess any of the medicinal qualities of the Valerians, and has nothing in common with them except in the shape of the leaves.

It is a common garden plant, with showy, blue flowers, and is called 'Jacob's Ladder,' from its successive pairs of leaflets. The name of the genus, *Polemonium*, is somewhat obscure – it is apparently derived from the Greek *polemos* (war), but its application is unexplained.

¶ *Description.* The plant is bright green and smooth, the upper portion generally clothed with short, gland-tipped hairs. The perennial root-stock is short and creeping, the stem 18 inches to 3 feet high, hollow and angular; the leaves, with very numerous pairs of entire leaflets, ½ to 1 inch long. The flowers are very numerous, terminating the stem of branches, slightly drooping, the corollas ¾ to 1 inch across, deep blue, with short tubes and five broad, spreading segments. The stamens, inserted at the throat of the tube, have yellow anthers.

A handsome form, frequent in gardens, has variegated leaves and white flowers.

¶ *Medicinal Action and Uses.* Culpepper says of it:

'It is under Mercury, and is alexipharmic, sudorific, and cephalic, and useful in malignant fevers and pestilential distempers; it helps in nervous complaints, headaches, trembling, palpitations of the heart, vapours, etc. It is good in hysteric cases, and epilepsies have been cured by the use of this herb.'

He tells us also, 'it is planted in gardens, and is found wild in some parts of Yorkshire.'

P. reptans (Linn.) (Abscess Root), known also as FALSE JACOB'S LADDER, is used in herbal medicine for its diaphoretic, astringent and expectorant qualities; an infusion of the root being considered useful in coughs, colds, and bronchial and lung complaints, producing copious perspiration; has been considered to have similar diaphoretic and astringent action to Jacob's Ladder.

See ABSCESS ROOT.

JALAP. *See* BINDWEED

JAMAICA DOGWOOD. *See* DOGWOOD

JAMBUL

Eugenia Jambolana (LANK.)
N.O. Myrtaceæ

Synonyms. Jambul. Jamum. Rose Apple. Java Plum. Syzygium Jumbolana
Part Used. Seeds, bark
Habitat. India, East Indies, Queensland

¶ *Description.* A tree from 20 to 30 feet high, with long narrow peach-like leaves; flowers a greeny-yellow colour, in terminal bunches, blooming in July; the fruit about the size of a hen's egg, varying from white to red and rose colour, in scent and taste like a ripe apricot. It was cultivated in England by Miller in 1768. The bark is dense and hard, pinky or reddy-brown colour, with a thick corky substance, whitish grey mottled, often ridged; the inner surface has a silky lustre; freshly fractured it shows a colour varying from fawn to a pinky purple, abruptly shortly fibrous; seeds are oval, ½ inch long and ¼ inch round, hard, heavy, blacky-grey colour, almost tasteless.

¶ *Constituents.* Essential oil, chlorophyll, fat, resin, gallic and tannic acids, albumen and in their seed ellagic acid.

¶ *Medicinal Action and Uses.* In India Jambul has long been used as a carminative in diarrhœa; stomachic and astringent. The fresh seeds have been found most effective in diabetes, as they quickly reduce sugar in the urine; also very beneficial in glycosuria. No poisoning or other harmful effects have been reported from its use.

¶ *Preparations and Dosages.* Van Morden advises: Fluid extract, ½ fluid ounce should be taken in 8 oz. hot water 1 hour before breakfast and before going to bed. Fluid extract, 1 to 2 drachms. Powdered seeds, 5 to 30 grains.

JASMINES

The Jasmine, or Jessamine (the name derived from the Persian *Yasmin*), belongs botanically to the genus *Jasminum*, of the natural order Oleaceæ, which contains about 150 species, mostly natives of the warmer regions of the Old World. About forty of these are cultivated in our gardens.

¶ *Description*. Their leaves are mostly ternate or pinnate; the flowers, usually white or yellow, with a tubular, five- or eight-cleft calyx, a cylindrical corolla-tube, with a spreading limb, two stamens enclosed in the corolla-tube and a two-celled ovary.

¶ *Habitat*. The COMMON WHITE JASMINE (*Jasminum officinale*), one of the best known and most highly esteemed of British hardy ligneous climbers, is a native of Northern India and Persia, introduced about the middle of the sixteenth century. In the centre and south of Europe it is thoroughly acclimatized.

Although it grows to the height of 12 and sometimes 20 feet, its stem is feeble and requires support. Its leaves are opposite, pinnate and dark green, the leaflets are in three pairs, with an odd one and are pointed, the terminal one larger with a tapering point. The fragrant flowers bloom from June to October; and as they are found chiefly on the young shoots, the plant should only be pruned in the autumn.

Varieties with golden and silver-edged leaves and one with double flowers are known.

¶ *Medicinal Action and Uses*. The roots of several species of *Jasminum* have had various ill-defined uses in medicine – that of *J. officinale* is mentioned by Millspaugh (*American Medicinal Plants*) as 'a proven plant' in the homœopathic sense, though he adds: 'the authority for the use of which I am unable to determine.'

The Dispensatory of the U.S.A. cites the case of a child, in 1861, being poisoned by the fruit of Jasmin,

'probably that of the common White species, *J. officinale*, the symptoms being coma, widely dilated pupil, snoring respiration, with cold, pale surface; slow, feeble pulse, followed by violent convulsions, with rigidity of muscle about head and throat.'

A palatable syrup can be prepared from the flowers. A preparation of the flowers has been employed medicinally. Green, in his *Universal Herbal* (1832), recommends :

'as an excellent medicine in coughs, hoarsenesses and other disorders of the breast, an infusion of five or six ounces of them picked clean from the leaves, in a quart of boiling water, being strained off and boiled in a syrup,

N.O. Oleaceæ and Jasminaceæ

with the addition of a sufficient quantity of honey.'

The SPANISH or CATALONIAN JASMINE (*J. grandiflorum*), a native of the north-west Himalayas, and cultivated in the Old and New World, is very like *J. officinale*, but differs in the size of the leaflets; the branches are shorter and stouter and the flowers very much larger and reddish beneath.

This is the Jasmine of the perfumery trade, one of the flowers most valued by perfumers, and grown at Grasse. Its delicate, sweet odour is so peculiar that it is without comparison one of the most distinct of all natural odours, and until quite recent years, it was believed that it was the only scent that could not be made artificially. A synthetic Otto of Jasmine now exists, however, its composition following more or less closely the constitution of the natural oil, containing benzyl acetate, a benzyl ester found in the natural oil of Jasmine, but the true perfume of Jasmine is not, however, exactly reproducible by any combination of chemical compounds or other natural products thus far known, and a proportion of the natural otto must be added to the mixture of synthetic substances to make the product satisfactory.

This Jasmine is very extensively cultivated at Cannes and Grasse. It is not grown on its own roots, but grafted on to two-year-old plants of *J. officinale*, an erect bush about 3 feet high being obtained, requiring no supports. The plants are set in rows, fully exposed to the sun, in a fresh, open soil, well sheltered from north winds, as they are very susceptible to cold and readily damaged by frost. They come into full bearing the second year after grafting. The blossoms, which are very large and intensely fragrant, are produced from July till the end of October, but those of August and September are the most odoriferous, the normal harvest being generally in full swing about the middle of August. The flowers open every morning at six o'clock and are culled after sunrise, as the morning dew would injure their fragrance. An acre of land will yield about 500 lb. weight of Jasmine blossoms.

A fungus, *Agaricus melleus*, is a plague of the Jasmine fields, attacking the roots of the grafted plants. When this mushroom has invaded a plantation, it is most difficult to combat, and the plants often have to be rooted out, causing much loss. It is not possible to grow Jasmine twice in succession on the same site, and the crop is replaced by roses or olives.

The perfume is extracted by the process

447

known as *enfleurage*, i.e. absorption by a fatty body, such as purified lard or olive oil. Jasmine flowers contain, when picked, only a portion of the perfume which they are capable of yielding, so fresh oil is developed by the flowers as the solvent removes what was originally present.

Square glass trays, framed with wood about 3 inches deep, are spread over with grease about ½ inch thick, in which ridges are made to facilitate absorption, and sprinkled with freshly-gathered flowers, which are renewed every morning during the whole time the plant remains in blossom. The trays are piled up in stacks to prevent the evaporation of the aroma and finally the pomade is scraped off the glass, melted at as low a temperature as possible and strained.

When oil is employed as the absorbent, coarse cotton cloths previously saturated with the finest olive oil are laid on wire-gauze frames, and are repeatedly covered in the same manner with fresh flowers. They are then squeezed under a press, yielding what is termed *huile antique au jasmin*. Three pounds of flowers will perfume 1 lb. of grease. This is extracted by maceration in 1 pint of rectified spirit to form the 'Extract.'

A small amount of Jasmine oil is prepared by extracting the blossoms with petroleum spirit and evaporating the solvent at a low temperature, but this treatment by killing the flower at once, stops the process of scent formation, so that the yield of oil is only one-fifth (some say one-ninth) of that extracted by fats in the enfleurage process. The Jasmine oil obtained by extraction with volatile solvents is a pale-brown liquid with a pleasant odour, which is quite distinct, however, from that of Jasmine pomade.

¶ *Constituents.* The essential oil of *J. grandiflorum* contains methyl anthranilate, indol, benzyl alcohol, benzyl acetate, and the terpenes linalol and linalyl acetate.

As essential oil is distilled from Jasmine in Tunis and Algeria, but its high price prevents its being used to any extent.

The East Indian oil of Jasmine is a compound, largely contaminated with sandal-wood-oil.

Syrup of Jasmine is made by placing in a jar alternate layers of the flowers and sugar, covering the whole with wet cloths and standing it in a cool place. The perfume is absorbed by the sugar, which is converted into a very palatable syrup.

The ZAMBAK, or ARABIAN JASMINE (*J. Sambac*), is an evergreen white-flowered climber, 6 or 8 feet high, introduced into Britain in the latter part of the seventeenth century. Two varieties introduced somewhat later are respectively three-leaved and double-flowered, and these, as well as that with normal flowers, bloom throughout the greater part of the year.

The Hindus string the flowers together as neck garlands for honoured guests. The flowers of one of the double varieties are held sacred to Vishnu and are used as votive offerings in Hindu religious ceremonies.

At Ghazipur, a town on the Ganges, Jasmine, there called *Chameli*, is used mainly for making perfumed hair oils by a process of enfleurage. The odour is absorbed in sesame seeds. The seeds are prepared by washing and rubbing, and when decorticated are dried. The prepared seeds and flowers are placed in alternate layers and allowed to remain for twelve to fourteen hours. The seeds are then separated from the flowers and repeatedly treated in the same way with fresh flowers. The spent flowers are used over and over again with fresh till seeds, these latter giving oil of an inferior quality. The oil obtained from seeds treated with fresh flowers only is the best. The perfumed seeds are pressed in an ordinary wooden country press borne by bullocks. The method is crude, wasteful, tedious and dirty. Some Otto of Jasmine is also made at Ghazipur.

In Borneo it is the custom among the women to roll up Jasmine blossoms in their well-oiled hair at night.

¶ *Medicinal Action and Uses.* An oil obtained by boiling the *leaves* of this Eastern Jasmine is used to anoint the head for complaints of the eye, and an oil obtained from the *roots* is used medicinally to arrest the secretion of milk.

In China JASMINUM PANICULATUM is cultivated. It is an erect shrub, valued for its flowers and known as *Sien-hing-hwa*, the flowers being used with those of *J. Sambac*, *Sambac-mo-le-hwa*, in the proportion of 10 lb. of the former to 30 lb. of the latter for scenting tea, 40 lb. of the mixture being required for 100 lb. of tea.

In Catalonia and in Turkey, the wood of the Jasmine is made into long, slender pipe-stems.

JASMINUM ANGUSTIFOLIUM, an Indian species, found in the Coromandel forest and introduced into Britain during the present century, is a beautiful evergreen climber, 10 to 12 feet high, its leaves of a bright shining green, its large, terminal flowers, white with a faint tinge of red, fragrant and in bloom throughout the year. Its bitter root, ground and mixed with the powdered root of *Acorus calamus*, the Sweet Sedge, is in India considered a valuable external application for ringworm.

In Cochin-China, a decoction of the leaves and branches of JASMINUM NERVOSUM is taken as a blood-purifier. The very bitter leaves of JASMINUM FLORIBUNDUM (called in Abyssinia, *Habbez-zelim*), mixed with kousso, is considered a powerful anthelmintic, especially for tapeworm; the leaves and branches are added to some fermented liquors to increase their intoxicating quality.

The distinguishing characters of the TRUE YELLOW JASMINE (*J. odoratissimum*), a native of the Canary Islands and Madeira, consist principally in the alternate, obtuse, ternate leaves, the three-flowered terminal peduncles and the five-cleft yellow corolla, with obtuse segments. The flowers have the advantage, when dry, of retaining their natural perfume, which is suggestive of a mixture of Jasmine, jonquil and orange-blossom.

Among other hardy species commonly cultivated in gardens are the low ITALIAN YELLOW-FLOWERED JASMINE (*J. humile*), an East Indian species, introduced into the south of Europe and now found wild there – an erect shrub, 3 or 4 feet high, with angular branches alternate and mostly ternate leaves, blossoming from June to September; JASMINUM FRUTICANS (Linn.) (*J. frutescens*, Gueldermeister), a native of Southern Europe and the Mediterranean region, a hardy, evergreen shrub, 10 to 12 feet high, with weak, slender stems, requiring support and bearing yellow, odourless flowers from spring to autumn, and JASMINUM NUDIFLORUM (Roth.) (*J. pubescens*, Willd.), of China, which bears its bright yellow flowers in winter before the leaves appear. It thrives in almost any situation and grows rapidly. The important medicinal plant known in America as the 'Carolina Jasmin' (*Gelsemium nitidum*) is not a true Jasmine, though often called 'Yellow Jasmine.' A more correct name for it is 'False Jasmine.'

The rhizome of *J. fruticans* is sometimes collected in the place of *Gelsemium*, but may be distinguished by the cells of the pith, which are thin-walled and full of starch, while those of *Gelsemium* are thick-walled and empty. *See* GELSEMIUM.

From the leaves of *J. fruticans*, the glucoside Jasminin has been isolated, and from the shoots of *J. nudiflorum*, the glucoside, Jasminiflorin.

Other plants called 'Jasmine,' but not related to it, are:

(i) The so-called American Jasmine (*Quamoclit coccinea*).

(ii) The Red Jasmine (*Plumiera rubra*), a shrubby tree, native to Central America, with delicately-scented flowers, which have obtained for it this name. Another member of the genus, *P. alba*, is known as the Frangipani plant, its scent having been characterized as 'the eternal perfume.'

(iii) The Cape Jasmine (*Gardenia florida*), with a strong, pleasant fragrance similar to that of Jasmine, much employed for 'buttonholes' and in wreaths, and in China, under the name of *Pak-Semahwa*, for scenting tea. Another Chinese species, *G. grandiflora*, is employed in dyeing the yellow robes of the mandarins. The fruit of *G. campanulata*, a species growing in the forests of Chittagong, is said to be used by the natives as acathartic and anthelmintic.

(iv) The Ground Jasmine (*Passerina stelleri*) is like the *Gardenia*, also a native of the Cape.

The WILD JASMINE or WHITE JASMINE OF JAMAICA (called there, 'Jamaica Wild Coffee'), with very fragrant white flowers, is a species of *Pavetta*. The Pavettas are shrubs inhabiting the tropical regions. The root of *P. Indica* is bitter and is employed as a purgative by the Hindus, the leaves being also used medicinally and for manuring; knife handles being made from the roots.

The leaves of the Indian Night Jasmine (*Nyctanthes arbortristis* – N.O. Jasminaceæ) are used in homœopathic medicine to make a tincture for rheumatism, sciatica and bilious fevers. – EDITOR.

JEQUIRITY. *See* INDIAN LIQUORICE

JEWELWEED

Impatiens aurea (MUHL.)
Impatiens biflora (WALT.)
N.O. Geraniaceæ

Synonyms. Wild Balsam. Balsam-weed. Impatiens pallida. Pale-touch-me-not. Spotted-touch-me-not. Slipperweed. Silverweed. Wild Lady's Slipper. Speckled Jewels. Wild Celandine. Quick-in-the-hand

Part Used. Herb

Habitat. Members of the genus *Impatiens* are found widely distributed in the north temperate zone and in South Africa, but the majority are natives of the mountains of tropical Asia and Africa

The flowers, purple, yellow, pink and white, sometimes a showy scarlet, are spurred and irregular in form and are borne in the leaf axils.

The name *Impatiens* is derived from the fact that the seed-pod, when ripe, discharges the seeds by the elastic separation and uncoiling of the valves.

Under the name of Jewelweed the herbage of *Impatiens aurea* and of *I. biflora* are largely employed in domestic practice and by homœopaths and eclectics.

¶ *Description.* The plants are tall and branching, tender and delicate succulent annuals, with swollen joints, growing in lowlying, damp, rather rich soil, beside streams and in similar damp localities.

They are smooth and somewhat glaucous, the stems somewhat translucent, the foliage showing a brilliant silvery surface when immersed in water, which will not adhere to the surface.

The leaves are thin, ovate oval, more or less toothed, of a tender green colour.

The slipper-shaped, yellow flowers, in bloom from July to September, have long recurved tails, those of the first-named species being of a uniform pale-yellow, those of the second species, orange-yellow, crowded with dark spots, hence its common name of Spotted-touch-me-not. The oblong capsules of both species when ripe explode under the slightest disturbance, scattering the seeds widely. Most of the popular names refer to this peculiarity, others to the shape of the flowers.

¶ *Medicinal Action and Uses.* The herbs have an acrid, burning taste and act strongly as emetics, cathartics and diuretics, but are considered dangerous, their use having been termed 'wholly questionable.'

¶ *Constituents.* The chemical constituents are not known, though the leaves apparently contain tannin, which causes them to be employed as an outward application for piles, proving an excellent remedy, the freshly gathered plants being boiled in lard and an ointment made of them.

The fresh juice of the herb appears to relieve cutaneous irritation of various kinds, especially that due to *Rhus* poisoning.

A yellow dye has been made from the flowers.

¶ *Other Species.*
The only species of *Impatiens* found wild in

Europe is *I. Noli-me-tangere*, an annual, succulent herb about a foot high, with yellow flowers, in bloom in July and August, the lateral petals spotted with red (by cultivation, changing often to pale yellow and purplish).

This is our native 'Touch-me-not' or 'Quick-in-hand.' Although uncommon, it is to be found wild in moist mountainous districts in North Wales, Lancashire and Westmorland and occasionally in moist, shady places and by the banks of rivulets in other counties.

The plant will grow in cultivation, delighting in a moist soil and partially-shaded situations; the seeds being sown in autumn, soon after they are ripe. When once established, the plant will scatter its own seeds.

The whole plant is rather acrid, so that no animal except the goat will touch it.

It was formerly considered to have diuretic and vulnerary properties and was given to relieve hæmorrhoids and strangury.

Boerhaave, the famous Dutch physician (1668–1738), considered it poisonous.

I. balsamin a, the Common Balsam of gardens, a well-known annual, is a native of India, China and Japan. It is one of the showiest of summer and autumn flowers and of comparatively easy cultivation.

In the East, the natives use the prepared juice for dyeing their nails red.

I. Roylei, a tall, hardy, succulent annual, with rose-purple flowers, a Himalayan species, is common in England as a self-sown garden plant or garden escape.

I. Sultani, a handsome plant, with scarlet flowers, a native of Zanzibar, is easily grown in a greenhouse throughout the summer, but requires warmth in winter.

I. Cornuta, the 'Horned Balsam,' has long nectaries to its flowers, the spurs being three times as long as the corollas. In Ceylon it is called the 'Swallow-leaf.'

The whole plant is fragrant and in Cochin-China, where it is a common garden weed, a decoction of the leaves is used as a hairwash, imparting a very sweet odour.

The 'Balsam Apple' is not related to the *Impatiens,* but is the fruit of *Momordica balsamina.*

JOHN'S BREAD

Ceratonia siliqua (LINN.)
N.O. Leguminosæ

Synonyms. Locust Pods. Carob. Algaroba (Spain). Bharout (Arabia). Sugar Pods
Part Used. Fruit
Habitat. Southern Europe, Africa and Asia – bordering on the Mediterranean

¶ *Description.* There was a tradition that this tree was the food of St. John in the wilderness, and the name is derived from the legend.

It is very common in the south of Spain, where it forms a small branching tree about 30 feet high, the wood of which has a pretty pinkish hue. Leaves pinnate in two or three pairs of oval blunt-topped leaflets, leathery texture, and colour shiny dark green. Flowers in small red racemes followed by flat pods 6 to 12 inches long and fully 1 inch wide, ¼ inch thick, a shiny dark browny purple colour. They do not split open when ripe; they contain a number of seeds in a line along the centre of the pods, each seed in a separate cell of fleshy pulp. This tree is much cultivated in dry parts because its long roots can grow deep enough in the ground to find moisture. The pods contain a large amount of mucilage and saccharine matter of pleasant flavour, and are largely employed for feeding all sorts of animals, and in time of scarcity for human consumption. In 1811 and 1812 they formed the principal food of the British cavalry during the War; they have been imported in considerable quantities for cattle food, though they do not contain much

nutritive property, the saccharine matter being carbonaceous, or heat-giving, the seeds alone being nitrogenous. These seeds are so small and hard they often escape mastication.

¶ *Constituents*. Similar to Cassia pods, it is not known to what constituents its laxative properties are due.

¶ *Medicinal Action and Uses*. Years ago the seeds were sold at a high price by chemists, as singers imagined they cleared the voice. By fermentation and distillation they give an agreeable spirit, which retains the flavour of the pod. The seeds were once used by jewellers as the original carat weight. Johannisbrod, so greatly esteemed in Germany, is made from the pulp of the Syrian *Ceratonia siliqua*. The fruit of John's Bread have similar constituents to those of Cassia pods and are also laxative and demulcent, with an odour somewhat like valerian.

¶ *Dosage*. Same as for Cassia pulp and pods.

JUJUBE BERRIES

Zizyphus vulgaris (LAMK.)
N.O. Rhamnaceæ

Synonyms. Zizyphus sativa. Brustbeeren. Judendornbeeren. Rhamnus Zizyphus
Part Used. Fruit
Habitat. Southern Europe

¶ *Habitat*. Originally a native of Syria, *Zizyphus vulgaris* was introduced into Italy in the reign of Augustus, and is now naturalized in Provence, and particularly in the islands of Hyères, where the berries are largely collected when ripe, and dried in the sun.

The trees average 25 feet in height and are covered with a rough, brown bark. They have many branches, with annual thorny branchlets bearing alternate, oval-oblong leaves of a clear green colour, with three to five strongly-marked, longitudinous veins. The small flowers are pale yellow and solitary. The fruit is a blood-red drupe, the size and shape of an olive, sweet, and mucilaginous in taste, slightly astringent. The pulp becomes softer and sweeter in drying, and the taste more like wine. They have pointed, oblong stones.

¶ *Constituents*. A full analysis has not yet been made, but the berries are valued for their mucilage and sugar.

¶ *Medicinal Action and Uses*. The Jujube is classed with the raisin, date, and fig as a pectoral fruit, being nutritive and demulcent. It is eaten both fresh and dried.

A syrup and a *tisane* were formerly made from it, but the berries are now little used in medicine.

Jujube paste, or 'Pâte de Jujubes,' is made of gum-arabic and sugar. It may be dissolved in a decoction of jujubes and evaporated, but is considered as good a demulcent without their addition. It is frequently merely mixed with orange-flower water.

A decoction of the *roots* has been used in fevers.

An astringent decoction of leaves and branchlets is made in large quantities in Algeria, and seems likely to replace the cachou.

¶ *Other Species*.
Z. Lotos, sometimes also called *Z. sativa*, of Northern Africa and *Z. Jujuba* of the East Indies possess similar properties, and are used in their respective countries. *Z. Lotos* is thought to have been one of the sources of the famous sweet fruits from which the ancient Lotophagi took their name, the liqueur prepared from which caused those who partook of it to forget even their native countries in its enjoyment. The Arabs call it *Seedra*. In Arabia a kind of bread is made of them by exposing them to the sun for a few days and then pounding them in a wooden mortar to separate the stones. The meal is mixed with water and formed into cakes which after drying in the sun resemble sweet gingerbread.

Z. Baclei is said to be used in the same way in Africa, and also for making a beverage.

Z. Jujuba is largely cultivated by the Chinese, in many varieties as a dessert fruit, some being called Chinese Dates, and it is also one of the main sources of stick-lac.

Z. *Œnoplia* of India has edible fruits, and the bark is esteemed as a vulnerary.

In Cochin-China the berries of *Z. agrestis* are eaten.

In Senegal the fruits of *Z. Barelei* are slightly styptic, and the negroes use the roots for gonorrhœa. It is probably the same species that is used there in venereal diseases.

A decoction of the dried leaves of *Z. Napeca* is said to be used for washing ulcers in Arabia.

Z. spina Christi, or *Rhamnus spina Christi*, of Ethiopia, is said to be the source of the crown of thorns placed on the Saviour's head. The Arabs call it *Nabka*.

JUNIPER BERRIES

Juniperus communis (LINN.)
N.O. Coniferæ

Synonyms. Genévrier. Ginepro. Enebro. Gemeiner Wachholder
Parts Used. The ripe, carefully dried fruits, leaves
Habitat. Europe. North Africa. North Asia. North America

¶ *Habitat*. The Juniper is a small shrub, 4 to 6 feet high, widely distributed throughout the Northern Hemisphere. It occurs freely on the slopes of the chalk downs near London, and on heathy, siliceous soils where a little lime occurs. It is a common shrub where bands of limestone occur, as on some of the Scotch mountains and on the limestone hills in the Lake district.

The *berries* are used for the production of the volatile oil which is a prime ingredient in Geneva or Hollands Gin, upon which its flavour and diuretic properties depend.

¶ *History*. Although these valuable berries are produced from a native shrub, the berries of commerce are chiefly collected from plants cultivated in Hungary. The oil distilled on the Continent, principally in Hungary, is chiefly from freshly-picked berries. It has, hitherto, not been possible to produce the oil competitively with Southern Europe because of the relative cheapness of labour and the vast tracts of land over which the trees grow wild. But the rise in the price of foreign oil of Juniper berries since the outbreak of war has directed attention to the possible extended production of the oil either in Great Britain or her northern colonies. Sunny slopes are likely to be the best places to cultivate the shrub for the berries. The yield of oil, however, varies considerably in different years.

There is a wide difference in the chemical and physical characters of the oil distilled on the Continent from fresh and that in England from imported berries, which in transit to this country have become partially dried.

Commercial oil of Juniper is obtained chiefly from the ripe fruit and is stated to be in all essential qualities superior to the oil of Juniper from the full-grown, unripe, green berries used medicinally, which occurs as a colourless or pale greenish-yellow, limpid liquid, possessing a peculiar terebinthic odour when fresh, and a balsamic, burning, somewhat bitter taste.

Juniper berries take two or three years to ripen, so that blue and green berries occur on the same plant. Only the blue, ripe berries are here picked. When collected in baskets or sacks, they are laid out on shelves to dry a little, during which process they lose some of the blue bloom and develop the blackish colour seen in commerce.

There is a considerable demand on the Continent for an aqueous extract of the berries called *Roob*, or Rob of Juniper, and the distilled oil is in this case a by-product, the berries being first crushed and macerated with water and then distilled with water and the residue in the still evaporated to a soft consistence. Much of the oil met with in commerce is obtained as a by-product in the manufacture of gin and similar products.

In Sweden a beer is made that is regarded as a healthy drink. In hot countries the tree yields by incision a gum or varnish.

¶ *Constituents*. The principal constituent is the volatile oil, with resin, sugar, gum, water, lignin, wax and salines. The oil is most abundant just before the perfect ripeness and darkening of the fruit, when it changes to resin. The quantity varies from 2·34 to 0·31 per cent. *Juniper Camphor* is also present, its melting-point being 1·65° to 1·66° C.

Adulteration by oil of Turpentine can be recognized by the lowering of the specific gravity.

The tar is soluble in Turpentine oil, but not in 95 per cent. acetic acid.

Junol is the trade name of a hydro-alcoholic extract.

¶ *Medicinal Action and Uses*. Oil of Juniper is given as a diuretic, stomachic, and carminative in indigestion, flatulence, and diseases of the kidney and bladder. The oil mixed with lard is also used in veterinary practice as an application to exposed wounds and prevents irritation from flies.

Spirit of Juniper has properties resembling Oil of Turpentine: it is employed as a stimulating diuretic in cardiac and hepatic dropsy.

The fruit is readily eaten by most animals, especially sheep, and is said to prevent and cure dropsy in the latter.

The chief use of Juniper is as an adjuvant to diuretics in dropsy depending on heart, liver or kidney disease. It imparts a violet odour to the urine, and large doses may cause irritation to the passages. An infusion of 1 oz. to 1 pint of boiling water may be taken in the course of twenty-four hours.

In France the berries have been used in chest complaints and in leucorrhœa, blenorrhœa, scrofula, etc. They are not given in substance.

The oil is a local stimulant.

¶ *Dosage.* Oil of Berries, B.P., 1 to 5 drops. Oil of Wood, 1 to 5 drops. Fluid extract, ½ to 1 fluid drachm. Spirit of Juniper, B.P. and U.S.P., 20 to 60 minims. Oil, 2 to 10 minims. Elixir of Potassium Acetate and Juniper as a diaphoretic, 4 fluid drachms. Comp. Spirit, U.S.P., 2 drachms. Solid extract, 5 to 15 grains.

¶ *Other Species.*

Gum Juniper is a name of Sandarac, the resinous product of *Thuja articulata* or *Callitris quadrivalvis.*

From dry distillation of the branches and heartwood of *Juniperus oxycedrus*, the Prickly Cedar or Medlar Tree, a large shrub, 10 to 12 feet high, with brownish-black berries the size of a hazel nut, native of the south of France, and occasionally from that of *J. communis*, is obtained the tarry, empyreumatic oil known as Cade Oil, or Juniper Tar Oil, used in the treatment of the cutaneous diseases of animals in France and other Continental countries, and for most of the purposes of Oil of Turpentine. It is a ready solvent for chemical drugs and is used externally for chronic eczema as oil, ointment, and soap.

J. virginiana, the American Juniper of Bermuda, known also as Red Cedar and Pencil Cedar, is only an ornamental tree in Britain, introduced in 1864, and growing 40 to 50 feet high. The smallness of the stem and slowness of growth render it unsuitable for planting here with a view to profit, but in America it is much used for cabinet-making, turnery, etc. The interior wood is of a reddish colour and highly valued on account of its great durability, being suitable for exposure to all weather. The highly-coloured and fragrant heartwood is largely used in the manufacture of the wood coverings of black-lead pencils, and also for pails, tubs, and various household utensils subjected to wettings. Boxes made of the wood are useful for the preservation of woollens and furs, it being an excellent insectifuge on account of the oil contained in it.

Red Cedar Oil is an article of commerce, obtained from the wood by distillation from the chips and waste wood, from 15,000 to 20,000 lb. of oil being annually produced in the United States. It is used in the preparation of insecticides and also in making liniments and other medicinal preparations and perfumed soaps. It is used generally in perfumery and was formerly one of the principal constituents of the popular Extract of White Rose.

The *berries* in decoction are diaphoretic and emmenagogue, like those of Common Juniper, and the *leaves* have diuretic properties.

KAMALA

Mallotus Philippinensis (MUELL.)
N.O. Euphorbiaceæ

Synonyms. Glandulæ Rotteleræ. Kamcela. Spoonwood. Röttlera tinctoria

Parts Used. Glands and hairs covering the fruits

Habitat. India, at the foot of the Madras hills, Malay Archipelago, Orissa, Bengal, Bombay, Abyssinia, Southern Arabia, China, Australia

¶ *Description.* A very common small Indian tree, named after the Rev. Dr. Röttler, the naturalist, who died in 1836. It is 20 to 30 feet high, trunk 3 or 4 feet in diameter, branches slender with pale bark, the younger ones covered with dense ferruginous tomentosum; leaves alternate, articulate petioles, 1 to 2 inches long; rusty tomentose, blade 3 to 6 inches long, ovate with two obscure glands at base, entire, coriaceous, upper surface glabrous, veins very prominent on under surface, flowers diœcious. Males three together in the axils of small bracts arranged in longer much-branched axillary branches to the females, both densely covered with ferrugineous tomentosum, flowering November to January. From the surface of the trilobed capsules of the plant, which are about the size of peas, a red mealy powder is obtained; this consists of minute glands and hairs coloured brick or madder red, nearly odourless and tasteless; it is much used by the Hindu silk dyers, who obtain from it by boiling in carbonate of soda, a durable flame colour of great beauty. The capsules are ripe February and March, when the red powder is brushed off and collected for sale; no other preparation is necessary to preserve it.

¶ *Constituents.* Rottlerin, yellow and red resins, wax, and a yellow crystalline substance, tannic acid, gum, and volatile oil.

¶ *Medicinal Action and Uses.* The root of the tree is used in dyeing, and for cutaneous eruptions, also used by the Arabs internally for leprosy and in solution to remove freckles and pustules. In this country it has been successfully used for an eruption in children known as wildfire, the powder is rubbed over the affected part with moist lint. Its greatest use, however, is in the use of tapeworm, being safer and more certain than other cures; the worm is passed whole and generally dead. The dose of Kamala for a robust person is 3 drachms, but only half that quantity for anyone of enfeebled health; the fluid extract is milder and acts with more certainty.

Kamala acts quickly and actively as a purgative, and often causes much griping and nausea, but seldom vomiting. It may be given in water mucilage or syrup; the worm is usually expelled at the third or fourth stool; if it fails to act, the dose is repeated after four hours, or a dose of castor oil is given. Kamala is largely used in India externally for cutaneous troubles, and is most effective for scabies. It has been successfully employed in herpetic ringworm (a disease very prevalent there), and as a tænifuge it has been used with good results, on the Continent, combined with Kousso and known as Kama-kosin.

Kamala is insoluble in cold water and boiling water has little effect on it. The resin is the most active constituent, and is dissolved by ether, chloroform, alcohol or benzol. When exposed to a flame it explodes with a flash resembling Lycopodium.

¶ *Preparations and Dosages.* Powdered Kamala, 2 to 4 drachms. Fluid extract, 2 to 4 drachms.

¶ *Adulterations.* Kamala is often grossly adulterated; its quality can be judged by throwing a little on the surface of water, when the adulterants, such as sand, ferric oxide, etc., will sink, and the pure drug float; stalks and leaves can be easily sifted out. Dyed starch is detected by microscope, also ground safflower by same means.

¶ *Other Species.* (N.O. Leguminosæ.)

Flemingia congesta, under the name of wurrus (contains a substance similar to Kamala), is a large shrub growing in India and Africa, gives a dull dark purplish powder and consists of single not grouped hairs and glands, the glands being in tiers not radiating; wurrus contains two resins, one dark and the other orange brown, an orange red crystalline substance, flemingin and homoflemingin, principles which while resembling Kamala are not identical with it, but largely used in India as a dye, giving silk a lovely golden colour.

Rottlera Schimfeeri, the bark of which has anthelmintic properties.

KAVA KAVA

Piper Methysticum (FORST.)
N.O. Piperaceæ

Synonyms. Ava. Intoxicating Pepper. Ava Pepper
Part Used. The peeled, dried and divided rhizome
Habitat. Polynesia, Sandwich Islands, South Sea Islands. Official in the Australian Colonies

¶ *Description.* An indigenous shrub several feet high, leaves cordate, acuminate, with very short axillary spikes of flowers; stem dichotomous, spotted. The natives prepare a fermented liquor from the upper portion of the rhizome and base of the stems; it is narcotic and stimulant and is drunk before important religious rites. The root of the plant, chewed and mixed with the saliva, gives a hot intoxicating juice; it is mixed with pure water or the water of the coco-nut. Its continued use in large doses causes inflammation of the body and eyes, resulting in leprous ulcers; the skin becomes parched and peels off in scales. Commercial Kava rhizome is in whitish or grey-brown roughly wedge-shaped fragments from which the periderm is cut off about 2 inches thick; the transverse section usually shows a dense central pith, surrounded by a clean ring of vascular bundles, narrow and radiating, separated by broadish light-coloured medullary rays. Fracture starchy, faint pleasant odour, taste bitter, pungent, aromatic; it yields not more than 8 per cent. of ash.

¶ *Constituents.* Oil cells often contain a greenish-yellow resin, termed kawine; it is strongly aromatic and acrid; the plant contains a second resin less active than the first, a volatile oil and an alkaloid, Kavaine Methysticcum yangonin, and abundance of starch.

¶ *Medicinal Action and Uses.* The effect on the nerve centres is at first stimulating, then depressing, ending with paralysis of the respiratory centre. The irritant action and insolubility of the resin has lessened its use as a local anæsthetic, but for over 125 years Kava root has been found valuable in the treatment of gonorrhœa both acute and chronic, vaginitis, leucorrhœa, nocturnal incontinence and other ailments of the genito-urinary tract. It resembles pepper in local action. A 20 per cent. oil of Kava resin in oil of Sandalwood, called gonosan, is used internally for gonorrhœa. Being a local anæsthetic it relieves pain and has an aphrodisiac effect; it has also an antiseptic effect on the urine. The capsules contain 0·3 gram; two to four can be given several times per day. As Kava is a strong diuretic

KIDNEYWORT

Synonyms. Wall Pennywort. Penny Pies.

The Kidneywort or Navelwort (*Cotyledon Umbilicus*) is a remarkably succulent plant, mostly to be found on moist rocks and walls in the high-lying districts in the west of England.

The whole plant is a pale bright green and very smooth. The rootstock from which it springs is a small, roundish tuber, varying according to the size of the plant, from the dimension of a small pea to that of a large nut. The leaves, most of which grow directly from the rootstock, are in shape somewhat like those of the garden Nasturtium, being circular, their stalks, 2 to 6 inches long, springing from about the centre of their under-surfaces, an arrangement that is termed botanically *peltate*. The succulent blades of the leaves are about 1 to 3 inches across, slightly concave, having a depression in the centre, where joined to the foot-stalk; and from this feature the generic name, *Cotyledon*, has been given, derived from the Greek *cotyle* (a cup). Some of the English names of the plant, Wall Pennywort, Wall Pennyroyal and Penny Pies, are references to the round form of the leaf suggesting a coin.

At the end of May or early in June, stout reddish flowering stems arise, decumbent for a greater or less distance at the base, but then growing very erect to the height of 6 to 18 inches or more. They bear leaves which pass by intermediate gradation from those of a round peltate form to a shortly stalked, wedge-shaped one, and are terminated by a long raceme, or spike, of numerous, pendulous, bell-shaped, yellow-green flowers, with corollas about half an inch long. The calyx is small and, like the corolla, is five-cleft. The plant is in blossom from June to August, and

KINOS

Kino is the inspissated juice of the Bastard Teak (*Pterocarpus marsupium*) obtained from incisions made in the trunk. The term Kino is also applied to the juice of other plants inspissated without artificial heat. The varieties commonly distinguished are:

it is useful for gout, rheumatism, bronchial and other ailments, resulting from heart trouble.

¶ *Dosages.* Fluid extract, ½ to 1 drachm. Powdered root, 1 drachm. Solid extract, 1 to 15 grains.

Cotyledon Umbilicus
N.O. Crassulaceæ
Wall Pennyroyal

the leaves often remain green most of the winter.

The juice and extract of the Kidneywort had an old reputation for epilepsy, especially among herb doctors in the west of England, where it is most frequently found; its use as a remedy in epilepsy was revived last century even in regular practice, but it has obtained no permanent reputation as a remedy.

It is applied by the peasantry in Wales to the eyes as a remedy in some diseases. The leaves, bruised to a pulp and applied as a poultice, are said to cure piles, and are also recommended as an application for slight burns or scalds. A decoction of the leaves is considered cooling and diuretic, and the juice when taken inwardly to be excellent for inflammation of the liver and spleen.

Culpepper tells us that

'the juice or distilled water being drunk is very effectual for all inflammations, to cool a fainting stomach, a hot liver or the bowels; the herb, juice or distilled water outwardly applied healeth pimples, St. Anthony's Fire (erysipelas) and other outward heats.'

He also recommends the juice or distilled water for ulcerated kidneys, gravel and stone, and an ointment made with it for 'painful piles' and pains of the gout and sciatia. In addition,

'it heals kibes or chilblains if they be bathed with the juice or anointed with ointment made hereof and some of the skin of the leaf upon them: it is used in green wounds to stay the blood and to heal them quickly.'

See STONECROPS.

Pterocarpus marsupium
Pterocarpus erinaceus
Butea frondosa
N.O. Leguminosæ

MALABAR or EAST INDIAN KINO obtained from *P. marsupium*.

AFRICAN or GAMBIA KINO from *P. erinaceus*.

BUTEA, BENGAL, or PALAS KINO from *Butea frondosa*.

BOTANY BAY, AUSTRALIAN or EUCALYPTUS KINO from different species of Eucalyptus.

WEST INDIAN or JAMAICA KINO from *Coccoloba uvifera.*

SOUTH AMERICAN or CARACAS KINO, which is identified with Columbian Kino and is believed to be obtained from the same plant that yields the West Indian Kino.

In the British Pharmacopœia Malabar or West Indian Kino is the only one recognized, and this is found in small, brittle glistening pieces, reddish-black in colour. They are odourless with a very astringent taste and stick to the teeth when chewed and make the saliva bright red.

Kino is almost entirely soluble in alcohol and entirely in ether and partly in water. Chemically it closely resembles catechu,

and is very like it in action, but it is less astringent and therefore less effective.

The Indian Pharmacopœia recognizes this kind and also Bengal Kino are recognized, and in the United States other kinds are official as well as these two.

¶ *Medicinal Action and Uses.* Astringent. Used whenever tannin is indicated. Internally in diarrhœa, dysentery, and pyrosis. Externally as a gargle and as an injection for leucorrhœa.

¶ *Preparations and Dosages.* Powdered gum, 5 to 20 grains. Comp. powder, B.P., 5 to 20 grains. Tincture, B.P. and U.S.P., ½ to 1 drachm.

See EUCALYPTUS.

KNAPWEED, BLACK

Centaurea nigra (LINN.)
N.O. Compositæ

Centaurea nigra, the Black Knapweed, is a perennial, with an unwinged, erect stem, 6 inches to 3 feet high, generally freely branched in the upper part. The leaves are very variable, both in breadth and degrees of division, the upper ones narrow and generally with entire margins, but the lower ones lobed, or at any rate with some coarse teeth. The whole plant is dull green,

rather rough with small hairs, the stems, like the preceding species, very tough. The flowers are without the spreading outer rays of the Greater Knapweed, the florets being all tubular, which makes the black fringes to the bracts of the involucre most noticeable, hence the name of the species. The florets are of a less bright purple in colour.

KNAPWEED, GREATER

Centaurea Scabiosa
N.O. Compositæ

Synonyms. Hardhead. Ironhead. Hard Irons. Churls Head. Logger Head. Horse Knops. Matte Felon. Mat Fellon. Bottleweed. Bullweed. Cowede. Boltsede

Parts Used. Root, seeds

Habitat. Frequent in the borders of fields and in waste places, being not uncommon in England, where it is abundant on chalk soil, but rare in Scotland

¶ *Description.* The plant is a perennial, the rootstock thick and woody in old plants. The stem is 1 to 3 feet high, generally branched, very tough. The leaves, which are firm in texture, are very variable in the degree of division, but generally deeply cut into, the segments again deeply notched. The lower leaves are very large, often a foot or even more in length, making a striking-looking rosette on the ground, from which the flowering stems arise. The whole plant is a dull green, sparingly hairy. It flowers in July and August. The flowers are terminal, somewhat similar to those of the Cornflower in general shape, though larger. All the florets are of the same colour, a rich purplish-crimson, the outer ray ones with the limb divided nearly to the base into narrow, strap-shaped segments. The flower-head is hard and solid, a mass of bracts lapping over each other like tiles, each having a central green portion and a black fringe-like edge. In some districts the plant is called from these almost round heads, 'Hardhead,' and

the ordinary English name, Knapweed, is based on the same idea, *Knap,* being a form of *Knop,* or *Knob.*

This larger species of Knapweed was in olden times called 'Matte Felon,' from its use in curing felons or whitlows. As early as 1440 we find it called 'Maude Felone,' or 'Boltsede.'

This species is very common and generally distributed in pastures, borders of fields and roadsides throughout Britain, and flowers from early June till well into September. Both species of Knapweed may readily be distinguished from Thistles by the absence of spines and prickles.

¶ *Medicinal Action and Uses.* The Knapweed was once in great repute as a vulnerary. It was included in the fourteenth-century ointment, *Save,* for wounds and for the pestilence, and was also used with pepper for loss of appetite.

The root and seeds are used. Its diuretic, diaphoretic and tonic properties are recognized.

It is good for catarrh, taken in decoction, and is also made into ointment for outward application for wounds and bruises, sores, etc.

KNAPWORT HARSHWEED

Synonym. Brown Radiant Knapweed

Centaurea Jacea, known to old writers as Knapwort Harshweed, its modern name being the Brown Radiant Knapweed, is a rare species.

It was also applied as a vulnerary and was used internally. Culpepper describes it as a mild astringent, 'helpful against coughs, asthma, and difficulty of breathing, and good for diseases of the head and nerves,' and tells us that 'outwardly the bruised herb is famous for taking away black and blue marks out of the skin.'

The botanical name of the species, *scabiosa*, signifying the Scabious-like Knapweed, is

Culpepper tells us: 'it is of special use for soreness of throat, swelling of the uvula and jaws, and very good to stay bleeding at the nose and mouth.'

Centaurea Jacea

given this species of *Centaurea* from its resemblance in general size, form of leaf and other features to the Scabious, another common plant also found in the chalk district, which obtains its name from the Latin word *scabies*, an irritating roughness of the skin, for which it has been employed as a remedy.

The medicinal qualities of the Greater Knapweed are similar to those of the Black Knapweed, a smaller variety, which is more generally collected for medicinal use, perhaps because more common.

See CENTAURY, GENTIAN, THISTLES

KNOTGRASS

Polyganum aviculare (LINN.)
N.O. Polygonaceæ

Synonyms. Knotgrass. Centinode. Ninety-knot. Nine-joints. Allseed. Bird's Tongue. Sparrow Tongue. Red Robin. Armstrong. Cowgrass. Hogweed. Pigweed. Pigrush. Swynel Grass. Swine's Grass

Part Used. Whole herb

Habitat. The entire globe

The Knotgrass is abundant everywhere, a common weed in arable land, on waste ground and by the roadside.

¶ *Description.* The root is annual, branched and somewhat woody, taking strong hold of the earth; the stems, ½ to 6 feet in length, much branched, seldom erect, usually of straggling habit, often quite prostrate and widely spreading. The leaves, alternate and often stalkless, are variable, narrow, lance-shaped or oval, ½ to 1½ inch long, issuing from the sheaths of the stipules or ochreæ, which are membraneous, white, shining, torn, red at the base and two-lobed. The flowers are minute, in clusters of two to three, in the axils of the stem, barely ⅛ in. long, usually pinkish, sometimes red, green, or dull whitish. In contrast to the other Polygonums, there is little or no honey or scent, so that the flowers are very rarely visited by insects and pollinate themselves by the incurving of the three inner stamens on to the styles. The remaining five stamens alternate with the perianth segments and bend outwards, thus ensuring cross-pollination in addition, should any insect visit the flower.

The plant varies greatly in size. When it grows singly in a favourable soil and clear of other vegetation, it will often cover a circle of a yard or more in diameter, the stems being almost prostrate on the ground and leaves

broad and large; but when growing crowded by other plants the stalks become more upright and all the parts are generally smaller.

The stems are smooth, with swollen joints, hence the common names, Nine-joints, Ninety-knots, etc., and when gathered it generally snaps at one of the joints.

It begins flowering in May and continues till September or October. Cleistogamic flowers (which do not open at all and in which therefore self-pollination is necessarily effected) are found under the ochrea, and this species is said also to possess subterranean cleistogamic flowers.

The specific name, *aviculare*, is from the Latin *aviculus*, a diminutive of *avis* (a bird), great numbers of our smaller birds feeding on its seeds. The seeds are useful for every purpose in which those of the allied Buckwheat are employed and are produced in great numbers, hence its local name – Allseed.

Some of the older herbals call it Bird's Tongue or Sparrow Tongue, these names arising from the shape of its little, pointed leaves. Its minute reddish flowers gained it the name of Red Robin. From the difficulty of pulling it up, it was called Armstrong, and from the fact that cattle and swine eat it readily, we find it called Cowgrass and Hogweed, Pigweed or Pigrush. Gerard tells us:

'It is given to swine with good successe when they are sicke and will not eat their meate, whereupon the country people so call it Swine's Grass and Swine's Skir. In the Grete Herball (1516) it is called Swynel Grass.'

Shakespeare (*Midsummer Night's Dream*) speaks of this plant as 'the hindering Knotgrass,' referring to the belief that its decoction was efficacious in retarding the growth of children and the young of domestic animals.

The larvæ of Geometer moths will eat the plant as a substitute for their usual food.

¶ *Medicinal Action and Uses*. The plant has astringent properties, rendering an infusion of it useful in diarrhœa, bleeding piles and all hæmorrhages; it was formerly employed considerably as a vulnerary and styptic.

It has also diuretic properties, for which it has found employment in strangury and as an expellant of stone, the dose recommended in old herbals being 1 drachm of the herb, powdered in wine, taken twice a day.

The decoction was also administered to kill worms.

The fresh juice has been found effectual to stay bleeding of the nose, squirted up the nose and applied to the temples, and made into an ointment it has proved an excellent remedy for sores.

Salmon stated:

'Knotgrass is peculiar against spilling of blood, strangury and other kidney affections, cools inflammations, heals wounds and cleanses and heals old filthy ulcers. The *Essence* for tertians and quartan. The *decoction* for colick; the *Balsam* strengthens weak joints, comforts the nerves and tendons, and is prevalent against the gout, being duly and rightly applied morning and evening.'

The fruit is emetic and purgative.

¶ *Other Species*.

P. Arifoleum, or Sickle-grass, Halbert-leaved Tear-thumb, Hactate Knotgrass. An infusion is a powerful diuretic, to be drunk freely in all urinary affections.

The Russian Knotgrass (*Polygonum erectum*, Linn.) possesses similar astringent properties, and an infusion of this herb is used in diarrhœa and children's summer complaints.

The Alpine Knotweed (*P. viviparum*, Linn.), a small perennial, only 4 to 8 inches high, found in British mountain alpine pastures, is peculiar in that its slender, spike-like raceme of white or pinkish flowers bears in its lower portion, in place of flowers, little red bulbs (as in certain species of *Lilium* and *Alium*), on which the plant depends for its propagation, its fruit rarely maturing.

This species is found in North America, being there the one nearest related to the Bistort, whose properties it shares.

See BISTORT.

KNOTGRASS, RUSSIAN

Polygonum erectum (LINN.)
N.O. Polygonacea

Synonym. Erect Knotgrass
Part Used. Whole herb
Habitat. British America, and Western and Middle States

¶ *Description*. This perennial herb was discovered in North America in 1790, but up to date it has not been largely utilized. It is a variety of the English one – *Polygonum aviculare*, and has similar properties. It has an upright smooth branched stem and grows from 1 to 3 feet high. Leaves are smooth, broadly obvate, rather obtuse – 1 to 2 inches long – and about half as broad – either sessile or petiolate. Flowers bloom June to September in bunches at axils of the leaves.

¶ *Medicinal Action and Uses*. It is highly astringent as an infusion or decoction; useful in diarrhœa as an injection and in children's summer complaints; also as a good gargle and a valuable remedy for inflammatory diseases of the tissues.

KOLA NUTS

Kola vera (SCHUM.)
N.O. Sterculiaceæ

Synonyms. Cola acuminata. Sterculia acuminata. Kola Seeds. Gurru Nuts. Bissy Nuts. Cola Seeds. Guru Nut
Part Used. Seeds
Habitat. Sierra Leone, North Ashanti near the sources of the Nile; cultivated in tropical Western Africa, West Indies, Brazil, Java

¶ *Description*. This tree grows about 40 feet high, has yellow flowers, spotted with purple; leaves 6 to 8 inches long, pointed at both ends.

The seeds are extensively used as a condiment by the natives of Western and Central tropical Africa, also by the negroes of the West Indies and Brazil, who introduced the trees to these countries.

In Western Africa these trees are usually

found growing near the sea-coast, and a big trade is carried on with the nuts by the natives of the interior – Cola being eaten by them as far as Fezzan and Tripoli. A small piece is chewed before each meal to promote digestion; it is also thought to improve the flavour of anything eaten after it and even to render putrid water palatable; the powder is applied to cuts.

There are several kinds of Cola seeds derived from different species, but the *Cola vera* are most generally used and preferred for medicinal purposes. Those from West Africa and West Indies supply the commercial drug. *C. acuminata*, or Gurru Nuts, are employed in the same way as *C. vera*; they are from a tree growing in Cameron and Congo, not esteemed so highly, but much in use as a caffeine stimulant; 600 tons are said to be sent yearly to Brazil for the negroes' use, who also employ the seeds of *S. Chica* and *S. Striata*. The Kola of commerce consists of the separated cotyledons of the kernel of the seed; when fresh it is nearly white, on drying it undergoes a fermentative change, turning reddish brown and losing much of its astringency. The dried cotyledons vary in size from 1 to 2 inches, are irregular in shape but roughly plano-convex, exterior reddy brown, interior paler, easily cut, showing a uniform section, odourless and almost tasteless. Large quantities of the fresh seeds are employed in Africa on account of their sustaining properties, where they form an important article of inland commerce.

¶ *Constituents.* The different varieties of nuts give a greater or lesser percentage of caffeine, which is only found in the fresh state. The seeds are said to contain a glucoside, Kolanin, but this substance appears to be a mixture of Kola red and caffeine. The seeds also contain starch, fatty matter, sugar, a fat decomposing enzyme acting on various oils.

¶ *Medicinal Action and Uses.* The properties of Kola are the same as caffeine, modified only by the astringents present. Fresh Kola Nuts have stimulant action apart from the caffeine content, but as they appear in European commerce, their action is indistinguishable from that of other caffeine drugs and Kola red is inert. Kola is also a valuable nervine, heart tonic, and a good general tonic.

¶ *Adulterations.* Male Kola (not to be confused with Kola) is the fruit of a small tree, Garcinia Kola, and contains no caffeine. The fruit is oblong, from 2 to 3 inches long and 1 inch broad; it is trigonal in section, reddish brown with nutmeg-like markings. Taste, bitter and astringent. Under microscope shows resinous masses, surrounded by cells full of starch. The seeds of *Lucuma Mammosa* are sometimes found mixed with Kola Nuts, but are easily detected by their strong smell of prussic acid. *Hertiera Litorales* seeds are also sometimes found mixed with Kola Nuts.

C. Ballayi (cornu) seeds are also used, but these are easily distinguished as the seeds have six cotyledons and contain little caffeine.

¶ *Preparations.* Fluid extract of Kola, 10 to 40 drops. Solid extract alc., 2 to 8 grains.

KOUSSO

Hagenia Abyssinica (WILLD.)
Brayera anthelmintica (KUNTH.)
N.O. Rosaceæ

Synonyms. Banksia Abyssinica. Kooso. Kusso. Kosso. Cossoo. Cusso.
Parts Used. Herb, unripe fruit, and the dried panicles of the pistillate flowers
Habitat. North-Eastern Africa, and cultivated in Abyssinia; official in United States of America

¶ *Description.* The tree is named after Dr. K. G. Hagen of Königsberg, a German botanist (*d.* 1829), and also after A. Brayera, a French physician in Constantinople, who wrote a monograph on the tree in 1823. It is a beautiful tree growing about 20 feet high, at an elevation of 3,000 to 8,000 feet. The flowers are unisexual, small, of a greenish colour, becoming purple. The dried flowers have a slight balsamic odour, and the taste is bitter and acrid; the female flowers are chiefly collected, although not exclusively so. 'Loose Kousso,' i.e. flowers stripped from their panicles, sometimes come into the market, often with some staminate flowers among it. These are much less active, easily distinguished by their greeny colour, fertile stamens and outer hairy sepals, whereas the female flowers are a dark reddish colour. As a medicine it is very apt to be adulterated, owing to its high price; therefore it is advisable to buy it in its unpowdered state.

¶ *Constituents.* A volatile oil, a bitter acrid resin, tannic acid, and a bitter principle called A Kosin and B Kosin, which is found in Kousso, but thought to be decomposition products. The principle constituent of Kousso is Koso-toxin, a yellow amorphous body, possibly closely allied to filicia acid, and Rottlerin; other inactive colourless bodies are crystalline Protokosin and Kosidin.

459

¶ *Medicinal Action and Uses.* Purgative and anthelmintic; the Abyssinians are greatly troubled with tapeworm, and Kousso is used by them to expel the worms. One dose is said to be effective in destroying both kinds of tapeworms, the *tænia solium* and *bothriocephalus latus*; but as it possesses little cathartic power the subsequent administration of a purgative is generally necessary to bring away the destroyed ectozoon. The dose of the flowers when powdered is from 4 to 5½ drachms, macerated in 3 gills of lukewarm water for 15 minutes; the unstrained infusion is taken in two or three doses following each other, freely drinking lemon-juice or tamarind water before and after the doses. It is advisable to fast twenty-four or forty-eight hours before taking the drug. The operation is usually safe, effective, and quick, merely causing sometimes a slight nausea, but it has never failed to expel the worm. Occasionally emesis takes place or diuresis, and collapse follows, but cases of this sort are extremely rare. It is said in Abyssinia that honey gathered from beehives immediately the Kousso plants have flowered is very effective in teaspoonful doses as a tænicide, its effect being to poison the worms.

¶ *Dosage.* Infusion of ½ oz. to 1 pint of boiling water is taken in 4 oz. doses, and repeated at short intervals. Fluid extract, 2 to 4 drachms.

LABRADOR TEA

Ledum latifolium (JACQ.)
N.O. Ericaceæ

Synonyms. St. James's Tea. Ledum Grœnlandicum
Parts Used. Leaves and tops
Habitat. Greenland, Labrador, Nova Scotia, Hudson's Bay

¶ *Description.* This evergreen shrub grows to a height of 4 to 5 feet, with irregular, woolly branches. The leaves are alternate, entire, elliptical or oblong, 1 to 2 inches long, the upper side smooth and woolly underneath, with the edges rolled back. The large, white, five-petalled flowers grow in flattened terminal clusters, opening in June and July. The plant grows in cold bogs and mountain woods. It is taller, more regularly formed, and has larger leaves than *L. palustre.* During the American War of Independence the leaves were much used instead of tea-leaves. They should be collected before flowering time, and the tops when the flowers begin to open.

Bees are much attracted by the flowers, but animals do not browse on the plants, which are said to be slightly poisonous.

Strewed among clothes, the leaves will keep away moths, and in Lapland the branches are placed among grain to keep away mice. In Russia the leaves are used for tanning leather.

¶ *Constituents.* There has been found in the leaves tannin, gallic acid, a bitter substance, wax, resin, and salts.

¶ *Medicinal Action and Uses.* The leaves are tonic, diaphoretic, and pectoral, having a pleasant odour and rather spicy taste. They yield their virtues to hot water or to alcohol. It is useful in coughs, dyspepsia, and irritation of the membranes of the chest. An infusion has been used to soothe irritation in infectious, feverish eruptions, in dysentery, leprosy, itch, etc. The strong decoction, as a wash, will kill lice. The leaves are also used in malignant and inflamed sore throat.

¶ *Dosage.* Of infusion, 2 to 4 fluid ounces, three to four times a day. Overdoses may cause violent headache and symptoms of intoxication.

¶ *Other Species.*

L. PALUSTRE (Marsh Tea, Marsh Cistus, Wild Rosemary, Wild Rosmarin, Rosmarinus[1] Sylvestris, Porsch, Sumpfporsch, Finne Thé) grows in swamps and wet places of northern Europe, Asia, and America, and on the mountains of southern districts. The leaves are reputed to be more powerful than those of *L. latifolium,* and to have in addition some narcotic properties, being used in Germany to make beer more intoxicating. The leaves contain a volatile oil, including *ledum camphor,* a stearopten, with valeric and volatile acids, ericolin, and ericinol. The tannin is called leditannic acid.

(*POISON*)
LABURNUM

Cytisus Laburnam (LINN.)
N.O. Leguminosæ

Synonym. Yellow Laburnum
Part Used. Seeds

The Laburnum, indigenous to the higher mountains of Europe, is cultivated throughout the civilized world for its flowers, which appear early in the spring, in rich, pendent, yellow clusters.

All parts of the plant are probably poisonous and children should be warned never to touch the black seeds which contain this highly poisonous alkaloid, as cases of poisoning after eating the seeds have been frequent.

---

[1] This species is used in Homœopathy. – EDITOR.

The Laburnum is a native of the mountains of France, Switzerland, and southern Germany, where it attains the height of 20 feet and upwards. It was introduced into England previously to 1597, at which time Gerard appears to have grown it in his garden under the names of Anagyris, Laburnum, and Bean Trefoil.

The heart-wood is of a dark colour, and though of a coarse grain it is very hard and durable, will take a polish, and may be stained to resemble ebony. It is much in demand among turners, and is wrought into a variety of articles which require strength and smoothness.

Cytisus purpurascens (Fr. *C. d'Adam*), the PURPLE LABURNUM, is a hybrid between *C. Laburnum* and *C. purpureus*. It was originated in Paris in 1828, by M. Adam, and has since been much cultivated in England. A curious result of hybridizing appears in this variety occasionally. The branches below the graft produce the ordinary yellow Laburnum flowers of large size; those above often exhibit a small purple Laburnum flower, as well as reddish flowers intermediate between the two in size and colour. Occasionally, the same cluster has some flowers yellow and some purple (Balfour).

Laburnum trees should not be allowed to overhang a field used as a pasture, for when cattle and horses have browsed on the foliage and pods, the results have proved deadly.

Symptoms of poisoning by Laburnum root or seeds are intense sleepiness, vomiting, convulsive movements, coma, slight frothing at the mouth and unequally dilated pupils. In some cases, diarrhœa is very severe and at times the convulsions are markedly tetanic.

In an article on the use of insecticides against lice, by A. Bacot, Entomologist to the Lister Institute of Preventive Medicine, in the *British Medical Journal* of September 30, 1916, the writer records the results of experiments with various reputedly insecticidal substances, but mainly with Cytisine, the alkaloid obtained from the seeds of the Gorse and Laburnum, the physiological properties of which resemble those of Nicotine. He found that while Cytisine is quite satisfactory from an experimental point of view, its use is contraindicated, because the degree of concentration required is such as to entail risk of absorption over a wide area of the body, with almost certain toxic consequences.

¶ *Constituents.* Cytisine was discovered in 1863 by Husemann and Marme, as one of the poisonous alkaloids present in the seeds of the Laburnum. It is a white, crystalline solid, of a bitter, somewhat caustic taste, with a very poisonous action. It has been recommended in whooping cough and asthma.

The same alkaloid has been isolated from the seeds of several leguminous plants. Plugge, in 1895, stated that he found it in eight species of the genus *Cytisus*, two of the genus *Genista*, two of the genus *Sophara*, two of the genus *Baptisia*, in *Anagyris fœtida*, and in other plants. He considered the Ulexine of Gerrard from *Ulex Europœa* (Linn.) to be identical with Cytisine.

LACHNANTHES

Lachnanthes tinctoria (ELL.)
N.O. Hæmodoraceæ

Synonyms. Gyrotheca capitata. Gyrotheca tinctoria. Wool Flower. Red Root. Paint Root. Spirit Weed

Parts Used. Root, herb

Habitat. The drug Lachnanthes is prepared from the entire plant, but especially from the rhizome and roots of *Lachnanthes tinctoria*, a plant indigenous to the United States of America, growing in sandy swamps along the Atlantic coast, from Florida to New Jersey and Rhode Island, and also found in Cuba, blossoming from June to September, according to locality

It was introduced into England as a greenhouse plant in 1812 and then propagated from seed

¶ *Description.* The plant is a perennial herb, 1½ to 2 feet high, the upper portion white-woolly, hence one of its local names: Woolflower. The rhizome is about 1 inch in length and of nearly equal thickness, and bears a large number of long, coarse, somewhat waxy, deep-red roots, yielding a red dye, to which its popular names of Paintroot and Redroot are due.

The leaves are mostly borne in basal rosettes and are somewhat succulent, ⅕ to ⅖ inch wide and reduced to bracts on the upper part of the stem. The flowers are in a close, woolly cyme, the ovary inferior, the perianth six-parted, the sepals narrower than the petals, the stamens three, alternately with the petals, on long filaments; the style is solitary, thread-like, its stigma slightly lobed; the fruit, a three-celled, many seeded, rounded capsule.

¶ *Constituents.* The root yields a fine red dye and a little resin, but so far no analysis determining the nature of its specific constituents has been made: they are, however, quite active, producing a peculiar form of cerebral stimulation or narcosis.

The drug has a somewhat acrid taste, but no odour.

¶ *Medicinal Action and Uses.*

'The root,' says Millspaugh, 'was esteemed an invigorating tonic by the American aborigines, especially by the Seminole tribe, who use it, it is said, to cause brilliancy and fluency of speech. A tincture of the root has been recommended in typhus and typhoid fevers, pneumonia, severe forms of brain disease, rheumatic wry-neck and laryngeal cough.'

Apart from its narcotic uses among the Indians, it has been used in the United States for dyeing purposes.

The drug is employed for various nervous disorders. A homœopathic tincture is prepared from the whole fresh plant, while flowering. Doses varying from a few drops of the tincture to a drachm, cause mental exhilaration, followed by ill-humour, vertigo and headache.

Fluid extract, 1 to 5 drops.

Although the drug is not related to the Solanaceæ, the effects of overdoses are said to resemble those of poisoning by Belladonna and other solanaceous drugs.

In the countries where it grows, there is a legend that the Paintroot plant is fatally poisonous to white pigs, but not injurious to black ones. Darwin, on the authority of Professor I. J. Wyman, cites the strange effect on albino pigs after eating the roots of this plant. In Virginia, where it grows abundantly, Professor Wyman noticed that all the pigs in this district were black, and upon inquiring of the farmers he found that all the white pigs born in a litter were destroyed, because they could not be reared to maturity. The roots of *Lachnanthes*, when eaten by white pigs, caused their bones to turn to a pink colour and their hoofs to fall off, but the black pigs, it was said, could eat the same plant with impunity. Heusinger has shown that white sheep and pigs are injured by the ingestion of certain plants, while the pigmented species may eat them without harm.

LADIES' BEDSTRAW. *See* BEDSTRAW

LADY'S MANTLE   Alchemilla vulgaris (LINN.)
                                                            N.O. Rosaceæ

Synonyms. Lion's Foot. Bear's Foot. Nine Hooks. Leontopodium. Stellaria
   (*French*) Pied-de-lion
   (*German*) Frauenmantle
Parts Used. Herb, root
Habitat. The Lady's Mantle and the Parsley Piert, two small, inconspicuous plants, have considerable reputation as herbal remedies. They both belong to the genus *Alchemilla* of the great order Rosaceæ, most of the members of which are natives of the American Andes, only a few being found in Europe, North America and Northern and Western Asia. In Britain, we have only three species, *Alchemilla vulgaris*, the Common Lady's Mantle, *A. arvensis*, the Field Lady's Mantle or Parsley Piert, and *A. alpina*, less frequent and only found in mountainous districts.
   The Common Lady's Mantle is generally distributed over Britain, but more especially in the colder districts and on high-lying ground, being found up to an altitude of 3,600 feet in the Scotch Highlands. It is not uncommon in moist, hilly pastures and by streams, except in the south-east of England, and is abundant in Yorkshire, especially in the Dales. It is indeed essentially a plant of the north, freely found beyond the Arctic circle in Europe, Asia and also in Greenland and Labrador, and only on high mountain ranges, such as the Himalayas, if found in southern latitudes

The plant is of graceful growth and though only a foot high and green throughout – flowers, stem and leaves alike, and therefore inconspicuous – the rich form of its foliage and the beautiful shape of its clustering blossoms make it worthy of notice.

¶ *Description.* The rootstock is perennial – black, stout and short – and from it rises the slender erect stem. The whole plant is clothed with soft hairs. The lower, radical leaves, large and handsome, 6 to 8 inches in diameter, are borne on slender stalks, 6 to

18 inches long and are somewhat kidney-shaped in general outline, with their margins cut into seven or mostly nine broad, but shallow lobes, finely toothed at the edges, from which it has obtained one of its local names: 'Nine Hooks.' The upper leaves are similar and either stalkless, or on quite short footstalks and are all actually notched and toothed. A noticeable feature is the leaf-like stipules, also toothed, which embrace the stem.

The flowers, which are in bloom from

June to August, are numerous and small, only about ⅛ inch in diameter, yellow-green in colour, in loose, divided clusters at the end of the freely-branching flower-stems, each on a short stalk, or pedicle. There are no petals, the calyx is four-cleft, with four conspicuous little bracteoles that have the appearance of outer and alternate segments of the calyx. There are four stamens, inserted on the mouth of the calyx, their filaments jointed.

The rootstock is astringent and edible and the leaves are eaten by sheep and cattle.

The common name, Lady's Mantle (in its German form, *Frauenmantle*), was first bestowed on it by the sixteenth-century botanist, Jerome Bock, always known by the Latinized version of his name: Tragus. It appears under this name in his famous *History of Plants*, published in 1532, and Linnæus adopted it. In the Middle Ages, this plant had been associated, like so many flowers, with the Virgin Mary (hence it is Lady's Mantle, not Ladies' Mantle), the lobes of the leaves being supposed to resemble the scalloped edges of a mantle. In mediæval Latin we also find it called *Leontopodium* (lion's foot), probably from its spreading root-leaves, and this has become in modern French, *Pied-de-lion*. We occasionally find the same idea expressed in two English local names, 'Lion's foot' and 'Bear's foot.' It has also been called 'Stellaria,' from the radiating character of its lower leaves, but this belongs more properly to quite another group of plants, with star-like blossoms of pure white.

A yellow fungus sometimes attacks the plant known as *Uromyces alchemillæ*, and has the curious effect of causing abnormal length of the leaf-stalk and rendering the blade of the leaf smaller and of a paler green colour; this fungus produces the same effect in other plants.

The generic name *Alchemilla* is derived from the Arabic word, *Alkemelych* (alchemy), and was bestowed on it, according to some old writers, because of the wonder-working powers of the plant. Others held that the alchemical virtues lay in the subtle influence the foliage imparted to the dewdrops that lay in its furrowed leaves and in the little cup formed by its joined stipules, these dewdrops constituting part of many mystic potions.

¶ *Part Used Medicinally.* The whole herb, gathered in June and July when in flower and when the leaves are at their best, and dried.

The root is sometimes also employed, generally fresh.

¶ *Medicinal Action and Uses.* The Lady's Mantle has astringent and styptic properties, on account of the tannin it contains. It is 'of a very drying and binding character' as the old herbalists expressed it, and was formerly considered one of the best vulneraries or wound herbs.

Culpepper says of it:

'Lady's Mantle is very proper for inflamed wounds and to stay bleeding, vomitings, fluxes of all sorts, bruises by falls and ruptures. It is one of the most singular wound herbs and therefore highly prized and praised, used in all wounds inward and outward, to drink a decoction thereof and wash the wounds therewith, or dip tents therein and put them into the wounds which wonderfully drieth up all humidity of the sores and abateth all inflammations thereof. It quickly healeth green wounds, not suffering any corruption to remain behind and cureth old sores, though fistulous and hollow.'

In modern herbal treatment, it is employed as a cure for excessive menstruation and is taken internally as an infusion (1 oz. of the dried herb to 1 pint of boiling water) in teacupful doses as required and the same infusion is also employed as an injection.

A strong decoction of the fresh root, by some considered the most valuable part of the plant, has also been recommended as excellent to stop all bleedings, and the root dried and reduced to powder is considered to answer the same purpose and to be good for violent purgings.

In Sweden, a tincture of the leaves has been given in cases of spasmodic or convulsive diseases, and an old authority states that if placed under the pillow at night, the herb will promote quiet sleep.

Fluid extract, dose, ½ to 1 drachm.

Horses and sheep like the plant, and it has therefore been suggested as a profitable fodder plant, but the idea has proved unpractical. Grazing animals will not eat the leaves till the moisture in them is dissipated.

¶ *Other Species.*

Alchemilla alpine, a mountain variety, found on the banks of Scotch rivulets. The leaves are deeply divided into five oblong leaflets and are thickly covered with lustrous silky hairs. A form of this plant in which the leaflets are connate for one-third of their length is known as *A. conjuncta*.

See PARSLEY PIERT

LADY'S SLIPPER. *See* AMERICAN VALERIAN

LADY'S TRESSES[1]

Spiranthes autumnalis (ORICH.)
N.O. Spiranthideœ

Part Used. Tuberous root

Habitat. Dry, hilly fields all over Europe – towards the Caucasus

¶ *Description.* This orchis takes its name from *speira* (a 'spiral') and *anthos* (a flower), in allusion to the spiral arrangement of the flowers. Rootstock produces every season two or three oblong tubers and a tuft of spreading, radical, ovate leaves about 1 inch long, a flowering stem 6 or 8 inches high by the side of the tuft of leaves. Blooms in autumn, flowers a greenish-white, smelling like almonds, in a close spiral spike about 2 inches long, diverging horizontally to one side – with the bracts erect on opposite side, in appearance not unlike lilies of the valley.

¶ *Medicinal Action and Uses.* Formerly used as an aphrodisiac.

A tincture of the root is used in homœopathy for skin affections, painful breasts, pain in the kidneys and eye complaints.

¶ *Other Species.*

Spiranthes diuretica, used in Chile in cases of ischury.

LARCH. *See* PINES

LARKSPUR, FIELD

Delphinium Consolida
N.O. Ranunculacæ

Synonyms. Lark's Heel. Lark's Toe. Lark's Claw. Knight's Spur

Part Used. Seed

Habitat. Europe

The Field Larkspur grows wild in cornfields throughout Europe. Though a doubtful native, it is found occasionally in England in considerable quantities in sandy or chalky cornfields, especially in Cambridgeshire.

¶ *Description.* It is an annual, with upright, round stems a foot high or more, pubescent and divided into alternate, dividing branches. The leaves are alternate, the lower ones with petioles ½ inch long, the upper ones sessile, or nearly so. The plant closely resembles some of the species commonly cultivated in gardens.

The flowers are in short racemes, pink, purple or blue, followed by glabrous follicles containing black, flattened seeds with acute edges and pitted surfaces. The seeds are poisonous, have an acrid and bitter taste, but are inodorous.

The active principle of the plant – Delphinine – is the same as in Stavesacre and is an irritant poison. Children should be warned against putting any part of this plant, or of its garden representatives, into their mouths. The seeds are especially dangerous, and cause vomiting and purging if eaten.

¶ *Medicinal Action and Uses.* As in Stavesacre, the part used medicinally is the seed, a tincture of which in like manner acts as a parasiticide and insecticide, being used to destroy lice and nits in the hair.[2]

The tincture, given in 10-drop doses, gradually increased, is also employed in spasmodic asthma and dropsy.

The expressed juice of the leaves is considered good as an application to bleeding piles, and a conserve made of the flowers was formerly held to be an excellent medicine for children when subject to violent purging.

The juice of the flowers and an infusion of the whole plant was also prescribed against colic.

The expressed juice of the petals with the addition of a little alum makes a good blue ink.

The name Delphinium, from *Delphin* (a dolphin), was given to this genus because the buds were held to resemble a dolphin. Shakespeare mentions the plant under the name of Lark's Heel.

The name Consolida refers to the plant's power of consolidating wounds.

See STAVESACRE

LAUREL (BAY)

Laurus nobilis (LINN.)
N.O. Lauraceæ

Synonyms. Sweet Bay. True Laurel. Bay. Laurier d'Apollon. Roman Laurel. Noble Laurel. Lorbeer. Laurier Sauce. Daphne

Parts Used. Leaves, fruit, oil

Habitat. Shores of the Mediterranean

¶ *Description.* The Sweet Bay is a small tree, growing in Britain to a height of about 25 feet, but in warmer climates reaching as much as 60 feet. The smooth bark may be olive-green or of a reddish hue. The luxurious, evergreen leaves are alternate,

---

[1] Lady's Tresses grow on the Sussex downs near Amberley. – EDITOR.

[2] During the Great War, when the men in the trenches took the trouble to use it, the results were said to be quite successful. – EDITOR.

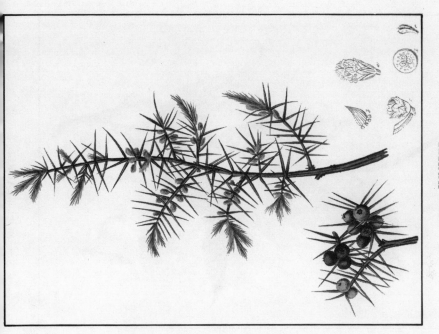

JUNIPER
Juniperus Communis

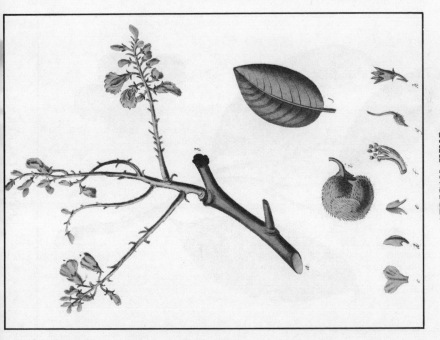

AFRICAN KINO
Pterocarpus Marsupium

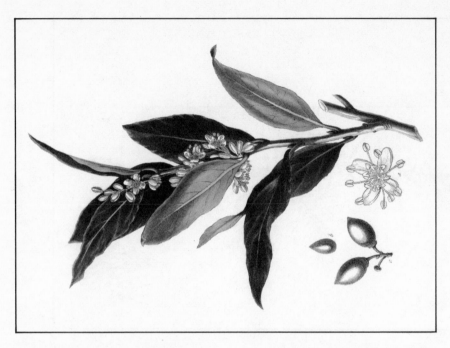

LAUREL.

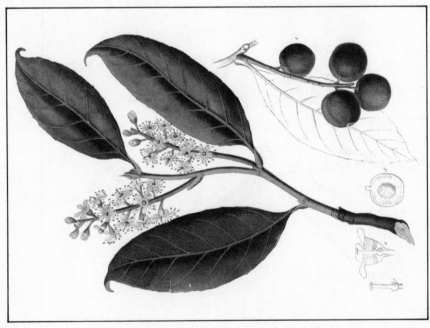

CHERRY LAUREL.

with short stalks, lanceolate, 3 to 4 inches long, the margin smooth and wavy. They are thick, smooth, and of a shining, dark green colour. The flowers are small, yellow and unisexual, and grow in small clusters. The shrub has been cultivated in Britain since the sixteenth century. It is the source of the ancients' crowns and wreaths for heroes and poets, and the modern term of 'bachelor,' given for degrees, is probably derived from *bacca-laureus*, or laurel-berry, through the French *bachelier*.

The Delphic priestesses are said to have made use of the leaves. It grows well under the shade of other trees if they are not too close, and is useful in evergreen plantations. The leaves are much used in cookery for flavouring. They are often packed with stick liquorice or dried figs. They are used fresh, and may be gathered all the year round.

The volatile oil is sometimes used in perfumery.

The dried, black, aromatic *berries* come from Provence, Spain, Italy and Morocco. They are ovoid, and the kernel of the seed is loose.

The *wood* is sweet-scented, and is used for marqueterie work.

Onguent de Laurier is prepared from the oil with *axonge* and the colouring and scenting principles of the leaves and fruit.

¶ *Constituents.* A greenish-yellow volatile oil is yielded by distillation from the leaves which contains a high percentage of oxygenated compounds. The berries contain both fixed and volatile oils, the former, known as *Oil of Bays*, includes *laurostearine*, the ether of *lauric acid*. *Laurin* can be extracted by alcohol.

A frequent substitute for the expressed oil is said to be lard-coloured with chlorophyll or indigo and turmeric, scented with the berries. Boiling alcohol, which dissolves the true oil, will detect this.

The volatile oil contains pinene, geraniol, eugenol, cineol, etc.

¶ *Medicinal Action and Uses.* Leaves, berries and oil have excitant and narcotic properties. The leaves are also regarded as a diaphoretic and in large doses as an emetic.

Except as a stimulant in veterinary practice the leaves and fruit are very rarely used internally. They were formerly employed in hysteria, amenorrhœa, flatulent colic, etc. The berries have been used to promote abortion.

Oil of Bays is used externally for sprains, bruises, etc., and sometimes dropped into the ears to relieve pain. The leaves were formerly infused and taken as tea, and the powder or infusion of the berries was taken to remove obstructions, to create appetite, or as an emmenagogue. Four or five moderate doses were said to cure the ague. The berries were formerly used in several French carminative preparations.

The following products are often mistaken for those of *Laurus nobilis*.

The fruits of *Cocculus Indicus* or *Anamirta paniculata.* They are odourless and kidney-shaped.

The oil of *Pimenta Acris*, from which *bay rum* is distilled in the West Indies, and which is also called oil of bay.

The leaves of *Prunus Laurocerasus*, or Cherry Laurel, to which the name of Laurel is now always applied. The margin of these short, strong serrations at intervals. Caution should be observed in distinguishing these, owing to their poisonous properties.

LAUREL, CHERRY

Prunus Laurocerasus (LINN.)
N.O. Rosaceæ

Synonyms. Laurocerasifolia. Cherry-Bay. Common Laurel. Laurier-armande. Laurier aux Crèmes. Laurier-cérise
Part Used. Fresh leaves
Habitat. A native of Asia Minor. Largely cultivated in Europe

¶ *Description.* This small, evergreen tree, growing to 20 feet in height, has spreading, slender branches, smooth, shining, and pale green. The leaves are thick, alternate, on short, thick stalks, oblong-ovate, from 5 to 7 inches long, growing narrower at each end, and with a slightly serrate margin. The dark green upper surface is smooth and shining and the under one much paler, dull, and the midrib very prominent. There are glandular depressions and hairs near the base.

The five-petalled, small white flowers grow in erect, oblong racemes. The fruit resembles black cherries, but grows in clusters like grapes. The leaves are without odour except when bruised and added to water, when they have the ratafia or almond odour of prussic acid. The taste is bitter, aromatic, and astringent.

The shrubs were introduced into Europe about 1580, and shortly afterwards into England.

The leaves are used for flavouring, but should be used with great care, owing to the risk of poisoning.

Cherry-Laurel Water has been used in Paris fraudulently to imitate the cordial called Kirsch.

The most active essence is reserved for perfumery.

There is difference of opinion as to the best season for gathering the leaves. Drying destroys the active principle.

The bruised leaves, like those of peach or almond, when rubbed within any vessel will remove the odour left by oil of cloves, balsam of copaiba, etc., if the grease has first been cleaned away with alcohol.

¶ *Constituents.* The leaves yield a volatile oil in the proportion of 40·5 grains to 1 lb. of leaves. This resembles oil of bitter almonds, and in Europe is sometimes sold for it, as flavouring, but the glucoside decomposes more slowly than crystallized amygdalin, and is liable to hold hydrocyanic acid, when it becomes poisonous. This glucoside was called Laurocerasin, or Amorphous amygdalin, and now Prulaurasin.

With emulsin and water, prulaurasin is decomposed, and yields benzaldehyde, hydrocyanic acid, and dextrose.

Cherry Laurel Water (Aqua Laurocerasi), according to the British Pharmacopœia, is prepared as follows:

'One pound of fresh leaves of cherry-laurel, 2½ pints of water. Chop the leaves, crush them in a mortar, and macerate them in the water for 24 hours; then distil 1 pint of liquid; shake the product, filter through paper, and preserve it in a stoppered bottle.'

In America, oil of Bitter Almonds is often substituted, owing to the variability of the above.

¶ *Medicinal Action and Uses.* The water is a sedative narcotic, identical in its properties, to a diluted solution of hydrocyanic acid, but of uncertain strength.

¶ *Dosage.* Water, B.P., ½ to 2 drachms.

Used for asthma, coughs, indigestion and dyspepsia, 1 drop of sulphuric acid added to a pint of Cherry Laurel Water will keep it unchanged for a year.

(POISON)
LAUREL, MOUNTAIN
Kalmia latifolia (LINN.)
N.O. Ericaceæ

Synonyms. Broad-leafed Laurel. Calico Bush. Spoon Wood. Ledum Floribus Bullates·
Cistus Chamærhodendros

Part Used. Leaves

Habitat. New Brunswick, Florida, Ohio, Louisiana, New Hampshire, Massachusetts, Alleghany Mountains

¶ *Description.* A beautiful evergreen shrub from 4 to 20 feet. When in full flower it forms dense thickets, the stems are always crooked, the bark rough. It was called Kalmia by Linnæus in honour of Peter Kalm, a Swedish professor. The hard wood is used in the manufacture of various useful articles. Leaves ovate, lanceolate, acute on each end, on petioles 2 to 3 inches long. Flowers numerous, delicately tinted a lovely shade of pink; these are very showy, clammy, interminal, viscid, pubescent, simple or compound heads, branches opposite, flowering in June and July. The flowers yield a honey said to be deleterious. The leaves, shoots and berries are dangerous to cattle, and when eaten by Canadian pheasants communicate the poison to those who feed on the birds. The fruit is a dry capsule, seeds minute and numerous.

¶ *Constituents.* Leaves possess narcotic poisoning properties and contain tannic acid, gum, fatty matter, chlorophyll, a substance resembling mannite, wax extractive, albumen, an acrid principle, Aglucoside-arbutin, yellow calcium iron.

¶ *Medicinal Action and Uses.* Indians are said to use the expressed juice of the leaves or a strong decoction of them to commit suicide. The leaves are the official part; powdered leaves are used as a local remedy in some forms of skin diseases, and are a most efficient agent in syphilis, fevers, jaundice, neuralgia and inflammation, but great care should be exercised in their use. Whisky is the best antidote to poisoning from this plant. An ointment for skin diseases is made by stewing the leaves in pure lard in an earthenware vessel in a hot oven. Taken internally it is a sedative and astringent in active hæmorrhages, diarrhœa and flux. It has a splendid effect and will be found useful in overcoming obstinate chronic irritation of the mucous surface. In the lower animals an injection produces great salivation, lachrymation, emesis, convulsions and later paralysis of the extremities and laboured respiration. It is supposed, but not proved, that the poisonous principle of this plant is Andromedotoxin.

¶ *Preparations and Dosages.* A saturated tincture of the leaves taken when plant is in flower, is the best form of administration, given in doses of 10 to 20 drops every two or three hours. Decoction, ½ to 1 fluid ounce of powdered leaves from 10 to 30 grains. Salve made from juice of the plant is an efficient local application for rheumatism.

¶ *Other Species.*

Kalmia augustifolia (Sheep's Laurel or Lambkill, or Narrow-leaved Laurel, so called because it poisons sheep, which feed on its leaves), this species is said to be the best for medicinal use. A decoction of its leaves, 1 oz. to 1 quart of water reduced to a pint, is used by the negroes as a wash for ulcerations between the toes. A poisonous glucoside is found in the leaves of this species called asebotoxin, and also in *K. latifolia.*

K. Glauca, or Swamp Laurel, has similar properties.

LAVENDERS

N.O. Labiatæ

Habitat. Lavender is a shrubby plant indigenous to the mountainous regions of the countries bordering the western half of the Mediterranean, and cultivated extensively for its aromatic flowers in various parts of France, in Italy and in England and even as far north as Norway. It is also now being grown as a perfume plant in Australia.

The fragrant oil to which the odour of Lavender flowers is due is a valuable article of commerce, much used in perfumery, and to a lesser extent in medicine. The fine aromatic smell is found in all parts of the shrub, but the essential oil is only produced from the flowers and flower-stalks. Besides being grown for the production of this oil, Lavender is widely sold in the fresh state as 'bunched Lavender,' and as 'dried Lavender,' the flowers are used powdered, for sachet making and also for pot-pourri, etc., so that the plant is a considerable source of profit.

Various species of Lavender are used in the preparation of the commercial essential oil, but the largest proportion is obtained from the flowers of *Lavandula vera,* the narrow-leaved form, which grows abundantly in sunny, stony localities in the Mediterranean countries, but nowhere to such perfection as in England.[1] English Lavender is much more aromatic and has a far greater delicacy of odour than the French, and the oil fetches ten times the price. The principal English Lavender plantations are at Carshalton and Wallington in Surrey, Hitchin in Herts, Long Melford in Suffolk, Market Deeping (Lincs) and in Kent, near Canterbury. Mitcham in Surrey used to be the centre of the Lavender-growing industry, but with the extension of London the famous Lavender plantations of Mitcham and surrounding districts have been largely displaced by buildings, and during the War the cultivation of Lavender was still further diminished to give place to food crops, so that in 1920 not more than ten acres under Lavender cultivation could be stated to be found in the whole of Surrey, though some of the oil is still distilled in the neighbourhood, and the finest products continue to be described as 'Mitcham Lavender Oil.'

¶ *Description.* ENGLISH LAVENDER (*Lavandula vera*), the common narrow-leaved variety, grows 1 to 3 feet high (in gardens, occasionally somewhat taller), with a short, but irregular, crooked, much-branched stem, covered with a yellowish-grey bark, which comes off in flakes, and very numerous, erect, straight, broom-like, slender, bluntly-quadrangular branches, finely pubescent, with stellate hairs. The leaves are opposite, sessile, entire, linear, blunt; when young, white with dense stellate hairs on both surfaces; their margins strongly revolute; when full grown, 1½ inch long, green with scattered hairs above, smoothly or finely downy beneath, and the margins only slightly revolute. The flowers are produced in terminating, blunt spikes from the young shoots, on long stems. The spikes are composed of whorls or rings of flowers, each composed of from six to ten flowers, the lower whorls more distant from one another. The flowers themselves are very shortly stalked, three to five together in the axils of rhomboidal, brown, thin, dry bracts. The calyx is tubular and ribbed, with thirteen veins, purple-grey in colour, five-toothed (one tooth being longer than the others) and hairy; shining oil glands amongst the hairs are visible with a lens. The majority of the oil yielded by the flowers is contained in the glands on the calyx. The two-lipped corolla is of a beautiful bluish-violet colour.

French Lavender oil is distilled from two distinct plants, found in the mountain districts of Southern France, both included under the name of *L. officinalis* by the sixteenth-century botanists, and *L. vera* by De Candolle. The French botanist Jordan has separated them under the name of *L. delphinensis,* the Lavender of Dauphine, and *L. fragrans.* The oils from the two plants are very similar, but the former yields oils with the higher percentage of esters.

[1] The Editor has often come across fields of French Lavender in bloom and the scent has been poor compared with English Lavender grown under the worst conditions. – EDITOR.

¶ *Description.* The SPIKE LAVENDER (*L. spica*, D.C., or *latifolia*, Vill.) is a coarser, broad-leaved variety of the Lavender shrub, also found in the mountain districts of France and Spain, though preferring alluvial ground which has been brought down by water from higher levels. In this country it cannot so easily be cultivated in the open as the common Lavender, to which it has a very close similarity, but from which it can be distinguished by the inflorescence, which is more compressed, by the bracts in the axils of which the flowers are placed being much narrower and by the leaves which are broader and spatula shaped. The flowers yield three times as much of the essential oil – known as Spike oil – as can be got from our narrow-leaved plant, but it is of a second-rate quality, less fragrant than that of the true Lavender, its odour resembling a mixture of the oils of Lavender and Rosemary.

Parkinson in his *Garden of Pleasure* says the *L. spica* 'is often called the Lesser Lavender or minor, and is called by some, Nardus Italica.' Some believe that this is the Spikenard mentioned in the Bible.

¶ *History.* Dr. Fernie, in *Herbal Simples*, says:

'By the Greeks the name Nardus is given to Lavender, from Naarda, a city of Syria near the Euphrates, and many persons call the plant "Nard." St. Mark mentions this as Spikenard, a thing of great value. . . . In Pliny's time, blossoms of the Nardus sold for a hundred Roman denarii (or £3 2*s*. 6*d*.) the pound. This Lavender or Nardus was called Asarum by the Romans, because it was not used in garlands or chaplets. It was formerly believed that the asp, a dangerous kind of viper, made Lavender its habitual place of abode, so that the plant had to be approached with great caution.'

L. SPICA and L. FRAGRANS often form hybrids, known as 'Bastard Lavender,' which grow in the mountain districts of France and Spain. Great care is necessary to avoid admixture in the still during distillation of Lavender, as Spike and the hybrids both injure the quality of the essential oil of true Lavender.

'White Lavender,' which is sometimes found in the Alps at extreme altitudes, is considered to be a form of *L. delphinensis*, the white flowers being a case of albinism. Attempts to propagate this form in this country rarely meet with much success.

¶ *Description.* Another species of LAVENDER, *L. Stœchas*, known also as French Lavender, forms a pretty little shrub, with narrow leaves and very small, dark violet flowers, terminated with a tuft of bright-coloured leaflets, which makes it very attractive. It is an inhabitant of the coast, but only occurs on sand or other crystalline rocks, and never on limestone. It is very abundant on the islands of Hyères, which the Ancient Romans called the 'Stœchades,' after this plant. This was probably the Lavender so extensively used in classical times by the Romans and the Libyans, as a perfume for the bath (whence probably the plant derived its name – from the Latin, *lavare*, to wash). It is plentiful in Spain and Portugal and is only used as a rule for strewing the floors of churches and houses on festive occasions, or to make bonfires on St. John's Day, when evil spirits are supposed to be abroad, a custom formerly observed in England with native plants. The odour is more akin to Rosemary than to ordinary Lavender. The flowers of this species were used medicinally in England until about the middle of the eighteenth century, the plant being called by our old authors, 'Sticadore.' It was one of the ingredients of the 'Four Thieves' Vinegar' famous in the Middle Ages. It is not used for distillation, though in France and Spain, the country people, in a simple manner extract an oil, used for dressing wounds, by hanging the flowers downwards in a closed bottle in the sunshine. The Arabs make use of the flowers as an expectorant and antispasmodic.

The Dwarf Lavender is more compact than the other forms and has flowers of a deeper colour. It makes a neat edging in the fruit or kitchen garden, where the larger forms might be in the way, and the flowers, borne abundantly, are useful for cutting.

All the forms of Lavender are much visited by bees and prove a good source of honey.

Lavender was familiar to Shakespeare, but was probably not a common plant in his time, for though it is mentioned by Spencer as 'The Lavender still gray' and by Gerard as growing in his garden, it is not mentioned by Bacon in his list of sweet-smelling plants. It is now found in every garden, but we first hear of it being cultivated in England about 1568. It must soon have become a favourite, however, for among the long familiar garden-plants which the Pilgrim Fathers took with them to their new home in America, we find the names of Lavender, Rosemary and Southernwood, though John Josselyn, in his *Herbal*, says that 'Lavender Cotton groweth pretty well,' but that 'Lavender is not for the Climate.'

Parkinson has much to say about Lavender:

'Of Sage and of Lavender, both the purple

468

and the rare white (there is a kinde hereof that beareth white flowers and somewhat broader leaves, but it is very rare and seene but in few places with us, because it is more tender and will not so well endure our cold Winters).'

'Lavender,' he says, 'is almost wholly spent with us, for to perfume linnen, apparell, gloves and leather and the dryed flowers to comfort and dry up the moisture of a cold braine.'

'This is usually put among other hot herbs, either into bathes, ointment or other things that are used for cold causes. The seed also is much used for worms.'

Lavender is of 'especiall good use for all griefes and paines of the head and brain,' it is now almost solely grown for the extraction of its essential oil, which is largely employed in perfumery.

Of French Lavender he says:

'The whole plant is somewhat sweete, but nothing so much as Lavender. It groweth in the Islands Staechades which are over against Marselles and in Arabia also: we keep it with great care in our Gardens. It flowreth the next yeare after it is sowne, in the end of May, which is a moneth before any Lavender.'

Lavender was one of the old street cries, and white lavender is said to have grown in the garden of Queen Henrietta Maria.

¶ *Cultivation.* Lavender is of fairly easy culture in almost any friable, garden soil. It grows best on light soil – sand or gravel – in a dry, open and sunny position. Loam over chalk also suits it. It requires good drainage and freedom from damp in winter.

The plant flourishes best on a warm, well-drained loam with a slope to the south or south-west. A loam that is too rich is detrimental to the oil yield, as excessive nourishment tends to the growth of leaf. Protection against summer gales by a copse on the south-west is also of considerable value, as these gales may do great damage to the crop by causing the tall flower-spikes to break away at their junction with the stem. Lavender also is liable to injury by frost and low-lying situations and those prone to become weather-bound in winter are to be avoided.

The founding of a Lavender plantation for the purpose of oil production is an enterprise which requires very careful consideration. The land should first be carefully cleaned of weeds in the autumn; these should be burnt, and the ashes distributed over the ground, together with some ordinary wood ashes if obtainable. The soil should then be pre-pared by 'trenching in' a quantity of short straw and stable refuse, but not much rich dung, and should lie fallow until the following spring, when any weeds remaining should be dealt with as before and the whole ploughed over. Towards late spring, the young plants should be dibbed in in rows running from north to south. Some growers plant out in rows 2 feet apart, leaving a foot between each plant. Another mode of planting favoured is to plant out 18 inches apart each way and when these plants have occupied the ground for one year, each intervening plant and those of every other row are taken out, leaving the land planted 36 inches by 36 inches, the wide spaces being judged to allow the plant full growth for flower-bearing, room for cutting flowers and for keeping the ground quite clear of weeds. The plants removed are utilized for planting up fresh ground, each being divided into about three.

The crop may be grown from seed, sown in April, but is mainly propagated by cuttings and layerings. It may also be propagated by division of roots. Cuttings of the young wood, or small branches, with a root or heel, pulled off the large plants, may be inserted in free, sandy soil, under hand-lights in August and September, and planted out during the following spring. The 'cuttings' are taken by pulling the small branches down with a quick movement, when they become detached with the desired 'heel' at their base. Cuttings root freely in April, also, in the open, protection being given in cold weather. They should be of young growths. A certain amount of watering will be required in dry weather until the cuttings are thoroughly established.

Young plants should as far as possible be kept from flowering during the first year by clipping, so that the strength of the plant is thrown into the lateral shoots to make it bushy and compact. A full picking is usually obtained from the second to the fifth year. After the third year, the bushes are apt to become straggly. They can be pruned in March and care should be taken to always have young plants ready to follow on, to take the place of exhausted, over-straggly bushes. In commercial practice, the bushes are seldom retained after their fifth year. It follows, therefore, that in order to keep up a continuous supply of bushes in their prime, planting and grubbing must, on an established plantation, be done every year. Most growers plant say a fifth portion of the ultimate area of Lavender aimed at in the first instance and this is repeated each year until the fifth year, when the area first planted is grubbed immediately after flowering, the old plants burnt, the ashes put upon the ground, and the land ploughed and manured and left fallow until the following spring, when re-stocking can commence.

At Mitcham, Lavender was grown for even six years in succession by judiciously removing worn plants and inserting young ones. Severe frost will often kill rows of plants and their place must be renewed.

During the last few years, plants have been subject to Lavender disease, caused by the fungus, *Phoma lavandulæ*; this causes a heavy loss, as the disease spreads rapidly. It can be eradicated, however, by eliminating and burning the infested plants. English Lavender is more robust in habit than the French plant.

A parasitic plant, *Cuscuta epithymum*, one of the Dodders, will attack and destroy the fine Lavenders, *delphinensis* and *fragrans*, but does not affect the less valuable 'Bastard' Lavender, which eventually survives by itself.

Insect pests are principally small caterpillars and similar animals, which feed upon the leaves of the plant.

¶ *Harvesting.* The bulk of the flowers are used for the distillation of the volatile oil, which is commonly distilled from the flowerstalks and flowers together, the spikes being cut with a small hook about 6 to 9 inches below the flowers, at the end of July or August, according to season. It will be necessary to provide a small distilling plant on the grower's premises, unless arrangements can be made for the distillation of the crop at a local distillery.

Cutting for distilling takes place generally about a week later than for market; the blooms must all be fully developed, because the oil at this time contains the maximum amount of esters.

Harvesting should be carried out rapidly – the cutting managed in a week if possible – so long as the weather is dry and there is no wind, the morning and evening of a fine day being particularly favourable to the flower gathering, on account of the fact that a certain amount of the ester portion of the oil is dissipated by a hot sun, as is easily seen by the fact that the Lavender plantations, and all fields of aromatic plants, are most highly perfumed about mid-day. Further, if there is any wind, the mid-day is the time when it will be hottest and most saturated with moisture, thus easily taking up the more volatile and more soluble particles of the essential oil. Very cold weather prevents the development of esters and rain is fatal for harvesting. If rain or fog appears, cutting should cease and not be resumed till the sun shines again. The cut Lavender should be laid on clean dry mats

and covered from sun scorch immediately. There must be no moisture in the stook, neither must it be dried up by wind or sun. The mats will be rolled up in the cool of the evening before the dew is falling and carted to the still. For some purposes, the stalks are shortened to about 6 inches before stilling, but, generally, the whole of the contents of the mat are placed carefully in the still right away.

If more flowers are cut than can be dealt with quickly in the still, the flowers should be stored in a closed shed so as to prevent them drying and losing a portion of the essential oil. Every effort should be taken to prevent the slightest fermentation of the flowers before distillation. Fermentation means a smaller yield and a poorer quality of oil.

In making the most refined Lavender oil, the blossoms are carefully stripped off the stalk previous to distillation and distilled alone, but this is necessarily a more expensive way of proceeding. The oil in the stalks has a much coarser odour. The British Pharmacopœia directs that Lavender oil for medicinal use should be thus distilled from the flowers after they have been separated from their stalks, and the oil distilled in Britain is alone official, as it is very superior to foreign oil of Lavender.

¶ *Distillation.* The stills usually employed by growers are of simple construction, any fault in the distillate being subsequently rectified by fractional distillation. The stills are constructed of copper, and generally built to take a charge of about 5 cwt. of flowers at a time. It is important to avoid burning, and the practice is to provide the stills with two chambers, with a perforated false bottom between, the lower chamber being filled with water which should be as soft as possible. Distillation is conducted by boiling the water beneath the charge with steam brought from a boiler to a coil, the top of which must be at least 1 foot beneath the bottom of the charge chamber. The oilflow from the condenser must be watched for, and complete distillation of the charge usually takes about six hours from commencement of the flow.

The yield of the oil is apt to vary considerably from season to season, as the age of the bushes and the weather will affect both the quantity and quality of the product. The amount of sunlight in the weeks before distillation has a great influence: the best oil is obtained after a hot, droughty season, heavy rains detract from the yield.

An acre of Lavender in its prime would in a favourable year yield from 15 to 20 lb. of oil, but taking the whole of the area planted as described above, an average yield of 12 lb. to the area would be a fair estimate.

The distillate should be left for several months to become quite clear and transparent before it is offered for sale.

At Hitchin, it has been calculated that 60 lb. of good flowers will yield on the average 16 fluid ounces of oil.

Growers not doing their own distilling, but preparing the flowers dry for market, should spread the stalks out in the open, on trays or sieves, in a cool, shady position, out of the sun, so that they may dry slowly. The trays should be raised a few feet from the ground, to ensure a warm current of air, and the stems must not be allowed to touch, or the flowers will be spoilt by the moist heat engendered. They must be taken indoors before there is any risk of them getting damp either by dew or showers. When dry, they should be stored in a dry place and made up into bundles. The flowers may also be stripped from the stalks and dried by a moderate heat. They have a greyish-blue colour when dried.

¶ *Constituents.* The principal constituent of Lavender is the volatile oil, of which the dried flowers contain from 1·5 to 3 per cent. fresh flowers yielding about 0·5 per cent. It is pale yellow, yellowish-green or nearly colourless, with the fragrant odour of the flowers and a pungent, bitter taste. The chief constituents of the oil are linalool and its acetic ester, linalyl acetate, which is also the characteristic ingredient of oil of bergamot and is present in English oil of Lavender to the extent of 7 to 10 per cent. Other constituents of the oil are cineol (in English oil, only a trace in French oils), pinene, limonene, geraniol, borneol and some tannin. Lavender oil is soluble in all proportions of alcohol.

It is principally to the esters that Lavender oil owes its delicate perfume. In the oil there are two esters which practically control the odour, of these the principal is linalyl acetate, the second is linalyl butyrate, and Lavender oil nowadays is very largely valued by chemical analysis, involving a determination of the esters. Many things influence the ester value of Lavender oil. In the first place, the preponderance of one or other of the varieties of Lavender used for distillation makes an appreciable difference; in cultivated material, the use of artificial manures not only increases the ester value of the oil, but also increases the yield. The gathering of the flowers when fully expanded and their rapid transport to the stills has considerable influence and the rapid distillation by steam shows a very marked advantage over water distillation. The proportion of esters in Lavender also depends on the period of development of the flower. In June, the esters are found disseminated throughout all the green parts of the plant. From this time onwards, as the plants develop, the esters commence to concentrate in the flowering spikes: the accumulation of oil in these spikes can be distinctly seen by the naked eye in brilliant sunshine, the tiny oil globules shining like little diamonds. The delicacy is completed by the concentration of the esters during the following month; in an ordinary year, the maximum odour is developed by the end of July. About the middle of August, the perfume commences to deteriorate. Oil distilled from the earliest flowers is pale and contains a higher proportion of the more valuable esters; oil distilled from the later flowers has a preponderance of the less valuable esters and is darker in colour. It is evident from these facts that the correct time of gathering is directly flowering is at the full, and English Lavender is always entirely harvested in under a week, and the flowers are distilled on the spot.

¶ *Medicinal Action and Uses.* Lavender was used in earlier days as a condiment and for flavouring dishes 'to comfort the stomach.' Gerard speaks of Conserves of Lavender being served at table.

It has aromatic, carminative and nervine properties. Though largely used in perfumery, it is now not much employed internally, except as a flavouring agent, occurring occasionally in pharmacy to cover disagreeable odours in ointments and other compounds.

Red Lavender lozenges are employed both as a mild stimulant and for their pleasant taste.

The essential oil, or a spirit of Lavender made from it, proves admirably restorative and tonic against faintness, palpitations of a nervous sort, weak giddiness, spasms and colic. It is agreeable to the taste and smell, provokes appetite, raises the spirits and dispels flatulence. The dose is from 1 to 4 drops on sugar or in a spoonful or two of milk.

A few drops of the essence of Lavender in a hot footbath has a marked influence in relieving fatigue. Outwardly applied, it relieves toothache, neuralgia, sprains, and rheumatism. In hysteria, palsy and similar disorders of debility and lack of nerve power, Lavender will act as a powerful stimulant.

'It profiteth them much,' says Gerard, 'that have the palsy if they be washed with the distilled water from the Lavender flowers, or are annointed with the oil made from the flowers and olive oil in such manner as oil of roses is used.'

Culpepper says that

'a decoction made with the flowers of Lavender, Horehound, Fennel and Asparagus root, and a little Cinnamon, is very profitably used to help the falling-sickness (epilepsy) and the giddiness or turning of the brain.'

Salmon in his *Herbal* (1710) says that

'it is good also against the bitings of serpents, mad-dogs and other venomous creature, being given inwardly and applied poultice-wise to the parts wounded. The spirituous tincture of the dried leaves or seeds, if prudently given, cures hysterick fits though vehement and of long standing.'

In some cases of mental depression and delusions, oil of Lavender proves of real service, and a few drops rubbed on the temple will cure nervous headache.

Compound Tincture of Lavender, sold under the name of Lavender drops, besides being a useful colouring and flavouring for mixtures, is still largely used for faintness. This tincture of red Lavender is a popular medicinal cordial, and is composed of the oils of Lavender and Rosmary, with cinnamon bark, nutmeg and red sandle wood, macerated in spirit of wine for seven days. A teaspoonful may be taken as a dose in a little water after an indigestible meal, repeating after half an hour if needed.

It has been officially recognized in the successive British Pharmacopœia for over 200 years. In the eighteenth century, this preparation was known as 'palsy drops' and as 'red hartshorn.' The formula which first appeared in the London Pharmacopœia at the end of the seventeenth century was a complicated one. It contained nearly thirty ingredients, and was prepared by distilling the fresh flowers of lavender, sage, rosemary, betony, cowslips, lily of the valley, etc., with French brandy; in the distillate such spices as cinnamon, nutmeg, mace, cardamoms were digested for twenty-four hours, and then musk, ambergris, saffron, red roses and red sanders-wood were tied in a bag and suspended in the spirit to perfume and colour it. The popularity of this remedy for two hundred and fifty years may be understood by referring to the statements made concerning its virtues when it was first made official. It was said to be useful

'against the Falling-sickness, and all cold Distempers of the Head, Womb, Stomach and Nerves; against the Apoplexy, Palsy, Convulsions, Megrim, Vertigo, Loss of Memory, Dimness of Sight, Melancholy, Swooning Fits and Barrenness in Women. It was given in canary, or the Syrup of the Juice of Black-cherries, or in Florence wine. Country people may take it in milk or fair water sweetened with sugar. . . . It is an excellent but costly medicine.'

In the London Pharmacopœia of 1746 a very drastic change was made in the recipe and practically no change has been made since that time.

A tea brewed from Lavender tops, made in moderate strength, is excellent to relieve headache from fatigue and exhaustion, giving the same relief as the application of Lavender water to the temples. An infusion taken too freely, will, however, cause griping and colic, and Lavender oil in too large doses is a narcotic poison and causes death by convulsions.

'The chymical oil drawn from Lavender,' to quote Culpepper, 'usually called Oil of Spike, is of so fierce and piercing a quality, that it is cautiously to be used, some few drops being sufficient to be given with other things, either for inward or outward griefs.'

Lavender oil is found of service when rubbed externally for stimulating paralysed limbs. Mixed with $\frac{3}{4}$ spirit of turpentine or spirit of wine it made the famous Oleum Spicæ, formerly much celebrated for curing old sprains and stiff joints. Fomentations with Lavender in bags, applied hot, will speedily relieve local pains.

A distilled water made from Lavender has been used as a gargle and for hoarseness and loss of voice.

Its use in the swabbing of wounds obtained further proof during the War, and the French Academy of Medicine is giving attention to the oil for this and other antiseptic surgical purposes. The oil is successfully used in the treatment of sores, varicose ulcers, burns and scalds. In France, it is a regular thing for most households to keep a bottle of Essence of Lavender as a domestic remedy against bruises, bites and trivial aches and pains, both external and internal.

Lavender oil is also used in veterinary practice, being very efficacious in killing lice and other parasites on animals. Its germicidal properties are very pronounced. In the south-east of France it is considered a useful vermifuge.

The oil is used in the embalming of corpses to a steadily increasing extent.

¶ *Preparations and Dosages.* Fluid extract, $\frac{1}{2}$ to 1 drachm. Compound Tincture, B.P., and U.S.P., $\frac{1}{2}$ to 1 drachm. Oil, 1 to 3 drops. Spirit, B.P. and U.S.P., 5 to 30 drops.

Adulteration of Lavender Oil. French oils containing less than 30 per cent. of esters are very often mixed with Spike or Bastard Lavender oils. Formerly adulteration used to be with oil of Turpentine, often mixed with coco-nut oil, but this has given place to various artificial esters prepared chemically, which are practically odourless and only added to make the oil appear to have a higher ester percentage than it really has. Recently, crude mixtures of Lavender oil with Petit-grain oil have been noticed on the market.

Spanish Lavender Oil, distilled in Spain and sold largely to England as Lavender oil, is not a genuine Lavender oil at all, but an oil practically free from esters, having the general character of Spike Lavender oil. The production of this oil now reaches about 40,000 kilos per annum.

Spike Lavender Oil is of a penetrating, camphoraceous odour and is never worth more than about one-fifth of the value of genuine Lavender oil. The oil is used in veterinary practice in considerable quantities, as a prophylactic in cases of incipient paralysis. It is also employed (together with that from *L. Stœchas*) in the manufacture of certain types of fine varnishes and lacquers, with oil of turpentine, and used by painters on porcelain. It is used to a very great extent in cheap perfumery and for scenting soaps, especially in England and the United States. The annual production of Spike Lavender oil in France is about 25,000 kilos.

This oil of Latifolia or Spica is said to admirably promote the growth of the hair when weakly or falling off. A decoction – Spike Water – can be made from the plant.

Dried Lavender flowers are still greatly used to perfume linen, their powerful, aromatic odour acting also as a preventative to the attacks of moths and other insects. In America, they find very considerable employment for disinfecting hotrooms and keeping away flies and mosquitoes, who do not like the scent. Oil of Lavender, on cotton-wool, tied in a little bag or in a perforated ball hung in the room, is said to keep it free from all flies.

Not only are insects averse to the smell of Lavender, so that oil of Lavender rubbed on the skin will prevent midge and mosquito bites, but it is said on good authority that the lions and tigers in our Zoological Gardens are powerfully affected by the scent of Lavender Water, and will become docile under its influence.

The flowers and leaves were formerly em-

ployed as a sternutatory and probably still enter into the composition of some snuffs.

In the East, especially in Turkey and Egypt, they are used, as of old, for perfuming the bath.

The 'straw,' completely freed from the flowers, is sold and used as litter and also for making ointment. If burnt, for deodorizing purposes, the stalks diffuse a powerful, but agreeable odour.

Lavender Water can easily be prepared at home. Into a quart bottle are put 1 oz. essential oil of Lavender, one drop of Musk and 1½ pint spirits of wine. These three ingredients are well mixed together by shaking. The mixture is left to settle, shaken again in a few days, then poured into little perfume bottles fitted with air-tight stoppers. This is another recipe from an old family book:

'Put into a bottle half a pint of spirit of wine and two drachms of oil of lavender. Mix it with rose-water, five ounces, orange-flower water, two ounces, also two drachms of musk and six ounces of distilled water.'

This is stated to be 'a pleasant and efficacious cordial and very useful in languor and weakness of the nerves, lowness of spirits, faintings, etc.'

Another recipe is to mix 2 oz. of refined essence of Lavender with ¾ pint of good brandy. This Lavender Water is so strong that it must be diluted with water before it is used.

Lavender Vinegar. A refreshing toilet preparation is made by mixing 6 parts of Rose-water, 1 part of spirits of Lavender and 2 parts of Orleans vinegar.

It can also be prepared from freshly-gathered flower-tops. These are dried, placed in a stoppered bottle and steeped for a week in Orleans vinegar. Every day the bottle must be shaken, and at the end of the week the liquid is drained off and filtered through white blotting paper.

Another delicious and aromatic toilet vinegar is made as follows: Dry a good quantity of rose leaves, lavender flowers and jasmine flowers. Weigh them, and to every 4 oz. of rose leaves allow 1 oz. each of lavender and jasmine. Mix them well together, pour over them 2 pints of white vinegar, and shake well, then add ½ pint of rose-water and shake again. Stand aside for ten days, then strain and bottle.

LAVENDER COTTON

Santolina Chamæcyparissus (LINN.)
N.O. Compositæ

Synonym. Santolina
Part Used. Herb

Lavender Cotton (also sometimes called French Lavender, like *L. Stœchas*) is botanically known as *Santolina Chamæcy-*

parissus. It is not a true Lavender at all, but has yellow, clustered buttons of composite flowers and finely-cut, grey, rather disagreeably-scented leaves, whose odour somewhat resembles Chamomile. It is used as a vermifuge for children. This plant was once also esteemed for its stimulant properties, and the twigs have been used for placing amongst linen, etc., to keep away moths. All the species of *Santolina* have a strong resemblance to one another, except *S. fragrantissima*, which differs in having the flowerheads in flat inflorescences termed corymbs, the flowers all being at the same level, instead of singly at the apex of the twigs.

The Arabs are said to use the juice of this plant for bathing the eyes. Culpepper tells us that Lavender Cotton 'resists poison, putrefaction and heals the biting of venomous beasts.' It is now chiefly used as an edging to borders, spreading like a silvery carpet close to the ground.

A perfume oil is also extracted from it.

LAVENDER, SEA, AMERICAN

Statice Caroliniana (WALT.)
N.O. Plumbaginaceæ

Synonyms. Statice Limonium. Ink Root. Sea Lavender. Marsh Rosemary
Part Used. Root
Habitat. America, Europe and England. A perennial maritime plant with a large, fleshy, fusiform, brownish-red root; limnal leaves in tufts – obovate, entire, obtuse, mucronate, smooth, and on long foot-stalks. Flowers, pale bluish-purple. Fruit an oblong utricle, one-seeded, enclosed in calyx, usually called Marsh Rosemary. It is common in the salt marshes of the Atlantic shore. Flowers August to October

¶ *Part Used* is the root. This is large, heavy, blackish, inodorous, with a bitter, saltish and very astringent taste.

¶ *Constituents.* Volatile oil, resin, gum, albumen, tannic acid, caoutchouc, extractive and colouring matter, woody fibre, and various salts. It has long been in use as a domestic remedy for diarrhœa, dysentery, etc., but is only used as an astringent tonic after the acute stage has passed. It is also very useful as a gargle or wash in ulcerations of mouth and throat, scarlatina, anguinosa, etc. The powdered root is applied to old ulcers, or made with a soothing ointment for piles. As an injection the decoction is very useful in chronic gonorrhœa, gleet, leucorrhœa, prolapsus of womb and anus, and in some ophthalmic affections. It can otherwise be used where astringents are indicated and may be applicable to all cases where kino and catechu are given. It is said to be a valuable remedy for internal and local use in cynanche maligna. Decoction is 1 ounce of powdered root to 1 pint, in wineglassful doses.

LEMON

Citrus Limonum (RISSO.)
N.O. Rutaceæ

Synonyms. Citrus medica. Citrus Limonum. Citronnier. Neemoo. Leemoo. Limoun. Limone
Parts Used. Rind, juice, oil
Habitat. Indigenous to Northern India. Widely cultivated in Mediterranean countries

¶ *Description.* The name *Limonum* is derived from the Arabic *Limun* or *Limu*, which in its turn probably comes from the Sanscrit *Nimbuka*. There are several varieties of *Citrus medica*, only differing in the character of their fruits. The principal ones are the lemon, citron or cedrat, and lime. The Bergamot is also closely related. The trees reached Europe by way of Persia or Media and were grown first in Greece and then in Italy in the second century.

The Lemon is a small, straggling tree about 11 feet high, irregularly branched, the bark varying in colour from clear grey on the trunk, green on the younger branches to a purplish colour on the twigs. The evergreen leaves are ovate-oval, about two inches long, the margin serrate with sharp spines in the axils of the stalks. The solitary, five-petalled flowers, white inside and tinged with deep pink outside, grow on stems in the axils. The well-known fruit is an ovoid berry, about three inches long, nipple-shaped at the end, smooth, bright yellow, indented over the oil-glands, having an acid, pale-yellow pulp. About forty-seven varieties are said to have been developed during the centuries of cultivation.

The finest fruits arrive wrapped separately in paper, cases of the Messina lemons containing 360, and of Murcia lemons 200. Those from Naples and Malaga are thought to be less fine. Inferior fruits, preserved in salt water, are packed in barrels. It is stated that they can be kept fresh for months if dipped in melted paraffin or varnished with shellac dissolved in alcohol.

The peel, *Limonis Cortex*, is white and spongy inside, varying much in thickness, and the yellow outer layer, formerly called the *flavedo*, has a fragrant odour and aromatic, bitter taste. Only the fresh rind is official.

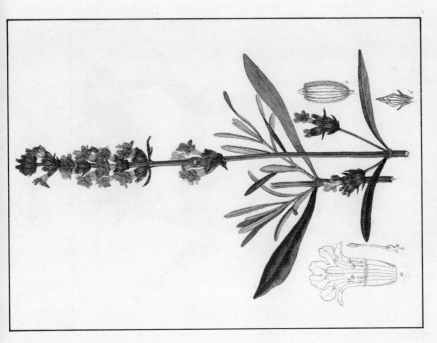

SPIKE LAVENDER
Lavandula Spica

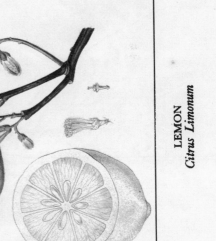

LEMON
Citrus Limonum

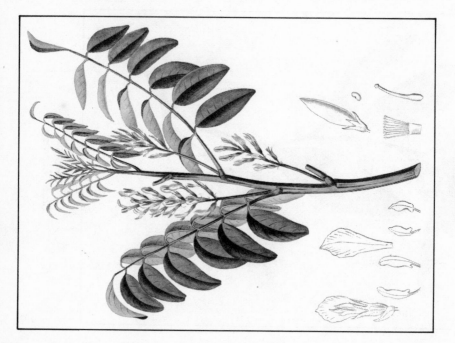

WILD LETTUCE
Lactuca Virosa

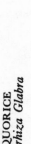

LIQUORICE
Glycyrrhiza Glabra

Candied lemon peel may be prepared by boiling the peel in syrup and then exposing it to the air until the sugar is crystallized.

The juice, *L. succus*, is largely imported as a source of citric acid, but is mixed with that of lime and bergamot. It does not keep well, and several methods are tried for preserving it, such as covering it with a layer of almond oil, mixing with alcohol and filtering, or adding sulphur dioxide, but none appear to be very satisfactory. The juice should be pressed fresh for pharmaceutical purposes, the amount of citric acid being greatest in December and January and least in August.

In Sicily, the pulp left after the production of the volatile oil is pressed for juice in large quantities and the solid matter left is used as cattle food.

The oil, *Oleum Limonis*, is more fragrant and valuable if obtained by expression than by distillation. It is usually prepared in Sicily and Calabria, and sometimes at Nice and Mentone, where the 'Essence de Citron distillée' is prepared by rubbing fresh lemons on a coarse, tin grater, and distilling the grated peel with water. The better 'Essence de Citron au zeste' is prepared with the aid of a saucer-shaped, pewter dish with a pouring lip at one side and a closed funnel sunk from the middle. In the bottom are sharp, strong brass pins on which the peel is rubbed. This vessel is called an *écuelle à piquer*, but a machine called *scorzetta* is gradually coming into use.

The method of expression in Sicily is that of squeezing large slices of peel against sponges fixed in the hand, the sponges when soaked being wrung into an earthen bowl with a spout, in which the oil separates from the watery liquid. The peel is afterwards pickled in brine and sold to manufacturers for candying.

The roots and wood are cut in winter. The latter takes a beautiful polish and is nicely veined.

The dried flowers and leaves are used in pharmacy in France.

The Lemon is widely used in cookery and confectionery. A thousand lemons yield between 1 and 2 lb. of oil. The immature fruit yields less and the quality is inferior.

Messina alone exported 155,000 kilos of oil in 1919.

¶ *Constituents.* Lemon Peel yields its virtues to alcohol, water, or wine. It contains an essential oil and a bitter principle. Crystals of the glucoside Hesperidin are deposited by the evaporation of the white, pulpy portion boiled in water. Diluted acids decompose it into Hesperitin and glucose.

Lemon Juice contains from 6·7 to 8·6 per cent. of citric acid. It is officially described as 'a slightly turbid yellowish liquor, possessing a sharp, acid taste and grateful odour.'

It contains also sugar, gum, and a very little potash. An imitation lemon juice has been made by dissolving tartaric acid in water, adding sulphuric acid and flavouring with oil of Lemon. It is useless therapeutically.

Oil of Lemon is dextrogyre. It contains 7 to 8 per cent. of *citral*, an aldehyde yielding geraniol upon reduction, a small amount of pinene and citronellal, etc. It is stated that citral, citronellal, and an ester of geraniol are all necessary for the true odour.

The oil is not very active, and is used chiefly for flavouring.

¶ *Medicinal Action and Uses.* Lemon juice is probably the best of all antiscorbutics, being almost a specific in scurvy. English ships are required by law to carry sufficient lemon or limejuice for every seaman to have an ounce daily after being ten days at sea. Its value in this direction has been stated to be due to its vitamines.

It is valuable as a cooling drink in fevers, and for allaying thirst. When unobtainable, a solution of 8 drachms of crystallized citric acid in 16 oz. of water, flavoured with oil of lemon, may be substituted.

The juice may be used in diaphoretic and diuretic draughts. It is highly recommended in acute rheumatism, and is sometimes given to counteract narcotic poisons, especially opium.

Locally, it is a good astringent, whether as a gargle in sore throat, in pruritis of the scrotum, in uterine hæmorrhage after delivery, or as a lotion in sunburn. It is said to be the best cure for severe, obstinate hiccough, and is helpful in jaundice and hysterical palpitation of the heart. The decoction has been found to be a good antiperiodic, useful as a substitute for quinine in malarial conditions, or for reducing the temperature in typhoid.

It is probable that the lemon is the most valuable of all fruit for preserving health.

The *oil*, externally, is a strong rubefacient, and taken internally in small doses has stimulating and carminative properties.

Preparations of the rind are used as an aromatic addition to tonics, and also the syrup of the fresh peel, and the juice.

¶ *Preparations and Dosages.* Fresh juice (for rheumatism), 4 to 6 fluid ounces. Oil, B.P., 3 to 5 minims. Juice, B.P., ½ to 4 drachms. Tincture, B.P. and U.S.P., ½ to 1 drachm. Syrup, B.P., ½ to 4 drachms.

¶ *Substitutes and Adulterations.* The most dangerous adulterant of the oil is *citrene*, the terpene left after extracting citral from oil of lemon which has been used in making terpeneless oil.

Fixed oils, alcohol, and purified oil of turpentine are sometimes found, the last causing a terebinthinate odour if evaporated from heated paper.

The pure oil should show scarcely any *pinene*.

Artificial lemon juice should not be used as an antiscorbutic.

¶ *Other Species.*

Lime juice, the product of *C. medica acida*, is recognized by the National Formulary under the name of *Succus Citri*.

Cedrat Lemon, or *C. medica cedra*, yields the essential oils of citron and cedra used in perfumery.

Lippia citriodora, yielding verbena oil, is commonly known as Lemon Verbena.

Java Lemon is *C. Javanica.* Median Lemon is a variety of *C. medica.* Pear Lemon is a variety of *C. Limetta.* Pearl Lemon is *C. margarita.* Sweet Lemon is *C. Lumia.* Water Lemon is *Passiflora laurifolia.* Wild Lemon or Ground Lemon is *Podophyllum peltatum.* Lemon Yellow is the name of Chrome Yellow, a neutral lead-chromate.

LETTUCE, WILD

Lactuca virosa (LINN.)
N.O. Compositæ

Synonyms. Lactucarium. Strong-scented Lettuce. Green Endive. Lettuce Opium. Laitue vireuse. Acrid Lettuce

Parts Used. The dried milk-juice (Lactuarium), the leaves

Habitat. Western and Southern Europe, including Britain

¶ *Description.* The name *lactuca* is derived from the classical Latin name for the milky juice, *virosa*, or 'poisonous.'

It is a biennial herb growing to a maximum height of 6 feet. The erect stem, springing from a brown tap-root, is smooth and pale green, sometimes spotted with purple. There are a few prickles on the lower part and short horizontal branches above. The numerous, large, radical leaves are from 6 to 18 inches long, entire, and obovate-oblong. The stem leaves are scanty, alternate, and small, clasping the stem with two small lobes. The heads are numerous and shortly-stalked, the pale-yellow corolla being strap-shaped. The rough, black fruit is oval, with a broad wing along the edge, and prolonged above into a long, white beak carrying silvery tufts of hair. The whole plant is rich in a milky juice that flows freely from any wound. This has a bitter taste and a narcotic odour. When dry, it hardens, turns brown, and is known as lactucarium.

¶ *Habitat.* The Wild Lettuce grows on banks and waste places, flowering in July and August. It is cultivated in Austria, France, Germany and Scotland. Collectors cut the heads of the plants and scrape the juice into china vessels several times daily until it is exhausted. By slightly warming and tapping, it is turned out of its cup mould, is cut into quarters and dried.

In the United States, after importation from Germany via England it is said to be used as an adulterant for opium. It is usually found in irregular, reddish-brown lumps the size of a large pea, frequently mouldy on the outside. In the United States the German and French *lactucarium* is considered inferior to the British product.

All lettuces possess some of this narcotic juice, *Lactuca virosa* having the most, and the others in the following order: *L. scariola*, or Prickly Lettuce, *L. altissima*, *L. Canadensis*, or Wild Lettuce of America, and *L. sativa*, or Garden Lettuce. Cultivation has lessened the narcotic properties of the last, but it is still used for making a lotion for the skin useful in sunburn and roughness. The Ancients held the lettuce in high esteem for its cooling and refreshing properties. The Emperor Augustus attributed his recovery from a dangerous illness to it; built an altar to it, and erected a statue in its honour.

Lactucarium is not easily powdered, and is only slightly soluble in boiling water, though it softens and becomes plastic.

Thridace, or the inspissated juice of *L. capitata*, is now regarded as inert.

A mild oil, used in cooking, is said to be obtained from the seeds in Egypt.

¶ *Constituents.* *L. virosa* has been found to contain lactucic acid, lactucopicrin, 50 to 60 per cent. lactucerin (lactucone) and lactucin. Lactucarium treated with boiling water and filtered is clear, but on cooling the filtrate becomes turbid. It is not coloured blue by iodine test solution. The usual constituents of latex are albumen, mannite, and caoutchouc.

The fresh juice reddens litmus paper.

¶ *Medicinal Action and Uses.* The drug resembles a feeble opium without its tendency to upset the digestive system. It is used to a small extent as a sedative and narcotic.

Dissolved in wine it is said to be a good anodyne.

Dr. Collins stated that twenty-three out of twenty-four cases of dropsy were cured by taking doses of 18 grains to 3 drachms of extract in twenty-four hours. It is used in Germany in this complaint, but combined with more active drugs. It is said to be also a mild diaphoretic and diuretic, easing colic, inducing sleep and allaying cough.

Water distilled from lettuce (*eau de laitre*) is used in France as a mild sedative in doses of 2 to 4 oz., and the fresh leaves boiled in water are sometimes used as a cataplasm.

Moderate doses given to the lower animals act as a narcotic poison, an injection having even caused death.

¶ *Dosages.* Of powder, 10 to 20 grains or more. Of tincture, 30 to 60 drops. Of alcoholic extract, 1 to 5 grains. Of Lactucarium, 5 to 20 grains. Of fluid extract leaves, ¼ to 1 drachm. Of syrup, U.S.P., 2 drachms. Tincture, U.S.P., 30 drops.

LIFE EVERLASTING (PEARL-FLOWERED)

Antennaria Margaritaceum
N.O. Compositæ

Synonyms. American Everlasting. Cudweed
Parts Used. Leaves, flowers, stalks
Habitat. North America, Kamschatka and in English gardens. Grows wild in Essex, near Bocking, and in Wales. Cultivated in Whin's Cottage garden by the writer

¶ *Medicinal Action and Uses.* Anodyne, astringent, pectoral, useful in diarrhœa, dysentery, pulmonary affections, as a poultice for sprains, bruises, boils, painful swellings. Said to produce sleep. When hops have failed, applied externally to the head, a decoction of the flowers and stalks used in America as a fomentation for pained and bruised limbs, and for bronchitis.

Leaves linear, lanceolate, acuminate; alternate stalk branched at top; corymbs fastigiate; root perennial, creeping, spreading, becoming almost a troublesome weed; stalks very downy, and white flowering branches form a flat broad bunch, each branch with numerous crowded heads, on short branched downy peduncles, the middle ones sessile; calyx scales bluntly ovate and white, but not downy, flowers July to September. Easily propagated by creeping roots. The plant is slightly fragrant.

See CATSFOOT, CUDWEED, GNAPHALIUM, WHITE BALSAM.

LIFE ROOT. *See* GROUNDSEL

LILACS (WHITE AND MAUVE)

Syringa vulgaris
N.O. Oleaceæ

Synonym. Common Lilac
Parts Used. Leaves, fruit
Habitat. Persia, mountainous regions of Eastern Europe

¶ *Description.* A shrub or small tree up to 20 feet in height producing a crowd of erect stems, occasionally a trunk over 2 feet in girth, clothed with spirally arranged flakes of bark. Shoots and leaves smooth, leaves heart-shape or ovate, 2 to 6 inches long, from ¾ to almost as much wide near the base; stalk ¾ to 1½ inch long. Panicles pyramidal, 6 to 8 inches long, usually in pairs from the terminal buds; flowers fragrant; corolla tube ⅓ to ½ inch long; lobes concave; calyx and flower-stalks have gland tipped down; seed vessels smooth, ⅝ inch long, beaked.

Introduced to Britain during time of Henry VIII, mentioned in an inventory taken at Norwich by Oliver Cromwell.

Syringa Baccifera is a synonym of *Mitchella repens* or Partridge Berry and *must not be confused* with *S. vulgaris*.

¶ *Medicinal Action and Uses.* Used as a vermifuge in America and as a tonic anti-periodic and febrifuge; may be used as a substitute for aloes and in the treatment of malaria.

LILIES

N.O. Liliaceæ

The Lilies belong to a genus consisting of less than 100 known species, occurring in all parts of the Northern Hemisphere. They are mostly found growing in fairly good soil in association with shrubs and other plants which shade their roots and help to keep the bulbs cool and in a uniform state as regards moisture.

¶ *Cultivation.* With some exceptions, Lilies grown as garden plants in this country are fairly hardy, especially if planted deep enough and in doubtful cases given protection with ashes or dry litter. The majority of Lilies require a soil fairly rich in humus or vegetable mould, and if it is desirable to plant Lilies in poor soil or in chalky districts, an area must be dug out 2 feet deep and filled in with kitchen garden soil mixed with fibrous loam and sand. Plant the bulbs fully 3 inches deep in most cases and surround them with an envelope of sand ½ inch thick; this allows excessive moisture to pass away freely; it acts also as a guard against the attacks of slugs, and, by reason of its sterility, as a barrier against the spread of such fungoid diseases as may infest the surrounding soil and which would be likely to destroy the bulbs if they gained access to them. The bulbs of all Lilies root quicker and with greater freedom if a few pieces of peat are placed beneath them when planted. Many cases of failure can be traced to the condition of the soil, as the bulbs rot during winter owing to the presence of stagnant moisture: it is useless to plant Lilies in very poor ground or in any position which is water-logged in winter. In their native countries they enjoy more sunshine in their growing season than we usually get and wet at the root during winter often proves fatal to many of them. When growing, however, all Lilies require plenty of moisture. If they are neglected in this respect they will not produce the glorious spikes of flowers they are capable of; moreover, a Lily once drought-stricken or in any way seriously checked in growth so as to produce debility, rarely recovers its health. Disappointment with Lilies is due often also to late planting, but if good home-grown bulbs of the different kinds are planted before the end of September, to give them time to make their natural autumn growth, they should, in suitable soil, flower well the next year.

A large number of varieties produce two distinct sets of root – those from the base of the bulb and others from the base of the stem, above the bulb. These are termed 'stem-rooting.'

In planting Lily bulbs, two points are essential to bear in mind: (1) Does the species relish lime or detest it? (2) Is it a stem-rooter, demanding in consequence to be deeply planted, or is it provided with basal roots only, requiring less depth in planting? *Lilium candidum, L. Martagon* and *L. tigrinum* succeed in well-drained sandy loam and may with advantage be planted in the herbaceous border, all except *candidum* being planted at least 6 to 8 inches in depth.

The best manure for all Lilies is wood ash, provided it has been carefully stored in a dry place, because its virtue consists in the potash it contains, which a single shower suffices to dissolve and wash to waste. The ash of twigs and leaves contains a larger percentage of potash than that of large branches and logs.

¶ *Propagation.* Lilies are propagated by means of division or offsets, which as such increase freely, but increase by seed and bulb-scales are the more usual methods.

L. tigrinum and some others produce little bulbs in the axils of the leaves, which form a ready means of increase and only need growing on under suitable conditions to produce flowering bulbs. *L. candidum* produces plenty of small bulbs around the parent bulb and thus affords a ready means of increase. For those that do not produce seeds or offsets readily, propagation by bulb-scales is resorted to, each healthy scale being capable of producing a new bulb at its base. The scales are pulled off and inserted in pans and boxes of sandy soil and stood in cold frames, when in about six months small bulbs are produced at the base of the scales.

All Lilies that do not afford a ready means of increase by bulbils or division, or bulb-scales should be grown by seeds, which is the only way to attain success in this country with many of them. Imported bulbs as a rule only grow for one or two years and then die; although immense consignments of beautiful Asiatic species of Lilies are annually imported, less than 50 per cent. of them survive to a second season, flowering, if at all, only once from nutriment stored within the bulb, the cause being probably want of care in raising and packing the bulb and the fact, also, that the great majority of bulbs on arrival are found to be infested with mites or fungus.

Lilies grown from seed take from two to six years to produce flowers. When raising from seed, a regular rotation should be maintained by sowing a quantity of seed each year. Many Lilies germinate exceedingly well in cold frames when sown in March, April or May. When the young seedlings have made their second or third leaf, they may be planted outdoors in a sheltered border during the spring, to get well-established before winter, the less hardy ones being grown in frames.

The mould *Botrytis cinerea*, which attacks so many garden plants, often attacks Lilies, especially *L. candidum*: it is usually the foliage that is attacked. On the first signs, the plants should be sprayed with a solution of sulphide of potassium, using an ounce to a gallon of warm water (temperature 100° to 120° F.), at the same time removing any affected leaves and burning them. If a little soft soap is dissolved with the mixture, it adheres much better to the foliage and is not so easily washed off by rain. In bad cases, the bulbs may be affected, in which case they should be thoroughly dusted with flowers of sulphur. Cut off and burn the diseased stems, lift the bulbs, place them in a large paper bag containing flowers of sulphur, give a good shaking to work the sulphur well into the scales and then replant in a fresh site. This precaution has often proved successful in warding off a subsequent attack of the disease.

The disease is a more or less mysterious one: it often appears in a virulent form in one garden, whereas in a neighbouring one the plants may be quite free from it. Once it finds foothold in the soil of a garden it remains there, potent for evil whenever the atmospheric conditions are favourable. In dull, chilly, damp summers, the disease becomes epidemic, and does widespread harm to many plants besides Lilies. The sun is the most powerful antidote against the fungus, which is spread by spores too minute for the eye to see.

It is often said that white Lilies in cottage gardens are exempt from attacks of the disease, but in an epidemic they are spared no more than are those in manor gardens. Spraying the foliage with a solution of potassium sulphide helps to keep the disease in check, but it is not a cure; no absolute remedy has yet been discovered, and those who plant this lily must not expect to have it in full beauty every year. This country has relied too much on other nations for its supply of bulbs in the past, and quantities of infected bulbs of *L. candidum* are imported annually from Central and Southern France, where *la Toile* – as the French call *B. cinerea* – has even more of a grip than it has here; and the rapid spread of the disease may well be due in some measure to that tainted source. All the bulbs needed in Great Britain could be grown here. The wild Grecian form of *L. candidum* seems more resistant to *Botrytis* than the cultivated forms.

Lilies are on the whole singularly free from insect and other pests, though wood-lice sometimes prove troublesome. On some soils, slugs are the chief menace; the grey slug attacks the stem and leaves, but the black slug is the more insidious, as it attacks the bulbs and working underground is difficult to deal with. The best means of keeping slugs in check are good cultivation and trapping. One mode of trapping that is much recommended is to place on the ground in the evening boards smeared on their under-

sides with a mixture of flour and stale beer. Examine the boards every morning and destroy the catch. Dry bran also catches many. Coarse, clean sand and small sifted cinders placed round the bulbs will also ward off attacks.

Mice will eat bulbs, especially *L. tigrinum*, and the edible Lilies of Japan.

In China, the dried scales of *L. japonicum* are considered nourishing and useful in diseases of the chest, as a substitute for Salep, the product of Orchis tubers.

L. Martagon (Linn.), the PURPLE TURK'S CAP LILY, is occasionally found growing wild in this country, but is rare, though it has been met with on chalk hills and in woody places in the south of England. It is, however, much cultivated, and is the hardiest of all Lilies, doing well in full sunshine, or in partial shade. It is a lime-lover, very easy to cultivate, usually increases very freely, and is easily raised from seed. It is strong-growing, but very graceful, producing twenty to thirty light spotted, purple flowers, on a tall stem, having reflexed petals, forming a sort of turban, the stamens appearing like a tuft of feathers at the top. The flowers give off their scent at night.

The Martagon group of Lilies, the form of whose flowers has led to their being called Turk's Cap, comprises many of our best known garden species whose habitats are in widely distant portions of the globe. From America have been introduced the so-called Swamp Lilies, *L. pardalinum*, the Panther Lily, *L. canadense* and *L. superbum*. *L. Hansoni* hails from Japan, and these with the Martagons proper carry their leaves in whorls, while in the best known of the remaining species the leaves are scattered on the stem. Of these may be mentioned the scarlet Turk's Cap (*L. chalcedonicum*) from Greece; *L. pyrenaicum* (straw-coloured) from the Pyrenees; *L. monadelphum* from the Caucasus; *L. pomponium verum* (yellow) from Italy.

The old Martagon is the commonest European species, being distributed throughout the whole of the southern and central portions of the Continent. It was mentioned by Gerard in his list of garden plants in 1596, and, though now out of favour, owing to its dull purple colour, has remained in cultivation, especially in cottage plots, ever since. Though interesting for its old associations, it is now superseded by the more striking forms. Although the purple Martagon bulbs are eaten in their native countries, they are too local here to be reckoned as one of our esculent herbs.

LILY, CROWN IMPERIAL

Fritillaria imperialis (LINN.)
N.O. Liliaceæ

Fritillaria imperialis (Linn.), the Crown Imperial Lily of Persia, is said to be there cultivated as a food plant, its bulb possessing poisonous properties when raw, but being wholesome when cooked.

There are two kinds of this handsome plant, associated with the earliest type of English gardens. They bear a circle of pendulous flowers – one blooms pure lemon yellow, the other deep orange red – and have a crown of foliage above them. The same name is given to this Lily in all European languages.

The bulbs have a fœtid odour, described as being like that of a fox, and are powerfully acrid and poisonous. Even honey from the flowers is said to be emetic.

Imperialine was isolated by Fragner in 1888, on extracting the bulbs with chloroform. This alkaloid and its salts are intensely bitter and are heart poisons.

No medicinal use is made of the plant.
See FRITILLARY.

LILY-OF-THE-VALLEY

Convallaria magalis (LINN.)
N.O. Liliaceæ

Synonyms. May Lily. Convallaria. Our Lady's Tears. Convall-lily. Lily Constancy. Ladder-to-Heaven. Jacob's Ladder. Male Lily

Parts Used. Flowers, leaves, whole herb

Habitat. It is a native of Europe, being distributed also over North America and Northern Asia, but in England it is very local as a wild flower. In certain districts it is to be found in abundance, but in many parts it is quite unknown. It is rare in Scotland and doubtfully native and only naturalized in Ireland. It grows mostly in the dryer parts of woods – especially ash woods – often forming extensive patches, and is by no means peculiar to valleys, though both the English and botanical names imply that it is so.

Culpepper reports that in his time these little Lilies grew plentifully on Hampstead Heath, but Green, writing about 100 years ago, tells us that 'since the trees on Hampstead Heath, near London, have been destroyed, it has been but sparingly found there.'

The Lily-of-the-Valley, with its broad leaves and fragrant little, nodding, white, bell-shaped flowers, is familiar to everyone.

¶ *Description.* In early spring days, the creeping rhizome, or underground stem, sends up quill-like shoots emerging from a scaly sheath. As they lengthen and uncoil, they are seen to consist of two leaves, their stalks sheathing one within the other, rising directly from the rhizome on long, narrowing foot-stalks, one leaf often larger than the other. The plain, oval blades, with somewhat concave surfaces, are deeply ribbed and slant a little backwards, thus catching the rain and conducting it by means of the curling-in base of the leaf, as though in a spout, straight down the foot-stalk to the root. At the back of the leaves, lightly enclosed at the base in the same scaly sheath, is the flower-stalk, quite bare of leaves itself and bearing at its summit a number of buds, greenish when young, each on a very short stalk, which become of the purest white, and as they open turn downwards, the flowers hanging, like a pearl of fairy bells, each bell with the edges turned back with six small scallops. The six little stamens are fastened inside the top of the bell, and in the centre hangs the ovary. There is no free honey in the little flowers, but a sweet, juicy sap is stored in a tissue round the base of the ovary and proves a great attraction to bees, who also visit the flower to collect its pollen and who play an important part in the fertilization of the flowers.

By September, the flowers have developed into scarlet berries, each berry containing vermilion flesh round a pale, hard seed. Though the plant produces fruit freely under cultivation, its propagation is mainly effected by its quickly-creeping underground stem, and in the wild state its fruit rarely comes to maturity. Its specific name, *Majalis*, or *Maialis*, signifies 'that which belongs to May,' and the old astrological books place the plant under the dominion of Mercury, since Maia, the daughter of Atlas, was the mother of Mercury or Hermes.

There is an old Sussex legend that St. Leonard fought against a great dragon in the woods near Horsham, only vanquishing it after a mortal combat lasting many hours, during which he received grievous wounds, but wherever his blood fell, Lilies-of-the-Valley sprang up to commemorate the desperate fight, and these woods, which bear the name of St. Leonard's Forest to this day, are still thickly carpeted with them.

Legend says that the fragrance of the Lily-of-the-Valley draws the nightingale from hedge and bush, and leads him to choose his mate in the recesses of the glade.

The Lily-of-the-Valley is one of the British-grown plants included in the Pharmacopœia, and its medicinal virtues have been tested by very long experience. Although not in such general use as the Foxglove, it is still prescribed by physicians with success. Its use dates back to ancient times, for Apuleius in his *Herbal* written in the fourth century, declares it was found by Apollo and given by him to Æsculapius, the leech.

In recent years it has been largely employed in experiments relating to the forcing of plants by means of anæsthetics such as chloroform and ether. It has been found that the winter buds, placed in the vapour of chloroform for a few hours and then planted, break into leaf and flower considerably before others not tested in this manner, the resulting plants being, moreover, exceptionally fine.

The leaves yield a green dye, with lime water.

¶ *Cultivation.* Lily-of-the-Valley is fairly easy to cultivate, preferring well-drained, rich, sandy loam, in moist situations.

Plant towards the end of September. The ground for Lily-of-the-Valley should be thoroughly stirred to a depth of 15 inches, early in September, laying it up rough for a few weeks, then breaking it down and adding some rotten manure, or if that cannot be obtained, some kind of artificial manure must be used, but this is better applied later on, hoeing it in just as growth appears. Plant the crowns about 6 inches apart and work fine, rich soil, with some leaf mould if possible, in between. Leave at least 9 inches between the rows. Keep the crowns well below the surface and above all plant firmly.

In some soils the plants will last longer in the best form than in others, but should be transplanted about every fourth year and in light, porous soils it may be necessary to do so every third year. Periodic transplanting, deep culture and liberal feeding produce fine blooms. Autumn is the best time for remaking beds, which are best done in entirely fresh soil. Cut the roots from the old bed out into tufts 6 inches or 9 inches square, and divide into pieces 3 inches square. Replant the tufts the original 6 inches apart. It is best to prepare the entire beds before replanting. Replanted by October, the crowns will be well settled in by winter rains, and the quality of the spikes will show a marked difference in early spring.

¶ *Parts Used Medicinally.* The whole plant, collected when in flower and dried, and also the root, herb and flowers separately. The inflorescence is said to be the most active part of the herb, and is preferred on that account, being the part usually employed.

The flowers are dried on the scape or flower-stalk, the whole stalk being cut before the lowermost flowers are faded. A good price is obtainable for the flowers, and in Lincolnshire, Derbyshire, Westmorland and other counties, where the plant grows freely wild, they would pay for collecting. During the process of drying, the white flowers assume a brownish-yellow tinge, and the fragrant odour almost entirely disappears, being replaced by a somewhat narcotic scent; the taste of the flowers is bitter.

If Lily-of-the-Valley flowers are thrown into oil of sweet almonds or olive oil, they impart to it their sweet smell, but to become really fragrant the infusion has to be repeated a dozen times with the same oil, using fresh flowers for each infusion.

¶ *Constituents.* The chief constituents of Lily-of-the-Valley are two glucosides, Convallamarin, the active principle, a white crystalline powder, readily soluble in water and in alcohol, but only slightly in ether, which acts upon the heart like Digitalin, and has also diuretic action, and Convallarin, which is crystalline in prisms, soluble in alcohol, slightly soluble in water and has a purgative action. There are also present a trace of volatile oil, tannin, salts, etc.

¶ *Medicinal Action and Uses.* Lily-of-the-Valley is valued as a cardiac tonic and diuretic. The action of the drug closely resembles that of Digitalis, though it is less powerful; it is used as a substitute and strongly recommended in valvular heart disease, also in cases of cardiac debility and dropsy. It slows the disturbed action of a weak, irritable heart, whilst at the same time increasing its power. It is a perfectly safe remedy. No harm has been known to occur from taking it in full and frequent doses, it being preferable in this respect to Digitalis, which is apt to accumulate in the blood with poisonous results.

It proved most useful in cases of poisonous gassing of our men at the Front.

It is generally administered in the form of a tincture. The infusion of ½ oz. of herb to 1 pint of boiling water is also taken in tablespoonful doses. Fluid extracts are likewise prepared from the rhizome, whole plant and flowers and the flowers have been used in powdered form.

A decoction of the flowers is said to be useful in removing obstructions in the urinary canal, and it has been also recommended as a substitute for aloes, on account of its purgative quality.

¶ *Preparations and Dosages.* Fluid extract, herb, 10 to 30 drops. Fluid extract, whole plant, 10 to 30 drops. Fluid extract, flowers, ½ to 1 drachm.

Russian peasants have long employed the Lily-of-the-Valley for certain forms of dropsy proceeding from a faulty heart.

Special virtues were once thought to be possessed by water distilled from the flowers, which was known as *Aqua aurea* (Golden Water), and was deemed worthy to be preserved in vessels of gold and silver. Coles (1657) gives directions for its preparation:

'Take the flowers and steep them in New Wine for the space of a month; which being finished, take them out again and distil the wine three times over in a Limbeck. The wine is more precious than gold, for if any one that is troubled with apoplexy drink thereof with six grains of Pepper and a little Lavender water they shall not need to fear it that moneth.'

Dodoens (1560) pointed out how this water 'doth strengthen the Memorie and comforteth the Harte,' and about the same time, Joachim Camerarius,[1] a renowned physician of Nuremberg, gave a similar prescription, which Gerard quotes, saying that

'a Glasse being filled with the flowers of May Lilies and set in an Ant Hill with the mouth close stopped for a month's space and then taken out, ye shall find a liquor in the glasse which being outwardly applied helps the gout very much.'

This spirit was also considered excellent as an embrocation for sprains, as well as for rheumatism.

We are told by old writers that a decoction of the bruised root, boiled in wine, is good for pestilential fevers, and that bread made of barley meal mixed with the juice is an excellent cure for dropsy, also that an ointment of the root and lard is good for ulcers and heals burns and scalds without leaving a scar.

Culpepper said of the Lily-of-the-Valley:

'It without doubt strengthens the brain and renovates a weak memory. The distilled water dropped into the eyes helps inflammations thereof. The spirit of the flowers, distilled in wine, restoreth lost speech, helps the palsy, and is exceedingly good in the apoplexy, comforteth the heart and vital spirits.'

The powdered flowers have been said to excite sneezing, proving serviceable in the relief of headache and earache; but to some sick people the scent of the flowers has proved harmful.

In some parts of Germany, a wine is still prepared from the flowers, mixed with raisins.

LILY, MADONNA

Lilium candidum (LINN.)
N.O. Liliaceæ

Synonym. White Lily
Part Used. The bulb
Habitat. Mediterranean countries

¶ *History.* When found in Palestine, *Lilium candidum* is sometimes pointed out as the 'Lily of the Field,' but this more probably was *L. chalcedonicum*, the brilliantly scarlet Martagon Lily, which is specially abundant about the Lake of Gennesaret on the plains of Galilee. The *Shushan*, or Lily of Scripture, had probably a very broad meaning and might refer to any striking blossom.

This white Lily was a popular favourite with the ancient Greeks and Romans. In the early days of Christianity it was dedicated by the Church to the Madonna (hence its popular name), probably because its delicate whiteness was considered a symbol of purity. It is employed on the 2nd July, in connection with the celebration of the Visitation of the Blessed Virgin.

It has been cultivated in this country for over three centuries, and no cottage garden was considered complete without this old favourite. Gerard, the famous apothecary, botanist and gardener of that period, says, 'Our English white lilie groweth in most gardens of England.'

It produces stiff, erect stems, 3 to 5 feet high, clothed with lance-shaped leaves. The flowers appear in June, flowering into July, and have a strong, sweet, penetrating perfume, so powerful as to be even annoying to some people. The honey is secreted in long grooves at the base of the white, floral leaves. There are several varieties, that with black stems, var. *peregrinum*, being the best for the garden.

¶ *Cultivation.* The Madonna Lily, when it is immune from disease, to which it is very prone, has a vigorous constitution, being so hardy that frost does not injure it. It will thrive in almost any soil and situation and is

---

[1] [Culpepper says it was *Gerard* who said this.–EDITOR.]

easily cultivated. Though it will do well in ordinary garden soil – especially in raised beds – one of the chief causes of disease is planting in low, badly-drained soil. It produces the finest flowers when growing in a rich, deep, moist loam, where its roots remain undisturbed for years. It is a lime-lover and failures to grow it can often be ascribed to absence of lime in the soil. No plant dislikes removal or digging near the roots more than this lily. This really is the secret of its thriving so well in cottage gardens. It should, therefore, be assigned a home where it can be left, so to speak, to the care of itself (if grown from the horticultural point of view), when it will flower and flourish for a number of years, but the bulbs should be dug up and replanted as soon as they show signs of deteriorating. So long as the plants continue to thrive, it is not advisable to disturb them, for cases have been known where they failed entirely after being transplanted, although they were in a perfect condition previous to shifting them, and they should never be moved more frequently than once in three years.

Planting or replanting should not be delayed beyond the end of August. The bulbs should not be planted more than 4 inches deep and not less than 6 inches apart, as the plants grow tall and spread very fast, being increased by offsets, which the bulbs send out in such plenty, as to make it necessary to take them off every other, or at most every third year, to prevent them weakening the principal bulb. The time for removing them, to ensure flowering next year, is the end of July to August, soon after the stalks decay.

Besides wood ash, an annual top dressing of decayed manure and a dusting of bone-meal in autumn have been found most beneficial to this Lily.

The bulbs are collected in August, and used both dry and fresh. Each bulb is composed of imbricated, fleshy scales, lanceolate and curved, about 1½ inch long and rather less than an inch broad at the widest part. It is odourless, with a slightly bitter and disagreeable taste. The scales should be stripped off separately for drying, and spread on shelves in a warm room for about ten days, then finished off by artificial heat.

The flowers of the Lily were formerly considered anti-epileptic and anodyne: a distilled water was employed as a cosmetic, and oil of Lilies was supposed to possess anodyne and nervine powers. But their odorous matter, though very powerful, is totally dissipated in drying and entirely carried off in distillation, either with spirit or water, so no essential oil can be obtained from them in this manner.

The petals communicate their fragrance to almond and olive oil, and also to lard, and have thus been employed in the past by perfumers.

¶ Uses. The *bulb*, only, is now employed for medicinal purposes, having highly demulcent and also somewhat astringent properties.

Bulbs are collected in August, and used both dried and fresh.

Each bulb is composed of imbricated, fleshy scales, lanceolate and curved, about 1½ inch long and rather less than ½ inch broad in the centre. It is without odour, but has a peculiar, disagreeable, somewhat bitter and mucilaginous taste.

To dry the scales, strip them off separately and spread them on shelves in a kitchen or other warm room for about ten days, then finish off more quickly in greater heat over a stove or gas fire, or in oven when the fire has just gone out.

The bulb contains a great deal of mucilage and a small proportion of an acrid principle, but the latter it loses by drying, roasting, or boiling; when cooked, the bulb is viscid, pulpy, sweet and sugary and is eaten by many people in the East. The Japanese are said to specially esteem the bulb of this species served with white sauce.

¶ *Medicinal Action and Uses.* Demulcent, astringent. Owing to their highly mucilaginous properties, the bulbs are chiefly employed externally, boiled in milk or water, as emollient cataplasms for tumours, ulcers and external inflammation and have been much used for this purpose in popular practice. The fresh bulb, bruised and applied to hard tumours, softens and ripens them sooner than any other application.

Made into an ointment, the bulbs take away corns and remove the pain and inflammation arising from burns and scalds, which they cure without leaving any scar.

The ointment also had the reputation of being an excellent application to contracted tendons. Gerard tells us:

'The root of the Garden Lily stamped with honey gleweth together sinewes that be cut asunder. It bringeth the hairs again upon places which have been burned or scalded, if it be mingled with oil or grease. . . The root of a white Lily, stamped and strained with wine, and given to drink for two or three days together, expelleth the poison of the pestilence.'

In the fresh state, the bulb is also said to have been employed with advantage in dropsy, for Culpepper (1652), besides confirming the uses of the Lily bulb which

Gerard gives, tells us 'the juice of it being tempered with barley meal baked is an excellent cure for the dropsy.'

Combined with Life Root (*Senecio aureus*), it is recommended in modern herbal practice for healing female complaints generally.

¶ *Dosage*. Of infusion, in water or milk, 3 tablespoonsful.

Country people sometimes steep the fresh blooms in spirit and use the liquid as a lotion for bruises in the same manner as *Arnica* or *Calendula*.

The bulbs of several other species of Lilies besides those of *L. candidum* are eaten, as those of *L. Kamschatcense*, *L. Martagon*, the Turk's Cap, and *L. Pomponium*, the Turban or Yellow Martagon, in Siberia. The Chinese and Japanese eat regularly the bulbs of *L. tigrinum*, the Tiger Lily and the Golden-rayed Lily of Japan, *L. auratum*.

LILY, TIGER

Lilium tigrinum
N.O. Liliaceæ

Parts Used. Leaves, stalks, flowers, collected when the plant is in full maturity
Habitat. China and Japan

¶ *Description*. The plant flowers in July and August; the bloom is orange colour and spotted. The upper leaves cordate and oval. It does not ripen seed in this country, but is propagated from the bulbils produced in the axils of the leaves which should yield flowering bulbs in three years from the time of planting.

¶ *Medicinal Action and Uses*. A tincture is made from the fresh plant and has proved of great value in uterine-neuralgia, congestion and irritation, also in the nausea and vomiting of pregnancy.

It relieves the bearing down pain accompanying uterine prolapse.

It is an important remedy in ovarian neuralgia. Poisoning by the pollen of the plant has produced vomiting, drowsiness and purging.

¶ *Dosage*. ⅛ to 5 drops of the tincture.

LILY, WHITE POND

Nymphæa odorata (SOLAND)
N.O. Nymphæaceæ

Synonyms. Sweet Water Lily. Sweet-scented Water Lily. Water Nymph. Large White Water Lily
Part Used. The fresh root
Habitat. Sluggish streams, ponds and marshes, in most parts of the United States, near the coast

¶ *Description*. Perennial aquatic herb, grows to the surface of the water from a thick horizontal root-stock, stem absent, flowers growing on long peduncles and the leaves on separate petioles. Stipules deltoid or nearly reniform, emarginate; leaves always floating orbicular, smooth, and shining, dark green above, wine-colour beneath. Flowers large white, showy and fragrant, often 6 inches in diameter; sepals four elliptical scaphoid, nearly free; petals numerous; stamens indefinite; ovary large globular, depressed, eighteen to twenty-four-celled. Fruit a depressed globular, fleshy body; seeds oblong, stipulate. The flowers open as the sun rises, after a few hours gradually closing, being entirely closed during the midday heat and at night.

¶ *Constituents*. The roots contain tannin, gallic acid and mucilage, starch, gum, resin, sugar, ammonia, tartaric acid, fecula, etc.

¶ *Medicinal Action and Uses*. The root is astringent, demulcent, anodyne, and anti-scrofulous, used in dysentery, diarrhœa, gonorrhœa, and leucorrhœa externally. The leaves and roots have been used in form of poultice to boils, tumours, scrofulous ulcers and inflamed skin; the infusion is used as a gargle for ulcers in the mouth and throat.

¶ *Dosage*. The powdered root, ½ drachm. Infusion up to 2 fluid ounces.

The virtues of the root are quickly imparted to water.

A poultice of leaves and roots relieves boils, tumours, ulcers, and inflamed skin. A complete cure of uterine cancer by a decoction and a vaginal injection is recorded.

The dose of the powdered root is ½ drachm in milk or sweetened water; but the best form is an infusion of 1 oz. in a pint of boiling water, macerated for thirty minutes, of which 2 to 4 fluid ounces may be given three or four times a day.

The EUROPEAN YELLOW POND-LILY (*Nuphar Advena* or *Nuphar luteum* – Spatterdock or Frog-lily) may be used as a substitute. It contains much nuphar-tannic acid.

484

LIME FRUIT

Citrus acida (ROXB.)
N.O. Rutaceæ

Synonyms. Citrus acris. Limettæ Fructus
Parts Used. The juice, the fruit
Habitat. West Indies, especially Montserrat. A native of Asia

¶ *Description.* The Lime is a small tree, crooked and prickly, only reaching as a rule a height of 8 feet. The leaves are ovate-oblong, and the stalk is not winged like that of the orange and lemon tree. The flowers are small and white and the fruit about half the size of a lemon, with a smoother, thinner rind, having a greenish tinge in its yellow. In Jamaica it is often planted for fences.

In London nurseries several varieties are found, the principal ones being the Chinese spreading, the West Indian, the Common, the broad-leaved and the weeping.

The juice is principally used in the manufacture of citric acid, and for medicinal purposes is often used indiscriminately with that of the lemon, although its flavour is not so popular.

Oil of Limes is used for flavouring purposes, especially in mineral waters and artificial lime-juice cordials, consisting of sweetened solutions of tartaric acid.

¶ *Constituents.* The National Formulary IV of America has defined and standardized Lime Juice as follows: the expressed juice of the ripe fruit of *Citrus medica acida*, contain-ing in each *one hundred mils* not less than 5 gm. nor more than 10 gm. of total acids, calculated as crystallized citric acid ($H_3C_6H_5O_7$ plus H_2O : 210·08). It is clear or slightly turbid, pale yellow or greenish-yellow, with the characteristic odour and taste of limes. Specific gravity 1·025 to 1·040 at 25° C.

It must be free from sulphuric acid, and may contain 0·04 gm. of SO_2 in each 100 mils, but no other preservatives nor artificial colours.

The *rind* contains a volatile oil including the terpene *limonene* and citral.

¶ *Medicinal Action and Uses.* Antiscorbutic. Used in dyspepsia with glycerine of pepsin.

¶ *Dosage.* Of 40 per cent. glycerite of pepsin and 60 per cent. Lime juice, 2 fluid drachms.

¶ *Other Species.*
C. Limetta, grown in Italy, yields an oil resembling oil of Bergamot, called Italian Limette oil. It contains 26 per cent. *ling* acetate. After standing it forms the yellow deposit *limettin*. It differs from the distilled West Indian oil of Limes.

See LEMON.

LIME TREE

Tilia Europœa (LINN.)
N.O. Tiliaceæ

Synonyms. Tilia vulgaris. Tilia intermedia. Tilia cordata. Tilia platyphylla. Linden Flowers. Linn Flowers. Common Lime. Flores Tiliæ. Tilleul
Parts Used. The flowers, the charcoal
Habitat. Northern Temperate Zone, especially British Isles

¶ *Description.* This tree will grow to 130 feet in height and when in bloom perfumes its whole neighbourhood. The leaves are obliquely heart-shaped, dark green above, paler below, from 2½ to 4 inches long and sharply toothed. The yellowish-white flowers hang from slender stalks in flattened clusters. They have five petals and five sepals. The original five stamens have each developed a cluster, and there is a spoon-shaped false petal opposite each true one.

Linden Tea is much used on the Continent, especially in France, where stocks of dried lime-flowers are kept in most households for making 'Tilleul.'

The honey from the flowers is regarded as the best flavoured and the most valuable in the world. It is used exclusively in medicine and in liqueurs.

The wood is useful for small articles not requiring strength or durability, and where ease in working is wanted: it is specially valu-able for carving, being white, close-grained, smooth and tractable in working, and admits of the greatest sharpness in minute details. Grinley Gibbons did most of his flower and figure carvings for St. Paul's Cathedral, Windsor Castle, and Chatsworth in Lime wood.

It is the lightest wood produced by any of the broad-leaved European trees, and is suitable for many other purposes, as it never becomes worm-eaten. On the Continent it is much used for turnery, sounding boards for pianos, in organ manufacture, as the framework of veneers for furniture, for packing-cases, and also for artists' charcoal making and for the fabrication of wood-pulp.

The *inner bark* or *bast* when detached from the outer bark in strands or ribands makes excellent fibres and coarse matting, chiefly used by gardeners, being light, but strong and elastic. Fancy baskets are often made of it. In Sweden, the inner bark, separated by maceration so as to form a kind of flax, has been employed to make fishing-nets.

The *sap*, drawn off in the spring, affords a considerable quantity of sugar.

The *foliage* is eaten by cattle, either fresh or dry. The leaves and shoots are mucilaginous and may be employed in poultices and fomentations.

¶ *Constituents.* The flowers contain a fragrant, volatile oil, with no colour, tannin, sugar, gum and chlorophyll.

The *bark* contains a glucoside, *tilicin*, and a neutral body, *tiliadin.*

The *leaves* exude a saccharine matter having the same composition as the manna of Mount Sinai.

¶ *Medicinal Action and Uses.* Lime-flowers are only used in infusion or made into a distilled water as household remedies in indigestion or hysteria, nervous vomiting or palpitation. Prolonged baths prepared with the infused flowers are also good in hysteria.

In the Pyrenees they are used to soothe the temporary excitement caused by the waters, and M. Rostan has used them with success against spasms. The flowers of several species of Lime are used.

Some doctors prefer the light charcoal of lime wood to that of the poplar in gastric or dyspeptic disturbances, and its powder for burns or sore places.

If the flowers used for making the tisane are too old they may produce symptoms of narcotic intoxication.

LINSEED. *See* FLAX

LIPPIA

Lippia dulcis (TREV.)
N.O. Verbenaceæ

Synonyms. Yerba dulce. Mexican Lippia
Part Used. Leaves

A dozen species of *Lippias* are utilized in medicine and in perfumery for their fragrant oils.

The drug *Lippia Mexicana* consists of the leaves and flowers of *L. dulcis*, an evergreen shrub, about 18 feet high, with rough bark, the branches and leaves in pairs, the flower-stalks in the axils of the leaves, bearing many pyramidal, scaly heads about the size of a small grey pea, in which are many small yellow flowers between the scales. The leaves are 1 to 1½ inch long, ovate, narrowed into the petiole, acute, finely-toothed above, veiny and glandular-hairy. They have a peculiar, sweet and very delightful, aromatic odour and taste.

¶ *Constituents.* In 1886, Podwisrotzki separated an essential oil from the leaves, resembling that of fennel, as well as a camphor-like substance which he named Lippiol. (According to Maish, however, the plant used was probably the *Cedronella Mexicana*.)

¶ *Medicinal Action and Uses.* The drug finds employment as a stimulating expectorant, the tincture, in doses of ½ to 1 fluid drachm, is given as a respiratory sedative in coughs. It acts as an alterative on the mucous membrane.

Lippiol, in doses of 4½ grains, causes warmth, flushing, diaphoresis and drowsiness.

¶ *Other Species.*

L. GRAVEOLENS (H. B.) is similarly employed in Mexico, where it is known as *Yerba dulce.*

L. ORIGANOIDES (Kunth) is used as a substitute for *origanum.*

The yellowish-green leaves of L. CYMOSA of Jamaica are scented like Pennyroyal.

L. NODIFLORA (Mx.) is employed in India under the names of Buccar, Vakhar, Ratolia; and in Chile it is called *Yerba de la Sainte Maria.*

In Brazil, L. PSEUDO-THEA (Schauer) is used as a substitute for tea and its fruit is eaten.

L. SCABERRIMA (Souder) is the South African shrub Benkess Boas, and its leaves yield about 0·25 per cent. of volatile oil, somewhat resembling lavender in its odour. It contains the crystalline alcohol, *Lippianol.*

The Lemon-scented Verbena of gardens (the *Verveine odorante* of the French), so much valued for the fragrance of its leaves, was once referred to the genus *Verbena*, under the name of *Verbena triphylla*. Lyons subsequently assigned it to the genus *Aloysia* (hence a gardener's popular name for it: Herb Louisa, a corruption of the Latin name, *Aloysia*), but it is now classed in the genus *Lippia* and named L. CITRIODORA (Kunth). It differs from *Verbena* in having two, not four, nutlets in the fruit.

See VERBENA, LEMON-SCENTED.

LIPPIA CITRIODORA. *See* VERBENA

LIQUORICE   Glycyrrhiza glabra (LINN.) and Other Species
                                                                    N.O. Leguminosæ

Synonyms. Liquiritia officinalis. Lycorys (thirteenth century).
    (*Welsh*) Lacris
    (*French*) Reglisse
    (*German*) Lacrisse
    (*Italian*) Regolizia
Part Used. Root
Habitat. The Liquorice plants are shrubs, natives of South-east Europe and South-west
Asia, as far as Persia, the *G. glabra* ranging more especially to the westward, the *G.
glandulifera* more to the eastward and being the source of the Eastern Liquorice root
of commerce

The Liquorice of medicine and commerce is derived from the sweet root of various species of *Glycyrrhiza*, a genus which contains about fourteen species, natives of warmer temperate countries in both the New and Old Worlds, ten of them having roots more or less sweet, but most of them not sufficiently so to be of use.

Hundreds of tons of Liquorice for commercial and medicinal purposes are imported annually from Spain, Russia, Germany, France and the East, most of our supply coming from Spain and Italy.

There are several well-marked species: *G. glabra, glandulifera, echinata,* etc. The chief source of the drug is *G. glabra,* which is cultivated in England, but is imported chiefly from Spain and Italy. There are several other varieties in commerce – Russian and Persian Liquorice – but these are not recognized by the British Pharmacopœia as suitable for medicinal purposes.

The use of the Liquorice plant was first learnt by the Greeks from the Scythians. Theophrastus (third century B.C.), in commenting on the taste of different roots (*Hist. Plant. lib.* IX. c. 13), instances the sweet Scythian root which grows in the neighbourhood of the Lake Mæotis (Sea of Azov), and is good for asthma, dry cough and all pectoral diseases.

Dioscorides, who names the plant Glyrrhiza (Greek *glukos*, sweet, and *riza*, a root), from his description of the plant possibly had in view *G. echinata,* as well as *G. glabra.*

The plant is often found under the name *Liquiritia officinalis.* The Latin name Liquiritia, whence is derived the English name Liquorice (Lycorys in the thirteenth century), is a corruption of Glycyrrhiza, as shown in the transitional form Gliquiricia. The Italian Regolizia, the German Lacrisse or Lakriz, the Welsh Lacris and the French Reglisse have the same origin.

The Roman writers, Celsus and Scribonius Largus, mention Liquorice as *Radix dulcis.* Pliny who describes it as a native of Cilicia, and Pontus makes no allusion to its growing in Italy.

Liquorice Extract was known in the times of Dioscorides and appears to have been in common use in Germany during the Middle Ages. In 1264, Liquorice (apparently the extract, not the root) is charged in the Wardrobe Accounts of Henry IV. Saladinus, who wrote about the middle of the fifteenth century, names it among the wares kept by the Italian apothecaries and it is enumerated in a list of drugs of the City of Frankfurt, written about the year 1450.

A writer in the first half of the sixteenth century notices the Liquorice plant as abundant in many parts of Italy, and describes the manner of making the Succus or Extract by crushing and boiling the fresh root.

The plant is described as being cultivated in Italy by Piero de Cresenzi of Bologna, who lived in the thirteenth century. As a medicine, the drug was well known in Germany in the eleventh century, and an extensive cultivation of the plant was carried on in Bavaria in the sixteenth century, but it is not mentioned in mediæval lists of plants.

Cultivation on a small scale has existed in England for a very long time. It appears from Turner's *Herbal* that it was cultivated in England in 1562, and Stow says 'the planting and growing of licorish began about the first year of Queen Elizabeth (1558).' Gerard, in 1597, tells us that he has plenty in his garden. It was known to and described by Culpepper who says: 'It is planted in fields and gardens, in divers places of this land and thereof good profit is made.'

John Parkinson grew Liquorice in his Holborn garden and John Josselyn gives the recipe for a beer which he used to brew for the Indians when they had bad colds. It was strongly flavoured with elecampane, liquorice, aniseed, sassafras and fennel.

Culpepper says:

'The English liquorice root shoots up several woody stalks, whereon are set, at several distances, many narrow, long green leaves, set together on both sides of the stalks and an odd one at the end, nearly resembling a young ash tree sprung up from the seed.

. . . This, by many years of continuance in a place without removal, and not else, will bring forth numerous flowers, standing together spike fashion, one above another upon the stalks in the form of pea-blossoms, but of a very pale blue colour, which turn into long, somewhat flat and smooth pods, wherein is contained small, round, hard seed. The root runneth down exceeding far into the ground, with divers smaller roots . . . they shoot out suckers in every direction, by which means the product is greatly increased.'

Liquorice is official in all pharmacopœias, which differ as to the variety or varieties recognized, as to the botanical name employed and as to the drug being peeled or unpeeled, dried Liquorice root being supplied in commerce either with or without the thin brown coat. In the latter state it is known as peeled or decorticated. The British Pharmacopœia requires that it be peeled, but others require that it be unpeeled.

¶ *Description.* The plants are graceful, with light, spreading, pinnate foliage, presenting an almost feathery appearance from a distance. The leaflets (like those of the False Acacia) hang down during the night on each side of the midrib, though they do not meet beneath it. From the axils of the leaves spring racemes or spikes of papilionaceous small pale-blue, violet, yellowish-white or purplish flowers, followed by small pods somewhat resembling a partly-grown pea-pod in form. In the type species *glabra*, the pods are smooth, hence the specific name; in others they are hairy or spiny.

The underground system, as in so many Leguminosæ, is double, the one part consisting of a vertical or tap root, often with several branches penetrating to a depth of 3 or 4 feet, the other of horizontal rhizomes, or stolons, thrown off from the root below the surface of the ground, which attain a length of many feet. These runners are furnished with leaf-buds and throw up stems in their second year. The perennial downward-running roots as well as the long horizontal stolons are equally preserved for use.

Various indications point to the habit of this plant of fixing atmospheric nitrogen, as do many others of the family.

In the species *glandulifera* (W. and K.) the pods are covered with thick, glandular spines, and the whole plant is pubescent or roughly glandular. The underground portion is not so spreading and produces a carrot-shaped root larger than the Spanish root derived from *G. glabra*. This species is indigenous to South-east Europe, Syria and Western Asia, and is both wild and cultivated in Russia.

Both the Russian and Persian Liquorice of commerce is derived from *G. glandulifera*, the Russian reaching this country is peeled or unpeeled: its taste although sweet, is accompanied by a more or less perceptible bitterness. It consists chiefly of roots, not runners.

Persian Liquorice root, collected in the valley of the Tigris and Euphrates, from *G. glandulifera*, and exported in bales from Bussorah, is usually unpeeled, and is in rather large, coarse pieces, closely resembling the Russian root. Both the Russian and Persian varieties are largely consumed in the United States; the root of *G. glandulifera* is equally official in the United States Pharmacopœia with that of *G. glabra*.

G. echinata, a native of Hungary, south Russia and Asia Minor, is the official German species. It has short globular heads of flowers and a small, ovoid pod with long spines. Probably a portion of the root from Italy and Sicily is the product of *G. echinata*, which grows wild in Apulia. The root is also somewhat bitter and there are contradictory statements concerning its quality, due perhaps to its having been confused with *G. glandulifera*.

Asiatic Liquorice is obtained from *G. uralensis* (Fisch.), found in Turkestan, Mongolia and Siberia, and little inferior to the best Russian Liquorice.

G. lepidota (Pursh), American Liquorice, is a species of the north-western United States. The rhizome is said to resemble that of Spanish Liquorice, but is smaller.

It is only grown now to a very limited extent in this country, being cultivated on a small scale near Pontefract in Yorkshire, though formerly it was extensively grown at Mitcham in Surrey, also at Godalming, and at Worksop (Notts).

The English Extract of Liquorice, made from the fresh home-grown root, sold in the lozenge form and known as Pontefract or Pomfrey cakes, is said to have a more delicate flavour than that imported, and it is considered that the cultivation of English Liquorice might well be extended, Essex and Surrey being suitable districts for its growth.

In southern Italy, large quantities of Liquorice root are grown, but it is chiefly converted into Extract, though some of the root is exported.

Spain and the south of France furnish quantities of carefully dried Liquorice root. Up to the year 1890, the cultivation of Spanish Liquorice was small or moderate in comparison with the wild collection. Owing, however, to the depletion of the natural supplies of root of good quality, this cultivation has grown rapidly in South and South-central Europe, where the climate is favourable.

Liquorice grows best on sandy soil near streams, usually not being found in the wild condition more than 50 yards from water.

It will not flourish on clay and prefers the rich, fine soil of bottom lands in river valleys, where there is an abundance of moisture during the growing period, but where the ground bakes hard during the hot, late summer months, when the dry heat is very favourable for the formation of the sweet constituents.

The plant succeeds most in a warm climate; not only can it not endure severe freezing, but cool weather interferes with the formation of its useful juice and renders it woody. It has been found that a climate particularly favourable to the production of the orange is favourable to that of Liquorice.

Owing to the depth to which the root penetrates and its ready propagation from detached pieces, the plant is a most persistent weed in cultivated grounds where it is indigenous and exceedingly difficult of extirpation. It is very healthy and robust and very little subject to disease, at the same time successfully occupying the ground to the exclusion of other plants. For this reason, the continuation of the natural supply may be considered as assured, though it is liable to suffer severe reduction from over-collection.

The supply of natural root has suffered severe fluctuations owing to the exhaustion of supplies in the districts previously worked, alternating with over-production from newly-opened districts. This fact, coupled with the operations of speculators, has resulted in equally great fluctuations in quality, the new districts yielding full-grown root of good quality, the older ones that which has not been allowed to develop properly.

The cultivation of Liquorice is easy, sure and profitable and, if properly conducted, conducive to the betterment of the soil.

On account of the depth to which the root strikes when the plant has room to flourish, the soil should have a good staple of mould 2 or 3 feet in depth and be manured if necessary.

The planting season is either October, or February and March; the latter is preferred. The plants are procured from old plantations, being waste from the harvesting process, consisting of those side roots or runners which have eyes or buds, cut into sections about 6 inches long. They are dibbled in, in rows 3 or 4 feet apart, about 4 inches underneath the surface and about 18 inches apart in the rows. In the autumn, the ground is dressed with farmyard manure, about 40 tons to the acre.

During the first two years the growth is slight, the plants not rising above a foot the first season, and in Calabria the intervening space is generally utilized for the production of potatoes, cabbages and similar crops. The soil being heavily fertilized for the production of Liquorice, these crops are usually very luxuriant. After the second year, the growing Liquorice plants cover the entire soil to the exclusion of other growth.

¶ *Harvesting and Preparation for Market.* Not until the end of the third season will the roots be ready to take up for use, but harvesting generally occurs only in the autumn of the fourth year. The soil is carefully removed from the space between the rows to a depth of 2 or 3 feet as required, thus exposing the roots and rhizomes at the side, the whole being then removed bodily. The earth from the next space is then removed and thrown into the trench thus formed and these operations are repeated continuously.

Every portion of the subterranean part of the plant is carefully saved, the drug consisting of both runners and roots, the former constituting the major part. The roots proper are washed, trimmed and sorted, and either sold in their entire state or cut into shorter lengths and dried, in the latter case the cortical layer being sometimes removed by scraping. The older or 'hard' runners are sorted out and sold separately; the young, called 'soft,' are reserved for propagation.

The average yield per acre is from 4 to 5 tons. The same ground yields a crop every three or four years, the fourth-year growth being the best. That of the third year and earlier is deficient in sweet substances, but immediately after the fourth year the texture begins to take on a tough, coarse and woody character. It is desirable also to collect the roots of those plants which have never borne fruit since that process exhausts the sweet substance of the sap.

English-grown Liquorice is dug up in late autumn and sold mostly in the fresh state for making extract, only a small amount being dried.

Fresh Liquorice (English) when washed is externally of a bright yellowish brown. It is very flexible, easily cut with a knife, exhibiting a light-yellow, juicy internal substance, which consists of a thick bark surrounding a woody column. Both bark and wood are extremely tough, readily tearing into long, fibrous strings. The root has a peculiar earthy odour and a strong, characteristic, sweet taste.

Most of the dried Liquorice root imported into this country comes from Spain and Russia, supplies of the official drug being drawn chiefly from Spain, the better quality of which comes from Tortosa and Alicante. Both Spanish and Russian Liquorice are usually exported in large bales or bundles, or rarely, in the case of the Spanish variety derived from Alicante, loose, or in bags. Spanish Liquorice root is in long, straight, nearly cylindrical, unpeeled pieces, several feet in length, varying in thickness from ¼ inch to about 1 inch, longitudinally wrinkled, externally greyish brown to dark brown, warty; internally tawny yellow; pliable, tough; texture coarsely fibrous; bark rather thick; wood porous, but dense, in narrow wedges; taste sweet, very slightly acrid. The underground stem which is often present has a similar appearance, but contains a thin pith. That from Alicante is frequently untrimmed and dirty in appearance, but that from Tortosa is usually clean and bright looking. When peeled, the pieces of root (including runners) are shorter, a pale yellow, slightly fibrous externally, and exhibit no trace of the small dark buds seen on the unpeeled runners here and there. Otherwise it resembles the unpeeled.

Nearly all the Russian Liquorice reaching this country has been peeled. It attains a much larger size than the Spanish, and the taste, although sweet, is accompanied by a more or less perceptible but not strong bitterness or acridity. It consists chiefly of roots, not runners, in long, often crooked pieces, about 2 inches in thickness, pale yellow externally and internally of a lighter yellow than the Spanish and softer. The size of all cells (when examined microscopically) is seen to be much larger than in the Spanish.

¶ *Extract*. The manufacture of Liquorice Juice, or *Extract*, is conducted on a liberal scale in Spain, southern France, Sicily, Calabria, Austria, southern Russia, Greece and Asia Minor, but the Extract with which England is supplied is almost exclusively the produce of Calabria, Sicily and Spain; Calabrian Liquorice is generally preferred. By far the larger part of the Italian and Sicilian crop is now manufactured there and exported in the form of Extract.

Spain formerly yielded most of the supply, hence the Extract is still termed 'Spanish Juice,' but that of the first grade has long since depleted to the point of scarcity.

The roots and runners of both wild and cultivated plants are taken up in late autumn and stacked through the winter in the cellars and yards of the factories. When required, they are crushed under millstones to a pulp, then transferred to boilers and boiled in water over a naked fire, the decoctions are run off and then evaporated in copper vessels over direct heat, till a suitable consistency is obtained, being constantly stirred to prevent burning. While warm, the mass is taken out and rolled into sticks, stamped and stacked on boards to dry. Vacuum pans and steam power have in some factories replaced the more simple methods.

The sticks vary in size, but are commonly about 1 inch in diameter and 6 or 7 inches in length and when imported are usually wrapped in bay leaves. At one end they are stamped with the maker's name or mark.

Stick Liquorice is very commonly impure, either from carelessness in its preparation, or from the fraudulent addition of other substances, such as starch, sand, carbonaceous matter, etc. Small particles of copper are also sometimes found in it.

Several varieties of Stick Liquorice are met with in English commerce, the most famous is the Solazzi Juice, manufactured at Corigliano, a small town of Calabria in the Gulf of Toranto.

The juice is also imported in a black form, having while warm and soft been allowed to run into the wooden cases of about 2 cwts. each, in which it is exported. This juice, known as *Liquorice Paste*, is largely imported from Spain and Asia Minor, but on account of a certain bitterness is unsuited for its use as a sweetmeat or in medicine, and is principally employed in the preparation of tobacco for chewing and smoking.

Extract of Liquorice in rolls has a black colour, is somewhat glossy and has a sharp and shining fracture. Some small cavities are found in the interior. The product of the different manufacturers of Stick Liquorice differ from one another not only in size, but often in the odour and taste; while some specimens are almost purely sweet, others are persistently acrid, rendering them unsuitable for medicinal purposes, for which they must be almost devoid of acridity.

Hard Extract of Liquorice, as described, is essentially different in composition and properties to the Extract of Liquorice of the British Pharmacopœia, which is entirely soluble in cold water, whereas the so-called Spanish Juice, when treated with cold water, leaves a large residue undissolved, retaining the shape of the stick. The amount soluble in cold water varies considerably and reaches in the best brands about 70 or 75 per cent. The United States and nearly all other Pharmacopœias recognize the commercial Extract of the root of *G. glabra*, but the British Pharmacopœia does not, and gives a process for making an extract which somewhat resembles the purified Extract of Liquorice of the United States Pharmacopœia. For the Liquid Extract of Liquorice, the British Pharmacopœia directs the exhaustion of the Liquorice root with two successive portions of cold water, using each time 50 fluid ounces for 20 oz. of the drug and allowing the mixture to macerate for 24 hours before expressing. The mixed infusions are heated to boiling point, strained through flannel and evaporated until the liquid has acquired, when cold, a specific gravity of 1·2, one-fourth of its volume of alcohol is added, and the mixture is set aside for 12 hours, after which it is filtered. It has a yellowish-brown colour and a pure sweet taste, free from all acridity.

¶ *Constituents*. The chief constituent of Liquorice root, to which its sweet taste is due, is Glycyrrhizin (6 to 8 per cent.), obtainable in the form of a sweet, white crystalline powder, consisting of the calcium and potassium salts of glycyrrhizic acid. The drug also contains sugar, starch (29 per cent.), gum, protein, fat (0·8 per cent.), resin, asparagin (2 to 4 per cent.), a trace of tannin in the outer bark of the root, yellow colouring matter, and 0·03 of volatile oil.

The amount of Glycyrrhizin present in Extract of Liquorice varies from 5 to 24 per cent., and the amount of moisture from 8 to 17 per cent. Upon ignition, the extract yields from 5 to 9 per cent. of ash.

The roots of *G. glandulifera* and *echinata* also contain in addition, Glycyrmarin, a bitter principle occurring mostly in the bark.

Glycyrrhizin, or a similar substance, has been obtained from other plants, viz. from the rhizome of *Polypodium vulgare*, the leaves of *Myrrhis odorata*, and the bark of *Lucuma glycyphlœa*.

¶ *Medicinal Action and Uses*. The action of Liquorice is demulcent, moderately pectoral and emollient.

It is a popular and well-known remedy for coughs, consumption and chest complaints generally, notably bronchitis, and is an ingredient in almost all popular cough medicines on account of its valuable soothing properties.

The Extract enters into the composition of cough lozenges and pastilles, with sedatives and expectorants. It is largely used in conjunction with infusion of linseed in the treatment of irritable cough, sore throat and laryngitis, and an infusion made by boiling 1 oz. of the bruised root deprived of its bark, with 1 pint of water for a few minutes, may be employed in the treatment of sore throat and in catarrhal conditions of the urinary intestinal tracts.

Beach mentions the following recipe as being used by the late Dr. Malone, of London, and speaks most highly of its efficacy:

'Take a large teaspoonful of Linseed, 1 ounce of Liquorice root, and ¼ lb. of best raisins. Put them into 2 quarts of soft water and simmer down to 1 quart. Then add to it ¼ lb. of brown sugar candy and a tablespoonful of white wine vinegar or lemon juice. Drink ½ pint when going to bed and take a little whenever the cough is troublesome.'

(N.B. – It is best to add the vinegar to that quantity which is required for immediate use.)

Fluid Extract of Liquorice is employed almost exclusively as a vehicle for disguising the taste of nauseous medicines, having a remarkable power of converting the flavour of acrid or bitter drugs, such as Mezereon, Quinine or Cascara.

The powdered root is useful in pill-making on account of its absorbent qualities, being used to impart stiffness to pill masses and to prevent the adhesion of pills.

As a remedial agent, powdered Liquorice root has been almost entirely replaced by the extract, though it is used in the well-known Compound Liquorice Powder, the mild laxative in which Senna and Fennel are the other ingredients. It is added mainly on account of its sweetness and emollient qualities, the action of the powder being mainly due to the Senna contained.

Liquorice was prescribed by early physicians from the time of Hippocrates, in cases of dropsy, to prevent thirst, for which it is an excellent thing, though probably the only sweet substance that has this effect. It is thought, however, that the property does not actually belong to the saccharine juice, but that if a piece of the root be chewed till all the juice is extracted, there remains a bitter, which acts on the salivary glands, and this may contribute to remove thirst.

The sugar of Liquorice may safely be taken by diabetic patients.

On the whole, Liquorice as a domestic medicine is far more largely used on the Continent than in Great Britain. It is much used in China and largely produced (both *L. glabra* and *L. echinata*) in some of the northern provinces, a variety of medicinal preparations being employed, not only as possessing tonic, alterative and expectorant properties, but also for the rejuvenating and highly nutritive qualities attributed to it.

It was recommended by Gervase Markham, a noted authority on husbandry and farriery in the early part of the seventeenth century, for the treatment of certain horses' ailments.

¶ *Preparations and Dosages*. Powdered root, ½ to 1 drachm. Fluid extract, 1 to 4 drachms. Comp. powder, B.P., 1 to 2 drachms. Solid extract, 1 drachm. Comp. lozenges, U.S.P. Solid extract in stick form, known as Liquorice Juice.

Liquorice is also largely used by brewers, being added to porter and stout to give thickness and blackness.

Block Liquorice is employed in the manufacture of tobacco for smoking and chewing.

According to the United States press, a new use for Liquorice Root has lately been discovered, the waste root being now utilized for the manufacture of boards for making boxes. After extraction of the Liquorice, the crushed root was formerly considered a waste product and destroyed by burning, but under a recently discovered process this refuse can now be made into a chemical wood pulp and pressed into a board that is said to have satisfactory resisting qualities and strength.

LIQUORICE, INDIAN

Abrus precatorius (LINN.)
N.O. Leguminosæ

Synonyms. Jequirity. Wild Liquorice. Prayer Beads (*Indian*) Gunga. (*Indian*) Goonteh. (*Indian*) Rati
Parts Used. Root, seeds

The root of an Indian leguminous plant, *Abrus precatorius* (Linn.), under the native names of Gunga or Goonteh, has been used as a demulcent. It contains Glycyrrhizin, and has been termed Indian Liquorice and used as a substitute for true Liquorice. Acrid resins, however, render the root irritant and poisonous.

An infusion and a paste of the seeds are included in the British Pharmacopœia. It has a strongly irritating effect upon the eyes and has been used both to produce and to allay certain ophthalmic diseases.

The hard, red, glossy seeds, nearly globular, with a large, black spot at one end, are known as Prayer Beads, or Jequirity seeds. The seeds, weighing about 1 carat each, have been used in India from very ancient times for the purpose of weighing gold, under the name of Rati. They are largely employed also for the making of rosaries and for ornamental purposes.

The weight of the famous Koh-i-noor diamond was ascertained by means of these seeds.

There is also a variety with perfectly white seeds.

Their medical importance is not great, but they have a notorious history in India as an agent in criminal poisoning. This practice has been directed chiefly against cattle and other live stock, but the poisoning of human beings has been not infrequent. That the attractive seeds form dangerous playthings for children has been proved by the records of a number of cases of poisoning which have occurred in this way.

The name Wild Liquorice has also been given to *Aralia nudicaulis* (Linn.), indigenous to Canada and the United States, and to the root of *Cephalanthus occidentalis*, a member of the Madder family, a large shrub, with rich, glossy foliage, growing in swamps almost throughout the United States and extending into Southern Canada, the bark and stem of which is used commercially.

Rest-Harrow has also been called Wild Liquorice.

LIQUORICE, WILD. *See* REST-HARROW, SARSAPARILLA

LITMUS

Roccella tinctoria (D. C.)
N.O. Lichenes

Synonyms. Lacmus. Orchella Weed. Dyer's Weed. Lacca cærulea. Lacca musica. Orseille. Persio. Rock Moss. Lichen Roccella. Roccella phycopsis. Roccella Pygmæa. Turnsole. Touresol. Laquebleu
Part Used. The whole plant, for its pigment
Habitat. Seashore rocks on all warm coasts and some mountain rocks

¶ *Description.* Various origins are ascribed to the name *Roccella*. It may be derived from *rocca* (a rock), or from the red colour produced by the plants. It occurs in an Italian *Natural History* of 1599.

Roccella tinctoria is a small, dry, perennial lichen, in appearance a bunch of wavy, tapering branched, drab-coloured stems from 2 to 6 inches high, springing from a narrow base. These bear nearly black warts at in- tervals, the *apothecia* or means of fructification peculiar to lichens. It is found principally on the Mediterranean coasts, but other species from other localities are also sources of commercial Litmus.

Blue and *Red Orchil* or *Archil* are used for dyeing, colouring and staining. The red is prepared by steeping the lichen in earthen jars and heating them by steam. The blue is similarly treated in a covered wooden vessel.

They are used as a thickish liquid for testing purposes.

Cudbear, prepared in a similar way, is also used as a dye. It is dried and pulverized, and becomes a purplish-red in colour.

The preparation of Litmus is almost exclusively carried on in Holland, the details being kept a secret. About nineteen kinds seem to be there, varying very much in value.

The lichens are coarsely ground with pearlashes, and macerated for weeks in wooden vessels in a mixture of urine, lime and potash or soda, with occasional stirring. In fermentation the mass becomes red and then blue, and is then moulded into earthy, crumbling cakes of a purplish-blue colour. The scent is like violets and indigo and the taste is slightly saline and pungent. Indigo is mixed with inferior kinds to deepen the colour.

Blue Litmus Paper is prepared by steeping unsized white paper in an infusion or Test Solution of Litmus, or by brushing the infusion over the paper, which must be carefully dried in the open air.

Red Litmus Paper is similarly prepared with an infusion faintly reddened by the addition of a small percentage of sulphuric or hydrochloric acid.

Vegetable red, much used in colouring foods, is a sulphonated derivative of orchil.

¶ *Constituents.* The lichen contains a brown resin, wax, insoluble and lichen starches, yellow extractive, gummy and glutinous matters, tartrate and oxalate of lime and chloride of sodium. The colouring princi-

ples are acids or acid anhydrides, themselves colourless but yielding colour when acted upon by ammonia, air and moisture.

The chief of these are Azolitmin and Erythro-litmin, sometimes called leconoric, orsellic and erythric acids.

The dye is tested by adding a solution of calcium hypochlorite to the alcoholic tincture, when a deep blood-red colour, quickly fading, should appear, or the plants can be macerated in a weak solution of ammonia, which should produce a rich violet-red.

¶ *Medicinal Action and Uses.* Demulcent and emollient. A decoction is useful in coughs and catarrhs.

Litmus is used officially as a test for acids and alkalis. Acids impart a red colour to blue Litmus and alkaloids cause reddened Litmus to return to its original blue. It may be used in solid or liquid forms as well as on the papers.

¶ *Adulterations.* Orchil is often adulterated with extracts of coloured woods, especially logwood and sappan wood.

¶ *Other Species.*

Two of the chief sources of Litmus are now *R. Montagnei* of Mozambique and *Dendrographa leucophœa* of California.

Lecanora Tartare, or Tartarean Moss, was formerly much used in Northern Europe.

R. pygmæa is found in Algeria.

R. fuciformis is larger, with flatter, paler branches.

R. phycopsis is smaller and more branched.

Inferior kinds of Litmus are prepared from species of *Variolaria, Lecanora* and *Parmelia.*

LIVERWORT, AMERICAN

Anemone hepatica (LINN.)
N.O. Ranunculaceæ

Synonyms. Hepatica triloba. Hepatica triloba, var. americana or obtusa. Round-leaved Hepatica. Noble Liverwort. Liverleaf. Liverweed. Trefoil. Herb Trinity. Kidneywort. Edellebere

Parts Used. Leaves and flowers

Habitat. Cooler latitudes of the North Temperate Zone

¶ *Description.* The name of the genus may be derived from *epatikos* (affecting the liver) or from *epar* (the liver), from a likeness in its appearance to that organ. The Hepaticas are distinguished by having carpels without feathery tails and by the involucre of three simple leaves being so close to the flower as to resemble a calyx.

The leaves are broad kidney or heart shaped, about 2 inches long and broad, with three broad, angular lobes, leathery, smooth and dark green above, almost evergreen, placed on long, slender foot-stalks growing direct from the root. In the wild state the flowers are generally blue, more rarely rose

or white, but in cultivation many other tints are to be found. There are numerous garden varieties, growing best in deep loam or clay, several having double flowers.

The leaves should be gathered during flowering time in March.

¶ *Constituents.* Liverwort contains tannin, sugar, mucilage, etc.; its value is due to its astringent principle. A full analysis has not been made.

¶ *Medicinal Action and Uses.* Demulcent, tonic, astringent, vulnerary. It has been described as 'an innocent herb which may be taken freely in infusion and in syrup.' It is a mild remedy in disorders of the liver, indigestion, etc., and possessing pectoral properties it is employed in coughs, bleeding of the lungs and diseases of the chest generally.

The infusion, made from 1 oz. of the dried herb to 1 pint of boiling water, is slightly astringent and mucilaginous. Frequent doses of ½ teacupful have been recommended in the early stages of consumption. In some countries the whole plant is regarded as a vulnerary and astringent. In cataplasms it is valued in hernia, affections of the urinary passages and skin diseases.

A distilled water is used for freckles and sunburn. Though in use from ancient days, its mild character has caused it to be little used.

¶ *Dosage.* 30 to 120 grains. Fluid extract, ½ to 2 drachms.

¶ *Other Species.*
Marchantia polymorpha is the true Liverwort.

The lichen *Pettigora canina* is known as English or Ground Liverwort. It was formerly regarded as a remedy for hydrophobia.

¶ *Cultivation.* Hepaticas are hardy, long-lived plants of a deep-rooting nature, preferring a rich, porous soil and a sheltered situation. They flourish best in a deep loam, but will thrive in clay: one condition of success is good drainage. It is not advisable to transplant them frequently; when left undisturbed for a few years, they form fine clumps.

The double varieties are propagated by division of roots. The strongest clumps should be lifted immediately after flowering and carefully divided into separate crowns, each division to have as many roots as can be secured to it. These must be at once planted in fresh soil and carefully closed in, and then lightly covered with some very fine earth. They will become established in the course of the season if the soil is well drained, care being taken to water when necessary. Being by nature woodside plants, they should not be exposed to long-continued sunshine.

The single varieties are raised by seed, which must be sown as soon as ripe in pans or shallow boxes, which should be filled with light rich, sandy loam, kept moist, and sheltered in a frame throughout the winter. Germination is very slow and the young plants will not appear till the end of September. Keep the seedlings in their seed-boxes, freely ventilated to prevent damping off, and in April remove them to a sheltered shady border. As the young plants make their proper leaves, carefully lift them out with a thin slip of wood and plant them in a border prepared for the purpose, where the soil must be sweet and sandy, without manure and a little shaded.

LIVERWORT, ENGLISH

Peltigera Canina (HOFFM.)
N.O. Lichenes

Synonyms. Lichen Caninus. Lichen Cinereus Terrestis. Ash-coloured Ground Liverwort
Part Used. Lichen
Habitat. Britain where the drainage is good; on mudwalls and molehills

¶ *Description.* The marginal disks of this lichen are at first veiled and project from the thallus, retaining fragments of the veil of the margin. The fronds are foliaceous, coriaceous, ascending, soft, underside is veined and attached to the ground or to whatever substance it grows upon – where they make handsome plants, especially when in fruit or studded with the little red parasite to which they are subject. The plant was formerly considered of great value in hydrophobia.

¶ *Medicinal Action and Uses.* Deobstruent, slightly purgative and held in esteem as a remedy for liver complaints.

¶ *Preparations and Dosages.* Infusion, 1 oz. to 1 pint of boiling water; take 4 oz. daily. Fluid extract, ½ to 2 drachms.

LOBELIA

Lobelia inflata (LINN.)
N.O. Lobeliaceæ

Synonyms. Rapuntium inflatum. Indian Tobacco. Pukeweed. Asthma Weed. Gagroot. Vomitwort. Bladderpod. Eyebright
Parts Used. The dried flowering herb, and seeds
Habitat. Dry places in the northern United States, Canada and Kamchatka. Grown in English gardens

¶ *Description.* The herb is named after the botanist Matthias de Lobel, a native of Lille, who died in London in 1616. It is an erect annual or biennial herb, 1 to 2 feet high; lower leaves and also flower are stalked, the latter being pale violet-blue in colour, tinted pale yellow within. Commercially, it is usually prepared in compressed, oblong packages, by the Shakers of New Lebanon for importation into England. The colour is a yellowish green, the odour irritating, the taste, after chewing, very like that of tobacco, burning and acrid, causing a flow of saliva. The powder has a greenish colour, but that of the seeds is brown, and stains paper with grease.

Several species are cultivated in English gardens for the splendour of their flowers, in every shade of scarlet, purple, and blue. *Lobelia Dortmanna* and *L. Urens* are British. The fixed oil, with constituents rather like that of linseed oil, possesses the drying qualities common to the fixed oils together with all the medicinal properties of the seed.

The plant was known to the Penobscot Indians and was widely used in New England long before the time of Samuel Thomson, who is credited with its discovery. It was brought into general professional use by Cutler of Massachusetts.

¶ *Constituents.* The activity of Lobelia is dependent upon a liquid alkaloid first isolated by Proctor in 1838 and named Lobeline. Pereira found a peculiar acid which he named Lobelic acid. Also, gum, resin, chlorophyl, fixed oil, lignin, salts of lime and potassium, with ferric oxide. Lobelacrine, formerly considered to be the acrid principle, is probably lobelate of lobeline. The seeds contain a much higher percentage of lobeline than the rest of the plant.

¶ *Medicinal Action and Uses.* Expectorant, diaphoretic, anti-asthmatic. It should not be employed as an emetic.[1] Some authorities attach great value to it as an expectorant in bronchitis, others as a valuable counter-irritant when combined with other ingredients in ointment form. It is sometimes given in convulsive and inflammatory disorders such as epilepsy, tetanus, diphtheria and tonsilitis. There is also difference of opinion with regard to its narcotic properties. Where relaxation of the system is required, as, for instance, to subdue spasm, Lobelia is invaluable. Relaxation can be counteracted by the stimulating and tonic infusion of capsicum. It may be used as an enema.

Externally, an infusion has been found useful in ophthalmia, and the tincture can be used as a local application for sprains, bruises, or skin diseases, alone, or in powder combined with an equal part of slippery elm bark and weak lye-water in a poultice. The oil of Lobelia is valuable in tetanus. One drop of oil triturated with one scruple of

sugar, and divided into from 6 to 12 doses, is useful as an expectorant, nauseant, sedative, and diaphoretic, when given every one or two hours.

¶ *Preparations and Dosages.* Powdered bark, 5 to 60 grains. Fluid extract, 10 to 20 drops. Acid tincture, 1 to 4 drachms. Tincture, U.S.P., 1 to 4 drachms. Etherial tincture, B.P., 5 to 15 drops. Syrup, 1 to 4 drachms. Solid extract, 2 to 4 grains. Oil of seed, 1 drop rubbed up with 20 grains of ginger and divided into 6 to 12 doses. Lobelin, $\frac{1}{4}$ to 3 grains.

Acetum Lobellæ (Vinegar of Lobelia). Lobelia seed powder, 4 oz. Diluted acetic acid, 2 pints. Macerate in a close glass vessel for seven days, then express the liquor, filter, and add to the filtered product alcohol, or concentrated acetic acid, 1 fluid ounce. The whole should measure 2 pints. This medicated vinegar may also be prepared by percolation. It is an emetic, nauseant, and expectorant, and a valuable relaxant in spasmodic affections. A good application in such skin diseases as salt-rheum, erysipelas, poisoning by rhus, etc. As an expectorant, 5 to 30 drops every half-hour in elm or flaxseed infusion. One part of Vinegar of Lobelia to 1 part of syrup forms a pleasant preparation for children.

¶ *Poisonous, if any, with Antidotes.* In excessive doses the effects are those of a powerful acro-narcotic poison, producing great depression, nausea, cold-sweats, and possibly death.[2] Poisonous symptoms may occur from absorption of it through the epidermis.

¶ *Other Species.*

L. Dortmanna. This is indigenous to Great Britain, and is rather similar in action to *L. inflata.* A tincture of the fresh plant cures headaches and noises in the ears.

L. Erinus. A tincture of the plant has been used in cancer and has produced absolute freedom from pain; is also used as a remedy in syphilis.

LOBELIA, BLUE (*L. Syphilitica*) and LOBELIA RED (*L. Cardinalia*). Both used in homœopathy. The first is diaphoretic, emetic and cathartic and has been used in dropsy, diarrhœa, syphilis and dysentery, the root being the part used. The Red Lobelia is said to be anthelmintic, nervine and antispasmodic.

L. Kalmit. Said to be used by the Indians in the cure of syphilis.

L. purpurascens. A tincture of the whole plant is used in paralysis of the lungs and tongue.

---

[1] Herbalists, who use lobelia far more than the ordinary practitioners, nearly always prescribe it in doses large enough to prove emetic, and regard it as of greater value thus used. – EDITOR.
[2] Herbalists also deny that it has poisonous properties and that it has ever caused death. – EDITOR.

LOGWOOD

Hæmatoxylon Campeachianum (LINN.)
N.O. Leguminosæ

Synonyms. Hæmatoxylon Lignum. Lignum Campechianum. Lignum Cœruleum. Peachwood. Bois de Campechey de Sang or d'Inde. Bloodwood
Part Used. The heart-wood, or duramen, unfermented
Habitat. Tropical America, especially the shores of the Gulf of Campeachy. Naturalized in West Indies and elsewhere

¶ *Description.* The name of the genus comes from the Greek and refers to the blood-red colour of the heart-wood. *Hæmatoxylon Campeachianum* is a crookedly-branched, small tree, the branches spiny and the bark rough and dark. The leaves have four pairs of small, smooth leaflets, each in the shape of a heart with the points towards the short stem. The flowers, small and yellow, with five petals, grow in axillary racemes.

The tree was introduced into Jamaica and other countries in 1715 and has been grown in England since 1730.

The average yearly import of logwood into the United Kingdom is about 50,000 tons, the four kinds recognized in the market, in order of value, being Campeachy, Honduras, St. Domingo and Jamaica.

The trees are felled in their eleventh year, the red heartwood, in 3-foot logs, being exported.

The principal value of logwood is in dyeing violet, blue, grey and black. For dyeing, the wood is chipped and fermented, thus rendering it unsuitable for medicinal use.

The many disputes and difficulties that arose over the rights of growing and cutting logwood are a matter of history. It is used also as a microscopical stain. The odour is faint and pleasant, the taste astringent and sweetish. It gives a reddish-violet tinge to water made alkaline with a solution of sodium hydroxide.

¶ *Constituents.* A volatile oil, an oily or resinous matter, two brown substances, quercitin, tannin, a nitrogenous substance, free acetic acid, salts, and the colouring principle Hæmatoxylin or Hæmatin (not the hæmatin of the blood). The crystals are colourless, requiring oxygen from the air and an alkaline base to produce red, blue, and purple.

Hæmatein, produced by extraction of two equivalents of hydrogen, is found in dark violet crystalline scales, showing the rich, green colour often to be seen outside chips of logwood for dyeing purposes.

¶ *Medicinal Action and Uses.* A mild astringent, especially useful in the weakness of the bowels following cholera infantum. It may be used in chronic diarrhœa and dysentery, in hæmorrhages from uterus, lungs, or bowels, is agreeable to take, and suitable whether or not there is fever. It imparts a blood-red colour to urine and stools. It is incompatible with chalk or lime-water. The patient should be warned of these two characteristics.

In large doses hæmatoxylin can produce fatal gastro-enteritis in lower animals.

The infusion, internally, combined with a spray or lotion, is said to have cured obstinate cases of fœtid polypus in the nose.

¶ *Preparations and Dosages.* Decoction, 2 to 4 fluid ounces. Decoction, B.P. 1895, ½ to 2 oz. Solid extract, B.P. 1885, 10 to 30 grains. Solid extract, U.S.P., 2 to 5 grains.

¶ *Other Species.*
'BASTARD LOGWOOD' from *Acacia Berteriana* and other species, contains no hæmatoxylin. It does not form a violet colour with alkalies, but yields a pure, yellowish-grey dye.

BRAZIL WOOD, a product of *Cæsalpinia*, is distinguished by forming a red colour with alkalis. It is now used only as a dye.

WEST INDIAN LOGWOOD is *Ceanothus Chloroxylon.*

LOOSESTRIFE, PURPLE

Lythrum salicaria
N.O. Lythraceæ

Synonyms. Lythrum. Purple Willow Herb. Spiked Loosestrife. Salicaire. Braune or Rother Weiderich. Partyke. Lysimaque rouge. Flowering Sally. Blooming Sally
Parts Used. Herb, root
Habitat. Europe, including Britain. Russian and Central Asia. Australia. North America

¶ *Description.* This handsome perennial, 2 to 4 feet in height, has a creeping rhizome, four to six angled, erect, reddish-brown stems, lanceolate leaves from 3 to 6 inches long, entire, sometimes opposite, sometimes in whorls clasping the stem, with reddish-purple or pink flowers in whorls forming terminal spikes. It grows in wet or marshy places, varying in different districts in the comparative lengths of stamens and styles, colour of flowers and pollen grains. It is odourless, with an astringent taste. It has been used in tanning leather.

The name Lythrum is from the Greek *luthron*, meaning 'gore,' from the colour of the flowers.

¶ *Constituents*. Mucilage and an astringent principle, but it has not been analysed.

¶ *Medicinal Action and Uses*. Although scarcely used at present, Loosestrife has been highly esteemed by many herbalists. It is well established in chronic diarrhœa and dysentery, and is used in leucorrhœa and blood-spitting. In Switzerland the decoction was used successfully in an epidemic of dysentery. It has also been employed in fevers, liver diseases, constipation and cholera infantum, and for outward application to wounds and sores.

It has been stated to be superior to Eyebright for preserving the sight and curing sore eyes, the distilled water being applied for hurts and blows on the eyes and even in blindness if the crystalline humour is not destroyed.

An ointment may be made with the water – 1 oz. to 2 drachms of May butter without salt, and the same quantity of sugar and wax boiled gently together. It cleanses and heals ulcers and sores, if washed with the water, or covered with the leaves, green or dry according to the season.

A warm gargle and drink cures quinsy or a scrofulous throat.

¶ *Dosages*. Of powder, a drachm two to three times a day. Of decoction of root, 2 fluid ounces.

¶ *Other Species*.

Lythrum hyssopifolia has similar properties.

L. verticillatum (Decodon or Swamp Willow-herb) has similar properties, and is said to cure abortion in mares and cows who browse on it.

A Mexican Salicaria, *Apanxaloa*, is regarded as an astringent and vulnerary.

Loosestrife is the common name of many members of the genus *Lysimachia*.

LOOSESTRIFE, YELLOW

Lysimachia vulgaris (LINN.)
N.O. Primulaceæ

Synonyms. Yellow Willow Herb. Herb Willow. Willow-wort. Wood Pimpernel
Part Used. Herb

The Yellow Loosestrife is a tall, handsome plant, from 2 to 3 or even 4 feet high, found as a rule on shady banks or crowning the herbage of the stream-side vegetation. It has a creeping root, which persists year after year, and every spring throws up afresh the tall, golden-topped stems, whose flowers are at their best in July and August.

¶ *Description*. Its stems are slightly branched and covered with a soft, fine down. Closely set upon them are a number of nearly stalkless leaves, sometimes in pairs, sometimes three or four springing from the same spot. They are rather large and broad, 3 to 6 inches long by about 1¼ inches broad, oblong or lance-shaped and sharply tapering at the top. Their edges are unbroken. The undersurfaces are downy with soft, spreading hairs, especially on the veins, and the upper surfaces are marked with black dots which are glands. Whatever arrangement we find in any given plant holds throughout: we do not find in the same plant some of the leaves in pairs and others in three. When the leaves are in pairs, the stem is quadrangular and the angles increase as the leaves increase in number.

At the top of the stem arise the flower-buds, in the axils of the leaves. Each becomes a short stalk carrying a terminal flower, below which other flowers on smaller stalks arise – the ends of the main stem thus becoming covered with a mass of golden blossoms. The flower stalks are somewhat viscid, or sticky, to the touch.

Each flower is about ¾ inch in diameter, forming a cup of five petals, quite distinct at their tips, but joined together near the base. When the flowers droop, the five-pointed calyx, whose edges are fringed with fine red hairs, are seen at the back of the petals. The five stamens look quite separate, but are joined together at the bottom by a fleshy band attached to the petals, so that they seem to stand on a little glandular tube. This tube has not, as one would expect, any honey, and, in fact, there is neither honey nor scent in any part of the flower. Nevertheless, the plant is visited by one particular kind of bee, *Macropsis labiata*, which will visit no other flower, hence where the Loosestrife does not grow the Macropsis does not seem to exist. Self-fertilization also takes place in smaller, less attractive-looking flowers, sometimes found among the others. As a result of fertilization, whether self or effected by insects, the ovary develops into a rounded capsule, which when dried opens at the top by five valves. The swaying of the stems by the wind jerks out the minute seeds.

The Yellow Loosestrife, which is in no way related to the Purple Loosestrife, has often been known as the Yellow Willow Herb, Herb Willow, or Willow Wort, as if it belonged to the true Willow Herbs (which are quite a different family – Onagraceæ). There is a superficial resemblance between them, especially with regard to the leaves. The Yellow Loosestrife belongs, however, to the same family as the Primrose and the Pimpernel.

The Purple Loosestrife, on the other hand, is more nearly allied to the Willow herbs.

¶ *Other Species.* Four species of Lysimachia are native in this country – the Yellow Loosestrife; the Moneywort – our familiar Creeping Jenny; the Yellow Pimpernel (or 'Wood Loosestrife'), which is remarkably like the Scarlet Pimpernel in general habit and in form, and the Tufted Lysimachia, a rare plant confined to the northern portions of this island.

Both the scientific and popular names of the Loosestrife have interesting origins. The name Lysimachia is supposed to have been given in memory of King Lysimachus of Sicily, who, as Pliny tells us, first discovered its medicinal properties and then introduced it to his people. A belief in these properties persisted for many centuries; it was 'a singular good wound herb for green wounds,' says one old herbalist, and it had a great reputation for stanching bleeding of any sort. It had the credit of being so excellent a vulnerary, that the young leaves bound about a fresh wound are said to immediately check the bleeding and perform a cure in a very short time.

Its common name of Loosestrife is a very old one, and refers to the belief that the plant would quieten savage beasts, and that in particular it had a special virtue 'in appeasing the strife and unruliness which falleth out among oxen at the plough, if it be put about their yokes.' The plant appears to be obnoxious to gnats and flies, and so, no doubt, placing it under the yoke, relieved the beasts of their tormentors, thus making them quiet and tractable. For the same reason, the dried herb used to be burnt in houses, so that the smoke might drive away gnats and flies. It was particularly valuable in marshy districts. Snakes and serpents were said to disappear immediately the fumes of the burning herb came near them.

Gerard speaks of the 'yellow pimpernel growing in abundance between Highgate and Hampstead.'

Coles's *Art of Simpling*, the only herbal which devotes a chapter to herbs useful for animals, refers to the belief that

'if loosestrife is thrown between two oxen when they are fighting they will part presently, and being tied about their necks it will keep them from fighting.'

Even in Pliny's days, it was suggested that the plant did not really derive its name from a more or less mythical king, but that it was compounded from the Greek words, signifying 'dissolving strife' – it being held that not only cattle at the plough, but also restive horses could be subdued by it.

The plants can be transferred to the garden if the soil be somewhat moist, and especially if a stream or a piece of water is available. They will grow and thrive, then, in their new quarters, creeping by their perennial roots, so that when once fairly established, they will flourish permanently.

¶ *Part Used.* The whole herb, collected from wild plants in July and dried.

The taste of the dried herb is astringent and slightly acid, but it has no odour.

¶ *Medicinal Action and Uses.* Astringent, expectorant. Loosestrife proves useful in checking bleeding of the mouth, nose and wounds, restraining profuse hæmorrhage of any kind.

It has demulcent and astringent virtues which render it useful in obstinate diarrhœa, and as a gargle it finds use in relaxed throat and quinsy.

For the cure of sore eyes, this herb has been considered equal, if not superior to Eyebright. Culpepper states:

'This herb has some peculiar virtue of its own, as the distilled water is a remedy for hurts and blows on the eyes, and for blindness, so as the crystalline humours be not perished or hurt. It cleareth the eyes of dust or any other particle and preserveth the sight.'

For wounds, an ointment was used in his days, made of the distilled water of the herb, boiled with butter and sugar. The distilled water was also recommended for cleansing ulcers and reducing their inflammation, and also, applied warm, for removing 'spots, marks and scabs in the skin.'

See MONEYWORT, YELLOW PIMPERNEL.

LOVAGE

Levisticum officinale (KOCH.)
N.O. Umbelliferæ

Synonyms. Ligusticum Levisticum (Linn.). Old English Lovage. Italian Lovage. Cornish Lovage

Parts Used. Root, leaves, seeds, young stems

Habitat. It is not considered to be indigenous to Great Britain, and when occasionally found growing apparently wild, it is probably a garden escape. It is a native of the Mediterranean region, growing wild in the mountainous districts of the south of France, in northern Greece and in the Balkans

The Garden Lovage is one of the old English herbs that was formerly very generally cultivated, and is still occasionally cultivated as a sweet herb, and for the use in herbal medicine of its root, and to a less degree, the leaves and seeds.

It is a true perennial and hence is very easy to keep in garden cultivation; it can be propagated by offsets like Rhubarb, and it is very hardy. Its old-time repute has suffered by the substitution of the medicinally more powerful Milfoil and Tansy, just as was the case when 'Elecampane' superseded Angelica in medical use. The public-house cordial named 'Lovage,' formerly much in vogue, however, owed such virtue as it may have possessed to Tansy. Freshly-gathered leafstalks of Lovage (for flavouring purposes) should be employed in long split lengths.

¶ *Description.* This stout, umbelliferous plant has been thought to resemble to some degree our Garden Angelica, and it does very closely resemble the Spanish *Angelica heterocarpa* in foliage and perennial habit of growth. It has a thick and fleshy root, 5 or 6 inches long, shaped like a carrot, of a greyish-brown colour on the outside and whitish within. It has a strong aromatic smell and taste. The thick, erect hollow and channelled stems grow 3 or 4 feet or even more in height. The large, dark green radical leaves, on erect stalks, are divided into narrow wedge-like segments, and are not unlike those of a coarse-growing celery; their surface is shining, and when bruised they give out an aromatic odour, somewhat reminiscent both of Angelica and Celery. The stems divide towards the top to form opposite whorled branches, which in June and July bear umbels of yellow flowers, similar to those of Fennel or Parsnip, followed by small, extremely aromatic fruits, yellowish-brown in colour, elliptical in shape and curved, with three prominent winged ribs. The odour of the whole plant is very strong. Its taste is warm and aromatic, and it abounds with a yellowish, gummy, resinous juice.

It is sometimes grown in gardens for its ornamental foliage, as well as for its pleasant odour, but it is not a striking enough plant to have claimed the attention of poets and painters, and no myths or legends are connected with it. The name of the genus, *Ligusticum*, is said to be derived from Liguria, where this species abounds.

¶ *Cultivation.* Lovage is of easy culture. Propagation is by division of roots or by seeds. Rich moist, but well-drained soil is required and a sunny situation. In late summer, when the seed ripens, it should be sown and the seedlings transplanted, either in the autumn or as early in spring as possible, to their permanent quarters, setting 12 inches apart each way. The seeds may also be sown in spring, but it is preferable to sow when just ripe. Root division is performed in early spring.

The plants should last for several years, if the ground be kept well cultivated, and where the seeds are permitted to scatter the plants will come up without care.

¶ *Parts Used.* The *root, leaves* and *seeds* for medicinal purposes.

The *young stems,* treated like Angelica, for flavouring and confectionery.

¶ *Constituents.* Lovage contains a volatile oil, angelic acid, a bitter extractive, resins, etc. The colouring principle has been isolated by M. Niklis, who gives it the name of Ligulin, and suggests an important application of it that may be made in testing drinking water. If a drop of its alcoholic or aqueous solution is allowed to fall into distilled water, it imparts to the liquid its own fine crimson-red colour, which undergoes no change; but if limestone water be substituted, the red colour disappears in a few seconds and is followed by a beautiful blue, due to the alkalinity of the latter.

¶ *Medicinal Action and Uses.* Formerly Lovage was used for a variety of culinary purposes, but now its use is restricted almost wholly to confectionery, the young stems being treated like those of Angelica, to which, however, it is inferior, as its stems are not so stout nor so succulent.

The leafstalks and stem bases were formerly blanched like celery, but as a vegetable it has fallen into disuse.

A herbal tea is made of the leaves, when previously dried, the decoction having a very agreeable odour.

Lovage was much used as a drug plant in the fourteenth century, its medicinal reputation probably being greatly founded on its pleasing aromatic odour. It was never an official remedy, nor were any extravagant claims made, as with Angelica, for its efficacy in numberless complaints.

The roots and fruit are aromatic and stimulant, and have diuretic and carminative action. In herbal medicine they are used in disorders of the stomach and feverish attacks, especially for cases of colic and flatulence in children, its qualities being similar to those of Angelica in expelling flatulence, exciting perspiration and opening obstructions. The leaves eaten as salad, or infused dry as a tea, used to be accounted a good emmenagogue.

An infusion of the root was recommended by old writers for gravel, jaundice and urinary troubles, and the cordial, sudorific nature of the roots and seeds caused their use to be extolled in 'pestilential disorders.' In the opinion of Culpepper, the working of the seeds was more powerful than that of the root; he tells us that an infusion 'being dropped into the eyes taketh away their redness or dimness. . . . It is highly recommended to drink the decoction of the herb for agues. . . . The distilled water is good for quinsy if the mouth and throat be gargled and washed therewith. . . . The decoction drunk three or four times a day is effectual in pleurisy. . . . The leaves bruised and fried with a little hog's lard and laid hot to any blotch or boil will quickly break it.'

Several species of this umbelliferous genus are employed as domestic medicines. The root of LIGUSTICUM SINENSE, under the name of KAO-PÂU, is largely used by the Chinese, and in the north-western United States the large, aromatic roots of LIGUSTICUM FILICINUM (OSHA COLORADO COUGH-ROOT) are used to a considerable extent as stimulating expectorants.

The old-fashioned cordial, 'Lovage,' now not much in vogue, though still occasionally to be found in public-houses, is brewed not only from the Garden Lovage, *Ligusticum levisticum*, but mainly from a species of Milfoil or Yarrow, *Achillea ligustica*, and from Tansy, *Tanacetum vulgare*, and probably owes its merit more to these herbs than to Lovage itself. From its use in this cordial, Milfoil has often been mistakenly called Lovage, though it is in no way related to the Umbellifer family.

Several other plants have been termed Lovage besides the true Lovage, and this has frequently caused confusion. Thus we have the SCOTCH LOVAGE, known also as Sea Lovage, or Scotch Parsley, and botanically as *Ligusticum scoticum*; the BLACK LOVAGE, or Alexanders, *Smyrnium Olusatrum*; BASTARD LOVAGE, a species of the allied genus, *Laserpitum*, and WATER LOVAGE, a species of the genus *Œnanthe*.

Laserpitum may be distinguished from its allies by the fruit having eight prominent, wing-like appendages. The species are perennial herbs, chiefly found in south-eastern Europe. Some of them are employed as domestic remedies, on account of their aroma.

The scent of the root of MEUM ATHAMANTICUM (Jacq.), SPIGNEL (also called *Spikenel* or *Spiknel*), MEU or BALD-MONEY, has much in common with that of both Lovage and Angelica, and the root has been eaten by the Scotch Highlanders as a vegetable. It is a perennial, smooth and very aromatic herb. The elongated root is crowned with fibres, the leaves, mostly springing from the root, are divided into leaflets which are further cut into numerous thread-like segments, which gives them a feathery appearance. The stem is about 6 or 8 inches high, and bears umbels of white or purplish flowers. The aromatic flavour of the leaves is somewhat like Melilot, and is communicated to milk and butter when cows feed on the herbage in the spring. The peculiar name of this plant, 'Baldmoney,' is said to be a corruption of *Balder*, the *Apollo* of the northern nations, to whom the plant was dedicated.

LOVAGE, BASTARD

Synonym. White Gentian

Bastard Lovage is not a native of Great Britain. The species respectively comprised in the genera *Laserpitum* and *Ligusticum*, have

Laserpitum latifolia (LINN.)
N.O. Umbelliferæ

much in common regarding foliage, manner of growth and aromatic odour.

LOVAGE, BLACK

Synonyms. Alexanders. Alisanders. Black Pot-herb
Part Used. Herb

Smyrnium Olisatrum (LINN.)

Black Lovage is in leaf and flower not unlike an Angelica, and amateur collectors have sometimes mistaken it for Wild Angelica.

Alexanders, to use its more common name, is a large perennial herb, growing 3 or 4 feet in height, with very large leaves, doubly and triply divided into three (ternate), with broad leaflets; the sheaths of the footstalks are very broad and membraneous in texture. The yellowish-green flowers are produced in numerous close, rounded umbels without involucres (the little leaves that are placed often at the spot where the various rays of the umbel spring). The whole herb is of a yellowish-green tint. The fruit is formed of two, nearly globular halves, with prominent ridges. When ripe, it is almost black, whence the plant received from the old herbalists the name of 'Black Pot-herb,' the specific name signifying the same. (*Olus*, a pot-herb, and *atrum*, black.)

LOVAGE, SCOTCH

Ligusticum Scoticum (LINN.)
N.O. Umbelliferæ

Synonym. Sea Lovage
Part Used. Root

The Scotch Lovage grows on cliffs and rocky shores in Scotland and Northumberland. It has a stout, branched rootstock, which is aromatic and pungent; a sparingly branched, erect, grooved stem, 1 to 3 feet high, and much cut-into dark green, shiny leaves, with three-lobed leaflets. The umbels of flowers, in bloom in July, are white or pink.

The leaves have been used in the Hebrides as a green vegetable, either boiled as greens, or eaten raw as salad, under the name of *Shunis*. The taste is strong and not very pleasant.

An infusion of the leaves in whey is used in Scotland as a purgative for calves, much valued, Green states in the *Universal Herbal*, in the Isle of Skye.

The root possesses aromatic and carminative properties; it has been applied in hysterical and uterine disorders.

When treated like celery, Sea Lovage proves quite inferior, though Angelica and Lovage have been thus used with a certain measure of success, even to the more fastidious modern palate.

This is one of the many cultivated plants that, escaping from gardens, have become apparently wild. It is now found rather abundantly in some parts of the sea-coast, on waste places near the mouth of rivers, especially in Scotland, and inland is occasionally seen in the neighbourhood of towns, or about the ruins of monasteries and other places where it was grown in olden times as a pot-herb and salad. It was formerly cultivated in the same manner as celery, which has now supplanted it, and boiled, was eaten by sailors returning from long voyages and suffering from scurvy. The young shoots and leaf-stalks eaten raw, have a rather agreeable taste, not very unlike that of celery, but more pungent. They were likewise used to flavour soups and stews, and some years ago were still so employed by the country people in parts where the plant abounds.

The seeds are sweetly aromatic and were formerly used as a carminative and stimulant medicine, and are still valued by herbalists for pleasantly flavouring confections of Senna and disguising the taste of other medicinal preparations.

(POISON)
LOVAGE, WATER

Œnanthe fistulosa (LINN.)
N.O. Umbelliferæ

Water Lovage is closely allied to Hemlock Water Dropwort (*Œnanthe crocata*, Linn.), and is by no means to be regarded as an edible plant. All the species of Water Dropwort are regarded as poisonous, and the Hemlock Water Dropwort should not be allowed to grow in places where cattle are kept, as instances are numerous in which cows have been poisoned by eating the roots, and it is equally poisonous to horses.

The genus *Œnanthe* is scattered throughout the whole of the Northern Hemisphere, but are rare in America; some of them are to be met with in Britain, and certain of them are very poisonous. *Œ. crocata* has been used with beneficial effect in certain skin-diseases; also in the form of poultices to ulcers, etc., as well as for the purpose of poisoning rats and moles.
See DROPWORT

LOVE LIES BLEEDING. *See* AMARANTHS

LUCERNE

Medicago sativa
N.O. Papilionaceæ

Synonyms. Purple Medicle. Cultivated Lucern
Part Used. Whole herb in flower
Habitat. Originally Medea, then old Spain, Italy, France; and cultivated in Persia and Peru

¶ *Description.* A deep-rooting perennial plant with numerous small clover-like spikes of blue or violet flowers of upright growth. Its herbage is green, succulent, and being an early crop is in a sense of some value as an agricultural plant. It yields two rather abundant green crops in the year – of a quality greatly relished by horses and cattle – it fattens them quickly and was much esteemed for increasing the milk of cows. One of the objections to growing it as a crop is the three to four years required before it attains full growth. When this plant is found in Britain growing wild it is merely an escape from cultivation. It may possibly have been a native of Europe; it is of great antiquity, having been imported into Greece from the East, after Darius had discovered it in Medea, hence its name. It is referred to by Roman writers, and is cultivated in Persia and Peru, where it is mown all the year round. It first came into notice in 1757 in Britain. Its chief characteristics are: herb, 1½ to 2 feet high; peduncled racemed; legumes contorted, twisted spirally, hairy; stem upright, smooth; leaves trifoliate; flowers in thick spikes, corolla purple.

To increase weight, an infusion of 1 oz. to the pint is given in cupful doses.

The root of Lucerne has sometimes been found as an adulterant of Belladonna root.

LUNGWORT

Sticta pulmonaria (LINN.)
N.O. Lichenes

Synonyms. Jerusalem Cowslip. Oak Lungs. Lung Moss
Part Used. Herb

Lungwort, a member of the Borage tribe, is found in woods and thickets, but is not common, and is by some only regarded as an escape from gardens, where it is cultivated now mostly for the sake of its ornamental leaves, which are curiously spotted with white.

¶ *Description.* The stem grows about a foot high, bearing rough, alternate, egg-shaped leaves, the lower ones stalked, and the flowers in a terminal inflorescence, red before expanding and pale purple when fully open.

The leaves of this plant, which are the part that has been used in medicine, have no peculiar smell, but when fresh have a slight astringent and mucilaginous taste, hence they have been supposed to be demulcent and pectoral, and have been used in coughs and lung catarrhs in the form of an infusion.

Its popular and Latin names seem to have been derived from the speckled appearance of the leaves resembling that of the lungs, and their use in former days was partly founded on the doctrine of signatures.

The Lungwort sold by druggists to-day is not this species, but a Moss, known also as Oak Lungs and Lung Moss.

The Lungwort formerly held a place in almost every garden, under the name of 'Jerusalem Cowslip'; and it was held in great esteem for its reputed medicinal qualities in diseases of the lungs.

Sir J. E. Smith says that

'every part of the plant is mucilaginous, but its reputation for coughs arose not from this circumstance, but from the speckled appearance of the leaves, resembling the lungs!'

¶ *Medicinal Action and Uses.* An infusion of 1 teaspoonful of the dried herb to a cup of boiling water is taken several times a day for subduing inflammation, and for its healing effect in pulmonary complaints.

Fluid extract, ½ to 1 drachm.

LUPINS

N.O. Leguminosæ

Synonyms. (*French*) Lupin. (*German*) Wolfsbohne
Parts Used. Seeds, herb

The *Lupinus* are a large genus of handsome plants, represented in Europe, Asia and North and South America, the poisonous properties of which are apparently very irregularly and unequally distributed.

A number of the species are cultivated only as ornamental plants, but others are grown for fodder, and if not over-fed, are found highly nutritive and wholesome. If the seeds of certain species are eaten in a more or less mature condition, poisoning is liable to occur, great numbers of animals sometimes being affected. These poisoning accidents have occurred in Europe and in the United States.

The species best known – as fodder – is the WHITE LUPIN of cultivation, *Lupinus albus* (Linn.) (French, *Lupin*; German, *Wolfs-* *bohne*), native of Southern Europe and adjacent Asia, a plant of about 2 feet high, with leaves cut palmately into five or seven divisions, 1 to 2 inches long, smooth above, and white, hairy, beneath. The flowers are in terminal racemes, on short footstalks, white and rather large, the pod 3 to 4 inches long, flattish, containing three to six white, circular, flattened seeds, which have a bitter taste.

¶ *History.* It is probably of Egyptian or East Mediterranean origin, and has been cultivated since the days of the ancient Egyptians. It is now very extensively used in Italy and Sicily, for forage, for ploughing-in to enrich the land, and for its seeds.

John Parkinson attributed wonderful virtues to the plant.

Many women, he says 'doe use the meale of Lupines mingled with the gall of a goate and some juyce of Lemons to make into a forme of a soft ointment.' He says that the burning of Lupin seeds drives away gnats.

Culpepper says they are governed by Mars in Ares:

'The seeds, somewhat bitter in taste, opening and cleansing, good to destroy worms. Outwardly they are used against deformities of the skin, scabby ulcers, scald heads, and other cutaneous distempers.'

This Lupin was cultivated by the Romans as an article of food. Pliny says:

'No kind of fodder is more wholesome and light of digestion than the White Lupine, when eaten dry. If taken commonly at meals, it will contribute a fresh colour and a cheerful countenance.'

Virgil, however, Dr. Fernie tells us (*Herbal Simples*, 1897), designated it '*tristis Lupinus*,' the sad Lupine. Dr. Fernie further states:

'The seeds were used as pieces of money by Roman actors in their plays and comedies, whence came the saying "nummus lupinus" – a spurious bit of money.'

The YELLOW LUPIN, also a native of Southern Europe and Western Asia, is called *Lupin luteus* from its yellow flowers. The BLUE-FLOWERED SPECIES of the North-eastern United States is *Lupinus perennis* (Linn.), the WILD or BLUE BEAN. In the Western United and southward into the Andes, the species are very numerous.

¶ *Cultivation*. If grown from seed, Lupins do not often come true to type, but if propagated, they will remain true. They must be isolated, owing to insects which might cross the pollen.

Lupins cross readily, hence isolation for propagation is absolutely necessary.

To intensify their colouring, sulphate of ammonia and sulphate of iron may both be employed.

Climatic conditions also more or less affect their colouring.

In a recent note in *The Western Gazette* (May 18, 1923) Lupins were spoken of as probably the best crop for light land, such as the poor land on the Suffolk coast, where Lupin growing is extending, as also on similar land in the northern part of Nottinghamshire.

In Suffolk the Blue Lupin is the local variety, and anyone travelling through that country in July will see whole fields devoted to it.

The great value of the plant lies in its capacity for growing luxuriantly on land which is so light and sandy that hardly anything else will thrive. Being a leguminous crop, it assimilates the free nitrogen of the air, greatly enriching the soil; and on light land it is probably quite the best plant we have for green manuring.

¶ *Constituents*. The bitter principle Lupinin is a glucoside occurring in yellowish needles. On boiling with dilute acids, it is decomposed into Lupigenin and a fermentable glucose.

Willstatter described the following alkaloids as occurring in the different species: Lupinine, a crystalline powder and Lupinidine, a syrupy liquid in LUPINUS LUTEUS and L. NIGER. Lupanine in L. ALBUS, L. ANGUSTIFOLIUS and L. PERENNIS, a pale yellow, syrupy fluid of an intensely bitter taste. E. Schmidt affirmed that the alkaloid of the seeds of *L. albus* is not the same as that of the herbage. A carbohydrate analogous to dextrin has been discovered in *L. luteus*.

According to Schwartz (1906) the seeds of LUPINUS ARABICUS contain a crystalline substance to which he gave the name of Magolan, which is a useful remedy in diabetes mellitus.

¶ *Medicinal Action and Uses*. The bruised seeds of White Lupine, after soaking in water, are sometimes used as an external application to ulcers, etc., and internally are said to be anthelmintic, diuretic and emmenagogue.

In 1917 a 'Lupin' banquet was given in Hamburg at a botanical gathering, at which a German Professor, Dr. Thoms, described the multifarious uses to which the Lupin might be put. At a table covered with a tablecloth of Lupin fibre, Lupin soup was served; after the soup came Lupin beefsteak, roasted in Lupin oil and seasoned with Lupin extract, then bread containing 20 per cent. of Lupin, Lupin margarine and cheese of Lupin albumen, and finally Lupin liqueur and Lupin coffee. Lupin soap served for washing the hands, while Lupin-fibre paper and envelopes with Lupin adhesive were available for writing.

¶ *Other Species*.

L. arboreus (the Tree Lupin), from California and Oregon, will, when well trained, produce a branching stem several feet in height that will live through four or five years, forming a trunk of light soft wood of the thickness of a man's arm.

L. polyphyllus and a few allied species from the same country are tall, erect, herbaceous perennials with very handsome richly-coloured spikes of flowers, which have become permanent inmates of our gardens.

MACE

Myristica fragrans (HONK.)
N.O. Myristicaceæ

Synonyms. Arillus Myristicæ. Myristica officinalis. Myristica moschata. Macis. Muscadier

Part Used. The dried arillus of the fruit or nutmeg

Habitat. Moluccas and Bandy Islands, New Guinea, West Indies, etc.

¶ *History.* The name is derived from a mediæval word for 'nut,' meaning 'suitable for an ointment.' The tree is a small evergreen, not more than 40 feet in height, with smooth, greyish-brown bark, green on the younger branches. The alternate leaves are oblong-ovate, acute, entire, smooth, and dark-green. The flowers are very small and unisexual. The fruits, smooth and yellow, resemble a pear grooved by a longitudinal furrow and contain a single erect seed about $1\frac{1}{4}$ inch long, the nucleus being the wrinkled 'nutmeg,' and the fleshy, irregular covering, scarlet when fresh and drying yellow and brittle, the 'mace.'

The principal harvest at Bencoolen is usually in the autumn, the smaller one in early summer. The fruits, which split open when ripe, are gathered with a long-handled hook and the products are separated. The mace when dried is often sprinkled with salt water to preserve it. If packed too moist it breeds worms.

Most of the supply comes from the Banda Islands by way of Java and Sumatra.

The 'blades,' 'bands,' or flattened, lobed pieces are about 25 mm. long, smooth, irregular, translucent, brittle or flexible, and if scratched or pressed exude an orange-coloured oil.

An inferior Mace is obtained from the long nutmeg, dark and very brittle and lacking the fragrant odour and aromatic taste of the official variety.

The medicinal properties resemble those of nutmeg, but it is principally used as a condiment.

¶ *Constituents.* The principal constituent is 7 to 9 per cent. of a volatile oil, protein, gum, resins, sugar and fixed oil. The volatile oil contains much pinene, and a little myristicin, which must be distinguished from the glyceride of myristic acid.

Two odorous fixed oils have been separated, a yellow one insoluble in boiling alcohol but soluble in ether, and a red one soluble in either.

The powder is brown or buff, orange-tinted.

Oil of Mace is practically identical with distilled oil of nutmeg or Nutmeg Butter.

¶ *Medicinal Action and Uses.* A flavouring agent, stimulant and tonic.

Both Mace and Nutmeg help digestion in stomachic weakness, but if used to excess may cause over-excitement. They increase circulation and animal heat. They have been employed in pestilential and putrid fevers, and with other substances in intermittent fevers, and enter into the composition of many French medicaments.

¶ *Dosage.* 5 to 20 grains.

¶ *Other Species.*

Myristica malabarica, yielding Bombay Mace, which is deficient in odour and taste. Several chemical tests provide means of detecting the substitution. It yields a much higher percentage of ether-soluble matter.

M. argentea, yielding Macassar Mace, which is of a dull brown colour with an odour like sassafras. It is too acrid for medicinal use.

M. otoba, yielding a Mace which, incorporated with fat, is used in gout and rheumatism.

See NUTMEG

MADDER

Rubia tinctorum (LINN.)
N.O. Rubiaceæ

Synonyms. Krapp. Dyer's Madder. Robbia
(*French*) Garance

Part Used. Root

Habitat. Southern Europe, including southern Britain, and Mediterranean countries

¶ *Description.* The stalks of the Madder are so weak that they often lie along the ground, preventing the plant from rising to its maximum height of 8 feet. The stalks are prickly, and the whorls of leaves at the joints have spines along the midrib on the underside, a feature that the French turn to advantage by using them for polishing metal-work.

The herb is used as fodder for animals.

The flower-shoots spring from the joints in pairs, the loose spikes of yellow, starry flowers blooming only in the second or third year, in June.

The thick, fleshy fibres that compose the perennial are about $\frac{1}{4}$ inch thick, and from their joining, or head, side roots run under the surface of the ground for some distance, sending up shoots. The main and side-roots are dried separately, their products being regarded as different, that of a young, parent root being the best. They are covered with a blackish rind, beneath which they are reddish, with a pale yellow pith. In France, after drying, the outer layer is threshed off and powdered and packed separately as an inferior product called *mall*. The stripped roots are again heated – excepting in hot climates – then powdered, and milled three times. The final product is packed in casks, which in Holland are stamped by sworn assayers.

The best European Madder is Dutch, but that from Smyrna is said to be even finer. The Turkey-red and other shades are adjective dyes, different mordants bringing many shades of red, pink, lilac, purple, brown, orange and black.

As a dye it colours milk, urine and bones, so that experiments in the growth of bones can be conducted with its help.

Rubia tinctoria differs very slightly from the Wild Madder or *R. peregrina*, and may be merely a variety.

¶ *Constituents*. The root contains rubian, rubiadin, ruberythric acid, purpurin, tannin, sugar and especially *alizarin. Pseudopurpurin* yields the orange dye and *xanthopurpurin* the yellow. The astringent taste, slight odour and red colour, are imparted to water or alcohol.

The most interesting of the colouring substances is the alizarin, and this is now termed dihydroscyanthraquinone. This occurs as orange-red crystals, almost insoluble in water, but readily soluble in alcohol, ether, the fixed oils and alkaline solutions. The alcoholic and aqueous solutions are rose-coloured, the ethereal, golden-yellow; the

alkaline, violet and blue when concentrated, but violet red when sufficiently diluted. A beautiful rose-coloured lake is produced by precipitating a mixture of the solutions of alizarin and alum.

Alizarin was recognized by Græbe and Liebermann, in 1868, as a derivative of anthracene – a hydrocarbon contained in coal-tar, and in the same year they elaborated a method for preparing it commercially from anthracene. Upon this arose rapidly a great chemical industry, and the cultivation of Madder has, of course, decreased correspondingly until it may be said that the coal-tar products have entirely displaced the natural ónes.

¶ *Medicinal Action and Uses*. Although not as a general rule employed medicinally, Madder has been reputed as effectual in amenorrhœa, dropsy and jaundice.

When taken into the stomach it imparts a red colour to the milk and urine, and to the bones of animals without sensibly affecting any other tissue. The effect is observed most quickly in the bones of young animals and in those nearest to the heart. Under the impression that it might effect some change in the nervous system, it has been prescribed in rachitis (rickets), but without noticeable favourable results. Dosage, ½ drachm three or four times daily.

¶ *Other Species*.
R. sylvestris, a nearly allied species, has been used as a remedy in liver diseases, jaundice, gall and spleen complaints. The root, leaves and seeds are all reputed as medicinally active.

R. cordifolia, or Bengal Madder, of India, yields the inferior dye called Munjeet.

In France it is thought that the root of *Galium cruciatum*, or Crosswort, might replace that of Madder.

MAGNOLIA

Magnolia acuminata
Magnolia virginiana (LINN.)
N.O. Magnoliaceæ

Synonyms. Cucumber Tree. Magnoliæ cortex. Blue Magnolia. Swamp Sassafras. Magnolia Tripetata
Parts Used. Bark of stem and root
Habitat. North America

¶ *Description*. The genus is named in commemoration of Pierre Magnol, a famous professor of medicine and botany of Montpellier in the early eighteenth century. All its members are handsome, with luxuriant foliage and rich flowers. The leaves of *Magnolia acuminata* are oval, about 6 inches long by 3 broad, and slightly hairy below, with a diameter of 6 inches, and the fruit or cone, about 3 inches long, resembles a small cucumber.

It is a large tree, reaching a height of 80 or more feet and a diameter of 3 to 5 feet, but only grows to about 16 feet in England. The wood is finely grained, taking a brilliant polish, and in its colour resembles that of the tulip or poplar, but it is less durable. It is sometimes used for large canoes and house interiors.

The bark of the young wood is curved or quilled, fissured outside, with occasional warts, and orange-brown in colour, being whitish and smooth within and the fracture short except for inner fibres. The older bark without the corky layer is brownish or whitish and fibrous. Drying and age cause the loss of its volatile, aromatic property.

¶ *Constituents.* The bark has no astringency. The tonic properties are found in varying degree in several species.

¶ *Medicinal Action and Uses.* A mild diaphoretic, tonic, and aromatic stimulant. It is used in rheumatism and malaria and is contra-indicated in inflammatory symptoms. In the Alleghany districts the *cones* are steeped in spirits to make a tonic tincture.

A warm infusion is laxative and sudorific, a cold one being antiperiodic and mildly tonic.

¶ *Dosage.* Fluid Extract. Frequent doses of ½ to 1 drachm, or the infusion in wineglassful doses.

¶ *Other Species.*
Both *M. virginiana* and *M. tripetala* were recognized as official with *M. acuminata.*

M. virginiana, or *M. glauca,* White Laurel, Beaver Tree, Swamp Sassafras, White Bay, Sweet Bay, Small or Laurel Magnolia, or Sweet Magnolia, is much used by beavers, who favour it both as food and building material. The light wood has no commercial use.

The bark and seed cones are bitter and aromatic, used as tonics, and in similar ways to *M. acuminata.* The leaves yield a green, volatile oil with a more pleasant odour than fennel or anise. There is probably also a bitter glucosidal principle.

M. tripetala, Umbrella Tree or Umbrella Magnolia. The fruit yields a neutral crystalline principle, Magnolin.

The bark, if chewed as a substitute for tobacco, is said to cure the habit.

MAIDENHAIR. *See* FERNS

MALABAR NUT

Adhatoda vasica (NEES)
N.O. Acanthaceæ

Synonyms. Justicia adhatoda (Linn.). Arusa. Adulsa Bakas
Parts Used. Leaves, flowers, fruit, root
Habitat. India

¶ *Description.* A common plant in India, the fresh leaves are 4 to 6 inches long, 2 inches wide, lanceolate entire, shortly petiolate, when dried dull brownish green, they become lighter when powdered, taste bitter and smell like strong tea. Its wood is soft and makes excellent charcoal for gunpowder.

¶ *Constituents.* The leaves contain a bitter crystalline alkaloid Vasicine, and an organic adhatodic acid, another alkaloid and an odorous volatile principle.

¶ *Medicinal Action and Uses.* In India the flowers, leaves, root and specially the fruit are considered a valuable antispasmodic for

asthma and intermittent fever; used with success also as an expectorant in cases of chronic bronchitis and phthisis; the leaves are dried and smoked as cigarettes to relieve asthma. Large doses irritate the alimentary canal and cause diarrhœa and vomiting.

Adhatodic acid is believed to exert a strong poisoning influence upon the lower forms of animals and vegetable life, though non-poisonous to the higher animals.

¶ *Dosages.* Liquid extract of Adhatoda, 20 to 60 minims. The freshly expressed juice, 1 to 4 fluid drachms. Tincture from ½ to 1 fluid drachm.

MALE FERN. *See* FERNS

MALLOWS

N.O. Malvaceæ

The large and important family of Mallows are most abundant in the tropical region, where they form a large proportion of the vegetation; towards the poles they gradually decrease in number. Lindley states that about a thousand species had been discovered, all of which not only contain much mucilage, but are totally devoid of unwholesome pro-

perties. Besides the medicinal virtues of so many species, some are employed as food; the bark of others affords a substitute for hemp; the cotton of commerce is obtained from the seed vessels of yet other species, and many ornamental garden flowers are also members of this group, the Hibiscus and our familiar Hollyhock among the number.

Synonyms. Mallards. Mauls. Schloss Tea. Cheeses. Mortification Root
(*French*) Guimauve
Parts Used. Leaves, root, flowers
Habitat. Marsh Mallow is a native of most countries of Europe, from Denmark south-ward. It grows in salt marshes, in damp meadows, by the sides of ditches, by the sea and on the banks of tidal rivers

     In this country it is local, but occurs in most of the maritime counties in the south of England, ranging as far north as Lincolnshire. In Scotland it has been introduced

¶ *Description.* The stems, which die down in the autumn, are erect, 3 to 4 feet high, simple, or putting out only a few lateral branches. The leaves, shortly petioled, are roundish, ovate-cordate, 2 to 3 inches long, and about 1¼ inch broad, entire or three to five lobed, irregularly toothed at the margin, and thick. They are soft and velvety on both sides, due to a dense covering of stellate hairs. The flowers are shaped like those of the common Mallow, but are smaller and of a pale colour, and are either axillary, or in panicles, more often the latter.

The stamens are united into a tube, the anthers, kidney-shaped and one-celled. The flowers are in bloom during August and September, and are followed, as in other species of this order, by the flat, round fruit called popularly 'cheeses.'

The common Mallow is frequently called by country people, 'Marsh Mallow,' but the true Marsh Mallow is distinguished from all the other Mallows growing in Britain, by the numerous divisions of the outer calyx (six to nine cleft), by the hoary down which thickly clothes the stems, and foliage, and by the numerous panicles of blush-coloured flowers, paler than the Common Mallow.

The roots are perennial, thick, long and tapering, very tough and pliant, whitish-yellow outside, white and fibrous within.

The whole plant, particularly the root, abounds with a mild mucilage, which is emollient to a much greater degree than the common Mallow. The generic name, *Althæa*, is derived from the Greek, *altho* (to cure), from its healing properties. The name of the order, Malvaceæ, is derived from the Greek, *malake* (soft), from the special qualities of the Mallows in softening and healing.

Most of the Mallows have been used as food, and are mentioned by early classic writers in this connexion. Mallow was an esculent vegetable among the Romans, a dish of Marsh Mallow was one of their delicacies.

The Chinese use some sort of Mallow in their food, and Prosper Alpinus stated (in 1592) that a plant of the Mallow kind was eaten by the Egyptians. Many of the poorer inhabitants of Syria, especially the Fellahs, Greeks and Armenians, subsist for weeks on herbs, of which Marsh Mallow is one of the most common. When boiled first and fried with onions and butter, the roots are said to form a palatable dish, and in times of scarcity consequent upon the failure of the crops, this plant, which fortunately grows there in great abundance, is much collected for food.

In Job xxx. 4 we read of Mallow being eaten in time of famine, but it is doubtful whether this was really a true mallow. Canon Tristram thinks it was some saline plant; perhaps the *Orache*, or Sea-Purslane.

Horace and Martial mention the laxative properties of the Marsh Mallow leaves and root, and Virgil tells us of the fondness of goats for the foliage of the Mallow.

Dioscorides extols it as a remedy, and in ancient days it was not only valued as a medicine, but was used, especially the Musk Mallow, to decorate the graves of friends.

Pliny said: 'Whosoever shall take a spoon-ful of the Mallows shall that day be free from all diseases that may come to him.' All Mal-lows contain abundant mucilage, and the Arab physicians in early times used the leaves as a poultice to suppress inflammation.

Preparations of Marsh Mallow, on account of their soothing qualities, are still much used by country people for inflammation, out-wardly and inwardly, and are used for lozenge-making. French druggists and Eng-lish sweetmeat-makers prepare a confec-tionary paste (*Pâté de Guimauve*) from the roots of Marsh Mallow, which is emollient and soothing to a sore chest, and valuable in coughs and hoarseness. The 'Marsh Mal-lows' usually sold by confectioners here are a mixture of flour, gum, egg-albumin, etc., and contain no mallow.

In France, the young tops and tender leaves of Marsh Mallow are eaten uncooked, in spring salads, for their property in stimu-lating the kidneys, a syrup being made from the roots for the same purpose.

¶ *Cultivation.* Marsh Mallow used always to be cultivated in gardens on account of its medicinal qualities. It is said to have been introduced by the Romans.

It can be raised from seed, sown in spring, but cuttings will do well, and offsets of the root, carefully divided in autumn, when the stalks decay, are satisfactory, and will grow of their own accord.

Plant about 2 feet apart. It will thrive in any soil or situation, but grows larger in moist than in dry land, and could well be cultivated on unused ground in damp localities near ditches or streams.

¶ *Parts Used.* Leaves, root and flowers. The leaves are picked in August, when the flowers are just coming into bloom. They should be stripped off singly and gathered only on a fine day, in the morning, after the dew has been dried off by the sun.

¶ *Constituents.* Marsh Mallow contains starch, mucilage, pectin, oil, sugar, asparagin, phosphate of lime, glutinous matter and cellulose.

¶ *Medicinal Action and Uses.* The great demulcent and emollient properties of Marsh Mallow make it useful in inflammation and irritation of the alimentary canal, and of the urinary and respiratory organs. The dry roots boiled in water give out half their weight of a gummy matter like starch. Decoctions of the plant, especially of the root, are very useful where the natural mucus has been abraded from the coats of the intestines, The decoction can be made by adding 5 pints of water to ¼ lb. of dried root, boiling down to 3 pints and straining: it should not be made too thick and viscid. It is excellent in painful complaints of the urinary organs, exerting a relaxing effect upon the passages, as well as acting curatively. This decoction is also effective in curing bruises, sprains or any ache in the muscles or sinews. In hæmorrhage from the urinary organs and in dysentery, it has been recommended to use the powdered root boiled in milk. The action of Marsh Mallow root upon the bowels is unaccompanied by any astringency.

Boiled in wine or milk, Marsh Mallow will relieve diseases of the chest, constituting a popular remedy for coughs, bronchitis, whooping-cough, etc., generally in combination with other remedies. It is frequently given in the form of a syrup, which is best adapted to infants and children.

RECIPES
Marsh Mallow Water

'Soak one ounce of marsh mallow roots in a little cold water for half an hour; peel off the bark, or skin; cut up the roots into small shavings, and put them into a jug to stand for a couple of hours; the decoction must be drunk tepid, and may be sweetened with honey or sugar-candy, and flavoured with orange-flower water, or with orange-juice. Marshmallow water may be used with good effect in all cases of inveterate coughs, catarrhs, etc.' (Francatelli's *Cook's Guide*.)

For Gravel, etc.

'Put the flower and plant (all but the root) of Marsh Mallows in a jug, pour boiling water, cover with a cloth, let it stand three hours – make it strong. If used for gravel or irritation of the kidney, take ½ pint as a Tea daily for four days, then stop a few days, then go on again. A teaspoonful of gin may be added *when there is no tendency to inflammation.*' (From a family recipe-book.)

The powdered or crushed fresh roots make a good poultice that will remove the most obstinate inflammation and prevent mortification. Its efficacy in this direction has earned for it the name of Mortification Root. Slippery Elm may be added with advantage, and the poultice should be applied to the part as hot as can be borne and renewed when dry. An infusion of 1 oz. of leaves to a pint of boiling water is also taken frequently in wineglassful doses. This infusion is good for bathing inflamed eyes.

An ointment made from Marsh Mallow has also a popular reputation, but it is stated that a poultice made of the fresh root, with the addition of a little white bread, proves more serviceable when applied externally than the ointment. The fresh leaves, steeped in hot water and applied to the affected parts as poultices, also reduce inflammation, and bruised and rubbed upon any place stung by wasps or bees take away the pain, inflammation and swelling. Pliny stated that the green leaves, beaten with nitre and applied, drew out thorns and prickles in the flesh.

The flowers, boiled in oil and water, with a little honey and alum, have proved good as a gargle for sore throats. In France, they form one of the ingredients of the *Tisane de quatre fleurs*, a pleasant remedy for colds.

¶ *Preparations and Dosage.* Fluid extract leaves, ½ to 2 drachms.

MALLOW, BLUE

Malva sylvestris (LINN.)

Synonym. Common Mallow
Parts Used. Flowers, leaves

The Common or Blue Mallow is a robust plant 3 or 4 feet high, growing freely in field, hedgerows and on waste ground. Its stem is round, thick and strong, the leaves stalked, roundish, five to seven lobed, downy, with stellate hairs and the veins prominent on the underside. The flowers are showy, bright mauve-purple, with dark veins. When they first expand in June, the plant is handsome, but as the summer advances, the leaves lose their deep green colour and the stems assume a ragged appearance.

Cattle do not appear to be fond of this plant, every part of which abounds with a mild mucilage.

¶ *Medicinal Action and Uses.* The use of this species of Mallow has been much superseded by Marsh Mallow, which possesses its valuable properties in a superior degree, but it is still a favourite remedy with country people where Marsh Mallow is not obtainable. The roots are not considered of much value compared with those of the Marsh Mallow, and as a rule the leaves and flowers are used only, mainly externally in fomentations and poultices. The infusion has been a popular remedy for coughs and colds, but the internal use of the leaves has fallen into disuse, giving place to Marsh Mallow root, though they are still employed as a decoction for injection, which, made strong, cures strangury and gravel.

The foliage when boiled, forms a wholesome vegetable. The seeds, or 'cheeses,' are also edible.

A tincture of the flowers, which turn blue in fading, forms a very delicate test for alkalis.

The flowers were used formerly on May Day by country people for strewing before their doors and weaving into garlands.

¶ *Preparation and Dosage.* Fluid extract, $\frac{1}{2}$ to 2 drachms.

MALLOW, MUSK

Malva meschata

Parts Used. Leaves, root, flowers

The Musk Mallow is not an uncommon plant in dry pastures and in hedgerows. It grows 2 feet high, with round, thick, erect stems, somewhat hairy, often purple-spotted. The foliage is light-green, the lower leaves kidney-shaped, five to seven lobed, those on the stem finely divided into numerous narrow segments. The handsome rose-coloured flowers are three times the size of the Common Mallow, crowded towards the summit of the stem. It emits from its leaves a faint, musky odour, especially in warm weather, or when drawn through the hand.

This Mallow is not common in Kent and other counties, but in Essex it is very abundant.

The root is white and is the part used. It has the same virtues as the Common Mallow, but is not quite as strong, and the leaves have similar properties.

MALLOW, DWARF

Malva rotundifolia

Part Used. Leaves

Habitat. The Dwarf Mallow is self-fertilizing, while the other kinds are insect-visited. It is common in most parts of Europe, including Britain, and in Western Asia. In Egypt, especially upon the banks of the Nile, it is extensively cultivated and used by the natives as a pot-herb

The Dwarf Mallow, a smaller variety than any of the other wild Mallows, is easily distinguishable by its prostrate stems and pale lilac flowers. Its leaves are heart-shaped and have also sometimes been used medicinally.

MALLOW, TREE SEA

Lavatera arborea

Part Used. Herb

The velvety leaves of the Sea Tree Mallow, a tall, handsome plant growing 5 or 6 feet high, on sea cliffs, on many parts of the coast, are used for sprains, steeped in hot water and laid on the injured spot.

See HOLLYHOCK.

MANACA

Brunfelsia hopeana (HOOK.)
N.O. Solanaceæ

Synonyms. Vegetable Mercury. Franciscea uniflora
Parts Used. Root, stem
Habitat. South America, West Indies, Brazil

¶ *Description.* Small trees, a name often given to the genus *Solanaceæ*, in honour of Brunfels, the German herbalist of the sixteenth century. The genus is known by a five-cleft calyx with rounded lobes, bilabiate in æstivation, four fertile and anthers confluent at the top, where it is divided into two stigmatic lobes, capsules fleshy or leathery, more rarely indehiscent and drupe-like, several large seeds embedded in pulp. Flowers large and some very fragrant, blue or white. In commerce the pieces of root vary from a few inches to 1 foot long, $\frac{1}{2}$ inch in diameter, very tough and woody, centre yellow, with a very thin outer bark; the stem has a small yellow pith.

¶ *Constituents*. Alkaloid Mannacine and a peculiar substance fluorescent and supposed to be identical with gelseminic acid.

¶ *Medicinal Action and Uses*. From experiments made on animals, Manaca acts on the spinal cord, stimulating, then abolishing the activities of the motor centres; stimulating specially the kidneys and all the other glands. In large doses it causes lassitude, perspiration and loose greenish discharges. It is highly recommended in the treatment of syphilis and chronic rheumatism of an arthritic nature.

¶ *Dosage*. Fluid extract, 10 to 30 minims three times daily.

¶ *Other Species*. *Franciscea uniflora* is the Brazilian name for Manaca, largely used for syphilitic complaints; root and leaves of this are used. It is a bitter purgative emetic, and in large doses poisonous.

MANDIOCA

Manihot utilissima
N.O. Euphorbiaceæ

Synonyms. Manioc. Yuca. Cassava. Farinha de Mandioca

Another food plant of enormous importance to tropical America in the present as well as in the past is *Manihot utilissima*, otherwise known as Manioc, Mandioca, or Yuca, from the tuberous root of which Cassava is prepared. It was, in fact, the plant of chief economic importance to the tribes of tropical South America east of the Andes, and its cultivation spread to the valley of Colombia, the Isthmus of Panama, and the West Indian Islands. Mandioca is a shrubby plant, with brittle stems, 6 feet to 8 feet high, large palmate leaves and green flowers. In the ordinary variety the tubers weigh up to 30 lb., and the juice, owing to the presence of hydrocyanic acid, is poisonous. A smaller nonpoisonous variety is also found.

The true native method of preparing it for food, followed with slight variation throughout the Southern Continent and islands, is as follows: The root is sliced, and grated on a board set with small stones, washed in water, and packed into a long cylindrical 'press' of basketwork with a loop at either end. This press is so made that when it is suspended by one loop and a weight applied to the other, it increases in length and decreases in diameter, and the juice is squeezed from the contents, and falls into a vessel placed below. The paste is then spread in thin layers on griddles of pottery or slate and cooked over a fire. The root is also eaten roasted, especially the sweet variety, though even in the case of the poisonous tuber, the unwholesome element is volatized by cooking. For this reason the juice is preserved and boiled, when it becomes wholesome, and is used as liquor for soup. If further inspissated by boiling, and sweetened in the sun, it is known as casareep, and is employed as a flavouring, especially in British Guiana, where it appears in almost every dish, and in the West Indies, where it is the foundation of the celebrated pepper pot. Casareep is highly antiseptic, and by its aid meat can be kept fresh for quite a long time.

An intoxicating drink can also be prepared from the Mandioca; the early West Indians fermented the sliced and grated tuber in water, adding a little chewed root or grated batata to assist the process. In British Guiana and North Brazil a similar process is still used; the chewed root is fermented in large wooden troughs of water, and the liquor is stored in gourds. At the present time Cassava flour, or *farinha de Mandioca*, is an important article of food throughout South America, and could be used much more extensively in Europe. The true starch of the Mandioca is known to commerce as Brazilian arrowroot, and this, after heating on hot plates and stirring with an iron rod, becomes tapioca. The cultivation is not difficult, the plant is propagated by cuttings, and the produce is at least six times that of wheat.

Sweet Cassava is nourishing, light and agreeable as a food for invalids, and infants during weaning.

See TAPIOCA.

MANDRAKE

Atropa mandragora
N.O. Solanaceæ

Synonyms. Mandragora. Satan's Apple
Part Used. Herb
Habitat. The Mandrake, the object of so many strange superstitions, is a native of Southern Europe and the Levant, but will grow here in gardens if given a warm situation, though otherwise it may not survive severe winters. It was cultivated in England in 1562 by Turner, the author of the *Niewe Herball*

The name *Mandragora* is derived from two Greek words implying 'hurtful to cattle.' The Arabs call it 'Satan's apple.'

¶ *Description*. It has a large, brown root, somewhat like a parsnip, running 3 or 4 feet deep into the ground, sometimes single and sometimes divided into two or three branches. Immediately from the crown of the root arise several large, dark-green leaves, which at first stand erect, but when grown to full size – a foot or more in length and 4 or 5 inches in width – spread open and lie upon the ground. They are sharp pointed at the apex and of a fœtid odour. From among these leaves spring the flowers, each on a separate foot-stalk, 3 or 4 inches high. They are somewhat of the shape and size of a primrose, the corolla bell-shaped, cut into five spreading segments, of a whitish colour, somewhat tinged with purple. They are succeeded by a smooth, round fruit, about as large as a small apple, of a deep yellow colour when ripe, full of pulp and with a strong, apple-like scent.

¶ *Medicinal Action and Uses.* The leaves are quite harmless and cooling, and have been used for ointments and other external application. Boiled in milk and used as a poultice, they were employed by Boerhaave as an application to indolent ulcers.

The fresh root operates very powerfully as an emetic and purgative. The dried bark of the root was used also as a rough emetic.

Mandrake was much used by the Ancients, who considered it an anodyne and soporific. In large doses it is said to excite delirium and madness. They used it for procuring rest and sleep in continued pain, also in melancholy, convulsions, rheumatic pains and scrofulous tumours. They mostly employed the bark of the root, either expressing the juice or infusing it in wine or water. The root finely scraped into a pulp and mixed with brandy was said to be efficacious in chronic rheumatism.

Mandrake was used in Pliny's days as an anæsthetic for operations, a piece of the root being given to the patient to chew before undergoing the operation. In small doses it was employed by the Ancients in maniacal cases.

A tincture is used in homœopathy to-day, made from the fresh plant.

Among the old Anglo-Saxon herbals both Mandrake and periwinkle are endowed with mysterious powers against demoniacal possession. At the end of a description of the Mandrake in the *Herbarium of Apuleius* there is this prescription:

'For witlessness, that is devil sickness or demoniacal possession, take from the body of this said wort mandrake by the weight of three pennies, administer to drink in warm water as he may find most convenient – soon he will be healed.'

Bartholomew gives the old Mandrake legend in full, though he adds: 'It is so feynd of churles others of wytches.' He also refers to its use as an anæsthetic:

'the rind thereof medled with wine . . . gene to them to drink that shall be cut in their body, for they should slepe and not fele the sore knitting.'

Bartholomew gives two other beliefs about the Mandrake which are not found in any other English Herbal – namely, that while uprooting it the digger must beware of contrary winds, and that he must go on digging for it until sunset.

In the *Grete Herball* (printed by Peter Treveris in 1526) we find the first avowal of disbelief in the supposed powers of the Mandrake. Gerard also pours scorn on the Mandrake legend.

'There have been,' he says, 'many ridiculous tales brought up of this plant, whether of old wives or runnegate surgeons, or phisick mongers, I know not, all which dreames and old wives tales you shall from henceforth cast out your bookes of memorie.'

Parkinson says that if ivory is boiled with Mandrake root for six hours, the ivory will become so soft 'that it will take what form or impression you will give it.'

Josephus says that the Mandrake – which he calls *Baaras* – has but one virtue, that of expelling demons from sick persons, as the demons cannot bear either its smell or its presence. He even relates that it was certain death to touch this plant, except under certain circumstances which he details. (*Wars of the Jews*, book vii, cap. vi.)

The roots of the Mandrake are very nearly allied to Belladonna, both in external appearance and in structure. The plant is by modern botanists assigned to the same genus, though formerly was known as *Mandragora officinalis*, with varieties *M. vernalis* and *M. autumnalis*. According to Southall (*Organic Materia Medica*, 8th edition, revised by Ernest Mann, 1915), the root

'contains a mydriatic alkaloid, Mandragorine ($C_{17}H_{27}O_3N$), which in spite of the name and formula which have been assigned to it, is probably identical with atropine or hyoscyamine.'

The roots of Mandrake were supposed to bear a resemblance to the human form, on account of their habit of forking into two and shooting on each side. In the old Herbals we find them frequently figured as a male with a long beard, and a female with a very bushy head of hair. Many weird superstitions collected round the Mandrake root. As an amulet, it was once placed on mantelpieces to avert misfortune and to bring prosperity and happiness to the house. Bryony roots were often cut into fancy shapes and passed off as Mandrake, being even trained to grow in moulds till they assumed the desired forms. In Henry VIII's time quaint little images made from Bryony roots, cut into the figure of a man, with grains of millet inserted into the face as eyes, fetched high prices. They were known as *puppettes* or *mammettes*, and were accredited with magical powers. Italian ladies were known to pay as much as thirty golden ducats for similar artificial Mandrakes.

Turner alludes to these 'puppettes and mammettes,' and says, 'they are so trymmed of crafty theves to mocke the poore people withall and to rob them both of theyr wit and theyr money.' But he adds:

'Of the apples of mandrake, if a man smell of them thei will make hym slepe and also if they be eaten. But they that smell to muche of the apples become dum . . . thys herbe diverse wayes taken is very jepardus for a man and may kill hym if he eat it or drynk it out of measure and have no remedy from it. . . . If mandragora be taken out of measure, by and by slepe ensueth and a great lousing of the streyngthe with a forgetfulness.'

The plant was fabled to grow under the gallows of murderers, and it was believed to be death to dig up the root, which was said to utter a shriek and terrible groans on being dug up, which none might hear and live. It was held, therefore, that he who would take up a plant of Mandrake should tie a dog to it for that purpose, who drawing it out would certainly perish, as the man would have done, had he attempted to dig it up in the ordinary manner.

There are many allusions to the Mandrake in ancient writers. From the earliest times a notion prevailed in the East that the Mandrake will remove sterility, and there is a reference to this belief in Genesis xxx. 14.

¶ *Cultivation.* Mandrake can be propagated by seeds, sown upon a bed of light earth, soon after they are ripe, when they are more sure to come up than if the sowing is left to the spring.

When the plants come up in the spring, they must be kept well watered through the summer and kept free from weeds. At the end of August they should be taken up carefully and transplanted where they are to remain. The soil should be light and deep, as the roots run far down – if too wet, they will rot in winter, if too near chalk or gravel, they will make little progress. Where the soil is good and they are not disturbed, these plants will grow to a large size in a few years, and will produce great quantities of flowers and fruit.

Culpepper tells us the Mandrake is governed by Mercury. The fruit has been accounted poisonous, but without cause. . . . The root formerly was supposed to have the human form, but it really resembles a carrot or parsnip.

See BELLADONNA.

MANDRAKE, AMERICAN

Podophyllum peltatum (LINN.)
N.O. Berberidaceæ

Synonyms. May Apple. Wild Lemon. Racoonberry. Duck's Foot. Hog Apple
Parts Used. Root, resin
Habitat. The American Mandrake is a small herb with a long, perennial, creeping rhizome, a native of many parts of North America, common in the eastern United States and Canada, growing there profusely in wet meadows and in damp, open woods

¶ *Description.* The root is composed of many thick tubers, fastened together by fleshy fibres which spread greatly underground, sending out many smaller fibres at the joints, which strike downward. The stems are solitary, mostly unbranched, 1 to 2 feet high, crowned with two large, smooth leaves, stalked, peltate in the middle like an umbrella, of the size of a hand, composed of five to seven wedge-shaped divisions, somewhat lobed and toothed at the apex. Between their foot-stalks, grows a solitary, drooping white flower, about 2 inches across, appearing in May. The odour of the flower is nauseous. When it falls off, the fruit that develops swells to the size and shape of the common rosehip, being 1 to 2 inches long. It is yellow in colour and pulpy. In taste it is sweet, though slightly acid and is edible. The leaves and roots are poisonous. The foliage and stems have been used as a pot-herb, but in some cases with fatal results.

The drug was well known to the North American Indians as an emetic and vermifuge. It was included in the British Pharmacopœia in 1864.

The Latin name is derived from *pous, podos* (a foot) and *phyllon* (a leaf), alluding to a fanciful resemblance in the palmate leaf to the foot of some web-footed aquatic bird. Hence one of the popular names of the plant – Duck's Foot.

¶ *Cultivation.* It grows in warm, sheltered spots, such as partially shaded borders, woods, and marshes, liking a light, loamy soil. It requires no other culture than to be kept clear of weeds, and is so hardy as to be seldom injured by frost.

Propagate (1) by sowing seeds, in sandy soil, planting out in the following spring or autumn; (2) by division of roots. It propagates so fast by its creeping roots that this mode of propagation is preferred. Every part of the root will grow. Divide either in autumn, when the leaves decay, or in spring, just before the roots begin to shoot, preferably the latter.

¶ *Part Used.* The dried rhizome, from which a resin is also extracted.

It must be carefully distinguished from English Mandrake (*Bryonia dioica*), which is sometimes offered as Mandrake root.

¶ *Constituents.* A neutral crystalline substance, podo-phyllotoxin, and an amorphous resin, podophylloresin, both of which are purgative. It also contains picro-podo-phyllin, a yellow colouring matter, quercetin, sugar, starch, fat, etc.

It yields about 3 per cent. of ash on incinceration.

Podophyllum rhizome is said to be most active when it is beginning to shoot. It is used almost entirely in the form of podophyllum resin.

The resin is prepared by making a tincture of the rhizome, removing from this the greater part of the spirit by distillation and pouring the remaining liquor into water acidified with hydrochloric acid. By this means the resin is precipitated, and may be collected and dried.

¶ *Medicinal Action and Uses.* Antibilious, cathartic, hydragogue, purgative.

Podophyllum is a medicine of most extensive service; its greatest power lies in its action upon the liver and bowels. It is a gastro-intestinal irritant, a powerful hepatic and intestinal stimulant. In congested states of the liver, it is employed with the greatest benefit, and for all hepatic complaints it is eminently suitable, and the beneficial results can hardly be exaggerated.

In large doses it produces nausea and vomiting, and even inflammation of the stomach and intestines, which has been known to prove fatal. In moderate doses, it is a drastic purgative with some cholagogue action. Like many other hepatic stimulants, it does not increase the secretion of bile so much when it acts as a purgative.

Podophyllum is a powerful medicine, exercising an influence on every part of the system, stimulating the glands to healthy action. It is highly valuable in dropsy, biliousness, dyspepsia, liver and other disorders. Its most beneficial action is obtained by the use of small doses frequently given. In such circumstances, it acts admirably upon all the secretions, removing obstructions, and producing a healthy condition of all the organs in the system. In still smaller doses, it is a valuable remedy in skin diseases.

It may either be given in infusion, decoction, tincture or substance, but it is not to be given warm.

It is often employed in combination with other purgatives, such as colocynth, aloes or rhubarb, and also administered in pills, with extract of henbane or belladonna, to prevent griping.

Externally applied, the resin, of podophyllum acts as an irritant. If incautiously handled, it often produces conjunctivitis, and in America it has on this account, when dissolved in alcohol, been used as a counter-irritant.

¶ *Preparations and Dosages.* Powdered root, 5 to 30 grains. Fluid extract, 5 to 30 drops. Tincture root, 5 to 30 drops. Tincture resin, B.P., 5 to 15 drops. Solid extract, 1 to 5 grains. Podophyllum resin, $\frac{1}{4}$ to 1 grain.

¶ *Substitutes. Podophyllum Emodi* (Indian Podophyllum), a native of Northern India. The roots are much stouter, more knotty, and about twice as strong as the American. It is not identical with, nor should it be substituted for, the American rhizome. It contains twice as much podophyllotoxin, and in other respects exhibits differences. Indian podophyllum is official in India and the Eastern Colonies, where it is used in place of ordinary podophyllum.

MANNA. *See* ASH

MANZANILLO

Hippomane mancinella (LINN.)
N.O. Euphorbiaceæ

Synonym. Manchineel
Parts Used. Juice of berries, leaves, bark
Habitat. South America, West Indian Islands, Venezuela, Panama

¶ *Description.* A tree growing to a height of 40 to 50 feet, mostly on sandy seashores, said to be so poisonous that men die under the shade of it; leaves shiny green, stalked, elliptical edges cut like saw teeth, a single gland on upper side where the stalk and leaf join, very small inconspicuous flowers (of separate sexes) on long slender spikes, the few females placed singly at base of the spike with a three-parted calyx, the males in little clusters on the upper part with a two-parted calyx and two or four stamens joined by their filaments, the females with a many-celled ovary crowned with from four to eight styles and reflexed stigmas. Fruit a rounded, fleshy, yellow-green berry.

¶ *Constituents.* A milky, very acrid juice both in the bark and the berries.

¶ *Medicinal Action and Uses.* A violent irritant and powerful cathartic, diuretic, vesicant. The least drop applied to the eye will cause blindness for some days; the smoke from the wood when burnt will also seriously affect the eyes. Much used in Cuba for tetanus. Indians use the juice to poison their arrows.

¶ *Dosage.* 2 minims as a cathartic.

See EUPHORBIAS.

MAPLES
N.O. Aceraceæ

Habitat. The Maples, belonging to the genus *Acer*, natural order Aceraceæ, are for the most part trees, inhabitants of the temperate regions of the Northern Hemisphere, particularly North America, Northern India and Japan

¶ *Description.* The leaves are long-stalked, placed opposite to one another, and palmately lobed; the flowers, in fascicles appearing before the leaves as in the Norway Maple, or in racemes appearing with, or later than, the leaves as in the Sycamore Some of the flowers are often imperfect.

The dry fruit, termed a 'samara,' is composed of two one-seeded cells, furnished with wings, which divide when ripe, the winged seeds being borne by the wind to a considerable distance.

The leaves of the Maples commonly exhibit varnish-like smears, of sticky consistence, known as *honey-dew*. This is the excretion of the aphides which live on the leaves; the insect bores holes into the tissues, sucks their juices and ejects a drop of honey-dew, on an average once in half an hour. In passing under a tree infested with aphides the drops can be felt like a fine rain. The fluid is rich in sugar. When the dew falls, the honey-dew takes it up and spreads over the leaf; later in the day evaporation reduces it to the state of a varnish on the leaf surface, which aids in checking transpiration. Many other trees exhibit this phenomenon, e.g. lime, beech, oak, etc.

Most of the Maples yield a saccharine juice from the trunk, branches and leaves. The wood of almost all the species is useful for many purposes, especially to the cabinet-maker, the turner and the musical instrument-maker, and for the manufacture of alkali the Maples of North America are of great value.

Many species with finely-cut or variegated leaves have been introduced, especially from Japan, as ornamental shrubs, most of them remarkable for the coppery-purple tint that pervades the leaves and younger growths.

The Common Maple (*Acer campestre*, Linn.) is the only species indigenous to Great Britain. This and the Sycamore, or Great Maple, were described by Gerard in 1597, the latter as 'a stranger to England.'

MAPLE, COMMON
Acer campestre

Though a native tree, *Acer campestre* is not often seen growing freely for the sake of its timber, being chiefly looked upon as a valuable hedge-tree, and is therefore frequently found in hedgerows.

When growing alone it is a small tree, seldom attaining more than 20 feet, but the wood is compact, of a fine grain, sometimes beautifully veined and takes a high polish. For this reason, it is highly praised by the cabinet-maker and has always been used much for tables, also for inlaying, and is frequently employed for violin cases. The wood makes excellent fuel and affords very good charcoal.

The wood of the roots is often knotted and is valuable for small objects of cabinet-work.

The young shoots, being flexible and tough, are employed in France as whips.

Sap drawn from the trees in spring yields a certain amount of sugar.

MAPLE, BIRD'S EYE
Acer saccharinum (LINN.)

Acer saccharinum (Linn.), the Sugar or Bird's Eye Maple, is an American species, introduced into Britain in 1735.

It bears a considerable resemblance to the Norway Maple, especially when young, but is not so hardy here as our native Maple and requires a sheltered situation.

So far it has only been grown as an ornamental tree, the vivid colours of its foliage in winter ranging from bright orange to dark crimson. Sometimes it attains a height of 70, or even 100 feet, though more commonly it does not exceed 50 or 60 feet. It is remarkable for the whiteness of its bark.

Where the tree is plentiful in America, the timber is much used for fuel and is extensively employed for house-building and furniture, used instead of Oak when the latter is scarce, being also employed for axle-trees and spokes, as well as for Windsor chairs, shoe-lasts, etc. The wood is white, but acquires a rosy tinge after exposure to light. The grain is fine and close and when polished has a silky lustre.

The wood of old trees is valued for inlaying mahogany. The name 'Bird's Eye Maple' refers to the twisting of the silver grain, which produces numerous knots like the eyes of birds. Considerable quantities of this Maple are imported from Canada for cabinet-making.

The wood forms excellent *fuel* and *charcoal*, while the ashes are rich in alkaline principles, furnishing a large proportion of the potash exported from Boston and New York.

Large quantities of sugar are made from the sap of this species of Maple. The sap is boiled and the syrup when reduced to a proper consistence is run into moulds to form cakes. Trees growing in moist and low situations afford the most sap, though the least proportion of sugar.

The trees are tapped in early spring, just before the foliage develops, either by making a notch in the stem, about 3 feet from the ground, with an axe, or by boring a hole about 2 inches deep and introducing a spout of sumach or elder, through which the sap flows into a trough below. The sap is purified and concentrated in a simple manner, the whole work being carried on by farmers, who themselves use much of the product for domestic and culinary purposes.

A cold north-west wind with frosty nights and sunny days tends to incite the flow, which is more abundant during the day than during the night. The flow ceases during a south-west wind and at the approach of a storm, and so sensitive are the trees to aspect and climatic variations that the flow of sap on the south and east sides has been noticed to be earlier than on the north and west sides of the same tree.

The sap continues flowing for five or six weeks, according to the temperature. A tree of average size yields 15 to 30 gallons of sap in a season, 4 gallons of sap giving about 1 lb. of sugar. The tree is not at all injured by the tapping operation.

The quality of Maple Sugar is superior to that of West Indian cane sugar: it deposits less sediment when dissolved in water and has more the appearance of sugar candy.

The profits of the Sugar Maple do not arise from the sugar alone: it affords good molasses and excellent vinegar. The sap which is suitable for these purposes is obtained after that which supplies the sugar has ceased to flow.

MAPLE, GREAT

Acer pseudo-Platanus (Linn.), the Sycamore or Great Maple (the Plane-tree of the Scotch), grows wild in Switzerland, Germany, Austria and Italy. It is remarkably hardy and will grow with an erect stem, exposed to the highest winds or to the sea-breezes, which it withstands better than most timber trees, being often planted near farmhouses and cottages in exposed localities for the sake of its dense foliage.

¶ *Description.* It is a handsome tree, of quick growth, attaining a height of 50 or 60 feet in 50 years. Though not a native, it has been cultivated here for four or five centuries, and has become so naturalized that self-sown examples are common.

The timber was formerly much used by Acer pseudo-Platanus (LINN.) the turner for cups, bowls and pattern blocks; and is still in repute by the saddle-makers and the millwright, being soft, light and tough.

In spring and autumn, if the trunk is pierced, it yields an abundance of juice, from which a good wine has been made in the Highlands of Scotland. Sugar is to a certain extent procured from it by evaporation, but 1 ounce to 1 quart of sap is the largest amount of sugar obtainable.

The leaves may be dried and given to sheep in winter.

The lobed shape of its leaf and its dense foliage caused it to be confounded with the True Sycamore (*Ficus sycamorus*) of Scripture.

MAPLE, NORWAY

Acer Platanoides, the Norway Maple, grows on the mountains of the northern countries of Europe, descending in some parts of Norway to the seashore. It abounds Acer Platanoides in the north of Poland and Lithuania, and is common through Germany, Switzerland, and Savoy.

It was introduced into Great Britain in

1683. It is a quick grower and on a tolerable soil it attains a large size (from 40 to 70 feet).

¶ *Description.* The leaves are smooth and of a shining green, as large or larger than those of the Sycamore, and are seldom eaten or defaced, because the tree is full of a sharp, milky juice disliked by insects. In the spring, when the flowers, which are of a fine yellow colour, are out, this tree has great beauty.

The wood is used for the same purposes as that of the Sycamore.

Sugar has been made from the sap in Norway and Sweden.

MAPLE, RED

Acer rubrum (LINN.)

Synonyms. Swamp Maple. Curled Maple

Acer rubrum (Linn.), the Red or Swamp Maple, is another American species, a middle-sized tree, introduced here in 1656, but so far only cultivated in England as an ornamental tree, for the sake of its striking bright scarlet flowers, which appear before the leaves in March and April, its red fruit and leaves rendering it very attractive also in autumn.

The wood is applicable to many purposes, such as the seats of Windsor chairs, turnery, etc. The grain of very old trees is sometimes undulated, which has suggested the name of 'Curled Maple': this gives beautiful effects of light and shade on polished surfaces.

The most constant use of Curled Maple is for the stocks of fowling pieces and rifles, as it affords toughness and strength, combined with lightness and elegance, but on the whole the wood is considered inferior to that of the Bird's Eye Maple, both in strength and as fuel.

Sugar has been made from the sap by the French Canadians, and also molasses, but the yield is only half as great as that from the Sugar Maple.

The inner bark is dusky red: on boiling, it yields a purple colour, which with sulphate of lead affords a black dye. It makes a good black ink.

¶ *Medicinal Action and Uses.* The bark has astringent properties and has been used medicinally as an application for sore eyes, a use which the early settlers learnt from the Red Indians.

It occurs in long quilled pieces 6 to 12 inches or more in length, $\frac{1}{4}$ to $\frac{3}{4}$ inch wide, externally blackish brown, slightly polished, with innumerable fine transverse lines and scattered, brownish, warts. The inner bark is in very tough and fibrous layers, pale reddish brown or buff. The bark has an astringent and slightly bitter taste.

The CHINESE SUGAR MAPLE is *Sorghum saccharatum* (known also as *Andropogon arundinaceus,* var. *saccharatus*), a cane-like plant containing sugary sap, belonging to the Grass family Graminaceæ.

It somewhat resembles Indian corn, or maize, from which it is distinguished by producing large heads of small grains.

It is cultivated in the United States to some extent as a forage crop, but is not used in the manufacture of sugar, owing to the difficulty of effecting its crystallization.

MARE'S TAIL

Hippuris vulgaris (LINN.)
N.O. Haloragaceæ

Synonyms. Female Horsetail. Marsh Barren Horsetail

The Mare's Tail (*Hippuris vulgaris*) must not be confused with the Horsetail (*Equisetum arvense*). The Mare's Tail is an aquatic flowering plant, the only British species of a group of plants found growing nearly all over Europe, Russia, Central Asia, and North America. It has a superficial resemblance to the Horsetails, having the same erect, many-jointed stems about as thick as a goosequill, unbranched, except at the base, and tapering to a point, crowded *in* the whole length by whorls of eight to twelve very narrow leaves $\frac{1}{2}$ to $1\frac{1}{3}$ inch long, closely set with hard tips.

The inconspicuous flowers are sessile, i.e. stalkless, in the axils of the upper leaves and consist of a minute calyx, forming an indistinctly two-lobed rim to the ovary, a solitary stamen, with red anthers and a single seed. Some of the flowers are often without stamens. They appear in June and July.

In stagnant water the plant grows erect, in running water it bends with the stream, swimming on the surface. The stems are as a rule about 2 feet long.

Culpepper, in common with the older herbalists, considered it of great value as a vulnerary:

'It is very powerful to stop bleeding, either inward or outward, the juice or the decoction being drunk, or the juice, decoction or distilled water applied outwardly. . . . It also heals inward ulcers. . . . It solders together the tops of green wounds and cures all ruptures in children. The decoction taken in wine helps stone and strangury; the distilled water drunk two or three times a day eases and strengthens the intestines and is effectual in a cough that comes by distillation from the head. The juice or distilled water used as a warm fomentation is of service in inflammations and breakings-out in the skin.'

The Mare's Tail is not uncommon in shallow ponds, the margins of lakes, etc. where there is a depth of mud and frost cannot reach the roots, which are stout and creeping. When the water is shallow, the upper part of the stem is stout and projects out of the water to a height of 8 inches to a foot or more. The submerged leaves, when the plant grows in deep streams, are often 2 to 3 inches long, paler and broader than those above water.

In some countries it is a troublesome weed in rivers and chokes up the ditches. It has been supposed to assist in purifying the putrid air of marshes by absorbing a great quantity of marsh gas. Goats are said to eat it, and in the north wild ducks to feed on it.

Gerard calls the plant Female Horsetail, and Parkinson Marsh Barren Horsetail. The name, *Hippuris*, is the Greek word for Mare's Tail.

See (WATER) MILFOIL.

MARIGOLD

Calendula officinalis (LINN.)
N.O. Compositæ

Synonyms. Caltha officinalis. Golds. Ruddes. Mary Gowles. Oculus Christi. Pot Marigold. Marygold. Fiore d'ogni mese. Solis Sponsa

Parts Used. Flowers, herb, leaves

The Common Marigold is familiar to everyone, with its pale-green leaves and golden orange flowers. It is said to be in bloom on the calends of every month, hence its Latin name, and one of the names by which it is known in Italy – *fiore d'ogni mese* – countenances this derivation. It was not named after the Virgin, its name being a corruption of the Anglo-Saxon *merso-meargealla*, the Marsh Marigold. Old English authors called it Golds or Ruddes. It was, however, later associated with the Virgin Mary, and in the seventeenth century with Queen Mary.

¶ *History*. It was well known to the old herbalists as a garden-flower and for use in cookery and medicine. Dodoens-Lyte (*A Niewe Herball*, 1578) says:

'It hath pleasant, bright and shining yellow flowers, the which do close at the setting downe of the sunne, and do spread and open againe at the sunne rising.'

Linnæus assigned a narrower limit to the expansion of its flowers, observing that they are open from nine in the morning till three in the afternoon. This regular expansion and closing of the flowers attracted early notice, and hence the plant acquired the names of *solsequia* and *solis sponsa*. There is an allusion to this peculiarity in the poems of Rowley:

'The Mary-budde that shooteth (shutteth) with the light.'

And in the *Winter's Tale*:

'The Marigold that goes to bed wi' th' sun, And with him rises weeping.'

It has been cultivated in the kitchen garden for the flowers, which are dried for broth, and said to comfort the heart and spirits.

Fuller writes: 'We all know the many and sovereign virtues in your leaves, the Herbe Generalle in all pottage.' (*Antheologie*, 1655.) Stevens, in *Maison Rustique, or the Countrie Farme* (1699), mentions the Marigold as a specific for headache, jaundice, red eyes, toothache and ague. The dried flowers are still used among the peasantry 'to strengthen and comfort the hart.' He says further:

'Conserve made of the flowers and sugar, taken in the morning fasting, cureth the trembling of the harte, and is also given in the time of plague or pestilence. The yellow leaves of the flowers are dried and kept throughout Dutchland against winter to put into broths, physicall potions and for divers other purposes, in such quantity that in some Grocers or Spicesellers are to be found barrels filled with them and retailed by the penny or less, insomuch that no broths are well made without dried Marigold.'

Formerly its flowers were used to give cheese a yellow colour.

In Macer's *Herbal* it is stated that only to look on Marigolds will draw evil humours out of the head and strengthen the eyesight.

'Golde [Marigold] is bitter in savour
Fayr and zelw [yellow] is his flowur
Ye golde flour is good to sene
It makyth ye syth bryth and clene
Wyscely to lokyn on his flowres
Drawyth owt of ye heed wikked hirores [humours].

. . . .

Loke wyscely on golde erly at morwe [morning]
Yat day fro feures it schall ye borwe:
Ye odour of ye golde is good to smelle.'

'It must be taken only when the moon is in the Sign of the Virgin and not when Jupiter is in the ascendant, for then the herb loses its virtue. And the gatherer, who must be out of deadly sin, must say three Pater Nosters and three Aves. It will give the wearer a vision of anyone who has robbed him.'

From Eleanour Sinclair Rohde's *Old English Herbals:*

'Of marygold we learn that Summe use to make theyr here yelow with the floure of this herbe, not beyng contēt with the naturall colour which God hath geven thē.'

Gerard speaks of:

'The fruitful or much-bearing marigold, . . . is likewise called Jackanapes-on-horsebacke: it hath leaves stalkes and roots like the common sort of marigold, differing in the shape of his floures; for this plant doth bring forth at the top of the stalke one floure like the other marigolds, from which start forth sundry other small floures, yellow likewise and of the same fashion as the first; which if I be not deceived commeth to pass per accidens, or by chance, as Nature often times liketh to play with other flowers; or as children are borne with two thumbes on one hande or such like; which living to be men do get children like unto others: even so is the seed of this Marigold, which if it be sowen it brings forth not one floure in a thousand like the plant from whence it was taken.'

Culpepper says it is a

'herb of the Sun, and under Leo. They strengthen the heart exceedingly, and are very expulsive, and a little less effectual in the smallpox and measles than saffron. The juice of Marigold leaves mixed with vinegar, and any hot swelling bathed with it, instantly gives ease, and assuages it. The flowers, either green or dried, are much used in possets, broths, and drink, as a comforter of the heart and spirits, and to expel any malignant or pestilential quality which might annoy them. A plaister made with the dry flowers in powder, hog's-grease, turpentine, and rosin, applied to the breast, strengthens and succours the heart infinitely in fevers, whether pestilential or not.'

¶ *Cultivation.* The Marigold is a native of south Europe, but perfectly hardy in this country, and easy to grow. Seeds sown in April, in any soil, in sunny, or half-sunny places germinate freely. They require no other cultivation but to keep them clean from weeds and to thin out where too close, leaving them 9 to 10 inches apart, so that their branches may have room to spread. The plants will begin to flower in June, and continue flowering until the frost kills them. They will increase from year to year, if allowed to seed themselves. The seeds ripen in August and September, and if permitted to scatter will furnish a supply of young plants in the spring.

Only the common deep orange-flowered variety is of medinical value.

¶ *Parts Used.* The flowers and leaves. *Leaves.* – Gather only in fine weather, in the morning, after the dew has been dried by the sun. *Flowers.* – The ray florets are used and need quick drying in the shade, in a good current of warm air, spread out on sheets of paper, loosely, without touching each other, or they will become discoloured.

¶ *Medicinal Action and Uses.* Marigold is chiefly used as a local remedy. Its action is stimulant and diaphoretic. Given internally, it assists local action and prevents suppuration. The infusion of 1 ounce to a pint of boiling water is given internally, in doses of a tablespoonful, and externally as a local application. It is useful in chronic ulcer, varicose veins, etc. Was considered formerly to have much value as an aperient and detergent in visceral obstructions and jaundice.

It has been asserted that a Marigold flower, rubbed on the affected part, is an admirable remedy for the pain and swelling caused by the sting of a wasp or bee. A lotion made from the flowers is most useful for sprains and wounds, and a water distilled from them is good for inflamed and sore eyes.

An infusion of the freshly-gathered flowers is employed in fevers, as it gently promotes perspiration and throws out any eruption – a decoction of the flowers is much in use in country districts to bring out smallpox and measles, in the same manner as Saffron. Marigold flowers are in demand for children's ailments.

The leaves when chewed at first communicate a viscid sweetness, followed by a strong penetrating taste, of a saline nature. The expressed juice, which contains the greater part of this pungent matter, has been given in cases of costiveness and proved very efficacious. Snuffed up the nose it excites sneezing and a discharge of mucous from the head.

The leaves, eaten as a salad, have been considered useful in the scrofula of children, and the acrid qualities of the plant have caused it to be recommended as an extirpator of warts.

A yellow dye has also been extracted from the flower, by boiling.

¶ *Preparations and Dosage.* Fluid extract, ¼ to 1 drachm. Tincture of Calendula,

MARIGOLD, BUR. *See* (WATER) AGRIMONY

MARIGOLD, MARSH

Caltha palustris (LINN.)
N.O. Ranunculaceæ

Synonyms. Kingcups. Water Blobs. Horse Blobs. Bull's Eyes. Leopard's Foot. Meadow Routs. Verrucaria. Solsequia. Sponsa solis
Parts Used. Whole plant, buds, leaves

The Marsh Marigold, a showy dark-green plant resembling a gigantic buttercup, is abundant in marshes, wet meadows, and by the side of streams, where it forms large tufts or masses.

¶ *Description.* It is a herbaceous perennial. The stems are about a foot in height, hollow, nearly round, erect, but at times creeping and rooting at intervals in the lower portions, which are generally of a purple colour.

Most of the leaves spring directly from the ground, on long stalks, kidney-shaped, large and glossy. The stem-leaves have very short stalks and are more pointed at the top.

It flowers from mid-March till the middle of June, the flowers being at the end of the stems, which divide into two grooved flower-stalks, each bearing one blossom, from 1 to 2 inches in diameter. The Marsh Marigold is closely allied to various species of buttercups, but the flower has no real corolla, the brilliant yellow cup being composed of the five petaloid sepals.

The generic name is derived from the Greek *calathos* (a cup or goblet), from the shape of its flowers; the specific name from the Latin *palus* (a marsh), in reference to its place of growth.

The English name Marigold refers to its use in church festivals in the Middle Ages, as one of the flowers devoted to the Virgin Mary. It was also used on May Day festivals, being strewn before cottage doors and made into garlands.

Shakespeare refers several times to the flower, 'Winking Marybuds begin to ope their golden eyes.'

It has been called *Verrucaria* because it is efficacious in curing warts; also *Solsequia* and *Sponsa solis* because the flower opens at the rising of the sun and closes at its setting.

¶ *Medicinal Action and Uses.* Every part of the plant is strongly irritant, and cases are on record of serious effects produced by rashly experimenting with it. Dr. Withering says:

'It would appear that medicinal properties may be evolved in the gaseous exhalations of plants and flowers, for on a large quantity of the flowers of Meadow Routs being put into the bedroom of a girl who had been subject to fits, the fits ceased.'

An infusion of the flowers was afterwards successfully used in various kinds of fits, both of children and adults.

A tincture made from the whole plant when in flower may be given in cases of anæmia, in small, well-diluted doses.

The buds have occasionally been used as capers, but rather inadvisedly; the soaking in vinegar may, however, somewhat remove the acid and poisonous character of the buds in their fresh state.

The leaves can be cooked and eaten like spinach.

The juice of the petals, boiled with a little alum, stains paper yellow, but the colour so produced is said not to be permanent.

¶ *Cultivation.* The Marsh Marigold is propagated by parting the roots in autumn. It should be planted in a moist soil and a shady situation. A double variety is cultivated in gardens.

See BUTTERCUP.

MARJORAM, SWEET

Origanum marjorana (LINN.)
N.O. Labiatæ

Synonyms. Knotted Marjoram. Marjorana hortensis
Parts Used. Herb, leaves

Sweet or Knotted Marjoram is not an annual, but is usually treated as such, as the plants – native to Portugal – will not stand the winter elsewhere, so must be sown every year.

Seeds may be sown, for an early supply, in March, on a gentle hot-bed and again, in a warm position, in light soil, in the open ground during April. Plants do well if sown in April, though they are long in germinating. The seed is small and should be sown either

in drills, 9 inches apart, or broadcast, on the surface, trodden, raked evenly and watered in dry weather. On account of the slowness of germination, care should be taken that the seedlings are not choked with weeds, which being of much quicker growth are likely to do so if not destroyed. They should be removed by the hand, until the plants are large enough to use the small hoe with safety. Seed may also be sown early in May. In common with other aromatic herbs, such as Fennel, Basil, Dill, etc., it is not subject to the attacks of birds, as many other seeds are. When about an inch high, thin out to 6 or 8 inches apart each way. It begins to flower in July, when it is cut for use, and obtains its name of Knotted Marjoram from the flowers being collected into roundish close heads like knots.

Marjoram has been cultivated on a small scale at Sfax, Tunis, for a long time, and is called by the natives 'Khezama' (the Arab name for lavender).

Before the War, the herb was bought by agents and exported to Marseilles and other places. The plant is suitable to the sandy soil of the country.

The Marjoram plants are obtained either by division of clumps in winter, or from seeds planted in parallel lines 2 metres apart, between the almond and olive trees; and the soil, being of necessity worked for cultivation of the trees, this also serves to fertilize the Marjoram. One cutting of plant-clumps is best, a second one weakens it. The stems are cut about 10 cms. from the ground, dried in the sun on earth which has been previously beaten slightly. The leaves are separated from the stems by being beaten with staves; they are discoloured by the sun, broken and mixed with the débris of stems of which the odour is less strong.

Drying in the shade obtains more aromatic and less broken leaves, with less impurities.

¶ *Medicinal Action and Uses.* The medicinal qualities of the oil extracted from Sweet Marjoram – *Oleum majoranæ* – are similar to that of the Wild Marjoram. Fifteen ounces of the oil are yielded by 150 lb. of the fresh herb. On being kept, it assumes a solid form. It is used as an external application for sprains, bruises, etc., and also as an emmenagogue. In powdered form the herb forms part of certain Sneezing Powders.

¶ *Other Species.* In addition to the species just mentioned, others are cultivated in this country as ornamental plants, such as *O.*

Dictamnus, the Dittany of Crete, which has roundish leaves thickly invested with white down, and flowers in drooping spikes; and *O. sipyleum*, which is similar, but taller and less woolly. These last are popularly called Hop Plants, and are often seen in cottage windows.

Aromatic Herbaceous Seasoning

Take of nutmegs and mace 1 oz. each, of cloves and peppercorns 2 oz. of each, 1 oz. of dried bay-leaves, 3 oz. of basil, the same of Marjoram, 2 oz. of winter savoury, and 3 oz. of thyme, ½ oz. of cayenne pepper, the same of grated lemon-peel, and 2 cloves of garlic; all these ingredients must be well pulverized in a mortar, and sifted through a fine wire sieve, and put away in dry corked bottles for use.

The following is from Halliwell's *Popular Rhymes and Superstitions*:

'On St. Luke's Day, says Mother Bunch, take marigold flowers, a sprig of *marjoram*, thyme, and a little wormwood; dry them before a fire, rub them to powder, then sift it through a fine piece of lawn, and simmer it over a slow fire, adding a small quantity of virgin honey and vinegar. Anoint yourself with this when you go to bed, saying the following lines three times, and you will dream of your future partner "that is to be":

St. Luke, St. Luke, be kind to me,
In dreams let me my true love see.

If a girl desires to obtain this information, let her seek for a green peascod in which there are full 9 peas, and write on a piece of paper –

Come in, my dear,
And do not fear;

which paper she must enclose in the peascod, and lay it under the door. The first person who comes into the room will be her husband.'

Shakespeare may allude to this in *As You Like It* (ii. iv.) when he talks about the wooing of a peascod.

MARJORAM, WILD

Origanum vulgare (LINN.)
N.O. Labiatæ

Parts Used. Herb, oil

Habitat. Generally distributed over Asia, Europe and North Africa; grows freely in England, being particularly abundant in calcareous soils, as in the south-eastern counties

The name *Origanum* is derived from two Greek words, *oros* (mountain) and *ganos* (joy), in allusion to the gay appearance these plants give to the hillsides on which they grow.

¶ *Description.* It is a perennial herb, with creeping roots, sending up woody stems about a foot high, branched above, often purplish. The leaves are opposite, petiolate, about an inch long, nearly entire, hairy beneath. The flowers are in corymbs, with reddish bracts, a two-lipped pale purple corolla, and a five-toothed calyx, blooming from the end of June, through August. There is a variety with white flowers and light-green stalks, another with variegated leaves. It is propagated by division of roots in the autumn.

When cultivated, the leaves are more elliptical in shape than the Wild Marjoram, and the flower-spikes thinner and more compact. Marjoram has an extensive use for culinary purposes, as well as in medicine, but it is the cultivated species, *Origanum Onites* (Pot Marjoram), *O. Marjorana* (Sweet or Knotted Marjoram), and *O. Heracleoticum* (Winter Marjoram) that are employed in cookery as a seasoning. They are little used for medicinal purposes for which the Wild Marjoram is employed.

¶ *History*. Marjoram has a very ancient medical reputation. The Greeks used it extensively, both internally and externally for fomentations. It was a remedy for narcotic poisons, convulsions and dropsy. Among the Greeks, if Marjoram grew on a grave, it augured the happiness of the departed, and among both the Greeks and Romans, it was the custom to crown young couples with Marjoram.

Either *O. Onites* or *O. Majorana* is supposed to be the plant called 'Amaracus' by Greek writers.

The whole plant has a strong, peculiar, fragrant, balsamic odour and a warm, bitterish, aromatic taste, both of which properties are preserved when the herb is dry. It yields by distillation with water a small quantity of a volatile oil, which may be seen in vesicles, on holding up the leaves between the eye and the light, and which is the chief source of its properties as a medicinal agent. 1 lb. of the oil is produced from about 200 lb. of the herb, which should be gathered when just coming into flower, early in July. Large quantities of it are still gathered and hung up to dry in cottages in Kent and other counties for making Marjoram tea.

The 'swete margerome' was so much prized before the introduction of various foreign perfumes that, as Parkinson tells us, 'swete bags,' 'swete powders' and 'swete washing water' made from this plant were widely used. Our forefathers also scoured their furniture with its aromatic juices, and it is one of the herbs mentioned by Tusser (1577) as used for strewing chambers.

The flowering tops yield a dye, formerly used in the country to dye woollen cloth purple, and linen a reddish brown, but the tint is neither brilliant nor durable. The tops are also sometimes put into table beer, to give it an aromatic flavour and preserve it, and before the introduction of hops they were nearly as much in demand for ale-brewing as the ground ivy or wood sage. It is said that Marjoram and Wild Thyme, laid by milk in a dairy, will prevent it being turned by thunder.

Goat and sheep eat this herb, but horses are not fond of it, and cattle reject it.

¶ *Medicinal Action and Uses*. Marjoram yields about 2 per cent. of a volatile oil, which is separated by distillation. This must not be confused with oil of Origanum, which is extracted from Thyme. Its properties are stimulant, carminative, diaphoretic and mildly tonic; a useful emmenagogue. It is so acrid that it has been employed not only as a rubefacient, and often as a liniment, but has also been used as a caustic by farriers. A few drops, put on cotton-wool and placed in the hollow of an aching tooth frequently relieves the pain. In the commencement of measles, it is useful in producing a gentle perspiration and bringing out the eruption, being given in the form of a warm infusion, which is also valuable in spasms, colic, and to give relief from pain in dyspeptic complaints.

Externally, the dried leaves and tops may be applied in bags as a hot fomentation to painful swellings and rheumatism, as well as for colic. An infusion made from the fresh plant will relieve nervous headache, by virtue of the camphoraceous principle contained in the oil.

¶ *Cultivation*. The Marjorams are some of the most familiar of our kitchen herbs, and are cultivated for the use of their aromatic leaves, either in a green or dried state, for flavouring and other culinary purposes, being mainly put into stuffings. Sweet Marjoram leaves are also excellent in salads. They have whitish flowers, with a two-lipped calyx, and also contain a volatile oil, which has similar properties to the Wild Marjoram.

Winter Marjoram is really a native of Greece, but is hardy enough to thrive in the open air in England, in a dry soil, and is generally propagated by division of the roots in autumn.

Pot Marjoram, a native of Sicily, is also a hardy perennial, preferring a warm situation and dry, light soil. It is generally increased by cuttings, taken in early summer, inserted under a hand-glass, and later planted out a space of 1 foot between the rows and nearly as much from plant to plant, as it likes plenty of room. It may also be increased by division of roots in April, or by offsets, slipping pieces off the plants with roots to them and planting with trowel or dibber, taking care to water well. In May, they grow quickly after the operation. May also be propagated by seed, sown moderately thin, in dry, mild weather in March, in shallow drills, about $\frac{1}{2}$ inch deep and 8 or 9 inches apart, covered in evenly with the soil. Transplant afterwards to about a foot apart each way. The seeds are very slow in germinating.

MARSHMALLOW. *See* MALLOW

MASTERWORT

Imperatoria ostruthium (LINN.)
N.O. Umbelliferæ

Part Used. Root

Masterwort, though rare in the wild state, was formerly cultivated in this country for use as a pot-herb and in medicine. It is sometimes found in moist meadows in the north of England and in Scotland, but is generally regarded as naturalized, having originally been a garden escape. Its native habitat is Central Europe.

¶ *Description.* It is a smooth, perennial plant, the stout, furrowed stem growing 2 to 3 feet high. The dark-green leaves, which somewhat resemble those of Angelica, are on very long foot-stalks and are divided into three leaflets, each of which is often again sub-divided into three. The umbels of flowers are large and many-rayed, the corollas white; the fruit has very broad wings.

¶ *Medicinal Action and Uses.* Stimulant, antispasmodic, carminative; of use in asthma, dyspepsia, menstrual complaints.

The root, to quote Culpepper,

'is the hottest and sharpest part of the plant, hotter than pepper, and (in his opinion) very available in cold griefs and diseases both of the stomach and body.'

He tells us that it was also used 'in a decoction with wine against all cold rheums, distillations upon the lungs or shortness of breath,' and also states that it was considered effectual in dropsy, cramp, falling sickness, kidney and uterine troubles and gout. Also, that 'it is of a rare quality against all sorts of cold poison, to be taken as there is a cause; it provoketh sweat.'

'But,' he advises, 'lest the taste hereof or of the seed, should be too offensive, the best way is to take the water distilled both from the herb and root.'

¶ *Preparation.* Fluid extract, 1 to 2 drachms.

MASTIC

Pistacia Lentiscus (LINN.)
N.O. Anacardiaceæ

Synonyms. Mastich. Lentisk
Part Used. Resin

¶ *Description and Habitat.* A shrub rarely growing higher than 12 feet, much branched, and found freely scattered over the Mediterranean region, in Spain, Portugal, France, Greece, Turkey, the Canary Islands, and Tropical Africa. It has been cultivated in England since 1664. It is principally exported from Scio, on which island it has been cultivated for several centuries. The trees there are said to be entire male.

The best Mastic occurs in roundish tears about the size of a small pea, or in flattened, irregular pear-shaped, or oblong pieces covered with a whitish powder. They are pale yellow in colour, which darkens with age. The odour is agreeable and the taste mild and resinous, and when chewed it becomes soft, so that it can easily be masticated. This char-

acteristic enables it to be distinguished from a resin called Sanderach, which it resembles, but which when bitten breaks to powder.

¶ *Constituents.* Mastic contains a small proportion of volatile oil, 9 per cent. of resin soluble in alcohol and ether, and 10 per cent. of a resin insoluble in alcohol.

¶ *Medicinal Action and Properties.* Stimulant, diuretic. It has many of the properties of the coniferous turpentines and was formerly greatly used in medicine. Of late years it has chiefly been used for filling carious teeth, either alone or in spirituous solution, and for varnishes, and in the East in the manufacture of sweets and cordials.

In the East it is still used medicinally in the diarrhœa of children and masticated to sweeten the breath.

MATICO

Piper angustifolium (R. and P.)
N.O. Piperaceæ

Synonyms. Artanthe elongata. Stephensia elongata. Piper granulosum. Piper elongatum. Yerba soldado. Soldier's Herb. Thoho-thoho. Moho-moho
Part Used. The dried leaves
Habitat. Peru

The classical name for the genus came originally from the Sanscrit *pippali.* 'Matico' is the name of the Spanish soldier who accidentally discovered the properties of the leaves when wounded in Peru.

The plant has spread over many moist districts of tropical America, and though grown as a stove-plant in English botanical gardens it does not flower there. It is a shrub of about 8 feet high, with many branches thickened at

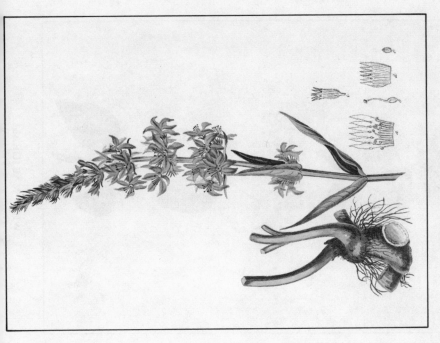

PURPLE LOOSETRIFE
Lythrum Salicaria

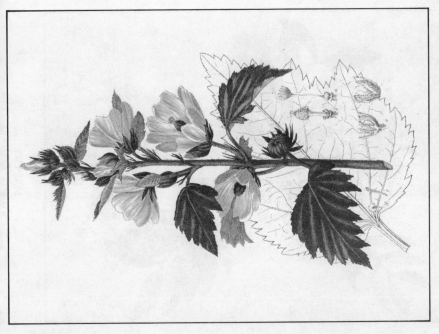

MARSH MALLOW
Althæa Officinalis

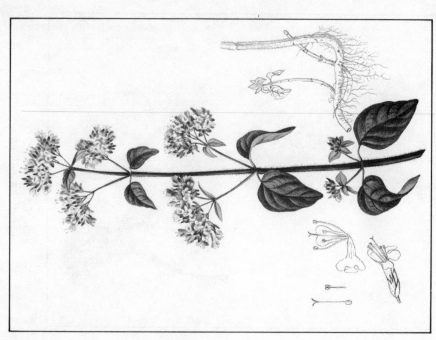

WILD MARJORAM
Origanum Vulgare

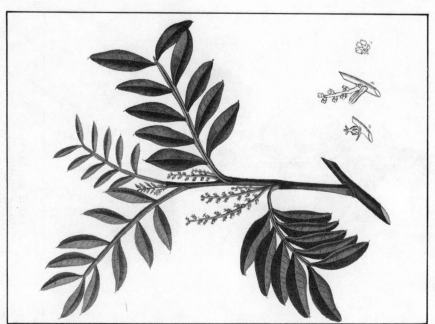

MASTIC
Pistacia Lentiscus

the joints, the younger ones thickly covered with hairs that fall off later. The alternate, bright green leaves are of distinctive shape, oblong-lanceolate with a broad, uneven base and a long, bluntly-tipped point. They are 5 to 7 inches long, entire and rather solid, with a fine network of sunken veins, hairy along the prominent veins of the underside.

The long, flexible spikes, 4 to 7 inches long, consist of tight rings of tiny yellow flowers packed round a fleshy axis. The seed fills the black fruit, which is about the size of a poppy-seed.

Two principal varieties in the shape of the leaves are recognized, the 'cordulatum' as described above, and the 'ossanum' with narrowed leaf-bases.

The drug is imported in bales, via Panama, the whole herb being pressed into a greenish-yellow mass. It is aromatic in taste and odour.

¶ *Constituents.* A volatile oil, slightly dextrogyrate, containing in some specimens Matico camphor. Some of the later specimens of oil are said to contain not camphor but asarol.

A crystallizable acid called artanthic acid and a little tannin and resin are also found.

¶ *Medicinal Action and Uses.* In South America Matico is used like cubeb. Its styptic properties are due to the volatile oil, and it is used for arresting hæmorrhages, as a local application to ulcers, in genito-urinary complaints, atonic diarrhœa, dysentery, etc.

In Peru it is considered aphrodisiac.

It is effective as a topical application to slight wounds, bites of leeches, or after the extraction of teeth. The under surface of the leaf is preferred to the powder for this purpose.

¶ *Dosages.* 45 to 75 grains. Of fluid extract, as intestinal astringent and diuretic, 1 fluid drachm.

¶ *Other Species.*

Piper aduncum, of Central America, yields a 'false matico'; the leaves are less tessellated above and hairy below, but the chemical properties are similar.

The name of Matico is also given to *Eupatorium glutinosum* and *Waltheria glomerata,* and possibly also to a species of Phlomis, but these are not recognized officially.

MATTE TEA. *See* PARAGUAY

MAYWEED

Anthemis cotula
N.O. Compositæ

Synonyms. Maroute. Maruta cotula. Cotula Maruta fœtida. Manzanilla loca. Dog Chamomile. Wild Chamomile. Camomille puante. Fœtid or Stinking Chamomile or Mayweed. Dog's Fennel. Maithes. Maithen. Mathor

Parts Used. Flowers, leaves

Habitat. Europe

¶ *Description.* This annual herb, growing freely in waste places, resembles the true Chamomile, having large, solitary flowers on erect stems, with conical, solid receptacles, but the white florets have no membraneous scales at their base. It is distinguished from the allied genera by its very fœtid odour, which rubbing increases.

The whole plant, including the fennel-like leaves, has this odour and is full of an acrid juice that has caused it to be classed among the vegetable poisons; it is liable to blister.

Its action resembles that of the Chamomiles, but it is weaker, and its odour prevents its general adoption.

Bees dislike it, and it is said to drive away fleas.

The flowers must not be gathered when wet, or they will blacken during drying.

¶ *Constituents.* The flowers have been found to contain volatile oil, oxalic, valeric and tannic acids, salts of magnesium, iron, potassium and calcium, colouring matter, a bitter extractive and fatty matter.

¶ *Medicinal Action and Uses.* The flowers are preferred for internal use, being slightly less disagreeable than the leaves. In hysteria it is used in Europe as an antispasmodic and emmenagogue. Applied to the skin fresh and bruised it is a safe vesicant. A poultice helpful in piles can be made from the herb boiled until soft, or it can be used as a bath or fomentation.

It is administered to induce sleep in asthma. In sick headache or convalescence after fever the extract may be used.

A strong decoction can cause sweating and vomiting. It is said to be nearly as valuable as opium in dysentery. It has also been used in scrofula, dysmennorrhœa and flatulent gastritis.

¶ *Dosage.* Of infusion, 1 to 4 fluid ounces.

¶ *Other Species.*

Anthemis tinctoria has similar properties and yields a yellow dye.

A. arvensis is considered in France to be one of the best indigenous febrifuges.

MAYWEED, SCENTLESS

Matricaria inodora
N.O. Compositæ

Synonym. Corn Feverfew
Part Used. Whole herb

The Scentless Mayweed owes its generic name to its reputed medicinal properties, which in a lesser degree resemble those of *Anthemis nobilis.*

It is an annual, commonly met with in fields, by the wayside, and on waste patches of ground, and flowers throughout the summer. The name 'Mayweed' is misleading, as it will be found in flower right up to the autumn. It is spreading and bunching in its growth, generally about 1 foot in height, but varying a good deal. The leaves, as in all the members of this group, are feather-like in character, springing direct from the main stems without leaf-stalks. The flower-heads are borne singly at the ends of long terminal flower-stems, the centre florets deep yellow on very prominent convex disks and the outer florets having very conspicuous white rays, much larger in proportion to the disk than in most of the allied species. Though compared with several of its allies, it may almost be termed 'scentless,' the term is not strictly appropriate as it yields slightly sweet and pleasant, aromatic odour.

The Finlanders use an infusion of this plant in consumption cases.

See CHAMOMILE.

MEADOWSWEET

Spiræa Ulmaria (LINN.)
N.O. Rosaceæ

Synonyms. Meadsweet. Dolloff. Queen of the Meadow. Bridewort. Lady of the Meadow
Part Used. Herb

¶ *Description.* The fragrant Meadowsweet is one of the best known wild flowers, decking our meadows and moist banks with its fernlike foliage and tufts of delicate, graceful, creamy-white flowers, which are in blossom from June to almost September. The leaves are dark green on the upper side and whitish and downy underneath, much divided, being interruptedly pinnate, having a few large serrate leaflets and small intermediate ones; the terminal leaflets are large, 1 to 3 inches long and three to five lobed. The stems are 2 to 4 feet high, erect and furrowed, sometimes purple. The flowers are small, clustered close together in handsome irregularly-branched cymes, and have a very strong, sweet smell. The whole herb possesses a pleasant taste and flavour, the green parts partaking of the aromatic character of the flowers.

A peculiarity of this flower is that the scent of the leaves is quite different from that of the flowers. The latter possess an almond-like fragrance; it is one of the fragrant herbs used to strew the floors of chambers. In allusion to this use, Gerard writes:

'The leaves and floures of Meadowsweet farre excelle all other strowing herbs for to decke up houses, to strawe in chambers, halls and banqueting-houses in the summer-time, for the smell thereof makes the heart merrie and joyful and delighteth the senses.'

Meadowsweet, water-mint, and vervain, were three herbs held most sacred by the Druids.

It is one of the fifty ingredients in a drink called 'Save,' mentioned in Chaucer's *Knight's Tale,* in the fourteenth century being called Medwort, or Meadwort, i.e. the mead or honey-wine herb, and the flowers were often put into wine and beer. It is still incorporated in many herb beers.

The name *Ulmaria* is given in allusion to the resemblance of its leaves to those of the Elm (*Ulmus*), being much wrinkled on the upper side.

Gerard says:

'It is reported that the floures boiled in wine and drunke do take away the fits of a quartaine ague and make the heart merrie. The distilled water of the floures dropped into the eies taketh away the burning and itching thereof and cleareth the sight.'

Culpepper says much the same and also: 'The leaves, when they are full grown, being laid on the skin will, in a short time, raise blisters thereon, as Tragus saith.' He also states that for acquiring the 'merry heart' (which Gerard mentions) 'some use the flowers and some the leaves.' He tells us that 'a leave hereof put into a cup of claret wine gives also a fine relish to it.'

¶ *Medicinal Action and Uses.* Aromatic, astringent, diuretic, and sub-tonic. It is a valuable medicine in diarrhœa, imparting to the bowels some degree of nourishment, as well as of astringency. It is also considered of some service as a corrector of the stomach, and not without some power as an alterative, and is frequently used in affections of the blood. It is a good remedy in strangury, dropsy, etc., and almost a specific in children's diarrhœa.

An infusion of 1 oz. of the dried herb to a pint of water is the usual mode of administration, in wineglassful doses. Sweetened with honey, it forms a very pleasant diet-drink, or beverage both for invalids and ordinary use.

The herb is collected in July, when in flower.

An infusion of the fresh tops produces perspiration, and a decoction of the root, in white wine, was formerly considered a specific in fevers.

Meadowsweet is visited by bees for the pollen.

¶ *Dosage.* Fluid extract, ½ to 1 drachm.

¶ *Other Species.*
Another member of the *Spiræa* is *Spiræa Filipendula* (Dropwort). A herb about a foot high, with short rhizome and nodulose rootlets; leaves interruptedly pinnate, leaflets cut into narrow serrated segments; flowers in crowded, erect, compound cymes, pink externally in bud; when open, white and scentless. Dry pastures on a limestone (or chalky) soil. Distinguished from *S. Ulmaria* by its elegantly cut foliage, pink buds, and whiter scentless blossoms. A double-flowered variety is common in gardens. Flowering time – June, July. Perennial.

Culpepper speaks of *Filipendula,* or Drop-wort, as being a good remedy for kidney affections, by 'taking the roots in powder or a decoction of them in white wine, with a little honey.' He adds that it

'is also very effectual for all the diseases of the lungs, as shortness of breath, wheezing, hoarseness of the throat; and to expectorate tough phlegm, or any other parts thereabout.'

WILLOW-LEAVED SPIRÆA (*S. salyciflora*), a shrub with simple ex-stipulate leaves and spike-like clusters of rose-coloured flowers, grows in moist woods in the north and in Wales; but it is not indigenous. It flowers in July and August. Perennial.

There are several foreign species of *Spiræa,* one from Japan being a beautiful shrub with pure white flowers, and leaves like those of the plum, hence its name, *S. prunifolia.*

There is another from Nepaul, *S. bella,* with rose-coloured flowers growing in lateral and terminal corymbs; another from Canada, *S. tomentosa,* with cottony leaves and pyramidal panicles of rose-coloured flowers; and *S. Fortunei* from China, with ovate, smooth, toothed leaves often tinged with purple, and rose-coloured flowers.

See HARDHACK, INDIAN PHYSIC.

MELILOT

Melilotus officinalis (LINN.)
Melilotus alba (DESV.)
Melilotus arvensis (LAMK.)
N.O. Leguminosæ

Synonyms. Yellow Melilot. White Melilot. Corn Melilot. King's Clover. Sweet Clover. Plaster Clover. Sweet Lucerne. Wild Laburnum. Hart's Tree
Part Used. Herb

The Melilots or Sweet Clovers – formerly known as Melilot Trefoils and assigned, with the common clovers, to the large genus *Trifolium,* but now grouped in the genus *Melilotus* – are not very common in Britain, being not truly native, though they have become naturalized, having been extensively cultivated for fodder formerly, especially the common yellow species, *Melilotus officinalis* (Linn.).

Although now seldom seen as a crop, having, like the Medick, given place to the Clovers, Sainfoin and Lucerne, Melilot seems, however, to have been a very common crop in the sixteenth century, seeding freely, spreading in a wild condition wherever grown, since Gerard tells us,

'for certainty no part of the world doth enjoy so great plenty thereof as England and especially Essex, for I have seen between Sudbury in Suffolke and Clare in Essex and from Clare to Hessingham very many acres of earable pasture overgrowne with the same; in so much that it doth not only spoil their land, but the corn also, as Cockle or Darnel and is a weed that generally spreadeth over that corner of the shire.'

¶ *Description.* The Melilots are perennial herbs, 2 to 4 feet high, found in dry fields and along roadsides, in waste places and chalky banks, especially along railway banks and near lime kilns. The smooth, erect stems are much branched, the leaves placed on alternate sides of the stems are smooth and trifoliate, the leaflets oval. The plants bear long racemes of small, sweet-scented, yellow or white, papilionaceous flowers in the yellow species, the keel of the flower much shorter than the other parts and containing much honey. They are succeeded by broad, black, one-seeded pods, transversely wrinkled.

All species of Melilot, when in flower, have a peculiar sweet odour, which by drying becomes stronger and more agreeable, somewhat like that of the Tonka bean, this similarity being accounted for by the fact that they both contain the same chemical principle, Coumarin, which is also present in new-mown hay and woodruff, which have the identical fragrance.

The name of this genus comes from the words *Mel* (honey) and *lotus* (meaning honey-lotus), the plants being great favourites of the bees. Popular and local English names are Sweet Clover, King's Clover, Hart's Tree or Plaster Clover, Sweet Lucerne and Wild Laburnum.

The tender foliage makes the plant acceptable to horses and other animals, and it is said that deer browse on it, hence its name 'Hart's Clover.' Galen used to prescribe Melilot plaster to his Imperial and aristocratic patients when they suffered from inflammatory tumours or swelled joints, and the plant is so used even in the present day in some parts of the Continent.

In one Continental Pharmacopœia of recent date an emollient application is directed to be made of Melilot, resin, wax, and olive oil.

Gerard says that

'Melilote boiled in sweet wine untile it be soft, if you adde thereto the yolke of a rosted egge, the meale of Linseed, the roots of Marsh Mallowes and hogs greeace stamped together, and used as a pultis or cataplasma, plaisterwise, doth asswge and soften all manner of swellings.'

It was also believed that the juice of the plant 'dropped into the eies cleereth the sight.'

Water distilled from the flowers was said to improve the flavour of other ingredients.

There are three varieties of Melilot found in England, the commonest being *Melilotus officinalis* (Linn.), the Yellow Melilot; *M. alba* (Desv.), the White Melilot, and *M. arvensis* (Lamk.), the Corn Melilot, which is found occasionally in waste places in the eastern counties, but is not considered indigenous.

The dried leaves and flowering tops of all three species form the drug used in herbal medicine, though the drug of the German Pharmacopœia is *M. officinalis*. Two yellow-flowered species are, however, often sold under this name, the common *M. officinalis*, which has hairy pods, and *M. arvensis*, which has small, smooth pods.

The White Melilot found in waste places in England, particularly on railway banks, is not uncommon, but apparently not permanently established in any of its localities. It differs from *M. officinalis* by its more

slender root and stems, which, however, attain as great a height, by its more slender and lax racemes and smaller flowers, which are about $\frac{1}{5}$ inch long and white. The standard is larger than the keel and wings, which alone would distinguish it from *M. officinalis*. The pods are smaller and free from the hairs clothing those of *M. officinalis*.

A new kind of Sweet Clover, an *annual* variety of *M. alba*, has been discovered in the United States. To distinguish it from the other Sweet Clovers, it is called Hubam, after Professor Hughes, its discoverer, and Alabama, its native state. Some five or six years ago, small samples were distributed by Professor Hughes among various experimental stations, with the result that the superiority of the plant has been generally recognized and its spread has been rapid, over 5,000 acres now being cultivated. The plant has specially valuable characteristics – great resistance to drought, adaptability to a wide variety of soils and climates, abundant seed production, richness in nectar and great fertilizing value to the soil, and has been grown successfully in the United States, Canada, Australia, Italy, and many other countries. The quantity of forage produced from a given acre is second to no other forage plant, and the quality, if properly handled, is excellent. It is of very quick growth and blooms in three to four months after sowing, producing an unusual wealth of honey-making blooms. The flowers remain in bloom for a longer period than almost any other honey-bearing plant, and in the matter of nectar production the quantity is surprising, equal to that of any other honey produced in the United States, and the quality compares favourably with the best honey produced either there or in Great Britain. It is considered that this annual Sweet Clover will one day stand at the head of the list of honey plants of the world, if the present rate of spreading continues.

¶ *Parts Used Medicinally.* The whole herb is used, dried, for medicinal purposes, the flowering shoots, gathered in May, separated from the main stem and dried in the same manner as Broom tops.

The dried herb has an intensely fragrant odour, but a somewhat pungent and bitterish taste.

¶ *Constituents.* Coumarin, the crystalline substance developed under the drying process, is the only important constituent, together with its related compounds, hydrocoumaric (melilotic) acid, orthocoumaric acid and melilotic anhydride, or lactone, a fragrant oil.

¶ *Medicinal Action and Uses.* The herb has aromatic, emollient and carminative properties. It was formerly much esteemed in medicine as an emollient and digestive and is recommended by Gerard for many complaints, the juice for clearing the eyesight, and, boiled with lard and other ingredients, as an application to wens and ulcers, and mixed with wine, 'it mitigateth the paine of the eares and taketh away the paine of the head.'

Culpepper tells us that the head is to be washed with the distilled herb for loss of senses and apoplexy, and that boiled in wine, it is good for inflammation of the eye or other parts of the body.

The following recipe is from the Fairfax Still-room book (published 1651):

'To make a bath for Melancholy. Take Mallowes, pellitory of the wall, of each three handfulls; Camomell Flowers, *Mellilot* flowers, of each one handfull, senerick seed one ounce, and boil them in nine gallons of Water untill they come to three, then put in a quart of new milke and go into it bloud warme or something warmer.'

Applied as a plaster, or in ointment, or as a fomentation, it is an old-fashioned country remedy for the relief of abdominal and rheumatic pains.

It relieves flatulence and in modern herbal practice is taken internally for this purpose.

The flowers, besides being very useful and attractive to bees, have supplied a perfume, and a water distilled from them has been used for flavouring.

The dried plant has been employed to scent snuff and smoking tobacco and may be laid among linen for the same purpose as lavender. When packed with furs, Melilot is said to act like camphor and preserve them from moths, besides imparting a pleasant fragrance.

'In Switzerland, Melilot abounds in the pastures and is an ingredient in the green Swiss cheese called *Schabzieger*. The Schabzieger cheese is made by the curd being pressed in boxes with holes to let the whey run out; and when a considerable quantity has been collected and putrefaction begins, it is worked into a paste with a large proportion of the dried herb Melilotus, reduced to a powder. The herb is called in the country dialect "Zieger kraut," *curd herb*. The paste thus produced is pressed into moulds of the shape of a common flowerpot and the putrefaction being stopped by the aromatic herb, it dries into a solid mass and keeps unchanged for any length of time. When used, it is rasped or grated and the powder mixed with fresh butter is spread upon bread.' (Syme and Sowerby, *English Botany*.)

MELONS

N.O. Cucurbitaceæ

The order Cucurbitaceæ (the sole representative of which in the British Islands is the familiar hedge-climbing, red-berried Bryony) contains many genera of economic importance: *Cucumis* affords cucumber and melon; *Cucurbita*, pumpkin and marrow; to the genus *Lagenaria* belong the gourds; the well-known bath-loofah is formed of the closely-netted vascular bundles in the fruit of *Luffa ægyptica*, another member of the order, the unripe fruit itself being used as a pickle by the Arabians; *Sechium edule*, a tropical American species, is largely cultivated for its edible fruit, *Choko*; *Citrullus vulgaris* is the Water Melon, which serves the Egyptians both as food, drink and physic; *Citrullus Colecynthis* furnishes the drug called Celocynth, and equally valuable medicinally is *Ecbalium Elaterium*, the Squirting Cucumber.

MELON, COMMON

Cucumis melo (LINN.)

Synonym. Musk Melon

Habitat. The Melon is a native of South Asia – from the foot of the Himalayas to Cape Comorin, where it grows wild – but is cultivated in the temperate and warm regions of the whole world

¶ *Description.* It is an annual, trailing herb, with large palmately-lobed leaves and bears tendrils, by which it is readily trained over trellises. Its flowers (which have bell-shaped corollas, deeply five-lobed) are either male or female, both kinds being borne on the one plant. The male flowers have three stamens, the ovary in the female flowers, three cells. The many varieties of Melon show great diversity in foliage and still more in the size and shape of the fruit, which in some kinds is as small as an olive, in others as large as the Gourd (*Cucurbita maxima*). Some are globular, others egg-shaped, spindle-shaped or serpent-like, the outer skin smooth or netted, ribbed or furrowed, and variously coloured; the flesh, white, green or orange when ripe, scented or scentless, sweet or insipid, some bitter and even nauseous.

¶ *History.* The cultivation of the Melon in Asia is of very ancient date. It was grown by the Egyptians, and the Romans and Greeks were familiar with it. Pliny describes Melons as *Pepones*, Columella as *Melones*. It began to be extensively cultivated in France in 1629. Gerarde in his *Herball* (1597) figured and described several kinds of Melons or Pompions, but included gourds under the same name. The Common Melon was commonly known as the Musk Melon.

To grow it to perfection, the Melon requires artificial heat, being grown on hot beds of fermenting manure, with an atmospheric temperature of 75°, rising with sun-heat to 80°.

MELON, CANTALOUP

Cucumis Cantalupensis (HABERL.)

The Cantaloups (*Cucumis Cantalupensis*, Haberl., so called from a place near Rome where it was long cultivated) is grown by the market gardeners round Paris and other parts of France, and has its origin in Persia and the neighbouring Caucasian region. It was first brought to Rome from Armenia in the sixteenth century. The netted species probably also originally came from Persia.

MELON, DUDAIM

Synonym. Queen Anne's Pocket Melon

Cucumis dudaim

The Dudaim Melon (*Cucunis dudaim*), Queen Anne's Pocket Melon, as it has been called, is also a native of Persia. It produces a fruit variegated with green and orange and oblong green spots of varying size. When fully ripe, it becomes yellow and then whitish. It has a very fragrant, vinous, musky smell, and a whitish, flaccid, insipid pulp. *Dudaim* is the Hebrew name of the fruit.

MELON, SERPENT

Synonym. Snake Cucumber

Cucumis flexuosum (LINN.)

Cucumis flexuosum (Linn.) is the Serpent Melon, or Snake Cucumber. It grows to a great length and may be used either raw or pickled.

The 'Cucumber' of the Scriptures (Isaiah i. 8) is considered to have been *Cucumis chate*, the Hairy Cucumber, a kind of wild Melon, which produces a fruit, the flesh of which is almost of the same substance as the Common Melon, its taste being somewhat sweet and as cool as the Water Melon. It is common both in Arabia and in Egypt, where a dish is prepared from the ripe fruit. Peter Forskäl, a contemporary of Linnæus, in his work on the plants of Egypt (*Flora ægyptiaco-arabica*, 1775), describes its preparation. The pulp is broken and stirred by means of a stick thrust through a hole cut at the umbilicus of the fruit: the hole is then closed with wax, and the fruit, without removing it from its stem, is buried in a little pit; after some days, the pulp is found to be converted into an agreeable liquor.

MELON, WATER

Parts Used. Seeds, juice

Citrullus vulgaris (LINN.)

Melons are a staple and refreshing fruit in Egypt and Palestine, especially the Water Melon (*Citrullus vulgaris*, Linn.), a native of tropical Africa and the East Indies, which grows to a great size, even attaining 30 lb. in weight. It refreshes the thirsty as well as the hungry. It has a smooth rind, and though generally oblong and about a foot and a half in length, varies much in form and colour, the flesh being either red or pale, the seeds, black or reddish. There is a succession of crops from May to November. For its cool and refreshing fruit, it has been cultivated since the earliest times in Egypt and the East and was known in Southern Europe and Asia before the Christian era. The banks of the Burlus Delta lake, east of the Rosetta channel of the Nile Delta, are noted for their Water Melons, which are yellow within, and come into season after those grown on the banks of the Nile. Of the plants found in the Kalahari Desert of South Africa, in Bechuanaland, the most remarkable is the Water Melon, present in abundance, which supplies both man and beast with water.

¶ *Medicinal Action and Uses.* The fruit should be eaten cautiously by Europeans, especially when taken in the heat of the day, but it is much used in the tropics and in Italy. In Egypt, it is practically the only medicine the common people use in fevers; when it is ripe, or almost putrid, they collect the juice and mix it with rosewater and a little sugar. The seeds have been employed to a considerable extent as a domestic remedy in strangury and other affections of the urinary passages, and are regarded as having diuretic properties. The Russian peasants use them for dropsy and hepatic congestion, also for intestinal catarrh.

The *Four Greater Cold Seeds* of the old materia medica were the seeds of the Pumpkin (*Cucurbita pepo*), the Gourd (*C. maxima*), the Melon and the Cucumber. These were bruised and rubbed up with water to form an emulsion, which was much used in catarrhal affections, disorders of the bowels and urinary passages, fever, etc.

The seeds of both the Water Melon and the Common or Musk Melon are good vermicides, having much the same constituents as those of the PUMPKIN (sometimes known as the Melon Pumpkin), which have long been a popular worm remedy and in recent years have also been used for tapeworm.

¶ *Constituents*. Pumpkin seeds contain 30 per cent. or more of a reddish, fixed oil, traces of a volatile oil, together with proteids, sugar, starch and an acrid resin, to which the anthelmintic properties appear to be due, though recent experiments have failed to isolate any substance of physiological activity, either from the kernels or shells of the seeds. The value of the drug is said to be due to its mechanical effect.

The seeds are employed when quite ripe and must not be used if more than a month old. A mixture is made by beating up 2 oz. of the seeds with as much sugar and milk or water added to make a pint, and this mixture is taken fasting, in three doses, one every two hours, castor oil being taken a few hours after the last dose. An infusion of the seeds, prepared by pouring a pint of boiling water on 1 oz. of seeds, has likewise been used in urinary complaints.

The Pumpkin or Pompion (its older name, of which Pumpkin is a corruption) is a native of the Levant. Many varieties are cultivated in gardens, both for ornament and also for culinary use. It is a useful plant to the American backwoods-farmer, yielding both in the ripe and unripe condition a valuable fodder for his cattle and pigs, being frequently planted at intervals among the maize that constitutes his chief crop. The larger kinds acquire a weight of 40–80 lb., but smaller varieties are in more esteem for garden culture.

In England, Pumpkins were formerly called English Melons, which was popularly corrupted to Millions. They are used cut up in soups and make excellent pies, either alone or mixed with other fruit, and their pulp is also utilized as a basis by jam manufacturers, as it takes the flavour of any fruit juice mixed with it, and adds bulk without imparting any flavour of its own.

The SQUASHES, which have such extensive culinary use in America, are a variety of the Pumpkin (*C. melopepo*), and another familiar member of the genus, *C. evifera*, a variety of *C. pepo*, is the Vegetable Marrow. While small and green the Pumpkin may be eaten like the Marrow.

¶ *Medicinal Action and Uses*. The *root* of the Common Melon is purgative, and in large doses (7 to 10 grains) is said to be a certain emetic, the active and bitter principle having been called Melon-emetin.

The MELON-TREE, so-called, is the PAPAW, or Papaya (*Carica Papaya*, Linn.), a native of tropical America, where it is everywhere cultivated for its edible fruit and digestive properties.

The dried juice is largely used in the treatment of indigestion, under various trade names, 'Papain,' a white powder, being administered in all digestive disorders where albuminoid substances pass away undigested.

¶ *Dosage*. Papain, 1 to 5 grains.

See PAPAW (APPLE, BITTER).

MERCURY, DOG'S

Mercurialis perennis (LINN.)
N.O. Euphorbiaceæ

¶ *Description*. Dog's Mercury, a perennial, herbaceous plant, sending up from its creeping root numerous, undivided stems, about a foot high, is common in woods and shady places throughout Europe and Russian Asia, except in the extreme north. It is abundant at Hythe in Sussex.

Each stem bears several pairs of rather large roughish leaves, and from the axils of the upper ones grow the small green flowers, the barren on long stalks, the fertile sessile, the first appearing before the leaves are quite out. The stamens and pistils are on different plants. The perianth is three-cleft to the base. The barren flowers have nine stamens or more, the fertile flowers two styles and two cells to the two-lobed ovary.

Male and female plants are rarely found intermixed, each usually growing in large patches. The female are less common than the male, and the plant increases more by the spreading of its creeping rootstocks and stems than by seed. It flowers from the end of March to the middle of May and seeds in the summer. The leaves of the male flowering plants are more pointed and less serrated than those on the female plants, which have longer stalks.

Dog's Mercury has a disagreeable odour and is extremely acrid, being poisonous to animals in the fresh state. It has been said, however, that heat destroys its harmfulness, and that it is innocuous in hay. Its chemical constituents have not been ascertained.

Dog's Mercury has proved fatal to sheep, and Annual Mercury to human beings who had made soup from it.

¶ *History.* We find it spoken of in the old herbals as possessing wonderful powers, but it has been abandoned as a dangerous remedy for internal use.

Culpepper speaks strongly of the 'rank poisonous' qualities of Dog's Mercury, and adds, with some contempt:

'The common herbals, as Gerarde's and Parkinson's, instead of cautioning their readers against the use of this plant, after some trifling, idle observations upon the qualities of Mercurys in general, dismiss the article without noticing its baneful effects. Other writers, more accurate, have done this; but they have written in Latin, a language not very likely to inform those who stand most in need of this caution.'

It derives its name from the legend that its medicinal virtues were revealed by the god Mercury. The Greeks called it Mercury's Grass. The French call it *La Mercuriale*, the Italians, *Mercorella*. The name Dog's Mercury or Dog's Cole, was probably given it because of its inferiority from an edible point of view, either to the Annual, or Garden Mercury, or to a plant known to the older herbalists as English Mercury, which was sometimes eaten in this country and some parts of the Continent as a substitute for that vegetable. The prefix 'Dog' was often given to wild-flowers that were lacking in scent or other properties of allied species – as, for instance, Dog Violet, Dog Rose, etc.

That Dog's Mercury has been eaten in mistake for Good King Henry, with unfortunate results, we know from the report of

MERCURY, ANNUAL

Annual Mercury (*Mercurialis annua*), known also to older writers as Garden Mercury and French Mercury, is a common weed in gardens.

It is taller than the Dog Mercury, and branched, and the leaves are smaller, perfectly smooth and of a light green hue.

Barren and fertile flowers are sometimes found on the same plant, the male flowers in peduncled axillary spikes.

It grows plentifully in waste places and seldom at any distance from inhabited districts.

Ray, one of the earliest of English naturalists, who relates that when boiled and eaten with fried bacon in error for this English spinach, it produced sickness, drowsiness and twitching. In another instance, when it was collected and boiled in soup by some vagrants, all partaking of it exhibited the ordinary symptoms of narcotic and irritant poisoning, two children dying on the following day.

The fact that some old books recommend Dog's Mercury as a good potherb arose probably from confusing it with the less harmful annual species, called by Gerard the French or Garden Mercury.

¶ *Medicinal Action and Uses.* Hippocrates commended this herb for women's diseases, used externally, as did also Culpepper, who says it is good for sore and watering eyes and deafness and pains in the ears. He advises the use of it, also, as a decoction, 'made with water and a cock chicken,' for hot fits of ague. It has been employed for jaundice and as a purgative.

The juice of the whole plant, freshly collected when in flower, mixed with sugar or with vinegar, is recommended externally for warts, and for inflammatory and discharging sores, and also, applied as a poultice, to swellings and to cleanse old sores.

A lotion is made from the plant for antiseptic external dressings, to be used in the same manner as carbolic.

The juice has also been used as a nasal douche for catarrh.

When steeped in water, the leaves and stems of the plant give out a fine blue colour, resembling indigo. This colouring matter is turned red by acids and destroyed by alkalis, but is otherwise permanent, and might prove valuable as a dye, if any means of fixing the colour could be devised. The stems are of a bright metallic blue, like indigo, and those that run into the ground have the most colouring matter.

Mercurialis annua (LINN.)
N.O. Euphorbiaceæ

It is in flower from July to October and increases so freely by the scattering of its rough seeds as to become a very troublesome weed in gardens, extremely hard to eradicate.

¶ *Medicinal Action and Uses.* The plant is mucilaginous and was formerly much employed as an emollient. The French made a syrup of the freshly-gathered herb, which was given as a purge, and the dried herb was used to make a decoction for injections, but as a herbal remedy it is now disregarded in England.

The seeds taste like those of hemp.

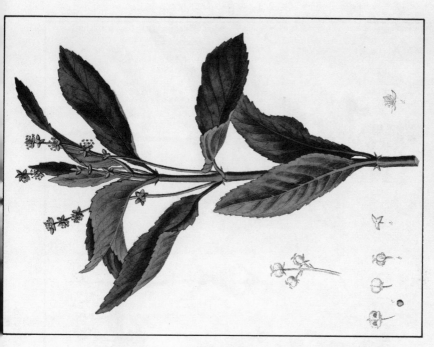
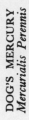

DOG'S MERCURY
Mercurialis Perennis

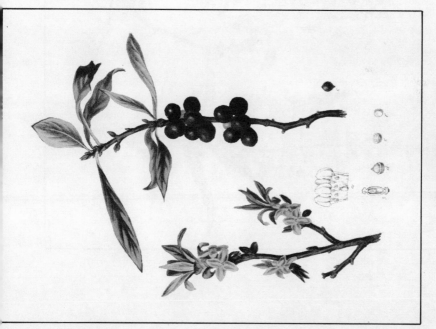

MEZEREON
Daphne Mezereum

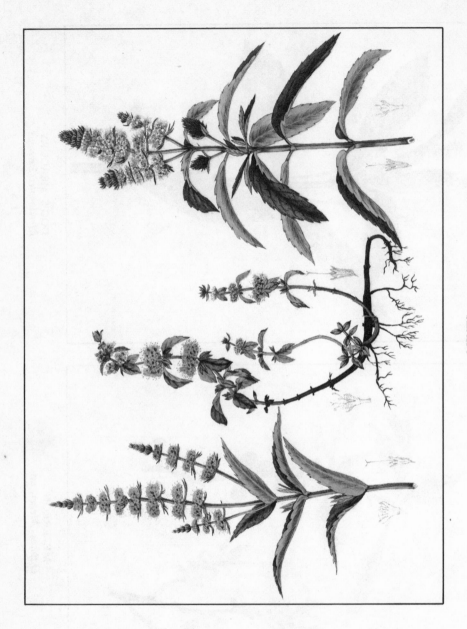

MINTS

Mentha Viridis, Mentha Pulegium, Mentha Piperita

As a pot-herb, this plant had some reputation, the leaves being boiled and eaten as spinach, and it is still eaten in this way in some parts of Germany, the acrid qualities being dissipated, it is believed, by boiling. Pigs have also been fed with it in France.

(POISON)
MESCAL BUTTONS

Anhalonium Lewinii (HENN.)
N.O. Cactaceæ

Synonyms. Lopophora Lewinii. Pellote. Muscal Buttons. Anhalonium Williamsii. Echinocactus Lewinii. Echinocactus Williamsii

Part Used. The tops, consisting of blunt leaves round a tuft of short, pale yellow hairs

Habitat. Mexico

¶ *Description.* These South American Cacti, formerly regarded as belonging to the *Anhalonium* genus, by the name of which they are chiefly known, were later attributed to the genus *Echinocactus* of the *Mammalaria* species, being spineless and flexible.

The principal species of *Williamsii* and *Lewinii*, found in the Rio Grande valley, grow to a height of only ½ inch, and the tops, or Mescal Buttons, are from 1 to 1½ inch across and ¼ inch thick. When dry they are hard and brittle, but become soft when moistened. The taste and smell are peculiar, bitter and disagreeable. The surface of *E. Lewinii*, or *Anhalonium Lewinii*, is crossed by thirteen irregular furrows, and that of *E. Williamsii* and *A. Williamsii* by eight regular ones. Small pink flowers are borne, but these do not appear in the drug.

The Kiowa Indians have used Mescal Buttons from ancient times for producing exaltation in their religious ceremonies.

¶ *Constituents.* Four alkaloids have been separated: Anhalonine, Mescaline, Anhalonidine, and Lophophorine, and two other bases, pellotine and anhalamine. Pellotine is said to be found only in the Williamsii variety, but this is always present in the commercial drug.

¶ *Medicinal Action and Uses.* Cardiac, tonic, narcotic, emetic. The value of the drug in practice is uncertain, but it is stated to be useful in neurasthenia, hysteria, and asthma, and has been recommended in gout, neuralgia and rheumatism.

Four to five buttons, or 215 to 230 grains of the drug will produce a strange cerebral excitement with visual disturbance, the visions being at first of varied beauty and later of gruesome shapes and monsters. The physical effects include dilatation of the pupil, muscular relaxation, loss of time sense, partial anæsthesia, wakefulness, and sometimes nausea and vomiting. The mental symptoms in some ways resemble those of Indian Hemp.

Pellotine, in doses of ⅛ to 1 grain, has been used in hypodermic injection in cases of insanity, producing sleep without undesirable reactions. Care is needed, as collapse is said to have been observed after a dose of $\frac{7}{10}$ of a grain. The uses of the various alkaloids are in the experimental stage.

¶ *Dosage.* Of the crude drug, 7 to 15 grains. Of fluid extract, 10 to 15 minims. Of 10 per cent. tincture, 1 to 2 teaspoonsful.

¶ *Other Species.*
There are also found in parcels of the tops specimens of *Mammalaria fissuratus*, *M. retusus*, and *A. jourdanianum*.

Mescal is a name given in Mexico to a liquor distilled from a number of species of Agave.

MEZEREON

Daphne mezereum (LINN.)
N.O. Thymelæaceæ

Synonyms. Mezerei Cortex. Mezerei officinarum. Dwarf Bay. Flowering Spurge. Spurge Olive. Spurge Laurel. Laureole gentille. Camolea. Kellerhals. Wolt schjeluke

Parts Used. The bark of root and stem, berries, roots

Habitat. Europe, including Britain, and Siberia. Naturalized in Canada and the United States

¶ *Description.* The mediæval name Mezereum is derived from the Persian *Mazariyun*, a name given to a species of Daphne. The barks of *Daphne laureola*, or Spurge Laurel, and *D. Gnidium* are also official in the British Pharmacopœia and United States.

Though a hardy shrub and indigenous to England, *D. mezereum* is not often found wild. The leaves appear at the ends of the branches after the flowers, and are alternate, lanceolate, entire, 2 to 3 inches long and dark green in colour. The small, purplish-pink, four-segmented flowers grow in little clusters, and the bright-red, fleshy, ovoid, bluntly-pointed fruits, about ⅜ inch long, appear close to the stem in July.

There are varieties with yellow fruit and white flowers.

Occasionally the bark is found in commerce in quills, but more often in tough, flexible, thin, long strips, rolled like tape, splitting easily lengthways but difficult to break horizontally. The inner surface is silky, and the thin, outer, corky layer, of a light greenish-brown colour, separates easily in papery fragments.

The unpleasant odour of the fresh bark diminishes with drying, but the taste is intensely burning and acrid, though sweetish at first. The root bark is most active, but inadequate supplies led to the recognition of the stem bark also.

¶ *Constituents.* The acridity of the bark is chiefly due to mezeen, a greenish-brown, sternutatory, amorphous resin. Mezereic acid, into which it can be changed, is found in the alcoholic and ethereal extracts, together with a fixed oil, a bitter, crystalline glucoside, daphnin, and a substance like euphorbone. Daphnin can be resolved into daphnetin and sugar by the action of dilute acids.

¶ *Medicinal Action and Uses.* Stimulant and vesicant. A moist application of the recent bark to the skin will cause redness and blisters in from twenty-four to forty-eight hours. It may be softened in hot vinegar and water and applied as a compress, renewed every twelve hours. It can be used for a mild, perpetual blister.

An ointment was formerly used to induce discharge in indolent ulcers.

The bark is used for snake and other venomous bites, and in Siberia, by veterinary surgeons, for horses' hoofs.

The official compound liniment of mustard includes an ethereal extract, and one of its rare internal uses in England is as an ingredient in compound decoction of sarsaparilla.

Authorities differ as to its value in chronic rheumatism, scrofula, syphilis and skin diseases. A light infusion is said to be good in dropsies, but if too strong may cause vomiting and bloody stools. Thirty berries are used as a purgative by Russian peasants, though French writers regard fifteen as a fatal dose.

In Germany a tincture of the berries is used locally in neuralgia.

Slices of the root may be chewed in toothache, and it is recorded that an obstinate case of difficulty in swallowing, persisting after confinement, was cured by chewing the root constantly and so causing irritation.

¶ *Dosages.* Ten grains. Of decoction, 1 to 3 fluid ounces. Of fluid extract, 2 to 10 drops.

¶ *Poisons and Antidotes.* In large doses it is an irritant poison, causing vomiting and hypercatharsis.

The berries have proved fatal to children.

¶ *Other Species.*

D. Gnidium, or *D. paniculata,* garou, sainbois, or Spurge Flax, deriving its name from its native Cnidos, is one of the official species. The leaves are numerous and very narrow, like those of flax.

D. Laureola, or Spurge Laurel, is less acrid. The leaves were formerly used as an emmenagogue, but may cause vomiting and purging. Both leaves and bark have been used to procure abortion.

D. Thymelœa, D. Tartonaira, D. pontica and *D. alpina* are used as substitutes.

AMERICAN MEZEREON is a name of *Dirca Palustris* or Leatherwood.

MILFOIL. *See* YARROW

MILFOIL, WATER

To the same natural order as the Mare's Tail (Haloragaceæ) belongs the Water Milfoil, which has the following varieties: SPIKED WATER MILFOIL (*Myriophyllum spicatum*), an aquatic plant forming a tangled mass of slender, much branched stems; leaves, four in a whorl, finely divided into numerous hair-like segments, the whole plant being submerged, except the spikes of inconspicuous greenish flowers, which rise a few inches above the surface.

MILKWEED. *See* ASCLEPIAS

MIMOSAS

Mimosa fragifolia is an acrid astringent.

M. linguis is a diuretic astringent.

M. humilis, Brazilian Mimosa or Sensitive Plant, so called because the leaves close at the least contact. Tincture of the leaves is used by homœopaths for swelling of ankles.

Cassia nictitans, or Wild Sensitive Plant, is used for certain forms of rheumatism.

N.O. Haloragaceæ

WHORLED WATER MILFOIL (*M. verticillatum*) differs from the preceding in having the flowers in whorls at the base of the leaves: alternate-flowered Water Milfoil (*M. alterniflorum*) has the barren flowers alternately arranged in a short leafless spike, with the fertile flowers about three together, in the axils of the leaves, at its base. Both species are rare.

See MARE'S TAIL.

N.O. Leguminosæ

MINTS

There are three chief species of mint in cultivation and general use: Spearmint (*Mentha viridis*), Peppermint (*M. piperita*),

N.O. Labiatæ

and Pennyroyal (*M. pulegium*), the first being the one ordinarily used for cooking.

The various species of mint have much in

common and have all been held in high medical repute. Dr. Westmacott, the author of a work on plants published in 1694, mentioning the different kinds of mint, states that they are well known to

'the young Botanists and Herb Women belonging to Apothecarys' shops. . . . In the shops are 1. The dry Herbs. 2ndly. Mint Water. 3rdly. Spirit of Mints. 4th. Syrup of Mints. 5th. The Conserve of the Leaves.

6th. The Simple Oyl. 7th. The Chemical Oyl.' He says 'the Mints have a biting, aromatick bitterish Sapor with a strong fragrant Smell abounding with a pungent Volatile Salt and a Subtil Sulphur which destroyeth Acids, and herein doth lodge the Causation of such medicinal Virtues in this Herb and others of the like Nature.'

All the Mints yield fragrant oils by distillation.

SPEARMINT

Mentha viridis (LINN.)
N.O. Labiatæ

Synonyms. Garden Mint. Mentha Spicata. Mackerel Mint. Our Lady's Mint. Green Mint. Spire Mint. Sage of Bethlehem. Fish Mint. Menthe de Notre Dame. Erba Santa Maria. Frauen Munze. Lamb Mint

Part Used. Herb

This common garden mint is not a native of these islands, though growing freely in every garden, but is originally a native of the Mediterranean region, and was introduced into Britain by the Romans, being largely cultivated not only by them, but also by the other Mediterranean nations. It was in great request by the Romans, and Pliny according to Gerard says of it: 'The smell of Mint does stir up the minde and the taste to a greedy desire of meate.' Ovid represents the hospitable Baucis and Philemon scouring their board with green mint before laying upon it the food intended for their divine guests. The Ancients believed that mint would prevent the coagulation of milk and its acid fermentation. Gerard, again quoting Pliny, says:

'It will not suffer milk to cruddle in the stomach, and therefore it is put in milk that is drunke, lest those that drinke thereof should be strangled.'

Many other references to it in old writings – among them, that of the payment by the Pharisees of tithes of Mint, Anise and Cumin – prove that the herb has been highly esteemed for many centuries. Mint is mentioned in all early mediæval lists of plants; it was very early grown in English gardens, and was certainly cultivated in the Convent gardens of the ninth century. Chaucer refers to 'a little path of mintes full and fenill greene.'

Turner states in his *Herball* (1568) that the garden mint of his time was also called 'Spere Mynte.' Gerard, in further praise of the herb, tells us that

'the smelle rejoiceth the heart of man, for which cause they used to strew it in chambers and places of recreation, pleasure and repose, where feasts and banquets are made.'

It has, in fact, been so universally esteemed, that it is to be found wild in nearly all the countries to which civilization has extended, and in America for 200 years it has been known as an escape from gardens, growing in moist soils and proving sometimes troublesome as a weed.

Parkinson, in his *Garden of Pleasure*, mentions 'divers sorts of mintes both of the garden and wilde, of the woods, mountain and standing pools or waters' and says:

'Mintes are sometimes used in Baths with Balm and other herbs as a help to comfort and strengthen the nerves and sinews. It is much used either outwardly applied or inwardly drunk to strengthen and comfort weak stomackes.'

The Ancients used mint to scent their bath water and as a restorative, as we use smelling salts to-day. In Athens where every part of the body was perfumed with a different scent mint was specially designated to the arms.

Gerard says of its medicinal properties:

'It is good against watering eies and all manner of breakings out on the head and sores. It is applied with salt to the bitings of mad dogs. . . . They lay it on the stinging of wasps and bees with good success.'

Culpepper gives nearly forty distinct maladies for which mint is 'singularly good.'

'Being smelled into,' he says, 'it is comfortable for the head and memory, and a decoction when used as a gargle, cures the mouth and gums, when sore.' Again, 'Garden Mint is most useful to wash children's heads when the latter are inclined to sores, and Wild Mint, mixed with vinegar is an excellent wash to get rid of scurf. Rose leaves and mint, heated and applied outwardly cause rest and sleep.'

In the fourteenth century, mint was used for whitening the teeth, and its distilled oil is still used to flavour tooth-pastes, etc., and in America, especially, to flavour confectionery, chewing gums, and also to perfume soap.

Mint ottos have more power than any other aromatic to overcome the smell of tobacco.

The application of a strong decoction of Spearmint is said to cure chapped hands.

Mice are so averse to the smell of mint, either fresh or dried, that they will leave untouched any food where it is scattered. As mice love Henbane and often prove very destructive to a crop, it has been suggested that their depredations might be checked if some mint were planted between the rows of Henbane.

It is probable that Spearmint was introduced by the Pilgrim Fathers when they landed in America, as it is mentioned among many other plants brought out from England, in a list given by John Josselyn. When in this country apparently found growing wild, it occurs in watery places, but is rather rare.

Professor Henslow (*Origin and History of our Garden Vegetables*) does not consider it truly native to any country. He says:

'The Garden Mint (*Mentha viridis*, Linn.) is a cultivated form of *M. sylvestris* (Linn.), the Horse Mint, which is recorded as cultivated at Aleppo. Either *M. sylvestris*, or some form approaching *M. viridis*, which is not known as a truly wild plant, was probably the mint of Scripture.'

Bentham also considers it not improbably a variety of *M. sylvestris*, perpetuated through its ready propagation by suckers, and though these two plants are sufficiently distinct as found in England, yet continental forms occur which bridge over their differences.

Its generic name, *Mentha*, is derived from the mythological origin ascribed to it, and was originally applied to the mint by Theophrastus. Menthe was a nymph, who because of the love Pluto bore her, was metamorphosed by Proserpine, from motives of jealousy, into the plant we now call mint.

¶ *Description.* From creeping root-stocks, erect, square stems rise to a height of about 2 feet, bearing very short-stalked, acute-pointed, lance-shaped, wrinkled, bright green leaves, with finely toothed edges and smooth surfaces, the ribs very prominent beneath. The small flowers are densely arranged in whorls or rings in the axils of the upper leaves, forming cylindrical, slender, tapering spikes, pinkish or lilac in colour. The little labiate flowers are fol-lowed by very few, roundish, minute brown seeds. The taste and odour of the plant are very characteristic.

There are several forms of Garden Mint, the true variety being of bold, upright growth, with fairly large and broad leaves, pointed and sharply serrated (or toothed) at the edges and of a rich, bright, green colour. Another variety, sometimes sold as Spearmint (*M. cardiaca*), is much smaller and less erect in growth, with darker leaves, the whorls of flowers distant and leafy, but possessing the same odour and flavour, and another has comparatively large, broad or rounded leaves. Yet another has soft hairs, but this, though distinct from what is known as Horse Mint, is inferior to the true Spearmint.

A form with its leaves slightly crisped is common in gardens under the name of *M. crispa*.

¶ *Cultivation.* A moist situation is preferable, but mint will succeed in almost any soil when once started into growth, though in dry, sandy soils it is sometimes difficult to grow, and should be planted in the coolest and dampest situations. Leaf mould, road scrapings, burnt ash and similar materials should, on the other hand, be used freely for lightening heavy, tenacious soils. It does best in a partially shaded position: if in a sheltered spot, it will start earlier in the spring than if exposed. Where a long or regular supply is required, it is a good plan to have at least one bed in a sunny and sheltered, and another in a shady position, where gatherings may be made both early and late.

As the plant is a perennial, spreading by means of its underground, creeping stems, propagation may be easily effected by lifting the roots in February or March, dividing them – every piece showing a joint will grow – and planting again in shallow trenches, covering with 2 inches of soil. Six inches apart in the rows and 8 inches between the rows are the right distances to allow. Cuttings in summer or offsets in spring may also be utilized for increasing a stock. Cuttings may be taken at almost any time during the summer, always choosing the young shoots, these being struck on a shady border of light soil and kept moist, or a better plan, if possible, is to insert them in a frame, keeping them close and moist till rooted. Cuttings or young shoots will also strike freely in good-sized boxes in a heated greenhouse, in the early spring, and after the tops have been taken off two or three times for use, the plants may be hardened off and planted outside.

The beds are much benefited by an annual top-dressing of rich soil, applied towards the close of autumn, when all remaining stalks should be cut down to the ground. A liberal top-dressing of short, decayed manure, such as that from an old hot-bed or mushroom bed, annually, either in the spring, when it commences to grow, or better still, perhaps, after the first or second cutting, will ensure luxuriant growth. Frequent cuttings of shoots constitute a great drain on the plants, and if not properly nourished they will fail, more or less. To have really good mint, the plantation should be re-made about every three years, or failing that, it is essential that a good top-dressing of rich soil be added.

A good stock should be kept up, so that plenty may be available for *forcing*. Cultivators having a greenhouse can easily force mint into an earlier development of new growth than would be in the open garden. Forcing is very easy, the only preparation being the insertion of a quantity of good roots in a box of light soil, which should be placed in a temperature of about 60° and watered freely as soon as growth starts. Cuttings may be made in two or three weeks. Forcing will generally be necessary from November to May – a succession being kept up by the introduction, at intervals of about three weeks, of an additional supply of roots, as forced roots soon decay. Often mint is so grown both upon and under the benches in greenhouses, and the demand for the young, tender stems and leaves during the winter is sufficient to make the plants pay well.

¶ *Mint Disease.* Unfortunately, mint is susceptible to a disease which in some gardens has completely destroyed it. This disease, which from its characteristic symptoms is known as Rust, is incurable. The fungus (*Puccinia Mentha*) which causes it develops inside the plant, and therefore cannot be reached by any purgicide, and as it is perennial, it cannot be got rid of by cutting off the latter. All that can be done is to prevent the spread of the disease by digging up all plants that show any sign of rust. The same ground should not be used again for mint for several years. Healthy stock should be obtained and planted in uninfected soil, some distance away. On account of this liability of mint to rust, it is advisable not to have it all in one bed, but to have several beds of it, placed at some distance from each other.

¶ *Harvesting.* When the plants are breaking into bloom, the stalks should be cut a few inches above the root, on a dry day, after the dew has disappeared, and before the hot sun has taken any oil from the leaves, and dried for culinary use for the winter. All discoloured and insect-eaten leaves should be removed and the stems tied loosely into bunches and hung to dry on strings in the usual manner directed for 'bunched' herbs. The bunches should be nearly equal in length and uniform in size to facilitate packing, if intended for sale, and placed when dry in airtight boxes to prevent re-absorption of moisture.

The leaves may also be stripped from the stems as soon as thoroughly dry and rubbed through a fine sieve, so as to be freed from stalks as much as possible, or pounded in a mortar and thus powdered, stored in stoppered bottles or tins rendered airtight. If preparing for market and not for home use, the rubbed herbs will, of course, command a higher price than the bunched herbs, and should be put up in tins or bottles containing a quantity of uniform weight.

When mint is grown commercially on a large scale, it has been estimated to yield from 4 to 5 tons per acre, from which 15 to 20 cwt. of dry should be obtained. Average yields per acre are, however, taken when crops are at maturity, and an estimate of the first cutting crop is hard to form, and is likely to be less profitable than succeeding years, on account of initial expenses.

If Spearmint is being grown as a *medicinal* herb, for the sake of the volatile oil to be extracted from it, the shoots should be gathered in August, when just coming into flower, and taken to the distillery as soon as possible after picking, the British Pharmacopœia directing that oil of Spearmint be distilled from the fresh, flowering plant. It is estimated that 350 lb. of Spearmint yield 1 lb. of oil. If the distillery is not on the ground or only a short distance away, and the crop has to be dispatched by train, the cutting should take place late in the afternoon on a fine day, before the dew falls, so as to be sent off by a night train to arrive at their destination next morning, having travelled in the cool, otherwise the leaves are apt to heat and ferment, losing colour.

¶ *Constituents.* The chief constituent of Spearmint oil is Carvone. There are also present Phellandrine, Limonene and dihydrocarveol acetate. Esters of acetic, butyric and caproic or caprylic acids are also present. (An Ester is a combination of an alcohol with an acid, the combination being associated with the elimination of water. The esters are highly important and in many cases dominant constituents of numerous essential oils, which owe their perfume largely, or in some cases entirely, to the esters contained. Many of the esters are used as flavouring or perfumery agents, and many are among the most important constituents of volatile salts.)

There are several different essential oils

known under the name of Spearmint oil, the botanical origin of the plant used for distillation differing with the country in which the plant is grown. In the United States and in this country several varieties of *M. viridis* are distilled. In Russia the plant distilled is *M. verticellata*, and in Germany either *M. longifolia*, or more generally *M. aquatica* var. *crispa* – a plant cultivated in Northern Germany, the oil (called there *Krausemünzöl*) being imported into this country as German Spearmint oil. It appears to be identical with that from *M. viridis*. Oil of Spearmint is little distilled in England, either German oil or American oil distilled from *M. viridis* being imported.

¶ *Medicinal Action and Uses.* Spearmint is chiefly used for culinary purposes. The properties of Spearmint oil resemble those of Peppermint, being stimulant, carminative and antispasmodic, but its effects are less powerful, and it is less used than Peppermint, though it is better adapted for children's maladies. From 2 to 5 drops may be given on sugar, or from ½ to 1 teaspoonful of spirit of Spearmint, with 2 tablespoonsful of water. Spearmint oil is added to many compounds on account of its carminative properties, and because its taste is pleasanter and less strong than Peppermint. A distilled water of Spearmint will relieve hiccough and flatulence as well as the giddiness of indigestion. For infantile trouble generally, the sweetened infusion is an excellent remedy, and is also a pleasant beverage in fevers, inflammatory diseases, etc. Make the infusion by pouring a pint of boiling water on an ounce of the dried herb; the strained-off liquid is taken in doses of a wineglassful or less. It is considered a specific in allaying nausea and vomiting and will relieve the pain of colic. A homœopathic tincture prepared from the fresh plant in flower has been found serviceable in strangury, gravel, and as a local application in painful hæmorrhoids. Its principal employment is for its febrifuge and diuretic virtues.

¶ *Preparations and Dosages.* Fluid extract, ¼ to 1 drachm. Water, B.P. and U.S.P., 4 drachms. Spirit, U.S.P., 30 drops.

When eaten with lamb, very finely chopped in sweetened vinegar, in the form of mint sauce, mint greatly aids the digestion, as it makes the crude, albuminous fibres of the immature meat more digestible. The volatile oil stimulates the digestive system and prevents septic changes within the intestines.

The fresh sprigs of mint are used to flavour green peas and also new potatoes, being boiled with them, and the powdered, dried leaves are used with pea soup and also in seasonings. On the Continent, especially in Germany, the powdered, dried mint is often used at table for dusting upon pea and bean purées, as well as on gravies.

A grating of mint is introduced sometimes into a potato salad, or into a fowl stuffing, and in Wales it is not unusual to boil mint with cabbage.

Mint Jelly can be used instead of mint sauce, in the same manner as red currant jelly. It may be made by steeping mint leaves in apple jelly, or in one of the various kinds of commercial gelatine. The jelly should be a delicate shade of green. A handful of leaves should colour and flavour about half a pint of jelly. Strain the liquid through a jelly bag to remove all particles of mint before allowing to set.

Mint Vinegar is made as follows: Fill a jar or bottle with young mint leaves picked from the stalks. Cover with cold vinegar and cork or cover the bottle. Infuse for 14 days, then strain off the vinegar.

This vinegar is sometimes employed in making Mint Jelly, as follows:

Take 1 pint of water, 1¼ oz. gelatine, the white and shell of an egg, ½ gill of Mint Vinegar, 1 dessertspoonful of Tarragon Vinegar, a bunch of herbs, 1 onion, 1 carrot, a stick of celery, 10 peppercorns, salt, 1 lemon. Peel the lemon very thinly, slightly whip the white of egg, wash and crush the shell. Put all the ingredients into a pan, strain in the juice of the lemon and whisk over the fire until just on boiling point. Boil up, then draw the pan to the side of the fire and simmer very gently for 20 minutes. Strain through a jelly bag until clear. Put into a mould to set. If liked, finely chopped mint may be added to the jelly after straining it, or more mint can be used and no Tarragon Vinegar.

To make *Mint Punch*: Pick a quart of fresh mint leaves, then wash and dry them by shaking them in a clean kitchen towel. Put them into a large jug and mash them with a wooden spoon till soft, when cover with freshly boiled water and infuse for ten minutes. Strain, cool, then set on ice till required. Add two cups of chilled grape juice and strained lemon juice to taste. Sweeten with castor sugar, stir till sugar is dissolved and then add a quart of ginger ale. Fill each tumbler to one-third with cracked ice and fill up with the punch.

The Garden Mint is also the basis of Mint Julep and Mint-water, the cordial distilled from the plant.

Mint Cake is a cake made of flour and dripping or lard, flavoured with sugar and chopped fresh mint and rolled out thin.

PEPPERMINT

Mentha piperita (SM.)
N.O. Labiatæ

Synonym. Brandy Mint
Part Used. Herb
Habitat. The plant is found throughout Europe, in moist situations, along stream banks and in waste lands, and is not unfrequent in damp places in England, but is not a common native plant, and probably is often an escape from cultivation. In America it is probably even more common as an escape than Spearmint, having long been known and grown in gardens

Of the members of the mint family under cultivation the most important are the several varieties of the Peppermint (*Mentha piperita*), extensively cultivated for years as the source of the well-known volatile oil of Peppermint, used as a flavouring and therapeutic agent.

¶ *Description.* The leaves of this kind of mint are shortly but distinctly stalked, 2 inches or more in length, and ¾ to 1½ inches broad, their margins finely toothed, their surfaces smooth, both above and beneath, or only very slightly, hardly visibly, hairy on the principal veins and mid-rib on the underside. The stems, 2 to 4 feet high, are quadrangular, often purplish. The whorled clusters of little reddish-violet flowers are in the axils of the upper leaves, forming loose, interrupted spikes, and rarely bear seeds. The entire plant has a very characteristic odour, due to the volatile oil present in all its parts, which when applied to the tongue has a hot, aromatic taste at first, and afterwards produces a sensation of cold in the mouth caused by the menthol it contains.

¶ *History.* Pliny tells us that the Greeks and Romans crowned themselves with Peppermint at their feasts and adorned their tables with its sprays, and that their cooks flavoured both their sauces and their wines with its essence. Two species of mint were used by the ancient Greek physicians, but some writers doubt whether either was the modern Peppermint, though there is evidence that *M. piperita* was cultivated by the Egyptians. It is mentioned in the Icelandic Pharmacopœias of the thirteenth century, but only came into general use in the medicine of Western Europe about the middle of the eighteenth century, and then was first used in England.

It was only recognized here as a distinct species late in the seventeenth century, when the great botanist, Ray, published it in the second edition of his *Synopsis stirpium britannicorum*, 1696. Its medicinal properties were speedily recognized, and it was admitted into the London Pharmacopœia in 1721, under *M. piperitis sapore*. The oldest existing Peppermint district is in the neighbourhood of Mitcham, in Surrey, where its cultivation from a commercial point of view dates from about 1750, at which period only a few acres of ground there were devoted to medicinal plants. At the end of the eighteenth century, above 100 acres were cropped with Peppermint, but so late as 1805 there were no stills at Mitcham, and the herb had to be carried to London for the extraction of the oil. By 1850 there were already about 500 acres under cultivation at Mitcham, and at the present day the English Peppermint plantations are still chiefly located in this district, though it is grown in several other parts of England – in Herts at Hitchin, and in Cambs at Wisbech, in Lincolnshire at Market Deeping and also at Holbeach (where the cultivation and distillation of English Peppermint oil, now carried on with the most up-to-date improvements was commenced over seventy years ago).

There is room for a further extension of its cultivation, owing to the great superiority of the English product in pungency and flavour.

Most of London's supplies are grown in a triangle with its base on a line Kingston to Croydon, and its apex at Chipstead in Surrey. This triangle includes Mitcham, still the centre of the Peppermint-growing and distilling industry, the district proving to be specially suited to the crop. There are large Peppermint farms at Banstead and Cheam.

On the Continent Peppermint was first grown in 1771 at Utrecht, but it is now grown in considerable amounts in several countries. In France it is cultivated in the Departments of the Yonne and du Nord, French Peppermint Oil being distilled at Grasse and Cannes, as well as in the Basses-Alpes, Haute-Garonne and other parts, though the French varieties of *M. piperita* are not identical with those cultivated in England. The variety cultivated in France is known as 'Red Mint' and can grow on certain soils where the true Peppermint does not grow. The 'Red Mint' can be cultivated for four or five years in the same field, but the true *M. piperita* can be cultivated in the same field for two years only. 'Red Mint' gives a higher yield of oil, but is of inferior quality. In the Siagne Valley, it is calculated that 300 kilos of fresh plant produce 1 kilo of essential oil, elsewhere a yield of 2 kilos to about 1,000 kilos of stems and green leaves is claimed. It has been proved by experience that all parts of the plant do not give the same proportion of oil, and it is more abundant when the plants have been grown in a hot region and have flowered to the best advantage.

The product of absolutely genuine English plants cultivated in French soil varies according to the district, for the soil has a very important influence upon the flavour of the oil and also the climate: badly-drained ground is known to give unfavourable results both as to the quantity and quality of the oil.

An oil very similar to Mitcham oil, and of an excellent quality, is distilled from English plants grown in Italy, mostly in Piedmont and also in Sicily. Next to the essential oils of lemon and orange, that obtained from Peppermint enjoys a high reputation among the numerous volatile oils produced by Italy. Vigone and Pancalieri are the centres of the cultivation and distillation of Peppermint in the province of Turin. This district, which has been designated the 'Mitcham of Italy,' yields annually about 11,000,000 kilograms of Peppermint, from which 25,000 to 27,000 kilograms of essential oil are obtained. A new variety of Peppermint, found at Lutra on the island of Tino, in the Grecian Archipelago, has been cultivated in the Royal Colonial Garden at Palermo.

A small amount of Peppermint oil of good quality is distilled from plantations in Germany, at Miltitz, in Saxony and near Leipzig, where the little town of Colleda, before the War, produced annually as much as 40,000 cwt. of the herb. Russia also produces some Peppermint, in the Ukraine and the Caucasus, but most of it is used in the country itself.

With regard to Hungarian oil of Peppermint, organized effort to secure improvement began in 1904 and has been greatly developed. Hungarian oil compares favourably with American oil of Peppermint as regards percentage of Menthol contained: Hungarian oil yielding 43 to 56 per cent. of free menthol, and 35 to 65 per cent. of total menthol; while American oil yields 40 to 45 per cent. free menthol and 60 per cent. total menthol.

Peppermint oil distilled in 1914 from Mitcham plants grown at Molo, in the highlands of British East Africa, possesses a most excellent aroma, quite free of bitterness, and a very high figure indeed for the menthol contained, and there is no question that this source of supply should be an important one in the future.

The United States, however, are now the most important producers of Peppermint oil, producing – mostly in Michigan, where its cultivation was introduced in 1855, Indiana, the western districts of New York State, and to a smaller extent in Ohio – rather under half of the world's total output of the oil. The whole of the Peppermint cultivation is confined to the north-east portion of the United States, and the extreme south of Canada, where some is grown in the province of Ontario. The first small distillery was erected in Wayne County, New York State, in the early part of last century, and at the present day the industry has increased to such an extent, that there are portions of Michigan where thousands of acres are planted with nothing else but Peppermint.

English oil is incomparably the best, but it fetches a very high price, and the French oil, though much inferior, is of finer quality than the American.

The problem is to obtain a strain of mint plants which would yield larger quantities of oil in our climate. It is possible that varieties yielding a more abundant supply of essential oils might be secured by persistent endeavour, without reducing our English standard of refinement. Also economy in harvesting and distilling should be studied. If our English oils could be reduced in price, they would replace the foreign to a greater or less extent depending upon the reduction in cost of production.

There are several varieties of Peppermint. The two chief, the so-called 'Black' and 'White' mints are the ones extensively cultivated. Botanically there is little difference between them, but the stems and leaves of the 'Black' mint are tinged purplish-brown, while the stems of the 'White' variety are green, and the leaves are more coarsely serrated in the White. The oil furnished by the Black is of inferior quality, but more abundant than that obtained from the White, the yield of oil from which is generally only about four-fifths of that from an equal area of the Black, but it has a more delicate odour and obtains a higher price. The plant is also more delicate, being easily destroyed by frost or drought; it is principally grown for drying in bundles – technically termed 'bunching,' and is the kind chiefly dried for herbalists, the Black variety being more generally grown for the oil on account of its greater productivity and hardiness. The variety grown at Mitcham is classified by some authorities as *M. piperita*, var. *rubra*.

¶ *Cultivation.* Both Peppermint and Spearmint thrive best in a fairly warm, preferably moist climate, and in deep soils rich in humus and retentive of moisture, but fairly open in texture and well drained, either naturally or artificially.

These conditions are frequently combined in effectively drained swamp lands, but the plants may also be commercially cultivated in well-prepared upland soils, such as would produce good corn, oil or potatoes. Though a moist situation is preferable, Peppermint will succeed in most soils, when once started into growth and carefully cultivated. It flourishes well in what are known in America as muck land, that is, those broad level areas, often several thousand acres in extent, of deep fertile soil, the beds of ancient lakes and swamps where the remains of ages of growths of aquatic vegetation have accumulated. In Michigan and Indiana, where there are large areas of such land, mint culture has become highly specialized, a considerable part of the acreage being controlled by a few well-equipped growers able to handle the product in an economical manner, who have of late years installed their own up-to-date distilling plants. The cultivation of Peppermint is a growing industry now also on the reclaimed lands of Louisiana.

The usual method of mint cultivation on these farms in America is to dig runners in the early spring and lay them in shallow trenches, 3 feet apart in well-prepared soil. The growing crop is kept well cultivated and absolutely free from weeds and in the summer when the plant is in full bloom, the mint is cut by hand and distilled in straw. A part of the exhausted herb is dried and used for cattle food, for which it possesses considerable value. The rest is cut and composted and eventually ploughed into the ground as fertilizer.

The area selected for Peppermint growing should be cropped for one or two years with some plant that requires a frequent tillage. The tillage is also continued as long as possible during the growth of the mint, for successful mint-growing implies clean culture at all stages of progress.

In one of our chief English plantations the following mode of cultivation is adopted. A rich and friable soil, retentive of moisture is selected, and the ground is well tilled 8 to 10 inches deep. The plants are propagated in the spring, usually in April and May. When the young shoots from the crop of the previous year have attained a height of about 4 inches, they are pulled up and transplanted into new soil, in shallow furrows about 2 feet apart, lightly covered with about 2 inches of soil. They grow vigorously the first year and throw out numerous stolons and runners on the surface of the ground. After the crop has been removed, these are allowed to harden or become woody, and then farmyard manure is scattered over the field and ploughed in. In this way the stolons are divided into numerous pieces and covered with soil before the frost sets in, otherwise if the autumn is wet, they are liable to become sodden and rot, and the next crop fails. In the spring the fields are dressed with Peruvian Guano.

¶ *Manuring*. Liberal manuring is essential, and the quantity and nature of the manure has a great effect on the characteristics of the oil. Mineral salts are found to be of much value. *Nitrate of Soda*, applied at the rate of 50 to 150 lb. to the acre both stimulates the growth of foliage and improves the quality of the essence. Half the total quantity should be applied a month before planting and the remainder a month before the harvest. *Potash*, also, is particularly useful against a form of chlorosis or 'rust' (*Puccinia menthœ*) due, apparently, to too much water in the soil, as it often appears after moist, heavy weather in August, which causes the foliage to drop off and leave the stems almost bare, in which circumstances the rust is liable to attack the plants. Some authorities have calculated that an acre of Peppermint requires 84 lb. of Nitrogen, 37 lb. of Phosphoric Acid and 139 lb. of Potash. Ground Bone and Lime do not seem to be of marked benefit. The top dressing of the running roots with fine loam either by ploughing as above described, or otherwise, is very essential before winter sets in.

In the south of France, sewage (1,300 lb. per acre) is extensively used, together with Sesame seeds from which the oil has been expressed. The latter are especially suited for light and limey soils, and are either worked in before planting or placed directly in the furrows with the plants. Up to 5,000 or 6,000 lb. per acre are applied, giving a crop of from 2,100 to 2,600 lb. per acre. The residues from the distillation of the crop are invariably used as manure. It is found, however, that although these manures supply sufficient nitrogen, they are deficient in phosphoric acid and potash. This shortage must be made up by chemical manures, otherwise the soil will become exhausted. Chemical manures *alone* are equally unsatisfactory in soils poor in organic matter. In conjunction with organic manures they give excellent results.

On suitable soil and with proper cultivation, yields of from 2 to 3 tons of Peppermint herb per acre may be expected, but large yields can only be expected from fields that are in the best possible condition. A fair average for well-managed commercial plantings may be said to be 30 lb. of oil per acre, but the yield of oil is always variable, ranging from only a few pounds to, in extremely favourable cases, nearly 100 lb. per acre. About 325 lb. of Peppermint, nearly 3 cwt., are required to produce a pound of oil in commercial practice, i.e. about 7 lb. of oil are generally obtained from 1 ton of the herb. The price varies as widely as the yield, the value depending upon the chemical composition.

The presence of weeds among the Peppermint, especially other species of *Mentha*, is an important cause of deterioration to the oil. *M. arvensis*, the Corn Mint, if allowed to settle and increase among the crop to such an extent as not to be easily separated, has been known when distilled to absolutely ruin the flavour of the latter. In new ground the Peppermint requires handweeding two or three times, as the hoe cannot be used without injury to the plant.

In America great detriment is occasioned by the growth of *Erigeron canadensis*, and newly cleared ground planted with Peppermint, is liable to the intrusion of another plant of the order Compositæ, *Erechtites hieracifolia*, which is also highly injurious to the quality of the oil.

¶ *Irrigation.* Peppermint requires frequent irrigation. In the south of France the crop is irrigated on the 15th of May, and thereafter every eight or ten days. When the plants are fully developed they are watered at least three times a week. It is important to keep the soil constantly moist, although well drained. Absorption of water makes the shoots more tender, thus facilitating cutting, and causes a large quantity of green matter to be produced.

A plantation lasts about four years, the best output being the second year. The fourth-year crop is rarely good. A crop that yields a high percentage of essential oil exhausts the ground as a rule, and after cropping with Peppermint for four years, the land must be put to some other purpose for at least seven years. In some parts of France the plantations are renewed annually with the object of obtaining vigorous plants.

Few pests trouble Peppermint, though crickets, grasshoppers and caterpillars may always do some damage.

¶ *Harvesting.* The herb is cut just before flowering, from the end of July to the end of August in England and France, according to local conditions. Sometimes when well irrigated and matured, a second crop can be obtained in September. With new plantations the harvest is generally early in September.

Harvesting should be carried out on a dry, sunny day, in the late morning, when all traces of dew have disappeared. The first year's crop is always cut with the sickle to prevent injury to the stolons. The herb of the second and third years is cut with scythes and then raked into loose heaps ready for carting to the stills.

In many places, the custom is to let the herb lie on the ground for a time in these small bundles or cocks. In other countries the herb is distilled as soon as cut. Again, certain distillers prefer the plants to be previously dried or steamed. The subject is much debated, but the general opinion is that it is best to distil as soon as cut, and the British Pharmacopœia directs that the oil be distilled from the fresh flowering plant. Even under the best conditions of drying, there is a certain loss of essential oil. If the herbs lie in heaps for any time, fermentation is bound to occur, reducing the quality and quantity of the oil, as laboratory experiments have proved. Should it be impossible to treat all the crop as cut, it should be properly dried on the same system as that adopted for other medicinal plants. The loss is then small. Variation in the chemical composition of the essence should be brought about by manuring, rather than by the system of harvesting, though in America the loss caused by partial drying in the field is not regarded by growers as sufficient to offset the increased cost of handling and distilling the green herb. Exposure to frost must, however, be avoided, as frozen mint yields scarcely half the quantity of oil which could otherwise be secured.

At Market Deeping the harvest usually commences in the beginning or middle of August, or as soon as the plant begins to flower and lasts for six weeks, the stills being kept going night and day. The herb is carted direct from the fields to the stills, which are made of copper and contain about 5 cwt. of the herb. Before putting the Peppermint into the still, water is poured in to a depth of about 2 feet, at which height a false bottom is placed, and on this the herb is then trodden down by men. The lid is then let down, and under pressure the distillation is conducted by the application of direct heat at the lowest possible temperature, and is continued for about $4\frac{1}{2}$ hours. The lid is then removed, and the false bottom with the Peppermint resting on it is raised by a windlass, and the Peppermint carried away in the empty carts on their return journey to the fields, where it is placed in heaps and allowed to rot, being subsequently mixed with manure applied to the fields in the autumn.

The usual yield of oil, if the season be warm and dry, is 1 oz. from 5 lb. of the fresh flowering plant, but if wet and unfavourable, the product is barely half that quantity.

If the cut green tops have some distance to travel to the distillery, they should be cut late in the afternoon, so as to be sent off by a night train to arrive at their destination next morning, or they would be apt to heat and ferment and lose colour.

Since the oil is the chief marketable product, adequate distilling facilities and a market for the oil are essential to success in the industry, and the prospective Peppermint grower should assure himself on these points before investing capital in plantations.

There is also a market, chiefly for herbalists, for the dried herb, which is gathered at the same time of year. It should be cut shortly above the base, leaving some leaf-buds, and not including the lowest shrivelled or discoloured leaves and tied loosely into bundles by the stalk-ends, about twenty to the bundle on the average, and the bundles of equal length, about 6 inches, to facilitate packing, and dried over strings as described for Spearmint. Two or three days will be sufficient to dry.

Peppermint culture on suitable soils gives fair average returns when intelligently conducted from year to year. The product, however, is liable to fluctuation in prices, and the cost of establishing the crop and the annual expenses of cultivation are high.

¶ *Constituents.* Among essential oils, Peppermint ranks first in importance. It is a colourless, yellowish or greenish liquid, with a peculiar, highly penetrating odour and a burning, camphorescent taste. It thickens and becomes reddish with age, but improves in mellowness, even if kept as long as ten or fourteen years.

The chief constituent of Peppermint oil is Menthol, but it also contains menthyl acetate and isovalerate, together with menthone, cineol, inactive pinene, limonene and other less important bodies.

On cooling to a low temperature, separation of Menthol occurs, especially if a few crystals of that substance be added to start crystallization.

The value of the oil depends much upon the composition. The principal ester constituent, menthyl acetate, possesses a very fragrant minty odour, to which the agreeable aroma of the oil is largely due. The alcoholic constituent, Menthol, possesses the well-known penetrating minty odour and characteristic cooling taste. The flavouring properties of the oil are due largely to both the ester and alcoholic constituents, while the medicinal value is attributed to the latter only. The most important determination to be made in the examination of Peppermint oil, is that of the total amount of Menthol, but the Menthone value is also frequently required. The English oil contains 60 to 70 per cent. of Menthol, the Japanese oil containing 85 per cent., and the American less than ours, only about 50 per cent. The odour and taste afford a good indication of the quality of the oil, and by this means it is quite possible to distinguish between English, American and Japanese oils.

Menthol is obtained from various species of *Mentha* and is imported into England, chiefly from Japan. The oils from which it is chiefly obtained are those from *M. arvensis*, var. *piperascens*, in Japan, *M. arvensis*, var. *glabrata* in China, and *M. piperita* in America.

Japan, and to a certain extent China, produce large quantities of Peppermint oil distilled from the plants just mentioned. The oils produced from these plants are greatly inferior to those distilled from *M. piperita*, but have the advantage of containing a large proportion of Menthol, of which they are the commercial source.

The Japanese Menthol plant is now being grown in South Australia, having been introduced there by the Germans from Japan.

Chinese Peppermint oil is largely distilled at Canton, a considerable quantity being sent to Bombay, also a large quantity of Menthol. Peppermint is chiefly cultivated in the province of Kiang-si.

M. incana, cultivated near Bombay as a herb, also possesses the flavour of Peppermint.

M. arvensis, var. *javanesa*, growing in Ceylon, has not the flavour of Peppermint, but that of the garden mint, while the type form of *M. arvensis*, growing wild in Great Britain, has an odour so different from Peppermint that it has to be carefully removed from the field lest it should spoil the flavour of the Peppermint oil when the herb is distilled.

The Japanese have long recognized the value of Menthol, and over 200 years ago carried it about with them in little silver boxes hanging from their girdles. The distillation of oil of Peppermint forms a considerable industry in Japan. The chief centre of cultivation is the province of Uzen, in the north-east of the island of Hondo, the largest of the Japanese Islands, and much is grown in the northern island of Hokkaido, but the best oil is produced in the southern districts of Okayama and Hiroshimo, the second largest Peppermint area in Japan, the yield of mint being yearly on the increase. The mint crop is a favourite one for farmers, owing to the distilling work it furnishes during the long and otherwise unprofitable winter.

The roots are planted at the end of November and beginning of December. The plant, which needs a light, well-drained soil, attains its full growth during the summer months and is cut in the latter part of July, during August and in the early part of September, three cuttings being made during the season. The third cutting yields the greatest percentage of oil and menthol crystals. The preliminary steps in the manufacture of Menthol are carried out by the farmers themselves, with the aid of stills of a simple design. The Peppermint plants are first dried in sheds, or under cover from the sun for thirty days. Then they are placed in the stills where they undergo a process of steaming. The resulting vapours are led off through pipes into cooling chambers, are condensed and deposited as crude Peppermint oil. This crude Peppermint is shipped to Yokohama and Kobe to the Menthol factories, of which there are over seventy in various parts of Japan, specially equipped for obtaining the full amount of Menthol. The residue of dementholized oil is further refined to the standard of purity required in the trade, and is known as Japanese Peppermint oil. The oil (known in Japan under the name of *Hakka no abura*) is exported from Hiogo and Osaka, but is frequently adulterated. The cheapest variety of Peppermint oil available in commerce is this partially dementholized oil imported from Japan, containing only 50 per cent. of Menthol.

Adulteration of American Peppermint oil with dementholized Japanese oil, known as Menthene, which is usually cheaper than American oil, is frequently practised. The failure of the mint crop in America in 1925 and the consequent scarcity and high price of the American oil caused this adulteration to be very extensive.

The Japanese oil, termed by the Americans Corn-Mint oil and not recognized by the United States Pharmacopœia, is at best only a substitute in confectionery and other products, such as tooth-pastes, etc. There are other varieties of so-called Peppermint oil on the market which are residues from Menthol-manufacture and are inferior even to the oil imported from Japan. These are not suitable for use in pharmacy.

As Japanese Peppermint oil, after being freed from Menthol crystals, is inferior both in taste and odour to English and American oil, experiments have been made in Japan with the cultivation of English and American Peppermint, but so far without success.

¶ *Adulterants.* Camphor oil is occasionally used as an adulterant of Peppermint oil, also Cedarwood oil and oil of African Copaiba. The oil is also often adulterated with one-third part of rectified spirit, which may be detected by the milkiness produced when the oil is agitated by water. Oil of Rosemary and oil of Turpentine are sometimes used for the same purpose. If the oil contains turpentine it will explode with iodine. If quite pure, it dissolves in its own weight of rectified spirits of wine.

In the form in which Menthol is imported, it bears some resemblance to Epsom Salts, with which it is sometimes adulterated.

Before the War about half the Menthol crystals exported from Japan were sent to Germany. During the War the United States became the largest purchaser of these crystals, followed in order by Great Britain, France and British India.

¶ *Medicinal Action and Uses.* Peppermint oil is the most extensively used of all the volatile oils, both medicinally and commercially. The characteristic anti-spasmodic action of the volatile oil is more marked in this than in any other oil, and greatly adds to its power of relieving pains arising in the alimentary canal.

From its stimulating, stomachic and carminative properties, it is valuable in certain forms of dyspepsia, being mostly used for flatulence and colic. It may also be employed for other sudden pains and for cramp in the abdomen; wide use is made of Peppermint in cholera and diarrhœa.

It is generally combined with other medicines when its stomachic effects are required, being also employed with purgatives to prevent griping. Oil of Peppermint allays sickness and nausea, and is much used to disguise the taste of unpalatable drugs, as it imparts its aromatic characteristics to whatever prescription it enters into. It is used as an infants' cordial.

The oil itself is often given on sugar and added to pills, also a spirit made from the oil, but the preparation in most general use is Peppermint Water, which is the oil and water distilled together.

Peppermint Water and spirit of Peppermint are official preparations of the British Pharmacopœia.

In flatulent colic, spirit of Peppermint in hot water is a good household remedy, also the oil given in doses of one or two drops on sugar.

Peppermint is good to assist in raising internal heat and inducing perspiration, although its strength is soon exhausted. In slight colds or early indications of disease, a free use of Peppermint tea will, in most cases, effect a cure, an infusion of 1 ounce of the dried herb to a pint of boiling water being employed, taken in wineglassful doses; sugar and milk may be added if desired.

An infusion of equal quantities of Peppermint herb and Elder flowers (to which either Yarrow or Boneset may be added) will banish a cold or mild attack of influenza within thirty-six hours, and there is no danger of an overdose or any harmful action on the heart. Peppermint tea is used also for palpitation of the heart.

In cases of hysteria and nervous disorders, the usefulness of an infusion of Peppermint has been found to be well augmented by the addition of equal quantities of Wood Betony, its operation being hastened by the addition to the infusion of a few drops of tincture of Caraway.

¶ *Preparations.* Fluid extract, ¼ to 1 drachm. Oil, ½ to 3 drops. Spirit, B.P., 5 to 20 drops. Water, B.P. and U.S.P., 4 drachms.

The following simple preparation has been found useful in insomnia:

1 oz. Peppermint herb, cut fine, ½ oz. Rue herb, ½ oz. Wood Betony. Well mix and place a large tablespoonful in a teacup, fill with boiling water, stir and cover for twenty minutes, strain and sweeten, and drink the warm infusion on going to bed.

A very useful and harmless preparation for children during teething is prepared as follows:

½ oz. Peppermint herb, ½ oz. Scullcap herb, ¼ oz. Pennyroyal herb. Pour on 1 pint of boiling water, cover and let it stand in a warm place thirty minutes. Strain and sweeten to taste, and given frequently in teaspoonful doses, warm.

Boiled in milk and drunk hot, Peppermint herb is good for abdominal pains. 'Aqua Mirabilis' is a term applied on the Continent to an aromatic water which is taken for internal pains. It is a water distilled from herbs, sometimes used in the following form:

Cinnamon oil, Fennel oil, Lavender oil, Peppermint oil, Rosemary oil, Sage oil, of each 1 part; Spirit, 350 parts; Distilled water, 644 parts.

Menthol is used in medicine to relieve the pain of rheumatism, neuralgia, throat affections and toothache. It acts also as a local anæsthetic, vascular stimulant and disinfectant. For neuralgia, rheumatism and lumbago it is used in plasters and rubbed on the temples; it will frequently cure neuralgic headaches. It is inhaled for chest complaints, and nasal catarrh, laryngitis or bronchitis are often alleviated by it. It is also used internally as a stimulant or carminative. On account of its anæsthetic effect on the nerve-endings of the stomach, it is of use to prevent sea-sickness, the dose being ½ to 2 grains. The bruised fresh leaves of the plant will, if applied, relieve local pains and headache, and in rheumatic affections the skin may be painted beneficially with the oil.

Oil of Peppermint has been recommended in puerperal fevers. 30 to 40 minims, in divided doses, in the twenty-four hours, have been employed with satisfactory results, a stimulating aperient preceding its use.

The local anæsthetic action of Peppermint oil is exceptionally strong. It is also powerfully antiseptic, the two properties making it valuable in the relief of toothache and in the treatment of cavities in the teeth.

Sanitary engineers use Peppermint oil to test the tightness of pipe joints. It has the faculty of making its escape, and by its pungent odour betraying the presence of leaks.

A new use for Peppermint oil has been found in connexion with the gas-mask drill on the vessels of the United States Navy.

Paste may be kept almost any length of time by the use of the essential oil of Peppermint to prevent mould.

Rats dislike Peppermint, a fact that is made use of by ratcatchers, who, when clearing a building of rats, will block up most of their holes with rags soaked in oil of Peppermint and drive them by ferrets through the remaining holes into bags.

See PENNYROYAL.

MINT, WILD

Mentha sativa (LINN.)
N.O. Labiatæ

Synonyms. Water or Marsh Mint. Whorled Mint. Hairy Mint
Part Used. Herb
Habitat. Common in Britain and found all over temperate and Northern Europe and Russian Asia

¶ *Description.* A rather coarse perennial 1 to 1½ feet high; leaves conspicuously stalked, ovate or oval-ovate, or oval-rounded or wedge-shaped at the base, subacute or acute serrate or crenate serrate, more or less hairy on both sides; flowers in whorls, usually all separate, beginning about or below the middle of the stem; bracts large, similar to leaves, sometimes the upper ones minute, uppermost ones often without flowers; bracteoles strap-shaped, subulate, hairy, shorter than flowers; pedicels hairy, rarely glabrous; calyx hairy, campanulate-cylindrical; teeth triangular, acuminate, half the length of tube, bristly, hairy; corolla scarcely twice as long as the calyx, hairy without and within; nucules rough with small points.

¶ *Medicinal and Other Uses.* The herb is considered to have emetic, stimulant, and astringent qualities, and is used in diarrhœa and as an emmenagogue. The infusion of 1 oz. of the dried herb to 1 pint of boiling water is taken in wineglassful doses.

MINT, CORN

Mentha arvensis
N.O. Labiatæ

Habitat. It is a perennial, the root-stock, as in all the Mints, creeping freely, so that when the plant has once taken hold of the ground it becomes very difficult to eradicate it, as its long creeping roots bind the soil together and ultimately overrun a considerable area. It is generally an indication that the drainage of the land has been neglected. It is abundantly distributed throughout Britain, though less common in the northern counties and flourishes in fields and moist ground, and Peppermint growers must be ever watchful for its appearance

The Corn Mint (*Mentha arvensis*) is the type species of the Japanese Menthol plant, but is not endowed with useful medicinal properties, great care indeed, as has been mentioned, having to be taken to eradicate it from Peppermint plantations, for if mingled with that valuable herb in distilling its strong odour affects the quality of the oil.

¶ *Description.* It is a branched, downy plant.

From the low, spreading, quadrangular stems that lie near the ground, the flowering stems are each year thrown up, 6 to 12 inches high. The leaves, springing from the stems, in pairs, are stalked, their outlines freely toothed. The upper leaves are smaller than the lower, and the flowers are arranged in rings (whorls) in their axils. The flowers themselves are small individually, but the delicacy of their colour and the dense clusters in which they grow, give an importance collectively, as ring after ring of the blossoms form as a whole a conspicuous head. The flowering season lasts throughout August and September.

This mint varies considerably in appearance in different plants, like all the other native species of mint, some being much larger than others, with a more developed foliage and a much greater hairiness of all the parts. It has a strong odour that becomes more decided still when the leaves are bruised in any way.

It is said that the effect of this plant, when animals eat it, is to prevent coagulation of their milk, so that it can hardly be made to yield cheese.

MINT, WILD WATER

Mentha aquatica (LINN.)
N.O. Labiatæ

Mentha aquatica, the Wild Mint, Water Mint or Marsh Mint in its many variations (of which *M. sativa*, the Hairy Mint, is by most botanists considered to be one, and not a distinct species), is the commonest of the Mints, growing abundantly 1 to 2 feet high, in extensive masses in wet places, banks of rivers and marshes, and well distinguished by its downy foliage and whorls of lilac flowers, which towards the summit of the stem are crowded into globose heads. The scent of the plant is strong and unpleasant to modern idea, but Dononæus says:

'The savour of scent of Mynte rejoiceth man, wherefore they sow and strow the wild Mynthe in this countrie in places where feasts are kept, and in Churches. The juyce of Mynte mingled with honied water cureth the payne of the eares when dropped therein, and taketh away the asperitie and roughness of the tongue when it is rubbed or washed therewith.'

The dried herb yields about 4 per cent. of essential oil, having an odour of Pennyroyal, the characters of which are not well determined. Russian Spearmint oil is derived from a form of this species.

¶ *Medicinal Action and Uses.* Emetic, stimulant and astringent. Used in herbal medicine in diarrhœa and as an emmenagogue, the infusion of 1 oz. of the dried herb to 1 pint of boiling water being taken in wineglassful doses.

In severe cold and influenza, or in any complaint where it is necessary to set up perspiration and in all inflammatory complaints, internal or external, the tea made from this plant may be taken warm as freely as the patient pleases. It can be used in conjunction with stomach remedies and in difficult menstruation. A strong infusion is inclined to be emetic.

A decoction of Water Mint prepared with vinegar is recommended to stop blood vomiting.

Pliny, describing the cultivation of mint, observes that the original name was *Mintha*, 'from which the Latin *Mentha* was derived, but of late it has been called Hedyosmon,' i.e. the sweet-scented. He speaks of 'a wild kind of Mint known to us as *Menastrum*.' This name was used in the fourteenth century for the Water Mint (*M. aquatica*).

Culpepper says it is good for the gravel, and in flatulent colics.

MINT, CURLED

Mentha acrispa

Mentha crispa, which has wavy, broad, sharply-toothed leaves, woolly beneath, is a variety of *M. aquatica*. It is sometimes found in Britain in gardens and has quite a different odour to that of the common Wild Water Mint.

MINT, BERGAMOT

Mentha citrata

Synonym. Mentha odorata

Mentha citrata (Ehr.), syn. *M. odorata*, the Bergamot Mint, by some botanists considered a separate species, is by others looked on as a variety of *M. aquatica*.

The whole plant is smooth, dotted with yellow glands and is of a dark green colour, generally tinged with purple, especially the margins of the leaves, which are finelly toothed. There are very conspicuous lines of yellow glands on the purple calyx.

This Mint has a very pleasant, aromatic, lemon-like odour, somewhat resembling that of the Bergamot Orange, or that of the Oswego Tea (*Monarda didyma*), also called Bergamot, and its leaves like those of the latter can be employed in pot-pourri.

It is found in wet places in Staffordshire and Wales, though very rarely, but is often cultivated in gardens.

MINT, ROUND-LEAVED

Mentha rotundifolia
N.O. Labiatæ

Synonym. Egyptian Mint

Mentha rotundifolia is a sturdy plant having the habit of *M. sylvestris*, but is more branched. The leaves are very broad, somewhat resembling those of Sage, dull green in colour and much wrinkled above, often densely woolly and whitish beneath. The flowers are pink or white, in tapering, terminal spikes.

This species has somewhat the flavour of Spearmint, but is stronger. It is frequently found on the ruins of monasteries, the monks having used it for the languor following epileptic fits, as it was considered refreshing to the brain. It is sometimes found cultivated in cottage gardens under the name of Egyptian Mint.

The American Horsemint (*Monarda punctata*, Linn.) is of considerable importance, as it may before long be available as a regular source of Thymol, which has hitherto been manufactured principally from Ajowan seeds. It yields from 1 to 3 per cent. of a volatile oil, which contains a large proportion of Thymol, up to 61 per cent. having been obtained; Carvacrol also appears to be a constituent. The oil has a specific gravity of 0·930 to 0·940 and on prolonged standing deposits crystals of Thymol.

In 1907, Horsemint was observed to occur in abundance as a common weed on the sandy lands of central Florida, and the preliminary examinations of the oil from the wild plants which were made at that time seemed to indicate that a promising commercial source of Thymol could be developed by bringing this plant under cultivation and selecting for propagation types of plants best suited for oil production.

The leaf area of the wild plants is rather small: the first problem, therefore, seemed to be to increase the leaf area and thus increase the yield of oil per acre.

During several years of experiment, selection was also made to increase the size of the plants in order that the tonnage of herb per acre might be increased. This was also successful and a considerably increased yield was noted year by year.

In 1912 a series of fertilizer experiments was carried out. It was found that although certain special methods of treatment had a marked effect on the percentage of yield of oil and of Thymol in the oil, the greatest yield was obtained by promoting the growth of the plant and thus securing the largest possible yield of herb per acre.

On the scarcity of Thymol becoming acute on the outbreak of the Great War, the United States Department of Agriculture took up the matter, entered thoroughly into the question of utilizing the native American plant for the source of the valued product, and carried out exhaustive experiments in 1914 and 1915 as to the cultivation of the plant, the extraction of Thymol, the yield per acre and the commercial prospects of the cultivation of the plant, the conclusions arrived at being that the use is now warranted of the improved form of the plant – its luxuriance increased by cultivation – being used for the commercial production of Thymol in the United States.

It has been shown that Horsemint can be grown on the lighter types of soil at comparatively little expense, and as the cost of transportation for the finished product, Thymol, is very low, it would seem that the production of this crop might be profitable when grown in connexion with other oil-yielding plants for which a distilling apparatus is required. Distillation of the Horsemint herb is carried on by the usual methods in practice for distilling such volatile oils as Peppermint and Spearmint.

HORSEMINT

Mentha sylvestris (LINN.)
N.O. Labiatæ

The English Horsemint (*Mentha sylvestris*) is a strong-scented plant, frequent in damp, waste ground, usually growing in masses, with downy, egg-shaped leaves tapering to a point, with finely toothed margins, their undersides very white with silky hairs. The flowers are in thick cylindrical spikes, which are often interrupted below; the corollas are lilac in colour and hairy.

The taste and odour of the plant resemble those of the Garden Mint.

The dry herb yields about 1 per cent. of essential oil, having carminative and stimulant properties.

Culpepper says:

'It is good for wind and colic in the stomach. . . . The juice, laid on warm, helps the King's evil or kernels in the throat. . . . The decoction or distilled water helps a stinking breath, proceeding from corruption of the teeth; and snuffed up the nose, purges the head. It helps the scurf or dandruff of the head used with vinegar.'

HORSEMINT, AMERICAN

Monarda punctata (LINN.)
N.O. Labiatæ

Synonyms. Monarda lutea. Spotted Monarda
Part Used. Whole herb

¶ *Description*. In 1569 a doctor of Seville, Nicolas Monardes, wrote a great book, in Spanish, making known the medicinal plants of the New World, and the genus *Monarda* was named in his honour.

Monarda punctata is a perennial herb, growing in dry, sandy places. It has a strong erect stem, reaching 2 feet or more in height, with lanceolate, opposite leaves, 2 to 4 inches long, dotted on the under-surface with glands. The flowers form dense whorls, one being terminal, and have a large yellow corolla, the upper lip being spotted with purple. A circle of large, leaf-like bracts, purplish-pink in colour, surrounds them.

The plant, which is hardy, was introduced into England in 1714. The odour is strong and aromatic, the taste pungent and slightly bitter.

Wild Basil (*Pycnanthemum incanum*) is said to be often substituted for it in the United States.

¶ *Constituents*. The active virtues depend on the abundant volatile oil, which has been found to contain a hydrocarbon, thymol, and higher oxygenated compounds. It yields its virtues to boiling water, but particularly to alcohol.

Oleum Monardæ or Oil of Horsemint is official in the United States.

¶ *Medicinal Action and Uses*. Rubefacient, stimulant, carminative. The infusion is used for flatulent colic, sickness, and as a diaphoretic and emmenagogue, or as a diuretic in urinary disorders.

The principal use is external, and in its pure state it may be a vesicant. It should be diluted with olive oil or soap liniment, two or four parts of either being added to one of oil of Monarda. It may be employed in chronic rheumatism, cholera infantum, or whenever rubefacients are required.

It may be taken like Hedeoma, or American Pennyroyal.

¶ *Dosage*. Two to 10 minims of oil.

¶ *Other Species*.
M. Didyma and *M. Squarrosa* may be used as substitutes.

M. Fistulosa (Wild Bergamot, or Oswego Tea) is an active diuretic.

M. citriodora, or Prairie Bergamot, contains a phenol and a citral.

SWEET HORSEMINT is a name of *Cunila origanoides*, the essential oil of which is a stimulant aromatic.

See BERGAMOT.

MISTLETOE

Viscum album (LINN.)
N.O. Loranthaceæ

Synonyms. Birdlime Mistletoe. Herbe de la Croix. Mystyldene. Lignum Crucis
Parts Used. Leaves and young twigs, berries

The well-known Mistletoe is an evergreen parasitic plant, growing on the branches of trees, where it forms pendent bushes, 2 to 5 feet in diameter. It will grow and has been found on almost any deciduous tree, preferring those with soft bark, and being, perhaps, commonest on old Apple trees, though it is frequently found on the Ash, Hawthorn, Lime and other trees. On the Oak, it grows very seldom. It has been found on the Cedar of Lebanon and on the Larch, but very rarely on the Pear tree.

When one of the familiar sticky berries of the Mistletoe comes into contact with the bark of a tree – generally through the agency of birds – after a few days it sends forth a thread-like root, flattened at the extremity like the proboscis of a fly. This finally pierces the bark and roots itself firmly in the growing wood, from which it has the power of selecting and appropriating to its own use, such juices as are fitted for its sustenance: the wood of Mistletoe has been found to contain twice as much potash, and five times as much phosphoric acid as the wood of the foster tree. Mistletoe is a true parasite, for at no period does it derive nourishment from the soil, or from decayed bark, like some of the fungi do – all its nourishment is obtained from its *host.* The root becomes woody and thick.

¶ *Description.* The stem is yellowish and smooth, freely forked, separating when dead into bone-like joints. The leaves are tongue-shaped, broader towards the end, 1 to 3 inches long, very thick and leathery, of a dull yellow-green colour, arranged in pairs, with very short footstalks. The flowers, small and inconspicuous, are arranged in threes, in close short spikes or clusters in the forks of the branches, and are of two varieties, the male and female occurring on different plants. Neither male nor female flowers have a corolla, the parts of the fructification springing from the yellowish calyx. They open in May. The fruit is a globular, smooth, white berry, ripening in December.

Mistletoe is found throughout Europe, and in this country is particularly common in Herefordshire and Worcestershire. In Scotland it is almost unknown.

The genus *Viscum* has thirty or more species. In South Africa there are several, one with very minute leaves, a feature common to many herbs growing in that excessively dry climate; one in Australia is densely woolly, from a similar cause. Several members of the family are not parasitic at all, being shrubs and trees, showing that the parasitic habit is an acquired one, and now, of course, hereditary.

Mistletoe is always produced by seed and cannot be cultivated in the earth like other plants, hence the ancients considered it to be an excrescence of the tree. By rubbing the berries on the smooth bark of the underside of the branches of trees till they adhere, or inserting them in clefts made for the purpose, it is possible to grow Mistletoe quite successfully, if desired.

The thrush is the great disseminator of the Mistletoe, devouring the berries eagerly, from which the Missel Thrush is said by some to derive its name. The stems and foliage have been given to sheep in winter, when fodder was scarce, and they are said to eat it with relish.

In Brittany, where the Mistletoe grows so abundantly, the plant is called *Herbe de la Croix*, because, according to an old legend, the Cross was made from its wood, on account of which it was degraded to be a parasite.

The English name is said to be derived from the Anglo-Saxon *Misteltan, tan* signifying twig, and *mistel* from *mist*, which in old Dutch meant birdlime; thus, according to Professor Skeat, Mistletoe means 'birdlime twig,' a reference to the fact that the berries have been used for making birdlime. Dr. Prior, however, derives the word from *tan*, a twig, and *mistl*, meaning different, from its being unlike the tree it grows on. In the fourteenth century it was termed '*Mystyldene*' and also *Lignum crucis*, an allusion to the legend just mentioned. The Latin name of the genus, *Viscum*, signifying sticky, was assigned to it from the glutinous juice of its berries.

¶ *History.* Mistletoe was held in great reverence by the Druids. They went forth clad in white robes to search for the sacred plant, and when it was discovered, one of the Druids ascended the tree and gathered it with great ceremony, separating it from the Oak with a golden knife. The Mistletoe was always cut at a particular age of the moon, at the beginning of the year, and it was only sought for when the Druids declared they had visions directing them to seek it. When a great length of time elapsed without this happening, or if the Mistletoe chanced to fall to the ground, it was considered as an omen that some misfortune would befall the nation.

The Druids held that the Mistletoe protected its possessor from all evil, and that the oaks on which it was seen growing were to be respected because of the wonderful cures which the priests were able to effect with it. They sent round their attendant youth with branches of the Mistletoe to announce the entrance of the new year. It is probable that the custom of including it in the decoration of our homes at Christmas, giving it a special place of honour, is a survival of this old custom.

The curious basket of garland with which 'Jack-in-the-Green' is even now occasionally invested on May-day is said to be a relic of a similar garb assumed by the Druids for the ceremony of the Mistletoe. When they had found it they danced round the oak to the tune of 'Hey derry down, down, down derry!' which literally signified, '*In a circle move we round the oak.*' Some oakwoods in Herefordshire are still called '*the derry*'; and the following line from Ovid refers to the Druids' songs beneath the oak:

'*Ad viscum Druidæ cantare solebant.*'

Shakespeare calls it 'the baleful Mistletoe,' an allusion to the Scandinavian legend that Balder, the god of Peace, was slain with an arrow made of Mistletoe. He was restored to life at the request of the other gods and goddesses, and Mistletoe was afterwards given into the keeping of the goddess of Love, and it was ordained that everyone who passed under it should receive a kiss, to show that the branch had become an emblem of love, and not of hate.

¶ *Parts Used Medicinally.* The leaves and young twigs, collected just before the berries form, and dried in the same manner as described for Holly.

¶ *Constituents.* Mistletoe contains mucilage, sugar, a fixed oil, resin, an odorous principle, some tannin and various salts. The active part of the plant is the resin, Viscin, which by fermentation becomes a yellowish, sticky, resinous mass, which can be used with success as a birdlime.

The preparations ordinarily used are a fluid extract and the powdered leaves. A homœopathic tincture is prepared with spirit from equal quantities of the leaves and ripe berries, but is difficult of manufacture, owing to the viscidity of the sap.

¶ *Medicinal Action and Uses.* Nervine, antispasmodic, tonic and narcotic. Has a great reputation for curing the 'falling sickness' – epilepsy – and other convulsive nervous disorders. It has also been employed in checking internal hæmorrhage.

The physiological effect of the plant is to lessen and temporarily benumb such nervous action as is reflected to distant organs of the body from some central organ which is the actual seat of trouble. In this way the spasms of epilepsy and of other convulsive distempers are allayed. Large doses of the plant, or of its berries, would, on the contrary, aggravate these convulsive disorders. Young children have been attacked with convulsions after eating freely of the berries.

In a French work on domestic remedies, 1682, Mistletoe (*gui de chêne*) was considered of great curative power in epilepsy. Sir John Colbatch published in 1720 a pamphlet on *The Treatment of Epilepsy by Mistletoe*, regarding it as a specific for this disease. He procured the parasite from the Lime trees at Hampton Court, and recommended the powdered leaves, as much as would lie on a sixpence, to be given in Black Cherry water every morning. He was followed in this treatment by others who have testified to its efficacy as a tonic in nervous disorders, considering it the specific herb for St. Vitus's Dance. It has been employed in convulsions, delirium, hysteria, neuralgia, nervous debility, urinary disorders, heart disease, and many other complaints arising from a weakened and disordered state of the nervous system.

Ray also greatly extolled Mistletoe as a specific in epilepsy, and useful in apoplexy and giddiness. The older writers recommended it for sterility.

The tincture has been recommended as a heart tonic in typhoid fever in place of Foxglove. It lessens reflex irritability and strengthens the heart's beat, whilst raising the frequency of a slow pulse.

Besides the dried leaves being given powdered, or as an infusion, or made into a tincture with spirits of wine, a decoction may be made by boiling 2 oz. of the bruised green plant with ½ pint of water, giving 1 tablespoonful for a dose several times a day. Ten to 60 grains of the powder may be taken as a dose, and homœopathists give 5 to 10 drops of the tincture, with 1 or 2 tablespoonsful of cold water. Mistletoe is also given, combined with Valerian Root and Vervain, for all kinds of nervous complaints, cayenne pods being added in cases of debility of the digestive organs.

Fluid extract: dose, ¼ to 1 drachm.

Country people use the berries to cure severe stitches in the side. The birdlime of the berries is also employed by them as an application to ulcers and sores.

It is stated that in Sweden, persons afflicted with epilepsy carry about with them a knife having a handle of Oak Mistletoe to ward off attacks.

MOMORDICA. *See* (BALSAM) APPLE

MONEYWORT

Lysimachia nummularia (LINN.)
N.O. Primulaceæ

Synonyms. Creeping Jenny. Creeping Joan. Wandering Jenny. Running Jenny. Wandering Tailor. Herb Twopence. Twopenny Grass. Meadow Runagates. Herbe 2 pence. Two Penigrasse. String of Sovereigns. Serpentaria

Part Used. Whole herb, dried or fresh

The Moneywort is far more often known by the familiar names of Creeping Jenny, Wandering Jenny, Running Jenny, Creeping Joan and Wandering Sailor – all names alluding to its rapid trailing over the ground. 'Meadow Runagates' has the same reference, and tells us also of its favourite home in damp pastures and by stream sides.

The earliest English Herbal, that of Turner, speaks of it as 'Herbe 2 pence' and 'Two penigrasse,' and it is still known in some localities as Herb Twopence and Twopenny Grass, the allusion here being to the leaves, which are set two and two on the stem, and rounded (though each has a short, sharp tip), and lying always faces turned to the sky, look like rows of pence. 'Moneywort' and 'Strings of Sovereigns,' though names based on the same idea, are probably suggested by the big golden flowers, rather than by the leaves. The leaves sometimes turn rose-pink in autumn. The specific name, *Nummularia*, is from the Latin *nummulus* (money).

¶ *Description.* The leaves and stems of the plant are all quite smooth, the stems being quadrangular. The flowers, which blossom through June and July, spring singly on slender stalks, just where each leaf joins the stem. Their five sepals are large, pale green and heart-shaped, somewhat 'frilly' round the base, perhaps as a protection against small creeping insects, which might otherwise make their way into the flowers, which are only just off the ground. The five petals are so deeply cut into that they appear separate, but are joined at the base to form a golden cup. The stamens, as in the Scarlet Pimpernel and others of this family, face their corresponding petals, instead of being alternate with them, and are also joined at their base to form a low ring. Their filaments, or little stalks, are covered with tiny golden hairs or knobs.

The ovary in the centre of the flower is so placed that the pollen from the stamens must fall on its stigma, but the flower is not only absolutely sterile to its own pollen, but also pollen from other Moneywort flowers seems to have little effect on its ovules, for as a rule no fruit follows the flowers. It has been thought, therefore, that the plant may not be a true native, and that there is something in our climate that does not suit it. It is probable, however, that it does not trouble to set seed, because it has adopted a simpler method of propagation. It frequently happens that plants which increase much in other ways seldom produce ripe seeds. This simple method of propagation lies in its trailing shoots – its 'stolons.' A stolon may be defined as a creeping stem which dies off every year, and is beset by leaves not very far apart. Close to the tip of each stolon, in the angle formed by little leaf-stalks, buds appear, which produce roots which pass into the ground. When winter comes, the stem and leaves die down between the old root and the new one, but when spring arrives, a new plant exists where the little roots entered the ground. In this way from a single plant which sends out stolons in various directions, many new plants appear by this so-called 'vegetative' method of reproduction.

In a damp situation, no plant thrives better in a garden, or requires less trouble to be taken with it.

¶ *Part Used.* The whole herb, used both dried and fresh. For drying, collect in June, and proceed as in Scarlet Pimpernel.

¶ *Medicinal Action and Uses.* The Moneywort in olden days was reputed to have many virtues. It was like the last species, one of the many 'best possible woundworts.' 'In a word, there is not a better wound-herb, no not tobacco itselfe, nor any other whatsoever,' said an old herbalist.

We are told by old writers that this herb was not only used by man, but that if serpents hurt or wounded themselves, they turned to this plant for healing, and so it was sometimes called 'Serpentaria.'

The bruised fresh leaves were in popular use as an application to wounds, both fresh and old, a decoction of the fresh herb being taken as a drink in wine or water, and also applied outwardly as a wash or cold compress to both wounds and inveterate sores. An ointment was made also for application to wounds.

The leaves are subastringent, slightly acid, and antiscorbutic. Boerhaave, the celebrated Dutch physician, recommended their use, dried and powdered, in doses of 10 grains in scurvy and hæmorrhages. Culpepper tells us:

'Moneywort is singularly good to stay all fluxes . . . bleeding inwardly or outwardly, and weak stomachs given to casting. It is very good for the ulcers or excoriations of the lungs.' Again, it was a specific for whooping-cough 'being boyled with wine or honey . . .

MONSONIA

Part Used. Plant, root
Habitat. Cape of Good Hope

¶ *Description.* Leaves oblong, subcordate, crenate, waved, flowers white axillary stalked, two on one peduncle, roots fleshy large, grown from seed.

¶ *Medicinal Action and Uses.* A valuable remedy for acute and chronic dysentery, specially of use in ulceration of the lower part of the intestines; the plant is not considered poisonous.

¶ *Dosage.* Saturated tincture, 1 to 2 fluid drachms, every three or four hours.

MORNING GLORY. *See* BINDWEED

MOSCHATEL, COMMON

Synonyms. Tuberous Moschatel. Musk Ranunculus

This plant, belonging to the natural order Caprifoliaceæ, is the only one of its species. The name *Adoxa* is from the Greek, signifying 'inglorious,' from its humble growth. It is an interesting little herbaceous plant, 4 to 6 inches high; stem four-angled; root-leaves long-stalked, ternate; leaflets triangular, lobed; cauline leaves or bracts two, smaller, with sheathing petioles; flowers arranged as if on five sides of a cube, small and pale green in colour; berry with one-seeded parchment-like chamber. Growing in hedgerows, local, but widely diffused, also in Asia and North America, even into the Arctic regions.

MOSQUITO PLANT. *See* THYME (WILD)

MOSS, AMERICAN CLUB

Synonym. American Ground Pine

The American Ground Pine is not a flowering plant, but one of the Club Mosses, which with the Ferns and Mosses belong to the great class of Cryptogams. The genus *Lycopodium* holds, as it were, an intermediate place between the Ferns and Mosses and includes only six British species, though there are about sixty-five distributed over the world.

Lycopodium complanatum, the American Club Moss, is a small mossy plant with aromatic, resinous smell and slightly turpentiny taste, the stalks hairy and the leaves close set, characteristics which have gained it the popular name of Ground Pine, as in

it prevaileth against that violent cough in children, commonly called the chinne-cough, but it should be chine-cough, for it doth make as it were the very chine-bone to shake.'

See PIMPERNEL (YELLOW), LOOSESTRIFE

Monsonia ovata (CAR.)
N.O. Geraniaceæ

The Pelargoniums belong to the same family, and all species have more or less astringent properties. Some have fragrant foliage, noticeably *Pelargonium roseum* and *P. capitatum*, from which a fragrant essential oil is extracted. In medicine they are used for dysentery and some for ulceration of the stomach and upper intestinal tracts. *P. Triste* has edible tubers.

See PELARGONIUMS

Adoxa Moschatellina
N.O. Caprifoliaceæ

The flowers, and indeed the whole plant, has a musk-like scent, which it emits towards evening when the dew falls – this scent, however, disappears if the plant is bruised. It flowers in April and May.

John Ray, in his early system of plant classification, placed the Moschatel amongst the berry-bearing plants. The early writers found considerable difficulty in classifying it botanically. One calls it the musk-ranunculus, whilst another classes it with the fumitories, probably because of its leaves.

Lycopodium complanatum (LINN.)
N.O. Lycopodiaceæ

the case of Yellow Bugle. The stem is long and creeping, only about ½ inch in diameter, yellowish-green, giving off at intervals erect, fan-shaped forked branches about 4 inches high, with minute scale-like leaves, leaving only the sharp tips free, the branches bearing fructification in the form of a stalked tuft of four to five cylindrical spikes, consisting of spore cases in the axils of minute bracts. The stem roots below at long intervals, the roots being pale, wiry and slightly branched.

¶ *Medicinal Action and Uses.* The whole plant is used, dried and powdered for infusion.

It has properties similar to the European Ground Pine, being a powerful diuretic, promoting urine and removing obstructions of the liver and spleen. It is, therefore, a valuable remedy in jaundice, rheumatism and most of the chronic diseases.

A decoction of this plant, combined with Dandelion and Agrimony, is a highly recommended herbal remedy for liver complaints and obstructions.

For EUROPEAN GROUND PINE, *see* (YELLOW) BUGLE.

MOSS, COMMON CLUB

Lycopodium clavatum (LINN.)
N.O. Lycopodiaceæ

Synonyms. Muscus Terrestris repens. Vegetable Sulphur. Wolf's Claw
Parts Used. The spores, the fresh plant

This species is found all over the world and occurs throughout Great Britain, being most plentiful on the moors of the northern counties.

Though this species of Club Moss occurs in Great Britain, the spores are collected chiefly in Russia, Germany and Switzerland, in July and August, the tops of the plants being cut as the spikes approach maturity and the powder shaken out and separated by a sieve. Probably the spores used commercially are derived also from other species in addition to *Lycopodium clavatum*.

¶ *Medicinal Action and Uses.* The part of the plant now employed is the minute spores which, as a yellow powder, are shaken out of the kidney-shaped capsules or sporangia growing on the inner side of the bracts covering the fruit spike. Under the names of *Muscus terrestris* or *M. clavatum* the whole plant was used, dried, by ancient physicians as a stomachic and diuretic, mainly in calculous and other kidney complaints; the spores do not appear to have been used alone until the seventeenth century, when they were employed as a diuretic in dropsy, a drastic in diarrhœa, dysentery and suppression of urine, a nervine in spasms and hydrophobia, an aperient in gout and scurvy and a corroborant in rheumatism, and also as an application to wounds. They were, however, more used on the Continent than in this country and never had a place in the London Pharmacopœia, though they have been prescribed for irritability of the bladder, in the form of a tincture, which is official in the United States Pharmacopœia.

The spores are still medicinally employed by herbalists in this country, both internally and externally, as a dusting powder in various skin diseases such as eczema and erysipelas and for excoriated surfaces, to prevent chafing in infants. Their chief pharmaceutical use is as a pill powder, for enveloping pills to prevent their adhesion to one another when placed in a box, and to disguise their taste. Dose, 10 to 60 grains. They have such a strong repulsive power that, if the hand is powdered with them, it can be dipped in water without becoming wet.

MOSS, CORSICAN

Fucus Helminthocorton (KÜTZ.)
N.O. Algæ

Synonym. Alsidium Helminthocorton
Part Used. Whole plant
Habitat. Mediterranean coast, specially Corsica

¶ *Description.* The drug is obtained from twenty to thirty species of Algæ, chiefly *Sphærococcus helminthocorton*. It is cartilaginous, filiform repeatedly forked, colour varies from white to brown, it has a nauseous taste, bitter and salt, odour rather pleasant.

¶ *Medicinal Action and Uses.* In Europe as an anthelmintic and febrifuge, it acts very successfully on lumbricoid intestinal worms. A decoction is made of it from 4 to 6 drachms to the pint. Dose, a wineglassful three times daily.
¶ *Dosage.* Ten to 60 grains in syrup or in infusion.

MOSS, CUP

Cladonia Pyxidata (FRIES.)
N.O. Lichenes

Part Used. Whole plant
Habitat. North-west America, but now a common weed in many counties in Britain

¶ *Description.* *Cladonia* is one of a numerous genus of lecidineous lichens. It grows abundantly in the woods and hedges and is a common species; it has no odour; taste sweetish and mucilagenous.

¶ *Medicinal Action and Uses.* Expectorant, a valuable medicine in whooping cough.
¶ *Dosage.* 2 oz. of the plant decocted and mixed with honey makes a good expectorant and a safe medicine for children's coughs.

¶ *Other Species.*
Cladonia rangiferina. The badge of the Clan McKenzie. Makes excellent food for reindeer.

C. sanguinea. In Brazil is rubbed down with sugar and water and applied in the thrush of infants.

MOSS, HAIR CAP

Polytrichium Juniperum (WILLD.)
N.O. Musci

Synonyms. Bear's Bed. Robin's Eye. Ground Moss. Golden Maidenhair. Female Fern Herb. Rockbrake Herb
Part Used. Whole herb
Habitat. High dry places, margins of woods, poor sandy soil

¶ *Description.* The genus have free veins, globose sort, and peltate indusia; only a few species are found in Britain. These are perennial, slender and reddish colour, from 4 to 7 inches high. Leaves lanceolate and spreading, fruit four-sided capsule, evergreen, darker in colour than other mosses.
¶ *Medicinal Action and Uses.* A very valuable remedy in dropsy as a powerful diuretic, and used with hydragogue cathartics of decided advantage. Very useful in urinary obstructions, gravel, etc., causing no nausea, can be given alone or combined with broom or wild carrot, and is excellent if it is necessary to give it indefinitely as an infusion, which is taken in 4-oz. doses.

MOSS, CELAND

Cetraria islandica (ACH.)
N.O. Lichenes

Synonyms. Cetraria. Iceland Lichen
Part Used. Lichen
Habitat. A common plant in northern countries and in the mountainous part of warmer countries

In spite of its name is not a Moss but a lichen. Found in Great Britain in barren stony ground, abundant in the Grampians, and in the Welsh hills, in Yorkshire, Norfolk, etc. It rarely fructifies but the thallus varies in size, amount of division and cusping as well as colour. It is sometimes much curled.

It contains about 70 per cent. of lichen starch and becomes blue on the addition of iodine. It also contains a little sugar, fumaric acid, oxalic acid, about 3 per cent. of cetrarin and 1 per cent. of licheno-stearic acid.
¶ *Medicinal Action and Properties.* Demulcent, tonic, and nutritive when deprived of its bitter principle. Excellent in chronic pulmonary troubles, catarrh, digestive disturbances, dysentery, advanced tuberculosis. Decoction, B.P. 1885, 1 to 4 oz. Ground, it can be mixed with chocolate or cocoa.

MOSS, IRISH

Chondrus crispus (STACKH.)
N.O. Algæ

Synonyms. Carrageen. Chondrus. Carrahan
Part Used. Plant, dried
Habitat. A perennial thallophyte common at low tide on all the shores of the North Atlantic, but remarkable for its extreme variability, the difference being mainly due to the great diversity in the width of the segments

¶ *Constituents.* It contains a large amount of mucilage with the presence of a big percentage of sulphur compounds.
¶ *Medicinal Action and Uses.* Demulcent, emollient, nutritive. A popular remedy made into a jelly for pulmonary complaints and kidney and bladder affections. Can be combined with cocoa. The decoction is made by steeping ½ oz. of the Moss in cold water for 15 minutes and then boiling it in 3 pints of milk or water for 10 or 15 minutes, after which it is strained and seasoned with liquorice, lemon or cinnamon and sweetened to taste. It can be taken freely.

MOSS, SPHAGNUM

Sphagnum Cymbifolium
N.O. Lichenes

Synonym. Bog Moss

Sphagnum Moss, commonly known as Bog Moss, is the only true Moss that has yet proved itself to be of appreciable economic value.

It is found in wet and boggy spots, preferably on peat soil, mostly near heather, on all our mountains and moors, in patches small or large, usually in water free from lime,

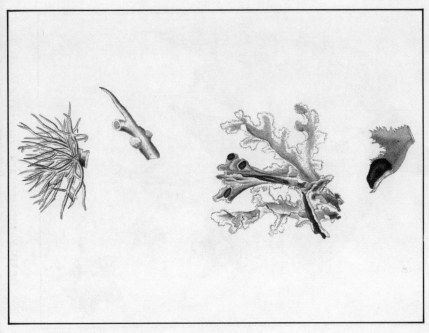

ICELAND MOSS
Cetraria Islandica

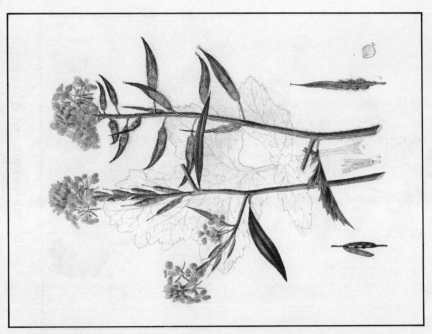

MUSTARDS, BLACK AND WHITE
Brassica Nigra and Brassica Alba

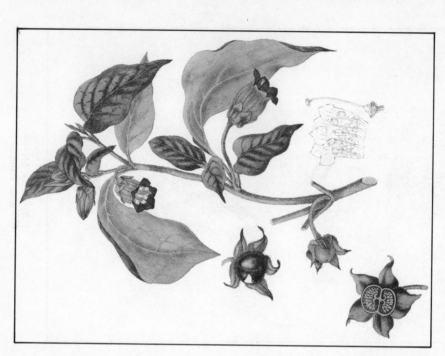

DEADLY NIGHTSHADE (BELLADONNA)
Atroba Belladonna

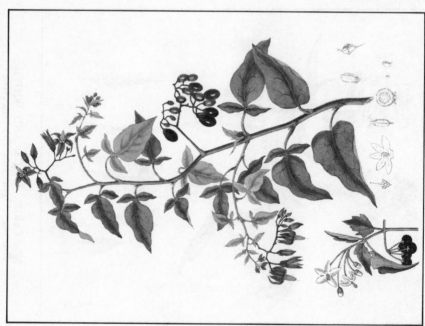

WOODY NIGHTSHADE (BITTERSWEET)
Solanum Dulcamara

growing so close together that it often forms large cushions or clumps. It is seldom found in woods; it grows best on heath moors, in water holes.

¶ *Description.* Sphagnum is easily distinguished from other mosses by its habit of growth, its soft thick fullness (each head resembling a full and elaborate bloom of *edelweiss*), and its vividly pale-green colour.

Its stem is densely beset with narrow, broken-up leaves, a branch being emitted at every fourth leaf; many of these are turned downwards and applied more or less closely to the stem.

Though the pale-green species is the most common, there are several others, large and small, varying in colour from the very light green (never dark green) to yellow, and all shades of pink to deep red and brown. The Moss often attracts attention by its display of beautiful shades of colour, such patches being avoided by wary persons, who do not wish to get their feet wet.

Every part of the moss is permeated with minute tubes and spaces, resulting in a system of delicate capillary tubes, having the effect of a very fine sponge. The cells readily absorb water and retain it. The water can be squeezed out, but the Moss does not collapse and is ready to take in fluid again.

The plant is not dependent on soil water, but also absorbs moisture from the atmosphere, and is laden throughout with water retained in its delicate cells.

The presence of these capillary cells makes Sphagnum economically useful. In horticulture, long before the war, this Moss had a marketable value, in combination with peat fibre, being widely used as a rooting medium for orchids, on account of the remarkable manner in which it retains moisture, a handful when wet being like a sponge, and when chopped and mixed with soil in pots preventing moisture passing too quickly through the soil.

In recent years, the light-brown layer of semi-decayed Sphagnum Moss deposits that lies above the actual peat on bogs and moors, has been largely employed as valuable stable litter in the place of straw, under the name of Moss Litter, entirely on account of its great absorptive powers.

On the outbreak of the late war a still wider economic use was found for this moss, as a dressing of wounds, and an interesting industry sprang up for war-workers living where this moss grows, mainly in Scotland, Ireland, Wales and Devon, much having also been collected from the Yorkshire moors, the Lake District and the Wye Valley.

Although this particular use of the moss is generally looked upon as an innovation, we owe the introduction of Sphagnum Moss as a modern surgical dressing to Germany, where its value for this purpose was quite accidentally discovered in the early eighties.

And though it is only in quite recent years that Sphagnum Moss has come to the fore in the dressing of wounds, bygone generations recognized its value for this purpose. A Gaelic Chronicle of 1014 relates that the wounded in the battle of Clontarf 'stuffed their wounds with moss,' and the Highlanders after Flodden stanched their bleeding wounds by filling them with bog moss and soft grass. Stricken deer are known to drag their wounded limbs to beds of Sphagnum Moss. The Kashmiri have used it from time immemorial and so have the Esquimaux. An old writer says:

'the Lapland matrons are well acquainted with this moss. They dry it and lay it in their children's cradles to supply the place of mattress, bolster and every covering, and being changed night and morning, it keeps the infant remarkable clean, dry and warm.'

The Lapps also use the moss for surgical purposes, and it has been used in Newfoundland as a dressing for wounds and sores from the earliest times.

For thirty years, Sphagnum Moss had been used as a surgical dressing in Germany.

The growing plant, with its underlying layers of withered stems and leaves, is collected, picked clean from other plants, pine-needles, etc., and dried. It is then lightly packed in bags of butter-muslin, which are sterilized before being placed on the wound.

Sphagnum Moss has important advantages (as an absorbent) over cotton-wool. Many materials, including other kinds of moss, are equally soft and light, but none can compare with it in power of absorption, due to its sponge-like structure. Prepared Sphagnum can absorb more than twice as much moisture as cotton, a 2-oz. dressing absorbing up to 2 lb. Even the best prepared cotton-wool lacks the power to retain discharges possessed by Sphagnum. A pad of Sphagnum Moss absorbs the discharge in lateral directions, as well as immediately above the wound, and holds it until fully saturated in all parts of the dressing before allowing any to escape. The even absorption of the moss is one of its chief virtues, for the patient is saved a good deal of disturbance, since the dressing does not require to be changed so frequently.

In civil hospitals, in times of peace, the deficiencies of cotton-wool are not so much noticed, the majority of wounds being those made by surgeons under ideal conditions, but for a variety of reasons the wounds of our men at the front were of such a suppurating character as to require specially absorbent dressings, and overworked doctors and nurses constantly expressed themselves thankful for a dressing that lasted longer than cotton-wool. Time and suffering are saved, as well as expense: the absorbent pads of moss are soft, elastic and very comfortable, easily packed and convenient to handle.

Fortunately the supply is practically an unlimited one; indeed, if the demand grew considerably, the artificial cultivation of Sphagnum for surgical purposes would be worth while. This Moss is easily propagated, as the stems and so-called leaves can be chopped up into fine particles and every morsel will grow and form a tassel-like head. Sphagnum only thrives in clean water and soil; it dislikes manure of any kind.

In gathering Sphagnum most people use their hands, though some employ a rake. The moss should be gathered as cleanly as possible, squeezed dry and carried home in sacks. The squeezing may be done with the hands, or with a towel or coarse sacking, further wringing being done at home, if necessary, with a laundry roller-wringer or mangle. Wringing or squeezing the moss does not harm it for surgical purposes, though it must not be allowed to dry in closely pressed pieces, because it tears when being opened up again. If squeezed with the hand, it must not be pressed into a hard ball. While still damp, all clumps should be separated out, as the moss, whether picked or not, must be sent to the workrooms in a loose state.

Cleaning or picking the moss is best done while still damp, though it may also be done when dry. The moss is spread out on a table and all other substances, such as grasses, twigs, bits of heather and other plants, and above all, pine-needles, must be carefully removed by hand. The moss itself must not be torn or broken into short pieces.

Drying is best done in the open air; artificial heat is apt to overheat the moss and diminish its elasticity, making it brittle and easily rubbed into dust.

An empty hayshed may also be employed, open on all sides, or the floors of an empty room, with windows open, wire netting being used to keep the moss from blowing away.

Where a moor produces large patches of coherent Sphagnum – cushions – the following method has been employed. Large cushions of the moss are taken out and placed on a drier area near by – a couple of workers can put out about a hundred of these in an hour. On the next visit, these are turned and another set put out. In favourable weather a few days' sun and wind will dry these thoroughly, as the cushions are too bulky to be scattered by the wind. Several big sacks can be filled on a final visit, and the carriage of perfectly dry moss is an easy matter.

¶ *Preparation of the Dressings.* The moss after being dried and carefully picked over is now ready for the dressings. All used in home hospitals is put up loosely in small, flat muslin bags, of a fairly close but very thin muslin, the bags only being loosely filled (as a rule 2 oz. of the moss to each bag, 10 inches by 14 inches), as allowance has to be made for the way in which the moss swells on being brought into contact with moisture.

Sphagnum Moss pads are supplied both plain and sterilized (sublimated), some hospitals preferring to sterilize them themselves, but a considerable proportion being sterilized at the depots and sent out ready for use. The filled bags are passed through a solution of corrosive sublimate by a worker in rubber gloves, squeezed through a little mangle and dried again, that they may return to the specified weight, for after the bath they are 2 oz. too heavy. The object of sublimating the moss is not for any antiseptic effect on a wound (as of course it does not come into direct contact with the skin) but to neutralize the discharge which may come through the inner dressings.

For use in field-hospitals, etc., the moss is packed in compressed cakes cut to a certain size, which are more conveniently packed for sending abroad than the soft dressings, these small slabs being also placed, each in a muslin bag, very much too large for the size of the dry cake put in them, for obvious reasons. There was a munition factory in Scotland, where much of the moss was sublimated and part of it compressed by hydraulic power into these cakes. The very hydraulic press which one hour was moulding shell bases, was in the next devoting its energy to compressing the healing cakes of Sphagnum Moss.

Sphagnum Moss was also used during the War in conjunction with Garlic, one of the best antiseptics. The Government bought up tons of the bulbs, which were sent out to the front; the raw juice expressed, diluted with water, was put on swabs of sterilized Sphagnum Moss and applied to wounds. Where this treatment was adopted there were no specific complications, and thousands of lives were thus saved.

¶ *Peat Tar.* In connexion with the uses of Spaghnum Moss as a dressing for wounds, mention should be made of the Tar extracted from the Peat on which the Moss is usually found growing.

The Peat Tar contains similar antiseptic and preservative properties as the Moss itself – conclusively demonstrated by the fact that bodies of animals have lain buried in peat bogs for years, and when accidentally disinterred have been found in a state of perfect preservation.

¶ *Medicinal Action and Uses.* Preparations of calcined peat have long been regarded as effective and cheap germicides, and as a valuable aid to sanitation; peat water possesses astringent and antiseptic properties, and the air in proximity to tracts of peat moss is invariably salubrious, owing probably to the absorption of hydrogen and the exhalation of oxygen by the mosses. Sphagnol, a distillate of Peat Tar, is authori-

tatively recognized as an extremely useful application in eczema, psoriasis, pruritus, hæmorrhoids, chilblains, scabies, acne and other forms of skin diseases, while it is very beneficial for allaying irritation arising from insect bites. For the latter purpose it is a preventative no less than a cure.

The manufacture of spinning material out of peat-fibre has been attempted in Sweden, and experiments have advanced so far that cloth as well as clothing has been made out of peat fibre mixed with other textile materials. This does not, however, appear likely to lead to any important industry, but absorptive material has been produced from white Sphagnum Moss and Wood Pulp. It has also lately been reported from Sweden that successful attempts have been made to extract alcohol from Sphagnum.

MOTHERWORT

Leonurus cardiaca (LINN.)
N.O. Labiatæ

Part Used. Herb

Motherwort, the only British representative of the genus *Leonurus*, is a native of many parts of Europe, on banks and under hedges, in a gravelly or calcareous soil. It is often found in country gardens, where it was formerly grown for medicinal purposes, but it is rare to find it truly wild in England, and by some authorities it is not considered indigenous, but merely a garden escape.

¶ *Description.* It is distinguished from all other British labiates by the leaves, which are deeply and palmately cut into five lobes, or three-pointed segments, and by the prickly calyx-teeth of its flowers. When not in flower, it resembles Mugwort in habit.

From the perennial root-stock rise the square, stout stems, 2 to 3 feet high, erect and branched, principally below, the angles prominent. The leaves are very closely set, the radical ones on slender, long petioles, ovate, lobed and toothed, those on the stem, 2 to 3 inches long, petioled, wedge-shaped; the lower roundish, palmately five-lobed, the lobes trifid at the apex, the upper three-fid, coarsely serrate, reticulately veined, the veinlets prominent beneath, with slender, curved hairs. The uppermost leaves and bracts are very narrow and entire, or only with a tooth on each side, and bear in their axils numerous whorls of pinkish, or nearly white, sessile flowers, six to fifteen in a whorl. The corollas, though whitish on the outside, are stained with paler or darker purple within. They have rather short tubes and nearly flat upper lips, very hairy above, with long, woolly hairs. The two front stamens are the longest and the anthers are sprinkled with hard, shining dots.

The plant blossoms in August. It has rather a pungent odour and a very bitter taste. It is a dull green, the leaves paler below, pubescent, especially on the angles of the stem and the underside of the leaves, the hairs varying much in length and abundance.

The name of the genus, *Leonurus*, in Greek signifies a Lion's tail, from some fancied resemblance in the plant.

¶ *Cultivation.* When once planted in a garden, Motherwort will soon increase if the seeds are permitted to scatter. It is perfectly hardy and needs no special soil, and the roots will continue for many years.

Seedlings should be planted about a foot apart.

¶ *Part Used.* The whole herb, dried, cut in August. The drying may be carried out in any of the ways described for Scullcap.

¶ *Medicinal Action and Uses.* Diaphoretic, antispasmodic, tonic, nervine, emmenagogue. Motherwort is especially valuable in female weakness and disorders (hence the name), allaying nervous irritability and inducing quiet and passivity of the whole nervous system.

As a tonic, it acts without producing febrile excitement, and in fevers, attended with nervousness and delirium, it is extremely useful.

Old writers tell us that there is no better herb for strengthening and gladdening the heart, and that it is good against hysterical complaints, and especially for palpitations of the heart when they arise from hysteric causes, and that when made into a syrup, it will allay inward tremors, faintings, etc.

There is no doubt it has proved the truth of their claims in its use as a simple tonic, not only in heart disease, neuralgia and other affections of the heart, but also in spinal disease and in recovery from fevers where other tonics are inadmissable.

In Macer's *Herbal* we find 'Motherwort' mentioned as one of the herbs which were considered all-powerful against 'wykked sperytis.'

The best way of giving it is in the form of a conserve, made from the young tops, says one writer. It may be given in decoctions, or a strong infusion, but is very unpleasant to take that way. The infusion is made from 1 oz. of herb to a pint of boiling water, taken in wineglassful doses.

¶ *Preparations and Dosages.* Powdered herb, ½ to 1 drachm. Fluid extract, ½ to 1 drachm. Solid extract, 5 to 15 grains.

MOUNTAIN ASH. *See* ASH

MOUNTAIN FLAX. *See* FLAX

MOUNTAIN GRAPE. *See* GRAPE

MOUNTAIN LAUREL. *See* LAUREL

MOUSE-EAR. *See* HAWKWEED

Culpepper wrote of Motherwort:

'Venus owns this herb and it is under Leo. There is no better herb to drive melancholy vapours from the heart, to strengthen it and make the mind cheerful, blithe and merry. May be kept in a syrup, or conserve, therefore the Latins call it cardiaca. . . . It cleansethe the chest of cold phlegm, oppressing it and killeth worms in the belly. It is of good use to warm and dry up the cold humours, to digest and disperse them that are settled in the veins, joints and sinews of the body and to help cramps and convulsions.'

And Gerard says:

'Divers commend it against infirmities of the heart. Moreover the same is commended for green wounds; it is also a remedy against certain diseases in cattell, as the cough and murreine, and for that cause divers husbandmen oftentimes much desire it.'

MUGWORT

Artemisia vulgaris (LINN.)
N.O. Compositæ

Synonyms. Felon Herb. St. John's Plant. Cingulum Sancti Johannis
Parts Used. Leaves, root

Mugwort abounds on hedgebanks and waysides in most parts of England. It is a tall-growing plant, the stems, which are angular and often of a purplish hue, frequently rising 3 feet or more in height. The leaves are smooth and of a dark green tint on the upper surface, but covered with a dense cottony down beneath; they are once or twice pinnately lobed, the segments being lance-shaped and pointed. The flowers are in small oval heads with cottony involucres and are arranged in long, terminal panicles; they are either reddish or pale yellow. The Mugwort is closely allied to the Common Wormwood, but may be readily distinguished by the leaves being white on the under-surfaces only and by the leaf segments being pointed, not blunt. It lacks the essential oil of the Wormwood.

The Mugwort is said to have derived its name from having been used to flavour drinks. It was, in common with other herbs, such as Ground Ivy, used to a great extent for flavouring beer before the introduction of hops. For this purpose, the plant was gathered when in flower and dried, the fresh herb being considered unsuitable for this object: malt liquor was then boiled with it so as to form a strong decoction, and the liquid thus prepared was added to the beer. Until recent years, it was still used in some parts of the country to flavour the table beer brewed by cottagers.

It has also been suggested that the name, Mugwort, may be derived not from 'mug,' the drinking vessel, but from *moughte* (a moth or maggot), because from the days of Dioscorides, the plant has been regarded, in common with Wormwood, as useful in keeping off the attacks of moths.

In the Middle Ages, the plant was known as *Cingulum Sancti Johannis*, it being believed that John the Baptist wore a girdle of it in the wilderness. There were many superstitions connected with it: it was believed to preserve the wayfarer from fatigue, sunstroke, wild beasts and evil spirits generally: a crown made from its sprays was worn on St. John's Eve to gain security from evil possession, and in Holland and Germany one of its names is St. John's Plant, because of the belief, that if gathered on St. John's Eve it gave protection against diseases and misfortunes.

Dr. John Hill extols its virtues, and says:

'Providence has placed it everywhere about our doors; so that reason and authority, as well as the notice of our senses, point it out for use: but chemistry has banished natural medicines.'

Dioscorides praises this herb, and orders the flowering tops to be used just before they bloom.

The dried leaves were, sixty or seventy years ago, in use by the working classes in Cornwall as one of the substitutes for tea, at a time when tea cost 7s. per lb., and on the Continent Mugwort is occasionally employed as an aromatic culinary herb, being one of the green herbs with which geese are often stuffed during roasting.

The downy leaves have been used in the preparation of *Moxas*, which the Japanese use to cure rheumatism. The down is separated by heating the leaves and afterwards rubbing them between the hands until the cottony fibres alone remain, these are then made up into small cones or cylinders for use. *Artemisia Moxa* and *A. sinensis* are mainly used in Japan. This cottony substance has also been used as a substitute for tinder.

Sheep are said to enjoy the herbage of the Mugwort, and also the roots. The plant may, perhaps, be the Artemesia of Pontos, which was celebrated among the ancients for fattening these animals. It is said to be good for poultry and turkeys.

A variegated variety of Mugwort also occurs.

¶ *Parts Used Medicinally.* The leaves, collected in August and dried in the same manner as Wormwood, and the root, dug in autumn and dried. The roots are cleansed in cold water and then freed from rootlets. Drying may be done at first in the open air, spread thinly, as contact may turn the roots mouldy. Or they may be spread on clean floors, or on shelves, in a warm room for about ten days, and turned frequently. When somewhat shrunken, they must be finished more quickly by artificial heat in a drying room or shed, near a stove or gas fire, care being taken that the heated air can escape at the top of the room. Drying in an even temperature will probably take about a fortnight, or more. It is not complete until the roots are dry to the core and brittle, snapping when bent.

Mugwort root is generally about 8 inches long, woody, beset with numerous thin and tough rootlets, 2 to 4 inches long, and about $\frac{1}{12}$ inch thick. It is light brown externally; internally whitish, with an angular wood and thick bark, showing five or six resin cells. The taste is sweetish and acrid.

¶ *Constituents.* A volatile oil, an acrid resin and tannin.

¶ *Medicinal Action and Uses.* It has stimulant and slightly tonic properties, and is of value as a nervine and emmenagogue, having also diuretic and diaphoretic action.

Its chief employment is as an emmenagogue, often in combination with Pennyroyal and Southernwood. It is also useful as a diaphoretic in the commencement of cold.

It is given in infusion, which should be prepared in a covered vessel, 1 oz. of the herb to 1 pint of boiling water, and given in $\frac{1}{2}$ teaspoonful doses, while warm. The infusion may be taken cold as a tonic, in similar doses, three times daily: it has a bitterish and aromatic taste.

As a nervine, Mugwort is valued in palsy, fits, epileptic and similar affections, being an old-fashioned popular remedy for epilepsy (especially in persons of a feeble constitution). Gerard says: 'Mugwort cureth the shakings of the joynts inclining to the Palsie;' and Parkinson considered it good against hysteria. A drachm of the powdered leaves, given four times a day, is stated by Withering to have cured a patient who had been affected with hysterical fits for many years, when all other remedies had failed.

The juice and an infusion of the herb were given for intermittent fevers and agues. The leaves used to be steeped in baths, to communicate an invigorating property to the water.

¶ *Preparations.* Fluid extract, $\frac{1}{2}$ to 1 drachm.

Culpepper directs that the tops of the plant are to be used fresh gathered, and says:

'a very slight infusion is excellent for all disorders of the stomach, prevents sickness after meals and creates an appetite, but if made too strong, it disgusts the taste. The tops with the flowers on them, dried and powdered, are good against agues, and have the same virtues with wormseed in killing worms. The juice of the large leaves which grows from the root before the stalk appears is the best against the dropsy and jaundice, in water, ale, wine, or the juice only. The infusion drank morning and evening for some time helps hysterics, obstruction of the spleen and weakness of the stomach. Its oil, taken on sugar and drank after, kills worms, resists poison, and is good for the liver and jaundice.

The root has a slow bitterness which affects not the head and eyes like the leaves, hence the root should be accounted among the best stomachics. The oil of the seed cures quotidians and quartans. Boiled in lard and laid to swellings of the tonsils and quinsy is serviceable. It is admirable against surfeits. . . . Wormwood and vinegar are an antidote to the mischief of mushrooms and henbane and the biting of the seafish called Draco marinus, or quaviver; mixed with honey, it takes away blackness after falls, bruises, etc. . . . With Pellitory of the Wall used as poultice to ease all outward pains. Placed among woolen cloths it prevents and destroys the moths.'

Another old writer affirmed that Mugwort was good 'for quaking of the sinews.'
See WORMWOOD, SOUTHERNWOOD.

MULBERRY, COMMON

Morus nigra (LINN.)
N.O. Artocapaceæ

The Common or Black Mulberry is not one of our native trees, but with several other members of its genus – which contains a dozen or more species – can be grown without protection in the south of Britain. There they are small bushy-headed trees, with large alternate, deciduous, toothed and often variously lobed leaves. It is by no means unusual for a Mulberry tree to produce leaves of several different shapes, or differing considerably in outline. As a rule, abnormal-shaped leaves are produced from stem-shoots or sucker growths, and frequently by very vigorous young branches. The Chinese White Mulberry (*Morus alba*, Linn.), cultivated in other countries as food for the silk-worm, is even more variable in leafage than the Common Mulberry, and quite a score of different forms of leaf have been gathered from a single tree and several from one shoot. Both species contain in every part a milky juice, which will coagulate into a sort of Indian rubber, and this has been thought to give tenacity to the filament spun by the silk-worm.

¶ *Description*. The Common Mulberry is a handsome tree, 20 to 30 feet high, of rugged, picturesque appearance, forming a dense, spreading head of branches usually wider than the height of the tree, springing from a short, rough trunk.

It bears unisexual flowers, the sexes in separate spikes, or catkins, which are small, more or less cylindrical and in no way beautiful. The oblong, short-stalked 'fruit,' which when ripe is about an inch long and of an intense purple, is really a fruit-cluster, composed of little, closely-packed drupes, each containing one seed and enclosed by the four enlarged sepals, which have become succulent, thus forming the spurious berry. By detaching a single fruit from the cluster, the overlapping lobes of the former perianth may be still discerned.

Mulberries are extremely juicy and have a refreshing, subacid, saccharine taste, but they are devoid of the fine aroma that distinguishes many fruits of the order Rosaceæ.

¶ *Habitat*. The tree grows wild in northern Asia Minor, Armenia and the Southern Caucasus region as far as Persia and is now cultivated throughout Europe. It ripens its fruits in England and also as far north as Southern Sweden and Gothland. It flourishes more in the southern part of Great Britain than in the northern counties, but is always of slow growth. Gerard describes it as 'high and full of boughes' and growing in sundry gardens in England, and he grew in his own London garden both the Black and the White Mulberry. Lyte also, before Gerard, in 1578, describes it. It is definitely known to have been cultivated in England since the early part of the sixteenth century, and possibly long before, it being considered probable that it was introduced into Britain by the Romans, being imported from Italy for the soldiers' use.

The Black Mulberry was known in the whole of Southern Europe from the earliest times, and it is presumed that it was introduced from Persia. It is mentioned by most of the early Greek and Roman writers.

The Romans ate Mulberries at their feasts, as we know from the *Satires* of Horace, who (*Sat. ii,*) recommends that Mulberries be gathered before sunset. We also find mention of the Mulberry in Ovid, who in the *Metamorphoses* refers to the legend of Pyramus and Thisbe, who were slain beneath its shade, the fruit being fabled to have thereby changed from white to deep red through absorbing their blood. By Virgil, the tree is termed *sanguinea morus*. Pliny speaks of its employment in medicine and also describes its use in Egypt and Cyprus. He further relates:

'Of all the cultivated trees, the Mulberry is the last that buds, which it never does until the cold weather is past, and it is therefore called the wisest of trees. But when it begins to put forth buds, it dispatches the business in one night, and that with so much force, that their breaking forth may be evidently heard.'

It has been suggested that the generic name of the Mulberry, *Morus*, has been derived from the Latin word *mora* (delay), from this tardy expansion of the buds, and as the wisest of its fellows, the tree was dedicated by the Ancients to Minerva. In alluding to the Black Mulberry, Pliny observes that there is no other tree that has been so neglected by the wit of man, either in grafting or giving it names. It abounded in Italy at that time, as a reference in Virgil's *Georgics* (II, v. 121) clearly shows. The excavations at Pompeii also bear witness to this, for, in the peristyle of the 'House of the Bull,' a Black Mulberry is represented. Mulberry leaves are also to be found in a mosaic from the 'House of the Faun.' Schouw, who wrote about the plants of Pompeii in 1854, considered that *M. alba* was unknown to the Pompeians. At the time of Virgil (who died in 19 B.C.) silk was held to be a product of the Mulberry leaves, the work of the silkworms not being understood. Silkworm culture was first introduced by Justinian from Constantinople – he ruled from A.D. 527–65. In Italy the Black Mulberry was employed for feeding the silkworm until about 1434, when *M. alba* was introduced from the Levant and has ever since been commonly preferred.

References in various old Chronicles show that the Mulberry was far more esteemed in ancient times than at present. It was included among the large number of useful plants ordered by Charlemagne (A.D. 812) to be cultivated on the imperial farm. The cultivation of the Mulberry in Spain is implied by a reference to the preparation of Syrup of Mulberries in the Calendar of Cordova of the year 961.

There are many famous Mulberry trees in England. Those of Syon House, Brentford, are of special historical interest and include what is reported to be the oldest tree of its kind in England, said to be introduced from Persia in 1548. It is this particular and venerable tree which forms the subject of an illustration in London's *Aboretum and Fruticetum*. Although a wreck compared to its former self, it is regarded as one of the largest Mulberry trees in the country. Its height is given by Loudon as 22 feet, and additional interest is attached to this tree, as it is said to have been planted by the botanist Turner. In 1608 James I, being anxious to further the silk industry by introducing the culture of the silkworm into Britain, issued an edict encouraging the cultivation of Mulberry trees, but the attempt to rear silkworms in England proved unsuccessful, apparently because the Black Mulberry was cultivated in error, whereas the White Mulberry is the species on which the silkworm flourishes. A letter was addressed by the King to the

'Lord Lieutenant of the several Shires of England urging them to persuade and require such as are of ability to buy and distribute in that County the number of ten thousand Mulberry plants which shall be delivered to them at our City of –, at the rate of 3 farthings the plant, or at 6s. the hundred containing five score plants.'

The following transaction is mentioned in the College accounts at Cambridge: 'Item for 300 mulberry plants, xviii. s.' This was in 1608–9, the date of Milton's birth, so that the old Mulberry tree growing in the grounds of Christ Church, Cambridge, still bearing excellent fruit, which is reputed to have been planted by Milton, is still older, probably the last of three hundred which cost the College 18s. in 1609.

There is another Mulberry tree still standing near the Vicarage at Stowmarket which, by tradition, is said to have been planted by Milton. A fine specimen of Mulberry tree is to be seen in front of the Head-master's house at Eton. It was measured in 1907, and found to be 30 feet high, with girth of 8 feet 3 inches, and there is a beautiful example in the Canons' old walled garden at Canterbury.

King James I not only issued his famous edict for introducing the culture of the silkworm into Britain, but he also planted largely himself, and directed payments to

'Master William Stallinge of the sum of £935 for the charge of 4 acres of land taken in for His Majesty's use, near to his Palace of Westminster, for the planting of Mulberry trees, together with the charge of walling, levelling and planting thereof with Mulberry trees.'

This plantation is the 'Mulberry Garden' often mentioned by the old dramatists and occupied the site of the present beautiful private grounds of Buckingham Palace, where one remaining Mulberry tree planted at that time is still to be seen. The tree still bears fruit, but is in no way remarkable either for size of its trunk or the spread of its branches.

'The Royal edict of James I,' writes Loudon, 'recommending the cultivation of silkworms and offering packets of Mulberry seeds to all who would sow them, no doubt rendered the tree fashionable, as there is scarcely an old garden or gentleman's seat throughout the country, which can be traced back to the seventeenth century, in which a Mulberry tree is not to be found. It is remarkable, however, that though these trees were expressly intended for the nourishment of silkworms, they nearly all belong to *M. nigra*, as very few instances exist of old trees of *M. alba* in England.' Shakespeare's famous Mulberry, of which there are descendants at Kew, is referable to this period. Shakespeare is said to have taken it from the Mulberry garden of James I, and planted it in his garden at New Place, Stratford-on-Avon, in 1609. This also was a Black Mulberry, 'cultivated for its fruit, which is very wholesome and palatable; and not for its leaves, which are but little esteemed for silkworms.'

'The tree,' Malone writes, 'was celebrated in many a poem, one especially by Dibdin, but about 1752, the then owner of New Place, the Rev. Mr. Gastrell, bought and pulled down the house and cut down Shakespeare's celebrated Mulberry tree, to save himself the trouble of showing it to those whose admiration of the poet led them to visit the ground on which it stood.'

The pieces were made into many snuffboxes and other mementoes of the tree, some of them being inscribed with the punning motto, 'Memento Mori.' Ten years afterwards, when the freedom of the city was presented to Garrick, the document was enclosed in a casket made from the wood of this tree. A cup was also made from it, and at the Shakespeare Jubilee, Garrick, holding the cup, recited verses, composed by himself, in honour of the Mulberry tree planted by Shakespeare. A slip of it was grown by Garrick in his garden at Hampton Court, and a scion of the original tree is now growing in Shakespeare's garden.

¶ *Cultivation.* Mulberry trees like a warm, well-drained, loamy soil, and *M. nigra* is especially worth growing for its luxuriant leafage and picturesque form. It can be increased by cuttings with the greatest ease – in February, cut off some branches of a fairly large size (the old writers say that pieces 8 feet long or more will grow) and insert a foot deep, where neither sun nor wind can freely penetrate. Envelop the stem above the ground level with moss, all but the upper pair of buds, in order to check evaporation. Branches broken down, but not detached, will usually take root if they touch the ground. Layers made in the autumn will root in twelve months, and cuttings of the young wood taken off with a heel and planted deeply in a shady border late in the year will root slowly, but more quickly and surely if put into gentle heat under glass. *M. alba* will also root from autumn or winter cuttings.

The Mulberry can also be increased by seeds, which, if sown in gentle heat, or in the open early in the year, will produce young seedlings by the autumn.

In a paper by Mr. J. Williams of Pitmaston, published in the Horticultural Transactions for 1813, is the statement:

'The standard Mulberry receives great injury by being planted on grass plots with a view of preserving the fruit when it falls spontaneously. No tree, perhaps, receives more benefit from the spade and the dunghill than the Mulberry; it ought therefore to be frequently dug about the roots and occasionally assisted with manure.'

Mulberry trees do not begin to bear fruit early in life, and few fruits can be expected from a tree before it is fifteen years of age. It is commonly said that the fruit of the oldest Mulberry trees is the best.

There are few trees better able to withstand the debilitating effects of the close atmosphere of small town gardens, and numerous fine examples are met with about London, several within the City boundaries, familiar examples of which are those in Finsbury Circus and many smaller ones in St. Paul's Churchyard.

Mulberry trees are not easily killed, and old examples that have been reduced to a mere shell have been rejuvenated by careful pruning and cultivation.

The WHITE MULBERRY (*M. alba*), a deciduous tree, 30 to 45 feet high, native of China, to which we have referred as the tree upon which the silkworm is fed, succeeds quite well in the south of England but is not often grown in this country.

The RED MULBERRY (*M. rubra*), a native of the United States of America, is very difficult to grow here.

The FRENCH MULBERRY (*Callicarpa Americana*) is a shrub 3 to 6 feet high, with bluish flowers and violet fruit, but the species is too tender for any but the mildest parts of Great Britain.

¶ *Constituents* of the Black Mulberry Fruit: Glucose, protein, pectin, colouring matter, tartaric and malic acids, ash, etc. This composition varies much, as in all fleshy fruits, with the ripeness and other conditions.

In amount of grape sugar, the Mulberry is surpassed only by the Cherry and the Grape.

¶ *Uses.* Mulberries are refreshing and have laxative properties and are well adapted to febrile cases. In former days, they used to be made into various conserves and drinks.

RECIPES

Mulberry Wine

On each gallon of ripe Mulberries, pour 1 gallon of boiling water and let them stand for 2 days. Then squeeze all through a hair sieve or bag. Wash out the tub or jar and return the liquor to it, put in the sugar at the rate of 3 lb. to each gallon of the liquor; stir up until quite dissolved, then put the liquor into a cask. Let the cask be raised a little on one side until fermentation ceases, then bung down. If the liquor be clear, it may be bottled in 4 months' time. Into each bottle put 1 clove and a small lump of sugar and the bottles should be kept in a moderate temperature. The wine may be used in a year from time of bottling.

Mulberries are sometimes used in Devonshire for mixing with cider during fermentation, giving a pleasant taste and deep red colour. In Greece, also, the fruit is subjected to fermentation, thereby furnishing an inebriating beverage.

Scott relates in *Ivanhoe* that the Saxons made a favourite drink, Morat, from the juice of Mulberries with honey, but it is doubtful whether the *Morum* of the Anglo-Saxon 'Vocabularies' was not the Blackberry, so that the 'Morat' of the Saxons may have been Blackberry Wine.

Mulberry Jam

Unless very ripe Mulberries are used, the jam will have an acid taste. Put 1 lb. of Mulberries in a jar and stand it in a pan of water on the fire till the juice is extracted. Strain them and put the juice into a preserving pan with 3 lb. of sugar. Boil it and remove the scum and put in 3 lb. of very ripe Mulberries and let them stand in the syrup until thoroughly warm, then set the pan back on the fire and boil them very gently for a short time, stirring all the time and taking care not to break the fruit. Then take the pan off and let them stand in the syrup all night. Put the pan on the fire again in the morning and boil again gently till stiff.

¶ *Medicinal Action and Uses.* The sole use of Mulberries in modern medicine is for the preparation of a syrup, employed to flavour or colour any other medicine. Mulberry Juice is obtained from the ripe fruit of the Mulberry by expression and is an official drug of the British Pharmacopœia. It is a dark violet or purple liquid, with a faint odour and a refreshing, acid, saccharine taste. The British Pharmacopœia directs that *Syrupus Mori* should be prepared by heating 50 fluid drachms of the expressed juice to boiling point, then cooling and filtering. Ninety drachms of sugar is then dissolved in the juice, which is warmed up again. When once more cooled, 6·25 drachms of alcohol is added: the product should then measure about 100 drachms (20 fluid ounces). The dose is 2 to 1 fluid drachm, but it is, as stated, chiefly used as an adjuvant rather than for its slightly laxative and expectorant qualities, though used as a gargle, it will relieve sore throat.

The juice of the American Red Mulberry may be substituted; it is less acid than the European, while that of the White Mulberry, native of China, is sweet, but rather insipid.

In the East, the Mulberry is most productive and useful. It is gathered when ripe, dried on the tops of the houses in the sun, and stored for winter use. In Cabul, it is pounded to a fine powder, and mixed with flour for bread.

The bark of *M. nigra* is reputed anthelmintic, and is used to expel tape worm.

The root-bark of *M. Indica* (Rumph) and other species is much used in the East under the name of San-pai-p'i, as a diuretic and expectorant.

The *Morinda tinctoria*, or Indian Mulberry, is used by the African aborigines as a remedial agent, but there is no reliable evidence of its therapeutic value.

A parasitic fungus growing on the old stems of Mulberry trees found in the island of Meshima, Japan, and called there *Meshimakobu*, brown outside and yellow inside, is used in Japan for medicine.

Gerard recommends the fruit of the Mulberry tree for use in all affections of the mouth and throat.

'The barke of the root,' he says, 'is bitter, hot and drie, and hath a scouring faculty: the decoction hereof doth open the stoppings of the liver and spleen, it purgeth the belly, and driveth forth wormes.'

With Parkinson, the fruit was evidently not in favour, for he tells us:

'Mulberries are not much desired to be eaten, although they be somewhat pleasant, both for that they stain their fingers and lips that eat them, and do quickly putrefie in the stomach, if they be not taken before meat.'

The Mulberry family, *Moraceæ*, formerly regarded, together with the *Ulmaceæ* (Elm family), as a division of the *Urticaceæ* (Nettle family), comprises upwards of 50 genera and about 900 species, of very diverse habit and appearance. Among them are the highly important food-plants *Ficus* (Fig) and *Artocarpus* (Bread fruit). *M. tinctoria* (Linn.), sometimes known as *Machura tinctoria* (D. Don), but generally now named *Chlorophora tinctoria* (Gaudich.), yields the dye-stuff Fustic, chiefly used for colouring wood of an orange-yellow colour. The tree is indigenous in Mexico and some of the West Indies, the wood being imported in logs of various sizes. This kind of fustic is known as old fustic, or Cuba fustic. Young fustic is a different product, obtained from *Rhus cotinus* (Linn.). It is known also as Venetian or Hungarian sumach, and is used in the Tyrol for tanning leather. The extract of fustic is imported as well as the wood. From *Maclura Brasiliensis* (Endl.) another important dye-wood is obtained. A yellow dye is also derived from the root of the Osage Orange (*Toxylon pomiferum*, Raf.), belonging to this order. The milky juice of *Brosimum Galactodendron* (Don) – the Cow or Milk-Tree of Tropical America – is said to be usable as cow's milk, and 'Bread-nuts' are the edible seeds of another member of this genus, *B. Alicastrum* (Swz.), of Jamaica. The famous deadly Upas Tree of the East Indies (*Antiaris toxicaria*, Lesc.) is a less useful member of this family.

The bast-fibres of many *Moraceæ* are tough and are used in the manufacture of cordage and paper. The Paper Mulberry (*Broussonetia papyrifera*, Vint.) is cultivated extensively in Japan. It is a native of China, introduced into Great Britain early in the eighteenth century and is a coarse-growing, vigorous shrub, or a tree up to 30 feet, forming a roundish, spreading head of branches. The young wood is thickly downy, soft and pithy, the leaves very variable in size and form, often shaped like fig-leaves, the upper surface dull, green and rough, the lower surface densely woolly. It is a diœcious plant, the male flowers in cylindrical, often curly, woolly catkins, the female flowers in ball-like heads, producing round fruits congregated of small, red, pulpy seeds. In Japan, the stems are cut down every winter, so that the shrub only attains a height of 6 or 7 feet, and the barks are stripped off as an important material for paper. *B. Kajinoki* (Sieb.) is a deciduous tree, wild in Japan, growing 29 to 30 feet high, similar to the Paper Mulberry and made use of in like manner, though inferior. The ripe fruits are beautifully red and sweet. Paper is also manufactured in Japan with the fibre of the bark of *B. kæmpferi* (Sieb.), a deciduous climber. A good paper may be manufactured from the bast of the *Morus alba*, var. *stylosa* (Bur.), Jap. 'Kuwa,' but as this plant is used especially for feeding silkworms, the paper made from the branches after the leaves are taken off for silkworms is of a very inferior quality.

MULLEIN, GREAT

Verbascum thapsus (LINN.)
N.O. Scrophulariaceæ

Synonyms. White Mullein. Torches. Mullein Dock. Our Lady's Flannel. Velvet Dock. Blanket Herb. Velvet Plant. Woollen. Rag Paper. Candlewick Plant. Wild Ice Leaf. Clown's Lungwort. Bullock's Lungwort. Aaron's Rod. Jupiter's Staff. Jacob's Staff. Peter's Staff. Shepherd's Staff. Shepherd's Clubs. Beggar's Stalk. Golden Rod. Adam's Flannel. Beggar's Blanket. Clot. Cuddy's Lungs. Duffle. Feltwort. Fluffweed. Hare's Beard. Old Man's Flannel. Hag's Taper

Parts Used. Leaves, flowers, root

Habitat. Verbascum thapsus (Linn.), the Great Mullein, is a widely distributed plant, being found all over Europe and in temperate Asia as far as the Himalayas, and in North America is exceedingly abundant as a naturalized weed in the eastern States. It is met with throughout Britain (except in the extreme north of Scotland) and also in Ireland and the Channel Islands, on hedge-banks, by roadsides and on waste ground, more especially on gravel, sand or chalk. It flowers during July and August

The natural order Scrophulariaceæ is an important family of plants comprising 200 genera and about 2,500 species, occurring mostly in temperate and sub-tropical regions, many of them producing flowers of great beauty, on which account they are frequently cultivated among favourite garden and greenhouse flowers. Of this group are the Calceolaria, Mimulus, Penstemon, Antirrhinum and Collinsia. Among its British representatives it embraces members so diverse as the Foxglove and Speedwell, the Mullein and Figworts, the Toadflax and the semi-parasites, Eyebright, Bartsia, Cowwheat, and the Red and Yellow Rattles.

Most of the flowers are capable of self-fertilization in default of insect visits.

Unlike the Labiatæ, to which they are rather closely related, plants belonging to this order seldom contain much volatile oil, though resinous substances are common. The most important constituents are glucosides, and many of them are poisonous or powerfully active.

A number of the Scrophulariaceæ are or have been valued for their curative properties and are widely employed both in domestic and in regular medicine.

The genus *Verbascum*, to which the Mullein belongs, contains 210 species, distributed in Europe, West and Central Asia and North Africa, six of which are natives of Great Britain. The Mulleins, like the Veronicas, are exceptions to the general character of the Scrophulariaceæ, having nearly regular, open corollas, the segments being connected only towards the base, instead of having the more fantastic flowers of the Snapdragon and others. They are all tall, stout biennials, with large leaves and flowers in long, terminal spikes.

¶ *Description.* In the first season of the plant's growth, there appears only a rosette of large leaves, 6 to 15 inches long, in form somewhat like those of the Foxglove, but thicker – whitish with a soft, dense mass of hairs on both sides, which make them very thick to the touch. In the following spring, a solitary, stout, pale stem, with tough, strong fibres enclosing a thin rod of white pith, arises from the midst of the felted leaves. Its rigid uprightness accounts for some of the plant's local names: 'Aaron's Rod,' 'Jupiter's' or 'Jacob's Staff,' etc.

The leaves near the base of the stem are large and numerous, 6 to 8 inches long and 2 to 2½ inches broad, but become smaller as they ascend the stem, on which they are arranged not opposite to one another, but on alternate sides. They are broad and simple in form, the outline rather waved, stalkless, their bases being continued some distance down the stem, as in the Comfrey and a few other plants, the midrib from a quarter to half-way up the blade being actually joined to the stem. By these 'decurrent' leaves (as this hugging of the stem by the leaves is botanically termed) the Great Mullein is easily distinguished from other British species of Mullein – some with white and some with yellow flowers. The leaf system is so arranged that the smaller leaves above drop the rain upon the larger ones below, which direct the water to the roots. This is a necessary arrangement, since the Mullein grows mostly on dry soils. The stellately-branched hairs which cover the leaves so thickly act as a protective coat, checking too great a giving off of the plant's moisture, and also are a defensive weapon of the plant, for not only do they prevent the attacks of creeping insects, but they set up an intense irritation in the mucous membrane of any grazing animals that may attempt to browse upon them, so that the plants are usually left severely alone by them. The leaves are, however, subject to the attacks of a mould, *Peronospora sordida*.

The hairs are not confined to the leaves alone, but are also on every part of the stem, on the calyces and on the outside of the corollas, so that the whole plant appears whitish or grey. The homely but valuable Mullein Tea, a remedy of the greatest antiquity for coughs and colds, must indeed always be strained through fine muslin to remove any hairs that may be floating in the hot water that has been poured over the flowers, or leaves, for otherwise they cause intolerable itching in the mouth.

Towards the top of the stalk, which grows frequently 4 or even 5 feet high, and in gardens has been known to attain a height of 7 or 8 feet, the much-diminished woolly leaves merge into the thick, densely crowded flower-spike, usually a foot long, the flowers opening here and there on the spike, not in regular progression from the base, as in the Foxglove. The flowers are stalkless, the sulphur-yellow corolla, a somewhat irregular cup, nearly an inch across, formed of five rounded petals, united at the base to form a very short tube, being enclosed in a woolly calyx, deeply cut into five lobes. The five stamens stand on the corolla; three of them are shorter than the other two and have a large number of tiny white hairs on their filaments. These hairs are full of sap, and it has been suggested that they form additional bait to the insect visitors, supplementing the allurement of the nectar that lies round the base of the ovary. All kinds of insects are attracted by this plant, the Honey Bee, Humble Bee, some of the smaller wild bees and different species of flies, since the nectar and the staminal hairs are both so readily accessible, though the supply of nectar is not very great. The three short hairy stamens have only short, one-celled anthers – the two longer, smooth ones have larger anthers. The pollen sacs have an orange-red inner surface, disclosed as the anthers open.

In some species, *Verbascum nigrum*, the Dark Mullein, and *V. blattaria*, the Moth Mullein, the filament hairs are purple. The rounded ovary is hairy and also the lower part of the style. The stigma is mature before the anthers and the style projects at the moment the flower opens, so that any insect approaching it from another blossom where it has got brushed by pollen, must needs strike it on alighting and thus insure cross-fertilization, though, failing this, the flower is also able to fertilize itself. The ripened seed capsule is very hard and contains many seeds, which eventually escape through two valves and are scattered round the parent plant.

¶ *History.* The down on the leaves and stem makes excellent tinder when quite dry, readily igniting on the slightest spark, and was, before the introduction of cotton, used for lamp wicks, hence another of the old names: 'Candlewick Plant.' An old superstition existed that witches in their incantations used lamps and candles provided with wicks of this sort, and another of the plant's many names, 'Hag's Taper', refers to this, though the word 'hag' is said to be derived from the Anglo-Saxon word *Hæge* or *Hage* (a hedge) – the name 'Hedge Taper' also exists – and may imply that the sturdy spikes of this tall hedge plant, studded with pale yellow blossoms, suggested a tall candle growing in the hedge, another of its countryside names being, indeed, 'Our Lady's Candle.' Lyte (*The Niewe Herball*, 1578) tells us 'that the whole toppe, with its pleasant yellow floures sheweth like to a wax candle or taper cunningly wrought.' 'Torches' is another name for the plant, and Parkinson tells us:

'Verbascum is called of the Latines Candela regia, and Candelaria, because the elder age used the stalks dipped in suet to burne, whether at funeralls or otherwise.'

And Gerard (1597) also remarks that it is 'a plant whereof is made a manner of lynke (link) if it be talowed.' Dr. Prior, in *The Popular Names of British Plants*, states that the word Mullein was Moleyn in Anglo-Saxon, and Malen in Old French, derived from the Latin *malandrium*, i.e. the malanders or leprosy, and says:

'The term "malandre" became also applied to diseases of cattle, to lung diseases among the rest, and the plant being used as a remedy, acquired its name of "Mullein" and "Bullock's Lungwort." '

Coles, in 1657, in *Adam in Eden*, says that

'Husbandmen of Kent do give it their cattle against the cough of the lungs, and I, therefore, mention it because cattle are also in some sort to be provided for in their diseases.'

The name 'Clown's Lung Wort' refers to its use as a homely remedy. 'Ag-Leaf' and 'Ag-Paper' are other names for it. 'Wild Ice Leaf' perhaps refers to the white look of the leaves. Few English plants have so many local names.

The Latin name *Verbascum* is considered to be a corruption of *barbascum*, from the Latin *barba* (a beard), in allusion to the shaggy foliage, and was bestowed on the genus by Linnæus.

Both in Europe and Asia the power of driving away evil spirits was ascribed to the Mullein. In India it has the reputation among the natives that the St. John's Wort once had here, being considered a sure safeguard against evil spirits and magic, and from the ancient classics we learn that it was this plant which Ulysses took to protect himself against the wiles of Circe.

The Cowslip and the Primrose are classed together by our old herbalists as Petty Mulleins, and are usually credited with much the same properties. Gerard recommends both the flowers and leaves of the primrose, boiled in wine, as a remedy for all diseases of the lungs and the juice of the root itself, snuffed up the nose, for megrim.

All the various species of Mullein found in Britain possess similar medicinal properties, but *V. thapsus*, the species of most common occurrence, is the one most employed.

For medicinal purposes it is generally collected from *wild* specimens, but is worthy of cultivation, not merely from its beauty as an ornamental plant, but also for its medicinal value, which is undoubted. In most parts of Ireland, besides growing wild, it is carefully cultivated in gardens, because of a steady demand for the plant by sufferers from pulmonary consumption.

Its cultivation is easy: being a hardy biennial, it only requires sowing in very ordinary soil and to be kept free from weeds. When growing in gardens, Mulleins will often be found to be infested with slugs, which can be caught wholesale by placing in borders slates and boards smeared with margarine on the underside. Examine in the morning and deposit the catch in a pail of lime and water.

¶ *Parts Used.* The leaves and flowers are the parts used medicinally.

Fresh Mullein leaves are also used for the purpose of making a homœopathic tincture.

¶ *Constituents.* The leaves are nearly odourless and of a mucilaginous and bitterish taste. They contain gum as their principal constituent, together with 1 to 2 per cent. of resin, divisible into two parts, one soluble in ether, the other not; a readily soluble amaroid; a little tannin and a trace of volatile oil.

The flowers contain gum, resin, a yellow colouring principle, a green fatty matter (a sort of chlorophyll), a glucoside, an acrid, fatty matter; free acid and phosphoric acid; uncrystallizable sugar; some mineral salts, the bases of which are potassia and lime, and a small amount of yellowish volatile oil. They should yield not more than 6 per cent of ash. Their odour is peculiar and agreeable: their taste mucilaginous.

¶ *Medicinal Action and Uses.* The Mullein has very markedly demulcent, emollient and astringent properties, which render it useful in pectoral complaints and bleeding of the lungs and bowels. The whole plant seems to possess slightly sedative and narcotic properties.

It is considered of much value in phthisis and other wasting diseases, palliating the cough and staying expectoration, consumptives appearing to benefit greatly by its use, being given in the form of an infusion, 1 oz. of dried, or the corresponding quantity of fresh leaves being boiled for 10 minutes in a pint of milk, and when strained, given warm, thrice daily, with or without sugar. The taste of the decoction is bland, mucilaginous and cordial, and forms a pleasant emollient and nutritious medicine for allaying a cough, or removing the pain and irritation of hæmorrhoids. A plain infusion of 1 oz. to a pint of boiling water can also be employed, taken in wineglassful doses frequently.

The dried leaves are sometimes smoked in an ordinary tobacco pipe to relieve the irritation of the respiratory mucus membranes, and will completely control, it is said, the hacking cough of consumption. They can be employed with equal benefit when made into cigarettes, for asthma and spasmodic coughs in general.

Fomentations and poultices of the leaves have been found serviceable in hæmorrhoidal complaints.

Mullein is said to be of much value in diarrhœa, from its combination of demulcent with astringent properties, by this combination strengthening the bowels at the same time. In diarrhœa the ordinary infusion is generally given, but when any bleeding of the bowels is present, the decoction prepared with milk is recommended.

On the Continent, a sweetened infusion of the *flowers* strained in order to separate the rough hairs, is considerably used as a domestic remedy in mild catarrhs, colic, etc.

A conserve of the flowers has also been employed on the Continent against ringworm, and a distilled water of the flowers was long reputed a cure for burns and erysipelas.

An oil produced by macerating Mullein flowers in olive oil in a corked bottle, during prolonged exposure to the sun, or by keeping near the fire for several days, is used as a local application in country districts in Germany for piles and other mucus membrane inflammation, and also for frost bites and bruises. Mullein oil is recommended for earache and discharge from the ear, and for any eczema of the external ear and its canal. Dr. Fernie (*Herbal Simples*) states that some of the most brilliant results have been obtained in suppurative inflammation of the inner ear by a single application of Mullein oil, and that in acute or chronic cases, two or three drops of this oil should be made to fall in the ear twice or thrice in the day.

Mullein oil is a valuable destroyer of disease germs. The fresh flowers, steeped for 21 days in olive oil, are said to make an admirable bactericide. Gerarde tells us that 'Figs do not putrifie at all that are wrapped in the leaves of Mullein.'

An alcoholic tincture is prepared by homœopathic chemists, from the fresh herb with spirits of wine, which has proved beneficial for migraine or sick headache of long standing, with oppression of the ear. From 8 to 10 drops of the tincture are given as a dose, with cold water, repeated frequently.

¶ *Preparation and Dosage.* Fluid extract, ½ to 1 drachm.

Formerly the flowers of several species of Mullein were officinal, but Mullein no longer has a place in the British Pharmacopœia, though Verbascum Flowers were introduced into the 4th Edition of the United States National Formulary, as one of the ingredients in pectoral remedies, and the leaves, in fluid extract of Mullein leaves, made with diluted alcohol were directed to be used as a demulcent, the dose being 1 fluid drachm.

In more ancient times, much higher virtues were attributed to this plant. Culpepper gives us a list of most extraordinary cures performed by its agency, and Gerard remarks that

'there be some who think that this herbe being but carryed about one, doth help the falling sickness, especially the leaves of the plant which have not yet borne flowers, and gathered when the sun is in Virgo and the moon in Aries, which thing notwithstanding is vaine and superstitious.'

A decoction of its roots was held to be an alleviation for toothache, and also good for cramps and convulsions, and an early morning draught of the distilled water of the flowers to be good for gout.

Mullein juice and powder made from the dried roots rubbed on rough warts was said to quickly remove them, though it was not recommended as equally efficacious for smooth warts. A poultice made of the seeds and leaves, boiled in hot wine, was also considered an excellent means to 'draw forth speedily thorns or splinters gotten into the flesh.' We also hear of the woolly leaves being worn in the stockings to promote circulation and keep the feet warm.

The flowers impart a yellow colour to boiling water and a rather permanent green colour with dilute sulphuric acid, the latter colour becoming brown upon the addition of alkalis. An infusion of the flowers was used by the Roman ladies to dye their hair a golden colour. Lyte tells us, 'the golden floures of Mulleyn stiped in lye, causeth the heare to war yellow, being washed therewithall,' and according to another old authority, Alexander Trallianus, the ashes of the plant made into a soap will restore hair which has become grey to its original colour.

The seeds are said to intoxicate fish when thrown into the water, and are used by poachers for that purpose, being slightly narcotic. According to Rosenthal (*Pharmaceutical Journal*, July, 1902), the seeds of *V. sinuatum* (Linn.), which are used in Greece as a fish poison, contain 6 to 13 per cent. of Saponin. Traces of the same substance were found in the seeds of *V. phlomoides* (Linn.) and *V. thapsiforme* (Schrad.), common in the south of Europe, which have been used for the same purpose. *V. pulverulentum* of Madeira (also used as a fish poisoner) and *V. phlomoides* are employed as tænicides (expellers of tapeworm).

MUSK SEED

Hibiscus Abelmoschus (LINN.)
N.O. Malvaceæ

Synonyms. Abelmoschus Moschatus. Semen Abelmoschi. Grana Moschata. Ambretta. Egyptian Alcée. Bisornkorner. Ambrakorner. Target-leaved Hibiscus. Ab-el-mosch. Bamia Moschata. Ketmie odorante. Galu gasturi. Capu kanassa
Part Used. Seeds
Habitat. Egypt, East and West Indies

¶ *Description.* This evergreen shrub is about 4 feet in height, having alternate, palmate leaves and large, sulphur yellow, solitary flowers with a purple base. The capsules are in the form of a five-cornered pyramid, filled with large seeds with a strong odour of musk. The capsules are used in soup and for pickles, and the greyish-brown, kidney-shaped seeds, the size of a lentil, with a strong aromatic flavour, are used by the Arabians to mix with coffee. They are used in perfumery for fats and oils, and for the adulteration of musk.

¶ *Constituents.* The seeds contain an abundance of fixed oil, and owe their scent to a coloured resin and a volatile, odorous body. They also contain albuminous matter.

¶ *Medicinal Action and Uses.* An emulsion made from the seeds is regarded as antispasmodic. In Egypt the seeds are chewed as a stomachic, nervine, and to sweeten the breath, and are also used as an aphrodisiac and insecticide. The seeds made into an emulsion with milk are used for itch.

¶ *Other Species.*
A variety is found in Martinique, of a lighter grey in colour and a more delicate odour.

Hibiscus esculentus or *A. esculentus*, okra, bendee, or gombo, is cultivated for its fruit, the abundant mucilage of which, called gombine, is used for thickening soup. The long roots have much odourless mucilage and when powdered are white, and are said to be better than marsh-mallow.

The bark is used for paper and cordage.

It is largely grown in Constantinople as a demulcent.

The leaves furnish an emollient poultice.

MUSTARDS

N.O. Cruciferæ

The Mustards, Black and White, are both wild herbs growing in waste places in this country, but are cultivated for their seeds, which are valuable medicinally and commercially. They were originally treated as members of a small genus of frequently cultivated European and Asiatic herbs named Sinapis, from the Greek *sinapi* (mustard), a name used by Theophrastus, but they are now generally included in the Cabbage genus, *Brassica*.

MUSTARD, WHITE

Brassica alba (BOISS.)

Synonym. Sinapis alba (LINN.)
Part Used. Seeds

The White Mustard, a native of Europe, common in our fields and by roadsides, and also largely cultivated, is an erect annual, about a foot or more in height, with pinnatifid leaves and large, yellow, cruciferous flowers. It closely resembles the Black Mustard, but is smaller. The fruit of the two plants differs considerably in shape, those of the White Mustard being more or less horizontal and hairy, while Black Mustard pods are erect and smooth. The pods of White Mustard are spreading, roundish pods, ribbed and swollen where the seeds are situated, and provided with a very large flattened, sword-shaped beak at the end. Each pod contains four to six globular seeds, about $\frac{1}{12}$ inch in diameter, yellow both on the surface and internally. The seed-coat, though appearing smooth, on examination with a lens, is seen to be covered with minute pits and to be finely reticulated. The inner seedcoats contain a quantity of mucilage, with which the seeds become coated when soaked in water, hence they are often employed to absorb the last traces of moisture in bottles which are not chemically dry. The cotyledons of the seeds contain oil and give a pungent but inodorous emulsion when rubbed with water.

The young seedling plants of White Mustard are commonly raised in gardens for salad, the seeds being usually sown with those of the garden cress and germinating with great rapidity. They may be grown all the year round, the seed readily vegetating under a hand-glass even in cold weather, if the ground is not absolutely frozen.

'When in the leaf,' wrote John Evelyn in 1699, in his *Acetaria*, 'Mustard, especially in young seedling plants, is of incomparable effect to quicken and revive the spirits, strengthening the memory, expelling heaviness, . . . besides being an approved antiscorbutic.'

In Gerard's time, a century earlier, White Mustard was not very common in England.

Both Mustards afford excellent fodder for sheep, and as they can be sown late in the summer are often used for this purpose after the failure of a turnip or rape crop, the White Mustard being more frequently employed, as it is less pungent, though equally nutritious. White Mustard makes a good catch crop, being ready for consumption on the land by sheep eight or nine weeks after being sown. It may be sown in southern counties after an early corn crop, about a peck of seed being sown broadcast to the acre. The plants are hoed sometimes to a distance of about 9 inches apart, if required for seed.

As *green manure*, both kinds of Mustard are employed, but the White Mustard is preferred for this purpose by English farmers, the seed being sown in August and September, and when the plants have attained a good size, about two months after sowing, they are ploughed in. Besides affording useful manure in itself, this green manure helps to prevent the waste of nitrates, which instead of being washed away in drainage water, which would probably happen if the soil were bare, are stored up in the growing plant.

The seeds of the Mustards retain their vitality for a great length of time when buried in the ground, so that after the plants have once been grown anywhere, it is difficult to get rid of them. It has been noticed in the Isle of Ely that whenever a trench was made, White Mustard sprang up from the newly-turned earth.

¶ *Part Used Medicinally.* The dried, ripe seeds are alone official. They possess rubefacient properties, and are mixed with Black Mustard seeds to produce mustard flour for preparing mustard poultices. The powder is not infrequently adulterated with farinaceous substances, coloured by turmeric.

¶ *Constituents.* The epidermal cells of the seed coat of White Mustard seeds contain mucilage, and the cotyledons contain from 23 to 26 per cent. of a fixed oil, which consists of the glycerides of oleic, stearic and erucic or brassic acids. The seeds also contain the crystalline glucoside Sinalbin and the enzyme Myrosin, which unite to form a volatile oil, called Sinalbin Mustard Oil, used for various purposes, though not so pungent as that of Black Mustard. This oil cannot be obtained by distillation, but is extracted by boiling alcohol after the seed has been deprived of its fixed oil. When cold, the volatile oil possesses only a faint, anise-like odour, but a pungent odour is given off on heating. The cake, after the oil is expressed, is pungent and therefore not well fitted for cattle food, but is used for manure.

¶ *Medicinal Action and Uses.* The seeds when ground form a pungent powder, but it is much inferior in strength to that prepared from the black-seeded species.

They have been employed medicinally from very early times. Hippocrates advised their use both internally and as a counter irritating poultice, made with vinegar. They have been administered frequently in disorders of the digestive organs. White Mustard seeds were at one time quite a fashionable remedy as a laxative, especially for old people, the dose being $\frac{1}{2}$ oz. in the entire state, but from the danger of their retention in the intestines, they are not very safe in large quantities, having in several cases caused inflammation of the stomach and intestinal canal.

An infusion of the seeds will relieve chronic bronchitis and confirmed rheumatism, and for a relaxed sore throat a gargle of Mustard Seed Tea will be found of service.

MUSTARD, BLACK

Brassica nigra (LINN.)
Sinapis nigra (LINN.)

Synonym. Brassica sinapioides (Roth.)
Part Used. Seeds
Habitat. The Black Mustard grows throughout Europe, except in the north-eastern parts, also in South Siberia, Asia Minor and Northern Africa, and is naturalized in North and South America. It is largely cultivated in England, Holland, Italy, Germany and elsewhere for the sake of the seed, used partly as a condiment, and partly for its oil

¶ *Description.* It is an erect annual, 3 feet or more in height, with smaller flowers than the White Mustard. The spear-shaped, upper leaves, linear, pointed, entire and smooth, and the shortly-beaked pods, readily distinguish it from the former species. The smooth, erect flattened pods, each provided with a short slender beak, contain about ten to twelve dark reddish-brown or black seeds, which are collected when ripe and dried. They are about half the size of White Mustard seeds, but possess similar properties. The seedcoat is thin and brittle and covered with minute pits. Like the White Mustard, the seeds are inodorous, even when powdered, though a pungent odour is noticeable when moistened with water, owing to the formation of volatile oil of Mustard, which is colourless or pale yellow, with an intensely penetrating odour and a very acrid taste.

¶ *History.* The ancient Greek physicians held this plant in such esteem for the medicinal use of its seeds that they attributed its discovery to Æsculapius.

When it was first employed as a condiment is unknown, but it was most likely used in England by the Saxons. Probably the Romans, who were great eaters of mustard, pounded and steeped in new wine, brought the condiment with them to Britain. Mustard gets its name from *mustum* (the must), or newly-fermented grape juice, and *ardens* (burning). It was originally eaten whole, or slightly crushed. Gerard in 1623 says that

'the seede of Mustard pounded with vinegar is an excellent sauce, good to be eaten with any grosse meates, either fish or flesh, because it doth help digestion, warmeth the stomache and provoketh appetite.'

Tusser mentions its garden cultivation and domestic use in the sixteenth century, and Shakespeare alludes more than once to it: Tewkesbury mustard is referred to in *Henry IV.* The herbalist Coles, writing in 1657, says:

'In Glostershire about Teuxbury they grind Mustard seed and make it up into balls which are brought to London and other remote places as being the best that the world affords.'

All mustard was formerly made up into balls with honey or vinegar and a little cinnamon, to keep till wanted, when they were mixed with more vinegar. It was sold in balls till Mrs. Clements, of Durham, at the close of the eighteenth century, invented the method of preparing mustard flour, which long went under the name of Durham Mustard. John Evelyn recommends for mustard-making 'best Tewkesbury' or the 'soundest and weightiest Yorkshire seeds,' and tells us that the Italians in making mustard as a condiment mix orange and lemon peel with the black seed. At Dijon, where the best Continental mustard is made, the condiment is seasoned with various spices and savouries, such as Anchovies, Capers, Tarragon and Catsup of Walnuts or Mushrooms.

The Black Mustard is said to have been employed by the Romans as a green vegetable. The young leaves may be eaten as salad in place of those of the White variety, but are more pungent.

The Mustard Tree of Scripture is supposed by some authorities to be a species of Sinapis, closely resembling the Black Mustard, but as the latter never attains the dimensions of a tree, it has been conjectured that the plant in question is the *Khardal* of the Arabs, a tree abounding near the Sea of Galilee, which bears numerous branches and has small seeds, having the flavour and properties of Mustard.

¶ *Cultivation.* Mustard is sown in spring, either broadcast or in drills, a foot or more apart, and ripens towards the end of summer, when, after it has stood in sheaves to dry, the seed is threshed out and dried on trays by gentle artificial heat. The crop is very liable to injury from wet. It is grown for market on rich, alluvial soil, chiefly in Lincolnshire and Yorkshire. In Durham, the cultivation of Mustard of an excellent quality has been pursued on a considerable scale for the last two hundred years. Before grinding, the husk is usually removed, the seeds are then passed between rollers and afterwards reduced to powder in a mortar. This is the system invented by Mrs. Clements, of Durham. The so-called London Mustard is almost always adulterated and

568

many samples consist of little but flour, coloured with turmeric and flavoured with pepper.

The only seeds resembling those of Black Mustard are Colchicum seeds, which are larger, rougher, harder, bitter and not pungent.

¶ *Constituents.* The virtues of Black Mustard depend on an acrid, volatile oil contained in the seeds, combined with an active principle containing much sulphur. The acridity of the oil is modified in the seeds by being combined with another fixed oil of a bland nature, which can be separated.

The epidermal cells of the seed-coat contain much less mucilage than those of White Mustard seeds, but the cotyledons of Black Mustard seeds contain from 31 to 33 per cent. of a fixed oil, which consists of the glycerides of Oleic, Stearic and Erucic or Brassic and Behenic acids. The seeds also contain the crystalline glucoside Sinigrin and the enzyme Myrosin. These substances are stored in separate cells. When brought together in water, the volatile Oil of Mustard is formed. It is distilled from the seeds that have been deprived of most of the fixed oil and macerated in water for several hours, and contains from 90 to 99 per cent. of the active principle, Allyl isothiocyanate, which is used as a counter irritant. It is on account of the abundant sulphur contained by this active principle that mustard discolours silver spoons left in it, black sulphuret of silver being formed.

Neither White nor Black Mustard seeds contain starch when ripe.

It was formerly supposed that Black Mustard was deficient in the enzyme Myrosin, and White Mustard was added to correct this and to secure the maximum pungency. It has been proved, however, that Black Mustard contains sufficient of the enzyme, and that no increase in the yield of the volatile oil is effected by adding White Mustard. The main object in using both Black and White Mustard for preparing mustard flour, is probably the production of a commercial article with a better flavour than could be obtained otherwise.

¶ *Medicinal Action and Uses.* Irritant, stimulant, diuretic, emetic. Mustard is used in the form of poultices for external application near the seat of inward inflammation, chiefly in pneumonia, bronchitis and other diseases of the respiratory organs. It relieves congestion of various organs by drawing the blood to the surface, as in head affections, and is of service in the alleviation of neuralgia and other pains and spasms.

Mustard Leaves, used instead of poultices,

consist of the mustard seeds, deprived of fixed oil, but retaining the pungency-producing substances and made to adhere to paper.

Oil of Mustard is a powerful irritant and rubefacient, and when applied to the skin in its pure state, produces almost instant vesication, but when dissolved in rectified spirit, or spirit of camphor, or employed in the form of the Compound Liniment of Mustard of the British Pharmacopœia, is a very useful application for chilblains, chronic rheumatism, colic, etc.

Hot water poured on bruised Black Mustard seeds makes a stimulating footbath and helps to throw off a cold or dispel a headache. It also acts as an excellent fomentation.

Internally, Mustard is useful as a regular and mild aperient, being at the same time an alterative. If a tablespoonful of Mustard flour be added to a glass of *tepid* water, it operates briskly as a stimulating and sure emetic. In cases of hiccough, a teaspoonful of Mustard flour in a teacupful of *boiling* water is effective. The dose may be repeated in ten minutes if needed.

The bland oil expressed from the hulls of the seeds, after the flour has been sifted away, promotes the growth of the hair and may be used with benefit externally for rheumatism.

Whitehead's Essence of Mustard is made with spirits of turpentine and rosemary, with which camphor and the farina of Black Mustard seed are mixed. This oil is very little affected by frost or the atmosphere, and is therefore specially prized by clock-makers and makers of instruments of precision.

Parkinson says that Mustard 'is of good use, being fresh, for Epilepticke persons . . . if it be applyed hot inwardly and outwardly.'

Culpepper considered Mustard good for snake poison if taken in time, and tells us that mustard seed powder, mixed with honey in balls, taken every morning fasting, will clear the voice, and that

'the drowsy forgetful evil, to use it both inwardly and outwardly, to rub the nostrils, forehead and temples, to warm and quicken the spirits . . . the decoction of the seeds . . . resists the malignity of mushrooms. . . . Being chewed in the mouth it oftentimes helps the tooth-ache. It is also used to help the falling *off* the hair. The seed bruised, mixed with honey, and applied, or made up with wax, takes away the marks and black and blue spots of bruises or the like . . . it helps also the crick in the neck. . . .'

¶ *Preparations.* Linament, B.P.

Mustard flour is considered a capital antiseptic and sterilizing agent, as well as an excellent deodorizer.

MUSTARD, FIELD   Sinapis arvensis
Synonyms. Charlock. Brassica Sinapistrum
Part Used. Seeds

Charlock is a troublesome weed on arable land throughout England, growing so abundantly that it can at a distance be mistaken for a legitimate crop. It grows from 1 to 2 feet high, the stems upright, branched, grooved and often clothed with short rough hairs. The leaves are rough, unequally cut and serrated, and the flowers, which are yellow and large, are followed by nearly erect, angular, knotty pods, longer than their flattened conical beak.

It is an annual, flowering in May and June, and may easily be eradicated if pulled up before seeding. The seeds form a good substitute for Mustard, but are not equal to them in quality. They yield a good burning oil, which was much commended by Dodoens, as a preferable substitute for the 'Traine Oyle.'

Charlock varies in appearance in different plants and under varying conditions of growth, that growing in corn is taller and less branched than when growing by the roadside. It is capable of being used when boiled as a green vegetable, and is so employed in Sweden and Ireland. It is much liked by cattle and especially by sheep, and might be a useful fodder plant, though is usually regarded merely as a noxious intruder.

Spraying with 4 per cent. solution of copper sulphate or 15 per cent. solution of iron sulphate is employed for the destruction of Charlock in cornfields. It requires 40 gallons of solution for each acre. The weed should not exceed 3 inches in height at the time of spraying, or the remedy may be ineffectual.

RAPE   Brassica napus
Synonym. Cole Seed
Habitat. It is not indigenous to this country, though almost naturalized in parts

Rape is cultivated for the sake of the oil pressed from its seeds, the refuse being used to make oil-cake, or rape-cake, for feeding cattle.

It is frequently grown instead of White Mustard as a crop, being rather milder in flavour. When grown for feeding cattle, it should be sown about the middle of June, 6 or 8 lb. of seed to the acre. The plants are thinned by hoeing when young, and by the middle of November are ready for the cattle to feed on.

The seeds are also sown in gardens for winter and spring salads, as it is one of the small salad herbs, though little used.

It is also cultivated in cottage gardens for spring greens – the tops being cut first, and afterwards the side shoots.

MUSTARD, COMMON HEDGE   Sisymbrium officinale
Synonyms. Singer's Plant. St. Barbara's Hedge Mustard. Erysimum officinale
Part Used. Whole plant

The Common Hedge Mustard grows by our roadsides and on waste ground, where it is a common weed, with a peculiar aptitude for collecting and retaining dust. The blackish-green stalks, slender but tough, are branched and rough, the leaves hairy, deeply-lobed, with their points turned backwards, the terminal lobe larger. The yellow flowers are small and insignificant, placed at the top of the branches in long spikes, flowering by degrees throughout July. The pods are downy, close pressed to the stem and contain yellow, acrid seeds.

This plant is named by the French the 'Singer's Plant,' it having been considered up to the time of Louis XIV an infallible remedy for loss of voice. Racine, in writing to Boileau, recommends him to try the syrup of Erysimum in order to be cured of voicelessness. A strong infusion of the whole plant used to be taken in former days for all diseases of the throat.

FLIXWEED   Sisymbrium sophia (LINN.)
Another plant of the same genus, *Sisymbrium Sophia*, a more slender plant, bears the name of Flixweed, or Fluxweed, from having been given in cases of dysentery. It was called by the old herbalists *Sophia Chirugorum*, 'The Wisdom of Surgeons,' on account of its vulnerary properties.

The juice, mixed with an equal quantity of honey or vinegar, has been recommended for chronic coughs and hoarseness, and ulcerated sore throats. A strong infusion of the herb has proved excellent in asthma, and the seeds formed a special remedy for sciatica.

Chemically, the Hedge Mustard contains a soft resin and a sulphuretted volatile oil. Combined with Vervain it is supposed to have been Count Mattaei's famous remedy, *Febrifugo.*

MUSTARD, GARLIC
Sisymbrium alliaria

Synonyms. Jack-by-the-Hedge. Sauce Alone
Parts Used. Seeds, herbs

Garlic Mustard is an early flowering hedge plant, with delicate green leaves and snow-white flowers. The leaves are broadly heart-shaped, stalked, with numerous broad teeth. The whole plant emits when bruised a penetrating scent of Garlic, from which it derives its Latin and English names.

¶ *Medicinal Action and Uses.* The leaves used to be taken internally as a sudorific and deobstruent, and externally were applied antiseptically in gangrenes and ulcers. The juice of the leaves taken alone or boiled into a syrup with honey is found serviceable in dropsy.

Country people at one time used the plant in sauces, with bread and butter, salted meat and with lettuce in salads, hence it acquired also the name of Sauce Alone. The herb, when eaten as a salad, warms the stomach and strengthens the digestive faculties.

When cows eat it, it gives a disagreeable flavour to the milk.

The seeds, when snuffed up the nose, excite sneezing.

MUSTARD, TREACLE HEDGE
Erysimum Cheiranthoides

Synonyms. Wormseed. Treacle Wormseed
Part Used. Seeds

The Treacle Hedge Mustard has round stalks about a foot high, quite entire, or only slightly toothed, lanceolate leaves and small yellow flowers with whitish sepals, produced at the tops of the branches. The blackish-brown seeds are produced on each side of a pouch parted in the middle, about eighteen to each cell. The seeds are intensely bitter, and have been used by country people as a vermifuge, hence the second name of Wormseed or Treacle Wormseed. The seeds have also been given in obstructions of the intestines, and in rheumatism and jaundice with success. When taken in small doses they are purgative, but care must be taken not to administer in too large doses.

This plant flowers from May to August, and is a native of most parts of Europe, though it is not very common in England.

The Hedge Mustards and Garlic Mustard were all formerly allocated to the same genus to which this plant belongs, *Erysimum.*

Another species, *Erysimum Orientale* (Hare's Ear Treacle Mustard), with smooth, entire leaves and cream-coloured flowers, grows on some parts of the coast of Essex, Suffolk and Sussex.

MUSTARD, MITHRIDATE
Thlaspi arvense

Synonym. Pennycress
Part Used. Seeds

Mithridate Mustard, *Thlaspi arvense*, grows higher than Treacle Mustard; the leaves are small and narrower, smooth, toothed, arrow-shaped at the base. The flowers are small and white, growing on long branches, the seed-vessels form a round pouch, flat, with very broad wings, earning for the plant its other name of Pennycress.

It was formerly an ingredient in the Mithridate confection, an elaborate preparation used as an antidote to poison, but no longer used in medicine.

MYRRH
Commiphora myrrha (HOLMES)
N.O. Burseraceæ

Synonyms. Balsamodendron Myrrha. Commiphora Myrrha, var. Molmol. Mirra. Morr. Didin. Didthin. Bowl
Part Used. The oleo-gum-resin from the stem
Habitat. Arabia, Somaliland

¶ *Description.* The bushes yielding the resin do not grow more than 9 feet in height, but they are of sturdy build, with knotted branches, and branchlets that stand out at right-angles, ending in a sharp spine. The trifoliate leaves are scanty, small and very unequal, oval and entire. It was first recognized about 1822 at Ghizan on the Red Sea coast, a district so bare and dry that it is called 'Tehama,' meaning 'hell.'

Botanically, there is still uncertainty about the origin and identity of the various species.

There are ducts in the bark, and the tissue between them breaks down, forming large cavities, which, with the remaining ducts, becomes filled with a granular secretion which is freely discharged when the bark is wounded, or from natural fissures. It flows as a pale yellow liquid, but hardens to a reddish-brown mass, being found in commerce

571

in tears of many sizes, the average being that of a walnut. The surface is rough and powdered, and the pieces are brittle, with a granular fracture, semi-transparent, oily, and often show whitish marks. The odour and taste are aromatic, the latter also acrid and bitter. It is inflammable, but burns feebly.

Several species are recognized in commerce. It is usually imported in chests weighing 1 or 2 cwts., and wherever produced comes chiefly from the East Indies. Adulterations are not easily detected in the powder, so that it is better purchased in mass, when small stones, senegal gum, chestnuts, pieces of bdellium, or of a brownish resin called 'false myrrh,' may be sorted out with little difficulty.

It has been used from remote ages as an ingredient in incense, perfumes, etc., in the holy oil of the Jews and the *Kyphi* of the Egyptians for embalming and fumigations. Little appears to be definitely known about the collection of myrrh. It seems probable that the best drug comes from Somaliland, is bought at the fairs of Berbera by the Banians of India, shipped to Bombay, and there sorted, the best coming to Europe and the worst being sent to China. The true myrrh is known in the markets as *karam*, formerly called *Turkey myrrh*, and the opaque bdellium as *meena harma*.

The gum makes a good mucilage and the insoluble residue from the tincture can be used in this way.

¶ *Constituents.* Volatile oil, resin (myrrhin), gum, ash, salts, sulphates, benzoates, malates, and acetates of potassa.

It is partially soluble in water, alcohol, and ether. It may be tested by a characteristic violet reaction if nitric acid diluted with an equal volume of water is brought into contact with the residue resulting from the boiling of 0·1 gramme of coarsely powdered myrrh with 2 c.c. of 90 per cent. alcohol, evaporated in a porcelain dish so as to leave a thin film.

The oil is thick, pale yellow, and contains myrrholic acid and heerabolene, a sesquiterpenene.

¶ *Medicinal Action and Uses.* Astringent, healing. Tonic and stimulant. A direct emmenagogue, a tonic in dyspepsia, an expectorant in the absence of feverish symptoms, a stimulant to the mucous tissues, a stomachic carminative, exciting appetite and the flow of gastric juice, and an astringent wash.

It is used in chronic catarrh, phthisis pulmonalis, chlorosis, and in amenorrhœa is often combined with aloes and iron. As a wash it is good for spongy gums, ulcerated throat and aphthous stomatitis, and the tincture is also applied to foul and indolent ulcers. It has been found helpful in bronchorrhœa and leucorrhœa. It has also been used as a vermifuge.

When long-continued rubefacient effect is needed, a plaster may be made with 1½ oz. each of camphor, myrrh, and balsam of Peru rubbed together and added to 32 oz. of melted lead plaster, the whole being stirred until cooling causes it to thicken.

Myrrh is a common ingredient of toothpowders, and is used with borax in tincture, with other ingredients, as a mouth-wash.

The Compound Tincture, or Horse Tincture, is used in veterinary practice for healing wounds.

Meetiga, the trade-name of Arabian Myrrh, is more brittle and gummy than that of Somaliland and has not its white markings.

The liquid Myrrh, or *Stacte*, spoken of by Pliny, and an ingredient of Jewish holy incense, was formerly obtainable and greatly valued, but cannot now be identified.

¶ *Dosages.* 10 to 30 grains. Of fluid extract, 5 to 30 minims. Tincture, B.P. and U.S.P., ½ to 1 drachm. Of tincture of aloes and Myrrh, as purgative and emmenagogue, 30 minims. Of N.F. pills of aloes and Myrrh, 2 pills. Of Rufus's pills of aloes and Myrrh, as stimulant cathartic in debility and constipation, or in suppression of the menses, 4 to 8 grains of Br. mass.

¶ *Other Species.*

Bissa Bôl, or perfumed bdellium of the Arabs, has an odour like mushrooms. Though it is sent from Arabian ports to India and China, it was formerly known as East Indian Myrrh. It is of a dark colour, and may be a product of *Commiphora erythræa*, var. *glabrescens*, of *B. Kalaf*, *A. Kafal*, *B. Playfairii* or *Hemprichia erythræa*.

B. Kua of Abyssinia has been found to yield Myrrh.

Mecca balsam, a product of *B.* or *C. Opobalsamum*, is said to be the Myrrh of the Bible, the Hebrew word *mar* having been confused with the modern Arabic *morr* or Myrrh in translation.

Bdellium, recognized as an inferior Myrrh and often mixed with or substituted for it, is a product of several species of *Commiphora*, according to American writers, or *Balsamodendron* according to English ones. Four kinds are collected in Somaliland, making sub-divisions of African Bdellium:

Perfumed Bdellium or Habaghadi,
African Bdellium,
Opaque Bdellium,
Hotai Bdellium.

These African bdelliums, said by some writers to be products of *Balsamodendron*

(*Heudelotia*) *Africanum*, are in irregular, hard, roundish tears about an inch in diameter, pale yellow to red-brown, translucent, the fracture waxy, taste and odour slight.

The product of *Ceradia furcata* is also called African Bdellium.

The commercial *Gugul*, or Indian Bdellium, is said by some writers to be a product of *Commiphora roxburghiana*, by others of *B. Mukul*, and by others again of *B. roxbhurghii*

NARCISSUS

The bulbs of plants belonging to the natural order Amaryllidaceæ are in many cases poisonous, though they are widely cultivated for the sake of their flowers.

The chief of these is the DAFFODIL, or Lent Lily (*Narcissus pseudo-narcissus*, Linn.). The botanical name of the genus, *Narcissus*, is considered to be derived, not as is often said, from the name of the classical youth who met with his death through vainly trying to embrace his image reflected in a clear stream, but from the Greek word *narkao* (to benumb), on account of the narcotic properties which the plant possesses. Pliny describes it as *Narce narcissum dictum, non a fabuloso puero*, 'named Narcissus from *Narce*, not from the fabulous boy.'

Socrates called this plant the 'Chaplet of the infernal Gods,' because of its narcotic effects. An extract of the bulbs, when applied to open wounds, has produced staggering, numbness of the whole nervous system and paralysis of the heart.

The popular English names Daffodowndilly, Daffodily Affodily, are a corruption of Asphodel, with which blossoms of the ancient Greeks this was supposed to be identical. It is in France the *fleur d'asphodèle*, also '*pauvres filles de Sainte Claire.*'

Herrick alludes in his *Hesperides* to the Daffodil as a portent of death, probably connecting the flower with the asphodel, and the habit of the ancient Greeks of planting that flower near tombs.

The bulbs of the Daffodil, as well as every other part of the plant are powerfully emetic, and the flowers are considered slightly poisonous, and have been known to have produced dangerous effects upon children who have swallowed portions of them.

The influence of Daffodil on the nervous system has led to giving its flowers and its bulb for hysterical affections and even epilepsy, with benefit.

A decoction of the dried flowers acts as an emetic, and has been considered useful for relieving the congestive bronchial catarrh of children, and also useful for epidemic dysentery.

·or *Amyris Bdellium*. It is more moist than Myrrh; is found in irregular, dark reddish-brown masses, with a waxy fracture; softens with the heat of the hand; adheres to the teeth when chewed; and smells slightly of Myrrh.

It is used in the East Indies in leprosy, rheumatism and syphilis, and in Europe for plasters.

¶ *Dosage.* 10 to 40 grains.

N.O. Amaryllidaceæ

In France, Narcissus flowers have been used as an antispasmodic.

A spirit has been distilled from the bulb, used as an embrocation and also given as a medicine and a yellow volatile oil, of disagreeable odour and a brown colouring matter has been extracted from the flowers, the pigment being Quercetin, also present in the outer scales of the Onion.

The Arabians commended the oil to be applied for curing baldness and as an aphrodisiac.

An alkaloid was first isolated from the bulbs of *N. pseudo-narcissus* by Gerard in 1578, and obtained in a pure state as Narcissine by Guérin in 1910. The resting bulbs contain about 0·2 per cent. and the flowering bulbs about 0·1 per cent. With cats, Narcissine causes nausea and purgation.

N. princeps also contains a minute quantity of this alkaloid.

A case of poisoning by Daffodil bulbs, cooked by mistake in the place of leeks, was reported from Toulouse in 1923. The symptoms were acute abdominal pains and nausea, which yielded to an emetic.

The bulbs of *N. poeticus* (Linn.), the POET'S NARCISSUS, are more dangerous than those of the Daffodil, being powerfully emetic and irritant. The scent of the flowers is deleterious, if they are present in any quantity in a closed room, producing in some persons headache and even vomiting.

The bulb is used in homœopathy for the preparation of a tincture.

From the fragrant flowers of the JONQUIL (*N. jonquilla*) and the CAMPERNELLA (*N. odorus*), a sweet-smelling yellow oil is obtained in the south of France, used in perfumery.

The ease with which most species of Narcissus can be grown in this country is remarkable, since, being mostly natives of Southern Europe and Northern Africa, they have to adapt themselves to very different conditions of soil and climate.

No genus of flowering plants is more readily cultivated and less liable to disease, and the presence in its leaves and roots of innumerable bundles of needle-shaped crystals of calcium oxalate, termed raphides, protect it from injury of browsing and gnawing animals, rendering the plants indigestible and possibly poisonous to cattle and smaller animals.

The Crocus and Lily are not thus equipped for defence against browsing animals. Rabbits often fall prey to it.

NASTURTIUM. *See* WATERCRESS

NETTLES

The Nettle tribe, Urticaceæ, is widely spread over the world and contains about 500 species, mainly tropical, though several, like our common Stinging Nettle, occur widely in temperate climates. Many of the species have stinging hairs on their stems and leaves. Two genera are represented in the British Isles, *Urtica*, the Stinging Nettles, and *Parietaria*, the Pellitory. Formerly botanists included in the order Urticaceæ the Elm family, *Ulmaceæ*; the Mulberry, Fig and Bread Fruit family, *Moraceæ*; and that of the Hemp and Hop, *Cannabinaceæ*; but these are now generally regarded as separate groups.

The British species of Stinging Nettle, belonging to the genus *Urtica* (the name derived from the Latin, *uro*, to burn), are well known for the burning properties of the fluid

The only insect enemy from which the Narcissus seems to suffer is the fly *Merodon equestris*, the grub of which lays an egg in or near the bulb, which then forms the food of the larva. This pest causes serious damage in Holland and the south of England.

See DAFFODIL.

. N.O. Urticaceæ

contained in the stinging hairs with which the leaves are so well armed. Painful as are the consequences of touching one of our common Nettles, they are far exceeded by the effects of handling some of the East Indian species: a burning heat follows the sensation of pricking, just as if hot irons had been applied, the pain extending and continuing for many hours or even days, attended by symptoms similar to those which accompany lockjaw. A Java species, *U. urentissima*, produces effects which last for a whole year, and are even said to cause death. *U. crenulato* and *U. heterophylla*, both of India, are also most virulent. Another Indian species, *U. tuberosa*, on the other hand, has edible tubers, which are eaten either raw, boiled or roasted, and considered nutritious.

NETTLE, GREATER

Urtica dioica (LINN.)

NETTLE, LESSER

Urtica urens (LINN.)
N.O. Urticaceæ

Synonyms. Common Nettle. Stinging Nettle
Parts Used. Herb, seeds

Our Common Nettle (*Urtica dioica*, Linn.) is distributed throughout the temperate regions of Europe and Asia: it is not only to be found in distant Japan, but also in South Africa and Australia and in the Andes.

A detailed description of this familiar plant is hardly necessary; its heart-shaped, finely-toothed leaves tapering to a point, and its green flowers in long, branched clusters springing from the axils of the leaves are known to everyone. The flowers are incomplete: the male or barren flowers have stamens only, and the female or fertile flowers have only pistil or seed-producing organs. Sometimes these different kinds of flowers are to be found on one plant; but usually a plant will bear either male or female flowers throughout, hence the specific name of the plant, *dioica*, which means 'two houses.'

The male flower consists of a perianth of four greenish segments enclosing an equal number of stamens, which bend inwards in

the bud stage, but when the flower unfolds spring backwards and outwards, the anthers, with the sudden uncoiling, exploding and scattering the pollen. The flowers are thus adapted for wind-fertilization. The perianth of the female flower is similar, but only contains a single, one-seeded carpel, bearing one style with a brush-like stigma. The male flowers are in loose sprays or racemes, the female flowers more densely clustered together.

The Nettle flowers from June to September. As a rule the stem attains a height of 2 to 3 feet. Its perennial roots are creeping, so it multiplies quickly, making it somewhat difficult of extirpation.

The whole plant is downy, and also covered with stinging hairs. Each sting is a very sharp, polished spine, which is hollow and arises from a swollen base. In this base, which is composed of small cells, is contained the venom, an acrid fluid, the active principle of which is said to be bicarbonate of ammonia. When, in consequence of pressure, the sting pierces the skin, the venom is instantly expressed, causing the resultant irritation and inflammation. The burning property of the juice is dissipated by heat, enabling the young shoots of the Nettle, when boiled, to be eaten as a pot-herb.

It is a strange fact that the juice of the Nettle proves an antidote for its own sting, and being applied will afford instant relief: the juice of the Dock, which is usually found in close proximity to the Nettle, has the same beneficial action.

'Nettle in, dock out.
Dock rub nettle out!'

is an old rhyme.

If a person is stung with a Nettle a certain cure will be effected by rubbing Dock leaves over the part, repeating the above charm slowly. Another version is current in Wiltshire:

Out 'ettle, in dock,
Dock zhall ha' a new smock;
'Ettle zhant ha' *narrun*! (none)

The sting of a Nettle may also be cured by rubbing the part with Rosemary, Mint or Sage leaves.

There are two other species of Nettle found in Britain, both annuals. The Lesser Nettle (*U. urens*) is widely distributed and resembles the Common Nettle in habit, but has smaller leaves and the flowers in short, mostly unbranched clusters, male and female in the same panicle. It is glabrous except for the stinging hairs, whereas *U. dioica* is softly hairy throughout. It rarely attains more than a foot in height and is a common garden weed.

The Roman Nettle (*U. pilulifera*), bearing its female flowers in little compact, globular heads, is not general and is considered a doubtful native. It is also smooth except for the stinging hairs, but these contain a far more virulent venom than either of the other species. It occurs in waste places near towns and villages in the east of England, chiefly near the sea, but is rare. It is supposed to have been introduced by the Romans. The antiquary Camden records in his work *Britannica* that this Nettle was common at Romney, saying that here or near it, Julius Cæsar landed and called it 'Romania,' from which Romney is a corruption. Camden adds:

'The soldiers brought some of the nettle seed with them, and sowed it there for their use to rub and chafe their limbs, when through extreme cold they should be stiff or benumbed, having been told that the climate of Britain was so cold that it was not to be endured.'

From their general presence in the neighbourhood of houses or spots where house refuse is deposited, it has been suggested that Nettles are not really natives, a supposition that to some extent receives countenance from the circumstance that the young shoots are very sensitive to frost. However that may be, they follow man in his migrations, and by their presence usually indicate a soil rich in nitrogen.

The common name of the Nettle, or rather its Anglo-Saxon and also Dutch equivalent, *Netel*, is said to have been derived from *Noedl* (a needle), possibly from the sharp sting, or, as Dr. Prior suggests, in reference to the fact that it was this plant that supplied the thread used in former times by the Germanic and Scandinavian nations before the general introduction of flax, *Net* being the passive participle of *ne*, a verb common to most of the Indo-European languages in the sense of 'spin' and 'sew' (Latin *nere*, German *na-hen*, Sanskrit *nah*, bind). Nettle would seem, he considers, to have meant primarily that with which one sews.

Its fibre is very similar to that of Hemp or Flax, and it was used for the same purposes, from making cloth of the finest texture down to the coarsest, such as sailcloth, sacking, cordage, etc. In Hans Andersen's fairy-tale of the Princess and the Eleven Swans, the coats she wove for them were made of Nettles.

Flax and Hemp bear southern names and were introduced into the North to replace it.

In the sixteenth and seventeenth century Nettle fibres were still used in Scotland for weaving the coarser household napery. The historian Westmacott says: 'Scotch cloth is only the housewifery of the nettle. In Friesland, also, it was used till a late period.' The poet, Campbell, complaining of the little attention paid to the Nettle in England, tells us:

'In Scotland, I have eaten nettles, I have slept in nettle sheets, and I have dined off a nettle tablecloth. The young and tender nettle is an excellent potherb. The stalks of the old nettle are as good as flax for making cloth. I have heard my mother say that she thought nettle cloth more durable than any other species of linen.'

After the Nettles had been cut, dried and steeped, the fibre was separated with instruments similar to those used in dressing flax or hemp, and then spun into yarn, used in manufacturing every sort of cloth, cordage, etc., usually made from flax or hemp. Green (*Universal Herbal*, 1832) says this yarn was particularly useful for making twine for fishing nets, the fibre of the Nettle being stronger than those of flax and not so harsh as those of hemps.

The fibre being, however, produced in less quantities than that of flax, and being somewhat difficult to extract, accounts, perhaps, for the fact that it is no longer used in Britain, though it was still employed in other countries in textile manufactures some sixty years ago. The greatest objection to its extensive employment is the necessity of growing it in rich, deep soil, for otherwise the fibre produced is short and coarse, and on land fitted for it flax can be grown at less cost compared to the value of the seed and fibre yielded. The most valuable sort of Nettle in regard to length and suppleness is most common in the bottom of ditches, among briars and in shaded valleys, where the soil is a strong loam. In such situations the plants will sometimes attain a great height, those growing in patches on a good soil, standing thick, averaging 5 to 6 feet in height, the stems thickly clothed with fine lint. Those growing in poorer soils and less favourable situations, with rough and woody stem and many lateral branches, run much to seed and are less useful, producing lint more coarse, harsh and thin.

When Germany and Austria ran short of cotton during the War, the value of the Nettle as a substitute was at once recognized, and the two ordinary species, *U. dioica* and *U. urens*, the great and the smaller Nettle, were specially selected for textiles.

Among the many fibrous plants experimented with, the Nettle alone fulfilled all the conditions of a satisfactory source of textile fibre, and it was believed that it would become an important factor in agriculture and in the development of the textile industry. Investigations and practical tests made in 1916 at Brünn and Reichenberg confirmed the hopes raised concerning the possibilities to be realized in Nettle fibre; the capabilities of the plant were thoroughly tested, and from the standpoint of the factory it was affirmed that goods woven from this fibre were for most purposes equal to cotton goods, so that it was believed that, for Central Europe at least, a large and increasing use of Nettle fibre seemed assured. Mixed with 10 per cent. cotton, it was definitely shown that underclothing, cloth, stockings, tarpaulins, etc., could be manufactured from the new fibre.

In 1915, 1·3 million kilograms of this material were collected in Germany, a quantity which increased to 2·7 million kilograms in 1916, and this without any attempt at systematic cultivation. The quantity of Nettles grown wild in Germany was estimated at 60,000 tons, but as time went on it was found that self-sown Nettles were insufficient in quantity for the need, and that their quality could be improved by cultivation, and great efforts were made to increase production, but the cultivation proved more difficult than was expected.

Cloth made from Nettle fibre was employed in many articles of army clothing. Forty kilograms were calculated to provide enough stuff for one shirt. In 1917 two captured German overalls, marked with the dates 1915 and 1916 respectively, were found to be woven of a mixed fibre consisting of 85 per cent. of the common Stinging Nettle and 15 per cent. of Ramie, the fibre of the Rhea, or Grass (*Boehmeria nivea*), a tropical member of the Nettle family, which is used in the manufacture of gas-mantles and is also valuable for making artificial silk and was largely employed in war-time in the making of gas-masks.

German army orders dated in March, April and May of 1918 give a good insight into the extent to which use was made of cloth woven from Nettle fibre. In these orders, Nettle is described as the only efficient cotton substitute.

In Austria, also, Nettles were cultivated on a large scale.

The length of the Nettle fibre varies from $\frac{3}{4}$ inch to $2\frac{1}{2}$ inches: all above $1\frac{3}{4}$ inch is equal to the best Egyptian cotton. It can be dyed and bleached in the same way as cotton, and when mercerized is but slightly inferior to silk. It has been considered much superior to cotton for velvet and plush.

The Textile Department of the Bradford Technical College exhibited in March, 1918, samples of Nettle fibre. It had a pleasing appearance to the eye, but when examined under the microscope, magnification showed that it had a glass-like surface, devoid of the serrations which endow wool as a fibre for textile production, and experts considered that its employment in Germany seemed to point to very straitened circumstances as the motive, rather than any recognition of a true textile value in the fibre.

These properties of the Nettle were recognized before the War, and considerable sums of money were spent in the endeavour to utilize that plant, but trouble was experienced in the separation of the fibres. Recently, great progress has been made and some fifty processes have been patented for attaining this separation. In 1917 some 70,000 hectares of Nettles were cultivated, and it is thought possible to plant a million hectares of lowlands, giving a yield of Nettle fibres that would cover about 18 per cent. of Germany's cotton requirements.

The by-products of the Nettle were also stated to be of enormous production, the Nettle not only supplying a substitute for cotton, but for such indispensable articles as sugar, starch, protein and ethyl alcohol.

Another use of great importance is the application of the fibres of Nettle to the manufacture of paper of various qualities. They used to be collected in France in considerable quantities for that purpose, and though, owing to the different ages of the fibre, the attempts to use it for paper-making have not always met with complete success, the subject deserves further attention.

From a *culinary* point of view the Nettle has an old reputation. It is one of the few wild plants still gathered each spring by country-folk as a pot-herb. It makes a healthy vegetable, easy of digestion.

The young tops should be gathered when 6 to 8 inches high. Gloves should be worn to protect the hands when picking them. They should be washed in running water with a stick and then put into a saucepan, dripping, without any added water, and cooked with the lid on for about 20 minutes. Then chopped, rubbed through a hair-sieve and either served plain, or warmed up in the pan again, with a little salt, pepper and butter, or a little gravy, and served with or without poached eggs. They thus form a refreshing dish of spring greens, which is slightly laxative. In autumn, however, Nettles are hurtful, the leaves being gritty from the abundance of crystals (*cystoliths*) they contain.

In Scotland it was the practice to force Nettles for 'early spring kail.' Sir Walter Scott tells us in *Rob Roy* how Andrew Fairservice, the old gardener of Lochleven, raised early Nettles under hand-glasses. By earthing up, Nettles may be blanched in the same way as seakale and eaten in a similar manner. They also make a good vegetable soup, and in Scotland are used with leeks, broccoli and rice to make Nettle pudding, a very palatable dish.

RECIPES
Nettle Pudding

To 1 gallon of young Nettle tops, thoroughly washed, add 2 good-sized leeks or onions, 2 heads of broccoli or small cabbage, or Brussels sprouts, and ¼ lb. of rice. Clean the vegetables well; chop the broccoli and

leeks and mix with the Nettles. Place all together in a muslin bag, alternately with the rice, and tie tightly. Boil in salted water, long enough to cook the vegetables, the time varying according to the tenderness or otherwise of the greens. Serve with gravy or melted butter. These quantities are sufficient for six persons.

Pepys refers to Nettle pudding in his *Diary*, February, 1661: 'We did eat some Nettle porridge, which was very good.'

Nettle Beer

The Nettle Beer made by cottagers is often given to their old folk as a remedy for gouty and rheumatic pains, but apart from this purpose it forms a pleasant drink. It may be made as follows: Take 2 gallons of cold water and a good pailful of washed young Nettle tops, add 3 or 4 large handsful of Dandelion, the same of Clivers (Goosegrass) and 2 oz. of bruised, whole ginger. Boil gently for 40 minutes, then strain and stir in 2 teacupsful of brown sugar. When lukewarm place on the top a slice of toasted bread, spread with 1 oz. of compressed yeast, stirred till liquid with a teaspoonful of sugar. Keep it fairly warm for 6 or 7 hours, then remove the scum and stir in a tablespoonful of cream of tartar. Bottle and tie the corks securely. The result is a specially wholesome sort of ginger beer. The juice of 2 lemons may be substituted for the Dandelion and Clivers. Other herbs are often added to Nettles in the making of Herb Beer, such as Burdock, Meadowsweet, Avens Horehound, the combination making a refreshing summer drink.

As an arrester of bleeding, the Nettle has few equals and an infusion of the dried herb, or alcoholic tincture made from the fresh plant, or the fresh Nettle juice itself in doses of 1 to 2 tablespoonsful is of much power inwardly for bleeding from the nose, lungs or stomach. Old writers recommended a small piece of lint, moistened with the juice, to be placed in the nostril in bad cases of nosebleeding. The diluted juice provides a useful astringent gargle. Burns may be cured rapidly by applying to them linen cloths well wetted with the tincture, the cloths being frequently re-wetted. An infusion of the fresh leaves is also soothing and healing as a lotion for burns.

Nettle is one of the best antiscorbutics. An infusion known as Nettle Tea is a common spring medicine in rural districts, and has long been used as a blood purifier. This tea made from young Nettles is in many parts of the country used as a cure for nettlerash. It is also beneficially employed in cases of gouty gravel, but must not be brewed too strong. A strong decoction of Nettle, drunk too freely, has produced severe burning over the whole body.

The homœopathic tincture, *Urtica*, is frequently administered successfully for rheumatic gout, also for nettlerash and chickenpox, and externally for bruises.

'Urtication,' or flogging with Nettles, was an old remedy for chronic rheumatism and loss of muscular power.

Young Nettles, mashed and pulped finely, mixed with equal bulk of thick cream, pepper and salt being added to taste, have been considered a valuable food for consumptives.

¶ *Medicinal Uses of the Nettle. Parts employed:* The whole herb, collected in May and June, just before coming into flower, and dried in the usual manner prescribed for 'bunched' herbs.

When the herb is collected for drying, it should be gathered only on a fine day, in the morning, when the sun has dried off the dew. Cut off just above the root, rejecting any stained or insect-eaten leaves, and tie in bunches, about six to ten in a bunch, spread out fanwise, so that the air can penetrate freely to all parts.

Hang the bunches over strings. If dried in the open, keep them in half-shade and bring indoors before there is any risk of damp from dew or rain. If dried indoors, hang up in a sunny room, and failing sun, in a well-ventilated room by artificial heat. Care must be taken that the window be left open by day so that there is a free current of air and the moisture-laden, warm air may escape. The bunches should be of uniform size and length, to facilitate packing when dry, and when quite dry and crisp must be packed away at once in airtight boxes or tins, otherwise moisture will be reabsorbed from the air.

The seeds and flowers are dried in the sun, or over a stove, on sheets of paper.

The Nettle is still in demand by wholesale herbalists, who stock the dried and powdered herb, also the seeds. Homœopathic chemists, in addition, employ the green herb for the preparation of a tincture.

¶ *Constituents.* The analysis of the fresh Nettle shows the presence of formic acid, mucilage, mineral salts, ammonia, carbonic acid and water.

It is the formic acid in the Nettle, with the phosphates and a trace of iron, which constitute it such a valuable food medicinally.

¶ *Action and Uses.* Although not prescribed by the British Pharmacopœia, the Nettle has still a reputation in herbal medicine, and is regarded in homœopathy as a useful remedy. Preparations of the herb have astringent properties and act also as a stimulating tonic.

Nettle is anti-asthmatic: the juice of the roots or leaves, mixed with honey or sugar, will relieve bronchial and asthmatic troubles and the dried leaves, burnt and inhaled, will have the same effect. The seeds have also been used in consumption, the infusion of herb or seeds being taken in wineglassful doses. The seeds and flowers used to be given in wine as a remedy for ague. The powdered seeds have been considered a cure for goitre and efficacious in reducing excessive corpulency.

In old Herbals the seeds, taken inwardly, were recommended for the stings or bites of venomous creatures and mad dogs, and as an antidote to poisoning by Hemlock, Henbane and Nightshade.

A quaint old superstition existed that a fever could be dispelled by plucking a Nettle up by the roots, reciting thereby the names of the sick man and also the names of his parents.

Preparations of Nettle are said to act well upon the kidneys, but it is a doubtful diuretic, though it has been claimed that incipient dropsy may be remedied by tea made from the roots.

A novel treatment for diabetes was reported by a sufferer from that disease in the daily press of April, 1926, it being affirmed that a diet of young Nettles (following a two days' fast) and drinking the brew of them had been the means of reducing his weight by 6 stone in three days and had vastly improved his condition.

An efficient Hair Tonic can be prepared from the Nettle: Simmer a handful of young Nettles in a quart of water for 2 hours, strain and bottle when cold. Well saturate the scalp with the lotion every other night. This prevents the hair falling and renders it soft and glossy. A good Nettle Hair Lotion is also prepared by boiling the entire plant in vinegar and water, straining and adding Eau de Cologne.

For stimulating hair growth, the old herbalists recommended combing the hair daily with expressed Nettle juice.

The homœopathic tincture of Nettle is made of 2 oz. of the herb to 1 pint of proof spirit.

The powder of the dried herb is administered in doses of 5 to 10 grains.

¶ *Preparations.* Fluid extract of herb, ½ to 1 drachm. Infusion, 1 oz. of the herb to a pint of boiling water.

¶ *Other Uses.* Nettles are of considerable value as fodder for live-stock, and might be used for this purpose where they occur largely. When Nettles are growing, no quadruped except the ass will touch them, on account of their stinging power, but if cut and allowed to become wilted, they lose their sting and are then readily cleared up by livestock. It is well known that when dried and made into hay, so as to destroy the poisonous matter of the stings, cows will relish them and give more milk than when fed on hay alone. In Sweden and Russia, the Nettle has sometimes been cultivated as a fodder plant, being mown several times a year, and given to milch cattle.

Nettles were much used as a substitute for fodder during the war, and instructions for their use were laid down by German military authorities. It was found that horses which had become thin and suffered from digestive troubles benefited from the use of Nettle leaves in their rations. When dried, the proportion of albuminoid matter in Nettles is as high as in linseed cake and the fat content is also considerable.

The Nettle is also of great use to the keeper of poultry. Dried and powdered finely and put into the food, it increases egg-production and is healthy and fattening. The seeds are also said to fatten fowls. Turkeys, as well as ordinary poultry, thrive on Nettles chopped small and mixed with their food, and pigs do well on boiled Nettles.

In Holland, and also in Egypt, it is said that horse-dealers mix the seeds of Nettles with oats or other food, in order to give the animals a sleek coat.

Although in Britain upwards of thirty insects feed solely on the Nettle plant, flies have a distaste for the plant, and a fresh bunch of Stinging Nettles will keep a larder free from them.

If planted in the neighbourhood of beehives, it is said the Nettle will drive away frogs.

The juice of the Nettle, or a decoction formed by boiling the green herb in a strong solution of salt, will curdle milk, providing the cheese-maker with a good substitute for rennet. The same juice, if rubbed liberally into small seams in leaky wooden tubs coagulates and will render them once more watertight.

A decoction of Nettle yields a beautiful and permanent green dye, which is used for woollen stuffs in Russia: the roots, boiled with alum, produce a yellow colour, which was formerly widely used in country districts to dye yarn, and is also employed by the Russian peasants to stain eggs yellow on Maundy Thursday.

The expressed seeds yield a burning oil, which has been extracted and used in Egypt.

The following passage from *Les Misérables* on the utilization of Nettles, shows how conversant Victor Hugo was with the virtues of this commonly despised 'weed':

'One day he (Monsieur Madeleine) saw some peasants busy plucking out Nettles; he looked at the heap of plants uprooted and already withered, and said – "They are dead. Yet it would be well if people knew how to make use of them. When the nettle is young, its leaf forms an excellent vegetable; when it matures, it has filaments and fibres like hemp and flax. Nettle fabric is as good as canvas. Chopped, the nettle is good for poultry; pounded it is good for cattle. The seed of the nettle mingled with fodder imparts a gloss to the coats of animals; its root mixed with salt produces a beautiful yellow colour. It is besides excellent hay and can be cut twice. And what does the nettle require? Little earth, no attention, no cultivation. Only the seed falls as it ripens, and is difficult to gather. That is all. With a little trouble, the nettle would be useful; it is neglected, and becomes harmful." '

Nettles are increasing all over the country, and for the benefit of those who desire their eradication, the Royal Horticultural Society, in their Diary for 1926, informed their members that if Nettles are cut down three times in three consecutive years, they will disappear.

NETTLE, WHITE DEAD-   Lamium album (LINN.)
                                              N.O. Labiatæ

Synonyms. Archangel. White Dead Nettle. Blind Nettle. Dumb Nettle. Deaf Nettle. Bee Nettle
Part Used. Herb

The White Dead-Nettle owes its name of Nettle to the fact that the plant as a whole bears a strong general resemblance to the Stinging Nettle, for which it may easily be mistaken in the early spring, before it is in bloom; but the flowers are absolutely different in the two plants, which are quite unrelated. It can, moreover, be always readily distinguished from the Stinging Nettle, even when not in flower, by the squareness and hollowness of its stem.

The 'Dead' in its name refers to its inability to sting. Lord Avebury points out that this resemblance is a clever adaption of nature.

579

'It cannot be doubted that the true nettle is protected by its power of stinging, and that being so, it is scarcely less clear that the Dead Nettle must be protected by its likeness to the other,'

the two species being commonly found growing together. The resemblance serves probably not only as a protection against browsing quadrupeds, but also against leaf-eating insects.

Many other country names refer to this false suggestion of stinging power. In some localities it is called White Archangel, or Archangel alone, probably because it first comes into flower about the day dedicated to the Archangel Michael, May 8, old style – eleven days earlier than our May 8.

This plant is also known as the Bee Nettle, because bees visit it freely for the honey which it provides lavishly. The flower is specially built to encourage bee visitors – especially the humble bee. In the axils of the leaves are whorls, or rings, of the flowers, each ring composed of six to twelve blossoms of a delicate creamy white; out of the spiky, green, five-pointed calyx rises the white petal tube, which expands into an erection of very irregular shape, composed of five petals, one forming the lip, two the hood, and two form the little wings.

Four stamens lie in pairs along the back of the flower, with their heads well up under the hood and their faces downwards. The long column from the ovary also lies with them, but its top, the stigma, hangs a little out beyond the pollen-bearing anthers of the stamens. At the bottom of the corolla-tube is a rich store of honey.

When a bee visits the flower, he alights on the lower lip, thrusts his proboscis down the petal tube, which is nearly ½ inch long, and reaches the honey, his back fitting meanwhile exactly into the conformation of the corolla, so that he first, as he settles on the lip, rubs

the projecting stigmas with the pollen already on his back (thus affecting the fertilization of the flower), and then presses on to the stamens and gets dusted with their pollen in exchange, and this is then passed on to the next flower he visits. Unless the insect visitor is a big one, his back will not fill the cavity and neither stigma nor stamens are touched. The honey is placed in such a position that only the big humble bees with their long probosces can reach it. The flower also guards against smaller insects creeping down its tube by placing a barrier of hairs round it just above the honey. Some insects, whose tongues are too short to reach the honey, get at it by biting through the wall of the white tube right down at its base, and sucking away the honey without taking any share in the fertilization of the flower.

When the flower fades, the green calyx still remains to protect the tiny nutlets. It is somewhat stiffened, and when the nutlets are ripe and ready for dispersal, any pressure upon it forces it back and on the pressure being removed, the nuts are shot out with some force.

The plant is to be found in flower from May almost until December. The heart-shaped leaves, with their saw-like margins, are placed on the square, hollow stems in pairs, each pair exactly at right angles to the one above and below. Both stems and leaves are covered with small rough hairs, and contain certain essential oils which probably make them distasteful to cattle, even after their powerlessness to sting has been discovered. When bruised, the whole plant has a strong, rather disagreeable smell.

The corners of the hollow stems are strengthened by specially strong columns of fibres. In the country, boys often cut the stems and make whistles out of them.

The generic name of the Dead Nettles, *Lamium*, is derived from the Greek word *laimos* (the throat), in allusion to the form of the blossom.

NETTLE, PURPLE DEAD-

Synonym. Purple Archangel

The Purple Dead-Nettle is a common weed in cultivated ground and by waysides, found in the same spots as the other species, but less conspicuous.

It has heart- or kidney-shaped leaves, blunt, not pointed as in the preceding species, and is distinguished by the purple tinge of its foliage, crowded upper leaves and small, reddish flowers, which have much shorter petal tubes than the Yellow and White Dead-Nettles, so that bees with shorter tongues

Lamium purpureum (LINN.)
N.O. Labiatæ

than the humble-bee, can reach its honey and fertilize it. It is, indeed, a favourite with bees, who find abundance of honey in its blossoms. The upper leaves are often densely clapped with silky hairs.

It flowers all the summer – from April to September and in mild seasons, both earlier and later. This species of Dead-Nettle is an annual, propagated by its seeds alone. It is one of the earliest weeds in gardens, but being an annual is easily eradicated.

The plant varies greatly in appearance, according to the situation in which it grows. On the open ground, it is somewhat spreading in habit, rarely more than 6 inches in height, whilst specimens growing in the midst of crowded vegetation are often drawn up to a considerable height, their leaves being of a dull green throughout, whereas those of the smaller specimens grown in the open are ordinarily more or less warm and rich in colour. At first glance the variation in the appearance of specimens grown under these different circumstances would leave the casual observer to suppose them to belong to different species.

¶ *Medicinal Action and Uses.* The herb and flowers, either fresh or dried, have been used to make a decoction for checking any kind of hæmorrhage.

The leaves are also useful to staunch wounds, when bruised and outwardly applied.

The dried herb, made into a tea and sweetened with honey, promotes perspiration and acts on the kidneys, being useful in cases of chill.

Linnæus reported that this species also has been boiled and eaten as a pot-herb by the peasantry in Sweden.

¶ *Other Species.*

The HENBIT DEAD-NETTLE (*Lamium amplexicaule*, Linn.), a small annual, fairly common on cultivated and waste ground, is not unlike the Purple Dead-Nettle, but somewhat lighter and more graceful. Its fine, deep rose-coloured flowers have a much slenderer tube, thrown out farther from the leaves.

The SPOTTED DEAD-NETTLE (*L. maculatum*), not considered a true wilding, but an escape from old-fashioned cottage gardens, is by some botanists regarded as a variety of the White Dead-Nettle, which it closely resembles, the flowers being, however, pale purple, instead of white and the foliage often marked by a broad, irregular streak of white down the centre of each leaf, with a few blotches on each side.

The HEMP NETTLE (*Galeopsis tetrahit*, Linn.) (named from *gale* (weasel) and *opsis* (a countenance), because of a fancied resemblance of its blossom to a weasel's face) is supposed to have been the source of one of Count Mattei's nostrums: *Pettorale.*

It is found on roadsides and borders of cornfields, tall-stemmed and erect, covered with long, dense bristles, the stem-joints thickened and the egg-shaped leaves hairy. The flowers, in dense whorls, are white, purple or yellow and are specially adapted for the visits of long-lipped bees, being much visited by the Humble Bee.

See DODDERS.

Gerard tells us:

'the White Archangel flowers compass the stalks round at certain distances, even as those of Horehound, whereof this is a kind and not of Nettle. The root is very threddy. The flowers are baked with sugar; as also the distilled water of them, which is said to make the heart merry, to make a good colour in the face, and to make the vital spirits more fresh and lively.'

Linnæus tells us that although refused by cattle, the leaves are eaten in Sweden as a pot-herb in the spring, in like manner as the True Nettle.

¶ *Part Used Medicinally.* The whole herb, collected in May and June, when just coming into flower and the leaves are in their best condition, and then dried in the manner directed for 'bunched' herbs.

The characteristic Dead-Nettle odour is lost in drying, but a slightly bitter taste remains.

The herb may be cultivated and propagated by means of seed sown in shallow drills, or by cuttings or division of roots – it spreads rapidly by means of its creeping, perennial roots, so that when once established, it is hard to get rid of it – but it would hardly pay for cultivation and is generally collected in the wild state.

¶ *Medicinal Action and Uses.* The whole plant is of an astringent nature, and in herbal medicine is considered of use for arresting hæmorrhages, as in spitting of blood and dysentery. Cotton-wool, dipped in a tincture of the fresh herb, is efficacious in staunching bleeding and a homœopathic tincture prepared from the flowers is used for internal bleeding, the dose being 5 to 10 drops in cold water.

As a blood purifier for rashes, eczema, etc., a decoction of Nettle flowers is excellent.

It has the reputation of being effectual in the healing of green wounds, bruises and burns.

This and the other species of Dead-Nettle have also been used in female complaints for their astringent properties.

Culpepper and the old herbalists tell us that the Archangel is an exhilarating herb, that it 'makes the heart merry, drives away melancholy, quickens the spirits, is good against the quartan agues, stauncheth bleeding at the mouth and nose if it be stamped and applied to the nape of the neck.'

It was used with great success in removing the hardness of the spleen, which was supposed to be the seat of melancholy, a decoction being made with wine and the herb applied hot as a plaster to the region of the spleen, the decoction also being used as a fomentation.

Bruised and mixed with salt, vinegar and lard, it has proved useful in the reduction of swellings and also to give ease in gout, sciatica and other pains in the joints and muscles.

NETTLE, YELLOW DEAD-

Lamium Galeobdolon (LINN.)
N.O. Labiatæ

Synonyms. Yellow Archangel. Weazel Snout. Dummy Nettle
Part Used. Herb

The closely-allied Yellow Archangel and the Purple Dead-Nettle (*Lamium purpureum*) have also been used medicinally for the same purposes as the White Dead-Nettle,⁴ Culpepper telling us that the Yellow Archangel is most to be commended of the three for healing sores and ulcers.

All three species have hollow, square stalks, with the leaves opposite, in pairs.

The Yellow Archangel resembles in habit the White Dead-Nettle, but its stems are straighter and more upright, the pairs of leaves farther apart, the leaves themselves, narrower, longer and more pointed. The flowers, which also grow in whorls, are a little longer. They are large and handsome; pale yellow, blotched with red, visited by both Humble- and Honey-bee.

It has a much shorter flowering season than either of the other Dead-Nettles, being only in flower for two months – mid-April to mid-June, or May to July, according to district.

The plant is not infrequent in damp woods and shady hedgerows, but is much more local in its habitat than either the White or Purple Dead-Nettle, being common in some localities and altogether absent from others.

Its specific name, *Galeobdolon*, is made up from two Greek words, *gale* (a weasel) and *bdolos* (a disagreeable odour), an allusion to the somewhat strong odour of the plant when crushed.

The whole herb was used medicinally, dried and employed in the same manner as the White Archangel.

(POISON)
NIGHTSHADE, BLACK

Solanum nigrum (LINN.)
N.O. Solanaceæ

Synonyms. Garden Nightshade. Petty Morel
Parts Used. Whole plant, fresh leaves

The Black Nightshade is an annual plant, common and generally distributed in the South of England, less abundant in the North and somewhat infrequent in Scotland. It is one of the most cosmopolitan of wild plants, extending almost over the whole globe.

In this country, it is frequently to be seen by the wayside and is often found on rubbish heaps, but also among growing crops and in damp and shady places. It is sometimes called the Garden Nightshade, because it so often occurs in cultivated ground.

¶ *Description.* It rarely grows more than a foot or so in height and is much branched, generally making a bushy-looking mass. It varies much according to the conditions of its growth, both as to the amount of its dull green foliage and the size of its individual leaves, which are egg-shaped and stalked, the outlines bluntly notched or waved. The stem is green and hollow.

The flowers are arranged in clusters at the end of stalks springing from the main stems at the intervals between the leaves, not, as in the Bittersweet, opposite the leaves. They are small and white, resembling those of Bittersweet in form, and are succeeded by small round berries, green at first, but black when ripe. The plant flowers and fruits freely, and in the autumn the masses of black berries are very noticeable; they have, when mature, a very polished surface.

On account of its berries, the Black Nightshade was called by older herbalists 'Petty Morel,' to distinguish it from the Deadly Nightshade, often known as Great Morel. Culpepper says: 'Do not mistake the deadly nightshade for this,' cautiously adding, 'if you know it not, you may then let them both alone.'

In the fourteenth century, we hear of the plant under the name of Petty Morel being used for canker and with Horehound and wine taken for dropsy.

¶ *Part Used.* The whole plant, gathered in early autumn, when in both flower and fruit and dried. Also the fresh leaves.

When the plant grows at all in a bunchy mass, strip off the stems singly and dry them under the same conditions as given above for Belladonna leaves, tying several stems together in a bunch, however, spread out fanwise for the air to penetrate to all parts, and hang the bunches over strings, rather than in trays. The bunches should be of uniform size.

¶ *Medicinal Action and Uses.* This species has the reputation of being very poisonous,

a fact, however, disputed by recent inquiries. In experimenting on dogs, very varying results have been obtained, which may be explained by the fact that the active principle, Solanine, on which the poisonous properties of this and the preceding species depend, and which exists in considerable quantity in the fresh herb, varies very much at different seasons.

The berries are injurious to children, but are often eaten by adults with impunity, especially when quite ripe, as the poisonous principle is chiefly associated with all green parts. Cattle will not eat the plant and sheep rarely touch it.

It is applied in medicine similarly to Bittersweet, but is more powerful and possesses greater narcotic properties.

According to Withering and other authorities, 1 or 2 grains of the dried leaves, infused in boiling water, act as a strong sudorific.

In Bohemia the leaves are placed in the cradles of infants to promote sleep. In the islands of Bourbon and Mauritius, the leaves are eaten in place of spinach: and the fruit is said to be eaten without inconvenience by soldiers stationed in British Kaffraria. (Lindley's *Treasury of Botany*.)

It has been found useful in cutaneous disorders, but its action is variable, and it is considered a somewhat dangerous remedy except in very small doses.

The bruised fresh leaves, used externally, are said to ease pain and abate inflammation, and the Arabs apply them to burns and ulcers. Their juice has been used for ringworm, gout and earache, and mixed with vinegar, is said to be good as a gargle and mouthwash.

Besides the above-mentioned species, others are used for medicinal, alimentary, and other purposes. Some are employed almost universally as narcotics to allay pain, etc.; others are sudorific and purgative. *Solanum toxicarium* is used as a poison by the natives of Cayenne. *S. pseudo-quina* is esteemed as a valuable febrifuge in Brazil. Among those used for food, are *S. Album* and *S. Æthiopicum*, the fruits of which are used in China and Japan. Those of *S. Anguivi* are eaten in Madagascar. *S. esculentum* and its varieties furnish the fruits known as Aubergines or Brinjals, which are highly esteemed in France, and may sometimes be met with in English markets; they are of the size and form of a goose's egg and usually of a rich purple colour. The Egg-plant, which has white berries, is only a variety of this. The Peruvians eat the fruits of *S. muricatum* and *S. quitoense*; those of *S. ramosum* are eaten as a vegetable in the West Indies. The Tasmanian Kangaroo Apple is the fruit of *S. laciniatum*; unless fully ripe this is said to be acrid. In Gippsland, Australia, the natives eat the fruits of *S. vescum*, which, like the preceding, is not agreeable till fully ripe, when it is said to resemble in form and flavour the fruits of *Physalis peruviana*. Of other species the leaves are eaten; as those of *S. oleraceum* in the West Indies and Fiji Islands, of *S. sessiflorum* in Brazil, etc.

Other species are used as dyes. *S. indigoferum*, in Brazil, cultivated for indigo. The juice of the fruit of *S. gnaphalioides* is said to be used to tint the cheeks of the Peruvian ladies, while their sisters of the Canary Isles employ similarly the fruits of *S. vespertilia*. The fruits of *S. saponaceum* are used in Peru to whiten linen in place of soap. *S. marginatum* is used in Abyssinia for tanning leather.

See POTATO, TOMATO, STRAMONIUM.

(POISON)
NIGHTSHADE, DEADLY

Atropa Belladonna (LINN.)
N.O. Solanaceæ

Synonyms. Belladonna. Devil's Cherries. Naughty Man's Cherries. Divale. Black Cherry. Devil's Herb. Great Morel. Dwayberry

Parts Used. Root, leaves, tops

Habitat. Widely distributed over Central and Southern Europe, South-west Asia and Algeria; cultivated in England, France and North America

Though widely distributed over Central and Southern Europe, the plant is not common in England, and has become rarer of late years. Although chiefly a native of the southern counties, being almost confined to calcareous soils, it has been sparingly found in twenty-eight British counties, mostly in waste places, quarries and near old ruins. In Scotland it is rare. Under the shade of trees, on wooded hills, on chalk or limestone, it will grow most luxuriantly, forming bushy plants several feet high, but specimens growing in places exposed to the sun are apt to be dwarfed, consequently it rarely attains such a large size when cultivated in the open, and is more subject to the attacks of insects than when growing wild under natural conditions.

¶ *Description.* The root is thick, fleshy and whitish, about 6 inches long, or more, and branching. It is perennial. The purplish-coloured stem is annual and herbaceous. It is stout, 2 to 4 feet high, undivided at the base, but dividing a little above the ground into three – more rarely two or four branches, each of which again branches freely.

The leaves are dull, darkish green in colour and of unequal size, 3 to 10 inches long, the lower leaves solitary, the upper ones in pairs alternately from opposite sides of the stem, one leaf of each pair much larger than the other, oval in shape, acute at the apex, entire and attenuated into short petioles.

First-year plants grow only about 1½ feet in height. Their leaves are often larger than in full-grown plants and grow on the stem immediately above the ground. Older plants attain a height of 3 to 5 feet, occasionally even 6 feet, the leaves growing about 1 to 2 feet from the ground.

The whole plant is glabrous, or nearly so, though soft, downy hairs may occur on the young stems and the leaves when quite young. The veins of the leaves are prominent on the under surface, especially the midrib, which is depressed on the upper surface of the leaf.

The fresh plant, when crushed, exhales a disagreeable odour, almost disappearing on drying, and the leaves have a bitter taste, when both fresh and dry.

The flowers, which appear in June and July, singly, in the axils of the leaves, and continue blooming until early September, are of a dark and dingy purplish colour, tinged with green (about an inch long), pendent, bell-shaped, furrowed, the corolla with five large teeth or lobes, slightly reflexed. The five-cleft calyx spreads round the base of the smooth berry, which ripens in September, when it acquires a shining black colour and is in size like a small cherry. It contains several seeds. The berries are full of a dark, inky juice, and are intensely sweet, and their attraction to children on that account, has from their poisonous properties, been attended with fatal results. Lyte urges growers 'to be carefull to see to it and to close it in, that no body enter into the place where it groweth, that wilbe enticed with the beautie of the fruite to eate thereof.' And Gerard, writing twenty years later, after recounting three cases of poisoning from eating the berries, exhorts us to 'banish therefore these pernicious plants out of your gardens and all places neare to your houses where children do resort.' In September, 1916, three children were admitted to a London hospital suffering from Belladonna poisoning, caused, it was ascertained, from having eaten berries from large fruiting plants of *Atropa Belladonna* growing in a neighbouring public garden, the gardener being unaware of their dangerous nature, and again in 1921 the Nor-

wich Coroner, commenting on the death of a child from the same cause, said that he had had four not dissimilar cases previously.

It is said that when taken by accident, the poisonous effects of Belladonna berries may be prevented by swallowing as soon as possible an emetic, such as a large glass of warm vinegar or mustard and water. In undoubted cases of this poisoning, emetics and the stomach-pump are resorted to at once, followed by a dose of magnesia, stimulants and strong coffee, the patient being kept very warm and artificial respiration being applied if necessary. A peculiar symptom in those poisoned by Belladonna is the complete loss of voice, together with frequent bending forward of the trunk and continual movements of the hands and fingers, the pupils of the eye becoming much dilated.

¶ *History.* The plant in Chaucer's days was known as Dwale, which Dr. J. A. H. Murray considers was probably derived from the Scandinavian *dool*, meaning delay or sleep. Other authorities have derived the word from the French *deuil* (grief), a reference to its fatal properties.

Its deadly character is due to the presence of an alkaloid, Atropine, $\frac{1}{10}$ grain of which swallowed by a man has occasioned symptoms of poisoning. As every part of the plant is extremely poisonous, neither leaves, berries, nor root should be handled if there are any cuts or abrasions on the hands. The root is the most poisonous, the leaves and flowers less so, and the berries, except to children, least of all. It is said that an adult may eat two or three berries without injury, but dangerous symptoms appear if more are taken, and it is wiser not to attempt the experiment. Though so powerful in its action on the human body, the plant seems to affect some of the lower animals but little. Eight pounds of the herb are said to have been eaten by a horse without causing any injury, and an ass swallowed 1 lb. of the ripe berries without any bad results following. Rabbits, sheep, goats and swine eat the leaves with impunity, and birds often eat the seeds without any apparent effect, but cats and dogs are very susceptible to the poison.

Belladonna is supposed to have been the plant that poisoned the troops of Marcus Antonius during the Parthian wars. Plutarch gives a graphic account of the strange effects that followed its use.

Buchanan relates in his *History of Scotland* (1582) a tradition that when Duncan I was King of Scotland, the soldiers of Macbeth poisoned a whole army of invading Danes by a liquor mixed with an infusion of Dwale supplied to them during a truce. Suspecting nothing, the invaders drank deeply and were easily overpowered and murdered in their sleep by the Scots.

According to old legends, the plant belongs to the devil who goes about trimming and tending it in his leisure, and can only be diverted from its care on one night in the year, that is on Walpurgis, when he is preparing for the witches' sabbath. The apples of Sodom are held to be related to this plant, and the name Belladonna is said to record an old superstition that at certain times it takes the form of an enchantress of exceeding loveliness, whom it is dangerous to look upon, though a more generally accepted view is that the name was bestowed on it because its juice was used by the Italian ladies to give their eyes greater brilliancy, the smallest quantity having the effect of dilating the pupils of the eye.

Another derivation is founded on the old tradition that the priests used to drink an infusion before they worshipped and invoked the aid of Bellona, the Goddess of War.

The generic name of the plant, *Atropa*, is derived from the Greek *Atropos*, one of the Fates who held the shears to cut the thread of human life – a reference to its deadly, poisonous nature.

Thomas Lupton (1585) says: 'Dwale makes one to sleep while he is cut or burnt by cauterizing.' Gerard (1597) calls the plant the Sleeping Nightshade, and says the leaves moistened in wine vinegar and laid on the head induce sleep.

Mandrake, a foreign species of *Atropa* (*A. Mandragora*), was used in Pliny's day as an anæsthetic for operations. Its root contains an alkaloid, Mandragorine. The sleeping potion of Juliet was a preparation from this plant – perhaps also the Mandrake wine of the Ancients. It was called Circæon, being the wine of Circe.

Belladonna is often confused in the public mind with dulcamara (Bittersweet), possibly because it bears the popular name of woody nightshade. The cultivation of Belladonna in England dates at least from the sixteenth century, for Lyte says, in the *Niewe Herball*, 1578: 'This herbe is found in some places of this Countrie, in woods and hedges and in the gardens of some Herboristes.' Though not, however, much cultivated, it was evidently growing wild in many parts of the country when our great Herbals were written. Gerard mentions it as freely growing at Highgate, also at Wisbech and in Lincolnshire, and it gave a name to a Lancashire valley. Under the name of *Solanum lethale*, the plant was included in our early Pharma-

copœias, but it was dropped in 1788 and reintroduced in 1809 as *Belladonna folia*. Gerard was the first English writer to adopt the Italian name, of which he makes two words. The root was not used in medicine here until 1860, when Peter Squire recommended it as the basis of an anodyne liniment.

Before the War, the bulk of the world's supply of Belladonna was derived from plants growing wild on waste, stony places in Southern Europe. The industry was an important one in Croatia and Slavonia in South Hungary, the chief centre for foreign Belladonna, the annual crop in those provinces having been estimated at 60 to 100 tons of dry leaves and 150 to 200 tons of dry root. In 1908 the largest exporter in Slavonia is said to have sent out 29,880 lb. of dry Belladonna root.

The Balkan War of 1912–13 interrupted the continuity of Belladonna exports from South Hungary. Stocks of roots and leaves made shorter supplies last out until 1914, when prices rose, owing to increasing scarcity roots which realized 45s. per cwt. in January, 1914, selling for 65s. in June, 1914. With the outbreak of the Great War and the consequent entire stoppage of supplies, the price immediately rose to 100s. per cwt., and soon after, from 300s. to 480s. per cwt. or more. The dried leaves, from abroad, which in normal times sold at 45s. to 50s. per cwt., rose to 250s. to 350s. or more, per cwt. In August, 1916, the drug Atropine derived from the plant had risen from 10s. 6d. per oz. before the War to £7 per oz.

¶ *Cultivation*. Belladonna herb and root are sold by analysis, the value depending upon the percentage of alkaloid contained. A wide variation occurs in the amount of alkaloid present. It is important, therefore, to grow the crop under such conditions of soil and temperature as are likely to develop the highest percentage of the active principle.

In connexion with specimens of the wild plant, it is most difficult to trace the conditions which determine the variations, but it has been ascertained that a light, permeable and chalky soil is the most suitable for this crop. This, joined to a south-west aspect on the slope of a hill, gives specially good results as regards a high percentage of alkaloids. The limits of growth of Belladonna are between 50° and 55° N. Lat. and an altitude of 300 to 600 feet, though it may descend to sealevel where the soil is calcareous, especially where the drainage is good and the necessary amount of shade is found. The question of suitability of soil is especially important. Although the cultivated plant contains less alkaloid than that which grows wild, this in reality is only true of plants transported to a soil unsuited to them. It has been found, on the contrary, that artificial aids, such as the judicious selection of manure, the cleansing and preparation of the soil, destruction of weeds, etc., in accordance with the latest scientific practice, have improved the plants in every respect, not only in bulk, but even in percentage weight of alkaloidal contents.

Authorities differ on the question of manuring. Some English growers manure little if the plants are strong, but if the soil is really poor, or the plants are weak, the crop may be appreciably increased by the use of farmyard manure, or a mixture of nitrate of soda, basic slag and kainit. Excellent results have been obtained in experiments, by treating with basic slag, a soil already slightly manured and naturally suited to the plant, the percentage of total alkaloid in dry leaf and stem from third-year plants amounting to 0·84. In this case, the season was, however, an exceptionally favourable one, and, moreover, the soil being naturally suited to the plant, the percentage of alkaloid obtained without added fertilizer was already high. Speaking from the writer's own experience, Belladonna grows in her garden at Chalfont St. Peter. The soil is gravelly, even stony in some parts, with a chalk subsoil – the conditions similar to those that the plant enjoys in its wild state. This neighbourhood, in her opinion, is a suitable one for growing fields of Belladonna as crops for medicinal purposes.

Notes and statistics taken from season to season, extending over nine years, have shown that atmospheric conditions have a marked influence on the alkaloidal contents of Belladonna, the highest percentage of alkaloid being yielded in plants grown in sunny and dry seasons. The highest percentage of alkaloid, viz. 0·68 per cent., was obtained from the Belladonna crop of 1912, a year in which the months May and June were unusually dry and sunny; the lowest, just half, 0·34 was obtained on the same ground in 1907, when the period May and June was particularly lacking in sunshine. In 1905, August and September proving a very wet season, specimens analysed showed the low percentages of 0·38 and 0·35, whereas in July and October, 1906, the intervening period being very fine and dry, specimens analysed in those months showed a percentage of 0·54 and 0·64 respectively.

There appears to be no marked variation in alkaloidal contents due to different stages of growth from June to September, except when the plant begins to fade, when there is

rapid loss, hence the leaves may be gathered any time from June until the fading of the leaves and shoots set in.

In sowing Belladonna seed, 2 to 3 lb. should be reckoned to the acre. Autumn sown seeds do not always germinate, it is therefore more satisfactory to sow in boxes in a cool house, or frame, in early March, soaking the soil in the seed-boxes first, with boiling water, or baking it in an oven, to destroy the embryo of a small snail which is apt, as well as slugs and various insects, to attack the seedlings later. Pieces of chalk or lime can be placed among the drainage rubble at the bottom of the boxes. Belladonna seed is very slow in germinating, taking four to six weeks, or even longer, and as a rule not more than 70 per cent. can be relied on to germinate. On account of the seeds being so prone to attack by insect pests, if sown in the open, the seed-beds should first be prepared carefully. First of all, rubbish should be burnt on the ground, the soil earthed up and fired all over, all sorts of burnt vegetable rubbish being worked in. Then thoroughly stir up the ground and leave it rough for a few days so that air and sun permeate it well. Then level and rake the bed fine and finally give it a thorough drenching with boiling water. Let it stand till dry and friable, add sharp grit sand on the surface, rake fine again and then sow the seed very thinly.

Considerable moisture is needed during germination. The seedlings should be ready for planting out in May, when there is no longer any fear of frost. They will then be about 1½ inch high. Put them in after rain, or if the weather be dry, the ground should be well watered first, the seedlings puddled in and shaded from the sun with inverted flower-pots for several days. About 5,000 plants will be needed to the acre. If they are to remain where first planted, they may be planted 18 inches apart. A reserve of plants should be grown to fill in gaps.

The seedlings are liable to injury by late frosts and a light top dressing of farmyard manure or leaf-mould serves to preserve young shoots from injury during sudden and dangerous changes of temperature. They do best in shade. In America, difficulties in the cultivation of Belladonna have been overcome by interspersing plants with rows of scarlet runners, which, shading the herb, cause it to grow rapidly. Healthy young plants soon become re-established when transplanted, but require watering in dry weather. Great care must be taken to keep the crop clean from weeds and handpicking is to be recommended.

By September, the single stem will be 1½ to 2½ feet high. A gathering of leaves may then be made, if the plants are strong; 'leaves' include the broken-off tops of the plants, but the coarser stems are left on the plant and all discoloured portions rejected, and the plants should not be entirely denuded of leaves.

Before the approach of winter, plants must be thinned to 2½ to 3 feet apart, or over-crowding will result in the second year, in which the plant will bear one or two strong stems.

The writer finds that the green tips and cuttings from side branches root well and easily in early summer, and that buds with a piece of the root attached can be taken off the bigger roots in April, this being a very successful way of rapid propagation to get big, strong plants.

In the second year, in June, the crop is cut a few inches above the ground, while flowering, and delivered to the wholesale buyer the same day it is cut.

The average crop of fresh herb in the second and third years is 5 to 6 tons per acre, and 5 tons of fresh leaves and tops yield 1 ton of dried herb. A second crop is obtained in September in good seasons.

The yield per acre in the first year of growth should average about 6 cwt. of *dry* leaves.

The greatest loss of plants is in wet winters. Young seedling plants unless protected by dead leaves during the winter often perish. On the lighter soils there is less danger from winter loss, but the plants are more liable to damage from drought in summer.

One of the principal insect pests that attack Belladonna leaves is the so-called 'flea-beetle.' It perforates the leaves to such an extent as to make them unfit for sale in a dried state. It is when the plants are exposed to too much sunlight in open spots that the attacks of the beetle are worst, its natural habitat being well-drained slopes, partly under trees. If therefore the ground around the plants is covered with a thick mulch of leaves, they are not so likely to be attacked. The caterpillars from which the beetles come feed on the ground, and as they dislike moisture, the damp leaves keep them away. If napthalene is scattered on the soil, the vapour will probably help to keep the beetles off. The only way to catch them is to spread greased sheets of paper below the plants, and whenever the plants are disturbed a number of beetles will jump off like fleas and be caught on the papers. This at best only lessens the total quantity, however, and the other methods of precaution are the best.

The plant is dug or ploughed up during the autumn in the fourth year and the root collected, washed and dried, 3 to 4 tons of fresh root yielding a little over 1 ton of dry root. In time of great scarcity, it would probably pay to dig the root in the third year.

Old roots must be replaced by a planting of young ones or offsets, and if wireworm is observed, soot should be dug in with replacements.

Although Belladonna is not a plant that can be successfully grown in every small garden, yet in a chalky garden a few plants might be grown in a shady corner for the sake of the seed, for which there is a demand for propagation. Those, also, who know the haunts of the plant in its wild state might profitably collect the ripe berries, which should then be put into thin cotton bags and the juice squeezed out in running water. When the water is no longer stained, wring the bag well and turn out the seeds on to blotting paper and dry in the sun, or in a warm room near a stove. Sieve them finally, when dry, to remove all portions of the berry skin, etc.

Belladonna has been successfully cultivated in the neighbourhood of Leningrad since 1914, and already good crops have been obtained, the richness of the stems in alkaloids being noteworthy. It is stated that in consequence of the success that has attended the cultivation of Belladonna in Russia, it will no longer be needful to employ German drugs in the preparation of certain alkaloids. Much is also being collected wild in the Caucasus and in the Crimea.

It is hoped that if sufficient stocks can be raised in Britain, not only will it be unnecessary to import Belladonna, but that it may be possible to export it to those of our Dominions where the climate and local conditions prevent its successful culture, though at present it is still included among the medicinal plants of which the exportation is forbidden.

The following note on the growth and cultivation of Belladonna is from the *Chemist and Druggist*, of February 26, 1921:

'Belladonna is a perennial, but for horticultural purposes it is treated as a biennial, or triennial plant. The root in 3 years has attained very large dimensions around Edinburgh; in fact, often so large as to make the lifting a very heavy, and therefore costly, matter, and in consequence 2 years' growth is quite sufficient. One-year-old roots are just as active as the three-year-old stocks, and to the grower it is merely a matter of expediency which crop he chooses to dig up. The aerial growth is very heavy, two-year-old plants making 5 to 6 feet in the season if not cut for first crop, and if cut in July they make a second growth of 2 to 3 feet by September. To obtain a supply of seeds certain plantations must be left uncut, so as to get a crop of seeds for the next season. Moisture is, from a practical point of view, a very important matter. A sample, apparently dry to the touch, but not crisp, may have 15 per cent. to 20 per cent. of moisture present. Therefore if a pharmacist was to use a sample of such Belladonna leaves, although assayed to contain 0·03 per cent. of alkaloids, he would produce a weaker tincture than if he had used leaves with, say, only 5 per cent. of water present. The alkaloidal factor of this drug is the index to its value. Both the British and the United States Pharmacopœias adopt the same standard of alkaloidal value for the leaves, but the British Pharmacopœia does not require a standard for the root, which is one of those subtle conundrums which this quaint book frequently presents! Plants grown in a hard climate, such as Scotland, give a good alkaloidal figure, which compares favourably with any others. For roots, the British Pharmacopœia as just stated, requires no standard, but United States Pharmacopœia standard is 0·45 per cent., and Scottish roots yielded 0·78 per cent. and 0·72 per cent. There is not a great deal of alkaloidal value in the stalks. About 0·08 in the autumn.'

¶ Constituents. The medicinal properties of Belladonna depend on the presence of Hyoscyamine and Atropine. The root is the basis of the principal preparations of Belladonna.

The total alkaloid present in the *root* varies between 0·4 and 0·6 per cent., but as much as 1 per cent. has been found, consisting of Hyoscyamine and its isomer Atropine, 0·1 to 0·6 per cent.; Belladonnine and occasionally, Atropamine. Starch and Atrosin, a red colouring principle, are also present in the root. Scopolamine (hyoscine) is also found in traces, as is a fluorescent principle similar to that found in horse-chestnut bark and widely distributed through the natural order Solanaceæ. The greater portion of the alkaloidal matter consists of Hyoscyamine, and it is possible that any Atropine found is produced during extraction.

The amount of alkaloids present in the *leaves* varies somewhat in wild or cultivated plants, and according to the methods of drying and storing adopted, as well as on the conditions of growth, soil, weather, etc.

The proportion of the total alkaloid present in the dried leaves varies from 0·3 to 0·7 per cent. The greater proportion consists of Hyoscyamine, the Atropine being produced during extraction, as in the root. Belladonnine and Apoatropine may also be formed during extraction from the drug. The leaves contain also a trace of Scopolamine, Atrosin and starch.

The British Pharmacopœia directs that the leaves should not contain less than 0·3 per cent. of alkaloids and the root not less than 0·45 per cent.

A standardized liquid extract is prepared, from which the official plaster, alcoholic extract, liniment, suppository, tincture and ointment are made. The green extract is prepared from the fresh leaves.

¶ *Medicinal Action and Uses.* Narcotic, diuretic, sedative, antispasmodic, mydriatic. Belladonna is a most valuable plant in the treatment of eye diseases, Atropine, obtained during extraction, being its most important constituent on account of its power of dilating the pupil. Atropine will have this effect in whatever way used, whether internally, or injected under the skin, but when dropped into the eye, a much smaller quantity suffices, the tiny discs oculists using for this purpose, before testing their patient's sight for glasses, being made of gelatine with $\frac{1}{5000}$ grain of Atropine in each, the entire disk only weighing $\frac{1}{50}$ grain. Scarcely any operation on the eye can safely be performed without the aid of this valuable drug. It is a strong poison, the amount given internally being very minute, $\frac{1}{200}$ to $\frac{1}{100}$ grain. As an antidote to Opium, Atropine may be injected subcutaneously, and it has also been used in poisoning by Calabar bean and in Chloroform poisoning. It has no action on the voluntary muscles, but the nerve endings in involuntary muscles are paralysed by large doses, the paralysis finally affecting the central nervous system, causing excitement and delirium.

The various preparations of Belladonna have many uses. Locally applied, it lessens irritability and pain, and is used as a lotion, plaster or liniment in cases of neuralgia, gout, rheumatism and sciatica. As a drug, it specially affects the brain and the bladder. It is used to check excessive secretions and to allay inflammation and to check the sweating of phthisis and other exhausting diseases.

Small doses allay cardiac palpitation, and the plaster is applied to the cardiac region for the same purpose, removing pain and distress.

It is a powerful antispasmodic in intestinal colic and spasmodic asthma. Occasionally the leaves are employed as an ingredient of cigarettes for relieving the latter. It is well borne by children, and is given in large doses in whooping cough and false croup.

For its action on the circulation, it is given in the collapse of pneumonia, typhoid fever and other acute diseases. It increases the rate of the heart by some 20 to 40 beats per minute, without diminishing its force.

It is of value in acute sore throat, and relieves local inflammation and congestion.

Hahnemann proved that tincture of Belladonna given in very small doses will protect from the infection of scarlet fever, and at one time Belladonnna leaves were held to be curative of cancer, when applied externally as a poultice, either fresh or dried and powdered.

Belladonna plasters are often applied, after a fall, to the injured or sprained part. A mixture of Belladonna plaster, Salicylic acid and Lead plaster is recommended as an application for corns and bunions.

¶ *Preparations and Dosages.* Powdered leaves, 1 to 2 grains. Powdered root, 1 to 5 grains. Fluid extract leaves, 1 to 3 drops. Fluid extract root, B.P., ¼ to 1 drop. Tincture, B.P., 5 to 15 drops. Alkaloid Atropine, Alcoholic extract, B.P., ¼ to 1 grain. Green extract, B.P., ¼ to 1 grain. Juice, B.P., 5 to 15 drops. Liniment, B.P. Plaster, B.P. and U.S.P. Ointment, B.P.

NIGHTSHADE, WOODY

Solanum Dulcamara (LINN.)
N.O. Solanaceæ

Synonyms. Bittersweet. Dulcamara. Felonwood. Felonwort. Scarlet Berry. Violet Bloom
Part Used. Twigs

The large and important natural order of Solanaceæ contains, besides Henbane and the Nightshades, some of the most poisonous of our native plants, such useful economic plants as the Potato, Tomato, Aubergine, Capsicum and Tobacco, also the medicinally valuable Thornapple (*Datura Stramonium*), the Winter Cherry and the Mandrake, which in earlier days was supposed to possess miraculous properties.

The prevailing property of plants belonging to the Nightshade tribe is narcotic, rendering many of them in consequence highly poisonous.

The genus *Solanum* – to which the older herbalists formerly assigned *Atropa Belladonna*, and to which the Potato and Aubergine belong, is represented in this country by two species: *Solanum nigrum* (Black or Garden Nightshade) and *S. Dulcamara* (Bittersweet or Woody Nightshade). The leaves bear a certain resemblance to those of Belladonna, and the flowers of both Bittersweet and Belladonna are purple, though totally distinct in shape, and both have berries, red in the case of Bittersweet, not black as in the Belladonna. Bittersweet is common throughout Europe and America. It abounds in almost every hedgerow in England, where it is rendered conspicuous in the summer by its bright purple flowers, and in autumn by its brilliant red berries. Belladonna for which it is often mistaken is rare.

¶ *Description.* It is a perennial, shrubby plant, quite woody at the base, but throws out long, straggling, slender branches, which trail over the hedges and bushes among which it grows, reaching many feet in length, when supported by other plants. They are at first green and hairy, but become woody and smooth as they grow older, with an ashy-green bark.

The flowers, which are open all the summer, are in loose, drooping clusters, on short stalks opposite the leaves. They are of a bluish purple tint, with reflexed petals when expanded, so as almost to appear drooping. Their bright yellow stamens project in a conical form around the pistil, or seed-bearing portion of the flower.

The leaves are chiefly auriculate on the upper stems, i.e. with little ears, having at their base from one to two (rarely three) wing-like segments, but are heart-shaped below. They are placed alternately on either side of the stem and arranged so that they face the light. The flower-clusters always face a different direction to the leaves. 'One may gather a hundred pieces of the Woody Nightshade, and this strange perversity is rampant in all,' remarks an observer of this very curious habit.

The berries are green at first, afterwards becoming orange and finally bright red, and are produced in constant succession throughout the summer and early autumn, many remaining on the plant long after the leaves have fallen.

The plant was called the Woody Nightshade by the old herbalists to distinguish it from the Deadly Nightshade. Its generic name *Solanum* is derived from *Solor* (I ease), and testifies to the medicinal power of this group of plants. The second name, *Dulcamara*, used to be more correctly written in the Middle Ages, *Amaradulcis*, signifying literally 'bittersweet,' the common country name of the plant, given to it in reference to the fact that the root and stem, if chewed, taste first bitter and then sweet. Another old name is Felonwood, probably a corruption of Felonwort, the plant for felons – felon being an old name for whitlow. We are told by an old writer that –

'the Berries of Bittersweet stamped with rusty Bacon, applied to the Joynts of the Finger that is troubled with a Felon hath been found by divers country people who are most subject thereto to be very successful for the curing of the same.'

In the days of belief in witchcraft, shepherds used to hang it as a charm round the necks of those of their beasts whom they suspected to be under the evil eye.

The older physicians valued Bittersweet highly and applied it to many purposes in medicine and surgery, for which it is no longer used. It was in great repute as far back as the time of Theophrastus, and we know of it being in use in this country in the thirteenth century.

Gerard says of it:

'The juice is good for those that have fallen from high places, and have been thereby bruised or beaten, for it is thought to dissolve blood congealed or cluttered anywhere in the intrals and to heale the hurt places.'

Boerhaave, the celebrated Dutch physician, considered the young shoots superior to Sarsaparilla as a restorative, and Linnæus, who at first had an aversion to the plant, later spoke of it in the highest terms as a remedy for rheumatism, fever and inflammatory diseases of all kinds. There are few complaints for which it has not been at some time recommended.

¶ *Part Used.* The limited demand for Bittersweet in modern pharmacy is supplied by the wild plant.

The dried young branches from indigenous plants, taken when they have shed their leaves, were the parts directed for use up to 1907, by the British Pharmacopœia, but it has been removed from the last two editions.

The shoots, preferably the extreme branches, are collected from two- to three-year-old branches, after the leaves have fallen in the autumn, cut into pieces about ½ inch long, with a chaff cutter, and then carefully dried by artificial heat. They require no other preparation. The peculiar unpleasant odour of the shoots is lost on drying.

An extract of the leaves or tops is frequently prepared also; 10 lb. of the dried shoots yield about 2 lb. of the extract. A decoction of the dried herb is likewise used.

The drug occurs in commerce in short, cylindrical pieces of a light greenish, or brownish-yellow colour, about ¼ inch thick, bearing occasional alternate scars where the leaves have fallen off, and are quite free from hairs, and more or less longitudinally furrowed and wrinkled. A thin, shining bark surrounds the wood, which is lined internally by a whitish pith, which only partially fills it, leaving the centre hollow.

The active properties of Bittersweet are most developed when it grows in a dry and exposed situation. The bitterness is more pronounced in the spring than in the autumn, and in America the shoots are gathered while still pliant, when the plant is just budding, though the British Pharmacopœia directs that they shall be collected in the autumn.

¶ *Constituents.* Bittersweet contains the alkaloid Solanine and the amorphous glucoside Dulcamarine, to which the characteristic bittersweet taste is due. Sugar, gum, starch and resin are also present.

Solanine acts narcotically; in large doses it paralyses the central nervous system, without affecting the peripheral nerves or voluntary muscles. It slows the heart and respiration, lessens sensibility, lowers the temperature and causes vertigo and delirium, terminating in death with convulsions.

¶ *Medicinal Action and Uses.* The drug possesses feeble narcotic properties, with the power of increasing the secretions, particularly those of the skin and kidneys. It has no action on the pupil of the eye.

It is chiefly used as an alterative in skin diseases, being a popular remedy for obstinate skin eruptions, scrofula and ulcers.

It has also been recommended in chronic bronchial catarrh, asthma and whooping-cough.

For chronic rheumatism and for jaundice it has been much employed in the past, an infusion of 1 oz. of the dried herb to ½ pint water being taken in wineglassful doses, two or three times daily. From the fluid extract made from the twigs, a decoction is prepared of 10 drachms in 2 pints of boiling water, boiled down to 1 pint, and taken in doses of ½ to 2 oz. with an equal quantity of milk.

The berries have proved poisonous to a certain degree to children.

Fluid extract, ½ to 2 drachms.

¶ *Other Species.*
The four following species are all used in Homœopathic medicine:

SOLANUM ARRABENTA
Part Used. Leaves.
Habitat. Rio Janeiro.
Medicinal Use. Apoplexy.

SOLANUM MAMMOSUM
Synonym. Apple of Sodom.
Part Used. Fresh ripe fruit.
Medicinal Use. Irritability and restlessness.

SOLANUM OLERACEÆ
Synonym. Jagueribo.
Part Used. Flowers.
Habitat. Shores of Rio Janeiro.
Medicinal Use. Acts specifically on the mammary glands.

SOLANUM PSEUDO-CAPSICUM
Synonym. Jerusalem Cherry.
Part Used. Fruit.
Medicinal Use. Somnolence.

NUTMEG

Myristica fragrans (HOUTT.)
ₗN.O. Myristicaceæ

Synonyms. Nux Moschata. Myristica officinalis (Linn.). Myristica aromata. Myristica
Part Used. Dried kernel of the seed
Habitat. Banda Islands, Malayan Archipelago, Molucca Islands, and cultivated in
Sumatra, French Guiana

¶ *Description.* The tree is about 25 feet high, has a greyish-brown smooth bark, abounding in a yellow juice. The branches spread in whorls – alternate leaves, on petioles about 1 inch long, elliptical, glabrous, obtuse at base – acuminate, aromatic, dark green and glossy above, paler underside and 4 to 6 inches long. Flowers diœcious, small in axillary racemes. Peduncles and pedicles glabrous. Male flowers three to five more on a peduncle. Calyx urceolate, thick and fleshy, covered with an indistinct reddish pubescence dingy pale yellow, cut into three erect teeth. Female flowers differ little from the male, except pedicel is often solitary. Fruit is a pendulous, globose drupe, consisting of a succulent pericarp – the mace arillus covering the hard endocarp, and a wrinkled kernel with ruminated endosperm. When the arillus is fresh it is a brilliant scarlet, when dry more horny, brittle, and a yellowish-brown colour. The seed or nutmeg is firm, fleshy, whitish, transversed by red-brown veins, abounding in oil. The tree does not bloom till it is nine years old, when it fruits and continues to do so for seventy-five years without attention. In Banda Islands there are three harvests, the chief one in July or August, the next in November, and the last in March or April. The fruit is gathered by means of a barb attached to a long stick. The mace is separated from the nut and both are dried separately. The nutmeg or kernel of the fruit and the arillus or mace are the official parts.

After the mace is removed, the nutmegs are dried on gratings, three to six weeks over a slow charcoal fire – but are often sun-dried for six days previously. The curing protects them from insects.

When thoroughly dried, they rattle in the shell, which is cracked with a mallet. The nutmegs are graded, 1st Penang, 2nd Dutch

(these are usually covered with lime to preserve them from insects), 3rd Singapore, and 4th long nutmegs.

Nutmegs have a strong, peculiar and delightful fragrance and a very strong bitter warm aromatic taste.

¶ *Constituents.* They contain lignin, stearin, volatile oil, starch, gum and 0·08 of an acid substance. By submitting nutmegs and water to distillation, a volatile oil is obtained. The small round heavy nutmeg is the best. Those that are larger, longer, lighter, less marbled, and not so oily, are inferior.

The powder of nutmegs, beaten to a pulp with water, then pressed between heated plates, gives from 10 to 30 per cent. of orange-coloured scented concrete oil erroneously called 'oil of mace' – an inferior oil is prepared in Holland from the spoiled or inferior nutmegs – and an artificial preparation is made by mixing together tallow, spermaceti, etc., colouring it with saffron and flavouring it with essential oil of nutmeg.

After the nutmegs have been collected, the outside fleshy pericarp is made into a preserve.

The mace of commerce should be somewhat flexible, cinnamon-yellow coloured, in single or double blades, with nutmeg-like smell and a warm, sharp, fatty, aromatic taste.

There is a large trade in wild nutmegs, which are known in commerce under the names of long, female, Macassar, Papua, Guinea, or Norse nutmegs. All these varieties have been traced to *Myristica argentea* of New Guinea, from whence they enter commerce as Macassar nutmegs.

There is much adulteration and fraud in the nutmeg trade. The essential oil has often been extracted before they are marketed – a fraud which can be detected by the light weight. This renders them more subject to attacks by insects.

Concrete oil of nutmeg, often erroneously termed 'oil of mace' or 'nutmeg butter,' is made by bruising the nuts and treating them with steam. The best nutmeg butter is imported from the East Indies in stone jars, or in blocks wrapped in palm leaves – it should be softly solid, unctuous to touch, orange yellow colour and mottled, with the taste and smell of nutmeg.

Holland prepares an inferior kind of oil sometimes offered for sale – it is said to be derived from nutmegs that have been deprived of their volatile oil by distillation. It is found in hard shining square cakes, light coloured and with less taste and smell than the East Indies oil. *Ucuhula* nut is the round or oval seed of *M. surinamensis*. It is distinguished by very large albuminous crystalloids, the seeds containing over 70 per cent. solid yellow fat. The Brazilian *M. officinalis* resembles the nutmeg in form and structure, it contains crystals like the preceding one, though less large; has a black shell covered with broad furrows and yields a fat or bicuhyba balsam very like the ordinary nutmeg, with a sharp sour taste, and a peculiar fatty acid, bicuhybastearic acid. From *M. otoba* otoba fat is procured. Almost colourless with a fresh smell of nutmeg, it contains myristin, olein, and otobite. The fruit of virola or *M. sebifera* also gives a fatty substance termed ocuba wax. The following are erroneously called nutmegs:

CALIFORNIAN NUTMEG. The seed of a coniferous tree, *Sorreya Californica* – its odour and taste terebinthinate.

JAMAICA or CALABACH NUTMEG. Obtained from *Monodora myristica*.

NEW HOLLAND or PLUME NUTMEG. Obtained from the *Atherosperma moschata*.

CLOVE NUTMEG. Obtained from *Agathophyllum aromaticum*.

Insects that attack nutmegs only extract the fat oil. They do not interfere in any way with the essential oil.

¶ *Medicinal Action and Uses.* The tonic principle is Myristicin. Oil of Nutmeg is used to conceal the taste of various drugs and as a local stimulant to the gastro-intestinal tract.

¶ *Uses of Nutmeg.* Powdered nutmeg is rarely given alone, though it enters into the composition of a number of medicines. The expressed oil is sometimes used externally as a gentle stimulant, and it was once an ingredient of the *Emplastrum picis*.

The properties of mace are identical to those of the nutmeg. Dose, 5 to 20 grains.

Both nutmeg and mace are used for flatulence and to correct the nausea arising from other drugs, also to allay nausea and vomiting.

Nutmeg is an agreeable addition to drinks for convalescents.

Grated nutmeg mixed with lard makes an excellent ointment for piles.

In some places roasted nutmeg is applied internally as a remedy for leucorrhœa. Dose of the powder, 5 to 20 grains. Fluid extract, 10 to 30 drops. Larger doses are narcotic and produce dangerous symptoms. Spirit, B.P., 5 to 20 drops.

See MACE.

(*POISON*)
NUX VOMICA

Strychnos Nux-vomica (LINN.)
N.O. Loganiaceæ

Synonyms. Poison Nut. Semen strychnos. Quaker Buttons
Part Used. Dried ripe seeds
Habitat. India, in the Malay Archipelago

¶ *Description.* A medium-sized tree with a short, crooked, thick trunk, the wood is white hard, close grained, durable and the root very bitter. Branches irregular, covered with a smooth ash-coloured bark; young shoots deep green, shiny; leaves opposite, short stalked, oval, shiny, smooth on both sides, about 4 inches long and 3 broad; flowers small, greeny-white, funnel shape, in small terminal cymes, blooming in the cold season and having a disagreeable smell. Fruit about the size of a large apple with a smooth hard rind or shell which when ripe is a lovely orange colour, filled with a soft white jelly-like pulp containing five seeds covered with a soft woolly-like substance, white and horny internally. The seeds are removed when ripe, cleansed, dried and

sorted; they are exported from Cochin, Madras and other Indian ports. The seeds have the shape of flattened disks densely covered with closely appressed satiny hairs, radiating from the centre of the flattened sides and giving to the seeds a characteristic sheen; they are very hard, with a dark grey horny endosperm in which the small embryo is embedded; no odour but a very bitter taste.

¶ *Constituents.* Nux Vomica contains the alkaloids, Strychnine and Brucine, also traces of strychnicine, and a glucoside Loganin, about 3 per cent. fatty matter, caffeotannic acid and a trace of copper. The pulp of the fruit contains about 5 per cent. of loganin together with the alkaloid strychnicine.

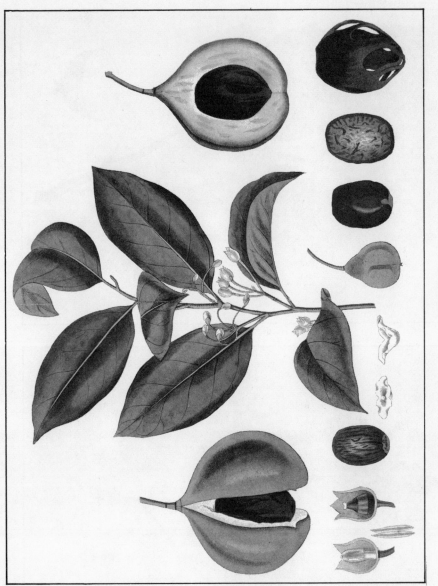

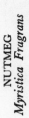

NUTMEG
Myristica Fragrans

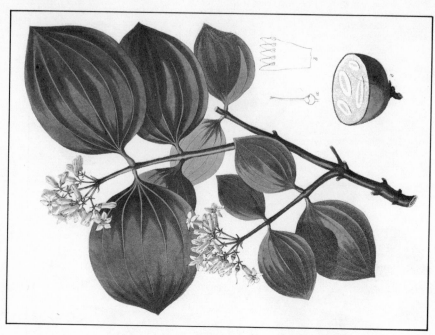

NUX VOMICA
Strychnos Nux-Vomica

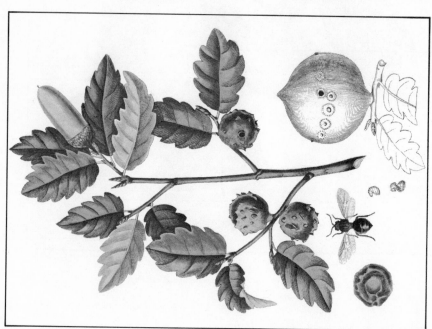

OAK GALLS
Quercus Infectoria

¶ *Medicinal Action and Uses.* The properties of Nux Vomica are substantially those of the alkaloid Strychnine. The powdered seeds are employed in atonic dyspepsia. The tincture of Nux Vomica is often used in mixtures – for its stimulant action on the gastro-intestinal tract. In the mouth it acts as a bitter, increasing appetite; it stimulates peristalsis; in chronic constipation due to atony of the bowel it is often combined with cascara and other laxatives with good effects. Strychnine, the chief alkaloid constituent of the seeds, also acts as a bitter, increasing the flow of gastric juice; it is rapidly absorbed as it reaches the intestines, after which it exerts its characteristic effects upon the central nervous system, the movements of respiration are deepened and quickened and the heart slowed through excitation of the vagal centre. The senses of smell, touch, hearing and vision are rendered more acute, it improves the pulse and raises blood pressure and is of great value as a tonic to the circulatory system in cardiac failure. Strychnine is excreted very slowly and its action is cumulative in any but small doses; it is much used as a gastric tonic in dyspepsia. The most direct symptom caused by strychnine is violent convulsions due to a simultaneous stimulation of the motor or sensory ganglia of the spinal cord; during the convulsion there is great rise in blood pressure; in some types of chronic lead poisoning it is of great value. In cases of surgical shock and cardiac failure large doses are given up to $\frac{1}{10}$ grain by hypodermic injection; also used as an antidote in poisoning by chloral or chloroform. Brucine closely resembles strychnine in its action, but is slightly less poisonous; it paralyses the peripheral motor nerves. It is said that the convulsive action characteristic of strychnine is absent in brucine almost entirely. It is used in pruritis and as a local anodyne in inflammations of the external ear.

¶ *Preparations and Dosages.* Strychnine should not be administered in liquid form combined with bromides, iodides or chlorides, there being a risk of formation of the insoluble hydrobromide, etc.

Nux Vomica, 1 to 4 grains. Extract of Nux Vomica, B.P., $\frac{1}{4}$ to 1 grain. Extract of Nux Vomica, B.P. 1885, $\frac{1}{4}$ to 1 grain. Extract of Nux Vomica, U.S.P., $\frac{1}{4}$ grain. Liquid extract of Nux Vomica, B.P., 1 to 3 minims. Fluid extract of Nux Vomica, U.S.P., 1 minim. Tincture of Nux Vomica, B.P., 5 to 15 minims. Tincture of Nux Vomica, B.P. 1885, 10 to 20 minims. Tincture of Nux Vomica, U.S.P., 10 minims. Strychnine, B.P., $\frac{1}{6}$ to $\frac{1}{15}$ grain. Hypodermic injection of strychnine. Solution of Strychnine Hydrochloride, B.P., 2 to 8 minims. Acid Strychnine Mixture, B.P.C., $\frac{1}{2}$ to 1 fluid ounce.

¶ *Poisoning and Antidotes.* In cases of poisoning by strychnine an emetic or the stomach pump should be used at once and tannin or potassium permanganate given to render the strychnine inactive. Violent convulsions should be controlled by administration of chloroform or large doses of chloral or bromide. Urethane in large doses is considered an antidote. Amyl nitrite is also useful owing to its rapid action during the convulsion, and in absence of respiration 3 to 5 minims may be hypodermically injected.

¶ *Other Species.*

Strychnos tieute, a clumbing shrub growing in Java, gives a juice termed Upas tieute, said to be used by the natives as an arrow poison; it produces death by violent convulsions, the heart stopping before respiration.

S. toxifera yields the deadly poison Curare (Woorari or Urari) used by the natives of British Guiana.

S. ligustrina, the wood of which contains brucine, as does the bark.

S. pseudo is found in the mountains and forests of India. It supplies the seeds known as clearing nuts. The fruit is black, the size of a cherry, containing only one seed; fruit and seeds are used medicinally in India and also to clear muddy water, the seeds being rubbed for a minute inside the vessel and the water then allowed to settle; their efficiency depending on their albumen and casein contents acting as a fining agent similar to those employed to clarify wine and beer.

S. innocua. The fruit and pulp are harmless and are eaten by the natives of Egypt and Senegal.

S. Ignatii is found in the Philippines, the seeds containing strychnine and brucine, strychnine being present in greater quantity than in Nux Vomica. A tincture made from the beans is official in the British Pharmacopœia Codex.

OAK, COMMON

Quercus robur
N.O. Cupuliferæ

Synonym. Tanner's Bark

The Common, or British Oak, for many centuries the chief forest tree of England, is intimately bound up with the history of these islands from Druid times. A spray of oak was for long engraved on one side of our sixpences and shillings, but is now superseded by the British lion. The Oak, although widely distributed over Europe, is regarded as peculiarly English.

The genus *Quercus* comprises numerous species, distributed widely over the Northern Hemisphere, and found also in Java, and the Mountains of Mexico and South America. One species from Guatemala, *Quercus Skinneri*, is remarkable for its resemblance to the Walnut (*Juglans*) in its lobed and wrinkled seed-leaves or cotyledons.

The Oak is subject to a good deal of variation; many species have been defined and many oaks of foreign origin are grown in our parks, the longest established being the Evergreen or Holm Oak (*Q. ilex*). There are two principal varieties of *Q. robur*, often regarded as separate species: *Q. pedunculata*, the Common Oak, which is distinguished by having acorns in ones and twos attached to the twigs by long stems, the leaves having scarcely any stalk at all; and *Q. sessiliflora*, the Durmast Oak, often included with the former, but distinct, the leaves being borne on long stalks, while the acorns 'sit' on the bough. This variety of oak is more generally found in the lower parts of Britain and in North Wales. It is not so long-lived as the Common Oak, and the wood, which has a straighter fibre and a finer grain, is generally thought less tough and more resisting.

Q. pedunculata and *Q. sessiliflora* make good timber, the latter being darker, heavier and more elastic. The wood of these trees when stained green by the growth of a peculiar fungus known as *Peziza œriginosa* is much valued by cabinet-makers.

¶ *Description.* The shape of the oak leaves is too familiar to need description. The flowers are of two kinds; the male, or barren, in long drooping catkins, 1 to 3 inches long, appearing with the leaves, and the leaves and the fertile flowers in distant clusters, each with a cup-shaped, scaly involucre, producing, as fruit, an acorn 1 to 1 inch long.

The Oak is noted for the slowness of its growth, as well as for the large size to which it attains. In eighty years the trunk is said not to exceed 20 inches in diameter, but old trees reach a great girth. The famous Fairlop Oak in Hainault Forest measured 36 feet in girth, the spreading boughs extending above 300 feet in circumference. The Newland Oak in Gloucestershire measures 46 feet 4 inches at 1 foot from the ground, and is one of the largest and oldest in the kingdom, these measurements being exceeded, however, by those of the Courthorpe Oak in Yorkshire, which Hooker reports as attaining the extraordinary girth of 70 feet. King Arthur's Round Table was made from a single slice of oak, cut from an enormous bole, and is still shown at Winchester.

Humboldt refers to an oak in the Département de la Charente-Inférieure measuring nearly 90 feet in circumference near the base; near Breslau an oak fell in 1857 measuring 66 feet in circumference at the base. These large trees are for the most part decayed and hollow in the interior, and their age has been estimated at from one to two thousand years.

The famous Oak of Mamre, Abram's Oak, was illustrated formerly in the *Transactions of the Linnean Society*, by Dr. Hooker. It is a fine specimen of the species *Q. Coccifera*, the prickly evergreen or Kermes Oak, a native of the countries bordering on the Mediterranean; the insect (*coccus*) from which it derives its name yielding the dye known as 'Turkey red.' Abram's Oak is 22 feet in circumference; it is popularly supposed to represent the spot where the tree grew under which Abraham pitched his tent. There is a superstition that any person who cuts or maims this oak will lose his firstborn son.

The oak of Libbeiya in the Lebanon measures 37 feet in girth, and its branches cover an area whose circumference measured over 90 yards. The Arab name is *Sindian*.

The Greeks held the Oak sacred, the Romans dedicated it to Jupiter, and the Druids venerated it.

In England the name Gospel Oak is still retained in many counties, relating to the time when Psalms and Gospel truths were uttered beneath their shade. They were notable objects as resting-places in the 'beating of the parish bounds,' a practice supposed to have been derived from the feast to the god Terminus.

The following is a quotation from Withers:

'That every man might keep his own possessions,
Our fathers used, in reverent processions,
With zealous prayers, and with praiseful cheere,
To walk their parish limits once a year;
And well-known marks (which sacrilegious hands
Now cut or breake) so bordered out their lands,
That every one distinctly knew his owne,
And brawles now rife were then unknowne.'

The ceremony was performed by the clergyman and his parishioners going the boundaries of the parish and choosing the most remarkable sites (oak-trees being specially selected) to read passages from the Gospels, and ask blessings for the people.

'Dearest, bury me
Under that holy oke, or Gospel Tree;
Where, though thou see'st not, thou may'st
think upon
Me, when you yearly go'st Procession.'

HERRICK

Many of these Gospel trees are still alive –
five in different parts of England.

An old proverb relating to the oak is still a
form of speculation on the weather in many
country districts.

'If the Oak's before the Ash,
Then you'll only get a splash;
If the Ash before the Oak,
Then you may expect a soak.'

The technical name of the Oak is said to be
derived from the Celtic *quer* (fine) and *cuez*
(tree).

A curious custom in connexion with wearing an oak-leaf (or preferably an *oak-apple*)
on May 29, still exists in some villages in
South Wilts. Each one has the right to collect fallen branches in a certain large wood in
the district. To *claim* this privilege each
villager has to bring them home shouting
'*Grovely, Grovely, and all Grovely!*' (this
being the name of the large wood).

After the Oak has passed its century, it
increases by less than an inch a year, but the
wood matured in this leisurely fashion is
practically indestructible. Edward the Con-
fessor's shrine in Westminster Abbey is of
oak that has outlasted the changes of 800
years. Logs have been dug from peat bogs,
in good preservation and fit for rough building purposes, that were submerged a
thousand years ago. In the Severn, break-
waters are still used as casual landing-places,
where piles of oak are said to have been
driven by the Romans.

As timber, the particular and most valued
qualities of the Oak are hardness and toughness; Box and Ebony are harder, Yew and
Ash are tougher than Oak, but no timber is
possessed of both these requisites in so
great a degree as the British Oak. Its elasticity and strength made it particularly advantageous in shipbuilding, and the oaks of
the Forest of Dean provided much material
for the 'wooden walls of England.' We read
that Philip of Spain gave special orders to
the Armada to burn and destroy every oak in
that forest, and a century later, during a
period of twenty-five years, nearly 17,000
loads of oak timber, of the value of £30,000,
were despatched to naval dockyards from this
forest. Nelson drew up a special memorial to
the Crown on the desirability of replanting
this forest with oak trees, and at that time no
forester dared to cut down a *crooked* tree
before maturity, because its knees and
twisted elbows were so desirable in ship-
building. A tree should be winter felled, if
perfection of grain is desired. Although not
employed as of old, for building ships of war,
it is in great request for peaceful land transit,
sharing with Ash in the making of railway
carriages and other rolling stock. The roots
were formerly used to make hafts for
daggers and knives.

Some of the American kinds also furnish
valuable timber. Such are *Q. alba*, the White
or Quebec Oak, the wood of which is used in
shipbuilding, and by wheelwrights and
coopers. *Q. virens*, the Live Oak, also yields
excellent timber for naval purposes. The
wood of *Q. ilex*, a Mediterranean species, is
said to be as good as that of the Common
Oak. *Q. cerris*, the Turkey Oak, supplies a
wood much in favour with wheelwrights,
cabinet-makers, turners, etc. There are also
several Japanese oaks, used for their excellent timber.

The False Sandalwood of Crete is the produce of *Q. abelicea*. This wood is of a reddish colour, and has an agreeable perfume.
The less valuable oaks furnish excellent
charcoal and firewood.

The bark is universally used to tan leather,
and for this purpose strips easily in April and
May. An infusion of it, with a small quantity
of copperas, yields a dye which was formerly
used in the country to dye woollen of a
purplish colour, which, though not very
bright, was said to be durable. The Scotch
Highlanders used it to dye their yarn. Oak
sawdust used also to be the principal indigenous vegetable used in dyeing fustian,
and may also be used for tanning, but is
much inferior to the bark for that purpose.
Oak apples have also been occasionally used
in dyeing as a substitute for the imported
Oriental galls, but the black obtained from
them is not durable.

In Brittany, tan compressed into cakes is
used as fuel. Oak-bark is employed for dyeing black, in conjunction with salts of iron.
With alum, oak-bark yields a brown dye;
with a salt of tin, a yellow colour; with a salt
of zinc, Isabella yellow. *Q. tinctoria*, a
North American species, yields *Quercitron
Bark*, employed for dyeing yellow; the
American Indians are said to dye their skins
red with the bark of *Q. prinus*. After the oak-
bark has been used for leather-tanning, it is
still serviceable to gardeners for the warmth
it generates and is largely used by them
under the name of Tan; it sometimes, however, favours the growth of certain fungi,
which are harmful to plants. Refuse tan is

also employed in the adulteration of chicory and coffee.

Acorns were of considerable importance formerly for feeding swine. About the end of the seventh century, special laws were made relating to the feeding of swine in woods, called pawnage, or pannage. In Saxon times of famine, the peasantry were thankful for a share of this nourishing, but somewhat indigestible food. The Board of Agriculture has lately issued a pamphlet, pointing out the use as fodder, which might be made both of the Acorn and of the Horse Chestnut. The analysis of the Acorn given by the *Lancet* is: water, 6·3 per cent.; protein, 5·2 per cent.; fat, 43 per cent.; carbohydrates, 45 per cent. The most important constituent of both the Acorn and the Horse Chestnut is the carbohydrate in the form of starch, while the Acorn should have further value on account of the substantial proportion of fat which it contains. The flavour of Acorns is improved if they are dried, and a flour with nourishing properties can be obtained by grinding the dried kernels.

In many country districts acorns are still collected in sacks and given to pigs; but these must be mixed with other vegetable food to counteract their binding properties.

Oak trees are more persistently attacked by insects than any other trees.

¶ *Medicinal Action and Uses.* The astringent effects of the Oak were well known to the Ancients, by whom different parts of the tree were used, but it is the *bark* which is now employed in medicine. Its action is slightly tonic, strongly astringent and antiseptic. It has a strong astringent bitter taste, and its qualities are extracted both by water and spirit. The odour is slightly aromatic.

Like other astringents, it has been recommended in agues and hæmorrhages, and is a good substitute for Quinine in intermittent fever, especially when given with Chamomile flowers.

It is useful in chronic diarrhœa and dysentery, either alone or in conjunction with aromatics. A decoction is made from 1 oz. of bark in a quart of water, boiled down to a pint and taken in wineglassful doses. Externally, this decoction has been advantageously employed as a gargle in chronic sore throat with relaxed uvula, and also as a fomentation. It is also serviceable as an injection for leucorrhœa, and applied locally to bleeding gums and piles.

¶ *Preparation and Dosage.* Fluid extract, ½ to 1 drachm.

Oak bark when finely powdered and inhaled freely, has proved very beneficial in consumption in its early stages. Working tanners are well known to be particularly exempt from this disease. A remedial snuff is made from the freshly collected oak bark, dried and reduced to a fine powder.

The bark is collected in the spring from young trees, and dried in the sun. It is greyish, more or less polished externally and brownish internally. The fracture is fibrous and the inner surface rough, with projecting medullary rays.

The older herbalists considered the thin skin that covers the acorn effectual in staying spitting of blood, and the powder of the acorn taken in wine was considered a good diuretic. A decoction of acorns and oak bark, made with milk, was considered an antidote to poisonous herbs and medicines.

The distilled water of the oak bud was also thought 'to be good used either inwardly or outwardly to assuage inflammation.'

Galen applied the bruised leaves to heal wounds.

OAK GALLS

Galls are excrescences produced in plants by the presence of the larvæ of different insects. The forms that they assume are many, and the changes produced in the tissues various. They occur in all parts of the plant and sometimes in great quantities.

The oak galls used in commerce and medicine are excrescences on the *Q. infectoria*, a small oak, indigenous to Asia Minor and Persia, and result from the puncture of the bark of the young twigs by the female Gall-wasp, *Cynips Gallæ-tinctoriæ*, who lays its eggs inside. This species of oak seldom attains the height of 6 feet, the stem being crooked, with the habit of a shrub rather than a tree.

The Common Oaks of this country are much affected by galls. They occur sometimes on the leaves, where they form the so-called 'Oak-apples,' sometimes on the shoots, where they do great mischief by checking and distorting the growth of the tree.

The young larva that hatches from the eggs feeds upon the tissues of the plant and secretes in its mouth a peculiar fluid, which stimulates the cells of the tissues to a rapid division and abnormal development, resulting in the formation of a gall.

The larva thus becomes completely enclosed in a nearly spherical mass, which projects from the twig, furnishing it with a supply of starch and other nutritive material.

The growth of the gall continues only so long as the egg or larva lives or reaches maturity and passes into a chrysalis, from which the fully-developed gall-wasp emerges and escapes into the air through a hole bored with its mandibles in the side of the gall.

The best Aleppo galls, collected in Asiatic Turkey, principally in the province of Aleppo, are collected before the insects escape.

Galls are also largely imported from Persia and to a lesser extent from Greece.

Aleppo Galls of good quality are hard and heavy, without perforations, dark bluish-green or olive green, nearly spherical in shape, 12 to 18 mm. in diameter (about ⅖ to ⅗ inch), and known in commerce as *blue* or *green* galls.

The Aleppo galls (from *Q. infectoria*) sometimes also called 'Mecca Galls,' are supposed to be the Dead Sea or Sodom Apples, 'the fruit that never comes to ripeness' – the fruit so pleasant to the eye, so bitter to the taste.

If collected after the insects have escaped, galls are of a pale, yellowish-brown hue, spongy and lighter in weight, perforated near the centre with a small hole. These are known in commerce as *white* galls.

On breaking a gall, it appears yellowish or brownish-white within, with a small cavity containing the remains of a larva of the Gall-wasp.

Galls have no marked odour, but an intensely astringent taste, and slightly sweet after-taste.

¶ *Constituents.* The chief constituents of *Aleppo* or Turkey Galls are 50 to 70 per cent. of gallotannic acid, 2 to 4 per cent. of gallic acid, mucilage, sugar, resin and an insoluble matter, chiefly lignin.

'White' galls contain less gallotannic acid than 'blue' or 'green.'

English Oak Galls, or Oak Apples, are smooth, globular, brown, usually perforated and much less astringent than Aleppo Galls, containing only 15 to 20 per cent. of gallo-tannic acid. They have no commercial value.

China Galls – produced by a species of Aphis on *Rhus semialata* – are used mainly for the manufacture of tannic and gallic acids, pyrogallol, ink, etc. They are not spherical, but of extremely diverse and irregular form, with a thick, grey, velvety down, making them a reddish-brown colour. They contain about 70 per cent of gallotannic acid.

Mecca Galls, from Bassorah, known as 'mala nisana,' are spherical in shape and surrounded about the centre by a circle of horned protuberances. They are not official.

¶ *Medicinal Action and Uses.* Galls are much used commercially in the preparation of gallic and tannic acid, and are extensively employed in tanning and dyeing, in the manufacture of ink, etc.

Medicinally, they are a powerful astringent, the most powerful of all vegetable astringents, used as a tincture internally, in cases of dysentery, diarrhoea, cholera, and as an injection in gonorrhœa, leucorrhœa, etc.

Preparations of gall are usually applied as a local astringent externally, mainly in Gall ointment (1 oz. powdered galls and 4 oz. benzoated lard), applied to painful hæmorrhoids, and also to arrest hæmorrhage from the nose and gums.

An infusion may be used also as a gargle in relaxed throat, inflamed tonsils, etc.

¶ *Preparations and Dosages.* Powdered gall, 5 to 20 grains. Fluid extract, 5 to 20 drops. Tincture, U.S.P., 1 drachm. Ointment, B.P. Compound ointment, B.P.

OAK, POLYPODY OF. *See* FERNS

OATS

Avena sativa (LINN.)
N.O. Graminaceæ

Synonyms. Groats. Oatmeal
Part Used. Seeds
Habitat. It is unknown when Oats were first introduced into Britain

¶ *Description.* There are about twenty-five varieties cultivated. The nutritive quality of Oats is less in a given weight than that of any other cereal grain. In the best Oats it does not exceed 75 per cent. *Avena sativa*, the Common Oat, has a smooth stem, growing up to 4 feet high, with linear lanceolate, veined rough leaves; loose striate sheaves; stipules lacerate; panicle equal, loose; spikelets pedunculate, pendulous, two-flowered, both perfect, lower one mostly awned; paleæ cartilaginous, embracing the caryopsis; root fibrous, annual. The Naked or Pilcorn Oat differs slightly from the other: calyces three-flowered, receptacle exceeding the calyx; petals awned at the back; the third floscule awnless; and the chief difference lies in the grains, which when ripe quit the husk and fall naked. The grains as found in commerce are enclosed in their pales and these grains divested of their paleæ are used for medicinal and dietary purposes; the grains when separated from their integuments are termed groats, and these when crushed are called Embden groats. Oatmeal is ground grain.

¶ *Constituents.* Starch, gluten, albumen and other protein compounds, sugar, gum oil, and salts.

¶ *Medicinal Action and Uses.* Nervine, stimulant, antispasmodic. Oats are made into gruel. This is prepared by boiling 1 oz. of oatmeal or groats in 3 pints of water till reduced to 1 quart, then straining it, sugar, lemons, wine, or raisins being added as flavouring. Gruel thus is a mild nutritious aliment, of easy digestion in inflammatory cases and fevers; it is very useful after parturition, and is sometimes employed in poisoning from acid substances. It is found useful also as a demulcent enema and boiled into a thick paste makes a good emollient poultice. Oatmeal is unsoluble in alcohol, ether, and the oils, but the two first move an oleoresinous matter from it. It is to be avoided in dyspepsia accompanied with acidity of the stomach. The pericarp of Oats con-

tains an amorphous alkaloid which acts as a stimulant of the motor ganglia, increasing the excitability of the muscles, and in horses causes excitement. A tincture is made by permeating 4 oz. of ground oatmeal to 1 pint diluted alcohol, keeping the first 5½ oz. (fluid), and evaporating the remainder down to ½ fluid ounce, and adding this to the first 5½ fluid ounces. The extract and tincture are useful as a nerve and uterine tonic.

Dosage.[1] Fluid extract, 10 to 30 drops in hot water.

OLEANDER. *See* PERIWINKLE

OLIBANUM. *See* FRANKINCENSE

OLIVE

Olea Europæa (LINN.)
N.O. Oleaceæ

Synonyms. Olea Oleaster. Olea lancifolia. Olea gallica. Olivier
Parts Used. The oil of the fruit, leaves, bark
Habitat. Asia Minor and Syria. Cultivated in Mediterranean countries, Chile and Peru, and South Australia

History. The high position held by the Olive tree in ancient as in modern days may be realized when it is remembered that Moses exempted from military service men who would work at its cultivation, and that in Scriptural and classical writings the oil is mentioned as a symbol of goodness and purity, and the tree as representing peace and happiness. The oil, in addition to its wide use in diet, was burnt in the sacred lamps of temples, while the victor in the Olympic games was crowned with its leaves.

Description. Olea europæa is a small, evergreen tree, averaging 20 feet or more in height. It has many thin branches with opposite branchlets and shortly-stalked, opposite, lanceolate leaves about 2¼ inches long, acute, entire and smooth, pale green above and silvery below. The bark is pale grey and the flowers numerous, small and creamy-white in colour.

The dark purple fruit is a drupe about ¾ inch long, ovoid and often pointed, the fleshy part filled with oil. The thick, bony stone has a blunt keel down one side. It contains a single seed.

Being hardier than the lemon, the Olive may sometimes produce fruit in England. The largest of the varieties under cultivation is produced in Spain, but probably Italy prepares most oil, the annual average being 33 million gallons.

The beautifully-veined wood not only takes a fine polish, but is faintly fragrant, and is much valued for small cabinet-work. It was in olden days carved into statues of gods.

For use as a dessert fruit the unripe olives

are steeped in water to reduce their bitterness. Olives *à la Picholine* are steeped in a solution of lime and wood ashes. They are bottled in an aromatic solution of salt.

In warm countries the bark exudes a substance called *Gomme d'Olivier*, which was formerly used in medicine as a vulnerary.

The large 'Queen Olives' grown near Cadiz are chiefly exported to the United States; the smaller 'Manzanillo' is principally consumed in Spain and Spanish America.

The trees bear fruit in their second year; in their sixth will repay cultivation, and continue as a source of wealth even when old and hollow, though the crop varies greatly from year to year.

The groves are cut until the beauty of the trees is lost.

The ripe fruits are pressed to extract the oil, the methods varying in the different countries.

Virgin Oil, greenish in tint, is obtained by pressing crushed fruit in coarse bags and skimming the oil from the tubs of water through which it is conducted. The cake left in the bags is broken up, moistened, and re-pressed. Sometimes the fruit is allowed to reach fermenting point before pressure, the quantity of oil being increased and the quality lessened. The product is called *Huile fermentée.*

Huile ordinaire is made by expression and mixture with boiling water.

Provence oil is the most valued and the most refined.

Official Olive *soap* is made from olive oil and sodium hydroxide.

Constituents. The exuding *gum-resin* contains benzoic acid and olivile. Mannite is

[1] The last dose at night should be taken in cold water instead of hot, or it may induce sleeplessness. – EDITOR.

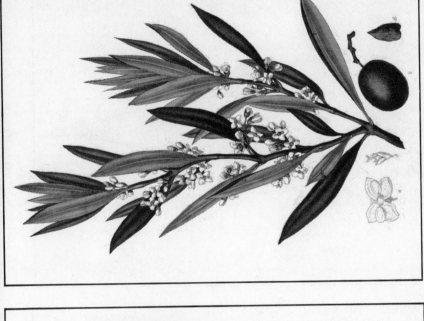

OLIVE
Olea Europaea

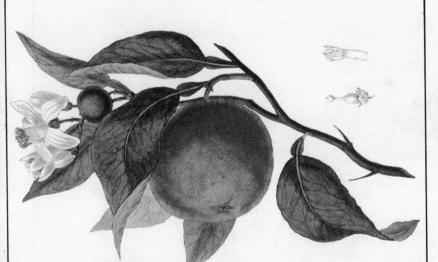

SWEET ORANGE
Citrus Aurantium

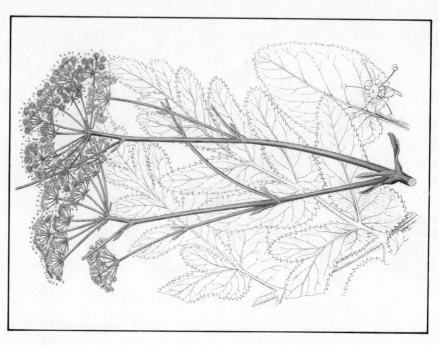

OPOPONAX
Opoponax Chi...

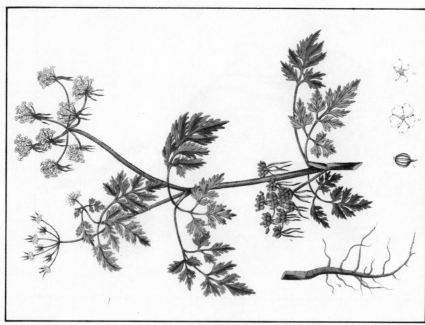

FOOLS' PARSLEY
Æthusa Cynapium

found in the green leaves and unripe fruit. The oil, *Oleum Olivæ*, non-drying, fixed, solidifies on treatment with nitrous acid or mercuric nitrate, is slightly soluble in alcohol, miscible with ether, chloroform or carbon disulphide. The specific gravity is 0·910 to 0·915 at 25° C. or 77° F. It is pale yellow or greenish-yellow, with a faint odour and bland taste, becoming slightly acrid. At a lower temperature than 10° C. or 50° F. it may become a soft, granular mass. Tripalmitin crystallizes and the remaining fluid is chiefly triolein. There are also arachidic esters and a little free oleic acid.

¶ *Medicinal Action and Uses.* The *leaves* are astringent and antiseptic. Internally, a decoction of 2 handsful boiled in a quart of water until reduced to half a pint has been used in the Levant in obstinate fevers. Both leaves and bark have valuable febrifugal qualities.

The *oil* is a nourishing demulcent and laxative. Externally, it relieves pruritis, the effects of stings or burns, and is a good

vehicle for liniments. With alcohol it is a good hair-tonic. As a lubricant it is valuable in skin, muscular, joint, kidney and chest complaints, or abdominal chill, typhoid and scarlet fevers, plague and dropsies. Delicate babies absorb its nourishing properties well through the skin. Its value in worms or gallstones is uncertain.

Internally, it is a laxative and disperser of acids, and a mechanical antidote to irritant poisons. It is often used in enemas. It is the best fat for cooking, and a valuable article of diet for both sick and healthy of all ages. It can easily be taken with milk, orange or lemon juice, etc.

¶ *Dosage.* As a laxative, 1 to 2 fluid ounces.

¶ *Adulterants.* Cotton-seed, rape, sesame, arachis and poppy-seed oils are the many adulterants found, and several official chemical tests are practised for their detection.

¶ *Other Species.* The flowers of *Olea fragrans* or Lanhoa give its odour to the famous Chulan or Schoulang tea of China.

ONION

Allium cepa (LINN.)
N.O. Liliaceæ

Part Used. Bulb

¶ *Medicinal Action and Uses.* Antiseptic, diuretic. A roasted Onion is a useful application to tumours or earache.

The juice made into a syrup is good for

colds and coughs. Hollands gin, in which Onions have been macerated, is given as a cure for gravel and dropsy.

ONION, POTATO

Allium cepa, var. aggregatum
N.O. Liliaceæ

Synonyms. The Underground Onion. Egyptian Onion
Part Used. Bulb

The Potato Onion, also known as the Underground Onion, from its habit of increasing its bulbs beneath the surface, is very prolific. It is a valuable vegetable because it furnishes sound, tender, full-sized bulbs at midsummer, three months before the ordinary Onion crop is harvested. The bulbs are rather large, of irregular shape, from 2 to over 3 inches in diameter and about 2 inches thick. The flesh of the bulb is agreeable to the taste and of good quality. The skin is thickish and of a coppery yellow colour.

In Lindley's *Treasury of Botany* this Potato Onion is called the 'Egyptian Onion,' and is stated to have been introduced from Egypt about the beginning of the nineteenth century. It is much cultivated in the West of England, being quite hardy, productive, and as mild in quality as the Spanish Onion.

This variety of Onion produces no seeds and is propagated by the lateral bulbs, which it throws out underground in considerable numbers. It requires a well-worked, moderately rich soil, and is largely grown in Devon-

shire, where in view of the mildness of the climate, the rule is to plant it in warm, sheltered situations in mid-winter, generally on the shortest day, with the hope of taking up the crop at mid-summer. In colder parts, however, the planting must be deferred until late winter, or early spring, yet the earlier it can be effected the better. The bulbs should be planted almost on the surface, in ground that has been previously well prepared and manured, and in rows 15 inches apart, with 6 to 10 inches space between the bulbs in the rows.

Each bulb will throw out a number of off-sets all round it, which grow and develop into full-sized bulbs, which are taken up and dried when ready for pulling, and then stored for use and for future propagation. If the plants attain full maturity each bulb will produce seven or eight bulbs of various sizes. The strongest of these will in their turn produce a number of bulbs, while the weaker ones generally grow into a single, large bulb. The largest bulbs do not always keep so well as the medium-sized ones.

ONION,[1] TREE

Allium cepa, var. proliferum

Synonym. L'oignon d'Egypte
Part Used. Bulb

The Tree Onion is a peculiar kind of Onion that produces at the top of a strong stem about 2 feet high, instead of seeds, a cluster of small bulblets, green at first, but becoming of a brownish-red colour, and about the size of hazel nuts, the stems bearing so heavily that they often require some support.

This singular variety of Onion was introduced into this country from Canada in 1820. The French call it 'l'oignon d'Egypte,' but there is no proof that it is a native of that country. It is quite probable that it is the common Onion introduced from France into Canada by the early colonists and changed by the climate. Besides the stem Onions, a few effects are also produced underground.

The Tree Onion is propagated from the little stem bulbs alone, which are set in February, 2 inches deep and 4 inches apart, in rows 8 inches asunder. When planted in spring, these small bulbs form large ones by the end of the year, but do not produce any bulblets until the following year. When the bulbs are matured, they can be preserved in a cool place after they have been allowed to dry in the sun for a brief period. They are flat and of a coppery colour, their flesh being considered tolerably agreeable to the taste, but rather deficient in flavour. The bulblets are excellent for pickling and keep very well, though the large bulbs do not always keep very long.

¶ *Other Species.* A variety of the Tree Onion, called the Catawissa Onion, or Perennial Tree Onion, was introduced from America thirty or forty years ago. It is distinguished from the Ordinary Tree Onion by the great vigour of its growth and the rapidity with which the bulblets commence to grow without being detached from the top of the stem. They have hardly attained their full size when they emit stems, which also produce bulblets, and in favourable seasons this second tier of bulblets will emit green shoots, leaves and barren stems, bringing the height of the plant up to over 2½ feet. Only a small number of bulblets, generally two or three on each stem, are thus proliferous. The rest do not sprout in the first year and can be used for propagation. The plant is perennial, with long fibrous roots, and may be propagated by division of the tufts, in the same manner as Chives. No offsets are produced underground. A small bed of these is growing at the Whins:[2] they are very hardy, having lived outdoors in open ground all through the severe weather experienced in the early part of 1917. Moles greatly dislike the smell of Onions, and if one is planted in each mole run as it shows up, the mole will leave the ground altogether.

OPOPONAX

Opoponax chironium
N.O. Umbelliferæ

Synonym. Pastinaca Opoponax
Part Used. Concrete juice from the base of stem
Habitat. Levant, Persia, South France, Italy, Greece, Turkey

¶ *Description.* A perennial, with a thick, fleshy root, yellowish in colour. It has a branching stem growing about 1 to 3 feet high, thick and rough near the base. Leaves pinnate, with long petioles and large serrate leaflets, the terminal one cordate, the rest deficient at the base, hairy underneath. The flowers, yellowish, are in large, flat umbels at the top of the branches. The oleo resin is procured by cutting into the stem at the base. The juice that exudes, when sun-dried, forms the Opoponax of commerce. A warm climate is necessary to produce an oleo gum resin of the first quality; that from France is inferior, for this reason. In commerce it is sometimes found in tears, but usually in small, irregular pieces. Colour, reddish-yellow, with whitish specks on the outside, paler inside. Odour, peculiar, strongly unpleasant. Taste, acrid and bitter. It is inflammable, burning brightly.

¶ *Constituents.* Gum-resin, starch, wax, gum, lignin, volatile oil, malic acid, a slight trace of caoutchouc.

¶ *Medicinal Action and Uses.* Antispasmodic, deobstruent. It is now regarded as a medium of feeble powers, but was formerly considered of service as an emmenagogue, also in asthma, chronic visceral affections, hysteria and hypochondriasis. It is employed in perfumery.

---

[1] Onions are a valuable disinfectant. Country people hang up a string of Onions as a protection against an infectious disease, and it has constantly been observed that the Onions will take the disease while the inmates remain immune. For this reason it is important to examine Onions before they are cooked, and to discard any which are imperfect. – EDITOR.

[2] The author's house at Chalfont St Peter. – EDITOR.

¶ *Dose.* 10 to 30 grains.

¶ *Other Species.* From some species of *Mulinum*, and *Bolax Gillesii* and *B. clebaria* (belonging to same order), a gum-resin similar to Opopanax is obtained, which is employed by the native Chilian practitioners.

ORANGE, BITTER

Citrus vulgaris (RISSO.)
var. Bigaradia

ORANGE, SWEET

Citrus Aurantium (LINN.)
var. dulcis
N.O. Rutaceæ

Synonyms. Citrus vulgaris. Citrus Bigaradia. Citrus aurantium amara. Bigaradier. Bigarade Orange. Bitter Orange. Seville Orange. (Sweet) Portugal Orange. China Orange. Citrus dulcis

Parts Used. Fruit, flowers, peel

Habitat. India, China. Cultivated in Spain, Madeira, etc.

¶ *Description.* Both common and official names are derived from the Sanskrit *nagaranga* through the Arabic *naranj*.

It is a small tree with a smooth, greyish-brown bark and branches that spread into a fairly regular hemisphere. The oval, alternate, evergreen leaves, 3 to 4 inches long, have sometimes a spine in the axil. They are glossy, dark green on the upper side, paler beneath. The calyx is cup-shaped and the thick, fleshy petals, five in number, are intensely white, and curl back.

The fruit is earth-shaped, a little rougher and darker than the common, sweet orange: the flowers are more strongly scented and the glands in the rind are concave instead of convex.

The first mention of oranges appears in the writings of Arabs, the time and manner of their first cultivation in Europe being uncertain.

The small, immature fruits are sometimes used under the name of *Orange berries* for flavouring Curaçoa. They are the size of a cherry and dark greyish-brown in colour. Formerly an essence was extracted from them.

The peel is used both fresh and dried. Much is imported from Malta, cut more thinly than that prepared in England.

In Grasse the blossoms are candied in large quantities.

Oil of petit grain is made from the leaves and young shoots.

The volatile oil of the bitter Orange peel is known as Oil of Bigarade, and Sweet Orange oil as Oil of Portugal. For methods of extraction, *see* LEMON.

Orange oil is one of the most difficult to preserve, the most satisfactory method being to add 10 per cent. of its volume of olive oil.

The flowers yield by distillation an essential oil known as 'Neroli,' which forms one of the chief constituents of Eau-de-Cologne. A pomade and an oil are also obtained from them by maceration.

The oil from Sweet Orange blossoms is found in commerce under the name of 'Neroli petalæ.' Being far less fragrant it only fetches half the price of neroli oil and on that account is frequently used to adulterate the true neroli oil.

The largest Bigarade-tree plantations are to be found in the South of France, in Calabria and in Sicily. The centre of the industry of neroli oil is the South of France, where the bitter Orange is extensively cultivated for that purpose alone. The tree requires a dry soil with a southern aspect. It bears flowers three years after grafting, increasing every year until it reaches its maximum, when it is about twenty years old. The quantity depends on the age and situation, a full-grown tree yielding on an average 50 to 60 lb. of blossoms. One hundred Orange trees, at the age of ten years, will occupy nearly an acre of land, and will produce during the season about 2,200 lb. of Orange flowers. The flowering season is in May and the flowers are gathered two or three times a week, after sunrise. When the autumn is mild and atmospheric conditions are favourable, flowering takes place in October, and this supplementary harvest lasts until January, or till a frosty morning stops the flowering. These autumn flowers have much less perfume than those of the spring and the custom is to value them at only one-half the price of May flowers. The Bitter Orange and Edible Orange trees bear a great resemblance to each other, but their leaf-stalks show a marked difference, that of the Bitter Orange being broadened out in the shape of a heart. The yield of oil is greatly influenced by the temperature and atmospheric conditions prevailing at the time of gathering. In warm weather it may amount to as much as 1,400 grams per 100 kilogrammes of flowers, but under adverse conditions, such as damp, cool and changeable weather, considerable diminution is experienced. Generally the largest yields are obtained at the end of the flowering season, on account of the warmer temperature.

The method most followed for extraction of the oil is by distillation, which yields a higher percentage of oil from the flowers than maceration or absorption in fats and volatile solvents. The flowers are distilled immediately after gathering, the essential oil rising to the surface of the distillate is drawn off, while the aqueous portion is sold as 'Orange Flower Water.' Orange flower water is being increasingly used in France by biscuit-makers to give crispness to their products, and some of the English biscuit-makers have also adopted it for this purpose.

There is a marked difference in the scent of the oils obtained by the different processes. Neroli obtained by distillation has quite a different odour from the fresh Orange flower; the oils obtained by solvents and by maceration and enfleurage are truest to the scent of the natural flower. From 100 kilogrammes of flowers 1,000 grams of oil are obtained; by volatile solvents, 600 grams; by maceration, 400 grams; and by enfleurage, only about 100 grams of oil.

Orange Flower Oil as obtained from pomatum, slightly modified with other extracts, can be employed to make 'Sweet Pea' and 'Magnolia' perfumes, the natural odours of which it slightly resembles.

The use of Orange-blossom as a bridal decoration is neither long-established nor indigenous, as it was introduced into this country from France only about a hundred years ago.

¶ *Constituents.* The peel of var. *Bigaradia* contains volatile oil, three glucosides, hesperidin, isohesperidin, an amorphous bitter principle, Aurantiamarin, aurantiamaric acid, resin, etc.

The ethyl ether of -naphthol, under the name of *nerolin,* is an artificial oil of neroli, said to be ten times as strong.

Oil of Orange Flowers is

'soluble in an equal volume of alcohol, the solution having a violet fluorescence and a neutral reaction to litmus paper. The specific

gravity is 0·868 to 0·880 at 25° C. (77° F.). When agitated with a concentrated solution of sodium bisulphate it assumes a permanent purple-red colour.'

It must not be coloured by sulphuretted hydrogen.

Oil of Sweet Orange Peel contains at least 90 per cent. δ-limonene, the remaining 10 per cent. being the odorous constituents, citral, citronellal, etc. It is a yellow liquid with the specific gravity 0·842 to 0·846 at 25° C. (77° F.).

Oil of Bitter Orange Peel, a pale yellow liquid, is soluble in four volumes of alcohol, the solution being neutral to litmus paper. The specific gravity is 0·842 to 0·848 at 25° C. (77° F.). The odour is more delicate than that of the Sweet Orange.

Fuming nitric acid gives a dark green colour to sweet peel and a brown to the bitter.

¶ *Medicinal Action and Uses.* The oil is used chiefly as a flavouring agent, but may be used in the same way as oil of turpentine in chronic bronchitis. It is non-irritant to the kidneys and pleasant to take.

On the Continent an infusion of dried flowers is used as a mild nervous stimulant.

The powdered Bitter Orange peel should be dried over freshly-burnt lime. For flavouring, the sweet peel is better, and as a tonic, that of the Seville or Bigaradia is preferred.

A syrup and an elixir are used for flavouring, and a wine as a vehicle for medicines.

The compound wine is too dangerous as an intoxicant, being mixed with absinthium, to be recommended as a tonic.

¶ *Preparations of Bitter Orange.* Syrup, B.P., ½ to 1 drachm. Tincture, B.P. and U.S.P., ½ to 1 drachm. Infusion of Orange, B.P., 4 to 8 drachms. Infusion of Orange Compound, B.P., 4 to 8 drachms. Compound spirit, U.S.P., 1 to 2 drachms. Syrup, B.P., ¼ to 1 drachm. Wine, B.P., a wineglassful.

¶ *Preparations of Sweet Orange.* Syrup, B.P. and U.S.P., ½ to 1 drachm. Tincture, U.S.P., ½ to 1 drachm.

ORCHIDS

N.O. Orchidaceæ
Orchis maculata
Orchis latifolia
Orchis mascula
Orchis Morio
Orchis militaris
Orchis saccifera
Orchis pyrimidalis
Orchis coriphora
Orchis conopea

Synonyms. Salep. Saloop. Sahlep. Satyrion. Levant Salep
Part Used. Root

Most of the Orchids native to this country have tuberous roots full of a highly nutritious starch-like substance, called Bassorin, of a

sweetish taste and with a faint, somewhat unpleasant smell, which replaces starch as a reserve material. In Turkey and Persia this has for many centuries been extracted from the tubers of various kinds of Orchis and exported under the name of *Sahlep* (an Arabian word, corrupted into English as Saloop or Salep), which has long been used, especially in the East, for making a wholesome and nutritious drink of the same name. Before coffee supplanted it, it used to be sold at stalls in the streets of London, and was held in great repute in herbal medicine, being largely employed as a strengthening and demulcent agent. The best English Salep came from Oxfordshire, but the tubers were chiefly imported from the East.

Charles Lamb refers to a 'Salopian shop' in Fleet Street, and says that to many tastes it has 'a delicacy beyond the China luxury,' and adds that a basin of it at three-halfpence, accompanied by a slice of bread-and-butter at a halfpenny, is an ideal breakfast for a chimney-sweep. Though Salep is no longer a popular London beverage, before the war it was regularly sold by street merchants in Constantinople as a hot drink during the winter.

Salep is collected in central and southern Europe and Asia. Most, if not all, of the species of *Orchis* and some allied plants found in Europe and Northern Asia, are provided with tubers which when duly prepared are capable of furnishing Salep. The varieties represent two forms, the one with branched, the other, and preferable one, with rounded and unbranched tubers. The tubers occur in pairs, one a little larger than the other.

Of those species actually used the following are the more important: *Orchis mascula* (Linn.), *O. Morio* (Linn.), *O. militaris* (Linn.), *O. ustulata* (Linn.), *O. pyramidalis* (Linn.), *O. coriophora* (Linn.), *O. longieruris* (Link.). These species, which have the tubers *entire*, are natives of the greater part of Central and Southern Europe, Turkey, the Caucasus and Asia Minor. The following species, with *palmate* or lobed tubers, are equally widely distributed: *O. maculata* (Linn.), *O. saccifera* (Brong.), *O. conopea* (Linn.), and *O. latifolia* (Linn.).

In the East, Salep is mostly obtained from *O. morio*, which is of frequent occurrence in this country in chalky soils, but it can be made here equally well from *O. mascula*, the Early Purple Orchis, *O. maculata* and *O. latifolia*, which are more common and very widely distributed throughout the country.

O. mascula (Linn.), the Early Purple Orchis, common in English woods, is in flower from mid-April to mid-June. A single flower-stem rises from the tuberous root, bearing flowers that as a rule are of a rich purple colour, mottled with lighter and darker shades, though often found of every tint from purple to pure white. Each flower has a long spur which turns upwards. The leaves are lance-shaped and do not rise far from the ground, giving a rosette-like effect, and are irregularly blotched with dark purple markings, which help to render the plant conspicuous. In woods and meadowland, the plant often attains a height of a foot or more, while on exposed and breezy downs it is seldom more than 6 inches high.

The blossoms are practically odourless in some specimens, whilst those of others are faintly fragrant, but in most cases the smell is not only strong, but offensive, especially in the evening. There is no honey in the flowers, but a sweet juice in the walls of the spur, which insects pierce with their probosces and suck out. The plant is provided with two fleshy, egg-shaped tubers, one serving to provide the necessities of the plant, shrinking as the plant reaches maturity, the other receiving the leaves' surplus supplies of foodstuffs to store for use in the following season.

Witches were supposed to use the tubers in their philtres, the fresh tuber being given to promote true love, and the withered one to check wrong passions. Culpepper speaks of them as 'under the dominion of Venus,' and tells us among other things, that 'being bruised and applied to the place' they heal the King's Evil.

This Early Purple Orchis in Northants is called 'Cuckoos,' because it comes into flower about the time when the cuckoo first calls. In Dorset it has the name of 'Granfer Griggles,' and the wild Hyacinth, which often flowers by its side, bears the name of 'Granny Griggles.'

O. Morio (Linn.), the Green-winged Meadow Orchis, is in flower about the same time as the Early Purple Orchis and resembles it in habit. It grows in meadows and is often very abundant. It is, however, a shorter plant, bearing fewer flowers in the spike, and is best distinguished by its two lateral sepals, which are bent upwards to form a kind of hood, being strongly marked with parallel green veins.

O. maculata (Linn.), the Spotted Orchis, receives its name from the blotches of reddish-brown, which mark the upper surfaces of the leaves similarly to those of *O. mascula*. The flowers, massed in spikes, about 3 inches long, on a stem about a foot high, with the leaves springing from it at distant intervals, vary in hue from pale lilac to rich purple, are curiously marked with dark lines and spots, and are very similar in structure to those of the Early Purple Orchis. It grows abundantly on heaths and commons, flowering in June and July.

In this species, the tubers are divided into two or three finger-like lobes, hence the plant has been known as 'Dead Men's Fingers' (*Hamlet*, IV, vii), Hand Orchis, or Palma Christi. Gerard calls it the 'Female Satyrion,' orchids being known in his time as Satyrions, from a legend that they were specially connected with the Satyrs. The plants were believed to be the food of the Satyrs, and to have incited them to excesses. Orchis, in the old mythology, was the son of a Satyr and a nymph, who, when killed by the Bacchanalians for his insult to a priestess of Bacchus, was turned, on the prayer of his father, into the flower that bears his name.

O. latifolia (Linn.), the March Orchis, is a taller plant than the last, but has also palmate roots. The broad leaves are very erect, the flowers rose-coloured or purple, the finely-tapering bracts being longer than the flowers. This species, in common with the three preceding ones, sometimes bears white flowers. It is very frequent in marshes and damp pastures, and will be found in bloom in June and July.

The Salep of commerce is prepared chiefly in the Levant, being largely collected in Asia Minor, but to some extent also in Germany and other parts of Europe. The European Salep is always smaller than the Oriental Salep. The drug found in English trade is mostly imported from Smyrna. That sold in Germany is partly obtained from plants growing wild in the Taunus Mountains, the Odenwald and other districts. Salep is also collected in Greece and used in that country and in Turkey in the form of a decoction, which is sweetened with honey and taken as an early morning drink. The Salep of India is mostly produced on the hills of Afghanistan, Beluchistan, Kabul and Bokhara, and also from the Nilgiri Hills and Ceylon.

The drug was known to Dioscorides and the Arabians, as well as to the herbalists and physicians of the Middle Ages, by whom it was mostly prescribed in the fresh state. Gerard (1636 edition) gives excellent figures of the various orchids, whose tubers, he says, 'our age useth.' Geoffrey (1740), having recognized the salep imported from the Levant to be the tubers of an Orchis, pointed out how it might be prepared from the species indigenous to France.

Levant Salep, as occurring in commerce, consists of tubers ½ inch to 1 inch in length, oblong in form, often pointed at the lower end and rounded at the upper, where is a depressed scar left by the stem; palmate tubers are infrequent. They are generally shrunken and contorted, covered with a roughly granular skin, pale brown, translucent, very hard and horny, practically inodorous and with an insipid, mucilaginous taste. After maceration in water for several hours the tubers regain their original form and size.

The branched or palmate Salep tubers (*Radix palmæ Christi*) are somewhat flattened and palmately two to five branched. The elongated mucilage cells are not so large as in the other form.

German Salep is more translucent and gummy-looking than that of the Levant, and more carefully prepared.

The Oriental Royal Salep, said to be much used as a food in Afghanistan, has been identified as the product of a bulbous plant related to the onion, *Allium Macleanii* (*Pharm. Journal*, Sept., 1889).

The Salep of the Indian bazaars, known as *Salib misri*, for fine qualities of which great prices are paid, is derived from certain species of *Eulophia*.

¶ *Collection and Preparation*. Tubers required for making Salep are taken up at the close of the summer, when the seed-vessels are fully formed, as the next year's tubers then contain the largest amount of starchy matter and are full and fleshy.

The shrivelled ones having been thrown aside, those which are plump are washed and then immersed for a short time in boiling water, this scalding process destroying their vitality and removing the bitterness of their fresh state and making them dry more readily. The outer skins are then rubbed off and the tubers are dried, either by exposure to the sun, or to a gentle artificial heat in an oven for ten minutes and heated to about bread-making temperature. On removing from the oven, their milky appearance will have changed to an almost transparent and horny state, though the bulk will not be reduced. They are then placed in the fresh air to dry and harden for a few days, when they are ready for use, or to be stored for as long as desired, as damp does not affect them. The dried tubers are generally ground to powder before using; it has a yellowish colour.

¶ *Constituents and Uses*. The constituents of Salep are subject to great variation, according to the season of collection. Raspail found the old tuber, collected in autumn, to be free from starch, while the young one was richly supplied with it.

The most important constituent is mucilage, amounting to 48 per cent. It also contains sugar (1 per cent.), starch (2·7 per cent.), nitrogenous substance (5 per cent.), and when fresh a trace of volatile oil. It yields

2 per cent. of ash, consisting chiefly of phosphates and chlorides of potassium and calcium.

Salep is very nutritive and demulcent, for which properties it has been used from time immemorial. It forms a diet of especial value to convalescents and children, being boiled with milk or water, flavoured and prepared in the same way as arrowroot. A decoction flavoured with sugar and spice, or wine, is an agreeable drink for invalids. Sassafras chips were sometimes added, or cloves, cinnamon and ginger.

From the large quantity of farinaceous matter contained in a small bulk, it was considered so important an article of diet as to constitute a part of the stores of every ship's company in the days of sailing ships and long voyages, an ounce, dissolved in 2 quarts of boiling water, being considered sufficient subsistence for each man per day, should provisions run short. In this form it is employed in some parts of Europe and Asia as an article of diet. It is to the mucilage contained in the tuber that Salep owes its power of forming jelly, only 1 part of Salep to 50 parts of boiling water being needed for the purpose.

To allay irritation of the gastro-intestinal canal, it is used in mucilage made by shaking 1 part of powdered Salep with 10 parts of cold water, until it is uniformly diffused, when 90 parts of boiling water are added and the whole well agitated. It has thus been recommended as an article of diet for infants and invalids suffering from chronic diarrhœa and bilious fevers. In the German Pharmacopœia, a mucilage of Salep appears as an official preparation.

OSIER, RED AMERICAN

Cornus sericea (LINN.)
N.O. Cornaceæ

Synonyms. Swamp's Dogwood. Red Willow. Silky Cornel. Female Dogwood. Blueberry. Kinnikinnik. Rose Willow.
(*French*) Cornouille
Parts Used. Root-bark and bark
Habitat. North America, Florida to Mississippi

¶ *Description.* A water-loving shrub, growing from 6 to 12 feet high. Branches spreading, dark purplish; branchlets silky downy; leaves narrowly ovate or elliptical, pointed, smooth above, silky downy below and often hairy upon ribs on petioles from half an inch to an inch long. Flowers yellowish white, small, disposed in large terminal, depressed and woolly cymes or corymbs. Berries globose, bright blue, stone compressed. It is found in moist woods and on the margins of rivers, flowering in June and July.
¶ *Constituents.* The active properties are similar to those found in Peruvian Bark, except that there is more gum mucilage and extractive matter and less resin quinine and tannin.
¶ *Medicinal Action and Uses.* It is tonic astringent and slightly stimulant, used in periodical and typhoid fever. Taken internally it increases the strength and frequency of the pulse, elevating the temperature of the body. It should be used in the dried state, the fresh bark being likely to upset the stomach.

The powdered bark has been used as tooth-powder, to preserve the gums and make the teeth white; the flowers have been used in place of chamomile.

OSIER, GREEN

Cornus circinata
N.O. Cornaceæ

Part Used. Fresh bark

A homœopathic tincture of the fresh bark is administered in ulcerated conditions of the mucous membranes and in liver complaints and jaundice.

OX-EYE DAISY. *See* DAISY

OX-TONGUE

Helminthia echioides

Part Used. Herb

Closely allied to the Sow Thistles and somewhat resembling them in general appearance is the Bristly Ox Tongue (*Helminthia echioides*), frequently met with in England on hedgebanks and on waste ground, especially on clay soil, but less common in Ireland and rare in Scotland.

¶ *Description.* It is somewhat stout and coarse, the sturdy stems attaining a height of from 2 to 3 feet, branching freely and covered with short, stiff hairs, each of which springs from a raised spot and is hooked at the end.

The lower leaves are much longer than the

upper, of lanceolate or spear-head form, with their margins coarsely and irregularly toothed and waved. The upper leaves are small and stalkless, heart-shaped and clasping the stem with their bases. All the leaves are of a grey-ish-green hue and very tough to the touch.

The flower-heads are ordinarily somewhat clustered together on short stalks and form an irregular, terminal mass at the ends of the main stems. The involucre, or ring of bracts from which the florets spring, is doubled – outside the ring of eight to ten narrow and nearly erect scales, simple in form and thin in texture, is an outer ring composed of a smaller number of spiny bracts of a broad heart-shape, in their roughness of surface and general character resembling the leaves of the plant. The combination of the inner and outer bracts may be roughly compared to a cup and saucer, and gives the plant a singular appearance.

The Ox Tongue is in blossom during June and July; all the florets of the flower-heads, as in the Dandelion, are of a rich golden yellow.

The generic name, *Helminthia*, is Greek in origin and signifies a small kind of worm. It is suggested that the name was bestowed

PÆONY

Synonym. Pæonia Corallina
Part Used. Root

The Pæony is not indigenous to Great Britain, and only grows wild on an island called the Steep Holmes, in the Severn, where it was probably introduced some centuries ago.

The varieties Female and Male Pæony have no reference to the sexes of the flowers. The roots of the Female or Common Pæony are composed of several roundish, thick knobs or tubers, which hang below each other, connected by strings. The stems are green (red when quite young) and about 2½ feet high. The leaves are composed of several unequal lobes, which are cut into many segments; they are of a paler green colour than those of the so-called Male Pæony, and the flowers are of a deeper purple colour. From this variety are derived the double garden Pæonies.

Many of the species have very fragrant flowers.

The roots of the Male Pæony – the kind found wild on the island in the Severn – are composed of several oblong knobs, hanging by strings fastened to the main head. The stems are the same height as in the preceding, and bear large single flowers, composed of five or six large roundish red (or sometimes white) petals. The flowers of both sorts

from the form of the fruit, but it seems more likely that the name may have been applied to the plant from some former belief in its power as a vermifuge. It has by some botanists been assigned to the genus *Picris*. The specific name, *echioides*, refers to the rough, prickly character of the stems and leaves.

In spite of its spiny character, the Ox Tongue was used as a pot-herb in the same manner as the Sow Thistles, but can only be eaten when young, when it is said to have a pleasant taste. The juice is milky, bitter, but not extremely acrid.

¶ *Other Species.*

The HAWKWEED OX-TONGUE (*Picris hieracioides*), a closely allied plant, has been similarly employed as a pot-herb. It is a rather slender plant, 2 to 3 feet high, the stems rough with hooked bristles, the stalkless leaves narrow, rough and toothed; flowers numerous and yellow. It is abundant on the edges of fields, especially in a gravelly or calcareous soil, and flowers from July to September. The name of the genus is derived from the Greek *picros* (bitter), from the bitter taste of the plant.

See (SOW) THISTLE.

Pæonia officinalis (LINN.)
N.O. Ranunculaceæ

open in May, the seeds ripening in the autumn.

The last-named variety is the kind formerly much cultivated for the roots, which were celebrated for their medicinal value in disorders of the head and nerves. It has been known also as *Pæonia Corallina*.

The genus is supposed to have been named after the physician Pæos, who cured Pluto and other gods of wounds received during the Trojan War with the aid of this plant.

The superstitions connected with the Pæony are numerous. In ancient times, it was thought to be of divine origin, an emanation from the moon, and to shine during the night, protecting shepherds and their flocks, and also the harvest from injury, driving away evil spirits and averting tempests. Josephus speaks of the Pæony as a wonderful and curious plant. He says – according to Gerard – that 'to pluck it up by the roots will cause danger to he that touches it, therefore a string must be fastened to it in the night and a hungry dog tied thereto, who being allured by the smell of roasted flesh set towards him may pluck it up by the roots.' Pliny and Theophrastus assert

'that of necessity it must be gathered in the

night, for if any man shall pluck of the fruit in the daytime, being seen of the woodpecker, he is in danger to lose his eyes.'

Gerard adds:

'But all these things be most vaine and frivolous, for the root of Peionne may be removed at any time of the yeare, day, or houre whatsoever.'

The seeds used to be strung as a necklace and worn as a charm against evil spirits.
Gerard says:

'The black graines (that is the seed) to the number of fifteene taken in wine or mead is a speciall remedie for those that are troubled in the night with the disease called the Nightmare, which is as though a heavy burthen were laid upon them and they oppressed therewith, as if they were overcome with their enemies, or overprest with some great weight or burthen; and they are also good against melancholie dreames.'

A drink called 'Pæony-water' made from the plant was once much used, and the kernels or seeds were used in cookery as a spice.
'Stick the cream with Pæony kernels,' *Mrs. Glasse's Cookery* (1796).

¶ *Cultivation.* Pæonies are extremely hardy and will grow in almost any soil or situation, in sun or shade. The best soil, however, is a deep, rich loam, which should be well trenched and manured, previous to planting. Propagation is by division of roots, which increase very quickly. The best season for transplanting is towards the end of August, or the beginning of September. In dividing the roots, care must be taken to preserve a bud upon the crown of each offset.

Single varieties are generally propagated from seeds, sown in autumn, soon after they are ripe, upon a bed of light soil, covering them with ½ inch of soil. Water well in dry weather and keep clear from weeds. Leave the young plants in this bed two years, transplanting in September.

¶ *Part Used.* The root, dried and powdered. It is dug in the autumn, from plants at least two years old. The roots should be cleansed carefully in cold water with a brush and only be allowed to remain in the water as short a time as possible. Then spread out on trays in the sun, or on the floor, or on shelves in a kitchen, or other warm room for ten days or more. When somewhat shrunken, roots may be finished off more quickly in greater heat over a stove or gas fire, or in an open oven, when the fire has just gone out. Dried roots must always be dry to the core and brittle.

Pæony root occurs in commerce in pieces averaging 3 inches long and ½ to ¾ inch in diameter, spindle-shaped, strongly furrowed and shrunken longitudinally, of a pinkish grey or dirty white colour, generally having been scraped. The transverse section is starchy and radiate, the rays more or less tinged with purple. The root has no odour, but its taste is sweet at first, and then bitter.

¶ *Medicinal Action and Uses.* Antispasmodic, tonic. Pæony root has been successfully employed in convulsions and spasmodic nervous affections, such as epilepsy, etc.

It was formerly considered very efficacious for lunacy. An old writer tells us: 'If a man layeth this wort over the lunatic as he lies, soon he upheaveth himself whole.'

The infusion of 1 oz. of powdered root in a pint of boiling water is taken in wineglassful doses, three or four times daily.

An infusion of the powdered root has been recommended for obstructions of the liver, and for complaints arising from such obstructions.

¶ *Other Species.*
Pæonia Albiflora, distinguished by its smooth recurved follicles, is a native of Siberia, and the whole of Northern Asia; the roots of this are sometimes boiled by the natives, and eaten in broth; they also grind the seeds and put them into their tea.

PAPAW

Carica Papaya (LINN.)
N.O. Cucurbitaceæ

Synonyms. Melon Tree. Mamæire. Papaya Vulgaris (D.C.)
Parts Used. Fruit juice, seeds, leaves – pawpain
Habitat. South America, West Indies, and cultivated in most tropical countries

¶ *Description.* A small tree seldom above 20 feet high, 1 foot in diameter, tapering to about 4 or 5 inches at its summit. It has a spongy soft wood, hollow in centre; leaves are as large as 2 feet in diameter, deeply cut into seven lobes, ending in sharp points and margins irregularly waived; foot-stalks 2 feet long, diverge horizontally from the stem;

fruit oblong, dingy green yellow colour, about 10 inches long, 3 or 4 broad with projecting angles, a rind like a gourd, thick and fleshy; the central cavity contains a quantity of black wrinkled seeds.

¶ *Constituents.* The seeds of the Papaw tree contain a glucoside, Caricin, which resembles Sinigrin, also the ferment Myrosin, and by reaction of the two a volatile, pungent body suggestive of mustard oil. From the leaves an alkaloid called carpaine has been obtained; physiologically this alkaloid has the same effect on the heart as digitalis. Papain is often adulterated with starch; in cases of acidity it is said to be much superior to pancreatin because its action is not affected to any extent by its contact with the acid. This plant must not be confounded with the custard apple, which is often called Papaw and botanically known as *Uvaria triloba*.

¶ *Medicinal Action and Uses.* The juice of the tree or an infusion of the leaves and fruit makes the toughest meat tender when rubbed with it or cooked in the leaves; if chickens and pigs are fed on the leaves it will make their flesh tender. The ripe fruit is refreshing and palatable; it is sometimes used as a sauce; the seeds cannot be detected from capers; it is sometimes preserved in sugar or boiled like turnips. The juice is used to remove freckles; it is also a strong vermifuge. The leaves are used as a substitute for soap; when the unripe fruit is pierced with a bone knife a milky juice exudes which is collected in a basin and allowed to coagulate; this is dried in the sun and contains a propeolytic enzyme which acts as a neutral or alkaline solution, and is given for impaired digestion. Pawpain is the dried white powdered unripe juice of Papaw, a ferment, and strongly suggests pepsin in odour, taste and appearance. It is said to dissolve the fibrinous membrane in croup and diphtheria, a solution over the pharynx painted every five minutes; when injected into the circulation in large doses it paralyses the heart; it is recommended to destroy warts and epithelioma, tubercules, etc.; is not caustic or astringent, but has the virtue of dissolving muscular and connective tissue.

The fresh leaves have been used as a dressing for foul wounds; internally the juice is useful in dyspepsia and catarrh of the stomach; the juice has a tendency to deteriorate by undergoing butyric fermentation, but this can be overcome by the addition of glycerine, which preserves it without impairing its digestive power.

See PAPAW SEEDS.

PAPAW SEEDS

Asimina triloba
N.O. Anonaceæ

Synonyms. Custard Apple. Uvaria triloba
Parts Used. Seeds, bark, and leaves
Habitat. Middle, Southern and Western States, also India, Africa, Asia

¶ *Description.* A small beautiful tree, growing up to 20 feet. The young shoots and leaves are at first clothed in a rusty down which soon becomes glabrous. The leaves are thin, smooth, entire, ovate, oblong, acuminate, 8 to 12 inches long by 3 broad, and tapering to very short petioles. Flowers dull purple, axillary, solitary; petals veiny, round, ovate, outer one orbicular, three or four times as large as the calyx. Flowers appear same time as leaves, March to June, and are about 1½ inches wide. Fruit, yellowish, ovoid oblong, pulpy pod about 3 inches long and 1 inch diameter, fragrant, sweet, ripe in autumn and contains about eight seeds; before fruit is ripe it has an unpleasant smell and when ripe after frost it is luscious and similar to custard; it is considered healthy to eat, being sedative and laxative; the seeds are the part used; these have a foetid smell like straminium; they are covered with an exterior coat which is tough and hard, light brown colour and smooth externally, wrinkled and lighter inside. It encloses a white kernel, deeply fissured on both sides and compressed, almost scentless, slightly bitter and sweet and dry and powdery when chewed; it leaves a faint, persistent, unpleasant sensation of sickness; seeds vary in shape, being flat ovoid, sometimes circular and somewhat reniform, with a depression along the centre of each flat surface, and frequently a ridge in place of the furrow.

¶ *Constituents.* Fixed oil, a resin, a resin insoluble in ether, glucose and extractive.

¶ *Medicinal Action and Uses.* Emetic, for which a saturated tincture of the bruised seeds is employed; dose, 10 to 60 drops. The bark is a bitter tonic and is said to contain a powerful acid, the leaves are used as an application to boils and ulcers.

¶ *Other Species.*

Uvaria Natrum. Root aromatic and fragrant, used in India in intermittent fevers and liver complaints. Bruised in salt water is used as an application to certain skin diseases. A fragrant greenish oil is distilled from it.

U. tripelaloidea. When incised, gives a fragrant gum.

U. febrifuga, so called by the Indians of Orinoco, who use its flowers for fevers.

U. longifolia. A perfume oil is extracted from the flowers in Bourbon and several other species are also fragrant.

U. Zeylandica and *U. cordata* have edible fruits.

PARADISE GRAINS. *See* PEPPER, HUNGARIAN

PARAGUAY TEA

Ilex Paraguayensis (A. ST. HIL).
N.O. Aquifoliaceæ

Synonyms. Paraguay Herb. Paraguay. Maté. Ilex Maté. Yerba Maté. Houx Maté. Jesuit's Tea. Brazil Tea. Gón gouha
Part Used. Leaves
Habitat. Brazil, Argentina, Paraguay

¶ *Description.* This large, white-flowered shrub grows wild near streams, but is largely cultivated in South America for the drink obtained by infusing the leaves. The leaves are alternate, large, oval or lanceolate and broadly toothed. The fruit is a red drupe the size of pepper grains. Its name of Yerba signifies the herb *par excellence,* and the consumption in South America is vast, as it is drunk at every meal and hour. 'Maté' is derived from the name of the vessel in which it is infused in the manner of tea, burnt sugar or lemon-juice being added. It is sucked through a tube, usually of silver, with a bulb strainer at the end, and the cup is passed round.

If the powder is dropped into water and stirred the mixture is called *cha maté.*

Large sums are paid to the Government for permission to gather the leaves, which are dried by heat and powdered. The season is from December to August. Paraguay exports 5 to 6 million pounds annually.

The tea is very sustaining, and sometimes it is the only refreshment carried for a journey of several days.

The odour is not very agreeable, but is soon unnoticed. The taste is rather bitter.

¶ *Constituents.* Fresh leaves dried at Cambridge were found to contain caffeine, tannin, ash and insoluble matter.

¶ *Medicinal Action and Uses.* Tonic, diuretic, diaphoretic, and powerfully stimulant. In large doses it causes purging and even vomiting. Fluid extract, $\frac{1}{2}$ to 1 drachm.

¶ *Other Species.*
In South America the infusion of leaves of different species are used, such as *Cassina paragua, Psoralea glandulosa* and a *Luxemburgia.*

Ilex vomitoria and *I. Dahoon,* Apalachin or Cassena and Dahoon holly, have emetic properties. A decoction is used by the North Carolina Indians as Yaupon, or ceremonial black drink, as well as in medicine.

PAREIRA

Chondrodendron tomentosum (RUIZ and P.)
N.O. Menispermaceæ

Synonyms. Pereira Brava. Cissampelos Pareira. Velvet Leaf. Ice Vine
Parts Used. Dried root, bark, bruised leaves
Habitat. West Indies, Spanish Main Brazil, Peru

¶ *Description.* A woody vine, climbing a considerable height over trees; very large leaves, often 1 foot long with a silky pubescence, on the inner side grey colour; flowers diœcious in racemes; in the female plant the racemes are longer than the leaves, bearing the flowers in spike fascicles; the berries, first scarlet, then black, are oval, size of large grapes in commerce. The root is cylindrical in varying lengths from $\frac{1}{2}$ inch to 5 inches in diameter and from 2 or 3 inches to several feet long; externally blackish brown, longitudinally furrowed, transversed knotty ridges; it is hard, heavy, tough, and when freshly cut has a waxy lustre; interior woody, reddy yellow; transversed section shows several successive eccentric and distinctly radiate concentric zones of projecting secondary bundles fibro-vascular. Stem deeply furrowed; colour grey and covered with patches of lichen; odour, slight, aromatic, sweetish flavour, succeeded by an intense nauseating bitterness, yielding its bitterness and active properties to water or alcohol.

¶ *Constituents.* A soft resin, yellow bitter principle, brown colouring, a nitrogenous substance, fecula, acid calcium malate, various salts and potassium nitrate.

¶ *Medicinal Action and Uses.* Tonic, diuretic, aperient; acts as an antiseptic to the bladder, chiefly employed for the relief of chronic inflammation of the urinary passages, also recommended for calculus affections, leucorrhœa, rheumatism, jaundice, dropsy, and gonorrhœa. In Brazil it is used for poisonous snake bites; a vinous infusion of the root is taken internally, while the bruised leaves of the plant are applied externally.

¶ *Dosages.* Infusion, 1 to 4 fluid ounces. Solid extract, 10 to 20 grains. Fluid extract, $\frac{1}{4}$ to 2 drachms.

¶ *Other Species.*
Cissampelos Glaberrima, growing in Brazil, appears to possess similar properties, Beberine chondrodine, some stearic acid, tannin and starch.

C. convolulaceum, called by the Peruvians the Wild Grape with reference to the form of the fruit and their acid and not unpleasant flavour; the bark is used as a febrifuge.

Arbuta rufescens, or White Pareira Brava, has a thick woody root which exhibits concentric layers, transversed by very distinct dark medullary rays, interradial spaces being white and rich in starch.

PARILLA, YELLOW

Menispermum Canadense (LINN.)
N.O. Menispermaceæ

Synonyms. Canadian Moonseed. Texas Sarsaparilla. Moonseed Sarsaparilla. Vine Maple

Parts Used. The rhizome and roots

Habitat. Canada and United States of America. Cultivated in Britain as a hardy, deciduous, ornamental shrub. A closely allied species is indigenous to the temperate parts of Eastern Asia

¶ *Description.* A climbing, woody plant, with a very long root of a fine yellow colour, and a round, striate stem, bright yellow-green when young; leaves, roundish, cordate, peltate, three to seven angled, lobed. Flowers small, yellow, borne in profusion in axillary clusters. Drupes, round, black, with a bloom on them, one-seeded. Seed, crescent-shaped, compressed, the name Moonseed being derived from this lunate shape of the seed. The rhizome is wrinkled longitudinally and has a number of thin, brittle roots; fracture, tough, woody; internally reddish; a thick bark encloses a circle of porous, short, nearly square wood wedges and a large central pith. The root is the official part; it has a persistent bitter, acrid taste and is almost inodorous.

¶ *Constituents.* Berberine and a white amorphous alkaloid termed Menispermum, which has been used as a substitute for Sarsaparilla, some starch and resin.

¶ *Medicinal Action and Uses.* In small doses it is a tonic, diuretic, laxative and alterative. In larger doses it increases the appetite and action of the bowels; in *full* doses, it purges and causes vomiting. It is a superior

The COMMON FALSE PAREIRA, botanical origin unknown. The arrangement of the woody zones is eccentric and the wavy appearance of true Pareira is absent. It contains no starch, and the root is much lighter and less waxy than the genuine variety.

laxative bitter; considered very useful in scrofula, cutaneous, rheumatic, syphilitic, mercurial and arthritic diseases; also for dyspepsia, chronic inflammation of the viscera and in general debility. Externally, the decoction has been applied as an embrocation in cutaneous and gouty affections.

¶ *Preparations and Dosages.* Powdered root, $\frac{1}{2}$ to 1 drachm. Fluid extract, $\frac{1}{2}$ to 1 drachm. Saturated tincture, $\frac{1}{2}$ to 1 drachm. Menispermum, 1 to 4 grains. Decoction, 1 to 4 fluid ounces, three times daily. Menisperine in powder is recommended as a nervine and is considered superior to Sarsaparilla, taken in doses of 1 to 3 grains, three times daily.

¶ *Other Species.*
Some of the species closely allied to *Menispermum* have narcotic properties and are very poisonous: *Anamirta paniculata* yields *Cocculus Indicus,* illegally used to impart bitterness to malt liquor; *Jateorhiza palmata* supplies bitter Columba root, used as a tonic; and *Cissampelos Pareira* is the tonic Pareira Brava.

See COLUMBA, COCCULUS, PAREIRA.

(*POISON*)
PARIS, HERB

Paris quadrifolia (LINN.)
N.O. Trilliaceæ

Synonyms. Herba Paris. Solanum quadrifolium. Aconitum pardalianches. True Love. One Berry

(*French*) Parisette

(*German*) Einbeere

Part Used. The entire plant, just coming into bloom

Habitat. Europe, Russian Asia, and fairly abundant in Britain, but confined to certain places

¶ *Description.* This singular plant gets its generic name of *Paris* from *par* (paris), equal on account of the regularity of its leaves. In olden times it was much esteemed and used in medicine, but to-day its use is almost confined to homœopathy. It is a

herbaceous perennial plant found in moist places and damp shady woods. It has a creeping fleshy rootstock, a simple smooth upright stem about 1 foot high, crowned near its top with four pointed leaves, from the centre of which rises a solitary greeny-white flower, blooming May and June with a fœtid odour; the petals and sepals remain till the purply-blackberry (fruit) is ripe, which eventually splits to discharge its seeds.

¶ *Constituents.* A glucoside called Paradin.

¶ *Medicinal Action and Uses.* Narcotic, in large doses producing nausea, vomiting, vertigo, delirium convulsions, profuse sweating and dry throat. The drug should be used with great caution; overdoses have proved fatal to children and poultry. In *small doses* it has been found of benefit in bronchitis; spasmodic coughs, rheumatism; relieves cramp, colic, and palpitation of the heart; the juice of the berries cures inflammation of the eyes. A cooling ointment is made from the seeds and the juice of the leaves for green wounds and for outward application for tumours and inflammations. The powdered root boiled in wine is given for colic. One or 2 scruples acts as an emetic in place of Ipecacuanha.

It has been used as an aphrodisiac – the seeds and berries have something of the nature of opium. The leaves in Russia are prescribed for madness. The leaves and berries are more actively poisonous than the root.

Herb Paris is useful as an *antidote* against mercurial sublimate and arsenic. A tincture is prepared from the fresh plant.

¶ *Other Species. Paris polyphylla*, which grows in Nepaul.

PARSLEY

Carum petroselinum (BENTH.)
N.O. Umbelliferæ

Synonyms. Apium petroselinum (Linn.). Petroselinum lativum (Hoffm.). Petersylinge. Persely. Persele

Parts Used. Root, seeds

Habitat. The Garden Parsley is not indigenous to Britain: Linnæus stated its wild habitat to be Sardinia, whence it was brought to England and apparently first cultivated here in 1548. Bentham considered it a native of the Eastern Mediterranean regions; De Candolle of Turkey, Algeria and the Lebanon. Since its introduction into these islands in the sixteenth century it has been completely naturalized in various parts of England and Scotland, on old walls and rocks

Petroselinum, the specific name of the Parsley, from which our English name is derived, is of classic origin, and is said to have been assigned to it by Dioscorides. The Ancients distinguished between two plants *Selinon*, one being the Celery (*Apium graveolens*) and called *heleioselinon* – i.e. 'Marsh *selinon*,' and the other – our parsley – *Oreoselinon*, 'Mountain selinon'; or *petroselinum*, signifying 'Rock selinon.' This last name in the Middle Ages became corrupted into *Petrocilium* – this was anglicized into Petersylinge, Persele, Persely and finally Parsley.

There is an old superstition against transplanting parsley plants. The herb is said to have been dedicated to Persephone and to funeral rites by the Greeks. It was afterwards consecrated to St. Peter in his character of successor to Charon.

In the sixteenth century, Parsley was known as *A. hortense*, but herbalists retained the official name *petroselinum*. Linnæus in 1764 named it *A. petroselinum*, but it is now assigned to the genus *Carum*.

The Greeks held Parsley in high esteem, crowning the victors with chaplets of Parsley at the Isthmian games, and making with it wreaths for adorning the tombs of their dead. The herb was never brought to table of old, being held sacred to oblivion and to the dead.

It was reputed to have sprung from the blood of a Greek hero, Archemorus, the forerunner of death, and Homer relates that chariot horses were fed by warriors with the leaves. Greek gardens were often bordered with Parsley and Rue.

Several cultivated varieties exist, the principal being the common plain-leaved, the curled-leaved, the Hamburg or broad-leaved and the celery-leaved. Of the variety *crispum*, or curled-leaved, there are no less than thirty-seven variations; the most valuable are those of a compact habit with close, perfectly curled leaves. The common sort bears close leaves, but is of a somewhat hardier nature than those of which the leaves are curled; the latter are, however, superior in every way. The variety *crispum* was grown in very early days, being even mentioned by Pliny.

Turner says, 'if parsley is thrown into fish-ponds it will heal the sick fishes therein.'

The Hamburg, or turnip-rooted Parsley, is grown only for the sake of its enlarged fleshy tap-root. No mention appears to have been made by the Ancients, or in the Middle Ages, of this variety, which Miller in his *Gardeners' Dictionary* (1771) calls 'the large-rooted Parsley,' and which under cultivation develops both a parsnip-like as well as a turnip-shaped form. Miller says:

'This is now pretty commonly sold in the London markets, the roots being six times as large as the common Parsley. This sort was many years cultivated in Holland before the English gardeners could be prevailed upon to sow it. I brought the seeds of it from thence in 1727; but they refused to accept it, so that I cultivated it several years before it was known in the markets.'

At the present day, the 'long white' and the 'round sugar' forms are sold by seed-growers and are in esteem for flavouring soups, stews, etc., the long variety being also cooked and eaten like parsnips.

Neapolitan, or celery-leaved, parsley is grown for the use of its leafstalks, which are blanched and eaten like those of celery.

The plain-leaved parsley was the first known in this country, but it is not now much cultivated, the leaves being less attractive than those of the curled, of a less brilliant green, and coarser in flavour. It also has too close a resemblance to Fool's Parsley (*Anthriscus cynapium*), a noxious weed of a poisonous nature infesting gardens and fields. The leaves of the latter, though similar, are, however, of a rather darker green and when bruised, emit an unpleasant odour, very different to that of Parsley. They are, also, more finely divided. When the two plants are in flower, they are easily distinguished, *Anthriscus* having three tiny, narrow, sharp-pointed leaflets hanging down under each little umbellule of the white umbel of flowers, whereas in the Garden Parsley there is usually only one leaflet under the main umbel, the leaflets or bracts at the base of the small umbellules only being short and as fine as hairs. *Anthriscus* leaves, also, are glossy beneath. Gerard called *Anthriscus* 'Dog's Parsley,' and says 'the whole plant is of a naughty smell.' It contains a peculiar alkaloid called Cynapium.

Stone Parsley (*Sison*), or Breakstone, is an allied plant, growing in chalky districts.

S. Amomum is a species well known in some parts of Britain, with cream-coloured flowers and aromatic seeds. The name is said to be derived from the Celtic *sium* (running stream), some of the species formerly included growing in moist localities.

Of our Garden Parsley (which he calls Parsele) Gerard says, 'It is delightful to the taste and agreeable to the stomache,' also 'the roots or seeds boiled in ale and drank, cast foorth strong venome or poyson; but the seed is the strongest part of the herbe.'

Though the medicinal virtues of Parsley are still fully recognized, in former times it was considered a remedy for more disorders than it is now used for. Its imagined quality of destroying poison, to which Gerard refers, was probably attributed to the plant from its remarkable power of overcoming strong scents, even the odour of garlic being rendered almost imperceptible when mingled with that of Parsley.

The plant is said to be fatal to small birds and a deadly poison to parrots, also very injurious to fowls, but hares and rabbits will come from a great distance to seek for it, so that it is scarcely possible to preserve it in gardens to which they have access. Sheep are also fond of it, and it is said to be a sovereign remedy to preserve them from footrot, provided it be given them in sufficient quantities.

¶ *Cultivation*. Parsley requires an ordinary, good well-worked soil, but a moist one and a partially-shaded position is best. A little soot may be added to the soil.

The seed may be sown in drills, or broadcast, or, if only to be used for culinary purposes, as edging, or between dwarf or short-lived crops.

For a continuous supply, three sowings should be made: as early in February as the weather permits, in April or early in May, and in July and early August – the last being for the winter supply, in a sheltered position, with a southern exposure. Sow in February for the summer crop and for drying purposes. Seed sown then, however, takes several weeks to germinate, often as much as a full month. The principal sowing is generally done in April; it then germinates more quickly and provides useful material for cutting throughout the summer. A mid-August sowing will furnish good plants for placing in the cold frames for winter use.

An even broadcast sowing is preferable, if the ground is in the condition to be trodden, which appears to fix the seed in its place, and after raking leaves a firm even surface.

The seed should be but slightly covered, not more than $\frac{1}{2}$ inch deep and thinly distributed; if in drills, these should be 1 foot apart.

It is not necessary, however (though usual), to sow the seed where the plants are to be grown, as when large enough, the seedlings can be pricked out into rows.

When the seedlings are well out of the ground – about an inch high – adequate thinning is imperative, as the plants dislike being cramped, and about 8 inches from plant to plant must be allowed: a well-grown plant will cover nearly a square foot of ground.

The rows should be liberally watered in dry weather; a sheltered position is preferred, as the plants are liable to become burnt up in very hot and dry summers. The rows should be kept clean of weeds, and frequent dressings may be applied with advantage.

If the growth becomes coarse in the summer, cut off all the leaves and water well. This will induce a new growth of fine leaves, and may always be done when the plants have grown to a good size, as it encourages a stocky growth.

Soon after the old or last year's plants begin to grow again in the spring, they run to flower, but if the flower stems are promptly removed, and the plants top dressed and watered, they will remain productive for some time longer. Renew the beds every two years, as the plant dies down at the end of the second season.

When sowing Parsley to stand the winter, a plain-leaved variety will often be found superior to the curled or mossy sorts, which are, perhaps, handsomer, but the leaves retain both snow and rain, and when frost follows, the plants soon succumb. A plain-leaved Parsley is far hardier, and will survive even a severe winter and is equally good for cooking, though not so attractive for garnishing. Double the trouble is experienced in obtaining a supply of Parsley during the winter, when only the curled-leaved varieties are given.

Where curled Parsley is desired and is difficult to obtain, because there is no sufficiently sheltered spot in the garden for it, it may often be saved by placing a frame-light over the bed during severe weather to protect the plants, or they may be placed altogether in cold frames. Care must be taken with all Parsley plants grown thus in frames, to pick off all decaying leaves directly noticed, and the soil should be stirred occasionally with a pointed stick between the plants, to prevent its becoming sour. Abundance of air should be given on all favourable occasions, removing the light altogether on fine days.

¶ *Medicinal Action and Uses.* The uses of Parsley are many and are by no means restricted to the culinary sphere. The most familiar employment of the leaves in their fresh state is, of course, finely-chopped, as a flavouring to sauces, soups, stuffings, rissoles, minces, etc., and also sprinkled over vegetables or salads. The leaves are extensively cultivated, not only for sending to market fresh, but also for the purpose of being dried and powdered as a culinary flavouring in winter, when only a limited supply of fresh Parsley is obtainable.

In addition to the leaves, the *stems* are also dried and powdered, both as a culinary colouring and for dyeing purposes. There is

a market for the seeds to supply nurserymen, etc., and the roots of the turnip-rooted variety are used as a vegetable and flavouring.

Medicinally, the two-year-old *roots* are employed, also the *leaves*, dried, for making Parsley Tea, and the *seeds*, for the extraction of an oil called Apiol, which is of considerable curative value. The best kind of seed for medicinal purposes is that obtained from the Triple Moss curled variety. The wholesale drug trade generally obtains its seeds from farmers on the East coast, each sample being tested separately before purchases are made. It has been the practice to buy second-year seeds which are practically useless for growing purposes: it would probably hardly pay farmers to grow for Apiol producing purposes only, as the demand is not sufficiently great.

¶ *Constituents.* Parsley Root is faintly aromatic and has a sweetish taste. It contains starch, mucilage, sugar, volatile oil and Apiin. The latter is white, inodorous, tasteless and soluble in boiling water.

Parsley fruit or 'seeds' contain the volatile oil in larger proportion than the root (2·6 per cent.); it consists of terpenes and Apiol, to which the activity of the fruit is due. There are also present fixed oil, resin, Apiin, mucilage and ash. Apiol is an oily, non-nitrogenous allyl compound, insoluble in water, soluble in alcohol and crystallizable when pure into white needles. The British Pharmacopœia directs that Apiol be prepared by extracting the bruised fresh fruits with ether and distilling the solvent. The residue is the commercial liquid Apiol. It exercises all the virtues of the entire plant. Crystallized Apiol, or Parsley Camphor, is obtained by distilling the volatile oil to a low temperature. The value of the volatile oil depends on the amount of Apiol it contains. Oil obtained from German fruit contains this body in considerable quantity and becomes semi-solid at ordinary temperature, that from French fruit is much poorer in Apiol. In France, only the crystalline Apiol is official, but three different varieties, distinguished as green, yellow and white, are in use.

Apiol was first obtained in 1849 by Drs. Joret and Homolle, of Brittany, and proved an excellent remedy there for a prevailing ague. It is greatly used now in malarial disorders. The name Apiol has also been applied to an oleoresin prepared from the plant, which contains three closely-allied principles: apiol, apiolin and myristicin, the latter identical with the active principle of oil of Nutmeg. The term 'liquid Apiol' is frequently applied to the complete oleoresin.

This occurs as a yellowish liquid with a characteristic odour and an acrid pungent taste. The physiological action of the oleoresin of Parsley has not been sufficiently investigated, it exercises a singular influence on the great nerve centres of the head and spine, and in large doses produces giddiness and deafness, fall of blood-pressure and some slowing of the pulse and paralysis. It is stated that the paralysis is followed by fatty degeneration of the liver and kidney, similar to that caused by myristicin.

Parsley has carminative, tonic and aperient action, but is chiefly used for its diuretic properties, a strong decoction of the root being of great service in gravel, stone, congestion of the kidneys, dropsy and jaundice. The dried leaves are also used for the same purpose. Parsley Tea proved useful in the trenches, where our men often got kidney complications, when suffering from dysentery.

A fluid extract is prepared from both root and seeds. The extract made from the root acts more readily on the kidneys than that from other parts of the herb. The oil extracted from the seeds, the Apiol, is considered a safe and efficient emmenagogue, the dose being 5 to 15 drops in capsules. A decoction of bruised Parsley seeds was at one time employed against plague and intermittent fever.

In France, a popular remedy for scrofulous swellings is green Parsley and snails, pounded in a mortar to an ointment, spread on linen and applied daily. The bruised leaves, applied externally, have been used in the same manner as Violet leaves (also Celandine, Clover and Comfrey), to dispel tumours suspected to be of a cancerous nature. A poultice of the leaves is said to be an efficacious remedy for the bites and stings of poisonous insects.

Culpepper tells us:

'It is very comfortable to the stomach . . . good for wind and to remove obstructions both of the liver and spleen . . . Galen commendeth it for the falling sickness . . . the seed is effectual to break the stone and ease the pains and torments thereof. . . . The leaves of parsley laid to the eyes that are inflamed with heat or swollen, relieves them if it be used with bread or meat. . . . The juice dropped into the ears with a little wine easeth the pains.'

Formerly the distilled water of Parsley was often given to children troubled with wind, as Dill water still is.

¶ *Preparations and Dosages.* Fluid extract root, ½ to 1 drachm. Fluid extract seeds, ½ to 1 drachm. Apiol (oil), 5 to 15 drops in capsule.

¶ *Preparation for Market.* The roots are collected for medicinal purposes in the second year, in autumn or late summer, when the plant has flowered.

To dry Parsley towards the close of the summer for culinary use, it may be put into the oven on muslin trays, when cooking is finished, this being repeated several times till thoroughly dry and crisp, when the leaves should be rubbed in the hands or through a coarse wire sieve and the powder then stored in tins, so that neither air nor light can reach it, or the good colour will not be preserved. In the trade, there is a special method of drying which preserves the colour.

The oil is extracted from the 'seeds' or rather fruits, when *fresh*, in which condition they are supplied to manufacturing druggists.

PARSLEY, FOOL'S

Æthusa cynapium (LINN.)
N.O. Umbelliferæ

Synonyms. Lesser Hemlock. Smaller Hemlock. Dog Parsley. Dog Poison
Part Used. Herb

¶ *Description.* This annual plant is not unlike both Parsley and Hemlock. Its leaves, which are very similar to those of Parsley, are more acute, of a darker green and when bruised emit a disagreeable odour. When in flower it is easily distinguished because it has no general involucre and the partial involucre is composed of three to five long pendulous bracts which are drawn to one side, also the flowers, instead of being yellow, are white. It differs from Hemlock in being smaller, having its stem unspotted and the ridges of its fruit not wavy, also in the odour of the leaves, which is less unpleasant than that of Hemlock.

¶ *Constituents.* The active principle is an alkaloid, Cynopine.

¶ *Medicinal Action and Uses.* Though poisonous, the plant is less so than Hemlock. Poisoning from Fool's Parsley showed symptoms of heat in the mouth and throat and a post-mortem examination showed redness of the lining membrane of the gullet and windpipe and slight congestion of the duodenum and stomach.

It is used medicinally as a stomachic and sedative for gastro-intestinal troubles in children, for summer diarrhœa and cholera infantum.

PARSLEY PIERT   Alchemilla arvensis (SCOP.)
                                                                  N.O. Rosaceæ
Synonyms. Parsley Breakstone. Parsley Piercestone. Field Lady's Mantle
Part Used. Herb

Parsley Piert is common in Great Britain everywhere, especially in dry soil, being abundant in fields and waste places, on the tops of walls and in gravel-pits.

It is widely distributed throughout Europe and North Africa and has been introduced into North America. Unlike the Common Lady's Mantle, it is not found in this country above an altitude of 1,600 feet.

Description. Parsley Piert is a smaller and even more inconspicuous plant than the Common Lady's Mantle. The stem is sometimes prostrate, but generally erect, and much branched from the base. It is rarely more than 4 inches high.

The leaves are of a dusky green colour, wedge-shaped, three-cleft, the lobes deeply cut, the whole leaf less than $\frac{1}{2}$ inch wide, narrowed into a short foot-stalk with leafy, palmately-cut stipules, sheathing and cleaving to the footstalk. The whole plant is downy with slender, scattered hairs.

The greenish, minute and stalkless flowers are crowded together in tufts almost hidden by the leaves and their large stipules. There is no corolla, the stamens, which have jointed filaments, being inserted at the mouth of the calyx, which is usually four-cleft, as in the preceding species. The plant is in bloom from May to August. It is an annual.

This species is still in high repute with herbalists, and has been used for many centuries for its action on stone in the bladder, on account of which it was given the name of 'Parsley Breakstone' and 'Parsley Piercestone,' which has been corrupted into Parsley Piert, the 'parsley' referring to the form of its cut-into leaves, not to any relationship to the true Parsley.

Part Used. The whole herb, either fresh or dried. It has an astringent taste, but no odour.

Medicinal Action and Uses. Diuretic, demulcent and refrigerant. Its chief employment is in gravel, stone, dropsy and generally for complaints of the bladder and kidneys. Acting directly on the parts affected, it is found very valuable, even in apparently incurable cases. It operates violently, but safely, by urine and also removes obstructions of the liver, being therefore useful in jaundice.

Fluid extract: dose, 1 drachm.

It is prescribed in the form of an infusion – a handful of the herb to a pint of boiling water – taken daily in half-teacupful doses, three or four times daily. When used alone, it forms a useful remedy in all these complaints; its best action is seen, however, when compounded with other diuretics, such as Broom, Buchu leaves, Wild Carrot, Juniper Berries, Parsley Root and Pellitory-of-the-Wall. To soothe and help the passage of the irritating substance, it is also often combined with a demulcent such as Comfrey, Marshmallow or Sweet Flagroot, Hollyhock or Mullein flowers, Gum Arabic, or Slippery Elm Bark.

Some of the older herbalists considered it best when fresh gathered. Culpepper, after telling us of its powers in expelling stone, tells us that

'it is a very good salad herb and it were well that the gentry would pickle it up as they pickle up Samphire for their use all the winter because it is a very wholesome herb, and may be kept either dried or in a syrup. You may take a drachm of the powder of it in sherry wine: it will bring away gravel from the kidneys insensibly and without pain. It cures strangury.'

See LADY'S MANTLE.

PARSNIP   Pastinaca sativa
                                                              N.O. Umbelliferæ
Synonyms. (*French*) Le Panais. (*German*) Die Pastinake
Part Used. Root
Habitat. The Wild Parsnip is a native of most parts of Europe, growing chiefly in calcareous soils, by the wayside and on the borders of fields

The food value of Parsnips exceeds that of any other vegetable except potatoes. It is easy of production and should be more extensively grown.

The Parsnip, together with the carrot, was cultivated by the Ancients, but the Roman horticulturists evidently knew nothing of the advantage of selecting seeds, by means of

which the best existing variety has been developed. Pliny tells us it was grown either from the root transplanted or else from seed, but that it was impossible to get rid of the pungent flavour. The finest strain raised by Professor Buckman, between 1848 and 1850, as a result of his experiments in selection, was named by him the 'Student,' and having been further improved, still takes the first rank. It differs in several respects from the wild plant.

According to Pliny, Parsnips were held in such repute by the Emperor Tiberius that he had them annually brought to Rome from the banks of the Rhine, where they were then successfully cultivated. They are dressed in various ways and are much eaten with salt-fish during Lent.

In Holland, Parsnips are used in soups, whilst in Ireland cottagers make a beer by boiling the roots with water and hops, and afterwards fermenting the liquor. A kind of marmalade preserve has also been made from them, and even wine which in quality has been said to approach the famed Malmsey of Madeira.

It has a tough, wiry root, tapering somewhat from the crown, from which arises the erect stem, 1 to 2 feet high, tough and furrowed. The leaf-stalks are about 9 inches long, the leaves divided into several pairs of leaflets, each 1 to 2 inches long, the larger, terminal leaflet, ¾ inch broad. All the leaflets are finely toothed at their margins and softly hairy, especially on the underside. The sheath at the base of the leaf-stalk is about 1½ inch long, the first pair of leaflets being 4 inches above it.

The modern cultivated Parsnip has developed a leaf-stalk 2 feet long, the first pair of leaflets being several inches above the sheath. The leaflets are oblong, about 2 inches across at the basal part and 4½ inches in length (more than double the size of those of the wild plant), and are entirely smooth and somewhat paler in colour. The flowers in each case are yellow and in umbels at the ends of the stems, like the carrot, though the umbels do not contract in seeding, like those of the carrot. The flowers of the cultivated Parsnip are of a deeper yellow colour than those of the wild plant. The Parsnip is a biennial, flowering in its second year, throughout June and August. The fruit is flattened and of elliptical form, strongly furrowed. Parsnip 'seeds' as the fruit is commonly called, are pleasantly aromatic, and were formerly collected for their medicinal value and sold by herbalists. They contain an essential oil that has the reputation of curing intermittent fever. A strong decoction of the root is a good diuretic and assists in removing obstructions of the viscera. It has been employed as a remedy for jaundice and gravel.

¶ *Medicinal Action and Uses.* Culpepper wrote:

'The wild Parsnip differeth little from the garden, but groweth not so fair and large,

nor hath so many leaves, and the root is shorter, more woody and not so fit to be eaten and, therefore, more medicinal. The Garden Parsnip nourisheth much and is good and wholesome, but a little windy, but it fatteneth the body if much used. It is good for the stomach and reins and provoketh urine. The wild Parsnip hath a cutting, attenuating, cleansing and opening quality therein. It easeth the pains and stitches in the sides and expels the wind from the stomach and bowels, or colic. The root is often used, but the seed much more, the wild being better than the tame.'

Gerard, speaking of its uses as a vegetable, observes:

'The Parsneps nourish more than do the Turneps or the Carrots, and the nourishment is somewhat thicker, but not faultie nor bad. . . . There is a good and pleasant foode or bread made of the rootes of Parsneps, as my friend Master Plat hath set foorth in his booke of experiments.'

Tournefort, in *The Compleat Herbal* (1730), wrote of Parsnips, that

'they are commonly boiled and eaten with butter in the time of Lent; for that they are the sweetest, by reason the juice has been concocted during the winter, and are desired at that season especially, both for their agreeable Taste and their Wholesomeness. For they are not so good in any respect, till they have been first nipt with Cold. It is likewise pretty common of late to eat them with salt-fish mixed with hard-boiled eggs and butter . . . and much the wholesomer if you eat it with mustard.'

John Wesley, in his *Primitive Physic*, says: '*Wild parsnips* both leaves and stalks, bruised, seem to have been a favorite application; and a very popular internal remedy for cancer, asthma, consumption and similar diseases.'

The roots are sweeter than carrots. They contain both sugar and starch, and for this reason beer and spirits are sometimes prepared from them. In the north of Ireland, they have been often brewed with malt instead of hops and fermented with yeast, the result being a pleasant drink, and Parsnip wine, when properly made, is esteemed by many people.

Parsnips are not only a valuable item of human food, but equal, if not superior to carrots for fattening pigs, making the flesh white, and being preferred by pigs to carrots. Washed and sliced and given with bran, horses eat them readily and thrive on them. In Brittany and the Channel Islands, they are largely given to cattle and pigs, and milch cows fed on them in winter are said to give as much and as good milk, and yield butter as well-flavoured as when feeding on grass in May and June.

¶ *Cultivation.* Parsnips require a long period of growth, and should be started, if possible, the latter part of February. In choosing the seed, the older varieties should be avoided, as there is no comparison between them and the newer and better kinds. The 'Student,' already mentioned, is suited in every way for the average small garden.

No specially good soil is required, though a strong soil is preferable to a sandy one; poorish or partially exhausted soil is no drawback, as there should be no recent manure in the top spit, for in common with carrots, its presence tends to form forked roots. The ground, however, should be deeply trenched and a slight dressing of manure may be buried deeply. Roots will be poor if grown in soil which has hardly been turned over, but if the land is deeply dug, plenty of lime, old mortar rubbish or wood ashes being mixed in, fine roots will be produced.

One ounce of Parsnip seed will sow a row 300 feet long. The seed is best sown in drills about 1 inch deep, as soon as the land is anything like dry enough to work. Drop three seeds together, 8 inches apart, and let the rows stand 15 inches asunder. After the plants appear, there is very little to do except to thin them and hoe, at intervals; no stimulants are needed. Thinning may be done as soon as they are well in their second leaf.

As the Parsnip is hardy, there is no need to lift the roots in autumn. The crop will be ready for use in September, but it may be left in the ground and be dug throughout the winter as required, and the remainder not finally raised till the middle or end of February, when the site the roots occupy has to be prepared for the crop of the ensuing summer.

PARSNIP, WATER

Synonym. Water Hemlock

Sium latifolium, the Broad-leaved Water Parsnip, is another of the umbelliferous plants sometimes called Water Hemlock. It occurs in watery places all over the British Isles. The long creeping root-stock of this and the somewhat smaller, closely allied species *S. angustifolium* is poisonous, but

To prepare *Parsnip Soup,* scrape and cut up 2 large Parsnips or 4 small ones, and wash them carefully. Peel 6 large potatoes and boil them with the Parsnips in a quart of water. When soft, mash and pass through a sieve. Boil up again in the water and pour on to slices of bread in the tureen, adding 2 oz. of butter. The addition of a little cream, in more favourable times, of course makes the soup more savoury.

Stewed Parsnips

Wash, peel and cut 3 Parsnips into slices, then boil them till they are nearly done, drain them and let them cool. Melt 2 or 3 oz. bacon fat in a stewpan; when hot, fry the Parsnips to a light brown colour. Next add a tablespoonful of flour and moisten with sufficient brown stock just to cover the Parsnips. Season with salt and pepper, and 1 or 2 tablespoonsful of tomato sauce. Bring to the boil and let the Parsnips simmer slowly for another 20 minutes. Dish up and serve with the prepared sauce.

Parsnip Cakes

Parsnips mashed with a little butter and pepper and salt, and then dipped into flour and formed into small, round cakes, are nice if fried in lard, dripping or bacon fat.

Parsnip Salad

Plainly-boiled Parsnips, when cold, make an excellent salad. Slice the Parsnips, not too thinly, and season with salt and pepper, and mix with a simple French oil and vinegar salad dressing.

Parsnip Wine

Take 15 lb. of sliced Parsnips, and boil until quite soft in 5 gallons of water; squeeze the liquor well out of them, run it through a sieve and add 3 lb. of coarse lump sugar to every gallon of liquor. Boil the whole for ¾ hour. When it is nearly cold, add a little yeast on toast. Let it remain in a tub for 10 days, stirring it from the bottom every day; then put it into a cask for a year. As it works over, fill it up every day.

Sium latifolium
N.O. Umbelliferæ

pigs and oxen eat the stem and leaves without harm. However, cows in milk should not be allowed to eat it, as it communicates a disagreeable taste to the milk.

Both species are easily recognized by their pinnate leaves, the leaf-stalks carrying about six to eight pairs of ovate, toothed leaflets.

The umbels of white flowers are flat and have a general involucre composed of broadish or lance-shaped bracts, and there is also an in-volucel. The fruit bears slender ribs. The erect, furrowed stems are from 3 to 6 feet high.

PASSION FLOWER

Passiflora incarnata (LINN.)
N.O. Passifloraceæ

Synonyms. Passion Vine. Granadilla. Maracoc. Maypops
Part Used. The dried herb, collected after some of the berries have matured
Habitat. Virginia

¶ *Description.* The Passion Flowers are so named from the supposed resemblance of the finely-cut corona in the centre of the blossoms to the Crown of Thorns and of the other parts of the flower to the instruments of the Passion of Our Lord. *Passiflora incarnata* has a perennial root, and the herbaceous shoots bear three-lobed, finely-serrated leaves and flesh-coloured or yellowish, sweet-scented flowers, tinged with purple. The ripe, orange-coloured, ovoid, many-seeded berry is about the size of a small apple; when dried, it is shrivelled and greenish-yellow. The yellow pulp is sweet and edible.

¶ *Constituents.* There appears to be no detailed analysis of this species, but its active principle, which has been called Passiflorine, would appear to be somewhat similar to morphine.

¶ *Medicinal Action and Uses.* The drug is known to be a depressant to the motor side of the spinal cord, slightly reducing arterial pressure, though affecting circulation but little, while increasing the rate of respiration. It is official in homœopathic medicine and used with bromides, it is said to be of great service in epilepsy. Its narcotic properties cause it to be used in diarrhœa and dysentery, neuralgia, sleeplessness and dysmenorrhœa.

¶ *Dosages.* 3 to 10 grains. Of Fluid extract, 10 to 20 minims.

¶ *Other Species.*
Many species yield edible fruits or are cultivated for their beauty and fragrance.

P. cærulea, the familiar Blue Passion Flower, hardy in southern districts of this country as a wall-climber, was introduced into England from Brazil in 1699.

P. quadrangularis, the Common Granadilla, a native of Jamaica and South America grown for its large edible fruit, the purple, succulent pulp of which is eaten with wine and sugar, has a root said to be very poisonous and a powerful narcotic; in small doses it is anthelmintic. It is used in Mauritius as a diuretic and emetic.

The fruit of *P. edulis* in colour and flavour resembles that of the orange, with a mixture of acid.

P. macrocarpa bears a gourd-like, oblong fruit, much larger than any of the other species, attaining a weight of 7 to 8 lb.

P. maliformis, the Apple-fruited Granadilla, the Sweet Calabash of the West Indies, has a fruit 2 inches in diameter, full of a pleasant gelatinous pulp. The juice of the leaves, and also of those of *P. pallida*, is used by the Brazilians against intermittent fevers.

P. laurifolia, the Water Lemon of the West Indies, is much cultivated throughout South America for its fruit, the aromatic juice of which quenches thirst, allays heat and induces appetite. Its bitter and astringent leaves are employed as an anthelmintic.

The roots of *P. contrayerva* and *P. normalis* are reputed to have counter-poison properties.

P. fœtida is used in hysteria, female complaints and as an expectorant, and the leaves as a poultice in skin inflammations.

The flowers of *P. rubra* yield a narcotic tincture.

P. capsularia is said to possess emmenagogue properties.

PATCHOULI

Pogostemon patchouli (PILL.)
N.O. Labiatæ

Synonym. Pucha-pat
Part Used. The herb, yielding a volatile oil by distillation
Habitat. East and West Indies and Paraguay

¶ *Description.* This fragrant herb, with soft, opposite, egg-shaped leaves and square stems, grows from 2 to 3 feet in height, giving out the peculiar, characteristic odour of patchouli when rubbed. Its whitish flowers, tinged with purple, grow in both axillary and terminal spikes. The crop is cut two or three times a year, the leaves being dried and packed in bales and exported for distillation of the oil. The best oil is freshly distilled near the plantations. That obtained from leaves imported into Europe, often damaged and adulterated even up to 80 per cent., is inferior. It is used in coarser perfumes and in 'White Rose' and 'Oriental' toilet soaps. Although the odour is objectionable to some, it is widely-used both in Asia and India. Sachets are made of the coarsely-powdered leaves, and before its common use in Europe, genuine Indian shawls and Indian ink were distinguished by the odour, which has the unusual quality of improving with age. Hence the older oil is preferred by perfumers and used to confer more lasting properties upon other scents.

¶ *Constituents.* Oil of Patchouli is thick, the colour being brownish-yellow tinted green. It contains cœrulein, the vivid blue compound found in matricaria, wormwood and other oils. It deposits a solid, or stearoptene, patchouli alcohol, leaving cadinene.

It is lævorotatory, with the specific

gravity of 0·970 to 0·990 at 15° C. (59° F.).

¶ *Medicinal Action and Uses.* Its use is said to cause sometimes loss of appetite and sleep and nervous attacks. The Chinese, Japanese and Arabs believe it to possess prophylactic properties.

¶ *Other Species and Adulterations.* *Java patchouli,* often grown in Indian gardens for home use, is a product of *Pogostemon Heyneanus.*

The inferior oil of Assam is from *Microtœna cymosa.*

Cubeb and cedar oils are said to be usual adulterants.

PAPYRUS. *See* SEDGES

PEACH

Prunus Persica (STOKES)
N.O. Rosaceæ

Synonyms. Amygdalis Persica (Linn.). Persica vulgaris Null
(*Chinese and Japanese*) 'Too'
Parts Used. Bark, leaves

The Peach is included by Hooker and other botanists in the genus *Prunus*, its resemblance to the plum being obvious. Others have classed it with the Almond as a distinct genus, *Amygdalus*, and others again have considered it sufficiently distinct to constitute it a separate genus, *Persica*.

As we now know it, the Peach has been nowhere recognized in the wild state. De Candolle attributes all cultivated varieties to a distinct species, probably of Chinese origin. Other naturalists, among them Darwin, look on the Peach as a modification of the Almond.

It has been cultivated from time immemorial in most parts of Asia, and appears to have been introduced into Europe from Persia, as its name implies. At what period it was introduced into Greece is uncertain. The Romans seem to have brought it direct from Persia during the reign of the Emperor Claudius.

When first introduced it was called *Malus persica,* or Persian Apple. The expedition of Alexander probably made it known to Theophrastus, 392 B.C., who speaks of it as a Persian fruit. It has no name in Sanskrit; nevertheless, the people speaking that language came into India from the Northwest, the country generally assigned to the species.

In support of the supposed *Chinese* origin, it may be added that the Peach-tree was introduced from China into Cochin-China, and that the Japanese call it by the Chinese name, *Too.*

The Peach is mentioned in the books of Confucius, fifth century before the Christian era, and the antiquity of the knowledge of the fruit in China is further proved by representations of it in sculpture and on porcelain.

It is said to have been first cultivated in England in the first half of the sixteenth century. Gerard describes several varieties as growing in his garden, and speaks of a 'double-flowered peach,' as a rarity, in his garden.

It is always cultivated here trained against walls or under glass. When growing naturally, it is a medium-sized tree, with spreading branches, of quick growth and not long-lived. The leaves are lance-shaped, about 4 inches long and 1½ inch broad, tapering to a sharp point, borne on long, slender, relatively unbranched shoots, and with the flowers arranged singly, or in groups of two or more at intervals along the shoots of the previous year's growth. The blossoms come out before the leaves are fully expanded, and are of a delicate, pink colour. They have a hollow tube at the base, bearing at its free edge five sepals, and an equal number of petals, usually concave, and a great number of stamens. They have very little odour.

The fruit is a drupe, like the plum, having a delicate, thin outer downy skin enclosing the flesh of the Peach, the inner layers becoming woody to form the large, furrowed, rugged stone, while the ovule ripens into the kernel or seed. This is exactly the structure of the plum and apricot, and differs from that of the almond, which is identical in the first instance, only in that the fleshy part of the latter eventually becomes dry and leathery, and cracks along a line called the suture, which is merely represented in the Peach by a furrow on one side.

In the South of France, and in other Continental countries possessing a similar climate, Peach-trees ripen their fruit very well as standards in the open air. In America, the

Peach grows almost without any care – extensive orchards, containing from 10,000 to 20,000 trees, being raised from the stones. At first, the trees there make rapid and healthy growth, and in a few years bear in great abundance; but they soon decay, their leaves becoming tinged with yellow even in summer, when they should be green. This is owing to their being grown on their own roots, for when that is the case in Britain the trees present a similar appearance. They require, therefore, to be budded on the plum or on the almond.

In America, the Peach is chiefly used for feeding pigs, and for making Peach Brandy.

¶ *Cultivation*. The soil best suited for the Peach is three parts mellow, unexhausted loam, mixed with vegetable mould or manure. Peaches require a lighter soil than pears or plums.

To perpetuate and multiply the choicer varieties, both the Peach and the newly-allied nectarine are budded upon plums or almond stocks. For dry soil, the almond stocks are preferable; for damp or clayey loam, it is better to use certain kinds of plums.

The fruit is produced on the ripened shoots of the preceding year, and the formation of young shoots in sufficient abundance, and of requisite strength, is the great object of peach training and pruning.

In cold soils and bleak situations, it is considered best to cover the walls upon which the trees are trained with a casing of glass, so that the trees may be under shelter during uncongenial spring weather.

Various kinds of *Aphis* and the *Acarus*, or Red Spider, infest the leaves of the Peach.

¶ *Medicinal Action and Uses*. The fruit is wholesome and seldom disagrees if eaten ripe, though the skin is indigestible. The quantity of sugar is only small.

All Peaches have in the kernel a flavour resembling that of noyau, which depends on the presence of prussic or hydrocyanic acid. Not only the kernels, but also the young branches and flowers, after maceration in water, yield a volatile oil, which is chemically identical with that of bitter almonds, and is the cause of this flavour. Infused in white brandy, sweetened with barley sugar, Peach leaves have been said to make a fine cordial, similar to noyau, and the flowers when distilled furnish a white liquor, which communicates a flavour resembling the kernels of the fruit.

The leaves, bark, flowers and kernels have medicinal virtue. Both the *leaves* and *bark* are still employed for their curative powers. They have demulcent, sedative, diuretic and expectorant action. An infusion of $\frac{1}{2}$ oz. of the bark or 1 oz. of the dried leaves to a pint of boiling water has been found almost a specific for irritation and congestion of the gastric surfaces. It is also used in whooping cough, ordinary coughs and chronic bronchitis, the dose being from a teaspoonful to a wineglassful as required.

The fresh leaves were stated by the older herbalists to possess the power of expelling worms, if applied outwardly to the body as a poultice. An infusion of the dried leaves was also recommended for the same purpose.

Culpepper informs us that a powder of the leaves 'strewed on fresh bleeding wounds stayeth their bleeding and closeth them.'

In Italy, at the present day, there is a popular belief that if fresh Peach leaves are applied to warts and then buried, the warts will fall off by the time the buried leaves have decayed.

A syrup and infusion of Peach *flowers* was formerly a preparation recognized by apothecaries, and praised by Gerard as a mildly acting efficient purgative. The syrup was considered good for children and those in weak health, and to be good against jaundice.

A tincture made from the flowers has been said to allay the pain of colic caused by gravel.

Culpepper recommends the milk or cream of the kernels applied to the forehead and temples as a means of procuring 'rest and sleep to sick persons,' and says 'the oil drawn from the kernels and the temples annointed therewith doth the like.' He tells us that 'the liquor that drops from the tree, being wounded,' added to coltsfoot, sweet wine and saffron, is 'good for coughs, hoarseness and loss of voice,' and that it 'clears and strengthens the lungs and relieves those who vomit and spit blood.' He concludes:

'If the kernels be bruised and boiled in vinegar until they become thick and applied to the head, it marvellously causes the hair to grow again upon any bald place or where it is too thin.'

'Peach cold' is an affection which prevails in some parts where Peach trees are largely cultivated, just as rose fever and rose catarrh are caused by roses in parts of America.

¶ *Collection*. The *bark* for medicinal purposes is stripped from the tree in the spring and taken from young trees. It is best dried in a moderate sun-heat, being taken indoors at night. The pieces of bark if thin are often threaded on strings and hung up in a warm current of air. They must not touch each other. Peach bark occurs in commerce in small, thin, pale-brown fragments, rarely exceeding $1\frac{1}{2}$ inch in length, and $\frac{1}{4}$ inch in thickness, having a smooth, dark brown skin and an inner surface with a faint network of fibres. It has a bitter, very astringent taste and slight odour.

Peach *leaves* should be collected for drying purposes in June and July, when at their best.

PEACH WOOD, known also as Nicaragua Wood, is in no way related to the fruit-tree, but is a much-used dyewood that dyes a delicate peach and cherry colour. It is obtained from the tree CÆSALPINIA ECHINATA, belonging to the Pea and Bean tribe, Leguminosae, and is imported into this country in blocks about 4 feet in length and 8 inches in diameter. We receive annually about 8,000 tons in normal times. That which comes from Peru yields the finest shades of colour, mainly tints of red and orange.

PELARGONIUMS

Pelargonium antidysentericum
And other Species
N.O. Geraniaceæ

Synonym. T'Namie
Part Used. Root
Habitat. Cape of Good Hope

¶ *Description.* This is a very extensive genus, and the greater number are natives of the Cape of Good Hope, most species possess astringent properties, and have been found valuable in dysentery (particularly *Pelargonium antidysentericum*), also for ulcerations of the stomach and upper part of the intestines.

¶ *Other Species.*
P. triste, native also of the Cape. This has yellow flowers with a purple spot, always open, but only fragrant after the sun has left them. The tuberous roots are eaten by the natives.

Others are cultivated for the distillation of a volatile oil (from the leaves) which is not unlike that from rose petals; *P. roseum* has very fragrant foliage; *P. capitatum* gives a good essential oil and yields Pelargonic fatty acid, this specie is often called rose geranium.

The oil of *P. odoratissimum* is much used as an adulterant to oil of Roses.

See MONSONIA.

PELLITORY

Anacyclus pyrethrum (D.C.)
N.O. Compositæ

Synonyms. Anthemis Pyrethrum. Pyrethrum officinarum. Pyrethrum. Pyrethri Radix. Roman Pellitory. Pellitory of Spain. Spanish Chamomile. Pyrethre. Matricaria Pyrethrum
Part Used. Root
Habitat. Algeria. Cultivated in Mediterranean countries

¶ *Description.* This perennial plant, in habit and appearance like the chamomile, has stems that lie on the ground for part of their length, before rising erect. Each bears one large flower, the disk being yellow and the rays white, tinged with purple beneath. The leaves are smooth, alternate, and pinnate, with deeply-cut segments.

The root is almost cylindrical, very slightly twisted and tapering and often crowned with a tuft of grey hairs. Externally it is brown and wrinkled, with bright black spots. The fracture is short, and the transverse section, magnified, presents a beautiful radiate structure and many oleoresin glands. The taste is pungent and odour slight.

¶ *Cultivation.* Planting may be done in autumn, but the best time is about the end of April. Any ordinary good soil is suitable, but better results are obtained when it is well-drained, and of a stiff loamy character, enriched with good manure. Propagation is done in three ways, by seed, by division of roots and by cuttings. If grown by *seed*, sow in February or March, thin out to 2 to 3 inches between the plants, and plant out early in June to permanent quarters, allowing a foot or more between the plants and 2 feet between the rows, selecting, if possible, a showery day for the operation. The seedlings will quickly establish themselves. Weeding should be done by hand, the plants when first put out being small, might be injured by hoeing. To propagate by *division*, lift the plants in March, or whenever the roots are in an active condition, and with a sharp spade, divide them into three or five fairly large pieces. *Cuttings* should be made from the young shoots that start from the base of the plant, and should be taken with a heel of the old plant attached, which will greatly assist their rooting. They may be inserted at any time from October to May. The foliage should be shortened to about 3 inches, when the cuttings will be ready for insertion in a bed of light, sandy soil. Plant very firmly, surface the bed with sand, and water in well. Shade is necessary while the cuttings are rooting.

¶ *Constituents.* Analysis has shown a brown, resinous, acrid substance, insoluble in potassium hydroxide and probably containing *pelletonin,* two oils soluble in potassium hydroxide – one dark brown and acrid, the other yellow – tannin, gum, potassium sulphate and carbonate, potassium chloride, calcium phosphate and carbonate, silica, alumina, lignin, etc.

An alkaloid, Pyrethrine, yielding pyrethric acid, is stated to be the active principle.

¶ *Medicinal Action and Uses.* Pellitory root is widely used because of its pungent efficacy in relieving toothache and in promoting a free flow of saliva. The British Pharmacopœia directs that it be used as a masticatory, and in the form of lozenges for its reflex action on the salivary glands in dryness of the mouth and throat. The tincture made from the dried root may be applied to relieve the aching of a decayed tooth, applied on cotton wool, or rubbed on the gums, and for this purpose may with advantage be mixed with camphorated chloroform. It forms an addition to many dentifrices.

A gargle of Pellitory infusion is prescribed for relaxed uvula and for partial paralysis of the tongue and lips. To make a gargle, two or three teaspoonsful of Pellitory should be mixed with a pint of cold water and sweetened with honey if desired. Patients seeking relief from rheumatic or neuralgic affections of the head and face, or for palsy of the tongue, have been advised to chew the root daily for several months.

Being a rubefacient and local irritant, when sliced and applied to the skin, it induces heat, tingling and redness.

The powdered root forms a good snuff to cure chronic catarrh of the head and nostrils and to clear the brain, by exciting a free flow of nasal mucous and tears.

Culpepper tells us that Pellitory 'is one of the best purges of the brain that grows' and is not only 'good for ague and the falling sickness' (epilepsy) but is 'an excellent approved remedy in lethargy.' After stating that 'the powder of the herb or root snuffed up the nostrils procureth sneezing and easeth the headache,' he goes on to say that 'being made into an ointment with hog's lard it taketh away black and blue spots occasioned by blows or falls, and helpeth both the gout and sciatica,' uses which are now obsolete.

In the thirteenth century we read in old records that Pellitory of Spain was 'a proved remedy for the toothache' with the Welsh physicians. It was familiar to the Arabian writers on medicine and is still a favourite remedy in the East, having long been an article of export from Algeria and Spain by way of Egypt to India.

In the East Indies the infusion is used as a cordial.

¶ *Dosages.* 20 grains. Tincture, B.P. and U.S.P., 20 to 30 drops.

¶ *Other Species.*

Anacyclus officinarum is indigenous to Africa, cultivated in Germany, and formerly official in the German Pharmacopœia. The roots are smaller and very pungent. It is also known as *A. pyrethrum, Pyrethrum germanicum* and German Pellitory.

P. umbelliferum is said to be used also, the Pyrethrum of Dioscorides being an Umbellifer.

Though dandelion and other roots, especially *Corrigiola littoralis* (Illecebraceæ), are named as adulterants, it is stated by French authorities that the roots of *A. pyrethrum* are often old when found in commerce, but are never mixed with others.

PELLITORY, DALMATIAN

PELLITORY, PERSIAN

Chrysanthemum cinerariæfolium (VIS.)

Chrysanthemum roseum (ADAM)
Pyrethrum roseum (BIEB.)
Chrysanthemum carneum
N.O. Compositæ

Synonyms. Insect Flowers. Insect Plants
Part Used. Closed flowers

The Insect Powder of commerce, used to stupefy and kill various small insects, especially the larvæ of Cochylis, which attacks the vine, was first known as Persian Insect Powder, or Persian Pellitory, being prepared from the closed flowers of *Pyrethrum roseum* and *P. carneum,* plants native to the north of Persia, where they flourish on the mountain slopes up to a height of 6,500 feet, and also in the Caucasus. These two species are familiar in this country as garden flowers, of which there are many varieties in cultivation, blossoming freely in May, the tufts of foliage of a dark green, much cut into, and the flowers of all shades of rose and crimson.

Some years ago, a Dalmatian species, *Chrysanthemum cinerariæfolium,* was found to be more active, and the Persian or Caucasian Insect Powder Plants are now seldom imported, being superseded by the Dalmatian species, which has white flowers, smaller than our Ox-Eye Daisy. It is cultivated both in Dalmatia and in California.

The cultivation of the Insect Powder plants has not yet been taken up on a commercial scale, either in Great Britain or the colonies, but it could be grown successfully in certain districts in this country.

There is a great demand for the flowers in commerce, and the flowers received from their usual source are so frequently adulterated by the addition of other composite flowers which are lacking in stupefying power, that the cultivation of the plant would be most desirable, either here or in our colonies. It can be profitably grown on dry, stony soil.

The conditions suiting the Dalmatian variety are sunny, pebbly, calcareous hillsides, dry, without irrigation, and in a fairly dry atmosphere. In ordinary garden soil, it does not flourish in shade and often dies off after flowering. All three species grown experimentally at Berne often succumbed during moist summers.

On the warmer southern and western coasts of Great Britain, the plant could easily be cultivated. It might be grown with success on the hilly slopes of oolite and limestone and chalk and on sandhills on the shore in Cornwall, Devon and Lancashire, or on the pebbly beach of Lydd, in Kent. In Jersey, on the pebbly and sandy shores, it would grow luxuriantly.

Attempts have already been made to cultivate the plant in Australia and South Africa.

Insect Powder is harmless to human beings. Besides being used as an insecticide in the form of a powder, it is also used as a lotion, a tincture of the flowers being prepared and used, diluted with 10 parts of water, to dab on the exposed skin to keep away insects. It is also employed as a fumigator. The smoke of the burnt flowers is as effective as the powder in keeping down insects, and might be valuable in Africa as a means against the tsetse-flies, and in sleeping sickness districts, if grown on the shores where they breed, and burnt when the flies emerge from the chrysalis.

In Dalmatia, the plant grows on the seashore, but it also grows well in the inland, mountainous districts of Herzegovina and Montenegro, the wild Montenegrin flowers being very highly esteemed. In the Adriatic islands, its cultivation is very remunerative.

¶ Cultivation. Sow seeds at the end of March on rich, light soil, in sunny situation and cover with ¼ to ½ inch of fine soil and then with dry leaves. If the autumn be mild, the seeds may also be sometimes sown in August, or early September, as soon as the seed is ripe, but then they need shading with canvas, placed about 6 inches above the soil, or more. Prick out the seedlings in the following March, or later, if sown in September. On the average only about half of the seedlings are fit for pricking out.

It is difficult to obtain seed that will germinate, the Dalmatian growers apparently dry the seeds by heat before disposing of them, to prevent germination.

Arrange the plants in deep furrows, prepared the previous autumn, about 15 to 20 inches apart, the seedlings 15 inches apart in the furrows. Of every 100 plants pricked out, fifteen to thirty generally die off and have to be replaced.

Weed several times during growth.

The plants begin to flower about the third week in May. The flower-buds are collected in the middle of May, or if it should then be damp, not till June. They must always be collected in dry weather.

A second gathering is made in August and September. The unopened flower-buds are kept separately, as they obtain the best price. The flower-heads are collected at different stages of development, the commercial varieties being known as 'closed,' 'half-closed' and 'open' flowers respectively. They are most active if collected when fully developed, but before they have expanded. They are cut off just below the involucre of bracts.

The flowers retain their insecticidal properties for an indefinite period, if kept under suitable condition, even if in the state of dry powder. It is the flowers alone that are active; the leaves have no insecticidal properties whatever.

The powder prepared from the Dalmatian flowers is distinguished from that of Persian flowers by numerous hairs. The better the quality of the powder, the larger will be the proportion of pollen and the smaller the proportion of stem issue.

One of the best tests of the quality of the powder is to keep a few house-flies under a tumbler with a little of the powder; they should be stupefied within a minute. Adulterated or less active powder will take about twenty minutes to effect this.

Each plant yields 80 to 100 flowers, and in one day 1,500 to 2,500 flowers can be gathered by one person. One hundred flowers weigh about 50 grammes (1⅘ oz.). One hundred kilos (220 lb.) of fresh flowers yield 25 to 33 kilos (55 to 72 lb.) of dried flowers.

In Dalmatia the flowers are dried in the shade on frames of cloth, in layers 1 to 1½ inch deep, turned over two or three times daily. The Persian flowers are dried first in the sun and then in the shade.

After harvesting, the land is tilled in the autumn and again in the spring, the soil being forked between the rows to keep it porous. Being a mountain plant, it requires

PELLITORY-OF-THE-WALL

Synonym. Lichwort
Part Used. Herb

Pellitory-of-the-Wall is a humble, inconspicuous plant belonging to the same group as the Stinging Nettle and the Hop. It is the only representative of its genus in Britain. The name of this genus, *Parietaria*, is derived from the Latin word *paries* (a wall), for it is very commonly found growing from crannies in dry walls, as its popular English name also tells us, and will frequently luxuriate in the midst of stony rubbish.

¶ *Description.* It is a much-branched, bushy, herbaceous, perennial plant, 1 to 2 feet high, with reddish, brittle stems and narrow, stalked leaves 1 to 2 inches long. The stems and veins of the under surface of the leaves are furnished with short, soft hairs, the upper surface of the leaves is nearly smooth, with sunken veins. The small, green stalkless flowers grow in clusters in the axils of the leaves and are in bloom all the summer. The filaments of their stamens are curiously jointed and so elastic that if touched before the expansion of the flower, they suddenly spring from their incurved position and scatter their pollen broadcast.

¶ *Constituents.* All parts of the plant contain nitre abundantly.

¶ *Medicinal Action and Uses.* Diuretic, laxative, refrigerant and slightly demulcent. Pellitory-of-the-Wall is a most efficacious remedy for stone in the bladder, gravel, dropsy, stricture and other urinary complaints. Its action upon the urinary calculus

a dry surface, well drained below. Sunlight and heat are necessary for luxuriant growth.

The plants live on the average for six years, but sometimes will remain healthy and strong for as much as twenty years.

Parietaria officinalis (LINN.)
N.O. Urticaceæ

is perhaps more marked than any other simple agent at present employed.

It is given in infusion or decoction, the infusion – the most usual form – 1 oz. to 1 pint of boiling water being taken in wineglassful doses. Frequently it is combined with Wild Carrot and Parsley Piert.

Fluid extract: dose, 1 drachm.

The decoction, says Gerard, 'helpeth such as are troubled with an old cough,' and 'the decoction with a little honey is good to gargle a sore throat.' He gives us many other uses:

'The juice held awhile in the mouth easeth pains in the teeth; the distilled water of the herb drank with sugar worketh the same effect and cleanseth the skin from spots, freckles, pimples, wheals, sunburn, etc. . . . 'The juice dropped into the ears easeth the noise in them and taketh away the pricking and shooting pains therein.'

In the form of an ointment he tells us it is capital for piles and a remedy for gout and fistula.

The leaves may be usefully applied as poultices.

The juice of the fresh herb, made into a thin syrup will stimulate the kidneys in the same way as the infusion of the dried herb. Ben Jonson says:

'A good old woman . . . did cure me With sodden ale and pellitorie o' the wall.'

PENNYROYAL

Mentha Pulegium (LINN.)
N.O. Labiatæ

Synonyms. Pulegium. Run-by-the-Ground. Lurk-in-the-Ditch. Pudding Grass. Piliole-rial
Part Used. Herb

This species of Mint, a native of most parts of Europe and parts of Asia, is the Pulegium of the Romans, so named by Pliny from its reputed power of driving away fleas – *pulex* being the Latin for flea, hence the Italian *pulce* and the French *puce*. This name given the plant in ancient times has been retained as its modern specific name. It is sometimes known to the country-people as 'Run by the Ground' and 'Lurk in the Ditch,' from its manner of growth.

It was formerly much used in medicine, the name Pennyroyal being a corruption of the old herbalists' name 'Pulioll-royall' (*Pulegium regium*), which we meet also in the Middle Ages as 'Piliole-rial.' It has been known to botanists since the time of Linnæus as *Mentha Pulegium*.

One of its popular names is 'Pudding Grass,' from being formerly used in stuffings for hog's puddings ('grass' being, like 'wort,' a word simply meaning 'herb'). It is still used abroad in various culinary preparations, but in this country it is now in disuse, as its taste and odour is too pronounced.

A famous stuffing was once made of Pennyroyal, pepper and honey.

¶ *Description.* Pennyroyal is the smallest of the Mints and very different in habit from any of the others. Two forms of the plant are met with in Great Britain: the commonest, the variety *decumbens*, has weak, prostrate stems, bluntly quadrangular, 3 inches to a foot long, which readily take root at the lower joints or nodes. The leaves are opposite, shortly stalked, more or less hairy on both sides, roundish oval, greyish green, about 1 to 1½ inch long and ½ inch broad. The flowers are in whorled clusters of ten or a dozen, rising in tiers one above the other at the nodes, where the leaves spring in pairs, beginning about the middle of the stem, their colour reddish purple to lilac blue, and in bloom during July and August. The seed is light brown, oval and very small. The other variety, *erecta*, has much stouter stems, not rooting at the nodes and not decumbent, but erect or sub-erect, 8 to 12 inches high. It is rarer, but the best for cultivation, as it can be reaped and tied up in bundles easily, whereas the stems of *decumbens* form a dense green turf, the flowering stems, sparingly produced, lying on the leafy cushions of the plant. There are other varieties on the Continent. The plant has been introduced into North and South America. It is mentioned in the Herbals of the New World as one of the plants the Pilgrim Fathers introduced.

It is found wild and naturalized throughout the civilized world in strong, moist soil on the borders of ponds and streams, and near pools on heaths and commons. Gerard speaks of it as found abundantly

'on a common at Mile End, near London, about the holes and ponds thereof, in sundrie places, from whence poore women bring plenty to sell in London markets.'

Turner says:

'It crepeth much upon the ground and hath many little round leves not unlyke the leves of mesierum gentil, but that they are a little longer and sharper and also little indented rounde about, and grener than the leves of mariurum ar. The leves grow in little branches even from the roote of certayn ioyntes by equall spaces one devyded from an other. Whereas the leves grow in little tuftes upon the over partes of the braunches. . . . Pennyroyal groweth much, without any setting, besyd hundsley (Hounslow) upon the heth beside a watery place.'

Like most of its near relatives, Pennyroyal is highly aromatic, perhaps even more so than any other Mint, containing an essential oil resembling in properties that of other mints, though less powerful. The flavour is more pungent and acrid and less agreeable than that of Spearmint or Peppermint.

Pennyroyal was in high repute among the Ancients. Both Pliny and Dioscorides described its numerous virtues. In Northern Europe it was also much esteemed, as may be inferred from the frequent references to it in the Anglo-Saxon and Welsh works on medicine.

'The boke of Secretes of Albertus Magnus of the vertues of Herbes, Stones and certaine Beastes' states that, by putting drowning flies and bees in warm ashes of Pennyroyal, 'they shall recover their lyfe after a little tyme as by ye space of one houre' and be revived.

Pennyroyal is often found in cottage gardens, as an infusion of the leaves, known as Pennyroyal Tea, is an old-fashioned remedy for colds and menstrual derangements.

¶ *Cultivation.* Locally, Pennyroyal grows abundantly, but being required by the hundredweight it has been cultivated to a certain extent in this country, on account of the difficulty of obtaining sufficient quantities from the widely separated localities in which it is found.

As a crop, it presents uncertainty, being diminished by drought, its natural habitat being on moist heaths and commons by the sides of pools. It is easily grown from seed and succeeds best in loamy soil, in a moist situation, but propagation is commonly by division of old roots in autumn or spring, March or April, like Spearmint, or more rarely by cuttings. The roots may be divided up in September where the winters are mild, in April where the winters are frosty.

In planting, allow a space of 12 inches between the rows and 6 inches between the plants in the row. Water shortly afterwards should the weather be at all dry. When a good stock of healthy roots has been obtained, Pennyroyal may be forced with advantage. The creeping underground roots grow in horizontal masses, as with the other mints, and if some of these are taken up at any time during the winter and laid out on a bed of good soil, covering them with 2 or 3 inches of the same, they will soon push up fresh shoots in quantity. They can be put in boxes in a moderately warm house or pit. If all the tops are not wanted they may be made into cuttings, each with four or five joints, and, inserted in boxes of light, sandy soil, will soon form roots in the same temperature, and after being duly hardened off, may be planted out in the open, in due course, and a healthy, vigorous stock thus be maintained. Towards the close of autumn all the stalks that remain should be cut down to the ground and the bed covered with fresh soil to the depth of 1 inch.

Plantations generally last for four or five years when well managed and on favourable soil, but frosts may cause the crop to die off in patches, so it is a safe plan to make new plantings yearly.

¶ *Harvesting.* Pennyroyal is mostly sold in the dry state for making tea, the stems being cut when the plant is just about to flower and dried in the usual manner.

¶ *Constituents.* The fresh herb yields about 1 per cent. of a volatile oil, oil of Pulegium, a yellow or greenish-yellow liquid, obtained by distillation, and having a strong aromatic odour and taste. The chief constituent is ketone pulegone.

A yield of 12 lb. of oil to the acre of crop is considered good.

¶ *Medicinal Action and Uses.* Pliny gives a long list of disorders for which Pennyroyal was a supposed remedy, and especially recommends it for hanging in sleeping rooms, it being considered by physicians as more conducive to health even than roses.

It was likewise thought to communicate its purifying qualities to water, and Gerard tells us: 'If you have Pennyroyale in great quantity dry and cast it into corrupt water, it helpeth it much, neither will it hurt them that drink thereof.' As a purifier of the blood, it was highly spoken of: 'Penny-royale taken with honey cleanseth the lungs and cleareth the breast from all gross and thick humours.'

It was deemed by our ancestors valuable in headaches and giddiness. We are told: 'A garland of Penny-royale made and worn about the head is of great force against the swimming in the head and the pains and giddiness thereof.'

Pennyroyal Water was distilled from the leaves and given as an antidote to spasmodic, nervous and hysterical affections. It was also used against cold and 'affections of the joints.'

Culpepper says of Pennyroyal:

'Drank with wine, it is good for venomous bites, and applied to the nostrils with vinegar revives those who faint and swoon. Dried and burnt, it strengthens the gums, helps the gout, if applied of itself to the place until it is red, and applied in a plaster, it takes away spots or marks on the face; applied with salt, it profits those that are splenetic, or liver-grown. . . . The green herb bruised and put into vinegar, cleanses foul ulcers and takes away the marks of bruises and blows about the eyes, and burns in the face, and the leprosy, if drank and applied outwardly. . . . One spoonful of the juice sweetened with sugar-candy is a cure for hooping-cough.'

Its action is carminative, diaphoretic, stimulant and emmenagogic, and is principally employed for the last-named property in disorders caused by sudden chill or cold.

It is also beneficial in cases of spasms, hysteria, flatulence and sickness, being very warming and grateful to the stomach.

The infusion of 1 oz. of herb to a pint of boiling water is taken warm in teacupful doses, frequently repeated, and the oil is also given on sugar, as well as being made up into pills and other preparations.

In France and Germany oil of Pennyroyal is also used commercially.

¶ *Preparations and Dosages.* Fluid extract, $\frac{1}{4}$ to 1 drachm. Essence, 5 to 20 drops. Oil, $\frac{1}{2}$ to 3 drops.

The following is reprinted by special permission from *Punch*:

PENNYROYAL. – A CAROL

'Far away in Sicily!'
    A home-come sailor sang this rhyme,
Deep in an ingle, mug on knee,
    At Christmas time.

In Sicily, as I was told,
    The children take them Pennyroyal,
The same as lurks on hill and wold
    In Cotsall soil.

The Pennyroyal of grace divine
    In little cradles they do weave –
Little cradles therewith they line
    On Christmas Eve.

And there, as midnight bells awake
    The Day of Birth, as they do tell,
All into bud the small buds break
    With sweetest smell.

All into bud that very hour;
    And pure and clean, as they do say,
The Pennyroyal's full in flower
    On Christmas Day.

Far away in Sicily!
    Hark, the Christmas bells do chime!
So blossom love in thee and me
    This Christmas time!
                                W. B.

December 19, 1917.

See MINTS.

PEPPER   Piper nigrum (LINN.)
                                    N.O. Piperaceæ

Synonyms. Black Pepper. Piper (United States Pharmacopœia)
Part Used. Dried unripe fruit
Habitat. In South India wild, and in Cochin-China; also cultivated in East and West Indies, Malay Peninsula, Malay Archipelago, Siam, Malabar, etc.

¶ *Description.* The best Pepper of commerce comes from Malabar. Pepper is mentioned by Roman writers in the fifth century. It is said that Attila demanded among other items 3,000 lb. of Pepper in ransom for the city of Rome. Untrained, the plant will climb 20 or more feet, but for commercial purposes it is restricted to 12 feet. It is a perennial with a round, smooth, woody stem, with articulations, swelling near the joints and branched; the leaves are entire, broadly ovate, acuminate, coriaceous, smooth, with seven nerves; colour dark green and attached by strong sheath-like foot-stalks to joints of branches. Flowers small, white, sessile, covering a tubular spadix; fruits globular, red berries when ripe, and surface coarsely wrinkled. The plant is propagated by cuttings and grown at the base of trees with a rough, prickly bark to support them. Between three or four years after planting they commence fruiting and their productiveness ends about the fifteenth year. The berries are collected as soon as they turn red and before they are quite ripe; they are then dried in the sun. In England, for grinding they mix Peppers of different origin. Malabar for weight, Sumatra for colour, and Penang for strength. Pepper has an aromatic odour, pungent and bitterish taste.

¶ *Constituents.* Piperine, which is identical in composition to morphia, volatile oil, a resin called Chavicin. Its medicinal activities depends mainly on its pungent resin and volatile oil, which is colourless, turning yellow with age, with a strong odour, and not so acrid a taste as the peppercorn; it also contains starch, cellulose and colouring.

The concrete oil is a deep green colour and very acrid.

¶ *Medicinal Action and Uses.* Aromatic, stimulant, carminative; is said to possess febrifuge properties. Its action as a stimulant is specially evident on the mucous membrane of the rectum, and so is good for constipation, also on the urinary organs; externally it is a rubefacient, useful in relaxed conditions of the rectum when prolapsed; sometimes used in place of cubebs for gonorrhœa; given in combination with aperients to facilitate their action, and to prevent griping. As a gargle it is valued for relaxed uvula, paralysis of the tongue. On account of its stimulant action it aids digestion and is specially useful in atonic dyspepsia and torbid condition of the stomach. It will correct flatulence and nausea. It has also been used in vertigo, paralytic and arthritic disorders. It is sometimes added to quinine when the stomach will not respond to quinine alone. It has also been advised in diarrhœa, cholera, scarlatina, and in solution for a wash for *tinea capititis.* Piperine should not be combined with astringents, as it renders them inert.

¶ *Dosages.* Black Pepper, 5 to 15 grains in powder. Piperine, 1 to 8 grains.

The root of the Pepper plant in India has been used by the natives as a cordial tonic and stimulant.

B.P. dose of Pepper, 1 to 2 drachms.

Oleoresin, U.S.P.: dose, ½ grain.

Heliotropin is recommended medicinally as an antiseptic and antipyretic. It is obtained by the oxidation of piperic acid and is used in perfumery. From the time of Hippocrates Pepper has been used as a medicine and condiment.

¶ *Adulteration of Pepper.* Linseed mustard seed, wheat and pea-flour, sago, ground rice. At one time when the duty levied on Pepper was very high, fictitious peppercorns were made of oil-cake, clay, with a little cayenne added.

¶ *Other Species Used.*
Piper trioicum, nearly allied to *P. nigrum,* is also used in commerce.

The female plant does not ripen properly, and is deficient in pungency, but the Peppers on plants with hermaphrodite flowers on same spike are very pungent, and equal to the best Malabar Pepper.

WHITE PEPPER (*Piper album*).

From the same plant as *P. nigrum,* White Pepper is ripe fruit, partially deprived of its pericarp by maceration in water, then rubbed and dried in the sun. It contains albuminous seed, having small starch grains, taste and smell like Pepper, more aromatic than black and not so pungent. Same as the black, but containing more starch and less ash. Sold as whole White Pepper or broken White Pepper. The removed hulls are sold separately as Pepper hulls, and form a brownish powder, very pungent in smell and flavour and containing a large quantity of oleoresin of Pepper, but no piperine.

Sometimes the hulls are mixed with the broken White Pepper; this mixture has more oleoresin in it and less piperine.

¶ *Medicinal Action and Uses.* Teaspoonful doses taken several times a day are recommended to overcome the obstinate constipation of dyspeptics.

LONG PEPPER (*Piper longum*).

Part Used. The dried, unripe spikes of *Pipers officinum* and *longum*.

Habitat. Java, India, Philippines, the best coming from Batavia, and Singapore.

P. officinarum is principally used and is considered the best; both are gathered when green, when they are hotter than when quite ripe. In *P. officinarum* the fruit is a dark grey colour with a weak aromatic odour and a very fiery pungent taste. In *P. longum* the fruits are shorter and thicker and the constituents almost identical with *P. nigrum*. It contains piperine, a soft green resin, a burning acridity, a volatile oil which possibly gives it its odour; it is inferior to *P. nigrum* and most used as its adulterant.

PIPER BETEL.

Habitat. East Indies.

The leaves are used to wrap round areca nut; rubbed with shell lime they are chewed by the Indians to sweeten their breath and strengthen the stomach. The trade in it forms considerable commerce. The Asiatic use of it amongst men destroys the teeth from the lime used with it. The women of the Malabar Coast, on the other hand, stain their teeth black with antimony, which preserves theirs to old age.

PIPER AMALAGO, or rough-leaved Pepper, a shrub growing up to 10 feet. It is called the small-grained Black Pepper, and grows on the hilly parts of Jamaica. The berries differ only in size from the East Indian Black Pepper, being only the size of mustard seed, good for seasoning, taste and flavour being the same as Black Pepper. It is picked when full-grown before it ripens, otherwise it loses its pungency and grows soft and succulent.

It is dried in the sun and often left on its stalks, which have the same flavour and pungency as the Peppers and are as easily ground in the mills.

¶ *Medicinal Action and Uses.* Leaves and tender shoots are used in discutient baths and fomentations and pounded for application to ulcers; root is warm and very useful as a resolutive and sudorific or diaphoretic, but best for infusions and decoctions; a good de-obstruent for dropsy.

PIPER PELLUCIDUM, or pellucoid-leaved Pepper.

Habitat. South America and West Indian Islands.

¶ *Description.* An annual found growing on moist, gravelly banks, etc.

Has very small berries each containing a small seed like dust. In Martinico the leaves are eaten with lettuce, vinegar and oil as a salad and called 'Cresson,' but they are too strong and hot for most Europeans.

PIPER ROTUNDIFOLIUM.

Habitat. Jamaica and Martinique.

A herbaceous plant living in close, moist woods covering the trunks of old trees and stones.

¶ *Description.* Leaves greasy, bright green, fragrant, reviving odour; good aromatics and cephalics, retaining perfume several years; water distilled from them smells deliciously of the plants.

PIPER UMBELLATUM.

Synonyms. Unbelled Pepper. Santa Maria Leaf.

Habitat. Jamaica.

This plant is a very common annual and found growing up to 4 feet high. Has large round leaves; the root is a warm, active remedy against poisons, and in many parts of the sugar colonies is made up into a syrup much used by the inhabitants for colds and catarrhs.

PEPPER, HUNGARIAN

Synonyms. Paprika. Sweet Pepper. Grains of Paradise

Paprika, or Hungarian Pepper, a tasteless cayenne, is recognized by the German Pharmacopœia, and in the United States is imported in three grades. The first grade is savoury and of a fine red colour; it is made of the selected pericarp, the stems and placenta removed, the seeds first washed, then ground. The second grade is made by grinding the entire pod with the stems. Third grade is all the waste and spoiled pods being ground together, the residue of other grades. This is a yellowish colour and much more pungent than the other. Paprika is generally made

from *Croton annum*, and sometimes called Sweet Pepper. It is mostly used to dilute the strength of other powdered chillies, and it is used by bird fanciers to improve the colour of canaries.[1]

Grains of Paradise, Guinea Grains, Melegueta or Mallaguetta Pepper, from *Ampelopsis Grana Paradisi*, or *Habzeli* of Ethiopia (Kanang of Ethiopia). Two kinds of these grains are known in the English markets, one plumper than the other. One may be that imported into America from West Africa, and into England from plants introduced into Deme-

---

[1] This is the paprika which flavours so many Hungarian dishes. – EDITOR.

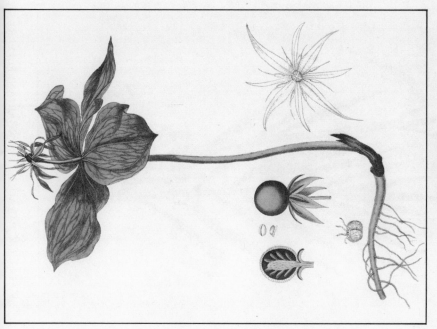

HERB PARIS
Paris Quadrifolia

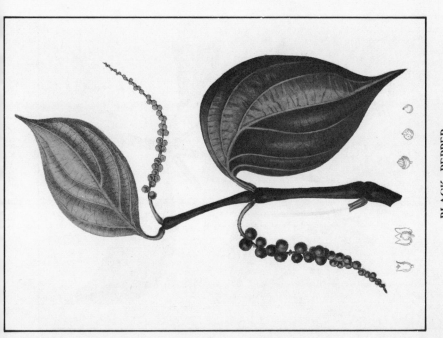

BLACK PEPPER
Piper Nigrum

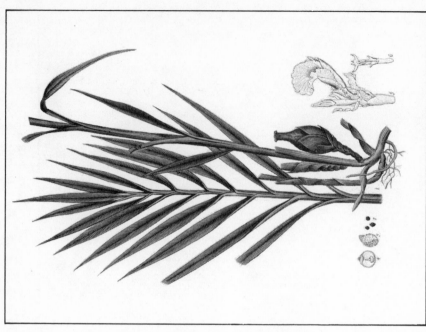

GRAINS OF PARADISE (HUNGARIAN PEPPER)

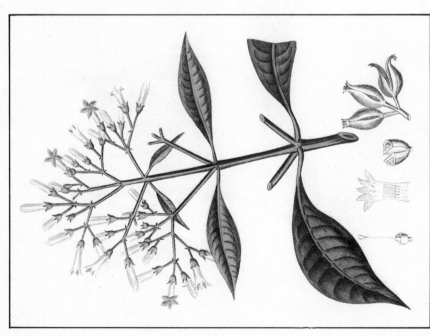

PERUVIAN BARK

rara, where they are thought to be a product of *A. Melegueta*. They resemble Pepper in their effects, but are seldom used except in veterinary practice and to give strength to spirits, wine, beer, and vinegar. The seeds have a rich reddish-brown colour.

PEPPERMINT. *See* MINTS

PERIWINKLES

GREATER PERIWINKLE (*Vinca major*, Linn.)

This is the species more generally used in herbal medicine, as an astringent and tonic, in menorrhagia and in hæmorrhages, also as a laxative, and gargle. Made into an ointment, useful for piles and inflammatory conditions of the skin.

LESSER PERIWINKLE (*Vinca minor*, Linn.)

Employed in homœopathy for preparation of a tincture used for hæmorrhages.

MADAGASCAR PERIWINKLE (*Vinca rosea*, Linn.)

A reputed cure for diabetes. (Synonym *Lochnera rosea*, Reichb.)

The well-known Periwinkles – both Greater and Lesser – familiar plants of our woods and gardens, are members of the genus *Vinca*, so named by Linnæus, which includes *five* in Europe, and the Orient, and three species native to the East Indies, Madagascar and America, assigned by a later botanist, Reichberg, to a separate genus, *Lochnera*, as they differ from Vinca in the stamens and head of the style not being hairy, though the main characteristics are the same.

Vinca is a genus of the natural order Apocynaceæ, which includes many tropical trees and shrubs with showy flowers, a large number of which are very poisonous, among these being the beautiful Oleander, so frequently grown in our greenhouses.

The Periwinkles are the only representatives of their order in our flora, and there is, in fact, considerable doubt among botanists whether the Periwinkle should be considered a true native of Great Britain. It was a familiar flower in the days of Chaucer, who refers to it as the 'fresh Pervinke rich of hew,' and it is now commonly found in woods and hedgerows, and, where it occurs, is generally in great profusion.

The plant is perennial and retains its glossy leaves throughout the winter. Occasionally, in the smaller kind, when cultivated in gardens, leaves occur with streaks of lighter green upon the dark rich colour that is characteristic of the rest of the foliage. The leaves are always placed in pairs on the stem, the flowers springing from their axils. In the Greater Periwinkle, the leaves are large and egg-shaped, with the margins minutely fringed. Those of the Lesser are much smaller, myrtle-like in form, their margins not fringed.

The plant seldom, if ever, ripens its seed, a

N.O. Apocynaceæ

fact that has been considered confirmatory of the theory that the Periwinkle is not truly indigenous, as in more southern countries it does so. It propagates itself by long, trailing and rooting stems, and by their means not only extends itself in every direction, but succeeds in obtaining an almost exclusive possession of the soil, since little or nothing else can maintain its ground against the dense mass of stems, which deprive other and weaker plants of light and air.

The flowers of the Periwinkle vary somewhat in intensity of colour, but the average colour is a deep purplish-blue. A white variety of the Lesser Periwinkle occurs in Devonshire and in gardens; it is often met with bearing purple, blue and white flowers, sometimes double.

The calyx is deeply cleft into five very narrow divisions. The corolla consists of a distinctly tubular portion terminating in a broad flat disk, composed of five broad lobes, twisted when in bud, curiously irregular in form, having the sides of the margin unequally curved, so that although the effect of the whole corolla is symmetrical, when each separate lobe is examined, it will be seen that an imaginary line from apex to the centre of the flower would divide it into two very unequal portions – very unusual in the petals of a flower. The whole effect is as if the lobes of the corolla were rotating round the mouth of its tube, and the movement had suddenly been arrested.

The mouth of the tube is angular and the tube closed with hairs, and the curiously curved anthers of the stamens, which are five in number, are inserted in the tube. The pistil of this flower, as well as of the smaller species, is a singularly beautiful object, resembling the shaft of a pillar with a double capital. The anthers stand above the stigmatic disk, but the stigma itself is on the under surface of the disk, so that self-fertilization is not caused as the insect's tongue enters the flowers.

The Lesser Periwinkle is not only smaller in all the parts, but has a more trailing habit of growth, matting itself together. The stems are very slender, only those bearing flowers being erect, growing to a height of 6 to 8 inches, the others trailing and rooting freely at intervals, so that a large space of ground is quickly monopolized by it.

Both the English and botanical names of the Periwinkle are derived from the Latin *vincio* (to bind), in allusion to these long, trailing stems that spread over and keep down the other plants where it grows. This is described by Wordsworth:

'Through primrose tufts in that sweet bower
The fair periwinkle trailed its wreaths.'

It is assumed that the *Vincapervinca* of Pliny is this plant.

¶ *History.* The old English form of the name, as it appears in early Anglo-Saxon Herbals, as well as in Chaucer, was 'Parwynke,' and we also find it called 'Joy of the Ground.' In Macer's *Herbal* (early sixteenth century) it is described:

'Parwynke is an erbe grene of colour
In Tyme of May he beryth blo flour,
His stalkys ain (are) so feynt and feye
Yet never more growyth he hey (high).'

And we are also told that 'men calle it ye Juy of Grownde.'

In more modern days it has locally been called 'Ground Ivy,' though that name is now generally assigned to quite another little, blue-flowered plant of the hedgerow, *Glechoma hederacea*. In Gloucestershire, we find the name 'Cockles' given locally to it; in Hampshire, its name is corrupted to 'Pennywinkle.' In some parts of Devonshire, the flowers from their use are known as 'Cut Finger,' and the more fanciful name of 'Blue Buttons' is also there given to it. In France, it has been known as *Pucellage*, or Virginflower, no doubt also from the madonnablue of its blossoms.

An old name, given both in reference to its colour and its use in magic, was 'Sorcerer's Violet' (corresponding to its old French name '*Violette des sorciers*'). It was a favourite flower with 'wise folk' for making charms and love-philtres. It was one of the plants believed to have power to exorcize evil spirits. In Macer's *Herbal* we read of its potency against 'wykked spirytis.'

Apuleius, in his *Herbarium* (printed 1480), gives elaborate directions for its gathering:

'This wort is of good advantage for many purposes, that is to say, first against devil sickness and demoniacal possessions and against snakes and wild beasts and against poisons and for various wishes and for envy and for terror and that thou mayst have grace, and if thou hast the wort with thee thou shalt be prosperous and ever acceptable. This wort thou shalt pluck thus, saying, "I pray thee, vinca pervinca, thee that art to be had for thy many useful qualities,

that thou come to me glad blossoming with thy mainfulness, that thou outfit me so that I be shielded and ever prosperous and undamaged by poisons and by water"; when thou shalt pluck this wort, thou shalt be clean of every uncleanness, and thou shalt pick it when the moon is nine nights old and eleven nights and thirteen nights and thirty nights and when it is one night old.'

These superstitions about the Periwinkle are of great age and are repeated by all the old writers. In *The Boke of Secretes of Albartus Magnus of the Vertues of Herbs, Stones and certaine Beastes*, we find:

'Perwynke when it is beate unto pouder with worms of ye earth wrapped about it and with an herbe called houslyke, it induceth love between man and wyfe if it bee used in their meales . . . if the sayde confection be put in the fyre it shall be turned anone unto blue coloure.'

In olden days it was used in garlands. An old chronicle tells us that when, in 1306, Simon Fraser, after he had been taken prisoner fighting for William Wallace, rode heavily ironed through London to the place of execution, a garland of Periwinkle was placed in mockery on his head.

The flower is called by the Italians *Centocchio*, or 'Hundred Eyes,' but it is also called 'The Flower of Death,' from the ancient custom of making it into garlands to place on the biers of dead children. To the Germans, it is the 'Flower of Immortality.' In France, the Periwinkle is considered an emblem of friendship, probably in allusion to Rousseau's recollection of his friend Madame de Warens, after a lapse of thirty years, by the sight of the Periwinkle in flower.

¶ *Uses.* Both species of Periwinkle are used in medicine for their acrid, astringent and tonic properties.

'The Periwinkle is a great binder,' said an old herbalist, and both Dioscorides and Galen commended it against fluxes. Culpepper says that it

'stays bleeding at the mouth and nose, if it be chewed . . . and may be used with advantage in hysteric and other fits. . . . It is good in nervous disorders, the young tops made into a conserve is good for the night-mare. The small periwinkle possesses all the virtues of the other kind and may very properly supply its place.'

It was considered a good remedy for cramp, Lord Bacon himself testifying that a limb suffering from cramp would be cured if bands of green Periwinkle were tied round it;

and William Coles, in his *Adam in Eden* (1657), gives a definite case of a friend who was

'vehemently tormented with the cramp for a long while which could be by no means eased till he had wrapped some of the branches hereof about his limbs.'

An ointment prepared from the bruised leaves with lard has been largely used in domestic medicine and is reputed to be both soothing and healing in all inflammatory ailments of the skin and an excellent remedy for bleeding piles.

Vinca major is used in herbal practice for its astringent and tonic properties in menorrhagia and in hæmorrhages generally. For obstructions of mucus in the intestines and lungs, diarrhœa, congestions, hæmorrhages, etc., Periwinkle Tea is a good remedy. In cases of scurvy and for relaxed sore throat and inflamed tonsils, it may also be used as a gargle. For bleeding piles, it may be applied externally, as well as taken internally.

A homœopathic tincture is prepared from the fresh leaves of *Vinca minor* and

'is given medicinally for the milk-crust of infants as well as for internal hæmorrhages, the dose being from 2 to 10 drops, three or four times in the day, with a spoonful of water.'

PERUVIAN BALSAM. *See* BALSAM

PERUVIAN BARK

The flowers of the Greater (and probably also of the Lesser) Periwinkle are gently purgative, but lose their effect on drying. If gathered in the spring and made into a syrup, they will impart thereto all their virtues, and this, it is stated, is excellent as a gentle laxative for children and also for overcoming chronic constipation in grown persons.

The bruised leaves put into the nostrils will, it is asserted, allay bleeding from the nose.

A still more important use has been found for another species, *V. rosea*, Linn. (synonym *Lochnera rosea*, Reichb.), sometimes known as the Madagascar Periwinkle, a small undershrub up to 3 feet high in its native habitat, the general appearance much resembling our English species, *V. major*, but with the stems more upright. It is widely spread in Tropical Africa and naturalized in the Tropics in general. It is not sufficiently hardy to stand our climate without protection, though it is often grown in conservatories in this country. The blossoms are a rich crimson.

In 1923, considerable interest was aroused in the medical world by the statement that this species of *Vinca* had the power to cure diabetes, and would probably prove an efficient substitute for Insulin, but *V. major* has long been used by herbalists for this purpose.

¶ *Preparation.* Fluid extract.

Cinchona succirubra (PAVON.)
N.O. Rubiaceæ

Synonyms. Red Bark. Jesuits' Powder. Cinchona Bark
Part Used. Bark dried from stem and branches
Habitat. South America, but cultivated in India, Java, Ceylon, etc.

¶ *Description.* The species most cultivated in India and elsewhere are *Cinchona succirubra*, or Peruvian Bark, and *C. officinalis*. These evergreen trees grow in the hottest part of the world and are said to constitute a twenty-ninth part of the whole flowering plants of the tropics. Peruvian bark was introduced to Europe in 1640, but the plant producing it was not known to botanists till 1737; a few years later it was renamed Cinchona after the Countess of Chinchon, who first made the bark known in Europe for its medicinal qualities. The history of Cinchona and its many vicissitudes affords a striking illustration of the importance of Government aid in establishing such an industry. It was known and used by the Jesuits very early in its history, but was first advertized for sale in England by James Thompson in 1658, and was made official in the London Pharmacopœia of 1677. The

bark is spongy, very slight odour, taste astringent and strongly bitter.

¶ *Constituents.* Alkaloids, quinine, cinchonidine, cinchonine, quinidine, hydrocinchonidine, quinamine, homocinchonidine, hydroquinine, quinic and cincholannic acids, bitter amorphous glucoside, starch and calcium oxalate. The history of the formation of the alkaloids, in different parts and age of the tree, is interesting. The process of 'mossing' introduced by Mr. M'Ivor, viz. the protection of the bark from light and air by layers of damp moss, increases the quantity of the alkaloids, allows of the periodical renewal of the bark, and increases the quantity of the alkaloid in the new bark.

¶ *Medicinal Action and Uses.* Febrifuge, tonic and astringent; valuable for influenza, neuralgia and debility. Large and too constant doses must be avoided, as they

631

produce headache, giddiness and deafness. The liquid extract is useful as a cure for drunkenness. The powdered bark is often used in tooth-powders, owing to its astringency, but not much used internally (except as a bitter wine); it creates a sensation of

PHEASANT'S EYE. *See* (FALSE) HELLEBORE

PICHI

Synonym. Fabiana
Parts Used. Dried leaf and twig
Habitat. Chile, Peru, Bolivia, and Argentine Republic

Fabiana imbricata (RUTZ. and PARON.)
N.O. Solanaceæ

¶ *Description.* A neat half-hardy shrub, very like a heath in general appearance. Fastigiate habit, has small branches covered with scale-like imbricated leaves, colour bluish green, leaves are smooth, entire, flowers solitary, terminal, corolla tubular, usually white, sometimes purple. A dwarf decorative plant; will grow in warmer parts of England; it needs a bright sheltered sunny spot, and would do well on a rockery. The fruit is a capsule containing a few sub-globular seeds. The odour of the drug is aromatic, the taste bitter, and terebinthinate.

¶ *Constituents.* Volatile oil, fat, resin, bitter fluorescent glucoside, and an alkaloid fabianine and tannin.

¶ *Medicinal Action and Uses.* Tonic, cholagogue, a valuable terebinthic diuretic,

warmth, but sometimes causes gastric intestinal irritation. Cinchona in decoction is a useful gargle and a good throat astringent.
¶ *Dosage.* 3 to 10 grains.

See CALISAYA.

largely used in acute vesical catarrh, giving very favourable results where urinary irritation is caused by gravel. Is said to ease the irritability and assist in the expulsion of renal, urethal or cystic calculi, very useful in the treatment of jaundice and dyspepsia due to lack of biliary secretion. Is contraindicated in organic disease of the kidneys, though cases of renal hæmorrhages from Bright's disease have been greatly benefited by its use; it has been used also for gonorrhœa and gonorrhœal prostatitis.

¶ *Dosage.* Solid extract, 2 to 10 grains. Fluid extract, 1 to 40 minims.

A strong tincture is made from the resinoid precipitate and is considered the best preparation of the drug.

PILEWORT. *See* CELANDINE

PIMPERNEL, SCARLET

Anagallis arvensis (LINN.)
N.O. Primulaceæ

Synonyms. Shepherd's Barometer. Poor Man's Weatherglass. Adder's Eyes
   (*Old English*) Bipinella
Parts Used. Leaves, herb
Habitat. The Scarlet Pimpernel grows on the roadside in waste places and on the dry sandy edges of corn and other fields; it is widely distributed, not only over Britain, but throughout the world, being found in all the temperate regions in both hemispheres

¶ *Description.* Its creeping, square stems, a foot in length at most, have their egg-shaped, stalkless leaves arranged in pairs. The edges of the leaves are entire (i.e. quite free from indentations of any sort), and in whatever direction the stem may run, either along the ground, or at an angle to it, the leaves always keep their faces turned to the light.

The Pimpernel flowers from May until late into August. The flowers appear singly, each on longish, thin stalks, springing from the junction of each leaf with the stem. The little flower-stalks are erect during flowering, but curved backward when the seed is ripening. The corolla is made up of five

petals, joined together at their base into a ring. A purple spot often appears in the centre of the flower. The petals are very sensitive, the flowers closing at once if the sky becomes overcast and threatens rain. Even in bright weather, the flowers are only open for a comparatively short time – never opening until between eight and nine in the morning and shutting up before three o'clock in the afternoon. As the petals are only brilliantly coloured on their upper faces, the flowers when closed disappear from view among the greenness of the leaves.

Inside the petals are five stamens, each standing exactly opposite to a petal. Upon the stamens are a number of delicate, violet hairs, which seem to serve as a bait to insects, taking the place, perhaps, of honey, of which the Pimpernel has none.

As the autumn comes on, the fruit in the centre of each flower swells and ripens. It is in the form of a little urn or capsule, full of tiny seeds. When the latter are quite ripe, the urn splits round its circumference into two halves – the upper half lifts up like a lid and the seeds are shaken out with every movement of the wind.

Propagation is entirely by seeds, as the plant is an annual, completely dying at the end of each season, both above and below ground.

A blue variety of an intense deep colour is occasionally found in Great Britain, and more commonly in central and southern Europe. A number of scientific experiments have been made on these blue and red Pimpernels by Darwin, Henslow and others. Henslow found that of the offspring of the blue, some had red and some blue petals, while Darwin discovered that by crossing the red and blue, some of the offspring were red, some blue, and some an intermediate colour. Gerard thought that the scarlet variety was the male plant, and that the blue was the female.

This blue variety (*Anagallis cerulea*) is described as growing in beautiful little tufts about the hills of Madeira.

The common variety (*A. arvensis*) is mentioned in lists of plants growing in Persia, Nepaul, China, New Holland, Mauritius, Cape of Good Hope, Japan, Egypt, Abyssinia, U.S.A., Mexico, and Chile. It is to be found in all the temperate regions in both hemispheres, but shuns the Arctic cold and hardly bears more than the sub-tropical heat.

Occasionally flesh-coloured and pure white blossoms have been found as varieties of this plant.

The plant appears in the Herbals and Vocabularies of the sixteenth century as 'Bipinella,' a name originally applied to the Great and Salad Burnet. It was much used as a cosmetic herb. Howard, in *The Old Commodore*, 1837, says: 'If she'd only used my pimpernel water, for she has one monstrous freckle in her forehead.' The plant was also said to be a remedy for the bites of mad dogs and to dispel sadness.

This plant once had a great reputation in medicine, and was used as a universal panacea.

'No heart can think, no tongue can tell
The virtues of the Pimpernel.'

Pliny speaks of its value in liver complaints, and its generic name *Anagallis* (given it by Dioscorides) is derived from the Greek *Anagelao*, signifying 'to laugh,' because it removes the depression that follows liver troubles.

The Greeks used it for diseases of the eye, and Gerard and Culpepper affirm that 'it helpeth them that are dim-sighted,' the juice being mixed with honey and dropped into the eyes.

It is 'a gallant, Solar herb, of a cleansing attractive quality, whereby it draweth forth thorns and splinters gotten into the flesh.'

'Used inwardly and applied outwardly,' Culpepper tells us, 'it helpeth also all stinging and biting of venomous beasts or mad dogs.'

And again, 'the distilled water or juice is much celebrated by French dames to cleanse the skin from any roughness, deformity or discolourings thereof.'

Another old writer says 'the Herb Pimpernel is good to prevent witchcraft, as Mother Bumby doth affirm.'

¶ *Part Used*. The whole herb, gathered in the wild condition, when the leaves are at their best, in June, and used both fresh and dried.

Pimpernel has no odour, but a bitter taste, which is rather astringent.

¶ *Constituents*. The plant possesses very active properties, although its virtues are not fully understood. It is known to contain Saponin, such as the Soapwort also specially furnishes.

The leaves are sufficiently inert to be eaten in salads, of which they often form a component part in France and Germany, but Professor Henslow tells us that caged birds have died from eating them instead of Chickweed, which it somewhat resembles.

Experiments have shown that it contains some injurious properties which neither drying nor boiling destroys. Though too small to be eaten in quantities by browsing animals, an extract made from it has been found to have a strong narcotic effect on them and to be of such a poisonous nature as to cause the deaths of some dogs to whom it was experimentally given in considerable doses.

¶ *Medicinal Action and Uses*. Diuretic, diaphoretic and expectorant. The ancient reputation of Scarlet Pimpernel has survived to the present day, especially in dealing with diseases of the brain. Doctors have considered the herb remedial in melancholy and in the allied forms of mental disease, the decoction or a tincture being employed.

John Hill (*British Herbal*, 1756) tells us that the whole plant, dried and powdered, is good against epilepsy, and there are well authenticated accounts of this disease being absolutely cured by it. The flowers alone have also been found useful in epilepsy, 20 grains dried being given four times a day.

It is of a cordial sudorific nature, and a strong infusion of it has been considered an excellent medicine in feverish complaints, which it relieves by promoting a gentle perspiration. It was recommended by Culpepper on this account as a preservative in pestilential and contagious diseases. The same simple preparation has also been much used among country people in the first stages of pulmonary consumption, it being stated to have often checked the disorder and prevented its fatal consequences.

The dried leaves may be given in powder, or an infusion made of the whole plant dried, but according to Green (*Universal Herbal*, 1832) nothing equals the infusion of the fresh plant.

The expressed juice has been found serviceable in the beginnings of dropsies and in obstructions of the liver and spleen. A tincture has also been used for irritability of the urinary passages, having been found effective in cases of stone and gravel.

In Gerard's days, a preparation of this herb, called 'Diacorallion,' was used for gout, and in California a fluid extract is given for rheumatism, in doses of 1 teaspoonful with water, three times a day.

Modern authorities consider that caution should be exercised in the use of this herb for dropsy, rheumatic affections, hepatic and renal complaints.

The tincture is made from the fresh leaves, in the proportion of 10 oz. to a pint of diluted alcohol; the dose is from 1 to 5 drops. A homœopathic tincture is also prepared from the flowers.

The powder of the dried leaves is given in 15 to 60 grain doses.

The seeds of the plant, which are very numerous, and enclosed in small capsules, are much eaten by birds.

¶ *Other Species*.

The BOG PIMPERNEL (*A. tenella*) is another of this species. Its blossoms are larger than those of the Scarlet Pimpernel, and of a pale rose colour, and the leaves which are numerous, are very small in proportion to the blossoms. It is found on marshy grounds, but is rare: it is a perennial; whereas the scarlet variety is an annual.

Gerard speaks of the '*pimpernel rose* in a pasture as you goe from a village hard by London called Knightsbridge unto Fulham, a village thereby.'

PINE

Various Species
N.O. Pinaceæ

Pines are among the most important commercial trees. Most of them have straight, unbranched, cylindrical trunks, which furnish large amounts of excellent saw timber. On account of the straight grain, strength, and other qualities of pine timber, it is used for nearly every sort of constructional work and the trade in it is enormous.

All the Pines yield *resin* in greater or smaller quantities, which is obtained by tapping the trees. The crude resin is almost entirely used for the distillation of *Oil of Turpentine* and *Rosin*, only small quantities being employed medicinally – for ointments, plasters, etc. When the Oil of Turpentine is entirely distilled off, the residuum is *Rosin* or *Colophony*, but when only part of the oil is extracted, the viscous mass remaining is known commercially as common *Crude Turpentine*.

Oil of Turpentine is a good solvent for many resins, wax, fats, caoutchouc, sulphur, and phosphorus, and is largely employed in making varnish, in oil-painting, etc. Medicinally, it is much employed in both general and veterinary practice as a rubefacient and vesicant, and is valuable as an antiseptic. It is used for horses and cattle internally as a vermifuge, and externally as a stimulant for rheumatic swellings, and for sprains and bruises, and to kill parasites.

Rosin is used not only by violinists, for rubbing their bows, but also in making sealing wax, varnish, and resinous soaps for sizing paper and *papier maché* and dressing hemp cordage, but one of its special uses is for making *brewer's pitch* for coating the insides of beer casks and for distilling resinous oils, when the *pitch* used by shoemakers is left as residuum. Pitch is also used in veterinary practice.

Tar is an impure turpentine, viscid and brown-black in colour, procured by destructive distillation from the roots of various coniferous trees, particularly from *Pinus sylvestris*. Tar is used medicinally, especially in veterinary practice, for its antiseptic, stimulant, diuretic and diaphoretic action. Tar-water is given to horses with chronic cough and used internally and externally as a cutaneous stimulant and antiseptic in eczema. Oil of Tar is used instead of Oil of Turpentine in the case of mange, etc.

A considerable industry has grown up in the United States in the distillation of Pine *wood* by means of steam under pressure. One of the products thus obtained, which has considerable commercial importance, is known as

Pine Oil. It has a pleasant odour, resembling that of caraway or Juniper Oil, and has been largely used for making paints which dry without gloss and as a 'flatting' material. It flows well under the brush and is a powerful solvent, and is useful for emulsion paints such as are now employed for inside work.

Pine resins are largely employed by the soap-maker for the manufacture of brown soaps.

The trade in resins was for many years almost exclusively a French industry, and only in France were the Pine forests turned to account for the production of resin on a commercial scale. Now, however, Switzerland, Sweden, Russia and North America furnish quantities, though, from the point of view of quality, the Pines which flourish near Bordeaux furnish a resin still much in request, and the turpentine extracted therefrom is abundant and one of the best qualities produced.

¶ *Medicinal Action and Properties.* Rubefacient, diuretic, irritant. A valuable remedy in bladder, kidney, and rheumatic affections and diseases of the mucous membrane and respiratory complaints; *externally* in the form of liniment plasters and inhalants.

¶ *Preparations and Dosages.* Oil of Turpentine. Spirits of Turpentine, B.P., 2 to 10 drops. As a vermifuge, 2 to 4 drachms. Tar, B.P., Pin. Sylv. Tar, U.S.P., Pin. Palust. Ointment Tar, B.P. Syrup Tar, U.S.P., 1 drachm.

See TAMARAC.

SPECIES OF PINES HAVING MEDICINAL PRODUCTS

Pinus balsamea. Abies canadensis. A. balsamea. Balsam Fir. Balm of Gilead Fir. Perusse. Hemlock Spruce.
Canada Turpentine. Pills for mucous discharge.
P. *Canadensis.* A. canadensis. Hemlock Spruce.
Pitch and Oil.
P. *Cedrus* of Mount Lebanon.
A false manna used in phthisis in Syria.
P. *Cembra* (Siberian Cedar or Tannenbaum). Europe and Asia.
Edible seeds eaten by Russians as nuts. Coniferin from the cambium.
P. *Cubensis.* Cuban Pine.
Turpentine.
P. *Damaris.* Agathis Damara.
Damara Turpentine that hardens into a hard rosin.
P. *Densiflora.* Japan.
An exudation called akamatsu. Timber.

P. *Echinata.* Short-leaved Pine.
Turpentine. Timber.
P. *Gerardiana.* Neosa Pine. N.W. India.
Edible seeds called neosa or chilgoza seeds.
P. *Halepensis.* Mediterranean countries.
Spirits of Turpentine.
P. *Heterophylla.* Eastern America.
Spirits of Turpentine. Timber.
P. *Khasya.* Burma.
Turpentine resembling French Oil.
P. *Larix.* Larix Europæa. A. larix. L. decidua. Larch.
Briançon manna, containing no mannite. Venice Turpentine.
P. *Maritima.* P. pinaster. Cluster Pine. Mediterranean countries.
Bordeaux Turpentine. Pitch. French Oil of Turpentine, 25 per cent.
P. *Merkusii.* Burma.
Turpentine resembling French Oil.
P. *Microcarpa.* P. pendula. L. Americana. Black or American Larch. Hackmatack. Tamarac.
A decoction of the bark used.
P. *Mughus.* Hungarian terebinth.
P. *Nigra.* Pieca Mariana. Black or Bog Spruce.
Decoction of young branches gives Essence of Spruce used for Spruce Beer.
P. *Palustris.* P. Australia. Long-leaved Pine. Yellow, Southern, Hard, Virginia.
Spirits of Turpentine, 17 per cent. oil. Carpets woven from leaves.
P. *Picea.* A. pectinata. Picea vulgaris. P. abies. A. vulgaris. A. alba. Spruce Fir. Norway Spruce.
Strassbourg Turpentine. Térébinthine au citron.
P. *Pinea.* Mediterranean countries.
Edible seeds. 'Pignons' or 'Pinocchi.'
P. *Ponderosa.* Heavy Pine. California.
Exudation is almost pure heptane; a chief constituent of American petroleum. Timber.
P. *Pumilio.* P. montana.
Volatile Oil from the leaves. Oil of Dwarf Pine Needles. Oil of Pine.
P. *Rigida.* Pitch Pine.
Tar.
P. *Roxburghii.* Himalayas.
Spirits of Turpentine.
P. *Sabiniana.* Nut or Digger Pine.
Turpentine, the oil being called abietene. Edible seeds.
P. *Scropica.*
Occasionally its Turpentine is used for American Rosin.
P. *Strobus.* P. alba. White Pine.
Coniferin from the Cambium Bark. Compound Syrup with Morphine. Timber.

P. Succinifera. Extinct.
Fossil resin or amber.
P. Sylvestris. Scotch Pine or Fir. Norway Pine.
Spirits of Turpentine, 32 per cent. of oil. Russian Turpentine. Finnan Turpentine is the oleoresin. Timber.

P. Toeda. Loblolly Pine. Old Field Pine. United States.
Occasionally its turpentine used for American rosin.
P. Teocoty. Mexican or Brea Turpentine.
P. Thunbergii. Japan.
Exudation called Kuromatsu. Timber.

PINE (LARCH)

Pinus larix (D.C.)
N.O. Coniferæ

Synonyms. Larix Europæa. Abies larix. Larix decidua. Laricis Cortex. Meleze. European Larch. Venice Turpentine
Part Used. The bark, deprived of its outer layer
Habitat. Central Europe

¶ *Description.* 'Larix' was the name given to Pine resin in the time of Dioscorides, and the term has been kept for these lofty trees. The leaves, bright green in spring, grow in small, spreading tufts like brushes. The male catkins, ½ inch long, are sessile and ovoid, with a cup of persistent bracts and inner, resinous, fringed, brown scales. The female cones, ¾ inch long, grow on short stalks, with hard, greyish-brown scales.

Larch is only indigenous to the hilly regions throughout Central Europe, where it forms large forests in the Alps, but it has for long been largely cultivated throughout Europe. It was first introduced into England in 1639.

It is one of the most valuable trees ever introduced into the country, both with respect to the rapidity of its growth (it grows six times quicker than Oak) and the value of its durable timber. Its wood is far tougher, stronger and more durable than that of any other conifer, excepting perhaps the Yew. Its durability makes it specially adapted for mining operations and there is also considerable demand for it for railway sleepers, because it lasts longer than any other kind of home-grown wood when under the wear and tear of traffic and the decomposing influence of damp, warmth, and fungi. It is also employed both in ship- and house-building, and in cabinet-work is capable of taking a very high polish. Gilding has a better effect on it than over almost any other, and it is a favourite for placing behind pictures, as it resists worm attacks. It is the one wood for which a ready sale can always be found in any part of the United Kingdom.

None of our forest trees is hardier than the Larch. The young trees establish themselves readily and soon grow rapidly. They are therefore, like the birch, used as 'nurses' for slow-growing and less hardy kinds of trees. The ground beneath a larch wood speedily improves in quantity and quality.

Large quantities of turpentine are collected from full-grown trees from May to October, holes being bored in the trunk and wooden tubes inserted. The exudation that flows is perfectly clear and needs no further preparation than straining through a coarse hair-cloth to free it from impurities. It was used in medicine and for making several kinds of varnish. In commerce it is known as 'Venice Turpentine,' being formerly exclusively exported from Venice. It is produced now mainly in the Tyrol, Switzerland, and Piedmont.

The frequently-found substitutes may be detected by their strong odour, and by drying into a hard varnish when painted on paper. The bark, which is not official in India or the United States, should be removed and stripped of its roughest outer portion in spring, and dried rapidly. In commerce it is found in flat pieces or quills of various sizes. The outer surface is rosy in colour, and the inner either yellowish or pinkish, easily separating into layers. It breaks with a close fracture, excepting the whitish fibres. The odour is a little like balsam and terebinth, and the taste astringent. The bark is sometimes used for tanning, but is inferior to oak, so that in Britain it is not always worth the cost of peeling and carriage.

¶ *Constituents.* The bark contains tannic acid, larixinic acid and turpentine. The larixin, a crystalline principle, resembles pyrogallol.

Briançon Manna is exuded from the leaves in summer. It is white and sweet, occurring in oblong tears and almost odourless. Its peculiar sugar is termed *Melezitose.* Its use is obsolete.

If the trees are burnt, a gum exudes from the trunk called *Gummi Orenbergense,* soluble in water like Gum Arabic.

¶ *Medicinal Action and Uses.* Stimulant, diuretic, astringent, balsamic and expectorant. As an external application it has been found useful in chronic eczema and psoriasis. Its chief official use is as a stimulant expec-

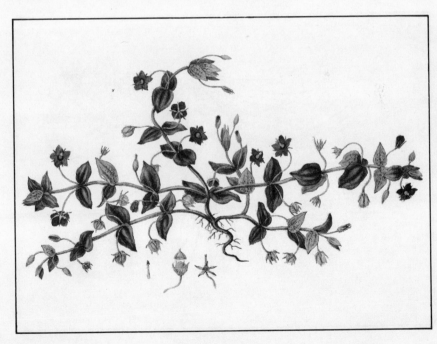

PELLITORY
Anacyclus Pyrethrum

SCARLET PIMPERNEL
Anagallis Arvensis

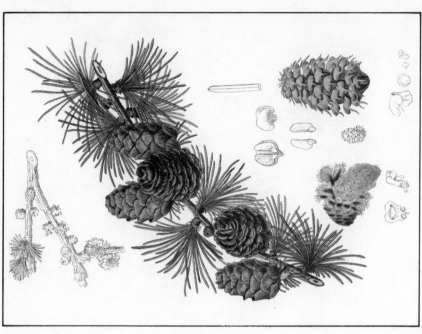

LARCH PINE
Pinus Larix

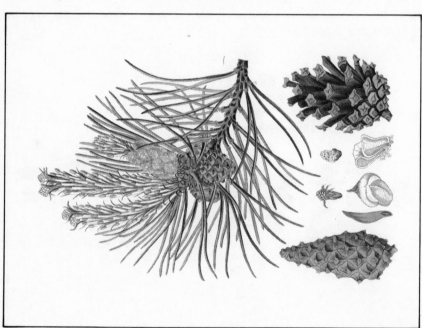

WILD PINE
Pinus Sylvestris

torant in chronic bronchitis, with much secretion. Its action is that of oil of turpentine.

It has also been given internally in hæmorrhage and cystitis.

The turpentine is used in veterinary practice. It has been suggested for combating poisoning by cyanide or opium, and as a disinfectant in hospital gangrene.

¶ *Dosage.* Of B.P. Tincture Laricis, 20 to 30 minims. Venice Turpentine.

See TAMARAC.

PINE, WHITE

Pinus strobus (LINN.)
N.O. Pinaceæ

Synonyms. Weymouth Pine. Pin du Lord. Pinus Alba
Part Used. Dried inner bark
Habitat. Eastern North America. Cultivated in Europe

¶ *Description.* The name of Weymouth Pine, common in Europe, refers to a Lord Weymouth who planted numbers of the trees shortly after their introduction in 1705. The French name is a similarly derived contraction.

In the United States it grows up to 200 feet in height, but rarely reaches half that stature in England. The wood is peculiarly adapted for the masts of ships, and in Queen Anne's reign legal measures were taken for the encouragement of its cultivation. The bark is very smooth, and the leaves grow in small bundles of five, the cylindrical cones being a little longer than these.

The bark is found in small, flattened pieces, the outer surface light, with a pinkish or yellowish tinge, sometimes patched with greyish-brown fragments, and the inner surface lighter or darker and finely striate. The tough, fibrous fracture shows yellowish and whitish layers. The odour is like terebinth, and the taste both bitter and sweet, astringent and mucilaginous.

¶ *Constituents.* The powder shows starch and resin. The bark yields a maximum of 3 per cent. of ash. It is a source of the terebinth of America. Coniferin is found in the cambium.

¶ *Medicinal Action and Uses.* Expectorant, demulcent, diuretic, a useful remedy in coughs and colds, having a beneficial effect on the bladder and kidneys.

The compound syrup contains sufficient morphine to assist in developing the morphine habit and should be used with caution.

¶ *Dosage.* Of Compound Syrup, 1 fluid drachm. Of Compound Syrup, with Morphine, 30 minims. Fluid Extract, ½ to 1 drachm.

(GROUND) PINE. *See* (YELLOW) BUGLE

PINE, AMERICAN GROUND. *See* (AMERICAN CLUB) MOSS

PINK ROOT

Spigelia Marylandica (LINN.)
N.O. Loganiaceæ

Synonyms. Indian Pink. Maryland Pink. Wormgrass. American Wormgrass. Carolina-, Maryland-, American-Wormroot. Starbloom
Parts Used. Dried rhizome and rootlets, or entire plant
Habitat. Southern United States of America

¶ *Description.* This herbaceous perennial plant has been known in commerce for many years and used to be collected by the Creek and Cherokee Indians for sale to the white traders. It is official in the United States Pharmacopœia. It has several smooth simple stems, arising from the same rhizome; these stems are rounded below and square above. Leaves, few, opposite, sessile, ovate-lanceolate, at apex acuminate, tapering at the base. The flowers are borne in a brilliant red-pink spike at top of the stem, the long corollas (terminating in spreading, star-like petals), externally red, yellow within, surrounding a double, many-seeded capsule. It grows in rich, dry soils on the edges of woods and flowers from May to July. The entire plant is collected in autumn and dried, but only the rhizome and rootlets are official in the United States Pharmacopœia, though in several other pharmacopœias on the Continent, in which Spigelia is official, a closely allied species is named and the flowering plant is specified. The rhizome is tortuous, knotty and dark-brown externally, with many thin, wiry motlets attached to it and the short branches on the upper side are marked with scars of the stems of former years; internally, the rhizome is whitish, with a dark-brown pith; the rootlets are lighter coloured than the rhizome, thin, brittle and long. Odour, aromatic; taste, bitter, sweetish, pungent and somewhat nauseous. It is usually powdered and then is of a greyish colour. Age impairs its strength. When imported from the Western United States, where it is very abundant, it is received in bales and casks.

¶ *Constituents.* A poisonous alkaloid, named Spigeline; also a bitter acrid principle, soluble in water or alcohol, but insoluble in ether; a small amount of volatile oil, a tasteless resin, tannin, wax, fat, mucilage, albumen, myricin, a viscid, saccharine substance, lignin, salts of sodium, potassium and calcium. The reactions of the poisonous alkaloid resemble those of nicotine, lobeline and coniine.

¶ *Medicinal Action and Uses.* Its chief use is as a very active and certain vermifuge, most potent for tapeworm and specially so for the round worm; its use was known among the Indians for worms long before America was discovered. It is a safe and efficient drug to give to children, if administered in proper doses and always followed by a saline aperient, such as magnesium sulphate, otherwise unpleasant and serious symptoms may occur, such as disturbed vision, dizziness, muscular spasms, twitching eyelids, increased action of the heart. In large doses, these are increased, both circulation and respiration being depressed and loss of muscular power caused, and cases have been known resulting, in children, in death from convulsions. It is also useful for children's fevers not caused by the irritation of vermin, such as those occurring from hydrocephalus.

¶ *Dosage.* The official U.S.P. preparation is the Fluid Extract: average dose, 1 fluid drachm.

It is also given in infusion and in powder.

It is often combined with a cathartic – Senna, Fennel and Manna – the narcotic ill-effects being thereby avoided.

Dose of powdered root for an adult: 1 to 2 drachms, morning and evening, for several successive days, followed by an active purgative. For children, 10 to 20 grains.

The infusion is made of ½ oz. troy of the bruised root to 1 pint boiling water. Dose for children, 1 tablespoonful, night and morning; for adults, a teacupful.

There is a preparation much in use called Worm Tea, composed of Spigelia, Savin, Senna and Manna, in the proportion of amounts to suit the individual need.

¶ *Adulterations.* Spigelia is frequently adulterated, so that an absolutely genuine and pure article is said to be the exception. The rhizomes are often extensively adulterated with those of *Ruellia ciliosa* (Acanthaceæ); they are, however, longer, straighter and thicker and the rootlets less wiry.

The rhizomes of species of Alpine Phlox, *Phlox ovata*, *P. Carolina* and *P. glaberrima*, are used in some localities and sometimes offered entirely as Spigelia. Those of *P. glaberrima* are somewhat darker and less ridged than *Ruellia* and more closely resemble Spigelia. Those of *P. Carolina* are rather coarse and straight, brownish-yellow, with a straw-coloured wood underneath and a readily removable bark.

The rhizomes of Golden Seal and *Caulophyllum* have often been found intermixed with the genuine Spigelia.

¶ *Other Varieties.*
The genus *Spigelia* comprises some thirty species, all American, mostly tropical, and several of them are employed like the official. Chief of these is *S. Anthelmia* (Linn.), native of the West Indies and northern South America, where it is abundant and is largely used as an anthelmintic. It is an annual, growing up to 2 feet high, of a similar habit to Pink Root, but the leaves, lanceolate below, and very broad, almost ovate, above, are mostly in whorls of four, the light reddish flowers only ½ inch long, the rhizome short, blackish externally, whitish internally and bearing numerous long, thin roots. The drug has a stronger narcotic and bitter taste than the official. It has been introduced into Europe and the Belgian Pharmacopœia specifically states that it is more active than the United States Pharmacopœia official species and directs that the flowering plant shall be employed. In large doses this is said to be a very powerful poison, causing death to animals and humans.

In cases of poisoning, the stomach should be emptied and stimulants administered, the patient being kept warm in bed. Artificial respiration with oxygen must be immediately resorted to if there are signs of respiratory failure. As an antidote, give strong tea or 15 to 20 grains of tannic acid in aqueous solution.

PINUS BARK. HEMLOCK SPRUCE

Tsuga Canadensis (CARR.)
N.O. Pinaceæ

Synonyms. Hemlock Pitch. Canada Pitch. Pix Canadensis. Hemlock Bark. Pinus Canadensis. Abies Canadensis. Hemlock Gum. Hemlock Spruce
Part Used. The bark encrusted with hardened juice
Habitat. North America

¶ *Description.* The flow of juice from incisions in the bark is much less than in most of the species, but at the time of late maturity a spontaneous exudation partly evaporates, hardening on the bark, which is stripped, broken in pieces, and boiled in water. The melted pitch is skimmed off and boiled for a second time. The product is of a dark reddish-brown colour, brittle, hard, opaque, almost tasteless, and with a very slight odour. It melts and softens at a low temperature.

An extract of the bark is used in tanning.

¶ *Constituents.* Besides resin, there is found a volatile oil, *oil of spruce* or *oil of hemlock,* and tannin.

¶ *Medicinal Action and Uses.* Canada Pitch is softer than Burgundy Pitch, so that even the temperature of the body makes it inconvenient to handle. It is a mild rubefacient, The liquid extract has been used as an astringent. It resembles rhatany in its action.

The volatile oil is used in veterinary liniments, and to procure abortion, but it is very dangerous for this purpose.

Hemlock or Canada Pitch Plaster can be made by melting together 90 parts of Canada Pitch to 10 parts of Yellow Wax, straining and stirring until it cools and thickens.

Fluid extract, ¼ to 1 drachm.

¶ *Other Species.*

Pseudotsuga tascifolia, the branches of which give out an emanation which, after being inhaled for some hours, is reported to have caused stupor, involuntary evacuation of urine, and collapse followed by psychic disturbance.

See PINES.

PIPSISSEWA

Chimaphila umbellata (LINN.)
N.O. Ericaceæ

Synonyms. Pyrola umbellata. Winter Green. Butter Winter. Prince's Pine. King's Cure. Ground Holly. Love in Winter. Rheumatism Weed

Parts Used. Dried leaves only are official, though the whole plant, including root, is used

Habitat. Europe, Asia, Siberia, America, and found in all parts of the United States

¶ *Description.* The name Chimaphila is derived from two Greek words meaning 'winter' and 'to love.' There are two varieties of this plant, *Chimaphila umbellata* and *C. maculata.* The former alone is the official plant, a small evergreen perennial with a creeping yellow rhizome, which has several creeping, erect or semi-procumbent stems, angular, marked with the scars of former leaves, and woody at the base. These are 4 to 8 inches high, with the leaves on upper surface, shiny, coriaceous, dark green and underside paler. Flowers corymbose, light purple colour, corolla five cream-coloured petals, fragrantly perfumed, purplish at base. Capsule erect, depressed five-celled, five-valved, numerous seeds, linear, chaffy. It flowers May till August; leaves when dried have only a slight odour, but when fresh and rubbed are sweet-smelling; taste astringently sweetish and not disagreeably bitter.

¶ *Constituents.* Leaves contain various crystalline constituents, Chimaphilin, etc., also arbutin gum, resin, starch, pectic acid, extractive fatty matter, chlorophyll tannic acid, sugar, potassa, lime, iron, magnesia, chloride of sodium, sulphuric phosphoric and silicic acids.

¶ *Medicinal Action and Uses.* Diuretic, astringent, tonic, alterative. The fresh leaves, when bruised and applied to the skin, act as vesicants and rubefacients, of great use in cardiac and kidney diseases, chronic rheumatism and scrofula. The decoction is advantageous for chronic gonorrhœa, strangury, catarrh of the bladder, and a good cure for ascites. It is said to diminish lithic acid in the

urine; for dropsy it is useful combined with other medicines; it is a substitute for uva-ursi and less obnoxious; said to be of value in diabetes, but this has not yet been confirmed; and it is very efficacious for skin diseases.

¶ *Dosage.* Decoction, 1 to 4 fluid ounces three times daily. Fluid extract, B.P.C., 15 to 45 grains. Fluid extract, B.P.C., 3 parts syrup to 1 part fluid extract. Fluid extract, 1 to 45 grains.

Syrup. – Macerate 4 oz. finely bruised leaves in 8 fluid ounces of water; let it stand 36 hours, strain till 1 pint of the fluid is obtained, evaporate to ½ pint, add ¾ lb. sugar; dose, 1 to 2 tablespoonsful.

Dose of Chimaphilin, 1 to 5 grains. This is very valuable for scrofulous complaints, hence its name, 'King's Cure'; also used externally in the form of a decoction to unhealthy scrofulous sores.

C. maculata, or Spotted Wintergreen, is very similar, but the leaves are a deep olive-green colour with greenish-white veins. When fresh and bruised they have a peculiar odour, which is lost on drying; taste pleasantly bitter, astringent and sweetish. A solution of perchloride of iron makes the infusion green colour. The leaves only are official, but all parts of the plant have active properties, and stem and leaves are often used together. The stem and root have a pungent taste and combine bitterness and astringency. Medicinal properties, diuretic with an antiseptic influence on the urine, occasionally prescribed for cystitis. The best preparation is the fluid extract.

See PYROLA, WINTERGREEN.

PITCHER PLANT

Sarracenia purpurea (LINN.)
N.O. Sarraceniaceæ

Synonyms. Sarazina Gibbosa. Sarracenie. Eve's Cups. Fly-catcher. Fly-trap. Hunts-man's Cup. Purple Side-saddle Flower. Side-saddle Plant. Water-cup. Nepenthes distillatoria

Parts Used. Root, leaves

Habitat. North America

¶ *Description.* A strange, perennial plant, the leaves of which form cups, often richly coloured, which become filled with water and small insects, and are covered by a lid in hot weather, due to the contraction of the fibres of the modified leaf-stalk. Water is sometimes present before opening. The insects gradually form a decaying mass, which emits a strong odour and probably serves as a fertilizer.

There appears to be little, if any, difference botanically between the American *Sarracenia* and the *Nepenthes distillatoria* of Ceylon, the East Indies and China. For lack of other definite information it may be concluded from the name that the latter is also used medicinally. (*Nepenthe,* from the Greek 'not' and 'grief.') In antiquity a magic potion, Nepenthe, is mentioned by Greek and Roman poets. It was said to cause forgetfulness of sorrows and misfortunes.

¶ *Cultivation.* The plant requires a moist, well-drained situation, and being a creeping plant needs trellis-work for support. The flowers are insignificant, with five petals shaped like a violin.

¶ *Constituents.* An alkaloid, Sarracenine resin, a yellow colouring principle (probably sarracenic acid) and extractive. 'Sarracenine is white, soluble in alcohol and ether, combines with acids to form salts, and with sulphuric acid forms handsome needles which are bitter, and communicate this taste to its members.'

¶ *Medicinal Action and Uses.* Tonic, laxative, stomachic, diuretic. Used in the southern United States in dyspepsia. The drug was unknown in Europe until a few years ago, when Mr. Herbert Miles introduced it as a specific for smallpox, as used by the North American Indians with great success, saving life and even the unsightly pitting. Some homœopaths confirm the value of the remedy, but allopaths do not appear to have been successful in its use, either in America, England or France.

Its principal value appears to be in torpid liver, stomach, kidney and uterus complaints.

¶ *Dosages.* Of tincture, 1 fluid drachm. Of fluid extract, 10 to 20 minims. Of powder, 10 to 30 grains.

PLANTAIN, COMMON

Plantago major (LINN.)
N.O. Plantaginaceæ

Synonyms. Broad-leaved Plantain. Ripple Grass. Waybread. Slan-lus. Waybroad. Snakeweed. Cuckoo's Bread. Englishman's Foot. White Man's Foot

(*Anglo-Saxon*) Weybroed

Parts Used. Root, leaves, flower-spikes

The Common Broad-leaved Plantain is a very familiar perennial 'weed,' and may be found anywhere by roadsides and in meadow-land.

¶ *Description.* It grows from a very short rhizome, which bears below a great number of long, straight, yellowish roots, and above, a large, radial rosette of leaves and a few long, slender, densely-flowered spikes. The leaves are ovate, blunt, abruptly contracted at the base into a long, broad, channelled footstalk (petiole). The blade is 4 to 10 inches long and about two-thirds as broad, usually smooth, thickish, five to eleven ribbed, the ribs having a strongly fibrous structure, the margin entire, or coarsely and unevenly toothed. The flower-spikes, erect, on long stalks, are as long as the leaves, ¼ inch thick and usually blunt. The flowers are somewhat purplish-green, the calyx four-parted, the small corolla bell-shaped and four-lobed, the stamens four, with purple

anthers. The fruit is a two-celled capsule, not enclosed in the perianth, and containing four to sixteen seeds.

The Plantain belongs to the natural order Plantaginaceæ, which contains more than 200 species, twenty-five or thirty of which have been reported as in domestic use.

The drug is without odour: the leaves are saline, bitterish and acrid to the taste; the root is saline and sweetish.

The glucoside Aucubin, first isolated in *Aucuba japonica,* has been reported as occurring in many species.

¶ *Medicinal Action and Properties.* Refrigerant, diuretic, deobstruent and somewhat astringent. Has been used in inflammation of the skin, malignant ulcers, intermittent fever, etc., and as a vulnerary, and externally as a stimulant application to sores. Applied to a bleeding surface, the leaves are of some value in arresting hæmorrhage, but they are useless in internal hæmorrhage, although they were formerly used for bleeding of the lungs and stomach, consumption and dysentery. The fresh leaves are applied whole or bruised in the form of a poultice. Rubbed on parts of the body stung by insects, nettles, etc., or as an application to burns and scalds, the leaves will afford relief and will stay the bleeding of minor wounds.

Fluid extract: dose, ½ to 1 drachm.

In the Highlands the Plantain is still called 'Slan-lus,' or plant of healing, from a firm belief in its healing virtues. Pliny goes so far as to state, 'on high authority,' that if 'it be put into a pot where many pieces of flesh are boiling, it will sodden them together.' He also says that it will cure the madness of dogs. Erasmus, in his *Colloquia*, tells a story of a toad, who, being bitten by a spider, was straightway freed from any poisonous effects he may have dreaded by the prompt eating of a Plantain leaf.

Another old Herbal says: 'If a wood hound (mad dog) rend a man, take this wort, rub it fine and lay it on; then will the spot soon be whole.' And in the United States the plant is called 'Snake Weed,' from a belief in its efficacy in cases of bites from venomous creatures; it is related that a dog was one day stung by a rattlesnake and a preparation of the juice of the Plantain and salt was applied as promptly as possible to the wound. The animal was in great agony, but quickly recovered and shook off all trace of its misadventure. Dr. Robinson (*New Family Herbal*) tells us that an Indian received a great reward from the Assembly of South Carolina for his discovery that the Plantain was 'the chief remedy for the cure of the rattlesnake.'

The Broad-leaved Plantain seems to have followed the migrations of our colonists to every part of the world, and in both America and New Zealand it has been called by the aborigines the 'Englishman's Foot' (or the White Man's Foot), for wherever the English have taken possession of the soil the Plantain springs up. Longfellow refers to this in 'Hiawatha.'

Our Saxon ancestors esteemed it highly, and in the old *Lacnunga* the Weybroed is mentioned as one of nine sacred herbs. In this most ancient source of Anglo-Saxon medicine, we find this 'salve for flying venom':

'Take a handful of hammer wort and a handful of maythe (chamomile) and a handful of *waybroad* and roots of water dock, seek those which will float, and one eggshell full of clean honey, then take clean butter, let him who will help to work up the salve, melt it

thrice: let one sing a mass over the worts, before they are put together and the salve is wrought up.'

Some of the recipes for ointments in which Plantain is an ingredient have lingered to the present day. Lady Northcote, in *The Book of Herbs* (1903), mentions an ointment made by an old woman in Exeter that up to her death about twenty years ago was in much request. It was made from Southernwood, Plantain leaves, Black Currant leaves, Elder buds, Angelica and Parsley, chopped, pounded and simmered with clarified butter and was considered most useful for burns or raw surfaces. A most excellent ointment can also be made from Pilewort (Celandine), Elder buds, Houseleek and the Broad Plantain leaf.

Decoctions of Plantain entered into almost every old remedy, and it was boiled with Docks, Comfrey and a variety of flowers.

A decoction of Plantain was considered good in disorders of the kidneys, and the root, powdered, in complaints of the bowels. The expressed juice was recommended for spitting of blood and piles. Boyle recommends an electuary made of fresh Comfrey roots, juice of Plantain and sugar as very efficacious in spitting of blood. Plantain juice mixed with lemon juice was judged an excellent diuretic. The powdered dried leaves, taken in drink, were thought to destroy worms.

To prepare a plain infusion, still recommended in herbal medicine for diarrhœa and piles, pour 1 pint of boiling water on 1 oz. of the herb, stand in a warm place for 20 minutes, afterwards strain and let cool. Take a wineglassful to half a teacupful three or four times a day.

The small mucilaginous seeds have been employed as a substitute for linseed. For 'thrush' they are recommended as most useful, 1 oz. of seeds to be boiled in 1½ pint of water down to a pint, the liquid then made into a syrup with sugar and honey and given to the child in tablespoonful doses, three or four times daily.

The seeds are relished by most small birds and quantities of the ripe spikes are gathered near London for the supply of cage birds.

Abercrombie, writing in 1822 (*Every Man his own Gardener*), giving a list of forty-four Salad herbs, includes Plantain.

Dr. Withering (*Arrangement of Plants*) states that sheep, goats and swine eat it, but that cows and horses refuse it.

It is a great disfigurement to lawns, rapidly multiplying if allowed to spread, each plant quite destroying the grass that originally occupied the spot usurped by its dense rosette of leaves.

Salmon's *Herbal* (1710) gives the following manifold uses for *Plantage major*:

'The liquid juice clarified and drunk for several days helps distillation of rheum upon the throat, glands, lungs, etc. Doses, 3 to 8 spoonsful. An especial remedy against ulceration of the lungs and a vehement cough arising from same. It is said to be good against epilepsy, dropsy, jaundice and opens obstructions of the liver, spleen and reins. It cools inflammations of the eyes and takes away the pin and web (so called) in them. Dropt into the ears, it eases their pains and restores hearing much decayed. Doses, 3 to 6 spoonsful more or less, either alone or with some fit vehicle morning and night. The powdered root mixed with equal parts of powder of Pellitory of Spain and put into a hollow tooth is said to ease the pain thereof. Powdered seeds stop vomiting, epilepsy, lethargy, convulsions, dropsy, jaundice, strangury, obstruction of the liver, etc. The liniment made with the juice and oil of Roses eases headache caused by heat, and is good for lunatics. It gives great ease (being applyed) in all hot gouts, whether in hands or feet, especially in the beginning, to cool the heat and repress the humors. The distilled water with a little alum and honey dissolved in it is of good use for washing, cleansing and healing a sore ulcerated mouth or throat.'

'Salmon also tells us that a good cosmetic is made with essence of Plantain, houseleeks and lemon juice.

Culpepper tells us that the Plantain is 'in the command of Venus and cures the head by antipathy to Mars, neither is there hardly a martial disease but it cures.' He also states that 'the water is used for all manner of spreading scabs, tetters, ringworm, shingles, etc.'

From the days of Chaucer onwards we find reference in literature to the healing powers of Plantain. Gower (1390) says: 'And of Plantaine he hath his herb sovereine,' and Chaucer mentions it in the *Prologue of the Chanounes Yeman.* Shakespeare, both in *Love's Labour's Lost, iii,* i, and in *Romeo and Juliet,* i, ii, speaks of the 'plain Plantain' and 'Plantain leaf' as excellent for a broken shin, and again in *Two Noble Kinsmen,* i, ii: 'These poore slight sores neede not a Plantin.' His reference to it in *Troilus and Cressida,* iii, ii: 'As true as steel, as Plantage to the moon,' is an allusion that is now no longer clear to us. Again, Shenstone in the *Schoolmistress:* 'And plantain rubb'd that heals the reaper's wound.'

PLANTAIN, BUCK'S HORN

Plantago Coronopus (LINN.)
N.O. Plantaginaceæ

Synonyms. Cornu Cervinum. Herba Stella. Herb Ivy. Buckshorne. Hartshorne
Parts Used. Whole plant, leaves
Habitat. It is an annual, found on sandy commons, waste places and chalky banks, especially near the sea, being fairly common and generally distributed in England.

The Buck's Horn Plantain is the only British species which has divided leaves more or less downy and usually prostrate. It is very variable in the size and in the lobing of the leaves, which are from 1 to 12 inches in length, one-ribbed, either deeply divided nearly to the base, or merely toothed and almost entire. The flower-spikes are slender, many-flowered, short or long, the bracts to the flowers have a long point and the sepals are strongly winged. The pale brown seeds are mucilaginous and adhere to the soil when they fall.

In Salmon's *Herbal* we find 'Our Common Buck's Horn Plantain' described thus:

'Root single, long and small, with several fibres. If sown or planted from seed, it rises up at first with small, long, narrow, hairy, dark-green leaves, almost like grass, without any division, but those that come after have deep divisions and are pointed at the end, resembling the snaggs of a Buck's Horn, from whence it took its name. When it is well grown, the leaves lie round about the root on the ground, resembling the form of a star and thereby called *Herba Stella.* There is also a prickly Buck's Horn Plantain, which is rougher, coarser and more prickly than the other. In Italy, they grow the first in their garden as a Sallet herb. The second grows on mountains and rocks. They both flower in May, June and July, their seeds ripening in the mean season and their leaves abide fresh and green in a manner all the winter. The qualities, specifications, preparation and virtues are the very same as those of Plantage major. The decoction in wine, if it is long drank, cureth the strangury and is profitable for such as are troubled with sand, gravel, stones, etc. The catasplasm of leaves and roots with bay salt applied to both wrists and bound on pretty hard (yet not too hard) cures agues admirably.'

¶ *Medicinal Action and Uses.* As a remedy for ague, the whole plant, roots included, was even hung round the neck as an amulet.

Gerard says: 'The leaves boyled in drinke and given morning and evening for certain days together helpeth most wonderfully those that have sore eyes, watery or blasted, and most of the griefs that happen unto the eyes.

PLANTAIN, HOARY

Plantago media (LINN.)
N.O. Plantaginaceæ

Part Used. Seeds

The Hoary Plantain is a common meadow species. The broadly-elliptical leaves, on short flat stalks, spread horizontally from the crown of the root and lie so close to the ground as to destroy all vegetation beneath and to leave the impression of their ribs on the ground. The flowers are in a close, cylindrical spike, shorter than in *Plantago major*, but growing on a longer stalk, which is downy. They are very fragrant, and are conspicuous by their light purple anthers, the filaments being long and pink or purplish.

¶ *Medicinal Action and Uses*. This species is a reputed cure for blight on fruit-trees. A few green leaves from the plant, if rubbed on the part of the tree affected, it has been recently discovered, will effect an instantaneous cure, and the wounds on the stem afterwards heal with smooth, healthy coverings. The plant is often found growing underneath the trees in orchards.

The medicinal virtues of this species were considered to be much the same as the preceding ones, the seeds, boiled in milk, being laxative and demulcent.

PLANTAIN, ISPAGHUL

Plantago ovata (FORSK.)
N.O. Plantaginaceæ

Synonyms. Ispaghula. Spogel Seed. Plantago Ispaghula. Plantago decumbens
Part Used. Dried seeds
Habitat. India, Persia, Spain, Canary Islands

¶ *Description*. The corolla gives attachment to four protruded stamina, ovary free with one or two cells, containing one or more ovules.

The style capillar, terminated by a single subulate stigma. The fruit is a small pyxidium covered by the persistent corolla; seeds composed of a proper integument which covers a fleshy endosperm at the centre of which is a cylindrical axile and a homotype embryo, boat-shaped, acute at one end $\frac{1}{12}$ to $\frac{1}{8}$ inch long and $\frac{1}{24}$ inch wide, pale-green brown with a darker elongated spot on the convex side; on concave side hilium is covered with the remains of a thin white membrane. It has no odour or taste, but the herbage is demulcent and bitter and somewhat astringent.

¶ *Constituents*. Mucilage contained in seed coat (sometimes used to stiffen linen), fixed oil, proteins.

¶ *Medicinal Action and Uses*. Useful in place of linseed or barley, also for diarrhœa and dysentery; the decoction is a good demulcent drink, or seeds mixed with sugar and taken dry invaluable in this form for reducing inflamed mucous membranes of the intestinal canal – a mild laxative. When roasted the seeds become astringent and are used for children's diarrhœa. In European medicine they are used chiefly for chronic diarrhœa and for catarrhal conditions of the genito-urinary tract. Dose, 2 to 2½ drachms of the seeds, mixed with sugar and taken dry. Decoction, ½ to 2 fluid ounces.

¶ *Other Species*. The seeds of the Indian species, *Plantago Amplexicaulis*, are sold in the bazaars as Ispaghula. They are of a darker colour than the official seeds, and are used in India as a demulcent in dysentery and other intestinal complaints.

P. decumbens (Forsk.), of South Africa, is regarded by some as the wild plant of which the preceding is a cultivated variety.

The seeds of *P. arenaria* (Waldst.), the SAND PLANTAIN, somewhat smaller, black and less glossy, and those of *P. Cynops* (Linn.), somewhat larger and lighter brown, are used similarly.

P. arenaria is an annual, with an erect, leafy, branched stem, bearing opposite, linear leaves and flowers in a spike, on long stalks, greenish-white. It flowers from June to September and grows in sandy, waste places, but in Britain has only been found on sandhills in one spot in Somerset and is not regarded as an indigenous species.

PLANTAIN, PSYLLIUM

Plantago Psyllium (LINN.)
N.O. Plantaginaceæ

Synonyms. Psyllium Seeds. Fleaseed. Psyllion. Psyllios
(*Barguthi*) Barguthi
Parts Used. Seeds, leaves

In Southern Europe, as well as in Northern Africa and Southern Asia, *Plantago Psyllium* (Linn.), Fleaseed is used similarly to *P. major*. The seeds are also used for their large yield of mucilage. *Semen psyllii* is the name given to the seeds of several species of European Plantago, but the best are those of *P. Psyllium*. They are dark brown on the convex side, shiny, inodorous and nearly tasteless, but mucilaginous when chewed. They are demulcent and emollient and may be used internally and externally in the same manner as flaxseed, which they closely resemble in medicinal properties.

P. Psyllium has once been found on ballast hills in Jersey, but has not permanently established itself.

PLANTAIN, RIBWORT

Plantago lanceolata
N.O. Plantaginaceæ

Synonyms. Snake Plantain. Black Plantain. Long Plantain. Ribble Grass. Ribwort. Black Jack. Jackstraw. Lamb's Tongue. Hen Plant. Wendles. Kemps. Cocks. Quinquenervia. Costa Canina

Parts Used. Leaves, seeds

Several of the wild Plantains have been used indiscriminately for *Plantago major*. Of these, the most important is *Plantago lanceolatus* (Linn.), the Ribwort Plantain.

¶ *Description.* This is a very dark green, slender perennial, growing much taller than *P. major*. Its leaf-blades rarely reach an inch in breadth, are three to five ribbed, gradually narrowed into the petioles, which are often more than a foot long. The flower-stalks are often more than 2 feet long, terminating in cylindrical blunt, dense spikes, $\frac{1}{2}$ to 3 or 4 inches long and $\frac{1}{3}$ to $\frac{1}{2}$ inch thick. It has the same chemical constituents as *P. major*.

When this Plantain grows amongst the tall grasses of the meadow its leaves are longer, more erect and less harsh, than when we find it by the roadside, or on dry soil. The leaves are often slightly hairy and have at times a silvery appearance from this cause, especially in the roadside specimens. The flower-stalks are longer than the leaves, furrowed and angular and thrown boldly up. The flower-head varies a good deal in size and form, sometimes being much smaller and more globular than others. The sepals are brown and paper-like in texture and give the head its peculiar rusty look. The corolla is very small and inconspicuous, tubed and having four spreading lobes. The stamens, four in number, are the most noticeable feature, their slender white filaments and pale yellow anthers forming a conspicuous ring around the flower-head.

In some old books we find this species called *Costa canina*, in allusion to the prominent veinings on the leaves that earned it the name of Ribwort, and it is this feature that caused it to receive also the mediæval name of *Quinquenervia*. Another old popular name was 'Kemps,' a word that at first sight seems without meaning, but when fully understood has a peculiar interest. The stalks of this plant are particularly tough and wiry, and it is an old game with country children to strike the heads one against the other until the stalk breaks. The Anglo-Saxon word for a soldier was *cempa*, and we can thus see the allusion to 'kemps.'

This species of Plantain abounds in every meadow and was brought into notice at one time as a possible fodder plant. Curtis, in his *Flora Londonensis*, says:

'The farmers in general consider this species of plantain as a favourite food of sheep and hence it is frequently recommended in the laying down of meadow and pasture land, and the seed is for that purpose kept in the shops.'

But its cultivation was never seriously taken up, for though its mucilaginous leaves are relished by sheep and to a certain extent by cows and horses, it does not answer as a crop, except on very poor land, where nothing else will grow. Moreover, it is very bitter, and in pastures destroys the more delicate herbage around it by its coarse leaves.

The seeds are covered with a coat of mucilage, which separates readily when macerated in hot water. The gelatinous substance thus formed has been used at one time in France for stiffening some kinds of muslin and other woven fabrics.

The leaves contain a good fibre, which, it has been suggested, might be adapted to some manufacturing purpose.

PLANTAIN, SEA

Plantago maritimo
N.O. Plantaginaceæ

Synonyms. Sheep's Herb
Part Used. Herb

The Sea Plantain has linear leaves grooved, fleshy and woolly at the base. It is common on the seashore and tops of mountains and is easily distinguished from the rest of the genus by its fleshy leaves.

It is so relished by sheep as food and considered so good for them, that in North Wales, where it has been cultivated, it is called Sheep's Herb, and the Welsh have two names for it, signifying 'the sheep's favourite morsel' and 'the suet producer.'

The RATTLESNAKE or NET-LEAVED PLANTAINS of the United States, *Peramium ripens* (Salisb.) (syn. *Goodyera ripens*, R. Br.), the White Plantain or Squirrel-ear, and *P. pubescens* (Willd.), peculiar little woodland herbs, their ovate leaves beautifully reticulated with white lines, are not allies of our common Plantains, but belong to the Orchid family.

The name WHITE PLANTAIN is also applied in the United States to *Antennaria plantaginifolia* (Linn.), the Ladies or Indian Tobacco, Spring Cudweed, or Life-Everlasting, to give several of its names, exceedingly common throughout Eastern North America, and one of the earliest blooming of spring plants in dry meadows, where it grows in patches.

It is used as a soothing expectorant with more or less marked stomachic properties.

PLANTAIN, WATER

Alisma Plantago
N.O. Alismaceæ

Synonym. Mad-Dog Weed
Part Used. Leaves

The Water Plantain, though its name suggests a similarity, is in fact widely different to the Plantago species, and belongs to another natural order, Alismaceæ. It is a water-plant, widely distributed in Europe, Northern Asia and North America and abundant in many parts of England, though only naturalized in Scotland. It grows freely around the margins of lakes or streams and in watery ditches, in company with the forget-me-not, brooklime, and other well-known waterside plants.

The name *Alisma* is said to be from the Celtic word for water, *alis*, in allusion to the aquatic habitat of the plant. The name *Plantago* was given by the early botanists because they were impressed with the similarity of form between the leaves of this plant and those of the plantain, and ignoring its dissimilarity in flower and fruit, etc., called it the 'Water Plantain.'

The roots of the Water Plantain are fibrous, but the base of the stem is swollen and fleshy, or tuberous and furnished with a tuft of numerous whitish hairs. The flower-stalk, which rises directly from it, is obtusely three-cornered, a form specially suitable to enable it to stem the current; it is from 1 to 3 feet in height. The flower-bearing branches that spring laterally from this at its upper extremity are thrown off in rings or whorls, and these branches are themselves branched in like fashion, the whole forming a loose pyramidal panicle. The large leaves, broad below, but tapering to a point, all spring directly from the root also and are borne on long, triangular stalks, growing in a nearly erect position. They are smooth in texture, their margins often more or less waved and are very strongly veined, the mid-rib and about three on each side being very conspicuous. The leaf-stems are deeply channelled, broadening out and sheathing at their bases. The flowers are attractive in form and colour. The calyx is composed of three ovate, concave, spreading sepals, while the corolla has three showy petals of a delicate, pale pink colour, somewhat round in form, slightly jagged at their edges. The stamens are six in number, their anthers being of a greenish tint. The fruit is composed of some twenty or more three-cornered, clustering carpels, each containing one seed.

¶ *Medicinal Action and Uses.* The Water Plantain has been considerably used medicinally, and is a drug of commerce. It contains a pungent, volatile oil and an acrid resin, to which all its virtues must be ascribed

The drug has diuretic and diaphoretic properties, and has been recommended by herbalists in renal calculus, gravel, cystitis, dysentery and epilepsy.

The powdered rhizome and leaves are employed by herbalists, also an infusion and a tincture prepared from the swollen rhizome, in its fresh state, is a homœopathic drug.

The powdered seeds were recommended by older herbalists as an astringent in cases of bleeding.

The bruised leaves are rubefacient and will inflame and sometimes even blister the skin, being injurious to cattle. They have been applied locally to bruises and swellings.

The roots formerly enjoyed some repute as a cure for hydrophobia (hence one of its names, formerly, Mad-Dog Weed), and have been regarded in Russia as a specific, but repeated experiments made with them in this country and a searching inquiry, have not confirmed their use as a remedy for this disease. Their acridity is lost in drying.

In America it has earned a reputation against the bite of the rattlesnake. The roots are also used medicinally in Japan, under the name of *Saji Omodaka*.

This group of plants, the Alismaceæ, in

645

general contains acrid juices, on account of which a number of species, besides the Water Plantain, have been used as diuretics and antiscorbutic.

PLANTAIN FRUIT

Musa paradisiaca
Musa sapientum
N.O. Musæ

Synonym. Bananas
Parts Used. Fruit, unripe and ripe, juice

The tropical fruit known as Plantain belongs to the genus *Musa*, which contains about forty species, widely distributed throughout the tropics of the Old World and in some cases introduced into the New World.

The great use of the family resides in the use of the unripe fruits as food and to a much less extent in that of the ripe fruit – Bananas. In many parts of the tropics they are as important to the inhabitants as are the grain plants to those living in cooler regions. The northern limit of their cultivation is reached in Florida, the Canary Islands, Egypt and Southern Japan, and the southern limit in Natal and South Brazil. There has been considerable discussion as to whether they were growing in America before the discovery of the New World.

The unripe fruit is rich in starch, which on ripening turns into sugar.

The most generally used fruits are derived from *Musa paradisiaca*, of which an enormous number of varieties and forms exist in cultivation. The sub-species, *sapientum*, formerly regarded as a distinct species (*M. sapientum*), is the source of the fruits generally known in England as Bananas and eaten raw, while the name Plantain is given to forms of the species itself which require cooking. The species is probably a native of India and Southern Asia.

Other species are *M. acuminata* in the Malay Archipelago, *M. Fehi*, in Tahiti, and *M. Cavendishii*, the so-called Chinese Banana, which has a thinner rind and is found in cooler countries.

Plantains often reach a considerable size. The hardly-ripe fruit is eaten (whole or cut into slices) roasted, baked, boiled, fried, as an ingredient of soups and stews, and in general as potatoes are used, possessing, like the potato, only a slight or negative flavour and no sweetness. They are also dried and ground into flour as meal, Banana meal forming an important food-stuff, to which the following constituents have been assigned: Water 10·62, albuminoids 3·55, fat 1·15, carbohydrates 81·67 (more than ⅔ starch), fibre 1·15, phosphates 0·26, other salts, 1·60. The sugar is chiefly cane-sugar.

Several species of *Sagittaria*, natives of Brazil, are astringent, and their expressed juice has been used in making ink.
See ARROWHEAD.

In East Africa and elsewhere an intoxicating drink is prepared from the fruit. The rootstock which bears the leaves is, just before the flowering period, soft and full of starch, and is sometimes used as food in Abyssinia, and the young shoots of several species are cooked and eaten.

The leaves cut into strips are plaited to form mats and bags; they are also largely used for packing and the finer ones for cigarette papers. The mature leaves of several species yield a valuable fibre, the best of which is 'Manila hemp.'

¶ *Medicinal Action and Uses.* The Banana family is of more interest for its nutrient than for its medicinal properties. Banana root has some employment as an anthelmintic and has been reported useful in reducing bronchocele.

The use of Plantain juice as an antidote for snake-bite in the East has been reported in recent years by the *Lancet*, an alleged cure at Colombo (reported in the *Lancet*, April 1, 1916), and again, in the same year, at Serampore:

'A servant of the Principal of the Government Weaving College was bitten by a venomous snake in the foot. The Principal applied a ligature eight inches above the bitten part and then cut it with a lancet and applied permanganate of potash, making the wound bleed freely. He then extracted some juice from a plantain tree and gave the patient about a cupful to drink. After drinking the plantain juice the man seemed to recover a little, and the wound was washed. He was made to walk up and down, and in the morning, when the ligature was removed, the man was declared cured.' – *Lancet*, June 10, 1916.

The BASTARD PLANTAIN (*Heliconia Bihai*) belongs to a genus containing thirty species, natives of tropical America. Although it belongs to the same order as the Banana, and has very large leaves, 6 to 8 feet long and 18 inches wide, it has quite different fruit, namely, small succulent berries, each containing three hard, rugged seeds, and is not employed economically.

PLEURISY ROOT
                                    Asclepias tuberose (LINN.)
                                    N.O. Asclepiadaceæ

Synonyms. Butterfly-weed. Swallow-wort. Tuber Root. Wind Root. Colic Root. Orange Milkweed

Part Used. Root

The genus *Asclepias* contains about eighty species, mostly natives of North America, a few being indigenous to South America and Africa.

Asclepias tuberosa, common from Canada southwards, growing from Ontario to Minnesota, most abundantly southward and southwestward, is known popularly as Pleurisy Root, from its medicinal use. Its stem forms an exception to Asclepias in general, by being almost or entirely devoid of the acrid milky juice containing caoutchouc, that distinguishes the rest of the genus and has gained them the name of Milkweeds.

¶ *Description.* It is a handsome, fleshy-rooted, perennial plant, growing 1 to 1½ foot high and bearing corymbs of deep yellow and orange flowers in September. When cultivated, it does not like being disturbed, and prefers good peat soil.

The rootstock, the part used medicinally, is spindle-shaped and has a knotty crown, slightly but distinctly annulate, the remainder longitudinally wrinkled.

The dried root as found in commerce is usually in cut or broken pieces of variable size, 1 to 6 inches long and about ¾ inch in thickness, externally pale orange-brown, becoming greyish-brown when kept long, internally whitish. It is tough and has an uneven fracture; the broken surface is granular; that of the bark is short and brittle. The wood is yellowish, with large white medullary rays. The drug is almost inodorous, but has a bitterish and disagreeable, somewhat acrid taste.

The powdered drug is yellowish brown and when examined under the microscope shows numerous simple or 2 to 4 compound starch grains, also calcium oxalate crystals.

The Western Indians boil the tubers for food, prepare a crude sugar from the flowers and eat the young seed-pods, after boiling them, with buffalo meat. Some of the Canadian tribes use the young shoots as a pot-herb, after the manner of asparagus.

¶ *Constituents.* The root contains a glucosidal principle, Asclepiadin, which occurs as an amorphous body, is soluble in ether, alcohol and hot water. It also contains several resins, and odorous fatty matter, and a trace of volatile oil. It yields not more than 9 per cent. of ash.

¶ *Medicinal Action and Uses.* Antispasmodic, diaphoretic, expectorant, tonic, carminative and mildly cathartic.

From early days this Asclepias has been regarded as a valuable medicinal plant. It is one of the most important of the indigenous American remedies, and until lately was official in the United States Pharmacopœia.

It possesses a specific action on the lungs, assisting expectoration, subduing inflammation and exerting a general mild tonic effect on the system, making it valuable in all chest complaints. It is of great use in pleurisy, mitigating the pain and relieving the difficulty of breathing, and is also recommended in pulmonary catarrh. It is extensively used in the Southern States in these cases, also in consumption, in doses of from 20 grains to a drachm in a powder, or in the form of a decoction.

It has also been used with great advantage in diarrhœa, dysentery and acute and chronic rheumatism, in low typhoid states and in eczema. It is claimed that the drug may be employed with benefit in flatulent colic and indigestion, but in these conditions it is rarely used.

In large doses it acts as an emetic and purgative.

A teacupful of the warm infusion (1 in 30) taken every hour will powerfully promote free perspiration and suppressed expectoration. The infusion may be prepared by taking 1 teaspoonful of the powder in a cupful of boiling water.

The decoction is taken in doses of 2 to 3 fluid ounces.

The dose of the fluid extract is ½ to 1 drachm; of Asclepin, 1 to 4 grains.

A much-recommended herbal recipe is: Essence of composition powder, 1 oz.; fluid extract of Pleurisy Root, 1 oz. Mix and take a teaspoonful three or four times daily in warm sweetened water.

It is often combined with Angelica and Sassafras for producing perspiration in fever and pleurisy and for equalizing the circulation of the blood.

More than a dozen other species have similar properties.

See ASCLEPIAN, CALOTROPIS and SWAMP MILKWEED.

PLOUGHMAN'S SPIKENARD. *See* SPIKENARD

PLUMBAGO

Plumbago Europæa (LINN.)
N.O. Plumbaginaceæ

Synonyms. Leadwort. Dentallaria
(*French*) Dentelaire
Parts Used. Root, herb
Habitat. China, Southern Europe, and cultivated in England in hot-houses

¶ *Description*. A half-hardy herbaceous climbing, half-shrubby plant, with large trusses of pale-blue flowers, which are in bloom continuously through the summer. This variety is also known under the name of *Plumbago Capensis*, and is greatly used in German gardening.

¶ *Constituents*. Plumbagin, a crystallizable acrid principle obtained from the root.

¶ *Medicinal Action and Uses*. It is acrid, and when chewed creates a free flow of saliva, particularly if root is used; said to be of benefit to relieve toothache, and has long been used in France for that purpose, hence its name, dentalaire; also useful for itch – a decoction of the root in olive oil is much used.

¶ *Other Species*. *P. Zeylanica* is said to be a strong diaphoretic.

POISON IVY
POISON OAK
See IVY

POKE ROOT

Phytolacca decandra (LINN.)
N.O. Phytolaccaceæ

Synonyms. Phytolacca Root. Phytolaccæ Radix. Phytolacca Berry. Phytolaccæ Bacca. Phytolacca Vulgaris. Phytolacca Americana. Blitum Americanum. Branching Phytolacca. Phytolaque. Garget. Pigeon Berry. Méchoacan du Canada. Bear's Grape. Poke Weed. Raisin d'Amérique. Red-ink Plant. American Spinach. Skoke. Crowberry. Jalap. Cancer-root. American Nightshade. Pocan or Cokan. Coakum. Chongras. Morelle à Grappes. Herbe de la Laque. Amerikanische scharlachbeere. Kermesbeere. Virginian Poke. Poke Berry
Parts Used. Dried root, berries
Habitat. Indigenous to North America. Common in Mediterranean countries

¶ *Description*. This is regarded as one of the most important of indigenous American plants, and one of the most striking in appearance. The perennial root is large and fleshy, the stem hollow, the leaves alternate and ovate-lanceolate, and the flowers have a white calyx with no corolla. The fruit is a deep purple berry, covering the stem in clusters and resembling blackberries.

The young shoots make a good substitute for asparagus, and poultry eat the berries, though large quantities give the flesh an unpleasant flavour, also causing it to become purgative, when eaten.

In Portugal the use of the juice of the berries to colour port wines was discontinued because it spoilt the taste. The stain of the juice is a beautiful purple, and would make a useful dye if a way of fixing it were found.

A decoction of the roots has been used for drenching cattle.

As found in commerce the roots are usually sliced either longitudinally or transversely, are grey in colour, hard and wrinkled. The fracture is fibrous. It is inodorous, and the taste is acrid and slightly sweet.

It is often used to adulterate belladonna, but may be recognized by the concentric

rings of wood bundles in the transverse section. The leaves are used for the same purpose, requiring microscopical identification.

¶ *Constituents*. Phytolaccic acid has been obtained from the berries, and tannin. In the root a non-reducing sugar, formic acid, and a small percentage of bitter resin have been found. The alkaloid Phytolaccin may be present in small quantities, but it has not been proved. A resinoid substance is called phytolaccin. The virtues are extracted by alcohol, diluted alcohol, and water. The powder is said to be sternutatory.

¶ *Medicinal Action and Uses*. A slow emetic and purgative with narcotic properties. As an alterative it is used in chronic rheumatism and granular conjunctivitis. As an ointment, in the proportion of a drachm to the ounce, it is used in psora, tinea capitis, favus and sycosis, and other skin diseases, causing at first smarting and heat.

The slowness of action and the narcotic effects that accompany it render its use as an emetic inadvisable. It is used as a cathartic in paralysis of the bowels. Headaches of many sources are benefited by it, and both lotion and tincture are used in leucorrhœa.

As a poultice it causes rapid suppuration in

felons. The extract is said to have been used in chronic rheumatism and hæmorrhoids.

Authorities differ as to its value in cancer. Great relief towards the close of a difficult case of cancer of the uterus was obtained by an external application of 3 oz. of Poke Root and 1 oz. of Tincture used in the strength of 1 tablespoonful to 3 pints of tepid water for bathing the part. It is also stated to be of undoubted value as an internal remedy in cancer of the breast.

The following prescription has been recommended: Fluid extracts of Phytolacca (2 oz.), Gentian (1 oz.) and Dandelion (1 oz.), with Simple Syrup to make a pint. One teaspoonful may be taken after each meal.

Infused in spirits, the fruit is used in chronic rheumatism, being regarded as equal to Guaicum.

It is doubtful if the root will cure syphilis without the help of mercury.

¶ *Dosages*. As emetic, 10 to 30 grains. As alterative, 1 to 5 grains. Of fluid extract of berries, ½ to 1 drachm. Of fluid extract of root, ¼ to ½ drachm; as an emetic, 15 drops; as an alterative, 2 drops. Phytolaccin, 1 to 3 grains.

¶ *Poisons and Antidotes*. In the lower animals convulsions and death from paralysis of respiration may be caused. Overdoses may produce considerable vomiting and purging, prostration, convulsions and death.

¶ *Other Species*. *Phytolacca drastica* of Chile is a violent purgative.

POLYPODY ROOT. *See* FERNS

POLYPORUS OF LARCH. *See* FUNGI

POMEGRANATE

Punica granatum (LINN.)
N.O. Lythraceæ

Synonyms. Grenadier. Cortex granati. Ecorce de Granade. Granatwurzelrinde. Melogranato. Malicorio. Scorzo del Melogranati. Cortezade Granada

Parts Used. The root, bark, the fruits, the rind of the fruit, the flowers

Habitat. Western Asia. Now grows widely in Mediterranean countries, China and Japan

¶ *History*. The Latin name of the tree was *Malus punica*, or *Punicum Malum*, the Lybian or Carthaginian apple; while the name of *granatum* was bestowed on account of its many seeds. Having no close relations, the tree has been placed by various authorities in different orders, some giving it an order of its own, Granateæ.

¶ *Description*. It is a small tree, not more than 15 feet high, with pale, brownish bark. The buds and young shoots are red, the leaves opposite, lanceolate, entire, thick, glossy and almost evergreen. The flowers are large and solitary, the crimson petals alternating with the lobes of the calyx. The fruit is the size of an orange, having a thick, reddish-yellow rind, an acid pulp, and large quantities of seeds.

The dried root bark is found in quills 3 to 4 inches long. It is yellowish-grey and wrinkled outside, the inner bark being smooth and yellow. It has a short fracture, little odour and a slightly astringent taste.

The rind of the fruit is in curved, brittle fragments, rough and yellowish-brown outside, paler and pitted within. It is called Malicorium.

The fruit is used for dessert, and in the East the juice is included in cooling drinks.

The flowers yield a red dye, and with leaves and seeds were used by the Ancients as astringent medicines and to remove worms.

The Pomegranate is mentioned in the Papyrus Ebers.

It is still used by the Jews in some ceremonials, and as a design has been used in architecture and needlework from the earliest times. It formed part of the decoration of the pillars of King Solomon's Temple, and was embroidered on the hem of the High-Priest's ephod.

There are three kinds of Pomegranates: one very sour, the juice of which is used instead of verjuice, or unripe grape juice; the other two moderately sweet or very sweet. These are (in Syria) eaten as dessert after being cut open, seeded, strewn with sugar and sprinkled with rosewater. A wine is extracted from the fruits, and the seeds are used in syrups and conserves.

The bark is used in tanning and dyeing, giving the yellow hue to Morocco leather.

The barks of three wild Pomegranates are said to be used in Java: the red-flowered *merah*, the white-flowered *poetih*, and the black-flowered *hitam*.

¶ *Constituents*. The chief constituent of the *bark* (about 22 per cent.) is called punicotannic acid. It also contains gallic acid, mannite, and four alkaloids, Pellètierine, Methyl-Pelletierine, Pseudo-Pelletierine, and Iso-Pelletierine.

The liquid pelletierine boils at 125° C., and is soluble in water, alcohol, ether and chloroform.

The drug probably deteriorates with age.

The *rind* contains tannic acid, sugar and gum.

Pelletierine Tannate is a mixture of the

tannates of the alkaloids obtained from the bark of the root and stem, and represents the tænicidal properties.

¶ *Medicinal Action and Uses.* The *seeds* are demulcent. The *fruit* is a mild astringent and refrigerant in some fevers, and especially in biliousness, and the bark is used to remove tapeworm.

In India the *rind* is used in diarrhœa and chronic dysentery, often combined with opium.

It is used as an injection in leucorrhœa, as a gargle in sore throat in its early stages, and in powder for intermittent fevers. The flowers have similar properties.

As a tænicide a decoction of the *bark* may be made by boiling down to a pint 2 oz. of bark that has been macerated in spirits of water for twenty-four hours, and given in wineglassful doses. It often causes nausea and vomiting, and possibly purging. It should be preceded by strict dieting and fol-lowed by an enema or castor oil if required. It may be necessary to repeat the dose for several days.

A hypodermic injection of the alkaloids may produce vertigo, muscular weakness and sometimes double vision.

The root-bark was recommended as a vermifuge by Celsus, Dioscorides and Pliny. It may be used fresh or dried.

¶ *Dosages.* Of rind and flowers in powder, 20 to 30 grains. Of pelletierine tannate, 3 to 5 grains. Of rind, 1 to 2 drachms.. Fluid extract, root-bark, ¼ to 2 drachms. Decoction, B.P., ½ to 2 oz. Of decoction of 4 oz. of bark to 20 of water, ½ a fluid ounce.

¶ *Adulterations.* The bitter but non-astrin-gent barks of Barberry and Box (*Boxux sempervirens*). Their infusion does not pro-duce the deep blue precipitate with a persalt of iron.

Pinana is a dwarf variety naturalized in the West Indies.

POPLAR

Populus tremuloides (MICHX.)
N.O. Salicaceæ

Synonyms. American Aspen. White Poplar. Quaking Aspen
Part Used. Bark
Habitat. North America

¶ *Description.* This tree does not grow well in Britain, but in America it grows up to 100 feet in height. It has a pale yellowish bark on the young trunk and main branches; broadly ovate finely-toothed leaves averaging 1¾ inch long and wide, and having fine hairs on the margin.

The bark should be collected in spring. It has a bitterish taste and no odour.

¶ *Constituents.* The bark probably has simi-lar properties to that of *Populus tremula* of Europe, i.e. salicin and populin.

¶ *Medicinal Action and Uses.* Febrifuge and tonic, chiefly used in intermittent fevers. It has been employed as a diuretic in urinary affections, gonorrhœa and gleet. The infusion has been found helpful in debility, chronic diarrhœa, etc. Is a valuable and safe substitute for Peruvian bark.

¶ *Dosages.* Fluid extract, 1 drachm. Of sali-cin, in intermittents, 10 to 30 grains. Of populin, 1 to 4 grains.

¶ *Other Species.*
P. grandidentata, the large Aspen, is said to have more activity and bitterness.

P. candicans is also used.

POPPY, PLUME

Bocconia cordata
N.O. Papaveraceæ

Synonym. Macleaya
Part Used. Juice of stems of leaves
Habitat. China, but grows freely in author's garden

¶ *Description.* This plant was named in honour of a Sicilian botanist. A handsome and vigorous perennial, growing in erect tufts up to 8 feet. Flowers in very large panicles; the inflorescence is a soft creamy to brown plume, not showy, but has a fine effect; the blue-green downy leaves are very effective and elegant; the plant is propagated by seeds and division of the root.

¶ *Constituents.* Protopine, homo-chilidonine chelerythrine and sanguinarine have been isolated from the plant.

¶ *Medicinal Action and Uses.* The liquid from the root and the juice of the stems of the leaves are a deep orange and stains the hands; the juice from the *stems of the leaves* is used for insect-bites.

It is considered probable that the various species of this genus may have active medi-cinal qualities.

¶ *Other Species.*
The Mexican (*Bocconia arborea*, Watson) has been found to contain two alkaloids, one of which is probably Sanguinarine, and the

leaves of other species are used in South America as purgatives and abortifacients.

B. frutescens and *B. integrifolia* are natives of the West Indies and Mexico, and are more tender than *B. cordata*, and are best protected or taken into greenhouse during the winter. It is easier to raise these by seeds than by cuttings.

POPPY, RED

Papaver Rhœas (LINN.)
N.O. Papaveraceæ

Synonyms. Corn Rose. Corn Poppy. Flores Rhœados. Headache
Parts Used. Flowers, petals

The Common Red Poppy, growing in fields and waste places, has petals of a rich scarlet colour when fresh, and is often nearly black at the base. They have the peculiar heavy odour of opium when fresh, but becomes scentless on drying.

There are several varieties, differing in the size of the lobes of the leaves and in the character of the fruit, which may be nearly cylindrical or globular, smooth or furnished with stiff hairs. The intensity of the scarlet colouring of the petals also varies. The fresh petals are used for preparing a syrup. The Red Poppy with petals having a dark spot at the base makes the deepest-coloured syrup; that with the oblong capsule should not be used, as it contains an alkaloid resembling Thebaine in action.

¶ *Collection*. The petals find a steady, though limited market, but must be collected in large quantities, by an organized band of collectors, to be of any use. Farmers might arrange to deliver the fresh petals to manufacturers. They can be collected by children in small muslin bags suspended from the neck, so that both hands are left free for gathering. The petals should not be taken out of the bags, but packed in them, among straw, and sent off the same day as collected, before they fade or lose their bright colour. All the collecting should be done in dry weather, and all handling possible should be avoided.

Although in this country the Field Poppy is only regarded as a weed, and only a limited amount of the petals are used, it is cultivated in Flanders and several parts of Germany for the sake of its seeds, which are not only used in cakes, but from which an excellent oil is made, used as a substitute for olive oil.

The foliage is said to have been used as a vegetable, and the syrup prepared from the petals has been employed as an ingredient in soups and gruels.

Attempts have also been made to utilize the brilliant red of the petals as a dye, but the colour has proved too fugitive to be of use. The syrup has, however, been used as a colouring matter for old ink.

¶ *Constituents*. *Papaver Rhœas* is very slightly narcotic. The chief constituent of the fresh petals is the red colouring matter, which consists of Rhœadic and Papaveric acids. This colour is much darkened by alkalis.

All parts of the plant contain the crystalline non-poisonous alkaloid Rhœadine. The amount of active ingredients is very small and rather uncertain in quantity. There is great controversy as to the presence of Morphine. Also it has not been determined whether Meconic Acid, which is present in opium, is a constituent.

(*POISON*)
POPPY, WHITE

Papaver somniferum (LINN.)
N.O. Papaveraceæ

Synonyms. Opium Poppy. Mawseed
Parts Used. Capsules, flowers
Habitat. The Opium Poppy (*Papaver somniferum*, var. *album*) is indigenous to Asia Minor, and is cultivated largely in European and Asiatic Turkey, Persia, India and China for the production of Opium

It has been observed growing on the cliffs between Folkestone and Dover.

The word opium is derived from the Greek *opos* (juice).

¶ *Description*. The plant is an erect, herbaceous annual, varying much in the colour of its flowers, as well as in the shape of the fruit and colour of the seeds. All parts of the plant, but particularly the walls of the capsules, or seed-vessels, contain a system of laticiferous vessels, filled with a white latex.

The flowers vary in colour from pure white to reddish purple. In the wild plant, they are pale lilac with a purple spot at the base of each petal. In England, mostly in Lincolnshire, a variety with pale flowers and whitish seeds is cultivated medicinally for the sake of the capsules. Belgium has usually supplied a proportion of the Poppy Heads used in this country, though those used for fomentations are mostly of home growth.

The capsules vary much in shape and size. They are usually hemispherical, but depressed at the top, where the many-rayed stigma occupies the centre; they have a swollen ring below where the capsule joins the stalk. Some varieties are ovoid, others again depressed both at summit and base. The small kidney-shaped seeds, minute and very numerous, are attached to lateral projections from the inner walls of the capsule and vary in colour from whitish to slate. The heads are of a pale glaucous green when young. As they mature and ripen they change to a yellowish brown, and are then cut from the stem if the *dried* poppy heads are required.

Opium is extracted from the poppy heads before they have ripened, and from Poppies grown in the East, those grown in Europe yielding but little of the drug. When the petals have fallen from the flowers, incisions are made in the wall of the unripe capsules, care being taken not to penetrate to the interior. The exuded juice, partially dried, is collected by scraping – the scrapings being formed eventually into cakes, which are wrapped in poppy leaves or paper and further dried in the sun, the white milky juice darkening during the drying.

The first poppies cultivated in this country for the purpose of extracting opium were grown by Mr. John Ball, of Williton, in 1794, but the production of opium has not become a home industry, as was expected at the time. The cultivation of the Opium Poppy has also been experimentally carried out in France and Germany, but the expense of the necessary labour and land has been too great to render it profitable. The British Pharmacopœia directs that opium, when used officially, must be obtained from Asia Minor. A certain amount is cultivated in Macedonia and exported from Salonica, and much of that cultivated in Persia is also sent to European markets. Chinese Opium is entirely consumed in the country and is not exported.

¶ *Constituents.* The most important constituents of opium are the alkaloids, which constitute in good opium about one-fifth of the weight of the drug. No fewer than twenty-one have been reported.

The principal alkaloid, both as regards its medicinal importance, and the quantity in which it exists, is Morphine. Next to this, Narcotine and Codeine are of secondary importance. Among the numerous remaining alkaloids, amounting in all to about 1 per cent. of the drug, are Thebaine, Narceine, Papaverine, Codamine and Rhœadine.

Meconic acid exists to the extent of about 5 per cent. combined with morphine. This acid is easily identified, and is important in toxicological investigation, as corroborative of the presence of opium.

Meconin and meconiasin exist in small quantity only. Mucilage, sugar, wax, caout-

chouc and salts of calcium, and magnesium are also contained in opium, and sulphuric acid is found in the ash. The presence of starch, tannin, oxalic acid and fat, common constituents of most plants, indicates adulteration, as these substances do not occur normally in the drug. Powdered poppy capsules stones, small shot, pieces of lead, gum, grape must, sugary fruits, and other mechanical impurities, have also been used as adulterants of opium. The drug should not contain more than $12\frac{1}{2}$ per cent. of moisture.

¶ *Medicinal Action and Uses.* Hypnotic, sedative, astringent, expectorant, diaphoretic, antispasmodic.

The drug was known in very remote times and the Greeks and Romans collected it. It is probable that the physicians of the Arabian school introduced the drug into India, as well as into Europe. It was originally used only as a medicine, the practice of opium eating having first arisen, probably in Persia. Opium is one of the most valuable of drugs, Morphine and Codeine, the two principal alkaloids, being largely used in medicine.

It is unexcelled as a hypnotic and sedative, and is frequently administered to relieve pain and calm excitement. For its astringent properties, it is employed in diarrhœa and dysentery, and on account of its expectorant, diaphoretic, sedative and antispasmodic properties, in certain forms of cough, etc.

Small doses of opium and morphine are nerve stimulants. The Cutch horsemen share their opium with their jaded steeds, and increased capability of endurance is observed alike in man and beast.

Opium and morphine do not produce in animals the general calmative and hypnotic effects which characterize their use in man, but applied locally, they effectually allay pain and spasm. Owing to the greater excitant action in veterinary patients, the administration of opium does not blunt the perception of pain as effectually as it does in human patients.

The British Pharmacopœia Tincture of Opium, popularly known as Laudanum, is made with 3 oz. of Opium and equal parts of distilled water and alcohol, and for immediate effects is usually preferable to solid Opium. Equal parts of Laudanum and Soap Liniment make an excellent anodyne, much used externally.

¶ *Preparations.* Syrup of Poppy, B.P., 1885. Syrup Papav. alba. Capsules, 1 to 2 drachms.

¶ *Antidotes.* Opium is not very quickly absorbed. When a poisonous dose has been swallowed, the stomach should be

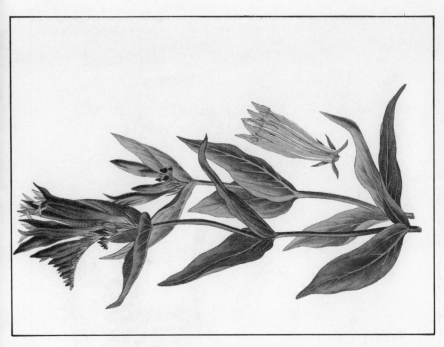

PINK ROOT
Spigelia Marilandica

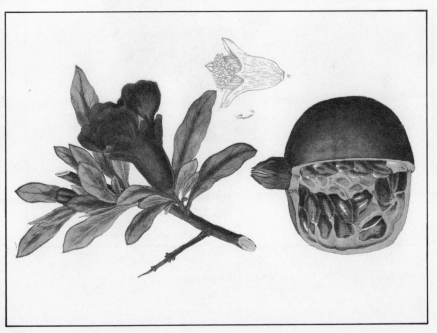

POMEGRANATE
Punica Granatum

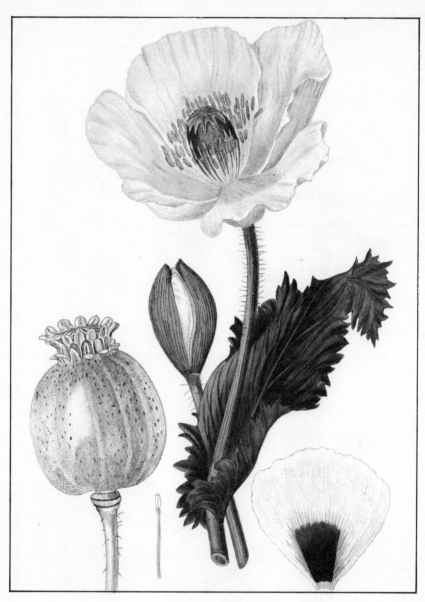

WHITE POPPY
Papaver Somniferum

emptied as soon as possible by the stomach pump and washed with a solution of potassium permanganate. Administration of nitrites and of small doses of atropine hypodermically maintain cardiac action, but the atropine must be used cautiously, as full doses are apt to intensify paralysis both of the heart and spinal cord. The lethal tendency is further combated by strychnine used hypodermically and by artificial respiration. Coma is prevented by giving strong coffee and stimulant enemata and keeping the patient moving. Tincture of gall and other chemical antidotes are of little avail.

The leaves of *Combretum Sundaicum*, a plant native to the Malay Peninsula and Sumatra, have been used in the form of a decoction of the roasted leaves, as a cure for the opium habit among the Chinese.

¶ *Cultivation.* The plants prefer rich, moist soil and much sun, and are often grown in succession to wheat and barley.

The land is manured and ploughed in autumn, to ensure a fine tilth in spring. Sowing is done at the end of March or in April – according to weather – allowing 1 lb. of seed per acre, and drilling in rows a foot apart. The whitest seeds are preferred.

Plants which are too forward are liable to be cut down by late frosts, while if the seed is sown too late, the seedlings may become dwarfed if dry weather sets in before they are well established. A light roller is sufficient to ensure the seeds being covered.

When the plants are 3 or 4 inches high, cut them with the hoe into clumps about 6 to 9 inches apart, and afterwards 'single' them, leaving a solitary strong plant from each group. Weeding is necessary, and a dressing of soot may be given if support appears to be needed.

Poppy heads of pale colour are most desired, but a week's rain, or even a few nights' heavy dew, may spoil the colour of the ripening fruit. High winds and heavy rains may cause much destruction, as the plants become top-heavy. The yield is very variable.

The capsules are left on the stems after the petals have fallen, until they cease to enlarge. The stems should then be bent in the middle and the capsules left on the plant until they are firm, which will be about September.

In India, when the flowers are in bloom, the first step is the removal of the petals, which are used in packing the prepared drug. After a few days, the imperfectly ripened capsules are scarified from above downwards by two or three knives tied together and called 'mushturs.' These make a superficial incision, or series of incisions, into the capsule, whereupon a milky juice exudes, which is allowed to harden and is then removed and collected in earthen pots. The time of day chosen for slicing the capsules is about two o'clock in the afternoon, when the heat of the sun causes the speedy formation of a film over the exuded juice; great attention is also paid to the weather, as all these causes modify the quantity, quality, or speediness of exudation of the opium.

The capsules are submitted to two or three slicing processes at intervals of a few days, and the drug is ultimately conveyed to the government factory where it is kneaded into a homogeneous mass by native workmen.

The capsules contain the principal constituents of opium, the most important of which is the alkaloid Morphine, which exists in combination with meconic and sulphuric acids. The seeds are free from morphine; their principle constituent is the pale yellow fixed oil, used as a drying oil by artists, as well as for culinary and various technical purposes.

The action of poppy capsules is the same as that of opium, anodyne and narcotic, but much weaker.

The crushed capsules are used as a poultice, together with chamomile.

A syrup is prepared from the capsules, prescribed as an ingredient in cough medicine. Syrup of Poppy is often employed to allay cough and likewise as an opiate for children; in the latter case it should be used with great caution.

Decoction of Poppy, made from the bruised capsules and distilled water, is not given internally, but is employed as an external application to allay pain and soothe.

The broken capsules are sold at a cheaper rate, for making fomentations.

The grey seeds are sold for birds' food, under the name of 'maw' seed, and are derived from the dark-red flowered form of *Papaver Somniferum*; the var. *album* having white seeds.

On the Continent the seeds are much used in special poppy cakes and are sprinkled on rolls, as also in India, where they are used in the native pancakes or 'chupaties.'

Anodyne, expectorant. The fresh petals are directed by the British Pharmacopœia for preparing a syrup, which may be given in 1 drachm doses, occasionally, as a mild astringent, but is principally employed as a colouring agent for mixtures and gargles.

Culpepper tells us that a syrup made of the leaves and flowers is effectual in pleurisy and erysipelas, or the green leaves can be applied outwardly, made into an ointment, but Gerard says these claims are without foundation and that 'it is only chance when persons are relieved by it.'

Culpepper also tells us :

'it is more cooling than any of the other Poppies, and therefore cannot but be as effectual in hot agues, frenzies, and other inflammations either inward or outward. Galen saith, The seed is dangerous to be used inwardly.'

There are other varieties of the Field Poppy – *P. Dubium*, frequently met with in some parts of the country, is a smaller, more slender plant than *P. Rhœas*, and may be at once distinguished by the capsule, which is

POTATO

Part Used. Edible tubers

The Potato is nearly related to the Nightshades, belonging to the same genus, *Solanum*. Its flowers are very similar in form, but larger and paler in colour than those of *Solanum Dulcamara*.

The stalks, leaves and green berries possess the narcotic and poisonous properties of the Nightshades, but the tubers we eat (which are not the root, but mere enlargements of underground stems, shortened and thickened, in which starch is stored up for the future use of the plant), not being acted on by light, do not develop the poisonous properties contained by that part of the plant above ground. The influence of light on the tubers can be observed if in spring-time young green potatoes are exposed to daylight, when it will be found that they become poisonous and have a disagreeable taste.

The Potato was introduced into Europe early in the sixteenth century, being brought to Spain from Peru, and was first brought into England in 1586 from North America, the colonists sent out by Sir Walter Raleigh bringing it back with them from Virginia.

Gerard, in his *Herbal* published in 1597, gives a figure of the Potato, under the name of 'Potato of Virginia' – to distinguish it from the Sweet Potato. The Herbal contains a portrait of himself on the frontispiece holding in his hand a spray of the Potato plant with flowers and berries.

Though Sir Walter Raleigh was the first to plant the Potato, on his estate at Youghall, near Cork, it is said that he knew so little about it that he tried to eat the berries, and on discovering their noxious character, ordered the plants to be rooted out. It is said that the gardener in doing so, first learnt the value of their wholesome tubers.

From Ireland, the Potato was soon after carried into Lancashire, but for some time Potatoes were only grown as a delicacy for the epicure, not as food for the people. Both

twice as long as broad, and by the bristles, which are flattened up against the stem. *P. hybridum* is less branched than the Field Poppy, which it greatly resembles, but differs in the filaments of the stamens, which are dilated from below upwards; and in the capsule, which, though globular, is covered with stiff bristles. This species is rare in this country.

P. Argemone is the smallest of the British Poppies; its capsule is in shape like that of *P. Dubium*, but it has a few stiff hairs or bristles which are directed upwards.

Solanum tuberosum (LINN.)
N.O. Solanaceæ

Gerard and Parkinson refer to them in this manner. The Puritans opposed their cultivation, because no mention of them could be found in the Bible, and it was not until the middle of the eighteenth century that potatoes became common in this country as a vegetable. As late as 1716, Bradley, in his *Historia Plantarum Succulentarum*, speaks of them as 'inferior to skirrets and radishes.'

The Potato is indigenous in various parts of South America, plants in a wild state having been found on the Peruvian coast, as well as on the sterile mountains of Central Chile and Buenos Aires. The Spaniards are believed to have first brought it to Europe, from Quito, in the early part of the sixteenth century. It afterwards found its way into Italy, and from thence it was carried to Mons, in Belgium, by one of the attendants of the Pope's legate. In 1598 it was sent from Mons to the celebrated botanist Clusius at Vienna, who states that in a short time it spread rapidly throughout Germany.

In the time of James I, potatoes cost 2s. a pound, and are mentioned in 1619 among the articles provided for the royal household. In 1633, when their valuable properties had become more generally known, they were noticed by the Royal Society, and measures were taken to encourage their cultivation in case of famine; but it was not till nearly a century after this that they were grown to any extent in England. In 1725 they were introduced into Scotland and cultivated with much success, first in gardens, and afterwards (about 1760), when they had become plentiful, in the open fields.

On the Continent, the adoption of the Potato as a vegetable met with considerable prejudice, and it did not become a general article of food for some time after it was in general use here. Gerard says: 'Bauhine saith that he heard that the use of these roots was forbidden in Burgundy for that they were persuaded the too frequent use of them caused the leprosie' – a belief without any foundation, for the disease is now confined to countries where the Potato is not grown, and its antiscorbutic properties have been proved.

Linnæus for some time objected to the use of the Potato on account of its connexion with the Deadly Nightshade and Bittersweet. Solanine, the poisonous active principle contained in the stalks, leaves and unripe fruit, is very powerful, and has not yet been fully investigated. It is also present in the peel of the tuber, but is dissipated and rendered inert when the whole potato is boiled and steamed, and is decomposed by baking.

¶ *Constituents.* The tuber is composed mainly of starch, which affords animal heat and promotes fatness, but the proportion of muscle-forming food is very small – it is said that $10\frac{1}{2}$ lb. of the tubers are only equal in value to 1 lb. of meat. The raw juice of the Potato contains no alkaloid, the chief ingredient being potash salts, which are present in large quantity. The tuber also contains a certain amount of citric acid – which, like Potash, is antiscorbutic – and phosphoric acid, yielding phosphorus in a quantity less only than that afforded by the apple and by wheat.

It is of paramount importance that the valuable potash salts should be retained by the Potato during cooking. If peeled and then boiled, the tubers lose as much as 33 per cent. of potash and 23 per cent. of phosphoric acid, and should, therefore, invariably be boiled or steamed with their coats on. Too much stress cannot be laid on this point. Peeled potatoes have lost half their food-value in the water in which they have been boiled.

The Potato is not only important as a valuable article of diet, but has many other uses, both medicinal and economic.

To carry a raw potato in the pocket was an old-fashioned remedy against rheumatism that modern research has proved to have a scientific basis. Ladies in former times had special bags or pockets made in their dresses in which to carry one or more small raw potatoes for the purpose of avoiding rheumatism if predisposed thereto. Successful experiments in the treatment of rheumatism and gout have in the last few years been made with preparations of raw potato juice. In cases of gout, rheumatism and lumbago the acute pain is much relieved by fomentations of the prepared juice followed by an application of liniment and ointment. Sprains and bruises have also been successfully treated by the Potato-juice preparations, and in cases of synovitis rapid absorption of the fluid has resulted. Although it is not claimed that the treatment in acute gout will cure the constitutional symptoms, local treatment by its means relieves the pain more quickly than other treatment.

Potato starch is much used for determining the diastatic value of malt extract.

Hot potato water has in years past been a popular remedy for some forms of rheumatism, fomentations to swollen and painful parts, as hot as can be borne, being applied from water in which 1 lb. of unpeeled potatoes, divided into quarters, has been boiled in 2 pints slowly boiled down to 1 pint. Another potato remedy for rheumatism was made by cutting up the tubers, infusing them together with the fresh stalks and unripe berries for some hours in cold water, and applying in the form of a cold compress. The potatoes should not be peeled.

Uncooked potatoes, peeled and pounded in a mortar, and applied cold, have been found to make a very soothing plaster to parts that have been scalded or burnt.

The mealy flour of baked potato, mixed with sweet oil, is a very healing application for frost-bites. In Derbyshire, hot boiled potatoes are used for corns.

Boiled with weak sulphuric acid, potato starch is changed into glucose, or grape sugar, which by fermentation yields alcohol – this spirit being often sold under the name of British Brandy.

A volatile oil – chemically termed Amylic alcohol, in Germany known as *Fuselöl* – is distilled by fermentation from potato spirit.

Although young potatoes contain no citric acid, the mature tubers yield enough even for commercial purposes, and ripe potato juice is an excellent cleaner of silks, cottons and woollens.

A fine flour is prepared from the Potato, and more used on the Continent than in this country for cake-making.

POTATO, PRAIRIE

Psoralea
N.O. Leguminosæ

Synonyms. Prairie Turnip. Tipsinah. Taahgu
Parts Used. Root, leaf, seeds
Habitat. United States. Other species of the genus in India and Europe

¶ *Description.* The tubers of *Psoralea esculenta* are eaten by the Indians and settlers of the North-western United States. The other species have various medicinal qualities. *P. pedunculata* or *P. melilotoides*, the Virginian variety, is also known as Congo

Root, Bob's Root, and Samson's Snake-root.

Leaflets of *P. obliqua*, bitter, and of a distinct odour, have been found to be mixed with Buchu.

¶ *Constituents.* Of the tuber, 70 per cent. starch and 5 per cent. of a new sugar not yet fully investigated. The root of the Virginian variety contains a volatile oil of pungent taste, and a bitter principle, not tannin. The Indian *P. corylifolia* yields a useful oleoresin.

¶ *Medicinal Action and Uses. P. glandulosa*, or yolochiahitl, has a leaf included in the Mexican Pharmacopœia as a tonic or anthelmintic, and an emetic root. *P. bituminosa* of Europe and *P. physodes* of California are tonic and emmenagogic. The root of the Virginian variety is a valuable, aromatic tonic, useful in chronic diarrhœa, while the Indian species is useful for leucoderma and other skin diseases.

POTATO, WILD

Convolvulus panduratus
N.O. Convolvulaceæ

Synonyms. Mechameck. Wild Jalap. Man-in-the-earth. Man-in-the-ground. Manroot. Now Ipomœa fastigiata, Sweet
Part Used. Root
Habitat. United States and a small amount in South America

¶ *Description.* The perennial, tapering root is very large, being from 2 to 8 feet in length, and 2 to 5 inches in diameter. It is brownish-yellow outside, whitish and lactescent within, having an acrid taste and disagreeable odour. It loses 75 per cent. of weight in drying. Usually it arrives in transverse, circular sections, not readily reducible to greyish powder. It is stated that the Red Indians can handle rattlesnakes with ease and safety after wetting their hands with the milky juice of the root. The leaves are 2 to 3 inches long, the flowers large and

white, and the fruit an oblong, two-celled capsule.

¶ *Constituents.* Unknown.

¶ *Medicinal Action and Uses.* Mildly cathartic and diuretic. It was formerly used in strangury and calculous diseases, and also slightly influences lungs, liver, and kidneys without excessive diuresis or catharsis. Probably the active principle would prove stronger than the crude root.

¶ *Dosage.* 40 grains of the dried root.

See BINDWEED, JALAP, POTATO (SWEET).

PRICKLY ASH. *See* ASH

PRIMROSE

Primula vulgaris (HUDS.)
N.O. Primulaceæ

Parts Used. Root, herb
Habitat. The plant is abundant in woods, hedgerows, pastures and on railway embankments throughout Great Britain, and is in full flower during April and May. In sheltered spots in mild winters it is often found in blossom during the opening days of the year

The Primrose possesses somewhat similar medicinal properties to those of the Cowslip. It has a root-stock, knotty with the successive bases of fallen leaves and bearing cylindrical, branched rootlets on all sides. The leaves are egg-shaped and oblong, about 5 inches long when fully developed, tapering into a winged stalk, about 1¼ inch broad in the middle, smooth above, the veins and veinlets prominent beneath and hairy, the margins irregularly toothed. The young leaf appears as a stout mid-rib, with the blade rolled on itself on either side into two crinkled coils laid tightly along it, in similar manner to the Cowslip.

The flowers are each on separate stalks.

There are two kinds of flowers, externally apparently identical, but inwardly of different construction. Only one kind is found on each plant, never both, one kind being known as 'pin-eyed' and the other as 'thrum-eyed.' In both, the green-tubed calyx and the pale yellow corolla of five petals, joined into a tube below and spreading into a disk above are identical, but in the centre of the pin-eyed flowers there is only the green knob of the stigma, looking like a pin's head, whereas in the centre of the thrum-eyed flowers there are five anthers, in a ring round the tube, but no central knob. Farther down the tube, there are in the pin-eyed flowers five anthers hanging on to the wall of the corolla tube, while in the thrum-eyed, at this same spot, is the stigma knob. At the bottom of the tube in both alike is the seed-case and round it the honey.

It was Darwin who first pointed out the reason for this arrangement. Only a long-tongued insect can reach the honey at the base of the tube and when he starts collecting the honey on a pin-eyed flower, pollen is rubbed on the middle part of his proboscis from the anthers midway down the tube. As he goes from flower to flower on the same plant, there is the same result, but when he visits another plant with thrum-eyed flowers, then the pollen on his proboscis is just in the right place to rub on the stigma which only reaches half-way up the tube, his head meanwhile getting pollen from the long stamens at the throat of the tube, which in turn is transferred to the tall stigmas of the next pin-eyed flower he ,may visit. Thus both kinds of flowers are cross-fertilized in an ingenious manner. It is also remarkable that the pollen of the two flowers differs, the grains of that in the thrum-eyed flower being markedly larger, to allow it to fall on the long stigmas of the pin-eyed flowers and to put out long tubes to reach to the ovary-sac far below, whereas the smaller pollen destined for the shorter stigmas has only to send out a comparatively short tube to reach the seeds waiting to be fertilized. This diversity of structure ensures cross-fertilization only by such long-tongued insects as bees and moths.

¶ *Parts Used Medicinally and Preparation for Market*. The whole herb, used fresh, and in bloom, and the root-stock (the so-called root) dried.

The roots of two- or three-year-old plants are used, dug in autumn. The roots must be thoroughly cleansed in cold water, with a brush, allowing them to remain in water as short a time as possible. All smaller fibres are trimmed off. Large roots may be split lengthwise to facilitate drying, but as a rule this will not be necessary with Primrose roots.

¶ *Constituents*. Both the root and flowers of the Primrose contain a fragrant oil and Primulin, which is identical with Mannite, whilst the somewhat acrid active principle is Saponin.

¶ *Medicinal Action and Uses*. Antispasmodic, vermifuge, emetic, astringent.

In the early days of medicine, the Primrose was considered an important remedy in muscular rheumatism, paralysis and gout.

Pliny speaks of it as almost a panacea for these complaints.

The whole plant is sedative and in modern days a tincture of the fresh plant in bloom, in a strength of 10 oz. to 1 pint of alcohol, in doses of 1 to 10 drops has been used with success in America in extreme sensitiveness, restlessness and insomnia. The whole plant has somewhat expectorant qualities.

An infusion of the flowers was formerly considered excellent against nervous hysterical disorders. 'Primrose Tea,' says Gerard, 'drunk in the month of May is famous for curing the phrensie.' The infusion may be made of 5 to 10 parts of the petals to 100 of water.

In modern herbal medicine the infusion of the root is generally taken in tablespoonful doses as a good remedy against nervous headaches. A teaspoonful of the powdered dry root serves as an emetic.

'Of the leaves of Primrose,' Culpepper tells us, 'is made as fine a salve to heal wound as any I know.'

The leaves are said to be eagerly eaten by the common silkworm.

In ancient cookery the flowers were the chief ingredient in a pottage called 'Primrose Pottage.' Another old dish had rice, almonds, honey, saffron, and ground Primrose flowers. (From *A Plain Plantain*.)

The Primrose family is remarkable for the number of hybrids it produces. The garden 'Polyanthus of unnumbered dyes,' as the poet Thomson calls it in 'The Seasons,' is only another form (probably of the Cowslip or Oxlip) produced by cultivation. The Oxlip is distinguished from the Primrose by its flowers being stalked umbels and of a deeper shade of yellow and by its leaves becoming suddenly broader above the middle. It varies from the Cowslip by its tubular, not bell-shaped calyx and flat, not concave corolla.

The following note is from the *Chemist and Druggist* (March 5, 1921):

'The Oxlip is of more interest to the botanist than to the pharmacist, though at one time it shared with its cousins the cowslip and primrose the name *Herba paralysis*, and had, like them, a considerable reputation as a remedy in several diseases. Our official books distinguished between *Herba paralysis* and *Primula veris*, and attributed different virtues to them.'

See COWSLIP, CYCLAMEN.

PRIMROSE, EVENING

Œnothera biennis (LINN.)
N.O. Onagraceæ

Synonym. Tree Primrose
Parts Used. Bark, leaves
Habitat. The Evening or Tree Primrose, though originally a native of North America, was imported first into Italy and has been carried all over Europe, being often naturalized on river-banks and other sandy places in Western Europe. It is often cultivated in English gardens, and is apparently fully naturalized in Lancashire and some other counties of England, having been first a garden escape

¶ *Description.* The root is biennial, fusiform and fibrous, yellowish on the outside and white within. The first year, many obtuse leaves are produced, which spread flat on the ground. From among these in the second year, the more or less hairy stems arise and grow to a height of 3 or 4 feet. The later leaves are 3 to 5 inches long, 1 inch or more wide, pointed, with nearly entire margins and covered with short hairs. The flowers are produced all along the stalks, on axillary branches and in a terminating spike, often leafy at the base. The uppermost flowers come out first in June. The stalks keep continually advancing in height, and there is a constant succession of flowers till late in the autumn, making this one of the showiest of our hardy garden plants, if placed in large masses. The flowers are of a fine, yellow colour, large and delicately fragrant, and usually open between six and seven o'clock in the evening, hence the name of Evening Primrose. From a horticultural point of view, the variety *grandiflora* or *Lamarkiana* should always be preferred to the ordinary kind, as the flowers are larger and of a finer colour, having a fine effect in large masses, and being well suited for the wild garden.

The generic name is derived from *oinos* (wine) and *thera* (a hunt), and is an old Greek name given by Theophrastus to some plant, probably an Epilobium, the roots of which were eaten to provoke a relish for wine, as olives are now; others say it dispelled the effects of wine.

The large, bright yellow, fragrant flowers are mostly fertilized by twilight-flying insects, especially in the early season. Later the plants keep 'open house' practically all day. In America it is considered a troublesome pest; in England it is not formidable.

The roots of the Evening Primrose are eaten in some countries in the spring, and the French often use it for garnishing salads.

¶ *Cultivation.* The Evening Primrose will thrive in almost any soil or situation, being perfectly hardy. It flourishes best in fairly good sandy soil and in a warm sunny position.

Sow the seeds an inch deep in a shady position out-doors in April, transplanting the seedlings when 1 inch high, 3 inches apart each way in sunny borders. Keep them free from weeds, and in September or the following March, transplant them again into the flowering positions. As the roots strike deep into the ground, care should be taken not to break them in removing.

Seeds may also be sown in cold frames in autumn for blooming the following year.

If the plants are once introduced and the seeds permitted to scatter, there will be a supply of plants without any special care.

¶ *Parts Used.* Bark and leaves. The bark is peeled from the flower-stems and dried in the same manner as the leaves, which are collected in the second year, when the flower-stalk has made its appearance.

¶ *Medicinal Action and Uses.* Astringent and sedative. The drug extracted from this plant, though not in very general use, has been tested in various directions, and has been employed with success in the treatment of gastro-intestinal disorders of a functional origin, asthma and whooping cough.

It has proved of service in dyspepsia, torpor of the liver, and in certain female complaints, such as pelvic fullness.

The dose ranges from 5 to 30 grains.

Henslow mentions another species, *Œnothera odorata*, which he states is found wild in the south of England, but only as a garden escape. It grows to 2 feet in height, with purplish stems and yellow flowers, 3 to 4 inches across. They are sweet-smelling, hence its specific name.

In *The Treasury of Botany* a large white-flowered species is also mentioned, said to have run wild over some parts of the Nilghiri Hills in India.

PRIMULAS

N.O. Primulaceæ

The leaves of some species produce irritation to face and hands resulting sometimes in a form of eczema. This is caused by a secretion in the glandular hairs and is termed primula dermatitis. The roots of *Primula grandiflora* give a crystalline polyatomic alcohol, 'primulite,' said to be identical with hepatomic alcohol 'volemite.' Two glucosides, Primverin and Primulaverin, and an enzyme, primverase, have also been isolated in it.

The Primrose family is remarkable for the number of hybrids it produces. The garden 'Polyanthus of unnumbered dyes,' as the poet Thomson calls it in 'The Seasons,' is only another form (probably of the Cowslip or Oxlip) produced by cultivation, and is one of the most favourite plants in cottage gardens, of endless variety and easy cultivation. The Oxlip is distinguished from the Primrose by its flowers being stalked umbels and of a deeper shade of yellow and by its leaves becoming suddenly broader above the middle. It varies from the Cowslip by its tubular, not bell-shaped calyx and flat, not concave corolla.

All the hardy varieties of Primula, whether Primrose, Cowslip, Polyanthus or Auricula, may be easily propagated by dividing the roots of old plants in autumn. New varieties are raised from seed, which should be sown as soon as ripe, in leaf-mould, and pricked out into beds when large enough.

Among the many splendid flowers that are grown in our greenhouses none shows more improvement under the fostering hand of the British florist than the Chinese Primula, which originally had small, inconspicuous flowers, but now bears trusses of magnificent blooms ranging from the purest white to the richest scarlet and crimson. The Star Primulas which have attained an even greater popularity in late years are considered perhaps even more elegant, being looser in growth and carrying their plentiful blossoms in more graceful, if not more beautiful trusses. Both varieties are among the most beautiful of our winter-flowering plants, the toothed and lobed, somewhat heart-shaped leaves being extremely handsome with their crimson tints.

Seeds of these greenhouse Primulas should be sown in the spring in gentle heat, the soil used being very fine and pleasantly moist. The seedlings must be pricked off and potted on as necessary, with a view to ensuring sturdy, healthy growth.

P. obconica is a slightly varying type of these greenhouse Primulas, the leaves approaching more the shape of those of the common Primrose; the plants are exceedingly floriferous and graceful, the full trusses of delicate lilac flowers are borne on tall slender stems and care must be used in the handling of it, as the leaves sometimes cause an eruption like eczema. Homœopaths make a tincture from this species.

The broad, thick leaves of the Auricula (*P. auricula*), a frequent garden plant in this country, though not native to Great Britain, are used in the Alps as a remedy for coughs.

See PRIMROSE, COWSLIP.

PRUNES

Prunus domestica (LINN.)
N.O. Rosaceæ

Synonym. Plum Tree
Part Used. Fruit, dried
Habitat. Asia and parts of Europe; best from Bordeaux

¶ *Description.* A small tree, 15 to 20 feet high, with numerous spreading branches without spines, young branches smooth, leaves small, alternate on longish petioles, provided with linear, fimbriated, pubescent stipules which are quickly deciduous, blade about 2 inches long, oval, acute at both ends, crenate-dentate, smooth above, more or less pubescent underneath, convolute in the bud, flowers appear before leaves. The cultivated plum has been developed from the wild plum, the thorns being lost in the process. Plums were known to the Romans in Cato's time.

¶ *Constituents.* Prunes have a faint peculiar odour and a sweetish slightly acidulous and viscid taste. The ripe fruit contains sugar, gum, albumen, malic acid, pectin, vegetable fibre, etc.

¶ *Medicinal Action and Uses.* Dried prunes are mildly laxative and are frequently employed in decoction. They form a pleasant and nourishing diet for invalids when stewed; they enter into the composition of Confection of Senna. A medicinal tincture is prepared from the fresh flower-buds of the Blackthorn. Some 20 per cent. of oil is obtainable by crushing the Plum kernel – this is clear, yellow in colour and has an agreeable almond flavour and smell. It is used for alimentary purposes. The residue after pressing is used in the manufacture of a brandy, which is largely consumed in Hungary.

PSYLLIUM SEEDS. *See* PLANTAIN

PULSATILLA. *See* ANEMONE

PUMPKIN. *See* MELON

PURSLANE, GREEN

Portulaca oleracea

PURSLANE, GOLDEN

Portulaca sativa
N.O. Caryophylleæ

Synonyms. Garden Purslane. Pigweed
Parts Used. Herb, juice, seeds
Habitat. The Purslanes are distributed all over the world. *Portulaca oleracea,* the Garden, or Green Purslane, is a herbaceous annual, native of many parts of Europe, found in the East and West Indies, China, Japan and Ascension Island, and though found also in the British Isles is not indigenous there

¶ *Description.* It has a round, smooth, procumbent, succulent stem, growing about 6 inches high, with small, oblong, wedge-shaped, dark-green leaves, thick and stalked, clustered together, destitute of the bristle in their axils which others of the genus have. The flowers are small, yellow, solitary or clustered, stalkless, placed above the last leaves on the branches, blooming in June and July, and opening only for a short time towards noon.

The growth of the plant somewhat resembles Samphire, and the rich red colour of the stems is very striking and most decorative in herb borders. The Golden Purslane (*Portulaca sativa*) is a variety of Purslane with yellow leaves, less hardy than the Green Purslane, but possessing the same qualities. The seeds of an individual plant have been known to produce both green and golden-leaved plants.

Purslane is a pleasant salad herb, and excellent for scorbutic troubles. The succulent leaves and young shoots are cooling in spring salads, the older shoots are used as a pot-herb, and the thick stems of plants that have run to seed are pickled in salt and vinegar to form winter salads. Purslane is largely cultivated in Holland and other countries for these purposes. It is used in equal proportion with Sorrel to make the well-known French soup *bonne femme.* Gerard said of this herb: 'Raw Purslane is much used in sallads, with oil, salt and vinegar. It cools the blood and causes appetite;' and Evelyn tells us that, 'familiarly eaten alone with Oyl and Vinegar,' moderation should be used, adding that it is eminently moist and cooling, 'especially the golden,' and is 'generally entertained in all our sallets. Some eate of it cold, after it has been boiled, which Dr. Muffit would have in wine for nourishment.'

Most of the plants in this order are mucilaginous. The root of one species, *Lewisia rediviva,* the Tobacco root, a native of North America, so called from its odour when cooked, possesses great nutritive properties. It is boiled and eaten by the Indians, and Hogg tells us that it proves most sustaining on long journeys, and that 2 or 3 oz. a day are quite sufficient for a man, even while undergoing great fatigue. *Claytonia tuberosa,* another plant belonging to the same order as the Purslanes, likewise a native of North America, has also an edible root.

Purslane in ancient times was looked upon as one of the anti-magic herbs, and strewn round a bed was said to afford protection against evil spirits. We are told that it was a sure cure for 'blastings by lightening or planets and burning of gunpowder.'

¶ *Medicinal Action and Uses.* It was highly recommended for many complaints. The expressed juice, taken while fresh, was said to be good for strangury, and taken with sugar and honey to afford relief for dry coughs, shortness of breath and immoderate thirst, as well as for external application in inflammation and sores.

It was supposed to cool 'heat in the liver' and to be excellent for 'hot agues,' and all pains in the head 'proceeding from the heat, want of sleep or the frenzy,' and also to stop hæmorrhages.

The herb, bruised and applied to the forehead and temple, was said to allay excessive heat, and applied to the eyes to remove inflammation. Culpepper says: 'The herb if placed under the tongue assuayeth thirst. Applied to the gout, it easeth pains thereof, and helps the hardness of the sinews, if it come not of the cramp, or a cold cause.'

The juice, with oil of Roses, was recommended for sore mouths and swollen gums and also to fasten loose teeth. Another authority declared that the distilled water took away pains in the teeth, both Gerard and Turner telling us too, that the leaves eaten raw are good for teeth that are 'set on edge with eating of sharpe and soure things.'

The seeds, bruised and boiled in wine, were given to children as a vermifuge.

¶ *Cultivation.* Sow the seeds in drills, on a bed of rich light earth, during any of the summer months, from May onwards. To have it early in the season, it should be sown upon a hot bed, at the end of March and planted out in a warm border in May. The Green Purslane is quite hardy, the Golden Purslane less so.

Keep the plants clear from weeds, and in dry weather water them two or three times a week. The Purslanes need rather more watering than most herbs.

In warm weather, they will be fit for use in six weeks. When the leaves are gathered, the plants must be cut low and then a fresh crop will appear.

To continue a succession, sow three or four times, at an interval of a fortnight or three weeks.

If the seeds are to be saved, leave some of the earliest plants for that purpose.

¶ *Other Species.*

Professor Hulme, in *Familiar Wild Flowers*, speaks of a variety which he calls the SEA PURSLANE (*Atriplex portulacoides*), common enough on the sea-shores of England and Ireland, though much less so in Scotland. It grows in saline marshes and muddy foreshores. It is a shrubby and much-branching plant, attaining to no great height, usually a foot to 18 inches – though occasionally to 2 feet. The lower portion of the stem is often somewhat creeping and rooting, which gives it a greater grip of the ground in view of fierce gales. The stems are often of a delicate purple colour, more or less covered with a grey bloom. The foliage is of pointed, lance-head form, thick and fleshy, and entirely silvery white in colour. The minute flowers are in little clusters that succeed one another at intervals on the short branches near the top of the plant and form a terminal head. The flowers are of two kinds: one is stamen-bearing, these stamens being five in number and within a five-cleft perianth; the other is pistil-bearing and consists of two flattened segments, closing somewhat like the leaves of a book, and contained within the ovary. After the flowering is over, this flattened perianth considerably enlarges. This construction of the seed-bearing flower is of some specific importance, for in the present species and the *A. pedunculata* the two segments are united nearly to the top, while in another species, the *A. rosea*, these segments are not joined above their centres; and in a third, the *A. hortensis*, they are not joined at all.

An entirely different plant, one of the great Pink family, the *Houckenya peploides*, is sometimes called the 'ovate-leaved Sea Purslane.' It is a common plant on sea-beaches, with large white five-petalled blossoms. Another name for it is 'ovate Sand-wort.'

The generic title of the Sea Purslane, *Atriplex*, is one of Pliny's plant names. It is derived from two Greek words signifying 'not to flourish,' the meaning of the word applied to the plant is obscure. The specific name, *Potrulacoides*, signifies 'resembling the purslane plant,' the *portulaca*. Another name for the Sea Purslane is 'Shrubby Orache.'

The origin of the name 'Purslane' is unknown. Turner calls the plant 'purcellaine,' and in the *Grete Herball*, 1516, it is 'procelayne.'

In the North American prairies Purslane is called 'Pussly.'

PYROLAS

N.O. Pyrolaceæ

The species are known by the common name of Wintergreen.

The name Pyrola is a diminutive of *Pyrus* (a pear tree), from the resemblance of its leaves to those of the pear.

WINTERGREEN

Pyrola secunda is known as Yevering Bells, from the resemblance of its flowers to little bells hung one above the other.

¶ *Description.* Low herbs, with a slender shortly creeping stock; orbicular or ovate, nearly radical leaves; and white or greenish, drooping flowers, either solitary or several in a short raceme, on leaflets, erect peduncles. Sepals five, small. Petals five, distinct or slightly joined at the base, forming at first a spreading corolla, which persists round the young capsule, assuming a globular shape. Stamens ten. Capsule five-celled, opening by slits in the middle of the cells.

Pyrola uniflora (one-flowered Winter-green), found in woods, in Northern and Arctic Europe, Asia and America, and along the high mountain ranges of Central Europe. In pine woods from Perth and Aberdeen northwards. Flowers in the summer.

P. media (Intermediate Wintergreen), not found in England south of Warwick and Worcester, whence it extends to Shetland; it also is found in the north and west of Ireland.

P. minor (Common Wintergreen). In woods and moist shady places in Europe, Northern Asia and the extreme north of America, becoming a mountain plant in Southern Europe and the Caucasus. Frequent in Scotland, northern England, more local in southern England. Rare in Ireland. Flowers in the summer.

P. secunda. Very local in Britain, found in Monmouthshire and from Yorkshire northward to Ross-shire. It is very rare in the north-east of Ireland only. Flowers in the summer.

Pyrola rotundifolia

Synonym. Round-leaved Wintergreen

¶ *Description.* A larger plant than *Pyrola minor*, with larger and whiter flowers and the petals more spreading, but chiefly distinguished from it by the long, protruding, much-curved style, usually at least twice as long as the capsule with a much smaller stigma, with short erect lobes.

¶ *Medicinal Action and Uses.* Astringent, diuretic, tonic, antispasmodic. The decoction much used in skin diseases and to eradicate a scropulous condition from the system. The decoction also valuable as a gargle and wash for ophthalmic eyes.

Used internally for epilepsy and other nervous affections.

Dose of decoction, 1 fluid ounce three times daily. Solid extract, 2 to 4 grains. The Germans use this plant in their wound drinks and in many ointments and plasters. A decoction of the leaves with the addition of a little cinnamon and red wine cures bloody stools, ulcers of the bladder and restrains the menses.

Salmon says:

'The liquid juice. It consolidates green wounds, uniting their lips speedily together; and taken inwardly 2 or 3 spoonfuls at a time in wine and water, it stops inward fluxes of the blood and cures inward wounds. It stops the overflowing of the Terms in women, cures spitting and vomiting of Blood, the Hepatick Flux, Bloody Flux and all other Fluxes of the Bowels. It is said to cure ulcers and wounds in the Reins and Bladder, Womb and other secret parts, as also ulcers and Fistulas in any other part of the Body, being inwardly taken and outwardly applied. The decoction in wine and water . . . has all the former virtues, but not altogether so powerful and may be given morning and night from 3 ounces to 6, sweetened with syrup of the juice of the same. . . . The Balsam or Ointment is made with Hog's Lard, or with oil olive, Bees Wax and a little Turpentine . . . heals cankers of the mouth and gums.'

See PIPSISSEWA, WINTERGREEN.

QUASSIA

Picræna excelsa (LINDL.)
N.O. Simarubeæ

Synonyms. Bitter Wood. Jamaica Quassia. Bitter Ash. Quassia Amara (Linn.). Quassia Lignum, B.P.
Part Used. Wood of trunks and branches
Habitat. Jamaica

¶ *Description.* A tree growing 50 to 100 feet, erect stem over 3 feet in diameter. Bark smooth and greyish. Leaves alternate, unequally pinnate, leaflets opposite, oblong, acuminate, and unequal at the base. Flowers small pale yellowish green, blooming October and November. Fruit three drupes size of a pea (maturing its fruit December and January), black, shining, solitary, globose, with a thin shell. The wood of this tree furnishes the Quassia of commerce. It is imported in large logs varying from a foot or more in diameter and 1 to 8 feet in length, occasionally much bigger, then it is split into quarters, retaining a friable and feebly attached cortex which has the same medicinal qualities as the wood, which is very tough, close grained and white, but changes to yellow on contact with the air. It is odourless and very bitter, the bark is thin and dark brown or thick greyish brown transversed by reticulating lines.

Quassia Amara, or Surinan Quassia, as found in commerce, is in much smaller billets than the Jamaica Quassia, and is used in its place on the Continent, and is easily recognized from the Jamaica one, which it closely resembles, by its medullary rays, which are only one cell wide, and contain no calcium oxalate.

¶ *Constituents of Jamaica Quassia.* Volatile oil, quassin, gummy extractive pectin, woody fibre, tartrate and sulphate of lime, chlorides of calcium, and sodium, various salts such as oxalate and ammoniacal salt, nitrate of potassa and sulphate of soda. Quassia, U.S.P., may be either Jamaica or Surinan Quassia.

¶ *Medicinal Action and Uses.* Quassia, found in the shops in the form of chips or raspings, has no smell but an intense bitter taste, which will always distinguish the pure drug from adulterations; the infusion of these by persalt of iron gives a bluish-black colour, but as the blue Quassia chips contain no tannic acid, no result is produced in the infusion. Quassia wood is a pure bitter tonic and stomachic; it is also a vermicide and slight narcotic; it acts on flies and some of the higher animals as a narcotic poison. It is a valuable remedy in convalescence, after acute disease and in debility and atonic

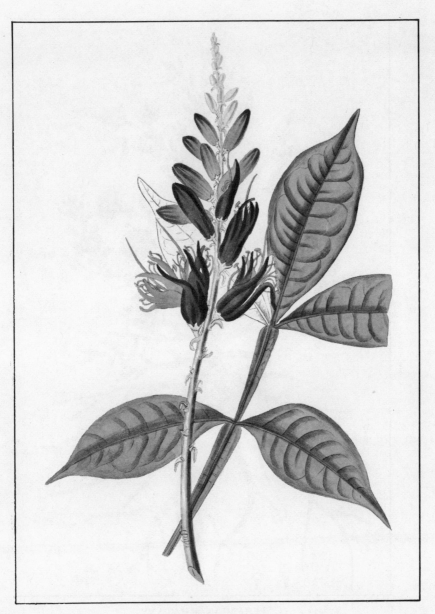

QUASSIA
Picræna Excelsa

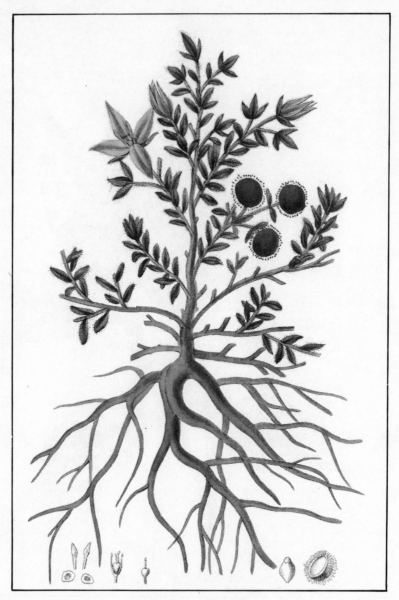

PERUVIAN RHATANY
Krameria Triandra

dyspepsia; an antispasmodic in fever. Having no tannic acid, it is frequently given with chalybeates and therefore can be prescribed with salts of iron; as an aromatic bitter stomachic it acts in the same way as calumba. In small doses Quassia increases the appetite; large doses act as an irritant and cause vomiting; its action probably lessens putrefaction in the stomach, and prevents the formation of acid substances during digestion. A decoction used as an injection will move ascarides; for an enema for this purpose, 3 parts Quassia to 1 part mandrake root are used, and to each ounce of the mixture, 1 fluid drachm of asafœtida or diluted carbolic acid is added; for a child up to three years, 2 fluid ounces are injected into the rectum twice daily. Cups made of the wood and filled with liquid will in a few hours become thoroughly impregnated and this drink makes a powerful tonic. The infusion is made by macerating in cold water for twelve hours 3 drachms of the rasped Quassia to 1 pint of cold water, 2 oz. of the infusion alone, or with ginger tea, taken three times a day, proves very useful for feeble emaciated people with impaired digestive organs. The extract can be made by evaporating the decoction to a pilular consistence, and taken in 1 grain doses, three or four times daily, this will be found less obnoxious to the stomach than the infusion or decoction. Quassia with sulphuric acid acts as a cure for drunkenness, by destroying the appetite for alcoholics.

¶ *Preparations and Dosages.* Fluid extract, 15 to 30 drops. Tincture, B.P. and U.S.P., $\frac{1}{2}$ to 1 drachm. Conc. Solut., B.P., $\frac{1}{2}$ drachm. Powdered Quassia, 30 grains. The infusion for killing flies should be sweetened with sugar.

See SIMARUBA.

QUEBRACHO

Aspidosperma quebracho-blanco
N.O. Apocynaceæ

Synonyms. Quebracho Bark. Quebracho-blanco
Part Used. Bark
Habitat. Chile and Argentina, Bolivia, Southern Brazil

¶ *History.* Quebracho is an evergreen tree which sometimes rises to 100 feet, with an erect stem and wide-spreading crown. The wood of all the species of this genus is valuable, and the name is due to its hardness, being derived from two Spanish words, *quebrar* and *hacha*, meaning 'the axe breaks.' It is used for tanning.

The bark was not introduced into Europe until 1878, though was for long used in South America as a febrifuge. Commercially, it is met with in large, thick pieces, covered on the outside with a very thick and rough, corky layer of a greyish-brown colour, and deeply divided by furrows and excavations. The inner bark is greyish or yellowish, smooth or somewhat fibrous, and often with small, black spots. The taste is very bitter, but there is scarcely any odour.

Two other plants are known as Quebracho: *Schinopsis Lorenzii*, the wood of which is sold in commerce as 'quebracho wood,' and *Iodina rhombifolia*, 'quebracho flojo,' the wood and bark of which are sometimes substituted for the 'quebracho colorado.'

¶ *Constituents.* Contains six alkaloids: Aspidospermine, Aspidospermatine, Aspidosamine, Quebrachine, Hypoquebrachine and Quebrachamine. All agree that quebrachine is the most active.

Two new sugars, quebrachite and lævogyrate inosite, tannin and starch have also been extracted.

¶ *Medicinal Action and Uses.* Tonic, febrifuge and anti-asthmatic.

When a preparation of Quebracho or Aspidosperma is injected into the circulation, the rate and depth of the respiration increases largely, apparently due to direct action on the respiratory centre, and the blood-pressure falls.

Aspidosperma is used in medicine for the relief of various types of dyspnœa, especially in emphysema and in asthma. It is not generally useful to interrupt the paroxysm, but, as a rule, if used continuously, it will reduce the frequency and severity of attacks.

Under the name of amorphous aspidospermine, a mixture of the various alkaloids has become known in commerce.

Quebracho Colorado, or *S. Lorenzii,* has been used as a substitute, but is essentially different, being probably a simple and gastrointestinal stimulant, though it has been said to be a much weaker form of quebracho-blanco.

¶ *Dosages.* Of amorphous aspidospermine, $\frac{1}{4}$ to 1 grain. Of crystalline aspidospermine, $\frac{1}{10}$ to $\frac{1}{20}$ grain. Of aspidospermine, 15 grains, but it is not used in the crude state. Fluid extract, $\frac{1}{4}$ to $\frac{1}{2}$ drachm.

QUEEN'S DELIGHT

Stillingia sylvatica (LINN.)
N.O. Euphorbiaceæ

Synonyms. Queen's Root. Silver Leaf. Also Sapium Sylvaticum Yaw Root
Part Used. Root
Habitat. In the southern United States of America from Virginia to Florida and westward to Texas

¶ *Description.* A perennial herb, with an angled glabrous stem, growing to 4 feet high, with a milky sap. The leaves are sessile, leathery and tapering at the base. Flowers yellow on terminal spike. Fruit a three-grained capsule. The plant was named after Dr. B. Stillingfleet. It flowers from April to July; a milky juice exudes from the plant or root when cut or broken. This should be used when fresh as it deteriorates if kept. As found in commerce, the root is 1 to 4 inches long and 1 inch or more thick, covered with a bark wrinkled longitudinally, greyish brown externally, and reddish-brown or rose-coloured internally, odour peculiar, oleaginous, taste bitter and unpleasant, followed by a persistent pungent acridity in mouth and throat. Fracture fibrous, short, irregular, and shows a pithy soft, yellowish-pink interior porous woody portion. The inner bark and medullary rays with brown resin cells, its best solvent is alcohol.

¶ *Constituents.* Its resinous acrid constituent is Sylvacrol, an acrid fixed oil, volatile oil, tannin, starch, calcium oxalate. Woody fibre, colouring matter extractive.

¶ *Medicinal Action and Uses.* In large doses it is emetic and purgative causing a disagreeable, peculiar, burning sensation in the stomach or alimentary canal with considerable prostration of the system; in smaller doses it is an excellent alterative, and influences the secretory functions; it has almost a specific action in the different forms of primary and secondary syphilis, also in skin diseases, scrofula and hepatic affections, acting with most successful results. The fluid extract combined with oils of anise or caraway, proves very beneficial in chronic bronchitis and laryngitis. Some pieces of fresh root chewed daily have permanently and effectually cured these troubles, it is also useful for leucorrhœa. The oil is too acrid for internal use uncombined with saccharine or mucilaginous substance, for internal use the fluid extract or syrup is sufficiently efficacious. As an external stimulating application in most cases the oil will be found very valuable. For croup 1 drop on the tongue three or four times daily, has been found successful for severe attacks. The dried root is said to be inferior in strength to the fresh one, but some chemists consider it more powerful. It may be given either alone or combined with sarsaparilla and other alteratives. It acts reflexly as a sialagogue and expectorant. It is often given for syphilitic complaints in place of mercury.

¶ *Dosages.* Tincture, $\frac{1}{2}$ to 2 drachms. Decoction, 1 to 2 fluid ounces. Powdered root, 6 to 10 grains. Solid extract, 2 to 5 grains. Stillingin, 1 to 3 grains. Fluid extract, 10 to 30 drops.

QUINCE

Pyrus Cydonia (LINN.)
N.O. Rosaceæ

Synonym. Cydonia vulgaris (PERS.)
Parts Used. Seeds, fruit

The Quince has been under cultivation since very remote times. It is a native of Persia and Anatolia and perhaps also of Greece and the Crimea, though it is doubtful if in the latter localities the plant is not a relic of former cultivation. It is certain that the ancient Greeks knew a common variety, upon which they grafted scions of a better variety, which they obtained from Cydon in Crete, from which place the fruit derived its name of *Cydonia*, of which the English name Quince is a corruption.

Botanically, the plant used to be called *Pyrus Cydonia*, but modern botanists now place it in the genus *Pyrus* and assign it to a separate genus, to which the former specific name *Cydonia* has been given.

In old English literature we find the fruit called a Coyne, as in the *Romaunt of the Rose* and the old English Vocabularies of the fourteenth and fifteenth centuries, this name being adapted from the French *coin*, whence Middle English *Coin, Quin*, the plural *quins*, becoming corrupted to the singular *Quince*.

The Quinces differ from the *Pyrus* genus in the twisted manner in which the petals are arranged in the bud and in the many-celled ovary, in which the numerous ovules are disposed horizontally, not vertically as in the Pears. They are much-branched shrubs, or small trees, with entire leaves and large, solitary, white or pink flowers, like those of a pear or apple, but with leafy calyx lobes.

The Quince as we know it in this country

is a different fruit to that of Western Asia and tropical countries, where the fruit becomes softer and more juicy. In colder climates, the fruit is of a fine, handsome shape, of a rich golden colour when ripe and has a strong fragrance, by some judged to be rather heavy and overpowering. The rind is rough and woolly and the flesh harsh and unpalatable, with an astringent, acidulous taste. In hotter countries, the woolly rind disappears and the fruit can be eaten raw. This is the case not only in Eastern countries, where it is much prized, but also in those parts of tropical America to which the tree has been introduced from Europe. This explains the fact that it figured so prominently in classical legends. It was very widely cultivated in the East and especially in Palestine, and many commentators consider that the *Tappuach* of Scripture, always translated Apple, was the Quince. It is also supposed to be the fruit alluded to in the *Canticles*, 'I sat down under his shadow with great delight and his fruit was sweet to my taste'; and in *Proverbs*, 'A word fitly spoken is like Apples of gold in pictures of silver.'

Pliny, who speaks at length of the medicinal virtues of the Quince, says that the fruit warded off the influence of the evil eye, and other legends connect it with ancient Greek mythology, as exemplified by statues on which the fruit is represented, as well as by representations in the wall-paintings and mosaics of Pompeii, where Quinces are almost always to be seen in the paws of a bear.

By the Greeks and Romans, the Quince was held sacred to Venus, who is often depicted with a Quince in her right hand, the gift she received from Paris. The 'golden Apples' of Virgil are said to be Quinces, as they were the only 'golden' fruit known in his time, oranges having only been introduced into Italy at the time of the Crusades.

The fruit, being dedicated to Venus, was regarded as the symbol of Love and Happiness, and Plutarch mentions the bridal custom of a Quince being shared by a married pair. Quinces sent as presents, or shared, were tokens of love. The custom was handed down, and throughout the Middle Ages Quinces were used at every wedding feast, as we may read in a curious book, *The Praise of Musicke*:

'I come to marriages, wherein as our ancestors did fondly and with a kind of doating, maintaine many rites and ceremonies, some whereof were either shadowes or abodements of a pleasant life to come, as the eating of a Quince Peare to be a preparative of sweet and delightful dayes between the married persons.'

Quinces are mentioned among the curious recipes in Manuscripts relating to domestic life in England. Wynkyn de Worde, in the *Boke of Kervynge*, speaks of 'char de Quynce,' and John Russell, in the *Boke of Nurture*, speaks of 'chare de Quynces' – the old name for Quince Marmalade. This preserve is now practically the only use made of the Quince as an article of food, though it is sometimes added to apple-tarts, to improve their flavour, but in Shakespeare's time, Browne spoke of the fruit as 'the stomach's comforter, the pleasing Quince,' and a little later, Parkinson says:

'There is no fruit growing in the land that is of so many excellent uses as this [the Quince], serving as well to make many dishes of meat for the table, as for banquets, and much more for their physical virtues.'

¶ *Cultivation.* The Quince is little cultivated in Great Britain, though it will thrive almost anywhere, but is best adapted to a damp spot, in a rich, high and somewhat moist soil. In Scotland, it seldom approaches maturity unless protected by a wall.

Propagation is generally by cuttings or layers, the former making the best plants, but taking longer to grow. The Quince forms a thick bush and is generally not pruned, unless required to form standard fruit-bearing trees, when it should be trained up to a single stem till a height of 5 or 6 feet is attained.

There are three principal varieties of the Quince: the Portugal, Apple-shaped and Pear-shaped. The Portugal is a taller and more vigorous grower than the others and has larger and finer fruit; the Apple-shaped, which is sometimes considered to have a finer flavour, has roundish fruit, is more productive and ripens under less favourable conditions than either of the others and earlier than the Pear-shaped variety and is therefore preferred to it.

The Quince is much used as a dwarfing stock for certain kinds of pears and for this purpose the young plants when bedded out in the quarters should be shortened back to about 18 to 20 inches. The effect is to restrain the growth of the tree, increase and hasten its fruitfulness and enable it to withstand the effects of cold.

¶ *Medicinal Action and Uses.* A syrup prepared from the fruit may be used as a grateful addition to drinks in sickness, especially in looseness of the bowels, which it is said to restrain by its astringency.

The seeds may be used medicinally for the sake of the mucilage they yield. When soaked in water they swell up and form a mucilaginous mass. This mucilage is analogous to, and has the same properties as, that which is formed from the seeds of the flax – linseed.

The seeds somewhat resemble apple-pips in size and appearance. They are of a dark brown colour, flattened on two sides, owing to mutual pressure and frequently adhere to one another by a white mucilage, which is derived from the epidermal cells of the seed-coats. The seed contains two firm, yellowish-white cotyledons, which have a faintly bitter taste resembling that of bitter almonds.

¶ *Chemical Constituents.* The cotyledons contain about 15 per cent. fixed oil and protein, together with small proportions of amygdalin and emulsion or some allied ferment. The chief constituent of the seed is about 10 per cent. mucilage, contained in the seed-coat. The pulp of the fruit contains 3 to 3·5 per cent. of malic acid.

Pereira considers the mucilage peculiar to this fruit; the chemists Tollens and Kirchner regard it as a compound of gum and cellulose. It differs from Arabin in not yielding a precipitate with potassium silicate and in being soluble both in hot and cold water. It is almost free from adhesive properties.

The seeds, on account of their mucilage, have soothing and demulcent properties and are used internally in the form of *Decoctum Cydoniæ*, an official preparation of the British Pharmacopœia. It is prepared by boiling 2 drachms of Quince seed in a pint of water in a tightly-covered vessel for 10 minutes and straining off. Large quantities of the decoction may be drunk in dysentery, diarrhœa and gonorrhœa and it is used in thrush and irritable conditions of the mucous membrane. The decoction also forms a usefu adjunct to boric-acid eye-lotions. On account of its mucilaginous character, it is not so readily washed away by the tears.

It is also used as an adjunct to skin lotions and creams.

It has been proposed to evaporate the decoction to dryness and powder the residue: 3 grains of this powder form a sufficiently consistent mucilage with an ounce of water. According to Grant (*Journal de Pharmacie et de Chénie*, Paris), 1 part communicates to a thousand parts of water a semi-syrupy consistence.

Mucilago Cydoniæ (Mucilage of Quince

QUINCE, JAPANESE

The Japanese Quince, familiar in our gardens, and formerly known as *Pyrus*

Seeds, B.P.) is stronger than the decoction and has similar properties. It forms a useful suspending agent for such liquids as tincture of Benzoin, when added to toilet preparations. When used for this purpose, it is sometimes prepared with rose-water.

Quince Marmalade

Pare and core the Quinces and cut them up, putting them into water as they are cored, to prevent them from blackening. Put them into a preserving pan with 1 lb. sugar and 1 pint water for every lb. of fruit. Boil over a gentle fire until soft. Then put through a sieve, or mash with a spoon, boil up again and tie down in the same way as any other preserve.

In France, before putting the marmalade into pots, a little rosewater and a few grains of musk, mixed together, are added. This is most delicious and among the French, by whom it is called *Cotiniat*, has a reputation for its digestive powers.

Quince and Apple Marmalade

Take equal quantities of Apple and Quinces. Put into an earthenware jar, 2 quarts of water and, as quickly as they can be pared and sliced, 4 lb. of Quinces. Stew them gently till soft and then strain them. They must not be boiled too long, or they will become red. Boil together, for ¾ hour, 4 lb. of sliced Apples, with the same weight of Quince juice. When it boils, take it off the fire and add 1½ lb. sugar. When dissolved, put it back on the fire and boil, together with the Quinces, for another 20 minutes, stirring all the time and removing the scum. Then pot.

Quince Jelly

Pare and core some ripe Quinces, cut them up, weigh them and put them at once into part of the water in which they will be cooked. Put the Quinces on the fire, with 1 pint water to each pound of fruit and let it simmer, but not long enough to change the colour to red – it should be quite pale. Strain through a jelly-bag. Weigh the juice the next day and put it in a preserving pan and boil it quickly for 15 minutes. Then take it from the fire and stir into it 12 oz. sugar for each lb. of juice. Boil for another 15 or 20 minutes, till cooked, stirring all the time, and remove the scum.

Quinces and Apples can be mixed, making a good combination.

Cydonia Japonica
Pyrus Japonica

Japonica, now usually described as *Cydonia Japonica*, is grown for the sake of its blossoms, which vary in colour from creamy white to rich red and are produced during the winter and early spring months. It is a handsome shrub, generally planted in a sheltered spot, often against a dwarf wall or a trellis, the brilliant flowers of the ordinary red variety being produced soon after the New Year. For the last hundred years it has been the chief spring ornament of English gardens and being quite hardy and easily grown is often seen covering the walls of cottages. A deep, moist loam suits it exactly. The flowers appear before the leaves, and later on in the year, old trees on warm walls will in a dry, hot summer produce a few fruits (Quinces), though it cannot be described as a fruitful tree in this coun-

try. They are nearly round and about the size of a tangerine orange, ripening off a dull green colour, very fragrant and as hard as flints. When cut up, they are found to be packed with large dark pips, around which is a broad rim of flesh of a most uninviting character and quite uneatable, the flavour being rough and styptic.

There are many varieties, differing chiefly in the colour of the flowers: there is often abundance of fruit on the white variety. *C. Maulei*, a more recently introduced shrub from Japan, bears a profusion of beautiful orange-red flowers, followed by fruit of a yellow colour and agreeable fragrance, so that when cooked with sugar, it forms a pleasant conserve.

QUINOA. *See* CHENOPODIUM

QUINSY-WORT
    Synonym. Squinancy-wort

Asperula cynanchica (LINN.)

Quinsy-Wort was formerly esteemed a remedy for the disorder the name of which it bears. The specific name, *cynanchica*, is derived from the Greek *Kunanchi* (dog strangle), from its choking nature.

Its roots, like those of the *Galiums* and *Rubia*, yield a red dye, which has been occasionally used in Sweden.

It is no longer applied in medicine.

This is not a common British plant, ex-

cept locally in dry pastures on a chalky or limehouse soil.

It is a small, smooth plant, 6 to 10 inches high, with very narrow, close-set leaves, four in a whorl, two of each whorl much smaller than the others.

The flowers are in loose terminal bunches, the corollas only $\frac{1}{6}$ inch in diameter, pink externally and white inside, and are in bloom during June and July.

RADISH

Raphanus sativus
N.O. Cruciferæ

    Parts Used. Root, seed-pods
    Habitat. Europe, especially Britain, and temperate Asia. A native of China, Cochin-China and Japan

¶ *Description.* The name of this familiar garden plant is suggested by its colour, being derived from the Saxon, *rude, rudo,* or *reod* (ruddy), or from the Sanskrit *rudhira,* meaning blood. The genus is distinguished by its elongated pod, which has no longitudinal partition when ripe, but contains several seeds separated by a pithy substance filling the pod. The actual plant is unknown in a wild state, but is supposed to have come from Southern Asia, and may be descended from the wild *Raphanus Raphanistrum* of the Mediterranean shores, the long roots developing seeds sown in a loose soil, and the turnip-rooted kinds in a stiff soil. In the days of the Pharaohs, the Radish was extensively cultivated in Egypt, but apparently it did not reach Britain until A.D. 1548. Gerard mentions four varieties as being recognized in 1597. The leaves are rough and partly divided into segments, the outer one being

larger and broader than the rest. The flower stem grows to about 3 feet in height, bearing medium-sized flowers that vary in colour from white to pale violet, with strongly-marked, dark veins. Structurally, it resembles the turnip, as the swollen, fleshy portion is really a stem which gradually passes downwards into the real root. Many kinds are named, the best known being (1) turnip-rooted, both red and white, including the white and black Spanish kinds; (2) olive-shaped, including the white, scarlet, and French breakfast forms; (3) the long, tapering varieties, like Long Red and Lady's Finger. The flesh is white, crisp, and tender, not specially nourishing, but valued as an antiscorbutic because of its quantity of nitrous juice. When too large for eating raw, they can be steamed for half an hour and served like asparagus. They should be well washed, but never peeled except when preparing the juice for medicinal purposes; in dry weather the bed should be watered the day before they are pulled. The young, green, seed-pods may be used for pickling, alone or with other vegetables, and are considered a fair substitute for capers.

¶ *Constituents.* Phenyl-ethyl isothiocyanite, a pungent, volatile oil, and an amylclytic enzyme.

¶ *Medicinal Action and Uses.* Radishes are an excellent food remedy for stone, gravel and scorbutic conditions. The juice has been used in the treatment of cholelithiasis as an aid in preventing the formation of biliary calculi. The expressed juice of white or black Spanish radishes is given in increasing doses of from ½ to 2 cupfuls daily. The 2 cupfuls are continued for two or three weeks. then the dose is decreased until ½ cupful is taken three times a week for three or four more weeks. The treatment may be repeated by taking 1 cupful at the beginning, then ½ daily, and later, ½ every second day.

The colouring matter is recommended as a sensitive indicator in alkalimetry.

¶ *Other Species.*

R. *Raphanistrum* (Wild Radish, or Jointed-podded Charlock). It was stated by Linnæus that in wet seasons this abounds as a weed among barley, in Sweden, and being ground with the corn, it is eaten in barley bread, causing violent convulsive complaints, or an epidemic, spasmodic disease. Other authorities say that it is harmless, liked by domestic animals and bees. It is bristly, and has rather large, straw-coloured flowers.

R. *Sibiricus*, or Siberian Radish, has cylindrical pods.

R. *caudatus*, the Java, or Rat's Tail Radish, a native of Final, furnishes long, edible pods, purple or violet in colour. They should be used half-grown. The root of this species is not used.

R. *maritimus* is an indigenous, seaside variety.

R. *Erucoides*, of Italy, has pods with a beak of their own length, and a simple, biennial root, scarcely thicker than the stem.

R. *Tenellus*, another native of Siberia, flowers in Britain in June and July, having awl-shaped, jointed, two-celled, smooth pods.

RAGWORT

Senecio Jacobæa (LINN.)
N.O. Compositæ

Synonyms. St. James-wort. Ragweed. Stinking Nanny. Staggerwort. Dog Standard. Cankerwort. Stammerwort
Part Used. Herb

¶ *Description.* Ragwort grows about 2 to 3 feet high, with a much branched, furrowed stem, without hairs, and deep, glossy, green leaves, irregularly divided and toothed. The root-leaves are broader, jagged at the base, those on the stalk deeply divided down to the rib. The flowers are arranged in rather large, flat-topped bunches (corymbs), into which the branches divide at the summit and are a beautiful bright yellow, ¾ to 1 inch across, with narrow rays, toothed at the outer edge. The plant is a perennial and abundant in most parts of the country, on dry roadsides and waste ground and pastures, often growing in large patches and flowering in July and August. It is distributed over Europe, Siberia and North-West India. In the Highlands it is found at a height of 1,200 feet above sea-level.

Ragwort was formerly much employed medicinally for various purposes. The leaves are used in the country for emollient poultices and yield a good green dye, not, however, permanent. The flowers boiled in water give a fair yellow dye to wool previously impregnated with alum. The whole plant is bitter and aromatic, of an acrid sharpness, but the juice is cooling and astringent, and

of use as a wash in burns, inflammations of the eye, and also in sores and cancerous ulcers – hence one of its old names, Cankerwort. It is used with success in relieving rheumatism, sciatica and gout, a poultice of the green leaves being applied to painful joints and reducing the inflammation and swelling. It makes a good gargle for ulcerated throat and mouth, and is said to take away the pain caused by the sting of bees. A decoction of the root has been reputed good for inward bruises and wounds. In some parts of the country Ragwort is accredited with the power of preventing infection.

In olden days it was supposed to be 'a certaine remedie to help the Staggers in Horses,' whence one of its popular names, Staggerwort. One of its other names, Stammerwort, probably indicates a belief in its efficacy as a remedy for impediment of speech.

Fluid extract, ½ to 1 drachm.

Ragwort is collected in August.

Culpepper says it is 'under the command of Dame Venus, and cleanses, digests, and discusses. In Sussex we call it Ragweed.'

Senecio aquaticus (MARSH RAGWORT) is a form of *S. Jacobæa*, common on the sides of rivers and ditches throughout the country, growing freely at an elevation of 1,500 feet above sea-level, in the Lake district and resembling the common Ragwort, but usually of laxer growth and readily distinguished by its less divided, longer-stalked leaves and larger heads of flowers, which are 1 to 1¼ inch in diameter.

All forms of this genus are not of beneficial use, and one at least has lately been found to be distinctly harmful, for Molteno disease, a cattle and horse disease prevalent in certain parts of South Africa, has been definitely traced to the presence of a poisonous alkaloid in *S. latifolius*, a near relative of the Common Groundsel.

Some botanists refer the genus *Cineraria* to the same order as the *Senecio*; these differ from *Senecio* in the achenes of the ray-florets being winged. The beautiful spring-flowering plants cultivated in greenhouses as *Cinerarias* belong, however, to *Senecio*, and have been obtained by horticulturists by intercrossing with each other a number of the Canary Island species, such as *S. populifolius, S. Tussilaginis*, etc. The deep blue colour of some of the garden varieties of these plants is singular in the genus, and not at all common in the family.

From the report of the Board of Agriculture's Chief Veterinary Officer (1917):

'It is not generally recognized that the common British Ragwort is *poisonous to cattle*. This probably arises from the fact that poisoning under natural conditions is a slow process, that is to say, an animal does not receive, and could not eat enough of the weed at one meal to cause acute poisoning. On the other hand, the poison is cumulative in its action; with continuous doses the amount of poison which becomes available is sufficient in time to cause very serious symptoms which often end in death. Much more attention has been given to the subject of poisoning by certain species of Ragwort in South Africa, Canada, and New Zealand, and in certain districts where it is commonly met with it was believed to be a disease of cattle until its actual cause was discovered. Thus, we find such names applied to it as Pictou, Winton, and Molteno disease. The following represent broadly the circumstances of the cases which have recently come to the notice of the Board. Pastures containing a considerable proportion of the weed were cropped in the hope that the comparatively early cropping might help to get rid of it. The crop was made into hay,

and owing to the prolonged spell of cold weather and the scarcity of other feeding stuffs, this was fed later and in considerable amount to animals at pasture.

'The actively poisonous agent in the plant seems to be one or two more alkaloids which have been extracted in more or less pure form from various species of Ragwort. . . . Some of the animals fed on the Ragwort died in a few days after the first appearance of definite symptoms. In others the symptoms continued for a month or more and deaths occurred at later dates. It would appear also that although animals which had received a toxic amount of Ragwort over a certain period may seem healthy at the time when feeding on the material is discontinued, they nevertheless develop active symptoms of poisoning and die at a later period. Thus in the cases investigated some of the animals did not show definite symptoms until twelve days or more after the feeding with Ragwort had been discontinued. In the early stages the animals have the appearance of being hide-bound. Later, they walk with a staggering gait, some appearing to be partially blind or heedless of where they go. Later, they may become very excitable, and will charge at anyone who approaches them. In some there may be diarrhœa, but usually constipation is so marked that it causes violent straining. The pulse is weak and rapid, but the temperature remains normal. . . . There is no cure, and prevention resolves itself into removing the Ragwort from the forage, or eradicating it from the pastures.'

McGovern makes the following recommendations for eradicating the weed:

'Ragwort may be exterminated by preventing the plant from seeding. This may be done in the following ways:

'(*a*) By grazing infested land with sheep in the winter and early spring.

'(*b*) By cutting the plants in the flowering stage either –

'(i) Twice, the first cut being made early in July, and the second about six weeks later, there being no necessity to gather up the cut portions; or

'(ii) Once only, cutting being done late in July or early in August. The cut portions of the plants must be gathered up at once and burnt.

'(*c*) By pulling the plants, if circumstances permit, preferably early in July, when there is no need to collect and burn the pulled plants. If pulled later the plants must be collected and burned to prevent seeding . . .

'It is not certain that sheep are absolutely immune to poisoning by Ragwort. Prob-

ably the flowering season – June, July, and early August – is when Ragwort is most actively poisonous.'

See GROUNDSEL, LIFE ROOT, CINERARIA MARITIME.

RAMPION

Campanula rapunculus (LINN.)
N.O. Campanulaceæ

Synonym. Ramps
Part Used. Herb
Habitat. The plant is found wild in England, on gravelly roadsides and hedgebanks and in open pastures, from Stafford southwards, but it is uncertain whether it should be held as a true native in the localities in southern England, where it is now established

The Rampion formerly regularly cultivated in English kitchen gardens, and much valued as a wholesome esculent vegetable, is seldom grown for use now, though its graceful flowers are sometimes seen to advantage in the borders as an ornamental plant.

The name Rampion is derived from its Latin specific name, *Rapunculus*, a diminutive of *rapa* (a turnip). It is still much cultivated in France, Germany and Italy, and occasionally here, for the roots which are boiled tender like parsnips and eaten hot with a sauce. They are sweetish, with a slight pungency, but though wholesome, are considered inferior to other roots now more widely grown for culinary use. The larger roots are reserved for boiling, sometimes the young roots are eaten raw with vinegar and pepper, and occasionally the leaves, as well as the roots, are eaten as a winter salad. The leaves can be used in the summer and autumn as a substitute for spinach. The young shoots may be blanched like asparagus and prepared in the same manner.

¶ *Description.* The roots are fleshy and biennial (but can be made perennial), the stems are 2 to 3 feet high, erect, stiff, though rather slender, generally simple, more or less covered with stiff, white hairs, which almost disappear when cultivated. The leaves are variable, 1 to 3 inches long, the radical leaves oblong or ovate, on long stalks and slightly crenate, the stem-leaves narrow and mostly entire, or obscurely toothed. The flowers, which bloom in July and August, are about ¾ inch long, reddish purple, blue or white, on short peduncles, forming long, simple or slightly branched panicles. The corolla is divided to about the middle into five lanceolate segments. The capsule is short and erect, opening in small lateral clefts, close under the narrow linear segments of the calyx.

Drayton names it among the vegetables and pot-herbs of the kitchen garden, in his poem *Polyolbion*, and there is a reference to it in the slang of Falstaff, showing how generally it was in cultivation in this country in Shakespeare's time.

There is an Italian tradition that the possession of a rampion excites quarrels among children. The plant figures in one of Grimm's tales, the heroine, Rapunzel, being named after it, and the whole plot is woven around the theft of rampions from a magician's garden. In an old Calabrian tale, a maiden, uprooting a rampion in a field, discovers a staircase that leads to a palace far down in the depths of the earth.

¶ *Cultivation.* Rampion is easily cultivated and will flourish in ordinary good soil, though a moist, sandy soil suits it best.

Seeds should be sown in shallow drills, a foot apart, in May, and thinned out to 5 or 6 inches in the rows. The young plants should be moderately watered at first.

If grown for culinary use, it must not be allowed to flower, and the roots should be earthed up several inches on each side in order to blanch them. They are fit for use in November, and should be lifted then and stored in a frost-proof place.

¶ *Medicinal Action and Uses.* Gerard tells us: 'Some affirme that the decoction of the roots are good for all inflammation of the mouth and almonds of the throte and other diseases happening in the mouth and throte, as the other Throte warts.'

An old writer states that the distilled water of the whole plant is excellent for the complexion and 'maketh the face very splendent.'

¶ *Other Species.*
Two other native species have been employed dietetically, *Campanula rapunculoides* and *C. persicifolia*, but they have fallen into disuse as culinary vegetables, though the latter is a favourite in the flower border.

All the plants of the genus have a milky juice, which is more or less acrid, though not sufficiently so to act poisonously.

RAPE SEED. *See* MUSTARD

RASPBERRY
Rubus Idæus (LINN.)
N.O. Rosaceæ

Synonyms. Raspbis. Hindberry. Bramble of Mount Ida
(*Danish*) Hindebar
(*Dutch*) Braamboss
(*German*) Hindbur
(*Saxon*) Hindbeer
Parts Used. Leaves, fruit

The well-known Raspberry, grown so largely for its fruit, grows wild in some parts of Great Britain. It is a native of many parts of Europe. The stems are erect and shrubby, biennial, with creeping perennial roots. It flowers in May and June.

¶ *Cultivation.* The plant is generally propagated by suckers, though those raised from layers should be preferred, because they will be better rooted and not so liable to send out suckers. In preparing these plants their fibres should be shortened, but the buds which are placed at a small distance from the stem of the plant must not be cut off, as they produce the new shoots the following summer. Place the plants about 2 feet apart in the rows, allowing 4 or 5 feet between the rows. If planted too closely, without plenty of air between the rows, the fruit will not be so fine.

The most suitable soil is a good, strong loam. They do not thrive so well in a light soil.

In October, cut down all the old wood that has produced fruit in the summer and shorten the young shoots to about 2 feet in length. Dig the spaces between the rows well and dress with a little manure. Beyond weeding during the summer, no further care is needed. It is wise to form new plantations every three or four years, as the fruit on old plants is apt to deteriorate.

¶ *Constituents.* The Raspberry contains a crystallizable fruit-sugar, a fragrant volatile oil, pectin, citric and malic acids, mineral salts, colouring matter and water. The ripe fruit is fragrant, subacid and cooling: it allays heat and thirst, and is not liable to acetous fermentation in the stomach.

Raspberry vinegar is an acid syrup made with the fruit-juice, sugar and white-wine vinegar, and when added to water forms an excellent cooling drink in summer, suitable also in feverish cases, where the acid is not an objection. It makes a useful gargle for relaxed, sore throat.

A home-made wine, brewed from the fermented juice of ripe Raspberries, is antiscrofulous, and Raspberry syrup dissolves the tartar of the teeth.

The fruit is also utilized for dyeing purposes.

¶ *Medicinal Action and Uses.* Astringent and stimulant. Raspberry Leaf Tea, made by the infusion of 1 oz. of the dried leaves in a pint of boiling water, is employed as a gargle for sore mouths, canker of the throat, and as a wash for wounds and ulcers. The leaves, combined with the powdered bark of Slippery Elm, make a good poultice for cleansing wounds, burns and scalds, removing proud flesh and promoting healing.

An infusion of Raspberry leaves, taken cold, is a reliable remedy for extreme laxity of the bowels. The infusion alone, or as a component part of injections, never fails to give immediate relief. It is useful in stomach complaints of children.

Raspberry Leaf Tea is valuable during parturition. It should be taken freely – warm.

¶ *Preparation.* Fluid extract, 1 to 2 drachms.

The Raspberry grows wild as far north as lat. 70°, and southward it appears to have been abundant on Mount Ida, in Asia Minor, lat. 39° 40′. It was known to the Ancients, and Linnæus retained the classic name of Ida, with which it was associated by Dioscorides. It was called in Greek *Batos Idaia*, and in Latin *Rubus Idæa*, the Bramble of Mount Ida. Gerard calls it Raspis or Hindberry, and Hindberry is a derivation of the Saxon name *Hindbeer*.

''Twas only to hear the yorling sing,
  And pu' the crawflower round the spring,
  The scarlet hep and the *hindberrie*,
  And the nut that hang frae the hazel tree.'

The Wild Raspberry differs from the cultivated variety mainly in its size.

RECIPES

Raspberry Wine

To every 3 pints of fruit, carefully cleared from mouldy or bad, put 1 quart of water; bruise the former. In 24 hours strain the liquor and put to every quart 1 lb. of sugar, of good middling quality, of Lisbon. If for white currants, use lump sugar. It is best to put the fruit, etc., into a large pan, and when, in three or four days, the scum rises, take that off before the liquor be put into the barrel. Those who make from their own gardens may not have a sufficiency to fill the barrel at once; the wine will not hurt if made in the pan in the above proportions, and added as the fruit ripens, and can be gathered in dry weather.

Keep an account of what is put in each time.

Raspberry Vinegar

Raspberry Vinegar is made either with malt vinegar or white vinegar (i.e. either white-wine vinegar or dilute acetic acid). Malt vinegar adds to the colour, which with white vinegar generally needs the addition of a little caramel to deepen it. When made from the fruit 2 lb. of raspberries is required to a pint of vinegar. Another method is to acidulate Raspberry-juice with acetic acid and sweeten with plain syrup.

Another Recipe for the Same

Put 1 lb. of fine fruit into a china-bowl, and pour upon it 1 quart of the best white-wine vinegar; next day strain the liquor on 1 lb. of fresh raspberries; and the following day do the same, but do not squeeze the fruit, only drain the liquor as dry as you can from it.

The last time pass it through a canvas, previously wet with vinegar, to prevent waste. Put it into a stone jar, with 1 lb. of sugar to every pint of juice, broken into large lumps; stir it when melted, then put the jar into a saucepan of water or on a hot hearth, let it simmer and skim it. When cold, bottle it.

This is one of the most useful preparations that can be kept in a house, not only as affording the most refreshing beverage, but being of singular efficacy in complaints of the chest. A large spoonful or two in a tumbler of water. Be careful to use no glazed nor metal vessels for it.

(Old Cookery-Book.)

Raspberry Brandy

Pick fine dry fruit, put it into a stone jar, and the jar into a kettle of water, or on a hot hearth, till the juice will run; strain, and to every pint add ½ lb. of sugar, give one boil and skim it; when cold, put equal quantities of juice and brandy, shake well and bottle. Some people prefer it stronger of the brandy.

(Old Cookery-Book.)

RATTLE, DWARF RED

Pedicularis sylvatica
N.O. Labiatæ

Synonyms. Red Rattle Grass. Lousewort. Lesser Red Rattle
Part Used. Herb

The Dwarf Red Rattle (*Pedicularis sylvatica*) and the Yellow Rattle or Cock's Comb (*Rhinanthus Crista-galli*) are very closely allied to the Eyebright. As remedies they have now fallen into disuse.

There are two Red Rattles, but the commoner and medicinal one is the Dwarf or Lesser Red Rattle, frequent in moist pastures and on swampy heaths. It is quite a small plant, generally nestling rather closely to the ground, the short root-stock sending up many prostrate and spreading, leafy stems, 3 to 10 inches long, branching a good deal at the base and rarely more than 3 or 4 inches high when in flower. The leaves are very deeply cut into numerous segments. The flowers are in terminal, loose spikes, the calyx smooth on the outside, but woolly inside at the mouth, broadly inflated and marked over with a fine network of veins, and at the top, cut into five unequal, leaf-like lobes. The lower portion of the corolla forms a tube hidden within the calyx, but then emerging projects boldly beyond it; it is labiate in form, like the Eyebright, the upper lip tall and dome-like, but compressed at the sides, the lower lip flatly expanded and cut into three

very distinct lobes. Both are of a bright rose colour and the whole flower is very striking and quaint. As the seeds ripen, they may be heard rattling in their capsule within the inflated calyx, hence the popular name Red Rattle. Another name for the plant is 'Lousewort,' from a belief that sheep eating it became diseased and covered with parasites, but when sheep do suffer in this manner after eating this plant, it is really because the presence of it in a pasture indicates a very bad and unsuitable pasture, since marshy land, the best suited to its growth, is the worst from the health point of view for the sheep. The generic name, *Pedicularis* (from the Latin *pediculus*=a louse), refers also to the supposititious vermin-producing qualities of the plant.

The old herbalists considered the Red Rattle a wound herb and styptic. Culpepper tells us that —

'The Red Rattle is accounted profitable to heal fistulas and hollow ulcers and to stay the flux of humours in them as also the abundance of the courses or any other flux of blood, being boiled in port wine and drunk.'

RATTLE, YELLOW

Rhinanthus Crista-galli
N.O. Labiatæ

Synonyms. Cock's Comb. Yellow Rattle Grass. Pennygrass
(*Welsh*) Crivell Melyn
(*French*) Crête-de-coq
(*Gælic*) Boden chloigin

The Yellow Rattle, a near relative of the Red Rattle, also obtains its name from the fact that the seeds rattle in the husky capsules when ripe. This is an erect, somewhat rigid plant, common in cultivated land, composed of a single stem, about a foot high, smooth and more or less spotted with purple, bearing pairs of stalkless, wedge-shaped leaves, with deeply notched margins and conspicuous veins, and terminated by a loose spike of yellow, labiate flowers, in which the calyx is large and very inflated (flattened so that its side view is much larger than its end view), of an uncommon pale green in colour and contracting at the mouth, where it is divided into four equal teeth. The upper lip of the corolla is very convex and ordinarily has a purple spot upon it; the lower lip is divided into three segments, the middle one being the largest. The stamens, which rest closely under the upper lip, have curious anthers, covered with little, bristly hairs.

Culpepper and other old writers call this plant Rattle Grass, like the preceding species, but Gerard gives also the name of 'Pennygrass,' an allusion to the flattened, fairly circular outline of the capsules. The generic name, *Rhinanthus*, is derived from the two Greek words signifying *nose* and *flower*, from the projecting beak of the upper portion of the corolla. The specific name, *Crista-galli*, means the crest or comb of a cock, because, according to Pliny, it has numerous leaves resembling a cock's comb. Parkinson, writing in 1640, also explains the name by saying the deeply-dented edges of the leaves 'resemble therein the crest or combe of a cocke,' but others have thought the name 'Coxcomb' refers rather to the notched calyx. In France it is called the 'Crête-de-coq.'

Both the Red Rattle and the Yellow Rattle are semi-parasites like the Eyebright, in similar manner extracting nourishment from the roots of the grasses among which they grow, the Yellow Rattle, however, to a more considerable degree than the others, impoverishing thereby the pastures in which it flourishes, and on the Continent it is often harmful to Rye crops, if not eradicated in time.

The Yellow Rattle was considered to have certain properties in common with Eyebright. Culpepper tells us that it 'is held to be good for those that are troubled with a cough or dimness of sight, if the herb being boiled with beans and some honey; put thereto be drunk or dropped into the eyes. The whole seed being put into the eyes draweth forth any skin, dimness or film from the sight without trouble or pain.'

RED CLOVER. *See* CLOVER

RED ROOT

Ceanothus Americanus (LINN.)
N.O. Rhamneæ

Synonyms. New Jersey Tea. Wild Snowball
Parts Used Root or bark of the root
Habitat. North America

¶ *History.* This is a half-hardy shrub growing to 4 or 5 feet high. It has downy leaves and stems and small ornamental white flowers in great numbers, coming into bloom June or July, followed by bluntly triangular seedvessels. It is usually called 'New Jersey Tea' in America because its leaves were used as a substitute for tea during the War of Independence. In Canada it is used to dye wool a cinnamon colour. It takes its name from its large red roots. Its wood is tough, pale brown red, with fine rays – taste bitter and astringent with no odour. Fracture hard, tough, splintering. Its bark is brittle, dark-coloured and thin.

¶ *Constituents.* The leaves are said to contain tannin, a soft resin and bitter extract, a green colouring matter similar to green tea in colour and taste, gum a volatile substance, lignin, and a principle called Ceanothine.

¶ *Medicinal Action and Uses.* Astringent, antispasmodic, anti-syphilitic expectorant and sedative, used in asthma, chronic bronchitis, whooping-cough, consumption, and dysentery; also as a mouth-wash and gargle, and as an injection in gonorrhœa, gleet and leucorrhœa.

¶ *Dosages.* Of the decoction, ½ oz. Fluid extract, 1 to 30 drops.

¶ *Other Species.* Mexican *Ceanothus azurea* (Desf.), a powerful febrifuge.

RED SAGE. *See* SAGE

REST-HARROW

Ononis arvensis
N.O. Leguminosæ

Synonyms. Wild Liquorice. Cammock. Stinking Tommy. Ground Furze. Land Whin
Part Used. Whole herb

¶ *Description*. A troublesome weed, with a root that affords a sweet, viscid juice. Common in arable land. Its long, thickly-matted root will arrest the progress of the harrow, hence its name.

It is a favourite food of the donkey, from which the generic name is derived, *onos* being the Greek word for an ass.

A tradition exists that this was the plant from which the crown of thorns was plaited for the Crucifixion.

The plant is obnoxious to snakes.

¶ *Medicinal Action and Uses*. The young shoots were much used at one time as a vegetable, being boiled, eaten in salad or pickled.

In medicine it was used for stone in the bladder and to subdue delirium.

RHATANY

Krameria triandra (R. and P.)
N.O. Polygaceæ

Synonyms. Rhatanhia. Ratanhiawurzel. Krameria Root. Peruvian Rhatany. Mapato. Pumacuchu. Raiz para los dientes. Red Rhatany
Part Used. Dried root
Habitat. Peru

¶ *Description*. A low shrub with large red flowers, growing on dry, sandy places on mountain-slopes, 3,000 to 8,000 feet above sea-level in several provinces of Peru, especially near the city of Huanuco. The root, as found in commerce, consists of long, cylindrical pieces, varying in thickness from ¼ to ½ inch or more (long Rhatany), or a short, thick portion, knotted, and as large as a man's fist (short, or stumpy Rhatany). The difference is caused by the diggers, the former being removed by them with care, and the latter torn up with force. The bark of the root is thin, readily separable, rough and scaly; of a dark, reddish-brown colour outside, and bright brownish-red within. It breaks with a somewhat fibrous fracture, is tough and difficult to powder, and has a strong, purely astringent taste, tingeing the saliva red when chewed. The central woody portion is very hard and almost tasteless. Neither bark nor wood has any marked odour. As the virtues of Rhatany reside in the bark, the smaller pieces are preferable.

A strong tincture of these roots in brandy is used in Portugal to impart roughness to port wines.

The genus *Krameria* was named after Kramer, a Hungarian physician and botanist. The name Rhatany is said to describe the creeping character of the plant, in the language used by the Peruvian Indians, while its Spanish name is derived from its dental properties.

The dried roots of two species besides the Peruvian are official: *Krameria Ixené*, or Savanilla Rhatany, and *Krameria Argentea*, known in commerce as Para or Brazilian Rhatany.

Krameria was dropped from the United States Pharmacopœia but retained in the British Pharmacopœia and National Formulary.

¶ *Constituents*. The essential constituent is a peculiar tannic acid, known as Rhatania-tannic acid or Krameria tannic acid, closely allied to catechu-tannic acid. By the action of dilute acid it is decomposed into a crystallizable sugar, and Rhatania-red. No gallic acid is present. Rhatanin is a homologue of tyrosine, and is identical with angelin, geoffrayin, and andirin. It appears to contain also lignin, and small quantities of gum, starch, saccharine matter, and a peculiar acid, krameric acid. The mineral acids and most of the metallic salts throw down precipitates with the infusion, decoction and tincture of Rhatany, and are incompatible in prescription.

Cold water extracts all the astringency of Rhatany.

Very inferior extracts of Rhatany are often sold. Its virtues may be considered as in proportion to its solubility.

¶ *Medicinal Action and Uses*. An active astringent, and slightly tonic. It has been found useful for internal administration in chronic diarrhœa, dysentery, menorrhagia, incontinence of urine, hæmaturia, and passive hæmorrhage from the bowels. In the form of an infusion it has been used locally in fissure of the anus, prolapsus ani, and leucorrhœa; as a gargle in relaxed, sore throat; and as an astringent wash for the mucous membrane of the eyes, nose, gums, etc.

The powder is also used as a dentifrice when mixed with equal parts of orris rhizome and charcoal, or with prepared chalk and myrrh.

¶ *Preparations and Dosages.* Tincture of 20 per cent. krameria and diluted alcohol, 1 fluid drachm. Syrup of 45 per cent. fluid extract of krameria and syrup – as an intestinal astringent – 1 fluid drachm. Of the powder (rarely used), 20 to 30 grains. Lozenges are also prepared, with cocaine. Powdered root, 10 to 30 grains. Fluid extract, 10 to 60 drops. Tincture, B.P., and U.S.P., ½ to 1 drachm. Infusion, B.P., ½ to 1 oz. Solid extract, U.S.P., 5 to 8 grains. Solid extract, B.P., 5 to 15 grains. Concentrated solution, B.P., ½ to 1 drachm.

Other Species.

A Rhatany from Guayaquil appeared on the London market, yielding a larger quantity of tannin than the Peruvian drug, but less than the other two species. A spurious Rhatany from Peru, of unknown botanical origin, has also been put on the market. The Krameria lanceolate (*Texan Rhatany*) of North America, is richer in tannin than the official drug. It takes a deep purple colour when treated with iron, while Para gives a dirty brown and Savanilla violet.

The powder is of a reddish-brown colour.

RHODODENDRON, YELLOW

Rhododendron Chrysanthum
N.O. Ericaceæ

Synonyms. Rosebay. Snow Rose. Rosage Alpenrose
Part Used. Leaves
Habitat. Mountains of Siberia

¶ *Description.* A small bush, stem 1 to 1½ foot high, spreading, much branched, often concealed by moss, tips of shoots only being visible. Leaves alternate like laurel, ovate, somewhat acute, tapering to stalk, reticulated, rough above, paler and smoother underneath. Flowers large, showy, nodding, on clustered terminal, loose peduncles emerging from large downy scales. Corolla campanulate, five cleft, rounded segments, three upper largest and streaked with livid dots next the tube, lower unspotted. Stamens ten, unequal deflexed; anthers oblong, incumbent, without appendages, opening by two terminal pores, capsule ovate, rather angular, five-celled, five-valved, septicidal; seeds numerous, minute. The leaves should be gathered directly the capsules have ripened. They have a faint odour when first gathered, and a bitter, acrid, astringent taste.

¶ *Constituents.* The leaves contain a stimulant narcotic principle, which they yield to water or alcohol.

¶ *Medicinal Action and Other Uses.*[1] Much used in Siberia as a remedy for rheumatism. Also useful in gout and syphilis.

¶ *Dosage.* 2 teaspoonsful of the infusion.

RHUBARBS

N.O. Polygonaceæ

Rhubarb is the root of different species of *Rheum*, growing in the mountains of the Western and North-western provinces of China and in the adjoining Thibetan terrtory.

Rhubarb occurs in commerce under various names: Russian, Turkey, East Indian and Chinese; but the geographical source of all species is the same, the commercial names of the drug indicating only the route by which it formerly reached the European market. Previous to 1842, Canton being the only port of the Chinese Empire holding direct communication with Europe, Rhubarb mostly came by overland routes: the Russian Rhubarb used to be brought by the Chinese to the Russian frontier town of Kiachta; the Turkey Rhubarb received its name because it came to us by way of Asiatic Turkey, through the Levant; East Indian came by way of Singapore and other East Indian ports, and Chinese Rhubarb was shipped from Canton. At the present day practically all is conveyed to Europe via Shanghai.

According to Lindley's *Treasury of Botany*, the technical name of the genus is said to be derived from *Rha*, the ancient name of the Volga, on whose banks the plants grow; other authorities derive the name from the Greek *rheo* ('to flow'), in allusion to the purgative properties of the root.

RHUBARB, TURKEY

Rheum palmatum
Rheum Rhaponticum

Synonyms. East Indian Rhubarb. China Rhubarb
Part Used. Root

¶ *Description.* The leaves of the Turkey Rhubarb are palmate and somewhat rough. The root is thick, of an oval shape, sending off long, tapering branches; externally it is brown, internally a deep yellow colour.

The stem is erect, round, hollow, jointed,

---

[1] In homœopathic medicine a tincture of the fresh leaves is said to be curative of diarrhœa, amenorrhœa, chorea, affections of the eyes and ears, and neuralgia. – EDITOR.

branched towards the top, from 6 to 10 feet high.

This species is distinguished from our familiar garden Rhubarb by its much larger size, the shape of its leaves, with their oblong, sharpish segments, and the graceful looseness of its little panicles of greenish-white flowers. The first buds which appear in spring are yellow, not red.

It was not until the year 1732 that botanists knew any species of Rheum from which the true Rhubarb seemed likely to be obtained. Then Boerhaave, the celebrated Dutch physician, procured from a Tartarian Rhubarb merchant the seeds of the plant which produced the roots he annually sold, and which were admitted at St. Petersburg to be the real Rhubarb. These seeds on being sown produced two distinct species: *Rheum Rhaponticum*, our Garden Rhubarb, and *Rheum* and *R. palmatum*, Turkey Rhubarb.

The Turkey Rhubarb grows remarkably quickly – a six-year-old plant was found to grow between April, when the stalk first emerged from the ground, to the middle of July, when it was at its greatest height, to 11 feet 4 inches. In one day it was observed to grow 3 inches and over 4 inches in one night. Many of its leaves were 5 feet long. The root, taken up in October, weighed 36 lb. when cleaned, washed and deprived of its small fibres.

'J. D. B. (31/10). – The rhubarb rhizome official in the British Pharmacopœia, 1914, must be collected in China and Thibet. English-grown rhubarb is inferior to the official rhubarb in medicinal qualities.'

We still depend upon Northern China and Thibet for Rhubarb; that grown in the English climate, near Banbury, does not command a high price in the market, although its medicinal properties are the same as those of the Chinese roots. If English growers would endeavour to produce a more marketable root by experimenting with different soils and methods of cultivation, the results might meet with success. It is possible that English roots are harvested when too young, and that not so much attention is paid to trimming the roots for market as is done by the Chinese. It is never collected from plants that are less than six years old.

It is said that the odour of the best samples is so delicate that the assistants in the wholesale drug-houses are not permitted to touch it without gloves.

¶ *Part Used.* The root, scraped or rasped, halved longitudinally when very large, and then cut into transverse pieces and strung on cords to dry in the sun, the drying afterwards being completed by stove heat. It is dug in October.

Chinese or Turkey Rhubarb occurs in commerce in brownish-yellow pieces of various size, usually perforated, the holes often containing a portion of the cord used to hang the sections of the root on during drying. The outer surface is generally powdery (the bark having been removed) and shows a network of white lines.

The taste is astringent and nauseous, and there is a characteristic odour.

The preparations used in medicine are: the powdered root, a fluid extract, a tincture, syrup, infusion and solution. It is also employed as a principal ingredient in compound powder (Gregory's Powder) and in compound pills.

¶ *Constituents.* The chemical constituents of Rhubarb root are not yet completely known. Recent investigations indicate that the most important constituents are a number of substances which may be divided into two groups, viz. tannoid constituents and purgative constituents, several of which have been isolated in a free state: the former are astringent and the latter laxative.

Three crystalline tannoids have been extracted. The purgative constituents apparently exist in the form of an unstable crystalline substance: Rheopurgarin. This splits up into four glucosides: two of these yield Chrysophanic acid (so named from its forming yellow crystals) and Rheochrysidin respectively. The other two glucosides have not yet been isolated, but they appear to yield Emodin and Rhein.

There are also several resinous matters, one of which, Phaoretin, is purgative, and mineral compounds are also present, especially Oxalate of Calcium. The astringency of Rhubarb is due to a peculiar tannic acid (Rheo-tannic), which is soluble in water and alcohol.

¶ *Medicinal Action and Uses.* Astringent, tonic, stomachic, aperient. In large doses, Rhubarb powder acts as a simple and safe purgative, being regarded as one of the most valuable remedies we possess, effecting a brisk, healthy purge, without clogging the bowels and producing constipation, too often consequent upon the use of the more active purgatives.

It is especially useful in cases of diarrhœa, caused by an irritating body in the intestines: the cause of irritation is removed and the after-astringent action checks the diarrhœa.

The following note from *The Chemist and Druggist* of March 31, 1923, supports this:

'*Rhubarb in Bacillary Dysentery.* – An in-

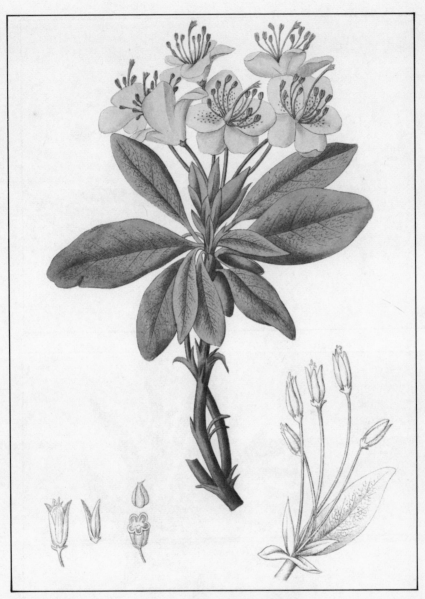

YELLOW RHODODENDRON
Rhododendron Chrysanthum

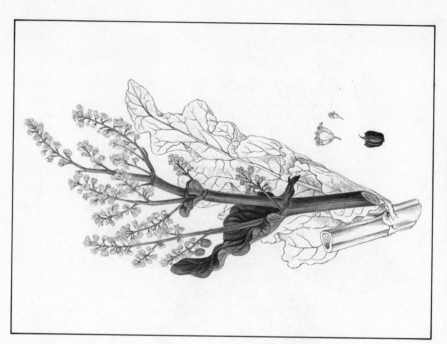

FRENCH RHUBARB
Rheum Undulatum

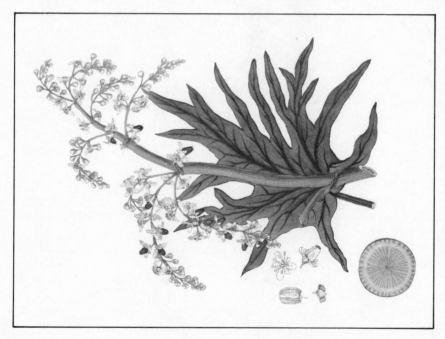

EAST INDIAN RHUBARB
Rheum Palmatum

vestigation was undertaken to determine the way in which rhubarb acts in this disease and which constituent was responsible for its action, one writer having stated in regard to the treatment of bacillary dysentery that no remedy in medicine has such a magical effect. (*Lancet*, I, 1923, 382.) A solution containing all the purgative constituents of rhubarb soluble in water (1 gr. of B.P. rhubarb extract) was allowed to act on *B. dysenterial Shiga and Flexner* of the bacillus No. 1 of Morgan without affecting growth in the broth tubes. Fresh undiluted ox bile has not distinct action on the bacilli, thus indicating that the therapeutic effect of rhubarb is not due to its cholagogue action. Neither does the serum of a rabbit treated with rhubarb have any germicidal action. The nature of the therapeutic effect of rhubarb in bacillary dysentery therefore still remains obscure.'

And again, September 3, 1921, in the *Lancet*, by Dr. R. W. Burkitt:

'In the former journal, Dr. R. W. Burkitt, of Nairobi, British East Africa, states that acute bacillary dysentery has been treated in that colony almost exclusively with powdered rhubarb for the past three years. The dose given has been 30 grains every two or three hours until the rhubarb appears in the stools. After a few doses the stools become less frequent, hæmorrhage ceases, and straining and the other symptoms of acute general poisoning, which characterize the disease, rapidly disappear. In children 5 grains is given every two hours for three doses only, as, if the administration is continued longer, the drug will cure the dysentery, but produce an obstinate simple diarrhœa. In both adults and children the thirst is combated by small, frequent doses of bicarbonate of soda and citrate of potash. Dr. Burkitt concludes: "I know of no remedy in medicine which has such a magical effect. No one who has ever used rhubarb would dream of using anything else. I hope others will try it in this dreadful tropical scourge." '

Rhubarb in small doses exhibits stomachic and tonic properties, and is employed in atonic dyspepsia, assisting digestion and creating a healthy action of the digestive organs, when in a condition of torpor and debility.

The tincture is chiefly used, but the powder is equally effective and reliable.

Rhubarb when chewed increases the flow of saliva.

¶ *Preparations and Dosages.* Powdered root, 3 to 30 grains. Comp. powder, B.P. (Gregory's), 20 to 60 grains. Comp. pill, B.P., 4 to 8 grains. Solid extract, U.S.P., 4 grains. Solid extract, B.P., 2 to 8 grains. Tincture comp., B.P., ½ to 4 drachms. Tincture, U.S.P., 1 drachm. Tincture aromat., U.S.P., ½ drachm. Fluid extract, 10 to 30 drops. Syrup, B.P., ½ to 2 drachms. Infusion, B.P., ½ to 1 oz. Syrup, B.P. and U.S.P., ½ to 2 drachms. Arom. syrup, U.S.P., 2 drachms. Rheum, 1 to 4 grains.

RHUBARB, ENGLISH

Rheum Rhaponticum (WILLD.)

Synonyms. Garden Rhubarb. Bastard Rhubarb. Sweet Round-leaved Dock

Parts Used. Root, stems

English Rhubarb is similar in action to Turkey or Chinese Rhubarb, though milder. It is derived from *Rheum Rhaponticum*, the ordinary Garden Rhubarb, and from *R. officinale.*

It has blunt, smooth leaves; large, thick roots, running deep into the ground, reddish-brown outside and yellow within, and stems 2 to 3 feet high, jointed and purplish. The flowers are white.

About 1777, Hayward, an apothecary, of Banbury, in Oxfordshire, commenced the cultivation of Rhubarb with plants of *R. Rhaponticum*, raised from seeds sent from Russia in 1762, and produced a drug of excellent quality, which used to be sold as the genuine Rhubarb, by men dressed up as Turks. The Society for the encouragement of Arts, Manufactures and Commerce exerted itself for many years in promoting the cultivation of Rhubarb, granting medals not only to this original pioneer, but also, some years later, to growers of Rhubarb in Somersetshire, Yorkshire and Middlesex, some of whom, it appears, attempted also to cultivate *R. palmatum*. When Hayward died, he left his Rhubarb plantations to the ancestor of the present cultivators of the Rhubarb fields at Banbury, where *R. officinale* is also now cultivated, from specimens first introduced into this country in 1873. Both *R. Rhaponticum* and *R. officinale* are at the present time grown, not only in Oxfordshire but also in Bedfordshire. Although specimens of *R. palmatum* were raised from seed as early as 1764, in the Botanical Gardens in Edinburgh, it is not grown now in this country for medicinal purposes, experiments having shown that it is the least easily cultivated of the rhubarbs, the main root in this climate being liable to rot. *R. officinale* and *R. Emodi* have to some extent been grown also as an ornamental plant, being also quite hardy and readily propagated.

¶ *Cultivation.* Rhubarb may be raised from seed, but it is better and more usual to obtain established roots. Seeds may be sown, however, in drills a foot or more apart, in the open, from March to April, and the young plants thinned out to 10 inches, transplanting them in the autumn, allowing about 4 feet every way to each plant.

Rhubarb roots may be planted at any time of the year, although mild weather in autumn or early spring is best; it should be planted on a clear, open spot, on good soil, which should be well trenched 3 feet deep, and before planting, a good substance of rotten manure should be worked into the soil.

When the plants are to be increased, it is merely necessary to take up large roots and divide them with a spade: every piece that has a crown to it will grow. Fresh plantations are generally made in February or March, but Rhubarb may still be divided early in May.

To ensure fine rhubarb for table use, a large dressing of well-rotted manure should be dug in about the roots as soon as the last of the leaves have been pulled. It is not right to wait until the winter, before the plants are dressed.

Old roots ought to be divided and replanted every fourth or fifth year, when the plants are grown for the use of the stems.

If Rhubarb be forced on the ground where it grows, nothing more is required than to cover with large pots, half casks, or boxes, round and over which should be placed plenty of stable manure. Roots forced in greenhouse or in frames do not need to have the light excluded from them. Such roots, however, require dividing and replanting in the spring out of doors.

¶ *Part Used Medicinally and Preparation.* The roots of English Rhubarb are generally taken from plants from four years old and upwards. They are dug up in October, washed thoroughly and the fibres taken away. The bark of English Rhubarb is not usually removed.

The roots of both *R. Officinale* and *R. Rhaponticum* are much smaller than those of the Chinese Rhubarb and are easily distinguished by their distinctly radiate structure. They are also more shrunken, more or less distinctly pink in colour, and have a diffuse circle of isolated star-spots on the transverse section. The roots of *R. officinale* cultivated in England resemble Chinese Rhubarb, but are more spongy, and shrink and wrinkle as they dry, and are softer to cut. They have a less rich colour than the Chinese, and have no network of white lines on the outer surface, the dark red and white lines usually running parallel to each other and the star-spots being less developed, fewer and more scattered.

The English Rhubarb from *R. Rhaponticum* shows red veins, that of *R. officinale* is usually in larger pieces and has blackish veins.

The root is used as a drug in powdered form.

¶ *Constituents. Root.* The constituents of *R. officinale* are similar to those of Chinese Rhubarb.

Rhapontic or Garden Rhubarb contains no emodine, rhein or rhabarberine, but has in it a crystalline body, rhaponticin.

Stem and Leaves of R. Rhaponticum. Potassium oxalate is present in quantity in Rhubarb *leaf-stems*, and certain persons who are constitutionally susceptible to salts of oxalic acid, show symptoms of irritant poisoning after eating rhubarb stewed in the ordinary manner. Many people of a gouty tendency do well to avoid it, and those subject to urinary irritation should take it very sparingly or not at all.

Rhubarb stems did not come into general use as a substitute for fruit till about 100 years ago. We hear of a pioneer grower, Joseph Myatt, of Deptford, sending, in 1810, five bunches of Rhubarb to the Borough Market and only being able to dispose of three. But he persevered in his efforts to make a market for Rhubarb, raised improved varieties, and a few years after, Rhubarb had become established in public favour as a culinary plant.

It was, however, soon realized that the use of Rhubarb as food was sometimes attended with some risk to health. Lindley, in his *Vegetable Kingdom,* 1846, remarks that oxalic acid exists in both Docks and Rhubarb, and that the latter contains also an abundance of nitric and malic acid, and goes on to say that whilst these give an agreeable taste to the Rhubarb when cooked, he considers them ill-suited to the digestion of some persons. The *Penny Cyclopædia,* 1841, warned persons subject to calculous complaints against eating Rhubarb stalks, owing to the presence of oxalic acid, stating that 'the formation of oxalate of lime, or mulberry calculus, may be the consequence of indulgence.'

The chemical constituents of Rhubarb *leaves* were till recently not fully ascertained, but the analysis has lately been undertaken under orders from the Home Office, in consequence of fatal and injurious effects having resulted from eating the leaves cooked as spinach. The report of the official analyist states that the leaves contain some 0·3 per cent. oxalates of potassium and calcium oxalates. It is possible that the recent cases of poisoning occurred in subjects specially susceptible to oxalic poisoning, as there are also many cases reported of no harm ensuing from a use of Rhubarb leaves as a vegetable.

In Maunders' *Treasury of Botany* Rhubarb leaves are mentioned as a pot-herb. Green (*Universal Herbal,* 1832) says: 'The leaves are also used by the French in their soups, to which they impart an agreeable acidity, like that of Sorrel.' Reference has recently been made in the press to a letter which appeared in the *Gardeners' Chronicle* for 1846, in which the gardener of the Earl of Shrewsbury at Alton Towers, Staffordshire, told how rhubarb leaves had been used there for many years as a vegetable. He also mentioned that the flower of the plant (before the leaves expanded) could be used like broccoli. A subsequent note by him makes it clear, however, that the leaf-stems were meant, for he then says:

'I have no experience in the eating of the leaves and think them nauseous to the taste and unpleasant to the smell. . . . I tasted them boiled and they did not appear to me to have one redeeming feature. . . .'

The flower of the plant, when in bud form, has been eaten as a pleasant substitute for broccoli; when cooked *au gratin*, with white sauce over it, the cheese quite obviates any bitterness of taste.

Further reference to the *Gardeners' Chronicle,* of 1847, shows records of the varying results of eating the young inflorescence, producing no ill-effects in some cases and serious illness in others, and a case is recorded of severe sickness attacking a whole family after partaking of the leaves boiled as a vegetable. In 1853 we find the question again raised. In 1872 we hear of deaths from eating the leaves in America, and in 1899 we find a revival of interest in Rhubarb leaves as a vegetable, quite opposite opinions being expressed in a correspondence in the gardening papers. In 1901 we hear of a man dying after eating stewed Rhubarb leaves, the verdict at the inquest being: 'Accidental death, caused by eating rhubarb-leaves.' It was stated then that the leaves were used as a vegetable in parts of Hampshire. The *British Medical Journal* in December, 1910, mentions several cases of rhubarb poisoning.

The leaves are sometimes made use of in the fabrication of fictitious cigars and tobacco. The shape of the hairs, however, as seen under a microscope, can enable the observer to detect the presence or absence of tobacco, but it is not so easy to determine the source of the fraudulent admixtures.

It is possible that the chemical composition of Rhubarb varies to some extent according to the variety and the soil on which it is grown. It has been stated that the amount of water present is less when the plants are grown on poor soil, while the acid principle is more abundant.

As regards the method of cooking, the *British Medical Journal* points out that hard water would precipitate the oxalate, while a soft water might leave it in the form of soluble oxalate, more readily assimilated into the systems of those susceptible to this kind of poisoning. In a recent case that terminated fatally, the leaves were well washed, drained, cut up and put into boiling water, in an iron saucepan, for 20 minutes. A little salt and kitchen soda were added, but nothing else. Being acid, the leaves should, of course, not be cooked in a copper vessel.

¶ *Medicinal Action and Uses.* Though the English Rhubarb root is milder as a purgative, it is more astringent, and has been considered a better stomachic than the foreign.

It is specially useful in infantile stomach troubles and looseness of the bowels.

In fairly large doses it acts as a laxative.

Dose of powdered root, 5 to 60 grains. The dose is entirely individual, 12 grains acting on some persons, as much as 20 on others of the same age. It has been held that 20 grains of the seed are equal to 30 of the root, as regards purgative power. The properties of the seeds are similar to those of the root.

A decoction of the seeds is supposed not only to ease pains in the stomach, but to strengthen it by increasing the appetite.

A strong decoction of the root has been employed as a good wash for scrofulous sores.

If a portion of the root be infused in water, and when strained a few grains of salt of tartar be added, a very beautiful red tincture results, which might prove valuable for the purposes of a dye.

Culpepper says of Rhubarb:

'If your body be anything strong, you may take 2 drams of it at a time being sliced thin and steeped all night in white wine, in the morning strain it out and drink the white wine; it purges but gently, it leaves a binding quality behind it, therefore dried a little by the fire and beaten into powder, it is usually given in Fluxes.'

RHUBARB, MONK'S

Synonym. Garden Patience

Monk's Rhubarb is, as Culpepper tells us, 'a Dock bearing the name of Rhubarb for some purging quality within.'

The root was formerly used medicinally, and the leaves as a pot-herb.

It is found on roadsides near cottages in the North of England and in Scotland, but is rare and naturalized.

The root-stock is very stout, of a yellow colour; the stem 2 to 4 feet high, bearing pale green leaves, broad and very long, the edges waved, but not cut into. The tops of the stems are divided into many small branches, bearing reddish or purple flowers, succeeded by angular seeds, as in other docks.

Rumex alpinus (LINN.)

The medicinal virtues of the root, when dried, are similar to the Garden or Bastard Rhubarb, but are not so strong.

Culpepper says:

'A dram of the dried root of Monk's Rhubarb with a scruple of Ginger made into powder, and taken fasting in a draught or mess of warm broth, purges choler and phlegm downwards very gently and safely without danger. . . . The distilled water thereof is very profitably used to heal scabs; also foul ulcerous sores, and to allay the inflammation of them. . . .'

See DOCKS.

RICE

Oryza sativa (LINN.)
N.O. Graminaceæ

Synonyms. Nivara. Dhan. O. montana. O. setegera. O. latifolia. Bras. Paddy
Part Used. The seeds
Habitat. East Indies. Most sub-tropical countries

¶ *Description.* Rice is an annual plant with several jointed culms or stems from 2 to 10 feet long, the lower part floating in water or prostrate, with roots at the nodes, the rest erect. The panicle is terminal and diffuse, bowing when the seed is weighty. It is probably indigenous to China, and certainly to India, where the wild form grows by tanks, ditches and rivers. It was early introduced into East Africa and Syria, and later into America, where it already appears as a native plant. In Europe, rice was brought into the Mediterranean basin from Syria by the Arabs in the Middle Ages, but is now grown largely only in the plain of Lombardy, and a little in Spain. In England it has been cultivated merely as a curiosity, and may be seen in the hothouses of most botanic gardens, treated as a water plant. The Cingalese distinguish 160 kinds, while 50 or 60 are cultivated in India, not including the wild form, from which the grain is collected, though it is never cultivated. Most kinds require irrigation, but some need little water, or can be grown on ordinary, dry ground.

Oryza (the classical name of the grain), or the husked seeds, is called Bras by the Malays, and Paddy when it is enclosed in the husk. Carolina and Patna rice are the most esteemed in England and the United States. The grain of the first is round and flat, and boils soft for puddings; the latter has a long and narrow grain that keeps its shape well for curries, etc.

The *flour* procured from the seeds is called Oryzæ Farina, or rice flour, commonly known as *ground rice.*

The granules of *rice starch* are the smallest of all known starch granules.

A kind of spirit called Arrack is sometimes distilled from the fermented infusion, but the name Arrack is usually applied to Palm wine or Toddy.

¶ *Medicinal Action and Uses.* The chief consumption of rice is as a food substance, but it should never be forgotten that the large and continued consumption of the white, polished rices of commerce is likely to be injurious to the health. The nations of which rice is the staple diet eat it unhusked as a rule, when it is brownish and less attractive to the eye, but much more nutritious as well as cheaper. Having no laxative qualities, rice forms a light and digestible food for those in whom there is any tendency to diarrhœa or dysentery, but it contains less potash and vegetable acids than potatoes.

A decoction of rice, commonly called *rice-water* is recommended in the Pharmacopœia of India as an excellent demulcent, refrigerant drink in febrile and inflammatory diseases, and in dysuria and similar affections. It may be acidulated with lime-juice and sweetened with sugar. This may also be used as an enema in affections of the bowels.

A poultice of rice may be used as a substitute for one of linseed meal, and finely-powdered rice flour may be used, like that of wheat flour, for erysipelas, burns, scalds, etc.

Rice starch may be used medicinally and in other ways in place of wheat starch.

A few years ago the injurious habit of chewing the raw white grains was practised by fashionable women and girls to produce a white velvety complexion.

ROCKET, GARDEN
Hesperis matronalis
N.O. Cruciferæ

Synonyms. Eruca sativa. Dame's Rocket. White Rocket. Purple Rocket. Rucchette. Roquette. Dame's Violet. Vesper-Flower
Part Used. Whole plant
Habitat. Central Europe

¶ *Description.* These biennial plants are natives of Italy, but are found throughout most of Central and Mediterranean Europe, and in Britain and Russian Asia as escapes from gardens. The stems are very erect, and grow from 2 to 3 feet in height, with spear-shaped, pointed leaves. The flowers, white purple, or variegated, are produced in a simple thyrse at the top of the stalk. Johnson wrote of a double-white variety in 1633. The Siberian Rocket is almost identical. The seeds are like those of mustard, but larger.

The leaves are very acrid in taste, and in many countries, especially in Germany, they are eaten like cress in salads.

In the language of flowers, the Rocket has been taken to represent deceit, since it gives out a lovely perfume in the evening, but in the daytime has none. Hence its name of Hesperis, or Vesper-Flower, given it by the Ancients.

For eating purposes, the plant should be gathered before flowering, but for medicinal use, when in flower.

¶ *Constituents.* The properties of the cultivated Rocket resemble those of the Cochlearea, but its taste is less acrid and piquant.

¶ *Medicinal Action and Uses.* In former days doctors combined with poets in attributing marvellous virtues to this plant. It is regarded principally as antiscorbutic.

A strong dose will cause vomiting, and may be taken in the place of ipecacuanha. Powdered, the effect is less strong than that of mustard.

¶ *Other Species.* The *Sea-Rocket* or *Cakile maritima*, *Eruca marina*, often found on sandhills, is very acrid, and can be used as an antiscorbutic, being prescribed in scrofulous affections, lymphatic disturbances, and the malaise that follows malaria. It is important not to confuse it with the real Rocket.

ROSEMARY
Rosmarinus officinalis (LINN.)
N.O. Labiatæ

Synonyms. Polar Plant. Compass-weed. Compass Plant. Rosmarinus coronarium
(*Old French*) Incensier
Parts Used. Herb, root

¶ *Description.* The evergreen leaves of this shrubby herb are about 1 inch long, linear, revolute, dark green above and paler and glandular beneath, with an odour pungently aromatic and somewhat camphoraceous. The flowers are small and pale blue. Much of the active volatile principle resides in their calyces. There are silver and gold-striped varieties, but the green-leaved variety is the kind used medicinally.

¶ *Cultivation.* Rosemary is propagated by seeds, cuttings and layers, and division of roots. (1) Seeds may be sown upon a warm, sunny border. (2) Cuttings, taken in August, 6 inches long, and dibbled into a shady border, two-thirds of their length in the ground, under a hand-glass, will root and be ready for transplanting into permanent quarters the following autumn. (3) Layering may be readily accomplished in summer by pegging some of the lower branches under a little sandy soil.

Rosemary succeeds best in a light, rather dry soil, and in a sheltered situation, such as the base of a low wall with a south aspect. On a chalk soil it grows smaller, but is more

fragrant. The silver- and gold-striped kinds are not quite so hardy.

The finest plants are said to be raised from seed.

¶ *History.* The Ancients were well acquainted with the shrub, which had a reputation for strengthening the memory. On this account it became the emblem of fidelity for lovers. It holds a special position among herbs from the symbolism attached to it. Not only was it used at weddings, but also at funerals, for decking churches and banqueting halls at festivals, as incense in religious ceremonies, and in magical spells.

At weddings, it was entwined in the wreath worn by the bride, being first dipped into scented water. Anne of Cleves, we are told, wore such a wreath at her wedding. A Rosemary branch, richly gilded and tied with silken ribands of all colours, was also presented to wedding guests, as a symbol of love and loyalty. Together with an orange stuck with cloves it was given as a New Year's gift – allusions to this custom are to be found in Ben Jonson's plays.

Miss Anne Pratt (*Flowers and their Associations*) says:

'But it was not among the herbalists and apothecaries merely that Rosemary had its reputation for peculiar virtues. The celebrated Doctor of Divinity, Roger Hacket, did not disdain to expatiate on its excellencies in the pulpit. In a sermon which he entitles "A Marriage Present," which was published in 1607, he says: "Speaking of the powers of rosemary, it overtoppeth all the flowers in the garden, boasting man's rule. It helpeth the brain, strengtheneth the memorie, and is very medicinable for the head. Another property of the rosemary is, it affects the heart. Let this rosmarinus, this flower of men, ensigne of your wisdom, love and loyaltie, be carried not only in your hands, but in your hearts and heads." '

Sir Thomas More writes:

'As for Rosmarine, I lett it runne all over my garden walls, not onlie because my bees love it, but because it is the herb sacred to remembrance, and, therefore, to friendship; whence a sprig of it hath a dumb language that maketh it the chosen emblem of our funeral wakes and in our buriall grounds.'

In early times, Rosemary was freely cultivated in kitchen gardens and came to represent the dominant influence of the house mistress. 'Where Rosemary flourished, the woman ruled.'

The *Treasury of Botany* says:

'There is a vulgar belief in Gloucestershire and other counties, that Rosemary will not grow well unless where the mistress is "master"; and so touchy are some of the lords of creation upon this point, that we have more than once had reason to suspect them of privately injuring a growing rosemary in order to destroy this evidence of their want of authority.'

Rosemary was one of the cordial herbs used to flavour ale and wine. It was also used in Christmas decoration.

'Down with the rosemary and so,
Down with the baies and mistletoe,
Down with the holly, ivie all
Wherewith ye deck the Christmas Hall.'
                                        HERRICK.

In place of more costly incense, the ancients used Rosemary in their religious ceremonies. An old French name for it was *Incensier*.

The Spaniards revere it as one of the bushes that gave shelter to the Virgin Mary in the flight into Egypt and call it *Romero*, the Pilgrim's Flower. Both in Spain and Italy, it has been considered a safeguard from witches and evil influences generally. The Sicilians believe that young fairies, taking the form of snakes, lie amongst the branches.

It was an old custom to burn Rosemary in sick chambers, and in French hospitals it is customary to burn Rosemary with Juniper berries to purify the air and prevent infection. Like Rue, it was placed in the dock of courts of justice, as a preventative from the contagion of gaol-fever. A sprig of Rosemary was carried in the hand at funerals, being distributed to the mourners before they left the house, to be cast on to the coffin when it had been lowered into the grave. In many parts of Wales it is still a custom.

One old legend compares the growth of the plant with the height of the Saviour and declares that after thirty-three years it increases in breadth, but never in height.

There is a tradition that Queen Philippa's mother (Countess of Hainault) sent the first plants of Rosemary to England, and in a copy of an old manuscript in the library of Trinity College, Cambridge, the translator, 'danyel bain,' says that Rosemary was unknown in England until this Countess sent some to her daughter.

Miss Rohde gives the following quotation from *Banckes' Herbal*:

'Take the flowers thereof and make powder thereof and binde it to thy right arme in a linnen cloath and it shale make *theee* light and merrie.

'Take the flowers and put them in thy chest among thy clothes or among thy Bookes and Mothes shall not destroy them.

'Boyle the leaves in white wine and washe thy face therewith and thy browes, and thou shalt have a faire face.

'Also put the leaves under thy bedde and thou shalt be delivered of all evill dreames.

'Take the leaves and put them into wine and it shall keep the wine from all sourness and evill savours, and if thou wilt sell thy wine thou shalt have goode speede.

'Also if thou be feeble boyle the leaves in cleane water and washe thyself and thou shalt wax shiny.

'Also if thou have lost appetite of eating boyle well these leaves in cleane water and when the water is colde put thereunto as much of white wine and then make sops, eat them thereof wel and thou shalt restore thy appetite againe.

'If thy legges be blowen with gowte, boyle the leaves in water and binde them in a linnen cloath and winde it about thy legges and it shall do thee much good.

'If thou have a cough drink the water of the leaves boyld in white wine and ye shall be whole.

'Take the Timber thereof and burn it to coales and make powder thereof and rubbe thy teeth thereof and it shall keep thy teeth from all evils. Smell it oft and it shall keep thee youngly.

'Also if a man have lost his smellyng of the ayre that he may not draw his breath, make a fire of the wood, and bake his bread therewith, eate it and it shall keepe him well.

'Make thee a box of the wood of rosemary and smell to it and it shall preserve thy youth.'

From the *Grete Herbal*:

'ROSEMARY. – For weyknesse of ye brayne. Against weyknesse of the brayne and coldenesse thereof, sethe rosemaria in wyne and lete the pacyent receye the smoke at his nose and keep his heed warme.'

¶ *Parts Used.* The oil of Rosemary, distilled from the flowering tops, as directed in the British Pharmacopœia, is a superior oil to that obtained from the stem and leaves, but nearly all the commercial oil is distilled from the stem and leaves of the wild plant before it is in flower.[1]

The upper portions of the shoots are taken, with the leaves on and the leaves are stripped off the portions of the shoots that are very wooden.

¶ *Constituents.* The plant contains some tannic acid, together with a resin and a bitter principle and a volatile oil. The chief constituents of the oil are Borneol, bornyl acetate and other esters, a special camphor similar to that possessed by the myrtle, cineol, pinene and camphene. It is colourless, with the odour of Rosemary and a warm camphoraceous taste. The chief adulterants of oil of Rosemary are oil of turpentine and petroleum. Rosemary yields its virtues partly to water and entirely to rectified spirits of wine.

From 100 lb. of the flowering tops, 8 oz. of the oil are usually obtained.

¶ *Medicinal Action and Uses.* Tonic, astringent, diaphoretic, stimulant. Oil of Rosemary has the carminative properties of other volatile oils and is an excellent stomachic and nervine, curing many cases of headache.

It is employed principally, externally, as *spiritus Rosmarini*, in hair-lotions, for its odour and effect in stimulating the hair-bulbs to renewed activity and preventing premature baldness. An infusion of the dried plant (both leaves and flowers) combined with borax and used when cold, makes one of the best hairwashes known. It forms an effectual remedy for the prevention of scurf and dandruff.

The oil is also used externally as a rubefacient and is added to liniments as a fragrant stimulant. Hungary water, for outward application to renovate the vitality of paralysed limbs, was first invented for a Queen of Hungary, who was said to have been completely cured by its continued use. It was prepared by putting $1\frac{1}{2}$ lb. of fresh Rosemary tops in full flower into 1 gallon of spirits of wine, this was allowed to stand for four days and then distilled. Hungary water was also considered very efficacious against gout in the hands and feet, being rubbed into them vigorously.

A formula dated 1235, said to be in the handwriting of Elizabeth, Queen of Hungary, is said to be preserved in Vienna.

Rosemary Wine when taken in small quantities acts as a quieting cordial to a weak heart subject to palpitation, and relieves accompanying dropsy by stimulating the kidneys. It is made by chopping up sprigs of green Rosemary and pouring on them white wine, which is strained off after a few days and is then ready for use. By stimulating the brain and nervous system, it is a good remedy for headaches caused by feeble circulation.

The young tops, leaves and flowers can be made into an infusion, called Rosemary Tea, which, taken warm, is a good remedy for removing headache, colic, colds and nervous diseases, care being taken to prevent the escape of steam during its preparation. It will relieve nervous depression. A conserve, made by beating up the freshly gathered tops with three times their weight of sugar, is said to have the same effect.

A spirit of Rosemary may be used, in doses of 30 drops in water or on sugar, as an antispasmodic.

Rosemary and Coltsfoot leaves are considered good when rubbed together and smoked for asthma and other affections of the throat and lungs.

Rosemary is also one of the ingredients used in the preparation of Eau-de-Cologne.

¶ *Preparations.* Oil, $\frac{1}{2}$ to 3 drops. Spirit, B.P., 5 to 20 drops.

ROSES

Roses are a group of herbaceous shrubs found in temperate regions throughout both hemispheres. All the Roses of the Antipodes,

N.O. Rosaceæ

South Africa and the temperate parts of South America have been carried there by cultivation.

---

[1] Rosemary is one of the plants like lavender which grows better in England than anywhere else, and English oil of Rosemary, though it is infinitely superior to that of other countries, is hardly found in commerce to-day. The bulk of the commercial oil comes from France, Dalmatia, Spain and Japan. – EDITOR.

The birthplace of the cultivated Rose was probably Northern Persia, on the Caspian, or Faristan on the Gulf of Persia. Thence it spread across Mesopotamia to Palestine and across Asia Minor to Greece. And thus it was that Greek colonists brought it to Southern Italy. It is beyond doubt that the Roses used in ancient days were cultivated varieties. Horace, who writes at length on horticulture, gives us an interesting account of the growing of Roses in beds. Pliny advises the deep digging of the soil for their better cultivation. In order to force their growth, it was the practice to dig a ditch round the plants and to pour warm water into the ditch just as the rose-buds had formed. The varieties were then very limited in number, but it would appear that the Romans, at all events, knew and cultivated the red Provins Rose (*Rosa gallica*), often mistakenly called the Provence Rose. The word *rosa* comes from the Greek word *rodon* (red), and the rose of the Ancients was of a deep crimson colour, which probably suggested the fable of its springing from the blood of Adonis.

The voluptuous Romans of the later Empire made lavish use of the blossoms of the Rose. Horace enjoins their unsparing use at banquets, when they were used not only as a means of decoration, but also to strew the floors, and even in winter the luxurious Romans expected to have petals of roses floating in their Falernian wine. Roman brides and bridegrooms were crowned with roses, so too were the images of Cupid and Venus and Bacchus. Roses were scattered at feasts of Flora and Hymen, in the paths of victors, or beneath their chariot-wheels, or adorned the prows of their war-vessels. Nor did the self-indulgent Romans disdain to wear rose garlands at their feasts, as a preventive against drunkenness: To them, the Rose was a sign of pleasure, the companion of mirth and wine, but it was also used at their funerals.

As soon as the Rose had become known to nations with a wide literature of their own, it was not only the theme of poets, but gave rise to many legends. Homer's allusions to it in the *Iliad* and *Odyssey* are the earliest records, and Sappho, the Greek poetess, writing about 600 B.C., selects the Rose as the Queen of Flowers. (The 'Rose of Sharon' of the Old Testament is considered to be a kind of Narcissus, and the 'Rose of Jericho' is a small woody annual, also not allied to the Rose.)

It was once the custom to suspend a Rose over the dinner-table as a sign that all confidences were to be held sacred. Even now the plaster ornament in the centre of a ceiling is known as 'the rose.' It has been suggested that because the Pretender could only be helped secretly, *sub rosa*, that the Jacobites took the white rose as his symbol. Although we have no British 'Order of the Rose,' our national flower figures largely in the insignia of other orders, such as the Garter, the order of the Bath, etc.

¶ *Constituents.* The essential oil to which the perfume of the Rose is due is found in both flowers and leaves, sometimes in one, sometimes in both, and sometimes in neither, for there are also scentless roses. In the flower, the petals are the chief secreting part of the blossom, though a certain amount of essential oil resides in the epidermal layers of cells, both surfaces of the petals being equally odorous and secretive. An examination of the stamens, which are transformed into petals in the cultivated roses, shows that the epidermal cells also contain essential oil.

More than 10,000 roses are known in cultivation and three types of odours are recognized, viz. those of the Cabbage Rose (*R. centifolia*), the Damask Rose (*R. damascena*) and the Tea Rose (*R. indica*), but there are many roses of intermediate character as regards perfume, notably the 'perpetual hybrid' and 'hybrid tea' classes, which exhibit every gradation between the three types and no precise classification of roses by their odour is possible.

The flowers adapted for the preparation of essence of roses are produced by several species of rose trees. The varieties cultivated on a large scale for perfumery purposes are *R. damascena* and *R. centifolia*. *R. damascena* is cultivated chiefly in Bulgaria, Persia and India: it is a native of the Orient and was introduced into Europe at the period of the Crusades. *R. centifolia* is cultivated in Provence, Turkey and Tunis; it has been found wild in the forests of the Caucasus, where double-flowered specimens are often met with.

Although the Rose was highly esteemed in the dawn of history, it does not appear that it was then submitted to the still, the method of preserving the aroma being to steep the petals in oil, or possibly to extract it in the form of a pomade. The *Oleum Rosarum, Ol. rosatum* or *Ol. rosacetum* of the Ancients was not a volatile oil, but a fatty oil perfumed with rose petals. The first preparation of rose-water by Avicenna was in the tenth century. It was between 1582 and 1612 that the oil or OTTO OF ROSES was discovered, as recorded in two separate histories of the Grand Moguls. At the wedding feast of the princess Nour-Djihan with the Emperor Djihanguyr, son of Akbar, a canal circling the whole gardens was dug and filled with rose-water. The heat of the sun separating the water from the essential oil of the Rose, was observed by the bridal pair when rowing on the fragrant water. It was skimmed off and found to be an exquisite perfume. The discovery was immediately turned to account and the manufacture of Otto of Roses was commenced in Persia about 1612 and long before the end of the seventeenth century the distilleries of Shiraz were working on a large scale. The first mention of Persian Otto or Attar of Roses is by Kampfer (1683), who alludes to the export to India. Persia no longer exports Attar of Roses to any extent, and the production in Kashmir and elsewhere in India – probably as ancient as that of Persia – practically serves for local consumption only.

Through the Turks, the manufacture was introduced into Europe, by way of Asia Minor, where it has long been produced. It is probable that the first otto was distilled in Bulgaria, then part of the Turkish Empire, about 1690 – its sale in Europe, at a high cost, is first alluded to in 1694 – but the importance of the Turkish otto industry is of comparatively late growth, and Turkish otto is not mentioned as an article of English commerce until the beginning of the last century.

A small amount of Otto of Roses has been produced in the South of France for at least 150 years, having been an established industry there before the French Revolution, but these earlier French ottos, almost entirely derived from *R. centifolia*, as a by-product in rose-water distillation, were consumed in the country itself. French roses were almost exclusively used for the manufacture of rose-pomade and of rose-water, the French rose-water having the reputation of being superior in odour to any that can be produced in England. In spite of their unrivalled delicacy of fragrance, which always commanded a high place in the estimation of connoisseurs, until recent years the high price and lack of body of French ottos did not enable them to compete for general purposes with the Balkan concrete oil. When, however, Bulgaria joined the Central Empires, the French seized their opportunity, and methods of distillation were modernized, improved stills were erected and many other blooms than those of *R. centifolia* were experimented with, until now French otto has made itself a place in perfumery. Large plantations of roses have been laid down, and the output of otto is increasing steadily, 10,000 to 20,000 oz. being at present the annual production. French chemists, botanists and horticulturists have studied the scientific aspect of the Rose, and in the new roses introduced, the chief object has been to improve the odour rather than the appear-

ance of tne flower. The variety of rose mostly cultivated is the *Rose de Mai*, a hybrid of *R. gallica* and *R. centifolia*, bearing recurved prickles on the flowering branches. Two types are grown in the Grasse district, one more spiny than the other. They are mingled in the plantations, but the more spiny is preferred for less irrigated ground and the one with fewer thorns for well-watered land. The bushes are planted half a metre apart, in rows one metre asunder. The first fortnight in May sees the rose harvest. The buds open gradually and are numerous, as each stalk bears a dense cluster and all the annual stems are well-covered. In the second half of May, after flowering, they are cut back and the complete pruning takes place in the following November. A rose plantation lasts from eight to ten years. Five thousand rose-trees will occupy about ½ acre of land and will produce about 2,200 lb. of flowers during the season. It is necessary to distil about 10,000 lb. of roses to obtain 1 lb. of oil. By the volatile solvents process a similar quantity will give anything up to 10 lb. of concrete. The rose-trees cultivated at Grasse in the last few years have been much attacked by disease, and in the opinion of some authorities the variety most grown hitherto would appear to be degenerating. The plantations are all more or less attacked by the rose rust parasite (*Pragmidium subcorticium*).

Quite recently a new and very promising rose has been introduced, known as the *Rose de Hai*, produced by crossing *R. damascena* with 'General Jacqueminot,' which in its turn is derived from *R. rugosa*, or the Japanese and Kamschatkan Rose. It has the advantage of not being so sensitive to heat and cold as the *Rose de Mai* and can be cultivated in the north of France, or as far south as Algeria. Its flowering period is much longer than that of the *Rose de Mai* and it gives more blooms and the oil is of almost equal quality. A certain amount of French otto is also distilled from garden roses. 'Ulrich Brunner,' distilled with other garden blooms, give a fair quality oil or concrete, known as 'Roses de France.' Other varieties which frequently enter into the composition of 'Roses de France' concretes are 'Grussan Teplitz,' 'Frau Karl Druschky,' Narbonnand, Van Houtte, Safrano, Paul Neyron, Madame Gabriel Luizet, Madame Caroline Testout, Baronne de Rothschild, Mrs. John Laing, Madame Maurice de Luze, François Juranville, Gerbe Rose and Gloire d'un Enfant d'Hiram.

Oil of Rose is light yellow in colour, sometimes possessing a green tint. It has a strong odour of fresh roses. When cooled, it congeals to a translucent soft mass, which is again liquefied by the warmth of the hand. The congealing point lies between 15° and 22° C., mostly between 17° and 21° C.

The composition of Rose oil is not quite uniform, the variation being due to a number of influences, the chief being the kind of flower and the locality in which it has been grown. The Rose oil from plants grown in colder climates contains a very high percentage of the waxy substance stearoptene, odourless and valueless as a perfume. This was the first constituent of Rose oil to be studied and was recognized as paraffin hydrocarbon by Fluckiger: it consists of a mixture of hydrocarbons. Sometimes this stearoptene is removed by large distillers and the resulting oil sold at a higher price as stearoptene-free Otto of Roses. Geraniol and Citronellol are the chief ingredients of Rose oil as regards percentage, though not the most characteristic as regards odour. Citronellol, a fragrant, oily liquid, forms about 35 per cent. of the oil. Geraniol, which may be present to the amount of 75 per cent., is a colourless liquid, with a sweet, rose-like odour. It is also found in Palmarosa or Turkish Geranium oil and in oils of Citronella, Lavender, Neroli, Petit Grain, Ylang Ylang, Lemongrass and some Eucalyptus oils. It is largely obtained industrially from the oils of Palmarosa and Citronella and is much used to adulterate Otto of Roses. The temptation to adulterate so expensive an oil is great and it is widely practised. Bulgaria usually exports from 30 to 60 per cent. more otto than is distilled in the country. This is due to the enormous amount of adulteration that takes place. This is so well done that a chemical analysis is imperative to ascertain the purity of the oil. The principal adulterant is Geraniol. The addition of this, or of Palmarosa oil, which contains it, either to the rose leaves before distillation, or to the product, reduces the congealing point, but this can be brought up to the normal standard by the addition of spermaceti. Hence in addition to the congealing point, the determination of the absence of spermaceti may become necessary. Another recent adulterant of importance, employed in Bulgaria, is the Guaiac Wood Oil, from *Bulnesia sarmienti*, which has an agreeable tea-rose-like odour. It can be recognized by the microscopic examination of the form of the crystals of guaicol, which separate from the oil on cooling. Guaicol forms needle-shaped crystals which are characterized by a channel-like middle-line. The crystals of the Rose oil paraffin are smaller and thinner and possess less sharply-outlined forms. The addition of Guaiac Wood oil to Rose oil raises the congealing point of the oil and increases the specific gravity and its presence may thus be detected.

A satisfactory artificial Otto of Rose cannot be obtained by the exclusive combination of aromatic chemicals, some of the natural oil must always enter into the composition of any artificial rose oil, or a purely synthetic oil may be distilled over a certain quantity of rose petals. A striking difference between synthetic and natural rose oils is that the former is almost entirely deodorized by iodine, while the latter is unaffected in this respect.

Apart from French Otto of Roses, the world's supply is mainly drawn from Bulgaria, the greater part being distilled by small peasant growers. The Bulgarian rose industry is confined to one special mountain district, having for its centre the town of Kazanlik. The rose district is about 80 miles long and about 30 miles wide and its average elevation about 1,300 feet above the sea-level. Attempts to extend the rose culture to other neighbouring districts in Bulgaria have proved a failure. The rose bush seems to thrive best in sandy soil, well exposed to the sun, protected from the cold winter winds and having perfect drainage. It is chiefly the mountain formation, the climatic peculiarities and the special sandy soil of the rose district which adapt it for this industry, in which, in addition to their other farm culture, about 180 villages are engaged. There are about 20,000 small proprietors of rose gardens, each one owning about 1 acre of rose plantation, which, when well tended, is calculated to yield at the average 100 lb. of flowers every day for three weeks.

Only two varieties of roses are cultivated in Bulgaria, the Damask Rose (*R. damascena*), light red in colour and very fragrant, with 36 petals, and the Musk Rose (*R. muscatta*), a snow-white rose, far less fragrant, yielding an oil of poorer quality, very rich in stearoptene, but containing very little otto. It is of more vigorous growth and is grown chiefly for hedges between the plantations to indicate the divisions of the rose fields. The rose bushes only yield one crop a year, the harvest beginning in the latter half of May and lasting from two to five weeks, according to the weather. The weather during the rose harvest has a great influence on the quality and quantity of the crop – should it be exceptionally dry and hot, the crop may only last two weeks and be poor, but if it be cool, with some rainfall, there is a rich yield, lasting over four or even six weeks. The weather during the budding season has also to be reckoned with, dry and hot weather causing the bushes to throw out only very small clusters of buds, while in favourable weather 13, 21 and even 18 buds will be found in the clusters. The flowers are gathered in the early morning, just before the sun rises and the picking should cease by ten or eleven o'clock, unless the day be cloudy, when it continues all day. The flowers are distilled on the same day. It takes 30 roses to make 1 drop of otto and 60,000 roses (about 180 lb. of flowers) to make 1 oz. of otto.

The small stills used by the farmers are very simple and primitive and are only capable of distilling at a time 24 lb. of flowers, but they are gradually being replaced by modern, improved, large steam stills, which obtain results immeasurably greater. In 1918, some far-sighted and influential rose-essence producers in Bulgaria combined to unite all parties interested in this industry into an association for mutual advantage. Of the membership of 5,000 nearly half were collective members, i.e. co-operative societies, so that the membership represents a very large number of growers. The objects of the association are: (1) to procure cheap credit for its members; (2) to prevent adulteration; (3) to organize joint distillation; (4) to provide the societies with the requisite apparatus for producing the otto.

The Bulgarian rose industry has developed steadily since 1885, though the Great War seriously handicapped it.

Bulgarian rose distillers do not obtain all their otto direct from the petals, but draw the greater part by treating the water. They charge the alembic with ten kills of flowers (about 25 lb.) and about 50 litres of water. They draw from this charge, 10 litres of distilled water, from which they gather a very small quantity of green concrete essence. When they have made four distillations, they carefully collect the 40 litres of water and re-distil, and obtain 10 or 15 litres of liquid. It is reckoned that 4,000 kilos of flowers yield 1 kilo of otto, of which only one-third – the green essence – comes from the first distillation and the other two-thirds – yellow – are the result of re-distilling the waters. This is the reason why in France, some 10,000 kilos of flowers are required for 1 kilo of oil, as French distillers do not re-distil the waters; these are sold separately. The product of the first operation is of markedly superior quality.

In 1919 the entire Bulgarian crop of Otto of Roses was taken over by the Government of that country in consequence of an agreement between the Bulgarian Government and the United States Food Administration, by which payment for food supplied to Bulgaria from America was to be made out of the proceeds of the Bulgarian otto crop.

¶ *Cyprus Otto of Roses.* In Cyprus, rose cultivation for Otto has of late years been keenly developed. It had been prepared since 1897 in a very small way with native stills at the village of Milikouri, where the Damask Rose is abundant, but no attempt had been made to extract the Rose oil by means of a modern still. The closing of the market for Bulgarian Otto of Roses, owing to the War, gave an impetus to the industry, and in the spring of 1917 the Department of Agriculture of Cyprus sent qualified officers to superintend the work at Milikouri and to carry out an experimental distillation. The samples of 1917 oil sent to the Imperial Institute were found to be similar to the Bulgarian article, though rather weaker.

¶ *Roses in Germany, Algiers and Morocco.* Otto of Roses is also prepared in Algiers to a limited extent and in Germany, from large rose plantations near Leipzig.

The cultivation of roses is already extensively practised in Morocco for the distillation of rose-water, which enters so largely into native perfumery, but there is no production of Otto of Roses on a commercial scale.

¶ *Indian Rose Otto.* The two main centres of the Rose industry in India are Ghazipore and Hathras, in Upper India. Rose plantations exist in the neighbourhood of both these places, but the industry is confined to the manufacture of rose-water and small quantities of Aytar – a mixture of Sandalwood oil and Otto of Roses.

¶ *Medicinal Action and Uses.* The petals of the dark red Rose, *R. gallica*, known as the Provins Rose, are employed medicinally for the preparation of an infusion and a confection. In this country it is specially grown for medicinal purposes in Oxfordshire and Derbyshire.

The petals of this rose are of a deep, purplish-red, velvety in texture, paler towards the base. They have the delicate fragrance of the Damask Rose and a slightly astringent taste.

The British Pharmacopœia directs that Red Rose petals are to be obtained only from *R. gallica*, of which, however, there are many variations, in fact there are practically no pure *R. gallica* now to be had, only hybrids, so that the exact requirements of the British Pharmacopœia are difficult to follow. Those used in medicine and generally appearing in commerce are actually any scented roses of a deep red colour, or when dried of a deep rose tint. The main point is that the petals suitable for medicinal purposes must yield a deep rose-coloured and somewhat astringent and fragrant infusion when boiling water is poured upon them. The most suitable are the so-called Hybrid Perpetuals, flowering from June to October, among which may be specially recommended the varieties:

Eugène Furst, deep dark red, sweet-scented.

General Jacqueminot, a fine, rich crimson, scented rose.

Hugh Dickson, rather a large petalled one, but of a fine, deep red colour and sweet-scented.

Ulrich Brunner, bright-red.

Richmond, deep crimson-red.

Liberty, scarlet-red.

¶ *Collection and Preparation.* When employed for the preparation of the drug, only flower-buds just about to open are collected, no fully-expanded flowers. They must only be gathered in dry weather and no petals of any roses that have suffered from effects of damp weather must be taken. The whole of the unexpanded petals are plucked from the calyx so that they remain united in small conical masses, leaving the stamens behind. Any stamens that may have come away with the petals should be shaken out. The lighter-coloured, lower portion is then cut off from the deep purplish-red upper part. The little masses, kept as entire as possible, are used in the fresh state for preparation of the 'confection,' but for making the infusion, they are dried carefully and quickly on trays in a good current of warm air. They are dried until crisp and while crisp packed in tins that the colour and crispness may be retained. If exposed to the air, they will re-absorb moisture and lose colour.

¶ *Constituents.* The important constituent of Red Rose petals is the red colouring matter of an acid nature. There have also been isolated two yellow crystalline substances, the glucoside *Quercitrin*, which has been found in many other plants and *Quercetin*, yielded when Quercitrin is boiled with a dilute mineral acid. The astringency is due to a little gallic acid, but it has not yet been definitely proved whether quercitannic acid, the tannin of oak bark, is also a constituent. The odour is due to a very small amount of volatile oil, not identical with the official *Ol. Rosæ*. A considerable amount of sugar, gum, fat, etc., are also present.

¶ *Preparations.* Red Rose petals are official in nearly all Pharmacopœias. Though formerly employed for their mild astringency and tonic value, they are to-day used almost solely to impart their pleasant odour to pharmaceutical preparations. The British

Pharmacopœia preparations are a Confection, Acid Infusion and a Fluid Extract. The *Confection* is directed to be made by beating 1 lb. of fresh Red Rose petals in a stone mortar with 3 lb. of sugar. It is mostly used in pill making. Formerly this was prescribed for hæmorrhage of the lungs and for coughs. The United States official confection is made by rubbing Red Rose petals, powdered, with heated rose-water, adding gradually fine, white sugar and heating the whole together till thoroughly mixed. The *Fluid Extract* is made from powdered Red Rose petals with glycerine and dilute alcohol. It is of a deep red colour, an agreeable odour of rose and of a pleasant, mildly astringent taste. The *Acid Infusion* is made from dried, broken-up, Red Rose petals, diluted with sulphuric acid, sugar and boiling water, infused in a covered vessel for 15 minutes and strained. It has a fine red colour and agreeable flavour and has been employed for its astringent effects in the treatment of stomatitis and pharyngitis. Its virtue is principally due to the aromatic sulphuric acid which it contains and the latter ingredient renders it a useful preparation, in the treatment of night-sweats resulting from depression. A *Simple* (non-acid) *Infusion* is mainly used as a flavouring for other medicines. It is also used as a lotion for ophthalmia, etc.

Syrup of Red Rose, official in the United States Pharmacopœia, is used to impart an agreeable flavour and odour to other syrups and mixtures. The syrup is of a fine red colour and has an agreeable, acidulous, somewhat astringent taste. *Honey of Roses*, also official in the United States Pharmacopœia, is prepared from clarified honey and fluid extract of roses. It is considered more agreeable than ordinary honey and somewhat astringent. In olden days, Honey of Roses was popular for sore throats and ulcerated mouth and was made by pounding fresh petals in a small quantity of boiling water, filtering the mass and boiling the liquid with honey. *Rose Vinegar*, a specific on the Continent for headache caused by hot sun, is prepared by steeping dried rose petals in best distilled vinegar, which should not be boiled. Cloths or linen rags are soaked in the liquid and are then applied to the head.

Two liqueurs made by the French also have rose petals as one of the chief ingredients. A small quantity of spirits of wine is distilled with the petals to produce 'Spirit of Roses.' The fragrant spirit, when mixed with sugar, undergoes certain preparatory processes and makes the liqueur called 'L'Huile de Rose.' It is likewise the base of another liqueur, called 'Parfait Amour.'

ROSA CENTIFOLIA.

The pale petals of the Hundred-leaved Rose or Cabbage Rose are also used in commerce. On account of its fragrance, the petals of this variety of rose are much used in France for distillation of rose-water. Though possessing aperient properties, they are seldom now used internally and preparations of them are not official in the British Pharmacopœia.

The roses grouped as varieties of *R. centifolia* have all less scent than *R. gallica.*

The best of them is the old Cabbage Rose. It is a large rose, sweet-scented, of a pink or pale rose-purple colour, the petals whitish towards the base. Its branches are covered with numerous nearly straight spines: the petioles and peduncles are nearly unarmed, but more or less clothed with glandular bristles and the leaves have five or sometimes seven ovate, glandular leaflets, softly hairy beneath. This species and its varieties have given rise to innumerable handsome garden roses.

The flowers are collected and deprived of the calyx and ovaries, the petals alone being employed. In drying, they become brownish and lose some of their delicious rose odour.

The *Constituents* of the Pink Rose are closely similar to those of the Red. The very little colouring matter is apparently identical with that of the Red Rose. A little tannin is present.

Rose-water. The British Pharmacopœia directs that it shall be prepared by mixing the distilled rose-water of commerce, obtained mostly from *R. damascena*, but also from *R. centifolia* and other species, with twice its volume of distilled water immediately before use. It is used as a vehicle for other medicines and as an eye lotion. *Triple rose-water* is water saturated with volatile oil of Rose petals, obtained as a by-product in the distillation of oil of Roses. The finest rose-water is obtained by distillation of the fresh petals. It should be clear and colourless, not mucilaginous, and to be of value medicinally must be free from all metallic impurities, which may be detected by hydrogen sulphide and ammonium sulphide, neither of which should produce turbidity in the water.

Ointment of rose-water, commonly known as *Cold Cream*, enjoys deserved popularity as a soothing, cooling application for chapping of the hands, face, abrasions and other superficial lesions of the skin. For its preparation, the British Pharmacopœia directs that $1\frac{1}{2}$ oz. each of spermaceti and white wax be melted with 9 oz. of Almond oil, the mixture poured into a warmed mortar and 7 fluid ounces of rose-water and 8 minims of oil of Rose then incorporated with it.

¶ *Medicinal Action and Uses.* The old herbalists considered the Red Rose to be more binding and more astringent than any of the other species:

'it strengtheneth the heart, the stomach, the liver and the retentive faculty; is good against all kinds of fluxes, prevents vomiting, stops tickling coughs and is of service in consumption.'

Culpepper gives many uses for the Rose, both white and red and damask.

'Of the Red Roses are usually made many compositions, all serving to sundry good uses, viz. electuary of roses, conserve both moist and dry, which is usually called sugar of roses, syrup of dry roses and honey of roses; the cordial powder called aromatic rosarum, the distilled water of roses, vinegar of roses, ointment and oil of roses and the rose leaves dried are of very great use and effect.'

'The electuary,' he tells us, 'is purging and is good in hot fevers, jaundice and joint-aches. The moist conserve is of much use both binding and cordial, the old conserve mixed with aromaticum rosarum is a very good preservative in the time of infection. The dry conserve called the sugar of roses is a very good cordial against faintings, swoonings, weakness and trembling of the heart, strengthens a weak stomach, promotes digestion and is a very good preservative in the time of infection. The dry conserve called the sugar of roses is a very good cordial to strengthen the heart and spirit. The syrup of roses cooleth an over-heated liver and the blood in agues, comforteth the heart and resisteth putrefaction and infection. Honey of roses is used in gargles and lotions to wash sores, either in the mouth, throat or other parts, both to cleanse and heal them. Red rose-water is well known, it is cooling, cordial, refreshing, quickening the weak and faint spirits, used either in meats or broths to smell at the nose, or to smell the sweet vapours out of a perfume pot, or cast into a hot fire-shovel. It is of much use against the redness and inflammation of the eyes to bathe therewith and the temples of the head. The ointment of roses is much used against heat and inflammation of the head, to anoint the forehead and temples and to cool and heal red pimples. Oil of roses is used to cool hot inflammation or swellings and to bind and stay fluxes of humours to sores and is also put into ointments and plasters that are cooling and binding. The dried leaves of the red roses are used both outwardly and inwardly; they cool, bind and are cordial. Rose-leaves and mint, heated and applied outwardly to the stomach, stay cast-ings, strengthen a weak stomach and applied as a fomentation to the region of the liver and heart, greatly cool and temper them, quiet the over-heated spirits and cause rest and sleep. The decoction of red roses made with white wine and used is very good for head-ache and pains in the eyes, ears, throat and gums.'

¶ *Preparations.* Rose-water, B.P., 1 to 2 oz. Fluid extract, ½ to 1 drachm. Confec., B.P. and U.S.P., 2 to 4 drachms. Infusion acid, B.P., ½ to 1 oz. Syrup, U.S.P. Oil, B.P.

In modern herbal medicine the flowers of the common Red Rose are given in in-fusions and sometimes in powder for hæmor-rhage. A tincture is made from them by pouring 1 pint of boiling water on 1 oz. of the dried petals, adding 15 drops of oil of Vitriol and 3 or 4 drachms of white sugar. The tinc-ture when strained is of a beautiful red colour. Three or four spoonsful of the tinc-ture taken two or three times a day are con-sidered good for strengthening the stomach and a pleasant remedy in all hæmorrhages.

Culpepper mentions a syrup made of the *pale* red petals of the Damask Rose by infus-ing them 24 hours in boiling water, then straining off the liquor and adding twice the weight of refined sugar to it, stating that this syrup is an excellent purge for children and adults of a costive habit, a small quantity to be taken every night. A conserve of the buds has the same properties as the syrup.

WILD ROSES.

The actual number of the roses indigenous to Great Britain is a subject open to dispute among botanists, as the roses found wild show many variations. Most authorities agree that there are only five distinct types or species: *R. canina*, the Dog Rose; *R. arvensis*, the Field Rose; *R. rubiginosa*, Sweet Briar; *R. spinosissima*, the Burnet Rose; and *R. villosa*, the Downy Rose.

The DOG ROSE (*R. canina*) is a flower of the early summer, its blossoms expanding in the first days of June and being no more to be found after the middle of July. The general growth of the Dog Rose is subject to so much variation that the original species defined by Linnæus has been divided by later botanists into four or five subspecies. The flowers vary very considerably in colour, from almost white to a very deep pink, and have a delicate but refreshing fragrance. The scarlet fruit, or hip (a name that has come down from the Anglo-Saxon *hiope*), is generally described as 'flask-shaped.' It is what botanists term a false fruit, because it is really the stalk-end that forms it and grows up round the central carpels, enclosing them as a case; the *real*

fruits, each containing one seed, are the little hairy objects within it. Immediately the flower has been fertilized, the receptacle round the immature fruits grows gradually luscious and red and forms the familiar 'hip,' which acts as a bait for birds, by whose agency the seeds are distributed. At first the hips are tough and crowned with the five-cleft calyx leaves, later in autumn they fall and the hips are softer and more fleshy. The pulp of the hips has a grateful acidity. In former times when garden fruit was scarce, hips were esteemed for dessert. Gerard assures us that 'the fruit when it is ripe maketh the most pleasante meats and bankettiing dishes as tartes and such-like,' the making whereof he commends 'to the cun-ning cooke and teethe to eate them in the riche man's mouth.' Another old writer says:

'Children with great delight eat the berries thereof when they are ripe and make chains and other pretty geegaws of the fruit; cookes and gentlewomen make tarts and suchlike dishes for pleasure.'

The Germans still use them to make an ordinary preserve and in Russia and Sweden a kind of wine is made by fermenting the fruit.

Rose hips were long official in the British Pharmacopœia for refrigerant and astringent properties, but are now discarded and only used in medicine to prepare the confection of hips used in conjunction with other drugs, the pulp being separated from the skin and hairy seeds and beaten up with sugar. It is astringent and considered strengthening to the stomach and useful in diarrhœa and dysentery, allaying thirst, and for its pectoral qualities good for coughs and spitting of blood. Culpepper states that the hips are 'grateful to the taste and a considerable re-storative, fitly given to consumptive persons, the conserve being proper in all distempers of the breast and in coughs and tickling rheums' and that it has 'a binding effect and helps digestion.' He also states that 'the pulp of the hips dried and powdered is used in drink to break the stone and to ease and help the colic.' The constituents of rose hips are malic and citric acids, sugar and small quan-tities of tannin, resin, wax, malates, citrates and other salts.

The *leaves* of the Dog Rose when dried and infused in boiling water have often been used as a substitute for tea and have a grate-ful smell and sub-astringent taste. The *flowers*, gathered in the bud and dried, are said to be more astringent than the Red Roses. They contain no honey and are visited by insects only for their pollen. Their scent is not strong enough to be of any practical use for distillation purposes.

Two explanations have been put forward for the popular name of this wild rose. The first is founded on an ancient tradition that the root would cure a bite from a mad dog (Pliny affirming that men derived their knowledge of its powers from a dream); and the other and more probable theory that it was the Dag Rose – 'dag' being a dagger – because of its great thorns, and like the 'Dogwood' (originally Dagwood) became changed into 'Dog' by people who did not understand the allusion.

The FIELD ROSE (*R. arvensis*) is generally a much more trailing rose than the Dog Rose, a characteristic which distinguishes it from all our other wild roses. It is widely distributed throughout England, but is much less common in Scotland and Ireland.

The leaves in general form are similar to those of the Dog Rose, but are often rather smaller and their surfaces more shining. The prickles, too, are somewhat smaller in size, but are more hooked. The flowers are white, much less fragrant than those of the Dog Rose and sometimes even scentless. Though occasionally occurring singly on the stem, they are generally in small bunches of three or four at the ends of the twigs, though only one of these at a time will as a rule be found expanded. This species generally comes into blossom rather later than the Dog Rose and continues in bloom a good deal longer. It is one of the chief ornaments of our hedge-rows, in the summer, from the profusion of its blossoms and long trailing stems; and in the autumn, by its scarlet hips, which are more globular in form than those of the Dog Rose. It has its styles united into a central column and not free or separate, as in the Dog Rose.

SWEET BRIAR (*R. rubiginosa*). The flowers of the Sweet Briar are a little smaller than those of the Dog Rose and generally of a deeper hue, though of a richer tint in some plants than in others. They are in bloom during June and July. The fruit is egg-shaped, its broadest part being uppermost or farthest from the stem.

The specific name *rubiginosa* signifies, in Latin, 'rusty,' the plant having been thus named as both stems and leaves are often of a brownish-red tint. It delights in open copses, though is sometimes found also in old hedge-rows and is more specially met with in chalk districts in the south of England.

Its fragrance of foliage is peculiarly its own and has led to it holding a cherished place in many old gardens. Under its older name of Eglantine its praises have been sung by poets.

It takes a shower to bring out the full sweetness of Sweet Briar, when its strong and refreshing fragrance will fill the air and be borne a long distance by the breeze. Though the leaves are so highly odorous, the flowers are almost entirely without scent.

Sweet Briar only obtains a place among perfumes in name, for like many other sweet-scented plants, it does not repay the labour of collecting its odour, the fragrant part of the plant being destroyed more or less under treatment. An Essence under this name is, however, prepared, compounded of various floral essences so blended as to resemble the spicy fragrance of the growing plant. In olden days the Sweet Briar was used medicinally.

Briarwood pipes are not made from the wood of either the Sweet Briar or of any wild rose, but from that of the Tree Heath (*Erica arborea*).

The BURNET ROSE (*R. spinosissima*), known also as the Pimpernel Rose, or Scotch Rose, is generally found on waste land near the sea, more rarely on dry, heath-clad hills inland. The whole plant rarely attains to more than a foot or so in height. Its stems are armed with numerous, straight thorns – hence its specific name, signifying in Latin 'exceedingly prickly.' The English name is given it from the fact that the general form of its small leaves, with seven or nine leaflets to each leaf, is very similar to those of the Burnet (*Poterium sanguisorba*) and the Burnet Saxifrage (*Pimpinella*).

The white or sulphur-tinted flowers are usually placed singly and are rather small. The roundish fruit is so deep a purple as to appear almost black. The juice of the ripe fruit has been used in the preparation of dye: diluted with water, it dyes silk and muslin of a peach colour and mixed with alum gives a beautiful violet, but is considered too fugitive to be of any real economic value.

This rose is frequently cultivated in gardens and a great many varieties have been raised from it. The first double variety was found in a wild state in the neighbourhood of Perth and from this one were produced about 50 others. The French have over 100 distinct varieties.

The DOWNY ROSE (*R. villosa*) is found only in England in the north and west, but is common in Scotland, Ireland and Wales. It receives its specific name from the downy texture of both sides of the leaves, the Latin word *villosa* meaning softly hairy.

This species is subject to many variations, five or six of which have been by some botanists considered separate species. The flowers are white or pale pink. The fruit, which is globular, is covered with fine prickles.

The stems of the various kinds of wild rose are often found tufted with little fluffy balls of what look like crimson moss. These are really galls and result from the puncture of a small insect, a kind of wasp – the *Rose Gall* – in a similar manner as Oak Galls are formed. The wasp punctures a leaf while it is yet undeveloped in the bud and there lays its eggs. Immediately the normal growth of the leaf alters and numerous larvæ are formed, which hatch out and creep further into the leaf tissues until the whole swells into the moss-like gall we know. In the Middle Ages these Rose Galls, under the name of Bedeguar, were held in high repute in medicine for their astringency and supposed power of inducing sleep if placed under the pillow at night.

POT-POURRI OF ROSES.

All varieties of both *R. gallica* and *R. centifolia* are used in the making of pot-pourri, the dried petals of all scented roses being valuable for the purpose as they retain their scent for a considerable time. Nearly every fragrant flower and scented leaf can be used as an ingredient of pot-pourri, blending with suitable spices to give charm to this favourite, old-fashioned sweet mixture, which in winter recalls so delightfully the vanished summer days. It must be understood that rose-petals should preponderate, and that the other component parts ought to be added in such proportions that the scent of one cannot kill the perfume of another.

There are two principal methods of making pot-pourri, the *dry* and the *moist*.

For the *dry* kind, the bulk of the rose-petals is fully dried and everything else – Sweet Geranium and Sweet Verbena leaves, Bay leaves and Lavender is also dried. The best way of drying is to spread out on sheets of paper in an airy room. Anything of lasting scent, such as cedar or sandalwood sawdust, or shavings, can be added. When all is ready, the spices and sweet gums, all in powder, are put together and the whole is thoroughly mixed. For two-thirds of a bushel of dried petals and leaves, the *spice mixture* is 2 oz. each of Cloves, Mace and Cinnamon, ½ oz. each of Coriander, Allspice, Gum Storax and Gum Benzoin, and 4 oz. Violet Powder.

The *moist* method of preparation takes more time and needs greater care. The rose leaves are not fully, but only partly dried, so that they lose a good half of their bulk and acquire a kind of tough, leathery consistency. To preserve them and to maintain them in this state, a certain proportion of salt is added. The salt is a mixture of half Bay salt and half common salt. Bay Salt is sold in lumps; these are roughly pounded, so that some of it is quite small and the larger pieces are about the size of a small hazel nut, and then mixed with the common salt. The roses must be absolutely dry when picked. The petals are stripped off and carefully separated and laid out to partially dry. The length of time depends on the temperature and atmospheric conditions, but they are usually ready the second day after picking. Large jars of glazed earthenware should be employed for storing the rose leaves, the most convenient being cylindrical, with lids of the same glazed ware and with flat leaded disks (supplied with handles), for pressing down the contents. Put two good handsful of the rose leaves in at a time and press them down with the handled rammer. Then sprinkle a small handful of the salt mixture, then more rose leaves and so on. Then weight down till the next batch is put in. Besides rose leaves, the other chief ingredient is leaves of the Sweet Geranium, torn into shreds, dried like the Roses and put into the jars in the same way, rammed, salted and pressed. Bay leaves, Sweet Verbena and Lavender are all of a drier nature and can be put into the jars and salted just as they are. When all is ready, the contents of the preparation jars are taken out and broken up small; the mass, especially of the rose-petals, will come out in thick flakes, closely compacted. It is then mixed with the spices and sweet powders. If the freshly made mixture be rammed rather tightly into a jar or wooden barrel and left for six months, or better still for a year, the quality is much improved by being thus matured.

Mr. Donald McDonald, in *Sweet-scented Flowers and Fragrant Leaves*, gives the following pot-pourri recipes.

I. Gather early in the day and when perfectly dry, a peck of Roses, pick off the petals and strew over them ¾ lb. common salt. Let them remain two or three days and if fresh flowers are added, some more salt must be sprinkled over them. Mix with the roses ½ lb. of finely powdered Bay salt, the same quantity of allspice, cloves and brown sugar, ¼ lb. gum benzoin, and 2 oz. Orris root. Add 1 gill of brandy and any sort of fragrant flowers, such as Orange and Lemon flowers, Lavender and lemon-scented Verbena leaves and any other sweet-scented flowers. They should be perfectly dry when added. The mixture must be occasionally stirred and kept in close-covered jars, the covers to be raised only when the perfume is desired in the room. If after a time the mixture seems to dry, moisten with brandy only, as essences too soon lose their quality and injure the perfume.

This mixture is said to retain its fragrance for fifty years.

II. Prepare 2 pecks of dry Rose leaves and buds, 1 handful each of Orange flowers, Violets and Jessamine, 1 oz. sliced Orris root and Cinnamon, ¼ oz. Musk, ¼ lb. sliced Angelica root, ¼ lb. of red part of Cloves (carnations), 2 handsful of Lavender flowers, Heliotrope and Mignonette, 1 handful each of Rosemary flowers, Bay and Laurel leaves, 3 sweet Oranges stuck full of cloves and dried in the oven and then powdered in a mortar, ½ handful of Marjoram, 2 handfuls of Balm of Gilead dried, 1 handful each of Bergamot, Balm, Pineapple and Peppermint leaves. Mix well together and put in a large china jar; sprinkle salt between the layers, add a small bottle of extract of New-Mown Hay and moisten with brandy. If the mixture becomes too dry, stir it, adding liquid or additional leaves when wanted for use. If the jar is tightly corked, the preparation will keep and be fragrant for many years.

III. Take the rind of 2 Lemons, cut thin, 1 lb. Bay salt, 1 oz. of powdered Orris root, 1 oz. Gum Benzoin, 1 oz. Cinnamon, ½ oz. Cloves, 1 oz. Nutmegs, 1 grain Musk, 12 Bay leaves, a few Sage leaves, Rosemary and Lavender, cut small, 1 oz. Lavender Water, 1 oz. Eau-de-Cologne, 1 oz. Bergamot oil. Mix all together in a pan and add sweet flowers in their natural state as they come into blossom, stir up frequently – at least once a day. It must be put into a covered stone pot, with a wooden spoon to stir it with. At the end of two or three months, this will be a sweet-scented mass ready to fill any number of Japanese rose jars. From time to time throw in fresh Rose petals.

Lady Rosalind Northcote in *The Book of Herbs* gives:

I. *A Devonshire Recipe*

'Gather flowers in the morning when dry and lay them in the sun till the evening:

Roses, Orange flowers, Jasmine, Lavender, Thyme, Sage, Marjoram, Bay, } in smaller quantities.

'Put them into an earthen wide jar or hand basin in layers. Add the following ingredients:

6 lb. Bay Salt
4 oz. Yellow Sandal Wood
4 oz. Acorus Calamus Root
4 oz. Cassia Buds
2 oz. Cinnamon
2 oz. Cloves

4 oz. Gum Benzoin
1 oz. Storax Calamite
1 oz. Otto of Rose
1 drachm Musk
½ oz. Powdered Cardamine Seeds.

'Place the rose leaves, etc., in layers in the jar. Sprinkle the Bay salt and other ingredients on each layer, press it tightly down and keep for two or three months before taking it out.'

II. *Sweet-Jar*

'½ lb. Bay salt, ¼ lb. saltpetre and common salt, all to be bruised and put on six baskets of rose-leaves, 24 bay leaves torn to bits, a handful of sweet myrtle leaves, 6 handfuls of lavender blossom, a handful of orange or syringa blossoms, the same of sweet violets and the same of the red of clove carnations. After having well stirred every day for a week add ½ oz. cloves, 4 oz. orris root, ½ oz. cinnamon and 2 nutmegs, all pounded; put on the roses, kept well covered up in a china jar and stirred sometimes.

'Put alternate layers of rose leaves and Bay salt in an earthern pot. Press down with a plate and pour off the liquor that will be produced, every day for six weeks, taking care to press as dry as possible. Break up the mass and add the following ingredients well pounded and mixed together: Nutmeg, ¼ oz.; cloves, mace, cinnamon, gum benzoin, orrisroot (sliced) 1 oz. each. Mix well with a wooden spoon. The rose leaves should be gathered on a dry, sunny afternoon, and the Bay salt roughly crushed before using. Orris root may be replaced with advantage by good violet powder.'

Besides the ingredients mentioned in these various recipes, the following may also be added: *leaves* of Basil, Bergamot, Mint, Lad's Love or Southernwood, Santolina, Costmary, Bog Myrtle, Anise and Sweet Woodruff and Cowslip and Agrimony *flowers*. The dried petals of Cornflower, Borage, Broom, Hollyhock and Marigold and any other bright petals that, though scentless, keep their colour when dried, are also often added to give a brighter and more attractive appearance to the mixture.

Sweet oils and essences played an important part in the recipes of a hundred years ago, as, for example, the following formula:

Four grains of Musk, 1 oz. of Pimento, crushed Cloves and powdered gum Benzoin, 80 drops of oil of Cassia, 6 drops of Otto of Roses, 150 drops of essence of Bergamot and the same quantity of oil of Lavender, the whole being thoroughly worked in and mixed with whatever petals are handy.

693

Another recipe (which was used by an old-fashioned Scottish chemist for some fifty years) was purely a liquid one, the essences consisting of Musk, Vanilla, Sandalwood, Patchouli, Verbena, Neroli and Otto of Roses. The mixture was bottled and sold under the all-bracing and appropriate title, 'A' the floers o' th' gairden in a wee bit bottle.'

RECIPE FOR CRYSTALLIZED ROSES

Choose a dry day for gathering the roses and wait until the dew evaporates, so that the petals are dry. Before gathering the roses, dissolve 2 oz. of gum-arabic in ½ pint of water. Separate the petals and spread them on dishes. Sprinkle them with the gum-arabic solution, using as many petals as the solution will cover. Spread them on sheets of white paper and sprinkle with castor sugar, then let them dry for 24 hours. Put 1 lb. of sugar (loaf) and ½ pint of cold water into a pan, stir until the sugar has melted, then boil fast to 250° F., or to the thread degree. This is ascertained by dipping a stick into cold water, then into the syrup and back into the water. Pinch the syrup adhering to the stick between the thumb and finger and draw them apart, when a thread should be formed. Keep the syrup well skimmed. Put the rose-petals into shallow dishes and pour the syrup over. Leave them to soak for 24 hours, then spread them on wire trays and dry in a cool oven with the door ajar. The syrup should be coloured with cochineal or carmine, in order to give more colour to the rose-petals.

Rose-petals have also been employed to flavour butter, for which the following recipe may be of interest:

Rose-Petal Sandwiches

Put a layer of Red Rose-petals in the bottom of a jar or covered dish, put in 4 oz. of fresh butter wrapped in waxed paper. Cover with a thick layer of rose-petals. Cover closely and leave in a cool place overnight. The more fragrant the roses, the finer the flavour imparted. Cut bread in thin strips or circles, spread each with the perfumed butter and place several petals from fresh Red Roses between the slices, allowing edges to show. Violets or Clover blossoms may be used in place of Roses.

ROSIN-WEED

Silphium Paciniatum (LINN.)
N.O. Compositæ

Synonyms. Compass Plant. Compass-weed. Polar Plant
Part Used. Root
Habitat. Western United States, especially Ohio

¶ *Description.* The plant is so closely allied to *Silphium laciniatum* (Compass Plant, Compass-weed, or Polar Plant) that some authorities identify them. Both are closely connected with *S. perfoliatum* (Indian Cup-Plant or Ragged Cup). They yield by exudation and incision a fragrant and bitter gumlike frankincense, white or amber colour, which is chewed by the American Indians to sweeten the breath. The taste of Compass-Plant roots is bitter and then acrid. They are odourless.

¶ *Constituents.* Rosin-weed yields an abundance of a resinous secretion, resembling mastic so closely that it might very well be used as an inexpensive substitute.

¶ *Medicinal Action and Uses.* Tonic, diaphoretic, alterative.

The resin has diuretic properties and imparts a strong, aromatic odour to the urine. The root has been used as an expectorant in cough and other pulmonary troubles. It is cut into slices, arranged in a dish in layers, each layer being strewn with sugar and the whole covered with brandy. It is then expressed and strained, and after standing for a few days is bottled.

Both Rosin-weed and Compass-weed are said to be emetic in decoction, and to have effected cures in intermittent fevers, and to have cured the heaves in horses. They are beneficial in dry, obstinate coughs, asthmatic affections, and pulmonary catarrhal diseases. A strong infusion or extract is said to be one of the best remedies for the removal of ague cake, or enlarged spleen, and for internal bruises, liver affections, and ulcers.

¶ *Dosage.* Of Silphium perfoliatum, 20 grains. Of fluid extract of Silphium laciniatum, ½ to 1 drachm.

See CUP PLANT.

RUE

Ruta graveolens (LINN.)
N.O. Rutaceæ

Synonyms. Herb-of-Grace. Herbygrass. Garden Rue
Part Used. Herb
Habitat. Southern Europe

Rue, a hardy, evergreen, somewhat shrubby plant, is a native of Southern Europe. The stem is woody in the lower part, the leaves are alternate, bluish-green, bi- or tri-pinnate, emit a powerful, disagreeable odour and have an exceedingly bitter, acrid and

694

nauseous taste. The greenish-yellow flowers are in terminal panicles, blossoming from June to September. In England Rue is one of our oldest garden plants, cultivated for its use medicinally, having, together with other herbs, been introduced by the Romans, but it is not found in a wild state except rarely on the hills of Lancashire and Yorkshire. This wild form is even more vehement in smell than the garden Rue. The whole plant has a disagreeable and powerful odour. The first flower that opens has usually ten stamens, the others eight only.

¶ *Cultivation.* The plant grows almost anywhere, but thrives best in a partially sheltered and dry situation. Propagation may be effected: (1) by seeds, sown outside, broadcast, in spring, raked in and the beds kept free from weeds, the seedlings, when about 2 inches high, being transplanted into fresh beds, allowing about 18 inches each way, as the plants become busy; (2) by cuttings, taken in spring and inserted for a time, until well rooted, in a shady border; (3) by rooted slips, also taken in spring. Every slip or cutting of the young wood will readily grow, and this is the most expeditious way of raising a stock.

Rue will live much longer and is less liable to be injured by frost in winter when grown in a poor, dry, rubbishy soil than in good ground.

Rue is first mentioned by Turner, 1562, in his *Herbal*, and has since become one of the best known and most widely grown simples for medicinal and homely uses.

The name *Ruta* is from the Greek *reuo* (to set free), because this herb is so efficacious in various diseases. It was much used by the Ancients; Hippocrates specially commended it, and it constituted a chief ingredient of the famous antidote to poison used by Mithridates. The Greeks regarded it as an antimagical herb, because it served to remedy the nervous indigestion they suffered when eating before strangers, which they attributed to witchcraft. In the Middle Ages and later, it was considered – in many parts of Europe – a powerful defence against witches, and was used in many spells. It was also thought to bestow second sight.

Piperno, a Neapolitan physician, in 1625, commended Rue as a specific against epilepsy and vertigo, and for the former malady, at one time, some of this herb used to be suspended round the neck of the sufferer.

Pliny, John Evelyn tells us, reported Rue to be of such effect for the preservation of sight that the painters of his time used to devour a great quantity of it, and the herb is still eaten by the Italians in their salads. It was supposed to make the sight both sharp and clear, especially when the vision had become dim through over-exertion of the eyes. It was with 'Euphrasy and Rue' that Adam's sight was purged by Milton's Angel.

At one time the holy water was sprinkled from brushes made of Rue at the ceremony usually preceding the Sunday celebration of High Mass, for which reason it is supposed it was named the Herb of Repentance and the Herb of Grace. 'There's rue for you and here's some for me; we may call it herb of grace o' Sundays.'

Gerard tells us: 'the garden Rue, which is better than the wild Rue for physic's use, grows most profitably, as Dioscorides said, under a fig tree.' But this is, probably, only a reference, originally, to the fact that it prefers a sheltered position.

Country-people boil its leaves with treacle, thus making a conserve of them. These leaves are curative of croup in poultry. It has also been employed in the diseases of cattle.

Shakespeare refers again to Rue in *Richard III*:

> 'Here in this place
> I'll set a bank of *rue*, sour herb of grace;
> Rue, even for ruth, shall shortly here be seen,
> In the remembrance of a weeping queen.'

The following is a quotation from Drayton:

> 'Then sprinkles she the juice of *rue*,
> With nine drops of the midnight dew
> From lunarie distilling.'

The latter was the Moonwort (*Lunaria*), often called 'honesty' – a common garden flower, with cross-shaped purple blossoms, and round, clear silvery-looking seed-vessels. Chaucer also calls it Lunarie.

Gerard says:

'If a man be anointed with the juice of rue, the poison of wolf's bane, mushrooms, or todestooles, the biting of serpents, stinging of scorpions, spiders, bees, hornets and wasps will not hurt him.'

Rue-water sprinkled in the house 'kills all the fleas,' says an old book.

The juice was used against earache.

Rue has been regarded from the earliest times as successful in warding off contagion and preventing the attacks of fleas and other noxious insects. It was the custom for judges sitting at assizes to have sprigs of Rue placed on the bench of the dock against the pestilential infection brought into court from gaol by the prisoner, and the bouquet still presented in some districts to judges at the assizes was originally a bunch of aromatic herbs, given to him for the purpose of warding off gaol-fever.

It is one of the ingredients in the 'Vinegar of the Four Thieves.'

Culpepper recommends it for sciatica and pains in the joints, if the latter be 'anointed' with it, as also for 'the shaking fits of agues, to take a draught before the fit comes.' He also tells us that

'the juice thereof warmed in a pomegranate shell or rind, and dropped into the ears, helps the pains of them. The juice of it and fennel, with a little honey, and the gall of a cock put thereunto, helps the dimness of the eyesight.'

In Saxony Rue has given its name to an Order. A chaplet of Rue, borne bendwise on bars of the Coat Armour of the Dukedom of Saxony, was granted by Frederick Barbarossa to the first Duke of Saxony, in 1181. In 1902 the King of Saxony conferred the Order of the Rautenkrone (Crown of Rue) on our present King, then Prince of Wales. Since the latter half of the seventeenth century, sprigs of Rue have been interlaced in the Collar of our Order of the Thistle.

¶ *Parts Used and Constituents*. The whole herb is used, the drug consisting of both the fresh and the dried herb. The tops of the young shoots contain the greatest virtues of any part of the plant. The shoots are gathered before the plant flowers.

The volatile oil is contained in glands distributed over the whole plant and contains caprinic, plagonic, caprylic and œnanthylic acids – also a yellow crystalline body, called rutin. Oil of Rue is distilled from the fresh herb. Water serves to extract the virtues of the plant better than spirits of wine. Decoctions and infusions are usually made from the fresh plant, or the oil may be given in a dose of from 1 to 5 drops. The dried herb – which is a greyish green – has similar taste and odour, but is less powerful. It is used, powdered, for making tea.

¶ *Medicinal Action and Uses*. Strongly stimulating and antispasmodic – often employed, in form of a warm infusion, as an emmenagogue. In excessive doses, it is an acro-narcotic poison, and on account of its emetic tendencies should not be administered immediately after eating.

It forms a useful medicine in hysterical affections, in coughs, croupy affections, colic and flatulence, being a mild stomachic. The oil may be given on sugar, or in hot water.

Externally, Rue is an active irritant, being employed as a rubefacient. If bruised and applied, the leaves will ease the severe pain of sciatica. The expressed juice, in small quantities, was a noted remedy for nervous nightmare, and the fresh leaves applied to the temples are said to relieve headache. Compresses saturated with a strong decoction of the plant, when applied to the chest, have been used beneficially for chronic bronchitis.

If a leaf or two be chewed, a refreshing aromatic flavour will pervade the mouth and any nervous headache, giddiness, hysterical spasm, or palpitation will be quickly relieved.

¶ *Preparations and Dosages*. Powdered herb, 15 to 30 grains. Fluid extract, ½ to 1 drachm.

RUE, GOAT'S

Galega officinalis (LINN.)
N.O. Leguminosæ

Synonyms. Herba ruta caprariæ. Italian Fitch
(*German*) Pestilenzkraut
Parts Used. Leaves, flowering tops

Goat's Rue, known in the old Herbals as *Herba rutæ caprariæ*, is a leguminous plant that in former times was much employed on account of its diaphoretic properties in malignant fevers and the plague, hence one of its German popular names of *Pestilenzkraut*.

'The leaves, gathered just as the plant is going into flower and dried, with the addition of boiling water, make an infusion which being drunk plentifully, excites sweating and is good in fevers.' (Hill's *Universal Herbal*, 1832.)

It was also used as a remedy for worms and recommended as a cure for the bites of serpents. Parkinson says it is 'good for fattening hens.'

This profuse-flowering, hardy perennial herb is a native of Southern Europe and the Mediterranean – Gerard calls it Italian Fitch – and it is widely cultivated in gardens in England.

¶ *Description*. From the several-headed root, rise erect stems, about 3 feet high, smooth and branched, bearing pinnate leaves with from six to eight pairs of lance-shaped leaflets, ¾ to 2 inches long, and an odd terminal one. The leaflets are bright green, smooth (or very slightly hairy), on short foot-stalks.

The small lilac, purplish or white flowers are in axillary racemes and produce narrow, almost cylindrical pods.

The plant is without scent, unless bruised, when it emits a disagreeable odour, whence perhaps its name of Goat's Rue.

It has a mucilaginous and somewhat bitter

and astringent taste. It colours the saliva yellowish-green, if chewed.

¶ *Cultivation.* Being pea-like in character, its chief requirements are deep soil and moisture. Given these it will grow strongly each season, producing great masses of flowers, and will grow undisturbed for many years. Autumn planting is best.

¶ *Constituents.* The constituents of Goat's Rue have not been investigated fully. It contains a bitter principle and tannin and yields not more than 12 per cent. of ash.

¶ *Medicinal Action and Uses.* Diaphoretic, galactagogue. The herb is official in the National Formulary IV attached to the United States Pharmacopœia; the dried flowering tops are made into a fluid extract with diluted alcohol.

In 1873 Gillet-Damitte, in a communication to the French Academy, stated that this plant when given to cows would increase the secretion of milk from 35 to 50 per cent., since which time, Cerisoli, Millbank and

several French physicians have affirmed that Goat's Rue is a powerful galactagogue. The best preparation is stated to be an aqueous extract prepared from the fresh plant. This almost black extract has a pronounced odour and is recommended to be given in doses of from 8 to 15 grains, from three to five times a day.

Culpepper says:

'A bath made of it is very refreshing to wash the feet of persons tired with over-walking. In the northern countries they use this herb for making their cheeses instead of Rennet, whence it is called also "Cheese-Rennet"; the flowers contain an acidity, which may be got by distillation. This plant is seldom used in the shops.'

The root of an American species of Goat's Rue (*Galega virginiana*, Linn.) is said to be diaphoretic and powerfully anthelmintic. It is given in decoction.

See BROOM, GORSE, MELILOT.

RUSHES. *See* SEDGES, GRASSES

RUPTUREWORT

Herniaria glabra (LINN.)
N.O. Caryophyllaceæ

Part Used. Herb

Habitat. Temperate and Southern Europe and Russian Asia, extending into Scandinavia, but not to high latitudes. A native of Britain, especially southern and central England

¶ *Description.* The *Herniaria* were formerly included in the *Illecebraceæ*. They are small annuals or undershrubs, with small green flowers crowding along the stems intermixed with leaves.

There are very few species of the genus.

H. hirsuta is a common Continental and west Asiatic species, and has been found near Christchurch, in Hampshire.

The taste is insipid and the plant is odourless.

¶ *Constituents.* A crystalline principle has been obtained, called Herniarine, which proved to be methylumbelliferone.

An alkaloid, Paronychine, has also been found.

¶ *Medicinal Action and Uses.* Very active diuretic properties have been attributed to Herniarine, which has been found successful in the treatment of dropsy, whether of cardiac or nephritic origin.

It is recommended for catarrh of the bladder.

SABADILLA

Veratrum sabadilla
N.O. Liliaceæ

Synonyms. Cevadilla. Schœnocaulon officinale. Melanthium sabadilla. Veratrum officinale. Helonias officinalis. Sabadilla officinarum. Asagræa officinalis. Sabadillermer

Parts Used. Seeds, dried fruit

Habitat. Southern North America, Guatemala and Venezuela

¶ *Description.* The name Schœnocaulon indicates the habit of the scape, meaning 'a rush' and 'a stem.' The name *Asagræa* commemorates Professor Asa Gray of Harvard University, the most distinguished of living American botanists. It is not quite certain whether the seeds are obtained from the *Veratrum Sabadilla*, a plant 3 or 4 feet high, or from the *V. officinale*, differing slightly in appearance and construction. The seeds are black, shining, flat, shrivelled and winged, odourless, with a bitter, acrid, persistent and

disagreeable taste, the pale grey, amorphous powder being errhine and violently sternutatory. The seeds were known in Europe as early as 1752, but officially only as the source of veratrine.

¶ *Constituents.* Sabadilla contains several alkaloids, the most important being Cevadine, yielding cevine on hydrolysis; Veratrine, obtained from the syrupy liquor from which the cevadine has crystallized; and Cevadilline or Sabadillie, obtained after the extraction of the veratrine with ether.

Two other alkaloids have been isolated: Sabadine, which is less sternutatory than veratrine, and Sabadinine, which is not sternutatory. Sabadilla yields about 0·3 per cent. of veratrine. The seeds also contain veratric acid, cevadic acid, fat and resin.

¶ *Medicinal Action and Uses.* Sabadilla, or cevadilla, is an acrid, drastic emeto-cathartic, in overdoses capable of producing fatal results. Cevine was found to be less poisonous than cevadine, though producing similar symptoms. The powdered seeds have been used as a vermifuge, and to destroy vermin in the hair, being the principal ingredient of the *pulvis capucinorum* used in Europe. Cevadilla was formerly used internally as an anthelmintic, and in rheumatic and neuralgic affections. The highly poisonous *veratria*, which is derived from it, has been given in minute doses internally in acute rheumatism

and gout, and in some inflammatory diseases, but it must be used with caution. Veratria is useful as an ointment in rheumatism and neuralgia, but is regarded as being less valuable than aconite. The ointment is also employed for the destruction of pedicule. Applied to unbroken skin it produces tingling and numbness, followed by coldness and anæsthesia. Given subcutaneously, it causes violent pain and irritation, in addition to the symptoms following an internal dose. The principal reason against its internal use is its powerful action on the heart, the contractions of the organ becoming fewer and longer until the heart stops in systole.

¶ *Dosage.* From 5 to 20 grains as a tænicide. Ointment veratrine, B.P.

¶ *Poisonous, if any, with Antidotes.* Large doses paralyse heart action and respiration, and its use is so dangerous that it is scarcely ever taken internally.

SAFFLOWER

Carthamus tinctorius
N.O. Compositæ

Synonyms. Dyer's Saffron. American Saffron. Fake Saffron. Flores Carthami. Bastard Saffron
Part Used. Flowers

This plant is not in any way related to Saffron, though the flowers are used similarly.[1]

The Safflower plant, known in India as Koosumbha and in China as Hoang-tchi, is extensively cultivated in India, China and other parts of Asia, also in Egypt and Southern Europe; but its native country is unknown. It grows about 2 to 3 feet high, with a stiff, upright whitish stem, branching near the top; and has oval, spiny, sharp-pointed leaves, their bases half-clasping the stem. Its fruits are about the size of barleycorns, somewhat four-sided, white and shining, like little shells.

Safflower contains two colouring matters, yellow and red, the latter being most valued.

It is chiefly used for dyeing silk, affording various shades of rose and scarlet. Mixed with finely-powdered talc it forms the well-known substance called 'rouge.' Another common use of Safflower is in adulterating Saffron. The seeds yield an oil much used in India for burning and for culinary purposes.

¶ *Medicinal Action and Uses.* The flowers are the part used, their action is laxative and diaphoretic. In domestic practice these flowers are used in children's and infants' complaints – measles, fevers, and eruptive skin complaints. An infusion is made of ½ oz. of the flowers to a pint of boiling water taken warm to produce diaphorasis.

SAFFRON

Crocus sativus
N.O. Iridaceæ

Synonyms. Crocus. Karcom. Krokos (*Arabian*) Zaffer
Part Used. Flower pistils

The true Saffron is a low ornamental plant with grass-like leaves and large lily-shaped flowers, inhabiting the European continent, and frequently cultivated for the sake of the yellow stigmas, which are the part used in medicine, in domestic economy and in the arts.

Saffron is the *Karcom* of the Hebrews (Song of Solomon iv. 14). The plant was also known to the ancient Greeks and Romans.

In the course of an inquest held in 1921 at

Poplar (London, E.), a medical witness testified to the prevalence of a domestic custom of giving Saffron 'tea' flavoured with brandy in cases of measles.

The *Emplastrum Oxycroceum* of the Edinburgh Pharmacopœia contained, in olden days, a large proportion of Saffron (from which – and vinegar – it derived its name), with the addition of colophony, gum ammoniacum, mastic and vinegar.

Saffron was imported to England from the

---

[1] It largely replaces the use of Saffron owing to the large price of the latter. – EDITOR.

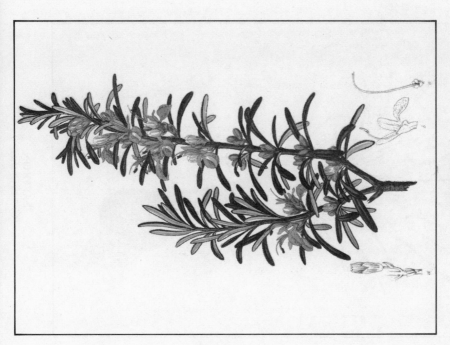

ROSEMARY
Rosmarinus Officinalis

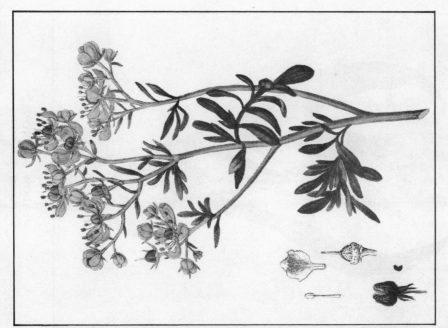

RUE
Ruta Graveolens

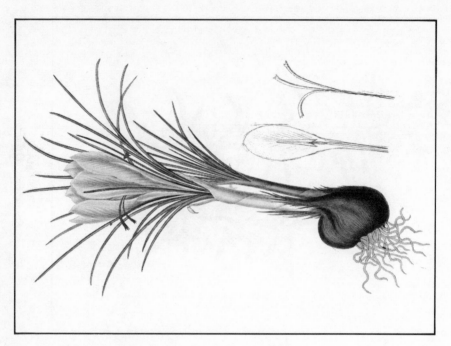

SAFFRON
Crocus Sativus

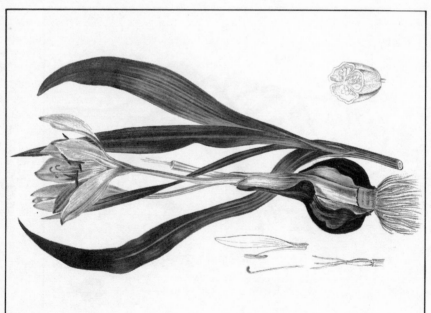

MEADOW SAFFRON
Colchicum Autumnale

East many centuries ago, and was once grown extensively round Saffron Walden, in Essex. One smoke-pervaded spot in the heart of London still bears the name of 'Saffron Hill.' It is a somewhat expensive product, the economic value residing in the *stigmas* of the flower, of which it is said 60,000 are needed to make 1 lb. of Saffron.

According to Dr. Pereira, a grain of good commercial Saffron contains the stigmas and styles of nine flowers, and consequently 4,320 flowers are required to yield 1 oz. of Saffron! English-grown Saffron is now very seldom met with in commerce; the best comes from Spain, while that imported from France is usually considered of second-rate quality. The quantity imported has been computed at between 5,000 and 20,000 lb. weight per annum. Saffron has a bitter taste and a penetrating aromatic odour.

Lately, Persian Saffron has made its appearance in the English market – although of rare occurrence – owing to the high and increasing price of the European article. It has long been known as a wild product of Persia, and was formerly sent from that country and Kashmir to Bombay, but was driven out of the market by the superior Saffrons of Europe.

Saffron was cultivated at Derbena and Ispahan in Persia in the tenth century. It differs a little in appearance from European Saffron in being rather more slender and in the unbranched part of the *style* being paler, but the characteristic odour is remarkably strong. On immersion in water it does not seem to give out so much colour as European Saffron, and could only compete with it if the price enabled it to be used in sufficient quantity to give a colour equal to that used in Europe. The wild Persian crocus is the variety *Hausknechtii*, which occurs on the Delechani and Sangur mountains between Kermanshah and Hamada in West Persia, and at Karput in Kurdistan, which is the most easterly point where any form of *Crocus sativus* occurs in the wild state.

It may be mentioned that five forms of *C. sativus* are known in the wild state. (1) Var. *Orsinii*, which may be regarded as the Italian form and is found at Ascoli, the most westerly point from which any wild form of the plant is recorded. It nearly resembles the cultivated type in purplish colour and habit, but the stigmas are erect and do not hang out between the segments of the perianth, as in the cultivated plant. (2) Var. *Cartwrightianus*, a Greek form common in the Piræus, in which the flowers are smaller and paler, but the stigma is erect and longer than the stamens, as in the cultivated plant. (3) Var. *Pallasii*, a still smaller form with pale flowers and smaller corms, the stigmas being nearly always shorter than the stamens. It is the commonest of the wild forms, extending through Bulgaria to the Crimea, and reaching Italy on the west. (4) Var. *Elwesii*. This is similar to the last, but has short stigmas and larger flowers, and occurs in Asia Minor. (5) Var. *Hausknechtii*. This, like Nos. 1 and 2, has long stigmas, but the perianth is usually white; it may be regarded as the Persian form, extending from West Persia to Kurdistan. But records of the collection of Saffron from the wild plants are wanting. Only Nos. 1, 2 and 5 are fitted for collection in having long stigmas, but the cultivated purple-flowered form with its stigmas hanging outside the flower would naturally be the easiest to collect, and it would only be the wild varieties from Italy, Greece and Persia that could be utilized. There is no doubt that the cultivated form is also grown from France to Kashmir, whence it was introduced from Persia, and also that it is largely cultivated in Burma (near the Youngaline River at Kuzeih, about ten miles from Pahun) and in China. But it is not always a paying crop, as it does not produce seeds unless cross-fertilized, and the corms are subject to disease if grown in the same ground too long.

In these circumstances it is quite likely that the Persian Saffron at present offered in commerce may have been derived from the wild Persian form, var. *Hausknechtii*; at all events, the pale, almost white, lower part of the styles gives it a characteristic appearance.

These details concerning the different forms are largely taken from the *Chemist and Druggist* of March 29, 1924.

¶ *Cultivation.* The corms are planted in rows, 6 inches apart from corm to corm, in a well-pulverized soil, neither poor nor a very stiff clay, and in the month of July. The flowers are collected in September and the yellow stigmas and part of the style are picked out and dried on a kiln between layers of paper and under the pressure of a thick board, to form the mass into cakes. Two pounds of dried cake is the average crop of an acre after the first planting, and 24 lb. for the next two years. After the third crop the roots are taken up, divided and transplanted.

The Arabs, who introduced the cultivation of the Saffron Crocus into Spain as an article of commerce, bequeathed to us its modern title of *Zaffer*, or 'Saffron,' but the Greeks and Romans called it *Krokos* and *Karkom* respectively.

To the nations of Eastern Asia, its yellow dye was the perfection of beauty, and its odour a perfect ambrosia. 'Saffron yellow shoes formed part of the dress of the Persian Kings,' says Professor Hehn. Greek myths and poetry exhibit an extravagant admiration of the colour and perfume. Homer sings 'the Saffron morn'; gods and goddesses, heroes and nymphs and vestals, are clothed in robes of Saffron hue. The Saffron of Lydia, Cilicia and Cyrene was much prized. The scent was valued as much as the dye; saffron water was sprinkled on the benches of the theatre, the floors of banqueting-halls were strewn with crocus leaves, and cushions were stuffed with it.

¶ *Medicinal Action and Uses.* Carminative, diaphoretic, emmenagogue. Used as a diaphoretic for children and for chronic hæmorrhage of the uterus in adults.

¶ *Preparations.* Powdered Saffron: Tincture, B.P., 5 to 15 drops.

(*POISON*)
SAFFRON, MEADOW

Colchicum autumnale (LINN.)
N.O. Liliaceæ

Synonym. Naked Ladies
Parts Used. Root, seeds
Habitat. Grows wild in meadows, especially on limestone

¶ *Description.* It has lanceolate leaves, dark green, glabrous, often a foot long. Flowers light purple or white, like crocus but for their six stamens; the ovaries remain underground until the spring after flowering, when they are borne up by the elongating peduncles and ripen. It flowers in September and October. The leaves and fruit are poisonous to cattle.

The root is called a *corm*, from which in autumn the light-purplish mottled flowers arise.

¶ *Cultivation.* Requires light, sandy loam, enriched with decayed manure or leafmould. Plant the bulbs 3 inches deep and 3 inches apart in July or August, in moist beds or rockeries, shrubbery, borders or lawns near shade of trees. The foliage dies down in June and July, and does not reappear until after the plant has flowered. It may also be propagated by seeds sown ⅛ inch deep in a bed of fine soil outdoors in August or September, or in pans or boxes of similar soil in cold frame at the same time, transplanting seedlings 3 inches apart when two years old; or by division of bulbs in August. Seedling bulbs do not flower till four or five years old.

¶ *Medicinal Action and Uses.* The Colchicum is valued for its medicinal properties. The parts used are the root and seeds, these being anti-rheumatic, cathartic, and emetic.

Its reputation rests largely upon its value in acute gouty and rheumatic complaints. It is mostly used in connexion with some alkaline diuretic; also in pill form. Overdoses cause violent purging, etc.

The active principle is said to be an alkaline substance of a very poisonous nature called Colchinine. It is acrid, sedative, and acts upon all the secreting organs, particularly the bowels and kidneys. It is apt to cause undue depression, and in large doses acts as an irritant poison. Dr. Lindley relates the case of a woman who was poisoned by the sprouts of Colchicum, which had been thrown away in Covent Garden Market and which she mistook for onions.

The Hermodactyls of the Arabians, formerly celebrated for soothing pains in the joints, are said to be this plant.

The corm or root is usually sold in transverse slices, notched on one side and somewhat reniform in outline, white and starchy internally, about ⅛ inch thick, and varying from ¾ to 1 inch in diameter. Taste sweetish, then bitter and acrid. Odour radish-like in fresh root, but lost in drying.

¶ *Preparations.* Powdered root, 2 to 5 grains. Extract, B.P., ¼ to 1 grain. Fluid extract (root), 1 to 10 drops. Fluid extract (seed), U.S.P., 1 to 10 drops. Tincture, B.P., 5 to 15 drops. Wine, B.P., 10 to 30 drops. Acetic solid extract, ¼ to 1 grain.

SAGES

Salvias
N.O. Labiatæ

SAGE, COMMON

Salvia officinalis (LINN.)
N.O. Labiatæ

Synonyms. (*Old English*) Sawge. Garden Sage. Red Sage. Broad-leaved White Sage. Narrow-leaved White Sage. Salvia salvatrix
Parts Used. Leaves, whole herb

The Common Sage, the familiar plant of the kitchen garden, is an evergreen undershrub, not a native of these islands, its natural habitat being the northern shores of the Mediterranean. It has been cultivated for culinary and medicinal purposes for many centuries in England, France and Germany, being sufficiently hardy to stand any ordinary winter outside. Gerard mentions it as being in 1597 a well-known herb in English gardens, several varieties growing in his own garden at Holborn.

¶ *Description*. Sage generally grows about a foot or more high, with wiry stems. The leaves are set in pairs on the stem and are 1½ to 2 inches long, stalked, oblong, rounded at the ends, finely wrinkled by a strongly-marked network of veins on both sides, greyish-green in colour, softly hairy and beneath glandular. The flowers are in whorls, purplish and the corollas lipped. They blossom in August. All parts of the plant have a strong, scented odour and a warm, bitter, somewhat astringent taste, due to the volatile oil contained in the tissues.

¶ *Habitat*. Sage is found in its natural wild condition from Spain along the Mediterranean coast up to and including the east side of the Adriatic; it grows in profusion on the mountains and hills in Croatia and Dalmatia, and on the islands of Veglia and Cherso in Quarnero Gulf, being found mostly where there is a limestone formation with very little soil. When wild it is much like the common garden Sage, though more shrubby in appearance and has a more penetrating odour, being more spicy and astringent than the cultivated plant. The best kind, it is stated, grows on the islands of Veglia and Cherso, near Fiume, where the surrounding district is known as the Sage region. The collection of Sage forms an important cottage industry in Dalmatia. During its blooming season, moreover, the bees gather the nectar and genuine Sage honey commands there the highest price, owing to its flavour.

In cultivation, Sage is a very variable species, and in gardens varieties may be found with narrower leaves, crisped, red, or variegated leaves and smaller or white flowers. The form of the calyx teeth also varies, and the tube of the corolla is sometimes much longer. The two usually absent upper stamens are sometimes present in very small-sterile hooks. The Red Sage and the Broad-leaved variety of the White (or Green) Sage – both of which are used and have been proved to be the best for medical purposes – and the narrow-leaved White Sage, which is best for *culinary* purposes as a seasoning, are classed merely as varieties of *Salvia officinalis*, not as separate species. There is a variety called Spanish, or Lavender-leaved Sage and another called Wormwood Sage, which is very frequent.

A Spanish variety, called *S. Candelabrum*, is a hardy perennial, the upper lip of its flower greenish yellow, the lower a rich violet, thus presenting a fine contrast.

S. Lyrala and *S. urticifolia* are well known in North America.

S. hians, a native of Simla, is hardy, and also desirable on account of its showy violet-and-white flowers.

The name of the genus, *Salvia,* is derived from the Latin *salvere*, to be saved, in reference to the curative properties of the plant, which was in olden times celebrated as a medicinal herb. This name was corrupted popularly to *Sauja* and *Sauge* (the French form), in Old English, 'Sawge,' which has become our present-day name of Sage.

In the United States Pharmacopœia, the leaves are still officially prescribed, as they were formerly in the London Pharmacopœia, but in Europe generally, Sage is now neglected by the regular medical practitioner, though is still used in domestic medicine. Among the Ancients and throughout the Middle Ages it was in high repute: *Cur moriatur homo cui Salvia crescit in horto?* ('Why should a man die whilst sage grows in his garden?') has a corresponding English proverb:

'He that would live for aye,
    Must eat Sage in May.'

The herb is sometimes spoken of as *S. salvatrix* ('Sage the Saviour'). An old tradition recommends that Rue shall be planted among the Sage, so as to keep away noxious toads from the valued and cherished plants. It was held that this plant would thrive or wither, just as the owner's business prospered or failed, and in Bucks, another tradition maintained that the wife rules when Sage grows vigorously in the garden.

In the Jura district of France, in Franche-Comte, the herb is supposed to mitigate grief, mental and bodily, and Pepys in his Diary says : 'Between Gosport and Southampton we observed a little churchyard where it was customary to sow all the graves with Sage.'

The following is a translation of an old French saying:

'Sage helps the nerves and by its powerful might
 Palsy is cured and fever put to flight,'

and Gerard says:

'Sage is singularly good for the head and brain, it quickeneth the senses and memory, strengtheneth the sinews, restoreth health to those that have the palsy, and taketh away shakey trembling of the members.'

He shared the popular belief that it was efficacious against the bitings of serpents, and says:

'No man need to doubt of the wholesomeness of *Sage Ale*, being brewed as it should be with Sage, Betony, Scabious, Spikenard, Squinnette (Squinancywort) and Fennell Seed.'

Many kinds of Sage have been used as substitutes for tea, the Chinese having been said to prefer Sage Tea to their own native product, at one time bartering for it with the Dutch and giving thrice the quantity of their choicest tea in exchange. It is recorded that George Whitfield, when at Oxford in 1733, lived wholesomely, if sparingly, on a diet of Sage Tea, sugar and coarse bread. Balsamic Sage, *S. grandiflora*, a broad-leaved Sage with many-flowered whorls of blossoms, used to be preferred to all others for making tea. An infusion of Speedwell (*Veronica officinalis*), Sage and Wood Betony is said to make an excellent beverage for breakfast, as a substitute for tea, Speedwell having somewhat the flavour of Chinese green tea. In Holland the leaves of *S. glutinosa*, the yellow-flowered Hardy Sage, both flowers and foliage of which exhale a pleasant odour, are used to give flavour to country wines, and a good wine is made by boiling with sugar, the leaves and flowers of another Sage, *S. sclarea*, the Garden Clary. The latter is known in France as 'Toute bonne' – for its medicinal virtues.

It was formerly thought that Sage used in the making of Cheese improved its flavour, and Gay refers to this in a poem:

'Marbled with Sage, the hardening cheese she pressed.'

Italian peasants eat Sage as a preservative of health, and many other country people eat the leaves with bread and butter, than which, it has been said, there is no better and more wholesome way of taking it.

A species of Sage, *S. pomifera*, the APPLE-BEARING SAGE, of a very peculiar growth, is common on some of the Greek islands. It has firm, fleshy protuberances of about ¾ inch thickness, swelling out from the branches of the plant and supposed to be produced in the same manner as oak apples, by the puncture of an insect of the *Cynips* genus. These excrescences are semi-transparent like jelly. They are called Sage Apples, and under that name are to be met with in the markets. They are candied with sugar and made into a kind of sweetmeat and conserve which is regarded by the Greeks as a great delicacy, and is said to possess healing and salutary qualities. It has an agreeable and astringent flavour. This plant is considerably larger than the common Sage of our gardens and its flavour and smell are much more powerful,

being more like a mixture of Lavender and Sage. It grows very abundantly in Candia, Syros and Crete, where it attains to the size of a small shrub. The leaves are collected annually, dried and used medicinally as an infusion, the Greeks being particular as to the time and manner in which they are collected, the date being May 1, before sunrise. The infusion produces profuse perspiration, languor, and even faintness if used to excess. There is a smaller Salvia in Greece, the *S. Candica*, without excrescences.

Another south European species, an annual, *S. Horminum*, the RED-TOPPED SAGE, has its whorls of flowers terminated by clusters of small purple or red leaves, being for this peculiarity often grown in gardens as an ornamental plant. The leaves and seed of this species, put into the vat, while fermenting, greatly increase the inebriating quality of the liquor. An infusion of the leaves has been considered a good gargle for sore gums, and powdered makes a good snuff.

Certain varieties of Sage seeds are mucilaginous and nutritive, and are used in Mexico by the Indians as food, under the name of *Chia*.

¶ *Cultivation.* The Garden Sage succeeds best in a warm and rather dry border, but will grow well almost anywhere in ordinary garden soil; it thrives in a situation somewhat shaded from sunshine, but not strictly under trees.

¶ *Description.* It is a hardy plant, but though a perennial, does not last above three or four years without degenerating, so that the plantation should be renewed at least every four years. It is propagated occasionally by seed, but more frequently by cuttings. New plantations are readily made by pulling off the young shoots from three-year-old plants in spring, generally in the latter end of April, as soon as they attain a sufficiency of hardness to enable them to maintain themselves on the moisture of the ground and atmosphere, while the lower extremities are preparing roots. If advantage be taken of any showery weather that may occur, there is little trouble in obtaining any number of plants, which may either be struck in the bed where they are to grow, inserting a foot apart each way, or in some other shady spot whence they may be removed to permanent quarters when rooted. The latter plan is the best when the weather is too bright and sunny to expect Sage to strike well in its ordinary quarters. See the young plants do not suffer from want of water during their first summer, and hoe the rows regularly to induce a bushy growth, nipping off the growing tips if shooting up too tall. Treat the ground with soot and mulch in winter with old manure. Cuttings may also be taken in the autumn, as soon as the plants have ceased flowering.

Sage is also often propagated by layers, in the spring and autumn, the branches of old plants being pegged down on the ground and covered with ½ inch of earth. The plant, being like other of the woody-stemmed garden herbs, a 'stem rooter,' each of the stems thus covered will produce quantities of rootlets by just lying in contact with the ground, and can after a time be cut away from the old plant and transplanted to other quarters as a separate plant.

Red Sage is always propagated by layering or by cuttings, as the seed does not produce a red-leaved plant, but reverts back to the original green-leaved type, though efforts are being made to insure the production of a Red Sage that shall set seed and remain true and develop into the red-leaved plant.

Sages backed by late-flowering Orange Lilies go very well together, and being in flower at the same time make an effective grouping. The calyces of Sage flowers remain on the plants well into late summer and give a lovely haze of reddish spikes; the smell of these seeding spikes is very distinct from the smell of the leaves, and much more like that of the Lemon-scented Verbena, pungent, aromatic and most refreshing.

At the present day, by far the largest demand for Sage is for culinary use, and it should pay to grow it in quantity for this purpose as it is little trouble. For this, the White variety, with somewhat pale green leaves should be taken.

In Dalmatia, where the collection of Sage in its wild condition forms an important cottage industry, it is gathered before blooming, the leaves being harvested from May to September, those plucked in midsummer being considered the best. The general opinion is that it should be gathered before the bloom opens, but the Austrian Pharmacopœia states that it is best when gathered *during* bloom.

¶ *Chemical Constituents.* The chief constituent of Sage and its active principle is a yellow or greenish-yellow volatile oil (sp. gr. 0·910 to 0·930) with a penetrating odour. Tannin and resin are also present in the leaves; 0·5 to 1·0 per cent. of the oil is yielded from the leaves and twigs when fresh, and about three times this quantity when dry.

The Sage oil of commerce is obtained from the herb *S. officinalis,* and distilled to a considerable extent in Dalmatia and recently in Spain, but from a different species of *Salvia.* A certain amount of oil is also distilled in Germany. The oil distilled in Dalmatia and in Germany is of typically Sage

odour, and is used for flavouring purposes. The botanical origin of Spanish Sage oil is now identified as *S. triloba,* closely allied to *S. officinalis,* though probably other species may also be employed. The odour of the Spanish oil more closely resembles that of Spike Lavender than the Sage oil distilled in Germany for flavouring purposes, and is as a rule derived from the wild Dalmatian herb, *S. officinalis.* The resemblance of the Spanish oil to Spike Lavender oil suggests the possibility of its use for adulterative purposes, and it is an open secret that admixture of the Spanish Sage oil with Spanish Spike Lavender oil does take place to a considerable extent, though this can be detected by chemical analysis. It is closer in character to the oil of *S. sclarea,* Clary oil, which has a decided lavender odour, although in the oil of *S. triloba,* the ester percentage does not appear to be as high as in the oil of the *S. sclarea* variety.

Pure Dalmatian or German Sage oil is soluble in two volumes of 80 per cent. alcohol, Spanish Sage oil is soluble in six volumes of 70 per cent. alcohol.

Sage oil contains a hydrocarbon called Salvene; pinene and cineol are probably present in small amount, together with borneol, a small quantity of esters, and the ketone thujone, the active principle which confers the power of resisting putrefaction in animal substances. Dextro-camphor is also present in traces. A body has been isolated by certain chemists called Salviol, which is now known to be identical with Thujone.

English distilled Sage oil has been said to contain Cedrene.

S. cypria, a native of the island of Cyprus, yields an essential oil, having a camphoraceous odour and containing about 75 per cent of Eucalyptol.

S. mellifer (syn. *Ramona stachyoides*) is a labiate plant found in South California, known as BLACK SAGE, with similar constituents, and also traces of formic acid.

¶ *Medicinal Action and Uses.* Stimulant, astringent, tonic and carminative. Has been used in dyspepsia, but is now mostly employed as a condiment. In the United States, where it is still an official medicine, it is in some repute, especially in the form of an infusion, the principal and most valued application of which is as a wash for the cure of affections of the mouth and as a gargle in inflamed sore throat, being excellent for relaxed throat and tonsils, and also for ulcerated throat. The gargle is useful for bleeding gums and to prevent an excessive flow of saliva.

When a more stimulating effect to the

throat is desirable, the gargle may be made of equal quantities of vinegar and water, ½ pint of hot malt vinegar being poured on 1 oz. of leaves, adding ¼ pint of cold water.

The infusion when made for *internal* use is termed Sage Tea, and can be made simply by pouring 1 pint of boiling water on to 1 oz. of the dried herb, the dose being from a wine-glassful to half a teacupful, as often as required, but the old-fashioned way of making it is more elaborate and the result is a pleasant drink, cooling in fevers, and also a cleanser and purifier of the blood. Half an ounce of fresh Sage leaves, 1 oz. of sugar, the juice of 1 lemon, or ¼ oz. of grated rind, are infused in a quart of boiling water and strained off after half an hour. (In Jamaica, the negroes sweeten Sage Tea with lime-juice instead of lemon.)

Sage Tea or infusion of Sage is a valuable agent in the delirium of fevers and in the nervous excitement frequently accompanying brain and nervous diseases and has considerable reputation as a remedy, given in small and oft-repeated doses. It is highly serviceable as a stimulant tonic in debility of the stomach and nervous system and weakness of digestion generally. It was for this reason that the Chinese valued it, giving it the preference to their own tea. It is considered a useful medicine in typhoid fever and beneficial in biliousness and liver complaints, kidney troubles, hæmorrhage from the lungs or stomach, for colds in the head as well as sore throat and quinsy and measles, for pains in the joints, lethargy and palsy. It will check excessive perspiration in phthisis cases, and is useful as an emmenagogue. A cup of the strong infusion will be found good to relieve nervous headache.

The infusion made strong, without the lemons and sugar, is an excellent lotion for ulcers and to heal raw abrasions of the skin. It has also been popularly used as an application to the scalp, to darken the hair.

The fresh leaves, rubbed on the teeth, will cleanse them and strengthen the gums. Sage is a common ingredient in tooth-powders.

The volatile oil is said to be a violent epileptiform convulsant, resembling the essential oils of absinthe and nutmeg. When smelt for some time it is said to cause a sort of intoxication and giddiness. It is sometimes prescribed in doses of 1 to 3 drops, and used for removing heavy collections of mucus from the respiratory organs. It is a useful ingredient in embrocations for rheumatism.

In cases where heat is required, Sage has been considered valuable when applied externally in bags, as a poultice and fomentation.

In Sussex, at one time, to munch Sage leaves on nine consecutive mornings, whilst fasting, was a country cure for ague, and the dried leaves have been smoked in pipes as a remedy for asthma.

In the region where Sage grows wild, its leaves are boiled in vinegar and used as a tonic.

Among many uses of the herb, Culpepper says that it is

'Good for diseases of the liver and to make blood. A decoction of the leaves and branches of Sage made and drunk, saith Dioscorides, provokes urine and causeth the hair to become black. It stayeth the bleeding of wounds and cleaneth ulcers and sores. Three spoonsful of the juice of Sage taken fasting with a little honey arrests spitting or vomiting of blood in consumption. It is profitable for all pains in the head coming of cold rheumatic humours, as also for all pains in the joints, whether inwardly or outwardly. The juice of Sage in warm water cureth hoarseness and cough. Pliny saith it cureth stinging and biting serpents. Sage is of excellent use to help the memory, warming and quickening the senses. The juice of Sage drunk with vinegar hath been of use in the time of the plague at all times. Gargles are made with Sage, Rosemary, Honeysuckles and Plantains, boiled in wine or water with some honey or alum put thereto, to wash sore mouths and throats, as need requireth. It is very good for stitch or pains in the sides coming of wind, if the place be fomented warm with the decoction in wine and the herb also, after boiling, be laid warm thereto.'

CULINARY RECIPES

Sage and Onion stuffing for ducks, geese and pork enables the stomach to digest the rich food.

From Warner's *Ancient Cookery*, 1791, for 'Sawgeat,' Sawge.

'Sawgeat

'Take Pork and seeth (boil) it wel and grinde it smale and medle (mingle) it with ayren (eggs) and ygrated (grated) brede (bread). Do thereto salt sprinkled and saffron. Take a close litull ball of it in foiles (leaves) of Sawge. Wet it with a bator (batter) of ayren, fry and serve forth.'

From *The Cook's Oracle*, 1821:

'Sage and Onion Sauce

'Chop very fine an ounce of onion and ½ oz. of green Sage leaves, put them in a stamper with 4 spoonsful of water, simmer gently for 10 minutes, then put in a teaspoonful of pepper and salt and 1 oz. of fine bread-crumbs. Mix well together, then pour to it ¼ pint of Broth, Gravy or Melted Butter, stir well together and simmer a few minutes longer. This is a relishing sauce for Roast Pork, Geese or Duck, or with Green Peas on Maigre Days.'

The same book gives:

'A Relish for Roast Pork or Goose

'2 oz. of leaves of Green Sage, an ounce of fresh lemon peel, pared thin, same of salt, minced shallot and ½ drachm of Cayenne pepper, ditto of citric acid, steeped for a fort-night in a pint of claret. Shake it well every day; let it stand a day to settle and decant the clear liquid. Bottle it and cork it close. Use a tablespoonful or more in ¼ pint of gravy or melted butter.'

Another modern Sage Sauce, excellent with Roast Pork is

Sagina Sauce

Take 6 large Sage leaves, 2 onions, 1 tea-spoonful of flour, 1 teaspoonful of vinegar, butter the size of a walnut, salt, pepper, and ½ pint of good, brown gravy. Scald the Sage leaves and chop them with the onions to a mincemeat. Put them in a stewpan with the butter, sprinkle in the flour, cover close and steam 10 minutes. Then add the vinegar, gravy and seasoning and simmer half an hour.

From Walsh's *Manual of Domestic Economy*, 1857:

'Sage Cheese

'Bruise the tops of young red Sage in a mortar with some leaves of spinach and squeeze the juice; mix it with the rennet in the milk, more or less, according to the pre-ferred colour and taste. When the curd is come, break it gently and put it in with the skimmer till it is pressed two inches above the vat. Press it 8 or 10 hours. Salt it and turn every day.'

MEDICINAL RECIPES

A Gargle for a Sore Throat

A small glass of port wine, a tablespoonful of Chile vinegar, 6 Sage leaves, and a dessert-spoonful of honey; simmer together on the fire for 5 minutes.

A Cure for Sprains

Bruise a handful of Sage leaves and boil them in a gill of vinegar for 5 minutes; apply this in a folded napkin as hot as it can be borne to the part affected.

SAGE, CLARY

Salvia sclarea
N.O. Labiatæ

Synonyms. Clary. Horminum. Gallitricum. Clear Eye. See Bright
(*German*) Muskateller Salbei
Parts Used. Herb, leaves, seeds
Habitat. The Common Clary, like the Garden Sage, is not a native of Great Britain, having first been introduced into English cultivation in the year 1562. It is a native of Syria, Italy, southern France and Switzerland, but will thrive well upon almost any soil that is not too wet, though it will frequently rot upon moist ground in the winter

Gerard describes and figures several varieties of Clary, under the names of *Horminum* and *Gallitricum*. He describes it as growing 'in divers barren places almost in every country, especially in the fields of Holborne neare unto Grayes Inne . . . and at the end of Chelsea.'

Salmon, in 1710, in *The English Herbal*, gives a number of varieties of the Garden Clary, which he calls *Horminum Hortense*, in distinction to *H. Sylvestre*, the Wild Clary, subdividing it into the Common Clary (*H. commune*), the True Garden Clary of Dioscorides (*H. sativum verum Dioscorides*), the Yellow Clary (*Calus Jovis*), and the Small or German Clary (*H. humile Germanicum* or *Gallitricum alterum Gerardi*). This last variety being termed *Gerardi*, indicates that Gerard classified this species when it was first brought over from the Continent, evidently taking great pains to trace its history, giving in his *Herbal* its Greek name and its various Latin ones. That the Clary was known in ancient times is shown by the second variety, the True Garden Clary, being termed *Dioscoridis*.

Another variety of *Horminum* is given in *The Treasury of Botany*, called *H. pyrenaicum*, and described as 'a tufted perennial herb, with numerous root-leaves, simple almost leafless stems and purplish-blue flowers which grow in whorls of six, all turned the same way. It is a native of the temperate parts of Europe, on the mountains.'

¶ *Description.* The Common Garden Clary is a biennial plant, its square, brownish stems growing 2 to 3 feet high, hairy and with few branches. The leaves are arranged in pairs, almost stalkless and are almost as large as the hand, oblong and heart-shaped, wrinkled, irregularly toothed at the margins and covered with velvety hairs. The flowers are in a long, loose, terminal spike, on which they are set in whorls. The lipped corollas, similar to the Garden Sage, but smaller, are of a pale blue or white. The flowers are interspersed with large coloured, membraneous bracts, longer than the spiny calyx. Both corollas and bracts are generally variegated with pale purple and yellowish-white. The seeds are blackish brown, 'contained in long, toothed husks,' as an old writer describes the calyx. The whole plant possesses a very strong, aromatic scent, somewhat resembling that of Tolu, while the taste is also aromatic, warm and slightly bitter.

According to Ettmueller, this herb was first brought into use by the wine merchants of Germany, who employed it as an adulterant, infusing it with Elder flowers, and then adding the liquid to the Rhenish wine, which converted it into the likeness of Muscatel. It is still called in Germany *Muskateller Salbei* (Muscatel Sage).

Waller (1822) states it was also employed in this country as a substitute for Hops, for sophisticating beer, communicating considerable bitterness and intoxicating property, which produced an effect of insane exhilaration of spirits, succeeded by severe headache. Lobel says:

'Some brewers of Ale and Beere doe put it into their drinke to make it more heady, fit to please drunkards, who thereby, according to their several dispositions, become either dead drunke, or foolish drunke, or madde drunke.'

In some parts of the country a wine has been made from the herb in flower, boiled with sugar, which has a flavour not unlike Frontiniac.

The English name Clary originates in the Latin name *sclarea*, a word derived from *clarus* (clear). Clary was gradually modified into 'Clear Eye,' one of its popular names, and from the fact that the seeds have been used for clearing the sight.

Sometimes we find the plant not only called 'Clear Eye,' but also 'See Bright' and even 'Eyebright,' though this name belongs to another plant – *Euphrasia officinalis*.

¶ *Cultivation.* Clary is propagated by seed, which should be sown in spring. When fit to move, the seedlings should be transplanted to an open spot of ground, a foot apart each way, if required in large quantities. After the plants have taken root, they will require no further care but to keep them free of weeds. The winter and spring following, the leaves will be in perfection. As the plant is a biennial only, dying off the second summer,

after it has ripened seeds, there should be young plants annually raised for use.

¶ *Parts Used.* The herb and leaves, used both fresh and dry, dried in the same manner as the Garden Sage. Formerly the root was used, dry, in domestic medicine, and also the seeds.

¶ *Constituents. Salvia sclarea* yields an oil with a highly aromatic odour, resembling that of ambergris. It is known commercially as Clary oil, or Muscatel Sage, and is largely used as a fixer of perfumes. Pinene, cineol and linalol have been isolated from this oil.

French oil of Clary has a specific gravity of 0·895 to 0·930, and is soluble in two volumes of 80 per cent. alcohol. German oil of Clary has a specific gravity of 0·910 to 0·960, and is soluble in two volumes of 90 per cent. alcohol.

¶ *Medicinal Action and Uses.* Antispasmodic, balsamic, carminative, tonic, aromatic, aperitive, astringent, and pectoral.

The plant has been used, both fresh and dry, either alone or with other herbs, as an infusion or a tincture.

It has mostly been employed in disordered states of the digestion, as a stomachic, and has also proved useful in kidney diseases.

For violent cases of hysteria or wind colic, a spirituous tincture has been found of use, made by macerating in warm water for 14 days, 2 oz. of dried Clary leaves and flowers, 1 oz. of Chamomile flowers, ½ ox. bruised Avens root, 2 drachms of bruised Caraway and Coriander seeds, and 3 drachms of bruised Burdock seeds, adding 2 pints of proof spirit, then filtering and diluting with double quantity of water – a wineglassful being the dose.

Culpepper says:

'For tumours, swellings, etc., make a mucilage of the seeds and apply to the spot. This will also draw splinters and thorns out of the flesh. . . . For hot inflammation and boils before they rupture, use a salve made of the leaves boiled with hot vinegar, honey being added later till the required consistency is obtained.' He recommends a powder of the dry roots taken as snuff to relieve headache, and 'the fresh leaves, fried in butter, first dipped in a batter of flour, egges, and a little milke, serve as a dish to the table that is not unpleasant to any and exceedingly profitable.'

The juice of the herb drunk in ale and beer, as well as the ordinary infusion, has been recommended as very helpful in all women's diseases and ailments.

In Jamaica, where the plant is found, it was much in use among the negroes, who considered it cooling and cleansing for ulcers, and also used it for inflammations of the eyes.

A decoction of the leaves boiled in coco-nut oil was used by them to cure the stings of scorpions. Clary and a Jamaican species of Vervain form two of the ingredients of an aromatic warm bath sometimes prescribed there with benefit.

SAGE, VERVAIN

Salvia Verbenaca
N.O. Labiatæ

Synonyms. Wild English Clary. Christ's Eye. Oculus Christi
Parts Used. Leaves, seeds.

The Wild English Clary, or Vervain Sage, is a native of all parts of Europe and not uncommon in England in dry pastures and on roadsides, banks and waste ground, especially near the sea, or on chalky soil. It is a smaller plant than the Garden Clary, but its medicinal virtues are rather more powerful.

¶ *Description.* The perennial root is woody, thicky and long, the stem 1 to 2 feet high, erect with the leaves in distinct pairs, the lower shortly stalked, and the upper ones stalkless. The radical leaves lie in a rosette and have foot-stalks 1½ to 4 inches long, their blades about the same length, oblong in shape, blunt at their ends and heart-shaped at the base, wavy at the margins, which are generally indented by five or six shallow, blunt lobes on each side, their surfaces much wrinkled. The whole plant is aromatic, especially when rubbed, and is rendered conspicuous by its long spike of purplish-blue flowers, first dense, afterwards becoming rather lax. The whorls of the spike are six-flowered, and at the base of each flower are two heart-shaped, fringed, pointed bracts. The calyx is much larger than the corolla. The plant is in bloom from June to August. The seeds are smooth, and like the Garden Clary, produce a great quantity of soft, tasteless mucilage, when moistened. If put under the eyelids for a few moments the tears dissolve this mucilage, which envelops any dust and brings it out safely. Old writers called this plant 'Oculus Christi,' or 'Christ's Eye.'

¶ *Medicinal Action and Uses.* 'A decoction of the leaves,' says Culpepper, 'being drank, warms the stomach, also it helps digestion and scatters congealed blood in any part of the body.'

This Clary was thought to be more efficacious to the eye than the Garden variety.

'The distilled water strengthening the eyesight, especially of old people,' says Culpepper, 'cleaneth the eyes of redness waterishness and heat: it is a gallant remedy for dimness of sight, to take one of the seeds of it and put it into the eyes, and there let it remain till it drops out of itself, the pain will be nothing to speak on: it will cleanse the eyes of all filthy and putrid matter; and repeating it will take off a film which covereth the sight.'

¶ *Other Species.*
Salvia pratensis, the MEADOW SAGE – our other native Sage – is a very rare plant, found only in a few localities in Cornwall, Kent and Oxfordshire, and by some authorities is considered hardly a true native.

It is common in some parts of Italy and the Ionian Islands.

It has the habit of *S. Verbenaca,* but is larger. The flowers are very showy, large and bright blue, arranged on a long spike, four flowers in each whorl, the corolla (about four times as long as the calyx) having the prominent upper lip much arched and compressed and often glutinous. The stem bears very few leaves.

Several plants, though not true Sages, have been popularly called 'Sage': *Phlomis fruticosa,* a hardy garden shrub, 2 to 4 feet high, with flowers either yellow or dusky yellow, was known as Jerusalem Sage; Turner (1548) terms it so and he is followed in this by Green (1832), whereas Lyte (1578) gives this name to *Pulmonaria officinalis,* the Common Lungwort, and Gerard (1597), describing *Phlomis fruticosa,* gives it another name, saying, 'The leaves are in shape like the leaves of Sage, whereupon the vulgar people call it French Sage.' Gerard gives the name of 'Sage of Bethlem' to *Pulmonaria officinalis;* in localities of North Lincolnshire, the name has been given to the Garden Mint, *Mentha viridis.* 'Garlick Sage' is one of the names quoted by Gerard for *Teucrium scorodonia,* which we find variously termed by old writers, Mountain Sage, Wild Sage and Wood Sage.
See GERMANDER.

ST. JOHN'S WORT

Hypericum perforatum (LINN.)
N.O. Hypericaceæ

Parts Used. Herb tops, flowers
Habitat. Britain and throughout Europe and Asia

¶ *Description.* A herbaceous perennial growing freely wild to a height of 1 to 3 feet in uncultivated ground, woods, hedges, roadsides, and meadows; short, decumbent, barren shoots and erect stems branching in upper part, glabrous; leaves pale green, sessile, oblong, with pellucid dots or oil glands which may be seen on holding leaf to light. Flowers bright cheery yellow in terminal corymb. Calyx and corolla marked with black dots and lines; sepals and petals five in number; ovary pear-shaped with three long styles. Stamens in three bundles joined by their bases only. Blooms June to August, followed by numerous small round blackish seeds which have a resinous smell and are contained in a three-celled capsule; odour peculiar, terebenthic; taste bitter, astringent and balsamic.

There are many ancient superstitions regarding this herb. Its name *Hypericum* is derived from the Greek and means 'over an apparition,' a reference to the belief that the herb was so obnoxious to evil spirits that a whiff of it would cause them to fly.

SALEP. *See* ORCHIDS and SAFFRON

SALSAFY

Tragopogon porrifolius (LINN.)
N.O. Compositæ

Synonyms. Purple Goat's Beard. Vegetable Oyster
(*French*) Salsifis des prés
Part Used. Root

The Salsafy, familiar as a kitchen-garden plant, is very similar to Goat's Beard, the main difference being the colour of the flowers – yellow in our native species, purple in the Salsafy.

Salsafy is often called the Purple Goat's Beard, from its likeness in general character to the Yellow Goat's Beard of the countryside. Some writers, again, invert this distinction and call the Yellow Goat's Beard, 'Meadow Salsafy.' The French call it '*Salsifis des prés.*'

Salsafy is a corruption of the old Latin name *solsequium*. This was derived from the Latin words *sol* (sun) and *sequens* (following), meaning the flower that followed the course of the sun.

It is a taller plant than the Goat's Beard, the stem being nearly 3 feet high. The leaves and flowers are similar in form, the flowers having the same peculiarity of closing at noon. The florets are of a delicate pale purple colour.

Though not a British species, it is occasionally found in moist meadows, having been originally a garden escape. It was formerly much cultivated for the sake of its fleshy, tapering roots.

¶ *Cultivation*. Salsafy is a very easy crop to grow and matures in a year.

A friable, open soil is preferable, though it will also grow on heavy soil. On a stony soil, or one made up of clay with flints scattered in it, it will not be a success, as the roots get

¶ *Medicinal Action and Uses*. Aromatic, astringent, resolvent, expectorant and nervine. Used in all pulmonary complaints, bladder troubles, in suppression of urine, dysentery, worms, diarrhœa, hysteria and nervous depression, hæmoptysis and other hæmorrhages and jaundice. For children troubled with incontinence of urine at night an infusion or tea given before retiring will be found effectual; it is also useful in pulmonary consumption, chronic catarrh of the lungs, bowels or urinary passages. Externally for fomentations to dispel hard tumours, caked breasts, ecchymosis, etc.

¶ *Preparations and Dosages*. 1 oz. of the herb should be infused in a pint of water and 1 to 2 tablespoonsful taken as a dose. Fluid extract, ½ to 1 drachm.

The oil of St. John's Wort is made from the flowers infused in olive oil.

coarse and forked. No manure should be added to the soil, as forking will also then result, but wood-ash, lime, soot, superphosphates, etc., may be used freely.

The seeds should be sown 1 inch or more deep, 4 inches apart, in drills 9 inches asunder, as early in March as possible, to give a long season for its growth.

The roots may be lifted in October and stored in the same way as Beet, Carrot, etc., or they may remain in the ground until the spring.

Salsafy seed frequently fails, unless kept wet from sowing time till the seedlings are well up.

¶ *Medicinal Action and Uses*. Culpepper says of Purple Goat's Beard:

'The virtues of this are the same as the other, only less pleasant, therefore more bitter, astringent, detersive and medicinal. This, however, may be eaten in great quantities, and so will be useful in chronic complaints. The roots are particularly specific in obstructions of the gall and the jaundice; the best way to use them is stewed like chardoons.'

It ranks as one of the most salubrious of culinary vegetables, being antibilious, cooling, deobstruent, and slightly aperient; but although it is deservedly esteemed as an esculent, it is nevertheless decidedly inferior to *Scorzonera* in properties, nor does it keep so well when taken out of the ground, as it soon becomes hardened, insipid, and difficult to cook properly.

See GOAT'S BEARD (YELLOW).

RECIPES

Baked Salsafy

Scrape 1 bundle of Salsafy, wash and cut into short pieces, and put into a basin of cold water containing lemon juice or vinegar. Drain and cook in stock or seasoned water till tender. Make a white sauce, put in the Salsafy previously drained and blend both carefully. Place on a buttered dish, pour over the sauce, sprinkle breadcrumbs over, add a few small pieces of butter and bake for 10 minutes in a sharp oven.

Salsafy with Cheese

Cook and drain and place a layer of Salsafy in a shallow dish. Sprinkle with grated cheese, then a layer of Bechamel sauce, again a layer of Salsafy, then more cheese and sauce, and sprinkle breadcrumbs over the top. Place in a quick oven to get well hot through and brown.

To serve plain boiled, the roots must be scraped lightly first, cut up into two or three portions, and placed in water, with a few drops of lemon juice or vinegar, to prevent them discolouring. Then boiled for an hour, quickly, in salt water till tender, drained and served with a white sauce.

SALVIAS. *See* SAGES

SAMPHIRE

Stewed Salsafy

Scrape about 20 heads of Salsafy, cut into pieces about 2 inches long, sprinkle them with salt and steep in water and milk. Cut a small onion, half a carrot, half a turnip and half a head of celery into small pieces. Put these on in a stewpan with ¼ lb. of lean bacon cut into pieces. Cook for 20 minutes. Mix 1 oz. flour with a little milk and stir in, fill up with a quart of stock or water, stir and bring to the boil. Put in the Salsafy and let it simmer till tender. Add a tablespoonful of cream, one of chopped parsley, and a little lemon juice. Season with pepper, grated nutmeg and castor sugar. Reheat and arrange the Salsafy neatly on a dish, garnish with button mushrooms, pour over the sauce and serve.

Salsafy Cream Soup

Scrape and wash a bundle of Salsafy. Cut it up small and place in a stewpan, with 3 oz. of butter and a finely-minced onion, and stir for a few minutes. Then moisten with about a quart of white stock, add also 1 oz. rice. When cooked, drain and pound with the rice and pass all through a fine sieve. Then put the purée with a stock, stir over the fire, boil up the soup, season with salt, pepper and nutmeg. At the last add half a gill of cream, 2 beaten-up yolks of eggs, but do not let the soup boil again.

Crithmum maritimum (LINN.)
N.O. Umbelliferæ

Synonyms. Sea Fennel. Crest Marine. Sampier
(*German*) Meerfenchel
(*Italian*) Herba di San Pietra. Sanpetra
Part Used. Herb

Occasionally we find the name SEA FENNEL given to a plant which is far more familiar under the name of SAMPHIRE, and which also belongs to the great order of umbelliferous plants, though not to the same genus as the fennel. In German, this plant is also given a name equivalent to sea-fennel: *Meerfenchel.*

Prior tells us that the name of this plant is more properly zas; it was formerly spelt Sampere, or Sampier, from Saint Pierre, and Herba di San Pietra (contracted to Sanpetra) is its Italian name. It is dedicated to the fisherman saint, because it likes to grow on sea-cliffs.

The Samphire is a succulent, smooth, much-branched herb, woody at the base, growing freely on rocks on the sea-shore moistened by the salt spray.

¶ *Description.* It is well distinguished by its long, fleshy, bright-green, shining leaflets (full of aromatic juice) and umbels of tiny, yellowish-green blossoms. The whole plant is aromatic and has a powerful scent.

The young leaves, if gathered in May, sprinkled with salt (after freeing them from stalks and flowers), boiled and covered with vinegar and spice, make one of the best pickles, on account of their aromatic taste.

On those parts of the coast where Samphire does not abound, other plants which resemble it in having fleshy leaves are sometimes sold under the same name, but are very inferior.

Samphire gathering is referred to in *King Lear* :

'Half-way down
Hangs one that gathers samphire; dreadful trade!'

At the present time it grows but sparingly

on the white cliffs of Dover, where Shakespeare described it, but in his days it was probably more abundant there. From his description of the perilous nature of the collection of Samphire, it might be assumed that it grows where none but the adventurous can reach it, but it is to be found growing freely in the clefts of the rocks, and is in many places easily accessible from the beach, and is even sometimes to be found in the salt marshes that in some districts fringe the coast.

Samphire is abundantly met with where circumstances are favourable to its growth, around the coasts of western or southern England, but is rarer in the north and seldom met with in Scotland.

The use of Samphire as a condiment and pickle, or as an ingredient in a salad is of ancient date. It used at one time to be cried in London streets as 'Crest Marine.'

SAMPHIRE, GOLDEN

Part Used. Herb

Inula crithmoides, popularly named Golden Samphire, is a species growing in salt marshes and on sea-cliffs, but rare, and in England only plentiful in the Isle of Sheppey.
¶ *Description.* It has narrow, fleshy leaves and large yellow flowers, growing singly at the extremity of the branches. Formerly, when Samphire (*Crithmum Maritimum*) was

¶ *Medicinal Action and Uses.* In Gerard's time it was in great reputation as a condiment. He wrote in 1597:

'The leaves kept in pickle and eaten in sallads with oile and vinegar is a pleasant sauce for meat, wholesome for the stoppings of the liver, milt and kidnies. It is the pleasantest sauce, most familiar and best agreeing with man's body.'

Culpepper, writing some fifty years later, deplores that it had in his days much gone out of fashion, for it is well known almost to everybody that ill digestions and obstructions are the cause of most of the diseases which the frail nature of man is subject to; both of which might be remedied by a more frequent use of this herb. It is a safe herb, very pleasant to taste and stomach.

In some seaside districts where Samphire is found, it is still eaten pickled by country people.

Inula crithmoides (LINN.)
N.O. Compositæ

sold in the London markets for a pickle, the young branches of this species were sometimes mixed with it, causing Green in his *Universal Herbal* (1832) to indignantly remark: 'but it is a villainous imposition because this plant has none of the warm aromatic taste of the true Samphire.'

See ELECAMPANE.

SANDALWOOD

Santalum album (LINN.)
N.O. Santalaceæ

Synonym. Sanders-wood
Parts Used. Wood, oil
Habitat. India

¶ *Description.* A small tree 20 to 30 feet high, with many opposite slender drooping branches, bark smooth grey-brown. Young twigs glabrous; leaves opposite, without stipules, petiole slender, about ½ inch long, blade 1½ to 2½ inches long, oval, ovate-oval or lanceolate, acute or obtuse at apex, tapering at base into petiole entire, smooth on both sides, glaucous beneath. Flowers small, numerous, shortly stalked in small pyramidal erect terminal and axillary, trichotomus paniculate, cymes panicle, branches smooth, bracts small passing into leaves below.

Perianth campanulate, smooth, about ⅕ inch long, divided into four (rarely five) triangular, acute, spreading segments, valvate, in bud rather fleshy, at first straw coloured, changing to deep reddish purple provided at the mouth with four erect, fleshy, rounded lobes. Stamens four, opposite, perianth segments, filaments short, in-

serted in mouth of perianth alternating with erect lobes. Anthers short, two-celled, introrse, ovary half, inferior, tapering, one-celled, an erect central placenta, rising from base and not reaching to the top, to the summit of which are attached three or four pendulous ovules without the usual coverings, style filiform, stigma small, three or four lobed on a level with anthers.

Fruit concealed about size of a pea, spherical, crowned by rim-like remains of perianth tube, smooth, rather fleshy, nearly black, seed solitary.

The trees are felled or dug up by roots; the branches are worthless, so are cut off. It is usual to leave the trunk on the ground for several months for the white ants to eat away the sap wood, which is also of no value; it is then trimmed and sawn into billets 2 to 2½ feet long and taken to mills in the forests, where it is again trimmed and sorted into grades. It is heavy, hard, but splits easily; colour light yellow, transverse sections yellow to light reddish brown, with alternating light and dark concentric zones nearly equal in diameter, numerous pores, and traversed by many very narrow medullary rays. Odour characteristic, aromatic, persistent; taste peculiar, strongly aromatic. Indian Sandalwood is a Government monopoly.

¶ *Medicinal Action and Uses.* Used internally in chronic bronchitis, a few drops on sugar giving relief; also in gonorrhœa and gleet; in chronic cystitis, with benzoic and boric acids. Much used as a perfume for different purposes. The wood is used for making fancy articles and is much carved.

Fluid extract, 1 to 2 drachms. Oil, 5 to 20 drops.

¶ *Adulterants.* Castor oil is often added, and on the Continent oil of cedar, made by distilling the chips remaining from the manufacture of lead pencils.

¶ *Other Species. Pterocarpus santalinus* or *Santalum rubrum (Red Sandalwood)*, solely used for colouring and dyeing. Other varieties come from the Sandwich Islands, Western Australia and New Caledonia.

SANDSPURRY, COMMON

Arenaria rubra (LINN.)
N.O. Caryophyllaceæ

Synonyms. Spergularia rubra. Sabline rouge. Tissa rubra. Birda rubra
Part Used. Herb
Habitat. Europe, Russia, Asia, North America, Australia

Common in Britain in sandy, gravelly heaths and waste places near the sea. Flowers all the summer. There are two marked varieties: the one growing inland has small flowers, thin leaves, short capsules, seeds rarely bordered. The other, often called *Spergularia Marina*, is larger in every respect and has fleshy leaves. For medicinal purposes the one most used is found in Malta, Sicily and Algiers, growing in dry sandy soil from Quebec to Virginia.

¶ *Description.* An annual or biennial plant, glabrous or with a short viscid down in the upper parts; numerous stems branching from the base forming prostrate tufts 3 to 6 inches long; leaves narrow, linear; very short conspicuous scarious stipules at the base. Flowers usually pink, sometimes white, but variable size; short pedicels in forked cymes, usually leafy at base. Petals shorter, rarely longer than the sepals. Seeds more or less flattened.

¶ *Medicinal Action and Uses.* Long used in bladder diseases. It contains a resinous, aromatic substance which presumably is its active principle. Very valuable for calculus diseases and acute and chronic cystitis.

¶ *Dosages.* Aqueous extract up to 30 grains, or of the fluid extract, 1 fluid drachm three or four times a day. Infusion, 1 oz. to 1 pint. Its taste is saline and slightly aromatic.

SANICLE, WOOD

Sanicula Europæa (LINN.)
N.O. Umbelliferæ

Synonyms. Poolroot. Self-Heal
Part Used. Herb
Habitat. Wood Sanicle is an umbelliferous perennial plant, common in woods and thickets and damp moist places, and generally distributed over the British Isles. It is most abundant in the middle and north of Europe and is found on the mountains of tropical Africa. It is the only representative in this country of the genus Sanicula, to which very few species are assigned

¶ *Description.* The root-stock (the short underground stem from which each year's new stalks grow upward) is shortly creeping and fibrous, with a few thick, brownish scales at the top, the remains of decayed leaf-stalks. The stem, erect, 8 inches to 2 feet high, is simple, often leafless or with a single leaf. The radical leaves are on stalks 2 to 8 inches long, the leaves themselves palmately three to five partite and divided nearly to the base of the leaf, the lobes, or divisions, often three-cleft again. The leaves are heart-shaped at the base near the stalk and toothed like a saw.

The flowers are in umbels. Each little group, or umbellule, forms a hemispherical head. The little stalks, each bearing a head of flowers, join together at one spot again to form what is termed a compound or general umbel, as in most plants of this order. In the case of the Sanicle, the umbel is said to be irregular, as the converging stalks forming these rays are often divided into two or three prongs. The flowers are pinkish-white, $\frac{1}{16}$ inch across, the outer flowers of the umbellules being without stamens; the inner, without pistils. They blossom in May and June and are succeeded in August by roundish seeds, which are covered with prickles, causing them to adhere to everything they touch.

The plant is glabrous and bright green, the leaves paler beneath and the stems often reddish.

The origin of the name of this genus is the Latin word *sano* (I heal or cure), in reference to the medicinal virtues.

In the Middle Ages the power of Sanicle was proverbial:

> Celuy qui sanicle a
> De mire affaire il n'a.

and

Qui a la Bugle et la Sanicle fait aux chirugiens la niche.

It was as a vulnerary that this plant gained its medical reputation. Lyte and other herbalists say that it will 'make whole and sound all wounds and hurts, both inward and outward.'

Wood Sanicle has locally often been known as Self-Heal, a name which belongs rightly to another quite distinct herb, *Prunella vulgaris*, belonging to the Labiate order.

¶ *Cultivation.* Sanicle is generally collected from wild specimens.

In a moist soil and a shady situation, Sanicle will thrive excellently, especially in rich soil.

Propagation may be effected by division of roots, any time from September to March, the best time for the operation being in the autumn. Plant from 8 to 9 inches apart each way.

¶ *Part Used.* The whole herb, collected in June and dried. Gather the herb only on a fine day, in the morning, when the sun has dried off the dew.

¶ *Constituents.* As yet no analysis has been made of this plant, but evidence of tannin in its several parts is afforded by the effects produced by the plant.

In taste it is at first very bitter and astringent, afterwards acrid, and probably partakes of the poisonous acridity which is so frequent in the Umbelliferæ. In the fresh leaves, the taste is very slight, but considerable in the dry leaves, and in the extract made from them.

¶ *Medicinal Action and Uses.* Astringent, alterative. Sanicle is usually given in combination with other herbs in the treatment of blood disorders, for which it is in high esteem.

As an internal remedy, it is of great benefit in all chest and lung complaints, chronic coughs and catarrhal affections, inflammation of the bronchii, spitting of blood, and all affections of the pulmonary organs.

As an alterative, it has a good reputation, and it is useful in leucorrhœa, dysentery, diarrhœa, etc.

It effectually cleanses the system of morbid secretions and leaves the blood healthier and in better condition. The infusion of 1 oz. to a pint of boiling water is taken in wineglassful doses.

Sanicle is used as a gargle in sore throat, quinsy, and whenever an astringent gargle is required. Culpepper mentions the use of Sanicle for disease of the lungs and throat, and recommends the gargle being made from a decoction of the leaves and root in water, a little honey being added.

In scald-head of children and all cases of rashes, the decoction or infusion forms an admirable external remedy.

Sanicle is popularly employed in France and Germany as a remedy for profuse bleeding from the lungs, bowels, and other internal organs and for checking dysentery, the fresh juice being given in tablespoonful doses.

¶ *Preparations.* Fluid extract, ½ to 1 drachm. A strong decoction of the leaves used to be a popular remedy for bleeding piles.

The root of an American species, *Sanicula marilandica*, contains resin and volatile oil, and has been used with alleged success in intermittent fever and in chorea, in doses of 10 to 60 grains.

American Bastard Sanicle belongs, not to this genus, but to the genus *Mitella*, and the Bear's Ear Sanicle (*Cortusa Matthiola*) is likewise not a true Sanicle, being related to the Primroses and Auriculas.

Yorkshire Sanicle is one of the names given sometimes to Butterwort, or Marsh Violet (*Pinguicula vulgaris*), a plant with violet-coloured flowers and thick plaintain-shaped leaves, which grow in a tuft or rosette on the ground, and to the touch are greasy, causing them to be used for application to sores and chapped hands.

SARSAPARILLA, AMERICAN

Aralia nudicaulis (LINN.)
N.O. Araliaceæ

Synonyms. False Sarsaparilla. Wild Sarsaparilla. Shot Bush. Small Spikenard. Wild Liquorice. Rabbit Root
Part Used. Root
Habitat. Canada to the Carolinas

¶ *Description.* A herbaceous perennial, with large, tortuous, fleshy, horizontal, creeping, long roots, externally yellowy brown, from which grows a large solitary compound leaf. Leaflets oval, obovate, acute, finely serrate. Flower-stem also comes from root, naked, about 1 foot high, terminating in three small many-flowered greenish umbels, no involucres. Fruit a small, black berry the size of elderberry. The root has a sweet spicy taste, and a pleasant aromatic smell.

¶ *Medicinal Action and Uses.* Alterative, pectoral, diaphoretic, sudorific. Used as a substitute for Smilax Sarsaparilla is useful in pulmonary diseases and externally as a wash for indolent ulcers and shingles. It is said to be used by the Crees under the name of Rabbit Root for syphilis and as an application to recent wounds. It contains resin, oil, tannin, albumen, an acid, mucilage and cellulose.

Fluid extract, ½ to 1 drachm.

SARSAPARILLA, CARACAO

Habitat. La Guayra

¶ *Description.* The radicals are often very amylaceous internally and in this respect is very like *Sarsaparilla papyracea*, but the plant has now almost been destroyed and is difficult to obtain. The roots contain large quantities of starch.

S. papyracea, native of Trinidad, French Guiana and North Brazil, is a near ally of *S. officinalis*, and like it, is only known by is leaf specimens; it is recognized by the old stems and lower branches, which instead of being cylindrical, as in most other species, always remain intensely quadrangular, their angles having very flat closely crowded prickles and leaves more membranaceous. The *Rio Negro Smilax* is an allied species *Smilax Spruceana*. This plant is known as affording *Guatemala Sarsaparilla* and is considered to be identical with *Sarsaparilla papyracea*. *Smilax syphilitica* is a native of New Grenada, has a smooth round stem, bearing at the knots two to four short, thick, straight prickles. Leaves 1 foot long, oblong, lanceolate, acuminate, shining, coriaceous, three nerved, ending in a long point.

Guayaquil Sarsaparilla grows in the valleys of the Western slopes of Equatorial Andes. It appears in commerce carelessly packed in bales. The rhizome and parts of the stem often mixed with the root, the stem is round and prickly, root dark, large and coarse, with much fibre. The bark furrowed thick and not mealy in the thinner portions of the root, which is near the foot-stalks. As the root gets thicker, the bark becomes thicker, smoother and amylaceous, showing when cut a pale yellow interior.

SARSAPARILLA, JAMAICA

Smilax ornata
N.O. Liliaceæ

Synonyms. Smilax Medica. Red-bearded Sarsaparilla
Part Used. Root
Habitat. Central America, principally Costa Rica

¶ *Description.* This plant derived its name from being exported to Europe through Jamaica. The word Sarsaparilla comes from the Spanish *Sarza*, meaning a bramble, and *parilla*, a vine, in allusion to the thorny stems of the plant. This is a non-mealy Sarsaparilla. It is a large perennial climber, rhizome underground, large, short, knotted, with thickened nodes and roots spreading up to 6 or 8 feet long. Stems erect, semi-woody, with very sharp prickles ½ inch long. Leaves large, alternate stalked, almost evergreen with prominent veins, seven nerved, mid-rib very strongly marked. Flowers and fruit not known. Cortex thick and brownish, with an orange red tint; when chewed it tinges the saliva, and gives a slightly bitter and mucilaginous taste, followed by a very acrid one; it contains a small proportion of starch, also a glucoside, sarsaponin, sarsapic acid, and fatty acids, palmitic, stearic, behenic, oleic and linolic.

Jamaica Sarsaparilla was introduced in the middle of the sixteenth century as a remedy for syphilis, and later came to be used for other chronic diseases, specially rheumatism. It is a mild gastric irritant due to its saponin content. The smoke of Sarsaparilla was recommended for asthma. It is also very useful as a tonic, alterative, diaphoretic and diuretic. Its active principle is a crystalline body, Parillin or Smilacin.

¶ *Preparations and Dosages.* Powdered root, ½ to 1 drachm. Fluid extract, U.S.P., ½ to 1 drachm. Fluid extract, B.P., 2 to 4 drachms. Solid extract, 10 to 20 grains. Compound solution, 2 to 8 drachms. Compound syrup, U.S.P., 4 drachms.

Smilax officinalis has a twining stem, angular and prickly; young shoots unarmed; leaves ovate, oblong, acute, cordate, smooth, 1 foot long; petioles 1 inch long, having tendrils above the base. This plant grows in New Granada, on the banks of Magdaline near Bajorgne. Commercially it consists of very long roots, with a thick bark, grey or brown colour. Almost odourless. Taste mucilaginous. The deep orange-tinted roots are the best.

¶ *Constituents*. Salseparin, starch, colouring matter, essential oil chloride of potassium, bassorin, albumen, pectic and ascitic acids, and salts of lime, oxide of iron, potassa and magnesia. It is said to be the source of *Honduras* Sarsaparilla and is considered the best of all Sarsaparillas. It is exported from the bay of Honduras in over 2 feet long roots folded into a sort of hank, with a few rootlets attached, grey or reddy brown, with mealy cortex. It has the same properties as the other varieties, but if alcohol is added to the infusions of the root it will greatly increase their medicinal qualities.

¶ *Medicinal Action and Uses*. Alterative, tonic. Used in chronic skin diseases, rheumatism, passive dropsy.

¶ *Dosages*. Powder, 20 grains. Infusion or syrup, 4 fluid ounces.

SARSAPARILLA, INDIAN

Hemidesmus Indica
N.O. Asclepiadaceæ

Synonyms. Hemidesmus. Periploca Indica. Nunnari Asclepias. Pseudosarsa
Part Used. Dried root
Habitat. All parts of India, the Moluccas, and Ceylon

¶ *Description*. A climbing slender plant with twining woody stems, and a rust-coloured bark, leaves opposite, petiolate, entire, smooth, shiny and firm, varying in shape and size according to their age. Flowers small green outside, deep purple inside, in axillary, sessile racemes, imbricated with flowers, followed with scale-like bracts. Fruit two long slender spreading follicles.

This plant has long been used in India as an antisyphilitic in place of Sarsaparilla, but was not introduced into England till 1831. The root is long, tortuous, rigid, cylindrical, little branched, consisting of aligneous centre, a brownish corky bark, furrowed and with annular cracks, odour aromatic, probably due to Coumarin and not unlike Sassafras or new-mown hay, with a bitter, sweetish, feeble aromatic taste. One side of the root is sometimes separated from the cork and raised above the cortex and transversely fissured, showing numerous laticiferous cells in the cortex.

¶ *Constituents*. Unknown. No satisfactory investigation has yet been made of the chemical properties. But a volatile oil has been found in it and a peculiar crystallizable principle, called by some Hemidesmine; others suggest that the substance is only a stearoptene. It also contains some starch, saponin, and in the suberous layer tannic acid.

¶ *Medicinal Action and Uses*. Alterative, tonic and diuretic. Useful for rheumatism, scrofula, skin diseases and thrush; it is used as an infusion, but not as a decoction as boiling dissipates its active volatile principle. Two oz. of the root are infused in 1 pint of boiling water and left standing for 1 hour then strained off and drunk in 24 hours.

It has been successfully used in the cure of venereal disease, proving efficacious where American Sarsaparilla has failed. Native doctors utilize it in nephritic complaints and for sore mouths of children.

Syrup, B.P., ½ to 1 drachm.

Particularly indicated for inveterate syphilis, pseudo-syphilis, mescurio-syphilis and struma in all its forms. Also valuable in gonorrhœal neuralgia and other depraved conditions of the system as well as for other diseases treated by other varieties.

Powder, 30 grains three times daily. Infusion or syrup, 4 fluid ounces.

An Alterative Mixture

1 lb. Rio Negro Sarsaparilla root, or in place of it Stillingia Sylvatica; 6 oz. rasped guaiac wood; aniseed and liquorice root bruised 2 oz. of each; 1 lb. molasses; 1 oz. Mezereon root-bark and 6 Cloves. Put all these into 2 gallons of boiling water and shake vessel well. When fermentation starts, take 4 fluid ounces three times daily.

SARSAPARILLA, WILD

Aralia nudicaulis (LINN.)
N.O. Araliaceæ

Synonyms. Bamboo Brier. Smilax Sarsaparilla
Part Used. Root
Habitat. A native of the southern United States and grows in swampy woods and thickets

¶ *Description*. It has a stout, flexuous and square stem, with a few hooked prickles above. Leaves unarmed, elliptical-ovate, cuspidate, abruptly contracted at each end; three strong veins, two lateral smaller secondary ones; underside glaucous, 3 inches diameter, on short margined petioles, with two long tendrils at their bases. Flowers

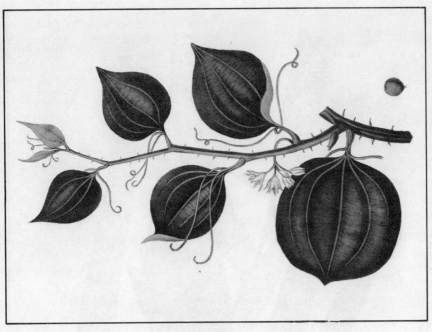

JAMAICA SARSAPARILLA
Smilax Ornata

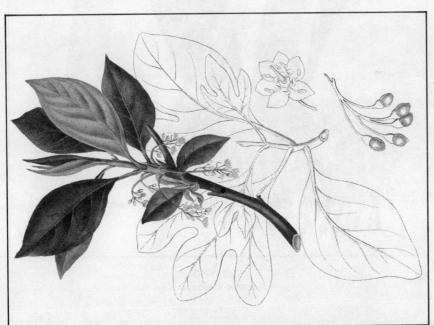

SASSAFRAS
Sassafras Officinale

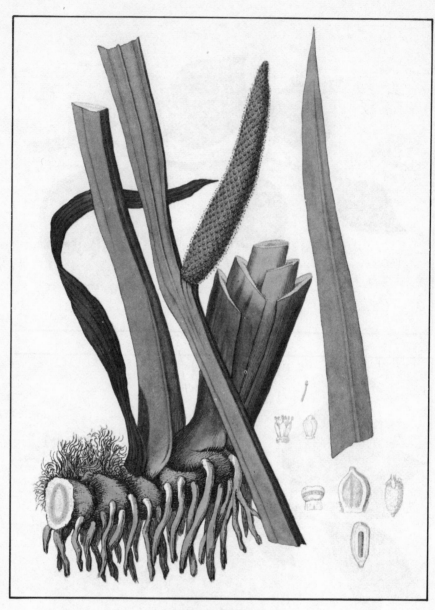

SWEET SEDGE
Acorus Calamus

yellowish-white, appearing May to August, in small thin umbels of three or four red or black berries, three-seeded.

¶ *Medicinal Action and Uses*. Alterative, tonic, antisyphilitic. Said to be inferior to all other Sarsaparillas. Much used by the American Indians. Used freely in decoction.

¶ *Other Species*.

Smilax Medica has an angular stem armed with straight prickles at joints, and a few hooked ones at intervals; paper-like leaves, bright green both sides, smooth, cordate, auriculate, shortly acuminate, five-nerved prominent veins underneath and otherwise variable in form. Mid-rib and petioles, when old, have straight, subulate prickles,

peduncles three lines to 1 inch; umbels twelve flowers; pedicle three lines long. Found growing in Papanta, Inspan, etc. Said to be similar to the Mexican or Vera Cruz Sarsapa of commerce, which may be derived from this species.

SARSAPARILLA MEXICAN (*Synonym.* Vera Cruz Sarsaparilla), as found in commerce, has a caudex with a number of long radicles which are smaller and have a thinner bark than the Honduras variety, contain little starch and have square endodermal cells with thickened walls, and more or less oval lumen. The taste is acrid and the plant contains the medical properties of other Sarsaparillas.

See SMILAX.

SASSAFRAS

Sassafras officinale (LEES and EBERM.)
N.O. Lauraceæ

Synonyms. Sassafras varifolium. Laurus Sassafras. Sassafrax. Sassafras radix
Parts Used. Bark-root and the root, pith
Habitat. Eastern United States, from Canada to Florida, and Mexico

¶ *Description*. The name 'Sassafras,' applied by the Spanish botanist Monardes in the sixteenth century, is said to be a corruption of the Spanish word for saxifrage. The tree stands from 20 to 40 feet high, with many slender branches, and smooth, orange-brown bark. The leaves are broadly oval, alternate, and 3 to 7 inches long. The flowers are small, and of an inconspicuous, greenish-yellow colour. The roots are large and woody, their bark being soft and spongy, rough, and reddish or greyish-brown in colour. The living bark is nearly white, but exposure causes its immediate discoloration. The roots are imported in large, branched pieces, which may or may not be covered with bark, and often have attached to them a portion of the lower part of the trunk. The central market for all parts is Baltimore. The entire root is official in the British Pharmacopœia, but only the more active bark in the United States, where wood and bark form separate articles of commerce. The bark without its corky layer is brittle, and the presence of small crystals cause its inner surface to glisten. Both bark and wood have a fragrant odour, and an aromatic, somewhat astringent taste.

The tree, which has berries like those of cinnamon, appears to have been cultivated in England some centuries ago, for in 1633 Johnston wrote: 'I have given the figure of a branch taken from a little sassafras tree which grew in the garden of Mr. Wilmot at Bon.' Probably it was discovered by the Spaniards in Florida, for seventy years earlier there is mention of the reputation of its roots in Spain as a cure for syphilis, rheu-

matism, etc., though its efficacy has since then been much disputed.

The fragrant oil distilled from the root-bark is extensively used in the manufacture of the coarser kinds of perfume, and for scenting the cheapest grades of soap. The oil used in perfumes is also extracted from the fruits. The wood and bark of the tree furnish a yellow dye. In Louisiana, the leaves are used as a condiment in sauces, and also for thickening soups; while the young shoots are used in Virginia for making a kind of beer. Mixed with milk and sugar, Sassafras Tea, under the name of 'Saloop,' could, until a few years ago, be bought at London street-corners in the early mornings.

SASSAFRAS PITH (*Sassafras medulla*) is only official in the United States. It is usually found in thin, cylindrical pieces, which are light and spongy, white and insipid. Its principal constituent is mucilage, which may be prepared by adding 60 grains of the pith to a pint of boiling water. This remains limpid when alcohol is added. It is used as a demulcent, especially for inflammation of the eyes, and as a soothing drink in catarrhal affection.

¶ *Constituents*. The root-bark contains a heavy and a light volatile oil, camphorous matter, resin, wax, a decomposition product of tannic acid called Sassafrid, tannic acid, gum, albumen, starch, lignin and salts. Sassafrid bears some analogy to cinchonic red. The bark yields from 6 to 9 per cent. of oil, of which the chief constituent is Safrol (80 per cent.). It is one of the heaviest of the volatile oils, and when cold deposits four- or six-sided prisms of Sassafras camphor, which retain the odour. It should be preserved in well-stoppered, amber-coloured bottles, away from the light. Three bushels of the root yield about 1 lb.

Safrol has been found to be one of those bodies which can exist either in a solid or a liquid condition long after freezing or melting-point. Chemically, it has been found to be the methylene ether of allyl-dioxibenene. It is found in many other species, is now commercially extracted from oil of Camphor, and could possibly be obtained from some members of the Cinnamomum family. Physiologically and therapeutically it is equivalent to oil of Sassafras.

Oil of Sassafras is *chiefly* used for flavouring purposes, particularly to conceal the flavour of opium when given to children. In the United States of America it is employed for flavouring effervescing drinks.

¶ *Medicinal Action and Uses.* Aromatic, stimulant, diaphoretic, alterative. It is rarely given alone, but is often combined with guaiacum or sarsaparilla in chronic rheumatism, syphilis, and skin diseases.

The oil is said to relieve the pain caused by menstrual obstructions, and pain following parturition, in doses of 5 to 10 drops on sugar, the same dose having been found useful in gleet and gonorrhœa.

Safrol is found to be slowly absorbed from the alimentary canal, escaping through the lungs unaltered, and through the kidneys oxidized into piperonalic acid.

A teaspoonful of the oil produced vomiting, dilated pupils, stupor and collapse in a young man.

It is used as a local application for wens and for rheumatic pains, and it has been praised as a dental disinfectant.

Its use has caused abortion in several cases.

Dr. Shelby of Huntsville stated that it would both prevent and remove the injurious effects of tobacco.

A lotion of rose-water or distilled water, with Sassafras Pith, filtered after standing for four hours, is recommended for the eyes.

¶ *Dosage.* Of fluid extract, ½ to 1 drachm. Of Sassafras bark, 1 to 2 drachms. Of oil of Sassafras, 1 to 5 drops. Mucilage, U.S.P., 4 drachms.

¶ *Poison and Antidotes.* The oil can produce marked narcotic poisoning, and death by causing widespread fatty degeneration of the heart, liver, and kidneys, or, in a larger dose, by great depression of the circulation, followed by a centric paralysis of respiration.

¶ *Other Species.* The name is also applied to the following:

BLACK SASSAFRAS, or *Oliveri Cortex* (Oliver's Bark), a substitute for cinnamon in Australia.

SWAMP SASSAFRAS, or *Magnolia glauca*, an aromatic, diaphoretic, tonic bitter.

AUSTRALIAN SASSAFRAS, or *Atherosperma moschatum*, a powerful poison, useful in rheumatism, syphilis and bronchitis.

SASSAFRAS GOESIANUM, or *Massoja aromatica*, yielding Massoi Bark.

CALIFORNIA SASSAFRAS, or *Umbellularia californica*, the leaves of which are employed in headache, colic and diarrhœa.

SASSY BARK

Erythrophlœum guineense (G. DON)
N.O. Leguminosæ

Synonyms. Nkasa. Mancona Bark. Doom Bark. Ordeal Bark. Casca Bark. Saucy Bark. Red Water Bark. Cortex erythrophlei
Part Used. Bark of the tree and branches
Habitat. Upper Guinea and Senegambia

¶ *Description.* The tree is large and spreading, and the bark very hard, breaking with a short, granular fracture. It varies in size and thickness according to the age of the stem or branch. It may be flat or curved, dull grey, red-brown, or almost black, with reddish warts or circular spots merging into bands running longitudinally. It is inodorous, with an astringent, acrid taste.

In West Africa the drug is used as an ordeal poison in trials for witchcraft and sorcery.

Possibly other species yield the Sassy Bark of commerce, differences being noticed in its properties at different periods.

¶ *Constituents.* Sassy Bark yields its properties to water. The poisonous principle Erythrophleine was obtained and confirmed in several experiments, possessing an action similar to that of digitalis. From this an acid called erythrophleic acid and a volatile alkaloid called Manzçonine were obtained by the action of hydrochloric acid. In contact with sulphuric acid and black manganese oxide, a violet colour is obtained, rather paler than that produced with strychnine. The bark also contains tannin and resin.

¶ *Medicinal Action and Uses.* Astringent, analgesic. The hydrochloride has been used in dental surgery. Erythrophleine causes a slow, strong pulse, with a rise in the arterial pressure. Purging is probably due to local action on peristalsis, and vomiting, the result of influence on the nerve centres, as it occurs when the alkaloid is given hypodermically. There has been much controversy concerning its anæsthetic powers. It has not yet been obtained in crystalline form, and needs fuller investigation.

Observations in West Africa about 1859 showed that Sassy Bark produced constriction in the fauces, with prickling, and later, numbness. It is asserted that it gives great relief in dyspnœa, but is uncertain as a heart tonic. The powder is strongly sternutatory.

It has been useful in mitral disease and dropsy, but disturbs the digestion even more than digitalis.

¶ *Dosages.* Of the alkaloid, $\frac{1}{40}$ to $\frac{1}{30}$ grain. Of the extract, $\frac{1}{4}$ to $\frac{1}{3}$ grain.

A solution of $\frac{1}{10}$ of 1 per cent. is used as an application to the cornea.

¶ *Poison with Antidotes.* An overdose causes stricture across the brow, severe pain in the head, coma, and death.

SAUNDERS, RED

Pterocarpus santalinus
N.O. Leguminosæ

Synonyms. Pterocarpi Lignum. Santalum rubrum. Lignum rubrum. Red Sandalwood. Rubywood. Rasura Santalum Ligni. Red Santal Wood. Sappan

Part Used. Wood

Habitat. Madras Presidency and Ceylon

¶ *Description.* A tree of 20 to 25 feet high, covered with rough bark resembling that of the Common Alder, and bearing spikes of yellow flowers. Plantations have been formed for its cultivation in Southern India, where it is very rare.

The name *Santalinus* refers to its name of red Sandalwood, which all its Indian titles signify, though it bears no relationship to *Santalum.* It is imported, usually from Ceylon, in the form of irregular logs or billets, without bark and sapwood, and about 3 to 5 feet in length. They are heavy, dense, reddish or blackish brown outside, and, if cut transversely, a deep blood-red inside, variegated with zones of a lighter red colour. In pharmacy the wood is in the form of chips, raspings, or coarse red powder. When rubbed, the wood has a faint peculiar odour, but is otherwise odourless, with a slight, astringent taste.

Gum Kino is obtained from other species of *Pterocarpus.* The chief use of Red Saunders wood is as a dye-stuff. In India it is employed mixed with sapan wood, for dyeing silk,

cotton and wool, the shade of red varying according to the mordant used.

¶ *Constituents.* The colouring principle, called Santalin, is readily soluble in alcohol (90 per cent.), but almost insoluble in water. Ether, alkalis, and three other crystalline principles have also been described as being present: Santal, Pterocarpin, and Homopterocarpin. A small quantity of tannin, probably kino-tannic acid, has also been found in the wood. The colouring principle is partially soluble in some of the essential oils, such as lavender, rosemary, cloves, and oil of bitter almonds, and as a colouring agent it forms part of the official Comp. Tincture of Lavender.

The colouring principles of the West African Barwood (*Pterocarpus angolensis*) and Camwood (*Baphia nitida*) are closely allied with that of Red Saunders, if not identical.

¶ *Medicinal Action and Uses.* Astringent, tonic. Chiefly used medicinally in India, and employed in pharmacy for colouring tinctures.

SAVINE

Sabina cacumina
N.O. Coniferæ

Synonyms. Savine Tops

Part Used. Fresh dried tops of Juniperas Sabina collected in spring from plants grown in Britain

Habitat. Britain. Indigenous to Northern States of America, Middle and Southern Europe

¶ *Description.* A shrub growing to a height of a few feet in Britain, but found as a tree in some Greek Islands, evergreen and compact in growth, spreads horizontally, branches round, tough, and slender; bark, when young, pale green, becoming rough with age on trunk; leaves small, ovate, dark green, in four rows, opposite, scale-like, ovate-lanceolate, having on back a shallow groove containing an oblong or roundish

gland. The fruit is a blackish purple berry, ovoid in shape, containing three seeds. Flowers unisexual; odour peculiar, terebinthinate; taste disagreeable, resinous and bitter.

¶ *Constituents.* Volatile oil, resin, gallic acid, chlorophyl extractive, lignin, calcareous salts, a fixed oil, gum and salts of potassia.

¶ *Medicinal Action and Uses.* Savine is an irritant when administered internally or locally; it is a powerful emmenagogue in large doses; it is an energetic poison leading to gastro enteritis collapse and death. It should never be used in pregnancy, as it produces abortion. It is rarely given internally, but is useful as an ointment and as a dressing to blisters in order to promote discharge; also applied externally to syphilitic warts, and other skin trouble. The powdered leaves mixed with an equal part of verdigris are used to destroy warts.

¶ *Adulterant.* Red Cedar (*Juniperus Virginiana*, Linn.) is often commonly referred to as Savin and is substituted commercially, the tops of *J. Phœnicæ* (Linn.), which contain volatile oil, are also admixed in Europe.

See CEDARS.

SAVORY, SUMMER

Satureia hortensis (LINN.)
N.O. Labiatæ

Part Used. Herb

The genus *Satureia* (the old Latin name used by Pliny) comprises about fourteen species of highly aromatic, hardy herbs or under-shrubs, all, except one species, being natives of the Mediterranean region.

Several species have been introduced into England, but only two, the annual Summer or Garden Savory and the perennial, Winter Savory are generally grown. The annual is more usually grown, but the leaves of both are employed in cookery, like other sweet herbs, the leaves and tender tops being used, with marjoram and thyme, to season dressings for turkey, veal or fish.

Both species were noticed by Virgil as being among the most fragrant of herbs, and on this account recommended to be grown near bee-hives. There is reason to suppose that they were cultivated in remote ages, before the East Indian spices were known and in common use. Vinegar, flavoured with Savory and other aromatic herbs, was used by the Romans in the same manner as mint sauce is by us.

In Shakespeare's time, Savory was a familiar herb, for we find it mentioned, together with the mints, marjoram and lavender, in *The Winter's Tale.*

In ancient days, the Savorys were supposed to belong to the Satyrs, hence the name Satureia. Culpepper says:

'Mercury claims dominion over this herb. Keep it dry by you all the year, if you love yourself and your ease, and it is a hundred pounds to a penny if you do not.'

He considered Summer Savory better than Winter Savory for drying to make conserves and syrups.

John Josselyn, one of the early settlers in America, gives a list of plants introduced there by the English colonists to remind them of the gardens they had left behind. Winter and Summer Savory are two of those mentioned.

¶ *Description.* Summer Savory is a hardy, pubescent annual, with slender erect stems about a foot high. It flowers in July, having small, pale lilac labiate flowers, axillary, on short pedicels, the common peduncle sometimes three-flowered. The leaves, about $\frac{1}{2}$ inch long, are entire, oblong-linear, acute, shortly narrowed at the base into petioles, often fascicled. The hairs on the stem are short and decurved.

¶ *Cultivation.* Summer Savory is raised from seeds, sown early in April, in shallow drills, 9 inches or a foot apart. Select a sunny situation and thin out the seedlings, when large enough, to 6 inches apart in the rows. It likes a rich, light soil.

The seeds may also be sown broadcast, when they must be thinned out, the thinned out seedlings being planted in another bed at 6 inches distance from each other and well watered. The seeds are very slow in germinating.

The early spring seedlings may be first topped for fresh use in June. When the plants are in flower, they may be pulled up and dried for winter use.

¶ *Uses.* As a *pot-herb,* Savory, which has a distinctive taste, though it somewhat recalls that of marjoram, is not only added to stuffings, pork pies and sausages as a wholesome seasoning, but sprigs of it, fresh, may be boiled with broad beans and green peas, in the same manner as mint. It is also boiled with dried peas in making pea-soup. For garnishing it has been used as a substitute for parsley and chervil.

¶ *Medicinal Action and Uses.* Savory has aromatic and carminative properties, and though chiefly used as a culinary herb, it may be added to medicines for its aromatic and warming qualities. It was formerly deemed a sovereign remedy for the colic and a cure for flatulence, on this account, and was also considered a good expectorant.

Culpepper tells us that

'The juice dropped into the eyes removes dimness of sight if it proceed from thin humours distilled from the brain. The juice heated with oil of Roses and dropped in the ears removes noise and singing and deafness: outwardly applied with wheat flour, it gives ease to them.'

He says:

'Keep it dry, make conserves and syrups of it for your use; for which purpose the Summer kind is best. This kind is both hotter and drier than the Winter kind. . . . It expels tough phlegm from the chest and lungs,

quickens the dull spirits in the lethargy, if the juice be snuffed up the nose; dropped into the eyes it clears them of thin cold humours proceeding from the brain . . . outwardly applied with wheat flour as a poultice, it eases sciatica and palsied members.'

Both the old authorities and modern gardeners agree that a sprig of either of the Savorys rubbed on wasp and bee stings gives instant relief.

SAVORY, WINTER

Satureia montana (LINN.)
N.O. Labiatæ

Part Used. Herb

Winter Savory is a dwarf, hardy, perennial, glabrous or slightly pubescent under shrub, also a native of Southern Europe, and it has been known in Great Britain since 1562.

The stems are woody at the base, diffuse, much branched. The leaves are oblong, linear and acute, or the lower ones spatulate or wedge-shaped and obtuse. The flowers, in bloom in June, are very pale-purple, the cymes shortly pedunculate, approximating to a spike or raceme.

¶ *Cultivation.* It is propagated either from seeds, sown at a similar period and in the same manner as Summer Savory, or from cuttings and divisions of root. It is woodier and more bushy than Summer Savory.

Cuttings formed of young side shoots, with a heel attached, may be taken in April or June, and will readily root under a hand-glass, or in a shady border outside.

Divisions of the roots should be made in March or April, and plants obtained in this way, or from cuttings, should be permanently inserted during a showery period in the latter part of summer, in rows, at the distance of 1 foot apart.

The plant grows better in a poor, stony soil than a rich one. In a rich soil, plants

take in too much moisture to stand the severity of our winter. In soil that suits it, Winter Savory makes a good-sized shrub. It will continue for several years, but when the plants are old the shoots are short and not so well furnished with leaves. It is, therefore, well to raise a supply of young plants every other year.

Parkinson tells us that Winter Savory used to be dried and powdered and mixed with grated bread-crumbs, 'to breade their meate, be it fish or flesh, to give it a quicker relish.' It is recommended by old writers, together with other herbs, in the dressing of trout.

When dried, it is used as seasoning in the same manner as Summer Savory, but is not employed medicinally.

Culpepper says that it is a good remedy for the colic.

¶ *Other Species.*

Satureia thymbra, which is used in Spain as a spice and is closely allied to the Savories grown in English kitchen gardens, yields an oil containing about 19 per cent. of thymal. Other species of *Satureia* contain carvacrol. The oil from wild plants of Winter Savory contains 30 or 40 per cent. of carvacrol, and that from cultivated plants still more.

SAW PALMETTO

Sarenoa serrulata (HOOK, F.)
N.O. Palmaceæ

Synonyms. Sabal. Sabal serrulata
Part Used. Partially-dried ripe fruit
Habitat. The Atlantic Coast from South Carolina to Florida, and southern California

¶ *Description.* The plant grows from 6 to 10 feet high, forming what is called the 'palmetto scrub.' It has a crown of large leaves, and the fruit is irregularly-spherical to oblong-ovoid, deep red-brown, slightly wrinkled, being from ½ to 1 inch long and about ½ inch in diameter. It contains a hard brown seed. The taste is sweetish and not agreeable, and the panicle containing it may weigh as much as 9 lb. It has no odour.

¶ *Constituents.* Volatile oil, fixed oil, glucose, about 63 per cent. of free acids, and 37 per

cent. of ethyl esters of these acids. The oil obtained exclusively from the nut is a glyceride of fatty acids, thick and of a greenish colour, without fruity odour. From the whole fruit can be obtained by pressure about 1½ per cent. of a brownish-yellow to dark red oil, soluble in alcohol, ether, chloroform and benzene, and partly soluble in dilute solution of potassium hydroxide. The fixed oil is soluble in alcohol, ether, and petroleum benzin. The presence of an alkaloid is uncertain.

The following formula will give elixir of sabal with terpinhydrate. Dissolve 1·75 gram of terpinhydrate in 40 mm. of fluid extract of sabal and 10 mm. of alcohol. Add 1 mm. of tincture of sweet orange peel, 0·2 mm. of solution of saccharin, 40 mm. of glycerin, and 100 mm. of syrup. This preparation will contain 8 grains of terpinhydrate and 184 grains of sabal in each fluid ounce.

¶ *Medicinal Action and Uses.* Diuretic, sedative, tonic. It is milder and less stimulant than cubeb or copaiba, or even oil of sandalwood. Like these, it has the power of affecting the respiratory mucous membrane, and is used for many complaints which are accompanied by chronic catarrh. It has been claimed that sabal is capable of increasing the nutrition of the testicles and mammæ in functional atony of these organs. It probably acts by reducing catarrhal irritation and a relaxed condition of bladder and urethra. It is a tissue builder.

¶ *Dosages.* Of fluid extract, ½ to 1 drachm. Of solid extract, 5 to 15 grains.

SAXIFRAGE, BURNET

Pimpinella Saxifraga (LINN.)
N.O. Umbelliferæ

Synonyms. Lesser Burnet. Saxifrage
Parts Used. Root, herb
Habitat. It grows abundantly in dry, chalky pastures, and is very generally distributed over the country

The Burnet Saxifrage, sometimes cultivated for kitchen use, is neither a Burnet nor a Saxifrage, but has obtained the latter name because supposed to break up stone in the bladder, and the former from the similarity of its leaves to the Greater and Lesser Burnets, though its umbels of white flowers mark the difference at the first glance.

¶ *Description.* The root-stock is slender, the stem also slender, round, striate, 9 inches to 3 feet high. The root-leaves are numerous, shortly stalked, pinnate, the leaflets oval or roundish, four to eight pairs, sometimes so deeply cut as to be bipinnate, sometimes merely serrated. The stem-leaves are few, with the petiole dilated, particularly in the uppermost ones, the leaflets narrower than in the radical leaves, and pinnatifid. The upper leaves are reduced to dilated sheaths, the leaflets represented by one or more linear lobes. The umbels are regular, flat-topped, the umbelules many-flowered, the individual flowers $\frac{1}{10}$ inch across, white, with notched petals. The whole plant is dark green, generally glabrous.

¶ *Parts Used.* The leaves and roots. The whole herb is cut in July and dried in the same way as the Burnets.

¶ *Medicinal Action and Uses.* Resolvent, diaphoretic, stomachic, diuretic. The root is very hot and acrid, burning the mouth like pepper. On drying, or on being kept long, its pungency is considerably diminished. It contains a bitter resin and a blue essential oil, which communicates that colour to water or spirit on distillation, and is said to be used in Germany for colouring brandy.

The oil and resin contained are useful to relieve flatulent indigestion.

The fresh root chewed is good for toothache and paralysis of the tongue. A decoction has the reputation of removing freckles. It is said to dissolve mucus, and on this account is used as a gargle in hoarseness and some cases of throat affection.

It is also prescribed in asthma and dropsy.

Small bunches of the leaves and shoots, tied together and suspended in a cask of beer impart to it an agreeable aromatic flavour, and are thought to correct tart or spoiled wines.

Cows which feed on this plant have their flow of milk increased.

Culpepper says:

'The whole plant is binding . . . it is a cordial. In the composition of the *Syrupus Altheæ* it is generally used instead of the Great Burnet Saxifrage.'

SAXIFRAGE, GREATER BURNET

Pimpinella magna
N.O. Umbelliferæ

Parts Used. Herb, seeds

The Greater Burnet Saxifrage is very like large specimens of *Pimpinella Saxifraga*, but larger in all its parts and of a paler green in colour, the root-stock much thicker and the stems generally 2 to 4 feet high, stouter and more angular. The leaflets are larger and broader, generally less deeply cut. The umbels and flowers are similar, though the styles are longer and more slender.

¶ *Medicinal Action and Uses.* This plant has much the same medicinal properties as the former species, and has been employed in a similar manner.

The root is very acrid, and is powerfully diuretic, having been prescribed with success, in strong infusion, in disorders arising from obstructions of the viscera. The seeds are carminative, and have been used in colic and for dispersing wind in the stomach, administered in powdered form.

The Aniseed of medicine and commerce is a foreign species of this same genus.

Culpepper says this plant

'has the properties of the parsleys but eases

pains and provokes urine more effectually. . . . The distilled water, boiled with castoreum, is good for cramps and convulsions, and the seed used in comfits (like carraway seeds) will answer the same purpose. The juice of the herb dropped into bad wounds in the head, dries up their moisture and heals them.'

SCABIOUS, FIELD

Knautia arvensis
N.O. Compositæ

Synonyms. Scabiosa arvensis
Part Used. Herb

¶ *Description.* There are several species of Scabious indigenous to these islands, of which the Field Scabious (*Knautia arvensis*) is the largest. It is abundant throughout Britain, flowering best, however, on chalk, and very frequent in meadows, hedgerows or amidst standing corn, where its large blossoms, of a delicate mauve, render it very conspicuous and attractive. The root is perennial, dark in colour and somewhat woody, and takes such a firm hold on the ground that it is only eradicated with difficulty. The stems are round and only slightly branched, 2 to 3 feet high, somewhat coarse with short, whitish hairs and rather bare of leaves, except at the base. The leaves vary in character in different plants and in different parts of the same plant; they grow in pairs on the stem and are hairy. The lowest leaves are stalked and very simple in character, about 5 inches long and 1 inch broad, lance-shaped, their margins cut into by large teeth. The upper ones are stalkless, their blades meeting across the main stem and cut into almost to the mid-rib, to form four or five pairs of narrow lobes, with a terminal big lobe. The flowers are all terminal and borne on long stalks. The heads are large and convex in outline, the inner florets are regularly cleft into four lobes or segments, the outer ones are larger and generally, though not always, with rays cut into very unequal segments. The florets when in bud are packed tightly, but with beautiful regularity. The fruit is rather large, somewhat four-cornered and crowned by several short, bristly hairs that radiate from its summit.

The generic name, *Knautia*, is derived

from a Saxon botanist of the seventeenth century, Dr. Knaut. The name Scabious is supposed to be connected with the word 'scab' (a scaly sore), a word derived from the Latin *scabies* (a form of leprosy), for which and for other diseases of a similar character, some of these species were used as remedies.

¶ *Medicinal Action and Uses.* Gerard tells us: 'The plant gendereth scabs, if the decoction thereof be drunke certain daies and the juice used in ointments.' We are told that this juice 'being drunke, procureth sweat, especially with Treacle, and atenuateth and maketh thin, freeing the heart from any infection or pestilence.' Culpepper informs us also that it is 'very effectual for coughs, shortness of breath and other diseases of the lungs,' and that the 'decoction of the herb, dry or green, made into wine and drunk for some time together,' is good for pleurisy. The green herb, bruised and applied to any carbuncle was stated by him to dissolve the same 'in three hours' space,' and the same decoction removed pains and stitches in the side. The decoction of the root was considered a cure for all sores and eruptions, the juice being made into an ointment for the same purpose. Also, 'the decoction of the herb and roots outwardly applied in any part of the body, is effectual for shrunk sinews or veins and healeth green wounds, old sores and ulcers.' The juice of Scabious, with powder of Borax and Samphire, was recommended for removing freckles, pimples and leprosy, the head being washed with the same decoction, used warm, for dandruff and scurf, etc.

SCABIOUS, LESSER

Scabiosa Columbaria
N.O. Compositæ

Part Used. Herb

The Lesser Scabious is not uncommon on a chalky soil, and is distinguished from the former by its smaller size. The foliage is of a light hue and the leaves very finely cut into. The flowers are lilac, but in nearly globular heads, not so convex, the corollas being five-cleft, not four-cleft, and the outer

florets larger than the inner, though not quite so large as in the Field Scabious. Its properties are similar to the larger species just described.

Scabious herb should be collected in July and August and dried. The root is no longer used.

SCABIOUS, DEVIL'S BIT

Scabiosa succisa (LINN.)
N.O. Compositæ

Synonyms. Ofbit. Premorse Scabious
Part Used. Herb

The Devil's Bit Scabious is almost as common a plant as the preceding species, but is more often to be found in open meadows and on heaths than in the hedgerow and the cornfield.

¶ *Description.* It is a slender, little-branched plant, with a hairy stem, few leaves, which are oblong and not cut into, and almost globular heads of deep purplish-blue flowers. It is to be found in bloom from July to October. The florets composing the head are all very much the same size, the outer ones being scarcely larger than the inner. The stamens of each floret, as in the other species of Scabious are a very conspicuous feature, the anthers being large and borne upon filaments or threads that are almost as long again as the corolla. The root is, when fully grown, nearly the thickness of a finger, and ends in so abrupt a way as almost to suggest that it had been bitten off, a peculiarity that has given it a place in legends. In the first year of the plant's existence the root is like a diminutive carrot or radish in shape; it then becomes woody and dies away, the upper part excepted; as it decays and falls away, the gnawed or broken look results. The portion left throws out numerous lateral roots, which compensate for the portion that has perished. The plant derives its common name from this peculiarity in the form of the root. Gerard tells us:

'The greater part of the root seemeth to be bitten away; old fantastick charmers report that the divel did bite it for envie, because it is an herbe that hath so many good vertues and it is so beneficial to mankinde.'

The legend referred to by Gerard tells how the devil found it in Paradise, but envying the good it might do to the human race, bit away a part of the root to destroy the plant, in spite of which it still flourishes, but with a stumped root. The legend seems to have been very widely spread, for the plant bears this name, not only in England but also on the Continent.

¶ *Medicinal Action and Uses.* This plant is still used for its diaphoretic, demulcent and febrifuge properties, the whole herb being collected in September and dried.

It makes a useful tea for coughs, fevers and internal inflammation. The remedy is generally given in combination with others, the infusion being given in wineglassful doses at frequent intervals. It purifies the blood, taken inwardly, and used as a wash externally is a good remedy for cutaneous eruptions. The juice made into an ointment is effectual for the same purpose. The warm decoction has also been used as a wash to free the head from scurf, sores and dandruff.

Culpepper assigned it many uses, saying that the root boiled in wine and drunk was very powerful against the plague and all pestilential diseases, and fevers and poison and bites of venomous creatures, and that 'it helpeth also all that are inwardly bruised or outwardly by falls or blows, dissolving the clotted blood,' the herb or root bruised and outwardly applied, taking away black and blue marks on the skin. He considered 'the decoction of the herb very effectual as a gargle for swollen throat and tonsils, and that the root powdered and taken in drink expels worms.' The juice or distilled water of the herb was deemed a good remedy for green wounds or old sores, cleansing the body inwardly and freeing the skin from sores, scurf, pimples, freckles, etc. The dried root used also to be given in powder, its power of promoting sweat making it beneficial in fevers.

The SHEEP'S (or SHEEP'S-BIT) SCABIOUS (*Jasione montana*) is not a true Scabious, though at first sight its appearance is similar. It may be distinguished from a Scabious by its united anthers, and it differs from a Compound Flower (Compositæ, to which the Scabious belongs) in having a two-celled capsule. It is a member of the Campanulaceæ, and is the only British species. The whole plant, when bruised, has a strong and disagreeable smell.

See CORNFLOWER, KNAPWEED, TEAZLE THISTLE.

SCAMMONY. *See* BINDWEED, CONVOLVULUS

SCOPOLIA

Scopola carniolica (JACQ.)
N.O. Solanaceæ

Synonyms. Scopolia atropoides. Scopola. Belladonna Scopola. Japanese Belladonna
Part Used. Dried rhizome
Habitat. Bavaria, Austro-Hungary, South-western Russia

¶ *Description.* The genus *Scopola* is a connecting link between *Atropa* and *Hyoscya-*mus, its leaf, flower and rhizome resembling the former, and the fruit the latter. The

Japanese *Scopola japonica* is so closely allied that it is doubtful if it can be regarded as a distinct species.

S. Carniolica grows in damp, stony places in hilly districts and resembles belladonna both in appearance and characteristics. It only grows to the height of 1 foot, and has thin leaves, its fruit being a transversely dehiscent capsule.

The rhizome is horizontal, curved, almost cylindrical, and somewhat flattened vertically. It is usually found in pieces from 2½ to 7½ cm. long and 0·8 to 1·6 cm. broad, often split before drying. The upper surface is marked with closely-set, large, cup-shaped stem-scars, and the colour varies from yellowish-brown to dark, brownish-grey; the fracture is short and sharp, showing a yellowish-white bark, its corky layer dark brown, or pale brown, the central pith being rather horny. It has scarcely any odour, and the taste is sweetish at first, but afterwards bitter and strongly acrid. The Japanese rhizome is larger, with circular scars, not whitish when broken, and having a slightly mousy, narcotic odour, and practically no bitterness in taste.

The bark of *S. Carniolica* is less thick than in belladonna and the starch grains smaller.

Scopolia is but little used in Britain, but has been used in America for many years in the manufacture of belladonna plasters.

¶ *Constituents.* The alkaloidal constituents are similar to those of Belladonna Root, hyoscine (scopolamine), however, predominating. Inactive scopolamine, also known as atroscine, is present, melting at 82° C. (179·6° F.) and yielding by hydrolysis tropic acid and scopoline. The result of an assay of many tons of the root of *Atropa Belladonna* and of the rhizome of Scopolia, each of the best qualities to be found in the American market, showed that while belladonna yielded on an average 0·50 per cent. of alkaloid, Scopolia yielded 0·58 per cent.

The root of *S. Carniolica* is official in the United States Pharmacopœia for the production of an extract and fluid extract. It should contain not less than 0·5 per cent. of alkaloids.

Scopolamine hydrobromide is recognized in the United States Pharmacopœia.

Scopolamine or hyoscine must be preserved in well-closed containers, protected from light. When pure, it forms a syrupy liquid. Great care must be used in tasting it, and then only in dilute solutions. When dried at 100° C. (212° F.) it loses about 12 per cent. of its weight. It is the same substance as Hyoscinæ Hydrobromicum. *Atro-scine* is an optically inert isomer of scopolamin and *Euscopol* is an optically inactive scopolaminum hydrobromicum.

¶ *Medicinal Action and Uses.* Narcotic and mydriatic. The medicinal properties are very like those of belladonna, but the crude drug has been scarcely used at all in internal medicine. Much of the hyoscine of commerce has been obtained from it during the last decade.

Many of the older investigations into the effects of scopolamine are contradictory because of the failure to realize the quantitative difference between *racemic* and *lævo-scopolamine*. The former, sometimes called *atrocine*, is very much less powerful in its effects upon the autonomic nerves, though its action upon the central nervous system is about equal.

Its most important use is as a cerebral sedative, especially in manias, hysteria, and drug habits, while in insomnias and epilepsy it increases the effects of other drugs, such as morphine and bromides. It is also useful to allay sexual excitement. In 1900 the use of a combination of morphine and scopolamine was introduced as a means of producing anæsthesia, under the name of 'Twilight Sleep,' either alone or as a preliminary to chloroform or ether, as its peculiar effect in large doses is to cause loss of memory, including that of pain. However, the anæsthesia has often been found to be unsatisfactory, while the mortality has been high.

¶ *Dosages.* Powdered extract, U.S.P., 1 to 5 grains. Of the drug, 1 to 2 grains. Of the fluid extract, U.S.P., 1 to 5 minims. Extract of Scopolia, ⅛ to ¼ grain. (Prepared by evaporating the fluid extract and assaying it so that it contains 2 per cent. of mydriatic alkaloids.) Of Scopolamine, $\frac{1}{200}$ to $\frac{1}{80}$ grain.

¶ *Poisonous, if Any, with Antidotes.* Many persons being very susceptible to the influence of the drug, the above doses of scopolamine may produce toxic symptoms, which are alarming, though the poisoning rarely ends fatally.

Sometimes there is disorientation, sometimes active delirium as in atropine poisoning. There may or may not be somnolence. The pupils may be dilated, the pulse rate accelerated and there is dryness of the mouth with a peculiar husky character of voice that appears to be due to laryngeal paralysis. If there should be serious difficulty in breathing, strychnine may be used. It is better not to give drugs for the relief of the delirium, but if very active, small doses of paraldehyde and bromides may be employed.

SCULLCAPS

Scutellarias
N.O. Labiatæ

Habitat. The Scullcaps, belonging to the genus *Scutellaria*, are herbaceous, slender, rarely shrubby, labiate plants, scattered over different parts of the world, in temperate regions and tropical mountains, being specially abundant in America. There are about ninety known species belonging to this genus, only two members of which are natives of Great Britain – *Scutellaria galericulata* and *S. minor*. Both are found on the banks of rivers and lakes, and in watery places generally, and are decumbent or spreading, seldom quite erect

N.O. Labiatæ

The generic name is from the Latin *scutella* (a little dish), from the lid of the calyx. The form of the latter is a peculiarity by which they can be recognized; it is bell-shaped, lipped, as Hooker describes it: 'the tube being dilated opposite to the posterior lip, with a broad, flattened hollow pouch, the lip and pouch being deciduous in fruit and the mouth closed after flowering.' Hooker adds: 'The only insect known to visit the first species is a butterfly.'

SCULLCAP, COMMON

Scutellaria galericulata (LINN.)

Synonyms. Greater Scullcap. Helmet Flower. Hoodwort.
(*French*) Toque
Part Used. Herb

The Common or Greater Scullcap is fairly common in England, though rare in Scotland and local in Ireland.

¶ *Description.* The root-stock is perennial and creeping. The square stems, 6 to 18 inches high, are somewhat slender, either paniculately branched, or, in small specimens, nearly simple, with opposite downy leaves, oblong and tapering, heart-shaped at the base, ½ to 2½ inches long, notched and shortly petioled.

The flowers are in pairs, each growing from the axils of the upper, leaf-like bracts, which are quite indistinguishable from the true leaves, and are all turned one way, the pedicels being very short. The corollas are bright blue, variegated with white inside, the tube long and curved, three or four times as long as the calyx, the lips short, the lower lip having three shallow lobes.

Soon after the corolla has fallen off, the upper lip of the calyx, which bulges outward about the middle, closes on the lower as if on a hinge, and gives it the appearance of a capsule with a lid. When the seed is ripe, the cup being dry, divides into two distinct parts, and the seeds, already detached from the receptacle, fall to the ground.

The plant is in flower from July to September. It is subglabrous, with the angles of the stem, the leaves and flowering calyx finely pubescent.

SCULLCAP, LESSER

Scutellaria minor (LINN.)

Part Used. Herb

The Lesser Scullcap, which grows chiefly in bogs, is not common, except in the western counties and in Ireland.

It has the habit of the preceding species, but is more slender and often much branched, and rarely attains 6 inches in height. The whole plant is more glabrous than *Scutellaria galericulata*.

The leaves are egg-shaped, the upper, quite entire, the lower ones often slightly toothed at the base. The flowers are small, dull pink-purple, the calyx having the same peculiarity as the larger species.

It flowers from July to October.

SCULLCAP, VIRGINIAN

Scutellaria lateriflora (LINN.)
N.O. Labiatæ

Synonyms. Mad-dog Scullcap. Madweed
Part Used. Herb

The American species, Virginian Scullcap, flowering in July, with inconspicuous blue flowers in one-sided racemes, is one of the finest nervines ever discovered.

Popularly this plant is known in America as Mad-dog Scullcap or Madweed, having the reputation of being a certain cure for hydrophobia.

The English species, *Scutellaria galericulata* and *S. minor*, possess similar nervine properties to the American, and with *S. integrifolia* and other American species with the flowers in one-sided terminal racemes, are often used as substitutes.

Among the cultivated species are *S. micrantha*, from Siberia and the north of China, a handsome species with spiked racemes of blue flowers; and *S. Coccinea*, from Mexico, with scarlet flowers.

The French name for this plant is *Toque*.

¶ *Cultivation.* The various species of *Scutellaria* will grow in any ordinary garden soil, preferring sunny, open borders, where they will live much longer and grow more strongly than on a rich soil, though they seldom continue more than two or three years.

Plant in March or April, 6 inches apart.

Propagation is mostly effected by seeds, sown in gentle heat in February or March or out of doors, in half-shady positions, in light soil in April. Transplant into permanent quarters in the autumn. No further care is necessary than weeding.

Propagation may also be effected by division of roots in March or April, but the roots are generally lifted, divided and replanted only when overgrown.

¶ *Part Used.* The whole herb, collected in June, dried and powdered.

¶ *Constituents.* A volatile oil, Scutellarin, and a bitter glucoside, yielding Scutellarein on hydrolysis. Also tannin, fat, some bitter principle, sugar and cellulose.

¶ *Medicinal Action and Uses.* Scullcap has strong tonic, nervine and antispasmodic action, and is slightly astringent.

In hysteria, convulsions, hydrophobia, St. Vitus's dance and rickets, its action is invaluable. In nervous headaches, neuralgia and in headache arising from incessant coughing and pain, it offers one of the most suitable and reliable remedies. The dried extract, given in doses of from 1 to 3 grains as a pill, will relieve severe hiccough.

Many cases of hydrophobia have been cured by this remedy alone.

It is considered a specific for the convulsive twitchings of St. Vitus's dance, soothing the nervous excitement and inducing sleep when necessary, without any unpleasant symptoms following.

Fluid extract, ½ to 1 drachm.

It may be prescribed in all disorders of the nervous system, and has been suggested as a remedy for epilepsy. Writing on this point in the *British Medical Journal*, 1915, Dr. William Bramwell says: 'Its efficacy appears to be partly due to its stimulating the kidneys to increased activity. . . .'

Overdoses of the tincture cause giddiness, stupor, confusion of mind, twitchings of the limbs, intermission of the pulse and other symptoms indicative of epilepsy, for which in diluted strength and small doses it has been successfully given.

The usual dose is an infusion of 1 oz. of the powdered herb to a pint of boiling water, given in half-teacupful doses, every few hours. Both fluid and solid extracts are prepared and Scutellarin is also administered in doses of 1 to 2 grains.

Fluid extract, ½ to 1 drachm.

The European species, *S. galericulata*, was at one time given for the tertian ague, and was said to have proved beneficial where the fits were more obstinate than violent, 1 to 2 oz. of the expressed juice, or an infusion of a handful or two of the herb, being given. In England, however, the remedy was not in use.

SCURVY GRASS

Cochlearia officinalis (LINN.)
N.O. Cruciferæ

Synonym. Spoonwort
Part Used. Herb
Habitat. Abundant on the shores in Scotland, growing inland along some of its rivers and Highland mountains and not uncommon in stony, muddy and sandy soils in England and Ireland, also in the Arctic Circle, sea-coasts of Northern and Western Europe and to high elevations in the great European mountain chains

¶ *Description.* It is a small, low-growing plant, annual or biennial, with thick, fleshy, glabrous, egg-shaped, cordate leaves (hence its name of spoonwort). The upper leaves are sessile – lower ones stalked, deltoid orbicular or reniform entire or toothed angularly. Flowers all summer in white short racemes – pods nearly globular – prominent valves of the mid-rib when dry. It has an unpleasant smell and a bitter, warm, acrid taste, very pungent when fresh.

¶ *Constituents.* Leaves abound in a pungent oil containing sulphur, of the butylic series.

¶ *Medicinal Action and Uses.* Formerly the fresh herb was greatly used on sea-voyages as a preventative of scurvey. It is stimulating, aperient, diuretic, antiscorbutic. The essential oil is of benefit in paralytic and rheumatic cases; scurvy-grass ale was a popular tonic drink.

The infusion of 2 oz. to a pint of boiling water is taken in frequent wineglassful doses.

SEA FENNEL. *See* FENNEL

SEA LAVENDER. *See* LAVENDER

SEAWEED. *See* BLADDERWRACK, (CORSICAN) MOSS, (IRISH) MOSS

SEDGE, SWEET   Acorus Calamus (LINN.)
                                                                N.O. Araceæ

Synonyms. Calamus. Sweet Flag. Sweet Root. Sweet Rush. Sweet Cane. Gladdon.
Sweet Myrtle. Myrtle Grass. Myrtle Sedge. Cinnamon Sedge
Part Used. Root
Habitat. Found in all European countries except Spain. Southern Russia, northern
Asia Minor, southern Siberia, China, Japan, northern United States of America,
Hungary, Burma, Ceylon and India

The Sweet Sedge is a vigorous, reed-like, aquatic plant, flourishing in ditches, by the margins of lakes and streams and in marshy places generally, associated with reeds, bull-rushes and bur-reed.

Its erect, sword-shaped leaves bear considerable resemblance to those of the Yellow Flag, hence its equally common popular name of 'Sweet Flag,' though it is not related botanically to the Iris, being a member of the Arum order, Araceæ. All parts of the plant have a peculiar, agreeable fragrance.

Formerly, on account of its pleasant odour, it was freely strewn on the floors of churches at festivals and often in private houses, instead of rushes. The specific name, *calamus*, is derived from the Greek *calamos* (a reed). The floors of Norwich Cathedral until quite recently were always strewn with calamus at great festivals.

As the Sweet Sedge did not grow near London, but had to be fetched at considerable expense from Norfolk and Suffolk, one of the charges of extravagance brought against Cardinal Wolsey was his habit of strewing his floors with fresh rushes.

Most species of this order give out a considerable amount of heat within the spathe at the time of flowering, so that the temperature rises noticeably above that of the external air. Many of the varieties also have lurid colouring and a fetid odour.

The generic name, *Acorus*, is from *Acoron*, the Greek name of the plant used by Dioscorides and said to be derived from *Coreon* (the pupil of the eye), diseases of which the Ancients used this plant to cure.

The rhizomes are an important commercial commodity and of considerable medicinal value.

Though now common throughout Europe, there is little doubt that the Sweet Flag is a native of eastern countries, being indigenous to the marshes of the mountains of India.

It is said to have been introduced into Poland by the Tartars, but not till 1588 is it recorded as abundant in Germany. Clusius, the famous botanist, first cultivated it at Vienna in 1574, from a root obtained from

Asia Minor and distributed it to other botanists in Belgium, Germany and France. It is readily propagated and rapidly becomes established. In England, it was probably introduced about 1596, being first grown by Gerard, who says that 'Anthony Coline the apothecarie sent him pieces from Lyons,' telling him that he had used it in his composition of Treacle. ('Treacle' was a term used by the old herbalists for a medicine composed of many herbal ingredients.) Gerard looked upon it as an Eastern plant, which he says is grown in many English gardens and might hence be fitly called the 'Sweet Garden Flag.'

Calamus was largely grown from time immemorial for its rhizomes in the East and the Indian rhizomes were imported extensively long after it was common in Europe. The Indian rhizome is said to have a stronger and more agreeable flavour than that obtained in Europe or the United States.

If the Calamus of the Bible is this plant, Exodus xxx. 23, Canticles iv. 14, and Ezekiel xxvii. 19, are the earliest records of its use.

The *Calamus aromaticus* of the Ancients is thought by some to be a plant belonging to the Gentian family, though the description of the plant '*Acoron*,' a native of Colchis, Galatia, Pontus and Crete, given by Dioscorides and Pliny, seems to refer to the Sweet Flag.

It is now found wild on the margins of ponds and rivers in most of the English counties, and is in some parts abundant, especially in the Fen districts. In Scotland it is scarce. It is found in all European countries except Spain, and becomes more abundant eastward and in southern Russia, northern Asia Minor and southern Siberia, China and Japan. It is also found in the northern United States of America, where it appears to be indigenous.

It is cultivated to a small extent in Hungary, Burma and Ceylon, and is common in gardens in India. In northern China another species is cultivated as an ornamental greenhouse plant, but the wild plant is that generally collected for use, especially in Russia, on the shores of the Black Sea. In 1724, Berlu (*Treasury of Drugs*) states that it was 'brought in quantities from Germany,' hence it may be inferred it was not collected in England until a later period, when the London market was supplied from the rivers and marshes of Norfolk, where it was cultivated in the Fen districts, and from the banks of the Thames, as much as £40 having been obtained for the year's crop of a single acre of the riverside land on which it naturally grows. But for many years now the native source has been neglected and the rhizomes for medicinal and commercial use are imported. In dry summers, large quantities are collected in the ditches in Germany, but the greater proportion of the imported drug is derived from southern Russia, via Germany.

In the districts in Norfolk where the plant flourishes the villagers call it 'Gladdon,' so the name would appear to apply to more than one species of the family. A few years since, the 'Gladdon harvest' was an important episode in the country of the 'Broads,' and many small boats might be seen laden with this plant, being brought to shore for marketing purposes. Some of the Norfolk churches in country districts are thatched with this 'reed.'

¶ *Description.* The Sweet Sedge is a perennial herb, in habit somewhat resembling the Iris, with a long, indefinite, branched, cylindrical rhizome immersed in the mud, usually smaller than that of the Iris, about the thickness of a finger and emitting numerous roots. The erect leaves are yellowish-green, 2 to 3 feet in length, few, all radical, sheathing at their bases (which are pink), sword-shaped, narrow and flat, tapering into a long, acute point, the edges entire, but wavy or crimped. The leaves are much like those of Iris, but may readily be distinguished from these and from all others by the peculiar crimped edges and their aromatic odour when bruised.

The scape or flower-stem arises from the axils of the outer leaves, which it much resembles, but is longer and solid and triangular. From one side, near the middle of its length, projecting upwards at an angle, from the stem, it sends out a solid, cylindrical, blunt spike or spadix, tapering at each end, from 2 to 4 inches in length, often somewhat curved and densely crowded with very small greenish-yellow flowers. Each tiny flower contains six stamens enclosed in a perianth with six divisions and surrounding a three-celled, oblong ovary with a sessile stigma. The flowers are sweet-scented and so formed that cross-pollination is ensured, but the plant is not usually fertile in the British Isles, as it is in Asia, the proper insects being absent here. The fruit, which does not ripen in Europe, is a berry, being full of mucus, which falls when ripe into the water or to the ground, and is thus dispersed, but it fruits sparingly everywhere and propagates itself mainly by the rapid growth of its spreading rhizome.

It is easily distinguished from all other British plants by its peculiar spadix, which appears in June and July, and by the fragrance of its roots, stems and leaves.

In most localities the flowers are not very abundantly produced: it never flowers unless actually growing in water.

¶ *Cultivation.* The plants can be propagated very readily by the division of the clumps or of the rhizomes in early spring, or at the commencement of autumn, portions of the rhizome being planted in damp, muddy spots, in marshes or on the margins of water, set 1 foot apart and well covered. It will succeed very well in a garden if the ground is moist, but a rich, moist soil is essential, or it has to be frequently watered.

¶ *Collection.* It is the root-stock or rhizome that is used for medicinal purposes, a digestive medicine being made from it which is official in the United States Pharmacopœia and in several others.

Calamus root has also value as a commercial commodity in various industries.

Experiments have lately been made with a distillation of the leaves, and if the fragrant volatile oil contained in them can be obtained successfully on economic conditions, this will create a trade.

The rhizomes are gathered when large enough, generally after two or three years, and before they lose their firmness and become hollow. Late autumn or early spring is the time chosen for collection.

If actually growing in water, the raft-like masses of interwoven roots and mud, which in a river or lake float about a foot below the surface of the water, are cut out in square sections, raked to the lake edge, the leaves stripped off and separated. Whether growing thus actually in water, or in moist ground, the rhizomes are next thoroughly washed in a trough, and then, deprived of the far less aromatic and brittle rootlets, which are 4 to 6 inches long, unbranched, but near the tip beset with soft, thin fibres.

The fresh root-stock is brownish-red, or greenish-white and reddish within and of a spongy texture, tolerably uniform in transverse section. It has an aromatic sweet odour and a bitterish, pungent taste.

The dried rhizome appears in commerce in tortuous, sub-cylindrical or flattened pieces, a few inches long and from $\frac{1}{2}$ to 1 inch in diameter; externally, yellowish-brown, with blackish patches; sharply longitudinally wrinkled, the upper surface obliquely marked with broad, dark, often fibrous leaf-scales, which are often broadly V-shaped and have sharply projecting margins, the lower surface is thickly pitted with a zigzag line of circular root-scars, which exhibit a low whitish rim and a dark depressed centre. The fracture is short, sharp, corky, whitish and starchy. The texture is spongy, exhibiting numerous oil-cells and scattered wood-bundles.

On drying, Calamus loses from 70 to 75 per cent. in weight, but improves in odour and taste. It deteriorates, however, after long keeping.

Since the oil-cells containing the aromatic essential oil are situated in the outer part, peeling the rhizomes before shipping or distilling, as is often done on the Continent, should not be resorted to. Most of the commercial article has the outer portion of the cortex removed, but the handsome, white peeled (German) Calamus of the market cannot be used in accordance with the official requirements of other pharmacopœias. The peeled rhizome is usually angular and often split. Though white when fresh, it turns pinkish on drying and is less aromatic and bitter than the unpeeled.

¶ *Constituents.* The properties of Calamus are almost entirely due to its volatile oil, obtained by steam distillation. The oil is contained in all parts of the plant, though in greatest quantity in the rhizome, the leaves yielding to distillation 0·2 per cent., the fresh root 1·5 to 3·5 per cent., the dried German root 0·8 per cent., and the Japan root as much as 5 per cent.

The oil is strong and fragrant, its taste warm, bitterish, pungent and aromatic. Its active principles are taken up by boiling water. It is a thick, pale yellow liquid. Little is known of its chemistry, though it possibly contains pinene and the chief aromatic constituent is asaryl aldehyde.

The rhizome also contains alkaloidal matter, mainly Choline (formerly thought to be a specific alkaloid, Calamine); soft resin, gum, starch and the bitter glucoside, Acorin, which is amorphous, semi-fluid, resinous, of neutral reaction, aromatic odour and bitter aromatic taste.

Calamus Oil is used in perfumery – an alcoholate is made with 3 kilos to 3·5 kilos of rhizome to 20 litres of 85 per cent. alcohol.

¶ *Medicinal Action and Uses.* Calamus was formerly much esteemed as an aromatic stimulant and mild tonic. A fluid extract is an official preparation in the United States and some other Pharmacopœias, but it is not now official in the British Pharmacopœia, though it is much used in herbal medicine as an aromatic bitter.

On account of the volatile oil which is present, it also acts as a carminative, removing the discomfort caused by flatulence and checking the growth of the bacteria which give rise to it.

It is used to increase the appetite and benefit digestion, given as fluid extract, infusion or tincture. Tincture of Calamus, obtained by macerating the finely-cut rhizome in alcohol for seven days and filtering, is used as a stomachic and flavouring agent. It has a brownish-yellow colour and a pungent, spicy taste.

The essential oil is used as an addition to inhalations.

The dried root may be chewed *ad libitum* to relieve dyspepsia or an infusion of 1 oz. to 1 pint of boiling water may be taken freely in doses of a teacupful. The dried root is also chewed to clear the voice.

Fluid extract, U.S.P., 15 to 60 drops.

Calamus has been found useful in ague and low fever, and was once greatly used by country people in Norfolk, either in infusion, or powdered, as a remedy against the fever prevalent in the Fens. Its use has been attended with great success where Peruvian bark has failed. It is also beneficial as a mild stimulant in typhoid cases.

The tonic medicine called Stockton Bitters, formerly in much esteem in some parts of England, is made from the root of this plant and that of *Gentiana campestris*.

Waller's *British Herbal* says:

'It is of great service in all nervous complaints, vertigoes, headaches and hypochondriacal affections. Also commended in dysentry and chronic catarrhs. The powdered root may be given, 12 grs. to ½ drachm. In an infusion of 2 drachms to a pint of water or of white wine, it is an agreeable stomachic, even to persons in health, to take a glass about an hour before dinner. When the root is candied with sugar, it is convenient to dyspeptic patients, who may carry it in a small box, in the pocket, and take it as they find occasion.'

On the Continent the candied rhizome is widely employed. The Turks use the candied rhizome as a preventive against contagion.

The rhizome is largely used in native Oriental medicines for dyspepsia and bronchitis and chewed as a cough lozenge, and from the earliest times has been one of the most popular remedies of the native practitioners of India. The candied root is sold as a favourite medicine in every Indian bazaar.

The powdered root is also esteemed in Ceylon and India as a vermifuge and an insecticide, especially in relation to fleas. Sprinkled round a tree attacked by white ants in Malay (Perak) it was found to destroy those that were near the surface and prevented others from attacking the tree.

In powder, Calamus root on account of its spicy flavour serves as a substitute for cinnamon, nutmeg and ginger.

It is said also to be used by snuff manufacturers and to scent hair-powders and in tooth-powders, in the same way as orris.

The highly aromatic volatile oil is largely used in perfumery.

The oil is used by rectifiers to improve the flavour of gin and to give a peculiar taste and fragrance to certain varieties of beer.

In the United States, Calamus was also formerly used by country people as an ingredient in making wine bitters.

In Lithuania, the root is preserved with sugar-like angelica.

The young and tender inflorescence is often eaten by children for its sweetness. In Holland, children use the rhizomes as chewing-gum and also make pop-gun projectiles of them.

The aroma that makes the leaves attractive to us, renders them distasteful to cattle, who do not touch the plant.

There is a seventeenth-century reference to broth 'flavoured with Angelica seed and *Calamus*.'

An extract from Salmon's *Herbal* (1710), giving no less than sixteen different preparations of Calamus, will show in how much greater esteem it was held in former days:

'It is a good stimulant and carminative. The preparations: The root only is of use, and you may have therefrom 1, A liquid Juice. 2, An Essence. 3, An Infusion of Wine. 4, A Decoction in Wine. 5, A Powder. 6, A Cataplasm. 7, A spirituous Tincture. 8, An acid Tincture. 9, An oily Tincture. 10, A Spirit. 11, A chemical Oil. 12, Potestates or Powers. 13, An Elixir. 14, A Collegium. 15, A Preserve. 16, A Syrup. The Liquid Juice, No. 1, was said "to prevail against the bitings of mad dogs and other venomous creatures." It is a peculiar thing against poison, the Plague and all contagious diseases.'

Culpepper says:

'The spicy bitterness of the root of this plant (which he calls the Bastard Flag) bespeaks it as a strengthener of the stomach and head and therefore may fitly be put into any composition of that intention. The root preserved may with good success be used by itself. The leaves, having a very grateful flavour, are by some nice cooks put into sauce for fish.'

¶ *Adulterations.* The rhizome of the Common Yellow Flag (*Iris pseudacorus*) is sometimes mixed with those of the Sweet Flag, when collected in this country, but is readily detected by its darker colour, different structure and want of aromatic odour and taste.

Calamus Draco (Willd.) (*Dæmonorops Draco*, Martius) is a slender palm of the East Indies, yielding the resin 'Dragon's Blood,' obtained from the fruit, used in former times as a mild astringent in diarrhœa, but now never given internally. It was formerly an ingredient of many plasters.

At present, it is mainly used as a colouring agent in pharmacy and the arts, to colour tooth-powders, tinctures and plasters and to impart a mahogany colour to varnishes and wood stains.

The term 'Dragon's Blood' has also been applied to the resin of *Dracæna draca* (Socotra), *Pterocarpus Draco* (West Indies) and *Croton Draco*.

See DRAGON'S BLOOD.

OTHER SEDGES

The Sedge family is of comparatively slight economic importance. The plants are distinguished from the true Grasses, which they closely resemble, by their solid stems, leaf-sheaths which are not connate, and the presence of but a single scale to each flower.

They are mostly coarse, harsh and indigestible, and not adapted for food purposes, though the rhizomes of several have been utilized as starchy foods.

Quite a number possess volatile oils and aromatic principles, while others are rich in astringents – chiefly the species indigenous to India and China.

N.O. Araceæ

Among the more important aromatics and carminatives are *Cyperus sanguinea-fuscus* (Nees), the Cure-pire of Paraguay, *C. elegans* (Rottb.) of Mexico; *C. pertenuis* (Roxb.), the Indian Nagar-motha or Koriak, whose roots, when dried and powdered, are used by the Indian ladies for perfuming their hair; and *C. tegetum* (Roxb.); *Adrue* or *Guinea Rush* is the rhizome of *C. articulatus* (Linn.), which, besides being used as a carminative, has a high repute in the East Indies for anti-emetic properties. The blackish tubers have a somewhat bitter, aromatic taste, resembling that of Lavender. A fluid extract is prepared from them used in herbal medicine. The aromatic properties of the drug cause a feeling of warmth to be diffused throughout the system and act as a sedative in dyspeptic disorders. It is common also in Jamaica and on the banks of the Nile.

Two Indian species of Sedge, *C. rotundus* and *C. scarious*, also possess fragrant roots, largely employed in Eastern perfumes, but they are little used in Europe.

The tubers of *C. hexastachys* are said to be successfully used by Hindu practitioners in cases of cholera. They call the plant 'Mootha.'

The tubers of *C. bulbosus* are said to taste like potatoes when roasted, and would be valuable for food if they were bigger.

The root of *C. odoratus* has a warm, aromatic taste, and is given in India in infusions as a stomachic.

The roots of the Sweet Cyperus or English Galingale (*C. longus*, Linn.) were once esteemed as an aromatic tonic, considered good as a stomachic and serviceable in the first stages of dropsy, but they have now fallen into disuse. This species is a native of France, Germany, Italy and Sicily, but very rare in this country, being only found in a few places in Dorsetshire and Wales. The plants throw up erect triangular stems, about 2 feet high, bearing three long, channelled, drooping leaves and a lax, compound umbel of flat flower-spikes, which renders it very ornamental when in flower.

C. esculentus is a native of Italy and Sicily and the Levant. Its roots are fibrous, with small round tubers hanging from them, of the size of peas, which taste like sweet filberts and are eaten in Italy, and sold in the markets.

The French call the tubers *Souchet comestible* or *Amande de terre*.

C. Papyrus is the Egyptian Papyrus, the fibrous stems of which provided the earliest form of paper known.

This plant had various economic uses, as Pliny and other writers have shown, though as the Egyptians cultivated other Sedges, it is probable that these became more exclusively used for food and fuel, sails and cordage, baskets and sieves, not to speak of punts or canoes to which the prophet Isaiah refers (Isaiah xviii. 2), where the Ethiopians are spoken of as sending ambassadors by the sea even in *vessels of bulrushes* upon the waters (the Hebrew word is *gome*). The papyrus was, in ancient times, carefully cultivated, especially in certain districts of Lower, and probably of Upper Egypt also, for the great and important purpose with which its name must ever be associated.

For this manufacture the rind was removed, the pith cut in strips and laid lengthwise on a flat board, their edges united by some glue or cement (Pliny says 'Nile water'), and the whole subjected to pressure, compacting the several strips into one uniform fabric. This material was well known to the Ancients, and continued to be used in Europe until the time of Charlemagne, when it was superseded by parchment. It is remarkable that although we have no trace in Scripture of the use of papyrus or other vegetable substance by the Jews for writing purposes, the plant has been found to exist in vast quantities in the Lake Merom at the northern end of the Lake of Tiberias, and in some of the streams which flow into the Mediterranean.

On the other hand, it has disappeared from Egypt, where it once grew in quantity. It is also grown in Sicily and Sardinia, but on a limited scale.

Of the Papyrus, or some allied species of Sedge, Heliodorus relates that the Ethiopians made swift-sailing wherries, capable of carrying two or three men; and the traveller Bruce refers to a similar use of this ancient plant among the modern Abyssinians.

Other writers give similar testimony, and it is highly probable that such light vessels were coated with bitumen, like the rude basket made by Jochabed for the infant Moses (Exod. ii. 3).

The stems of the Papyrus were likewise used for ornamenting Egyptian temples, and crowning the statues of their gods.

This plant, if grown in Britain, requires the aid of a stove to grow it properly, and then it must have a good supply of water.

Scirpus lacustris, the Great Club-Rush or Common Bulrush, is used for making chair seats, mats and hassocks, being imported dried, in large bundles from Holland. The roots are astringent and diuretic and were formerly employed in medicine, but are now no longer used.

S. capillaris is used in Spanish America under the name of Espartillo, as a pectoral.

Other British species are the chocolate-headed Club-Rush (*S. pauciflorus*), Deer's-hair (*S. cæspitosus*), Dwarf Club-Rush (*S. nanus*), Floating Mud-Rush (*S. fluitans*), Savi's Mud-Rush (*S. cernuus*), Bristle-like Mud-Rush (*S. sætaceus*), Round-headed Mud-Rush (*S. Holoschœuus*), and eight others of the genus *Scirpus*.

Kyllingia monocephala is used in Paraguay as a substitute for Calamus.

Carex arenaria (Linn.), the Sand Sedge, is a familiar seaside species of Sedge, which is very widely distributed and common on sandy coasts, growing on sand-dunes and elsewhere at high-water mark, amongst grasses and herbage, helping to bind it together.

The plant is perennial, propagating itself rapidly in loose sand, on which account it is planted on dykes in Holland for the purpose of binding the sand by means of its long and interlacing underground stems, which penetrate horizontally about 4 inches below the surface, thus helping to prevent the incursions of the sea. It has been used for this purpose also on the British East Coast.

The rhizomes have been used medicinally in Germany as a substitute for Sarsaparilla, in the same way that Couch Grass is here employed, having diuretic and sudorific properties.

C. vulpinoides, an allied species to *C. vulpina* (Great or Fox Sedge), is a North American plant, but has been found on the banks of the Thames near Kew.

There are sixty-nine species of *Carex* given by Johns (*Flowers of the Field*), besides those mentioned above; some only grow in Scotland, and none have medicinal or practical uses. *Eriophorum angustifolium* (Cotton Grass),

with its long white tufts of hair, is very decorative on our bogs and mosses in the middle of summer. The down is used in moorland districts for stuffing pillows, and attempts have been made to employ it as a substitute for cotton, under the name of 'Arctic Wool,' thread having been spun from it, but the fibres are more brittle than those of cotton and do not bear twisting as well. Candles and lamp wicks have been made from the down by country people.

In former days the leaves and roots had some reputation in northern countries as a medicine in diarrhœa, as like most members of the Sedge family, they possess considerable astringency.

The name *Eriophorum* is from the Greek *erion* (wool) and *phero* (I bear).

Culpepper approved of the use of 'Bulrushes' and 'some of the smoother sorts,' but considered they should be 'given with caution,' as they were apt to 'cause head-ache, and provoke sleep. The root, boiled in water, to the consumption of one-third, helps the cough.'

See GRASSES.

SELF-HEAL
Prunella vulgaris (LINN.)
N.O. Labiatæ

Synonyms. Prunella. All-Heal. Hook-Heal. Slough-Heal. Brunella. Heart of the Earth. Blue Curls
Part Used. Herb
Habitat. Common throughout the British Isles and Europe

The Self-Heal holds an equal place with Bugle in the esteem of herbalists.

¶ *Description.* It may at once be distinguished from other members of the great Labiate order because on the top of its flowering stalks, the flowers – to quote Culpepper – are 'thicke set together like an eare or spiky knap.' No other plant is at all like it. Immediately below this ear are a pair of stalkless leaves standing out on either side like a collar. The flowers and bracts of this spike or 'ear' are arranged in most regular tiers or whorls, each tier composed of a ring of six stalkless flowers, supported by a couple of spreading, sharp-pointed bracts. The number of whorls varies from half a dozen to a dozen. The flower-spike is at first very short, compact and cylindrical, but then opens out somewhat, maintaining much the same size throughout its length, not tapering as in the flower spikes of most other flowers. The flowers do not come out simultaneously in any one ring, so that a somewhat ragged-looking head of flowers is produced.

Each flower consists of a two-lipped calyx, the upper lip very wide and flat, edged with three blunt teeth, the lower lip much nar-

rower and with two long, pointed teeth. Both lips have red margins and carry hairs. The two-lipped corolla is of a deep purple hue, the upper lip strongly arched, on the top of the arch many hairs standing on end, and the lower lip of much the same length, spreading out into three holes. Under the roofing upper lip are two pairs of stamens, one pair longer than the other, their filaments ending in two little branches, one of which carries an anther, the other remaining a little spike. Through the centre of the two pairs of stamens the long style runs, curving so as to fit under the lip, its lower end set between four nutlets. Honey lies at the bottom of the corolla tube, protected from tiny insects by a thick hedge of hairs placed just above it. The flower is adapted by this formation, like the rest of the Labiate group, for fertilization by bees, who alight on the lower lip and in thrusting their probosces down the tube for the honey, dust their heads with the pollen from the anthers and then on visiting the next flower, smear this pollen on the end of the curving style that runs up the arch of the upper lip and thus effect fertilization. After fertilization is effected, the corolla falls out of the sheath-like calyx, which, however, remains in place, as do also the two bracts supporting each whorl. When all the purple corollas have fallen and only the rings of the persistent calyces remain, the resemblance to an ear of corn, which Culpepper points out, is very marked.

The plant does not rely wholly for its propagation on the four little nutlets that ripen within the continually reddening calyx, even though the flowering season is particularly long, lasting through all the summer months, for its creeping stems can throw out roots at every point, new plants thus being formed, as in the case of the Bugle. It is from the creeping stems that the flowering spikes arise, standing upright among the herbage, 3 inches to a foot in height.

The leaves, oblong in form and blunt, about an inch long and ½ inch broad, grow on short stalks in pairs down the square stem, from which they stand out boldly, and are often roughish on the top, with scattered, close hairs, their mid-rib at the back also carrying hairs and their margins fringed with tiny hairs. Their outline is either one continuous line, or they are slightly indented along their margins.

¶ *Habitat.* Self-Heal is a very common plant throughout Britain and all over Europe, abundant in pastures and on waste ground. In open and exposed situations, the plant is diminutive, while in more sheltered spots it is larger in all its parts. It branches freely, lateral stems being thrown out in pairs at almost every node, from which the leaves spring. The main stem is often deeply grooved and rough to the touch, the lower parts tinted with reddish purple.

Self-Heal is one of those common wildflowers that have found their way to North America, tending even to oust the native flowers. It is known there as 'Heart of the Earth' and 'Blue Curls.'

Cole, in *Adam in Eden* (1657), says:

'It is called by modern writers (for neither the ancient Greek nor Latin writers knew it) Brunella, from Brunellen, which is a name given unto it by the Germans, because it cureth that inflammation of the mouth which they call "die Breuen," yet the general name of it in Latin nowadays is Prunella, as being a word of a more gentile pronunciation.'

Cole further explains that the disease in question 'is common to soldiers when they lye in camp, but especially in garrisons, coming with an extraordinary inflammation or swelling, as well in the mouth as throat, the very signature of the Throat which the form of the Floures so represent signifying as

much' – an instance of the doctrine of signatures of which William Cole was such a ready exponent.

'There is not a better Wound herbe,' says Gerard, 'in the world than that of Self-Heale is, the very name importing it to be very admirable upon this account and indeed the Virtues doe make it good, for this very herbe without the mixture of any other ingredient, being onely bruised and wrought with the point of a knife upon a trencher or the like, will be brought into the form of a salve, which will heal any green wounde even in the first intention, after a very wonderful manner. The decoction of Prunell made with wine and water doth join together and make whole and sound all wounds, both inward and outward, even as Bugle doth. To be short, it serveth for the same that the Bugle serveth and in the world there are not two better wound herbs as hath been often proved.'

¶ *Constituents.* The chemical principles of Bugle and Self-Heal resemble those of the other Labiate herbs, comprising a volatile oil; some bitter principle, not yet analysed; tannin, to which its chief medicinal use is due; sugar and cellulose.

¶ *Part Used.* The whole herb, collected when in best condition in mid-summer.

¶ *Medicinal Action and Uses.* Astringent, styptic and tonic.

Self-Heal is still in use in modern herbal treatment as a useful astringent for inward or outward use.

An infusion of the herb, made from 1 oz. to a pint of boiling water, and taken in doses of a wineglassful, is considered a general strengthener. Sweetened with honey, it is good for a sore and relaxed throat or ulcerated mouth, for both of which purposes it also makes a good gargle. For internal bleeding and for piles, the infusion is also used as an injection.

Culpepper, explaining the name 'Self-Heal whereby when you are hurt, you may heal yourself,' tells us that

'it is an especial herb for inward or outward wounds. Take it inwardly in syrups for inward wounds, outwardly in unguents and plasters for outward. As Self-Heal is like Bugle in form, so also in the qualities and virtues, serving for all purposes, whereunto Bugle is applied with good success either inwardly or outwardly; for inward wounds or ulcers in the body, for bruises or falls and hurts. If it be combined with Bugle, Sanicle and other like wound herbs, it will be more effectual to wash and inject into ulcers in the parts outwardly. . . . It is an especial remedy for all green wounds to close the lips of them and to keep the place from further inconveniences. The juice used with oil of roses to annoint the temples and forehead is very effectual to remove the headache, and the same mixed with honey of roses cleaneth and healeth ulcers in the mouth and throat.'

SENEGA

Polygala Senega (LINN.)
N.O. Polygaleæ

Synonyms. Snake Root. Senegæ Radix. Seneca. Seneka. Polygala Virginiana. Plantula Marilandica. Senega officinalis. Milkwort. Mountain Flax. Rattlesnake Root
Part Used. Dried Root
Habitat. North America

¶ *Description.* This perennial herb, about a foot high, grows throughout central and western North America, in woods, and on dry, rocky soil. The leaves are small alternate, and narrowly lanceolate, and the numerous, small pinky-white flowers are crowded on to a narrow, terminal spike from 1 to 2 inches long.

The name of the genus, *Polygala*, means 'much milk,' alluding, to its own profuse secretions and their effects. 'Senega' is derived from the Seneca tribe of North American Indians, among whom the plant was used as a remedy for snake-bites.

The root, varying in colour from light yellowish grey to brownish grey, and in size from the thickness of a straw to that of the little finger, has as its distinguishing mark a projecting line, along its concave side. It is usually twisted, sometimes almost spiral, and has at its upper end a thick, irregular, knotty crown, showing traces of numerous, wiry stems. It breaks with a short fracture, the wood often showing an abnormal appearance, since one or two wedge-shaped portions may be replaced by parenchymatous tissue, as if a segment of wood had been cut out. The keels are due to the development of the bast, and not to any abnormality in the wood. The odour and taste resemble that of Wintergreen.

About 1735, Dr. John Tennent, a Scottish physician living in Pennsylvania, was introduced to the use of the root by the Seneca Indians for curing rattlesnake-bite. As the symptoms were similar to those of pleurisy and the latter stages of pleuropneumonia, he experimented with it in those diseases with success, and as a result the drug was accepted in Europe and cultivated in England in 1739. The roots should be gathered when the leaves are dead, and before the first frost. From carelessness in collection other roots are often found mixed with it, but not for intentional adulteration. The root of commerce is obtained from *Polygala latifolia* also, this species being several inches taller and having larger leaves than *P. Senega.* The dried roots, usually in broken pieces, are brought into market in bales weighing from 50 to 400 lb. They vary a little in appearance according to their locality. The official Senega is the small Southern Senega, 400 to 500 of the dried roots of which are required to make a pound. Manitoba Senega is larger and darker, often with purple markings near the crown. The Northern, White, False, or Large Senega, comes from Wisconsin, Minnesota, and farther west. About 80 to 100 of its roots will make a pound. It is stated that it is not possible to distinguish the two when powdered.

¶ *Constituents.* The root contains polygalic acid, virgineic acid, pectic and tannic acids, yellow, bitter, colouring matter, cerin fixed oil, gum, albumen, woody fibre, salts, alumina, silica, magnesia and iron. The powder is yellowish-grey to light yellowish-brown.

The active principle, contained in the bark, is Senegin (which some authorities regard as another name for polygalic acid, while others differentiate between the two). It is a white powder easily soluble in hot water and alcohol, forming a soapy emulsion when mixed with boiling water. It is almost identical with the saponin of *Saponaria officinalis* and *Quillaria Saponaria.* Thus its influence counteracts, or can be counteracted, by digitalis.

Another analysis, in 1889, gives fixed oil and resin, traces of volatile oil (a mixture of valeric ether and methyl salicylate), 7 per cent. sugar, from 2 to 5 per cent. senegin, yellow colouring-matter, and malates.

It is advisable to use an alkali in small proportion in making galenical preparations of senega.

Oil of Senega is bitter, rancid, and disagreeable, with the consistency of syrup and an acid reaction. It is not Seneca oil.

¶ *Medicinal Action and Uses.* A stimulating expectorant, diuretic and diaphoretic. The Ancients regarded its action as identical with that of ipecacuanha, but in doses of three times the strength. It should be used when the power to expectorate is small – very useful in the second stage of acute bronchial

733

catarrh or pneumonia. It is of little value when the expectoration is tough and scanty, but very helpful in chronic pneumonia or bronchitis or dropsy dependent on renal disease. Spirit of chloroform will lessen its disagreeable taste. It has been used also in croup, whooping-cough, and rheumatism.

As it stimulates most of the secretions, it is also useful as a sialagogue and emmenagogue. In active inflammation its use is contra-indicated.

In large doses it is emetic and cathartic.

¶ *Dosages.* Powdered root, 5 to 20 grains. Fluid extract, 10 to 20 drops. Of infusion, B.P., 4 to 8 drachms. Of syrup, U.S.P., 1 drachm. Of tincture, B.P., ½ to 1 drachm. Conct. Solut., B.P., ½ to 1 drachm.

¶ *Poisons and Antidotes.* In overdose it can act as an irritant or general protoplasmic poison, with violent vomiting and purging. A dose of from 10 minims of the tincture to a scruple of the powdered root will cause heaviness and vertigo, dazzling vision, sneez-

ing, inflammation of the œsophagus, with constriction, thirst, nausea, mucous vomiting, colic, scalding, frothy urine, irritation of the larynx, and general debility. Like saponin, it causes a paresis of the muscles of the respiratory tract and the vaso-motor system in general, resulting in capillary congestions followed by rapid exosmosis.

¶ *Adulterations and Other Species.*
Panax quinquefolium, or American Ginseng Root, is the most common admixture. It is larger and has no ridge.

Various species of *Gillenia*, *Asclepias Vincetoxicum*, or Swallow-wort, *Triosteum perfoliatum*, and the rhizome of *Cypripedium pubescens* have also been found in parcels. They have a different taste and odour, and show no ridge.

P. Boykinii or *P. Alba* resemble *P. Senega*, but have no ridge and are much less acrid.

Arnica, Valerian, Serpentary and Green Hellebore roots resemble it, but have no keel.

SENNA

Cassia Acutifolia (DELL.)
N.O. Leguminosæ

Synonyms. Alexandrian Senna. Nubian Senna. Cassia Senna. Cassia lenitiva. Cassia Lanceolata. Cassia officinalis. Cassia æthiopica. Senna acutifolia. Egyptian Senna. Sēnē de la palthe. Tinnevelly Senna. Cassia angustifolia. East Indian Senna
Parts Used. Dried leaflets, pods
Habitat. Egypt, Nubia, Arabia, Sennar

¶ *Description.* Several species of *Cassia* contribute to the drug of commerce, and were comprised in a single species by Linnæus under the name of *Cassia Senna*. Since his day, the subject has been more fully investigated, and it is known that several countries utilize the leaves of their own indigenous varieties in the same way. The two most widely exported and officially recognized are *C. acutifolia* and *C. angustifolia* (India or Tinnevelly Senna).

C. acutifolia, yielding the finest and most valuable variety of the drug is a small shrub about 2 feet high. The stem is erect, smooth, and pale green, with long, spreading branches, bearing leaflets in four or five pairs, averaging an inch long, lanceolate or obovate, unequally oblique at the base, veins distinct on the under surface, brittle, greyish-green, of a faint, peculiar odour, and mucilaginous, sweetish taste. The form of the base, and freedom from bitterness, distinguish the Senna from the Argel leaves, which are also thicker and stiffer. The flowers are small and yellow. The pods are broadly oblong, about 2 inches long by ⅞ inch broad, and contain about six seeds.

Senna is an Arabian name, and the drug was first brought into use by the Arabian physicians Serapion and Mesue, and Achi-

arius was the first of the Greeks to notice it. He recommends not the leaves but the fruit, and Mesue also prefers the pods to the leaves, thinking them more powerful, though they are actually less so, but they do not cause griping.

The leaves of *C. acutifolia* are collected principally in Nubia. Ignatius Pallme, who travelled much in Africa, wrote:

'Senna is found in abundance in many parts of Kardofan, but the leaves are not collected on account of the existing monopoly. The Government draws its supplies from Dongola in Nubia.'

Two crops are collected annually in Nubia, the more abundant in September, after the rains, the other in April, in dry seasons a very bad one. The plants are cut down, exposed on the rocks in hot sunshine until thoroughly dry, then stripped, and packed in palm-leaf bags, being sent thus on camels to Essouan and Darao, and by the Nile to Cairo, or via Massowah and Suakin on the Red Sea. It is made up at Boulak, near Cairo, under the superintendence of the Egyptian Government, though much adulteration takes place there. The leaves are loosely packed, and as they curl when drying, often present this appearance, while Indian

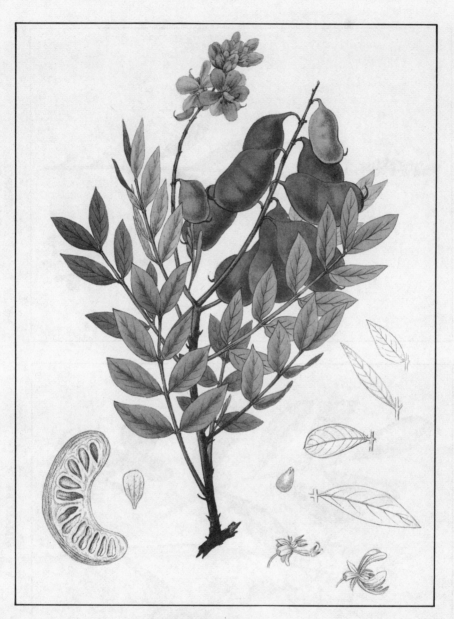

SENNA
Cassia Acutifolia

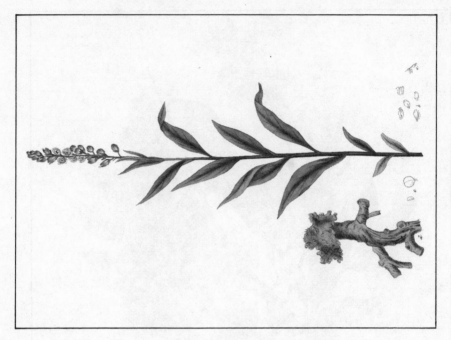

SENEGA
Polygala Senega

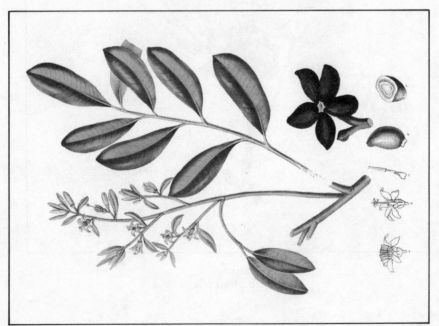

SIMARUBA
Simaruba Amara

Senna is packed tightly, and the leaves come out flat.

Senna appears to have been cultivated in England about 1640. By keeping the plants in a hot-bed all the summer, they frequently flowered; but rarely perfected their seeds.

Commercial Senna is prepared for use by *garbling*, or picking out the leaflets and rejecting the lead-stalks, impurities, and leaves of other plants. The amount annually exported is about 8,000 bales of each of the varieties, and the price is high, owing to the failure of the crops at certain seasons. Good Senna may be known by the bright, fresh, yellowish-green colour of the leaves, with a faint and peculiar odour rather like green tea, and a nauseous, mucilaginous, sweetish, slightly bitter taste. It should be powdered only as wanted, because the powder absorbs moisture, becomes mouldy, and loses its value. Boiling destroys its virtues, unless it be in *vacuo*, or in a covered vessel.

¶ *Constituents*. Water and diluted alcohol extract the active principles of Senna. Pure alcohol only extracts them imperfectly. The leaves yield about one-third of their weight to boiling water.

The purgative constituents are closely allied to those of Aloes and Rhubarb, the activities of the drug being largely due to anthraquinone derivatives and their glucosides. It contains rhein, aloe-emedin, kæmpferol, isormamnetin, both free and as glucosides together with myricyl alcohol, etc. The ash amounts to about 8 per cent., consisting chiefly of earthy and ashy carbonates.

The active purgative principle was discovered in 1866. It is a glucoside of weak acid character, and was named Cathartic Acid. By boiling its alcoholic solution with acids it yields Cathartogenic Acid and sugar. There were also found Chrysophanic Acid, Sennacrol and Sennapicrin, and a peculiar non-fermentable saccharine principle which was named Cathartomannite or Sennit.

The conclusions reached after experimenting with Senna leaves washed with alcohol were as follows:

(1) Strong spirit does not remove any of the active principle from Senna leaves.

(2) The therapeutic action of cathartic acid is assisted by one or more of the constituents yielded by Senna to strong alcohol, though these constituents produce no purgative effect when taken alone.

(3) Senna exhausted by alcohol is a reliable and pleasant purgative, but somewhat weaker in its action than the unexhausted leaves.

Many substances produce precipitates with the infusion of Senna, but they may remove only inert ingredients, and not be really incompatible medicinally. Cathartic acid is precipitated by infusion of galls and solution of lead subacetate. Lead acetate and tartar emetic, which disturb the infusion, have no effect upon a solution of this substance.

Cathartin is the name of a mixture of the salts of cathartic acid which may be used in doses of from 3 to 6 grains.

Sennax is the name applied to the water-soluble glucoside of Senna, marketed in tablets containing 0·075 gram each.

¶ *Medicinal Action and Uses*. Purgative. Its action being chiefly on the lower bowel, it is especially suitable in habitual costiveness. It increases the peristaltic movements of the colon by its local action upon the intestinal wall. Its active principle must pass out of the system in the secretions unaltered, for when Senna is taken by nurses, the suckling infant becomes purged. It acts neither as a sedative nor as a refrigerant, but has a slight, stimulating influence. In addition to the nauseating taste, it is apt to cause sickness, and griping pains, so that few can take it alone; but these characteristics can be overcome or removed, when it is well adapted for children, elderly persons, and delicate women. The colouring matter is absorbable, and twenty or thirty minutes after the ingestion of the drug it appears in the urine, and may be recognized by a red colour on the addition of ammonia.

The addition of cloves, ginger, cinnamon, or other aromatics are excellent correctives of the nauseous effects. A teaspoonful of cream of tartar to a teacupful of the decoction of infusion of Senna, is a mild and pleasant cathartic, well suited for women if required soon after delivery. Some practitioners add neutral laxative salts, or saccharine and aromatic substances. The purgative effect is increased by the addition of pure bitters; the decoction of guaiacum is said to answer a similar purpose. Senna is contraindicated in an inflammatory condition of the alimentary canal, hæmorrhoids, prolapsus, ani, etc. The well-known 'black draught' is a combination of Senna and Gentian, with any aromatic, as cardamom or coriander seeds, or the rind of the Seville orange. The term 'black draught,' it is stated, should never be used, as mistakes have been made in reading the prescriptions, and 'black drop' or vinegar of opium has been given instead, several deaths having been caused in this way.

SENNA PODS, or the dried, ripe fruits, are official in the British Pharmacopœia, though the quantity is restricted, as an adulterant, in the United States Pharmacopœia.

They are milder in their effects than the leaflets, as the griping is largely due to the resin, and the pods contain none, but have about 25 per cent. more cathartic acid and emodin than the leaves, without volatile oil. From 6 to 12 pods for the adult, or from 3 to 6 for the young or very aged, infused in a claret-glass of cold water, act mildly but thoroughly upon the whole intestine.

The fluid extract was formerly treated with alcohol for the removal of the griping principles, but the process was deleted from the United States Pharmacopœia. The fluid extract is a dark, blackish, thick and somewhat turbid liquid, with a strong flavour of Senna. It is well adapted for exhibition with saline cathartics, such as Epsom salt or cream of tartar. In this case not more than half the full dose should be given at once. The British Pharmacopœia 1898 'Liquor Sennæ Concentratus' was more like a concentrated infusion than a fluid extract, but had the same strength as the latter, the menstrum being distilled water; tincture of ginger and alcohol being added.

The infusion of Senna, or Senna Tea, consists of 100 grams of Senna leaves, 5 grams of sliced Ginger, 1,000 millilitres of distilled water, boiling. Infuse in a covered vessel for fifteen minutes, and strain, while hot. The United States Pharmacopœia prefers coriander to ginger. The infusion deposits, on exposure to air, a yellowish precipitate, so it is advisable to make it in very small quantities, as the deposit aggravates its griping tendency. It is usual to prescribe manna and one of the saline cathartics with it. The cold infusion is said to be less unpleasant in taste, and equal in strength to the hot.

SYRUP OF SENNA is prepared by mixing 8 fluid ounces, 218 minims of fluid extract of Senna, with 81 minims of oil of Coriander and sufficient syrup to make 33 fluid ounces (6½ fluid drachms).

The Aromatic Syrup includes also jalap, rhubarb, cinnamon, clove, nutmeg, oil of lemon, sugar, and diluted alcohol.

The Compound Syrup includes rhubarb, frangula, methyl salicylate, alcohol, and syrup.

¶ *Dosages.* Powdered leaves, 1 drachm. Conct. solution, B.P., ½ to 1 drachm. Of compound or aromatic syrup, 2 fluid drachms. Of U.S.P. syrup, for an adult, 1 to 4 fluid drachms. Of B.P. syrup, 1 to 2 fluid drachms. Of Senna, ½ to 2 drachms. Of compound mixture, B.P., 4 to 16 drachms. Of infusion, B.P., ½ to 2 fluid ounces. Of fluid extract, for an adult, ½ to 2 fluid drachms. Of confection, B.P., 1 to 2 drachms.

¶ *Adulterations and Other Species Used.* Owing to the high price, what is known as 'broken Senna' is found on the market and sold for the genuine article with government sanction in the United States of America. Also, 'Senna siftings,' containing sand and other foreign matter have been offered for sale, causing trouble to government inspectors.

Formerly there was an intentional mixture of 5 parts of *C. acutifolia*, 3 of *C. obovata*, and 2 of *Cynanchum*, but now Alexandrian Senna is more uniform. It is often called in the French Pharmacopœia *séné de la palthe*, because of the duty formerly laid upon it by the Ottoman Porte. A parcel of Alexandrian Senna in the market formerly consisted of (1) leaflets of *C. acutifolia*, (2) leaflets of *C. obovata*, (3) the pods, broken leaf-stalks, flowers, and fine fragments of either, (4) leaves of *Cynanchum oleofolium*. The last are larger, thicker, regular at the base, and have no lateral nerves visible on their undersurface. They must be regarded as an adulteration.

C. angustifolia or *Tinnevelly Senna, Senna Indica, C. elongata*, is an annual growing in the Yemen and Hadramaut provinces of Arabia Felix, in Somaliland, Mozambique, Scind, and the Punjab. In Southern India it is cultivated and grows to a larger size. In the German and Swiss Pharmacopœias, the official drug is restricted to Tinnevelly Senna, and also in the British Pharmacopœia and the Pharmacopœia of India. *Senna Indica* also includes the variety known as Arabian, Mocha, Bombay, or East Indian Senna. Both varieties, as well as Alexandrian Senna, are official in the United States Pharmacopœia.

There is a certain difference in the qualities and also in the names of the species imported into Britain and America. The fine Tinnevelly Senna goes from Madras or Tuticorin to Britain. The leaflets are unbroken, from 1 to 2 or more inches long, thin, flexible, and green.

It has been stated that it contains only two-thirds as much of the active principle as the Alexandrian.

The other, or Arabian variety, comes via Mocha and Bombay, and is less pure and less carefully prepared. The leaflets are long and narrow, pike-like, so are called in France *séné de la pique*. Leaflets resembling these were brought by Livingstone from Southeast Africa. *Mecca Senna*, also known in America as Arabian or Bombay Senna, is obtained from both the wild and the cultivated kinds of *C. angustifolia*. The best comes from British India. The variety has sometimes a yellowish or tawny colour, more like the Indica than the Alexandrian, and may be the product of *C. lanceolata* of Forskhal. *C. obovata, C. obtusa* or *Senna obtusa* is usually a perennial, found wild in Egypt, Nubia, Abyssinia, Tripoli, Senegal and Benguella, Arabia and India. It was the first kind of Senna known, and being brought by the Moors into Europe, was formerly cultivated in Northern Italy, Spain, and Southern France, and called *S. italica*. It is official in the British Pharmacopœia and the Pharmacopœia of India as one of the botanical sources of Alexandrian Senna, but now few of its leaflets are included. It is called by the Arabs *S. baladi*, i.e. indigenous or wild Senna, to distinguish it from *C. acutifolia, S. jebeli*, or Mountain Senna. It is common in Jamaica, where its cultivation has been suggested, and where it is called Port Royal Senna or Jamaica Senna.

C. Marilandica or *American Senna, Wild Senna, Poinciana pulcherima*, formerly *Maryland Senna*, is a common perennial from New England to Northern Carolina. Its leaves are compressed into oblong cakes like other herbal preparations of the Shakers. It acts like Senna, but is weaker, and should be combined with aromatics. The dose in powder is from $\frac{1}{2}$ to $2\frac{1}{2}$ drachms. For the infusion, add 1 ounce of the leaves and 1 drachm of coriander seeds to 1 pint of boiling water. Macerate for an hour in a covered vessel, and strain. Dose: 4 to 5 fluid ounces. These leaves are also found mixed with or substituted for Alexandrian Senna.

C. Chamæcrista, Prairie Senna, Partridge Pea, Dwarf Cassia, or *Sensitive Pea*, found on the Western Prairies, is an excellent substitute for the above.

C. fistula, or *Purging Cassia, C. Stick, Pudding Pipe-Tree*, or *Alexandrian Purging Cassia*, is a tree rising to 40 feet in height, the pulp of the pods being used in the electuary of Senna. It is found in Egypt, the Indies, China, etc.

Colutea arborescens, or *Bladder-Senna (see* SENNA, BLADDER), *Baguenaudier, Séné Indigène*, the *Sutherlandia frutescens* of the Cape, formerly often met with as a substitute, is now usually replaced by *Globularia Turbith* or *Alypum*, the leaves of which are milder, so that a double dose may be taken. It is the Wild Senna of Europe.

Coriaria Myrtifolia is a Mediterranean shrub and highly poisonous, so that it should be recognized when present. The leaves are green, very thin, and soft, three veined, ovate-lanceolate, and equal at the base. It grows wild in Southern Europe, and its leaves are used as a black dye. It is also used to adulterate sweet marjoram. Deaths are recorded from eating the small, black berries. A Mexican drug, Tlolocopetale, containing coriarin and coriamurtin, is said to be a product. Other names are *Currierts Sumach* and *Redoul*.

Argel leaves (Solenostemma or *Cynanchum Argel)*, from Nubia, are paler in colour, have less conspicuous veins, and an equal base.

Tephrosia leaflets and legumes (*Tephrosia Apollinea*), from the banks of the Nile, are silky or silvery, equal at the base and usually folded longitudinally on their mid-rib.

Jaborandi Leaflets (Bilocarpus Microphyllus) have been imported under the name of Senna.

Aden Senna is believed to be obtained from *C. holosericeæ*.

C. montana yields a false Senna from Madras, partly resembling the Tinnevelly Senna, though the colour of the upper surface of the leaves is browner.

It must be remembered that the Senna leaf contains no tannic acid and does not alter a ferric solution, while most of those encountered as adulterations precipitate ferric-chloride.

Other varieties used in their native countries, of which little appears to be known, are also:

C. cathartica, C. rugosa, C. splendida, C. lævigata, C. multijuja, Coronilla Emerus or Scorpion Senna, *C. obovata* or Senegal Senna.

SENNA, BLADDER

Colutea arborescens
N.O. Leguminosæ

Part Used. Leaves

Habitat. Indigenous to Southern Europe, Mediterranean region, said to be the sole vegetation found growing on the crater of Vesuvius

¶ *Description.* Cultivated in Britain as a decorative shrub, flowers yellow, papilionaceous, specially characterized by membraneous, bladder-like pods, which when pressed go off with a loud bang, hence its name of Bladder Senna. The plant grows well in the author's garden.

¶ *Medicinal Action and Uses.* The leaflets are purgative and on the Continent are often substituted for Senna leaves, but they are much milder in action than the true Senna. Taken in the form of an infusion, 1 or 2 drachms of the seeds will excite vomiting.

SENSITIVE PLANT. *See* MIMOSAS

SHALLOT. *See* GARLIC, ONION

SHEEP'S SORREL. *See* SORREL

SHEPHERD'S PURSE

Capsella bursa-pastoris (MEDIC.)
N.O. Cruciferæ

Synonyms. Shepherd's Bag. Shepherd's Scrip. Shepherd's Sprout. Lady's Purse. Witches' Pouches. Rattle Pouches. Case-weed. Pick-Pocket. Pick-Purse. Blindweed. Pepper-and-Salt. Poor Man's Parmacettie. Sanguinary. Mother's Heart. Clappedepouch (*Irish*)
(*French*) Bourse de pasteur
(*German*) Hirtentasche
Part Used. Whole plant
Habitat. All over the world, outside the tropics. It is probably of European or West Asiatic origin, and is abundant in Britain, flowering all the year round

Shepherd's Purse is so called from the resemblance of the flat seed-pouches of the plant to an old-fashioned common leather purse. It is similarly called in France *Bourse de pasteur*, and in Germany *Hirtentasche.*

The Irish name of 'Clappedepouch' was given in allusion to the begging of lepers, who stood at cross-roads with a bell or clapper, receiving their alms in a cup at the end of a long pole.

It is a common weed of the Cruciferous order, said to be found all over the world and flourishing nearly the whole year round.

A native of Europe, the plant has accompanied Europeans in all their migrations and established itself wherever they have settled to till the soil. In John Josselyn's *Herbal* it is one of the plants named as unknown to the New World before the Pilgrim Fathers settled there.

It will flourish and set seed in the poorest soil, though it may only attain the height of a few inches. In rich soil it luxuriates and grows to 2 feet in height.

¶ *Description.* The plant is green, but somewhat rough with hairs. The main leaves, 2 to 6 inches long, are very variable in form, either irregularly pinnatifid or entire and toothed. When not in flower, it may be distinguished by its radiating leaves, of which the outer lie close to the earth.

The slender stem, which rises from the crown of the root, from the centre of the rosette of radical leaves, is usually sparingly branched. It is smooth, except at the lower part, and bears a few, small, oblong leaves, arrow-shaped at the base, and above them, numerous small, white, inconspicuous flowers, which are self-fertilized and followed by wedge-shaped fruit pods, divided by narrow partitions into two cells, which contain numerous oblong yellow seeds.

When ripe, the pod separates into its two boat-shaped valves.

The odour of the plant is peculiar and rather unpleasant, though more cress-like than pungent.

It has an aromatic and biting taste, but is less acrid than most of the Cruciferæ, and was formerly used as a pot-herb, the young radical leaves being sold in Philadelphia as greens in the spring. It causes taint of milk when freely eaten by dairy cattle.

¶ *Part Used.* In modern herbal medicine the whole plant is employed, dried and administered in infusion, and in fluid extract.

A homœopathic tincture is prepared from the fresh plant.

¶ *Constituents.* During the summer, the plant has a sharp, acrid taste, due to the stimulating principle.

Several partial analyses have been made of it, but no characteristic principle has been definitely separated. The active constituent is said to be an organic acid, which Bombelon, a French chemist, termed bursinic acid. He also found a tannate and an alkaloid, Bursine, which resembles sulphocyansinapine.

A peculiar sulphuretted volatile oil, closely similar to, if not identical with oil of mustard, as well as a fixed oil, have been determined and 6 per cent. of a soft resin.

¶ *Medicinal Action and Uses.* Shepherd's Purse is one of the most important drug-plants of the family Cruciferæ.

When dried and infused, it yields a tea which is still considered by herbalists one of the best specifics for stopping hæmorrhages of all kinds – of the stomach, the lungs, or the uterus, and more especially bleeding from the kidneys.

Its hæmostyptic properties have long been known and are said to equal those of ergot and hydrastis. During the Great War, when these were no longer obtainable in German commerce, a liquid extract of *Capsella bursa-*

pastoris was used as a substitute, the liquid extract being made by exhausting the drug with boiling water. Bomelon found the herb of prompt use to arrest bleedings and flooding, when given in the form of a fluid extract, in doses of 1 to 2 spoonfuls.

Culpepper says it helps bleeding from wounds – inward or outward – and

'if bound to the wrists, or the soles of the feet, it helps the jaundice. The herb made into poultices, helps inflammation and St. Anthony's fire. The juice dropped into ears, heals the pains, noise and matterings thereof. A good ointment may be made of it for all wounds, especially wounds in the head.'

It has been used in English domestic practice from early times as an astringent in diarrhœa; it was much used in decoction with milk to check active purgings in calves.

It has been employed in fresh decoction in hæmaturia, hæmorrhoids, chronic diarrhœa and dysentery, and locally as a vulnerary in nose-bleeding, which is checked by inserting the juice on cotton-wool. It is also used as an application in rheumatic affections, and has been found curative in various uterine hæmorrhages, especially those with which uterine cramp and colic are associated, and also in various passive hæmorrhages from mucous surfaces.

It is a remedy of the first importance in catarrhal conditions of the bladder and ureters, also in ulcerated conditions and abscess of the bladder. It increases the flow of urine. Its use is specially indicated when there is white mucous matter voided with the urine; relief in these cases following at once.

Its antiscorbutic, stimulant and diuretic action causes it to be much used in kidney complaints and dropsy; other similar stimulating diuretics such as Couch Grass may be combined with it.

Dr. Ellingwood, in his valuable work on Therapeutics, says of Shepherd's Purse:

'This agent has been noted for its influence in hæmaturia . . . soothing irritation of the renal or vesical organs. In cases of uncomplicated chronic menorrhagia (excessive menstruation) it has accomplished permanent cures, especially if the discharge be persistent. The agent is also useful where uric acid or insoluble phosphates or carbonates produce irritation of the urinary tract. Externally, the bruised herb has been applied to bruised and strained parts, to rheumatic joints, and where there was ecchymosis, or extravasations within or beneath the skin.

'The herb is rather unpleasant to take, but it is valuable mixed with Pellitory of the Wall, and a little Spirits of Juniper much disguises the flavour. A small quantity of Nitrate of Potash will further disguise it, and not detract from its medicinal value. The infusion may be taken in wineglassful doses, four times a day.'

The medicinal infusion should be made with an ounce of the plant to 12 oz. of water, reduced by boiling to ½ pint, strained and taken cold.

The fluid extract is given in doses of ½ to 1 drachm. In the United States, the fluid extract is given for dropsy in doses of ½ to 1 teaspoonful in water.

Shepherd's Purse was said to be the principal herb in the blue 'Electric Fluid' used by Count Matthei to control hæmorrhage.

Small birds are fond of the seeds of Shepherd's Purse: chaffinches and other wild birds may often be observed feeding on them, and they form valuable food for all caged birds.

When poultry have fed freely on the green plant in the early spring, it has been noticed that the egg yolks become dark in colour, a greenish brown or olive colour, and stronger in flavour.

SIEGESBECKIA

Siegesbeckia orientalis (LINN.)
N.O. Compositæ

Synonym. The Holy Herb
Parts Used. Juice, leaves, and whole plant
Habitat. Isle of Bourbon

¶ *Description.* A small composite plant or small shrub growing in hot climates. The heads are small with an involucre of five bracts covered with very sticky glandular hairs. The secretion continues till after the fruit is ripe and aids in its distribution, the whole head breaking off and attaching itself to some passing animal. In China it is a common weed. The drug contains a white crystalline body resembling salicylic acid.

¶ *Medicinal Action and Uses.* Used by Creoles as a protective covering for wounds, burns, etc. The juice when applied to the skin leaves a coating similar to that of collodion. Creoles call it 'Colle Colle' – Stick Stick.

In China it is used as a remedy for ague,

rheumatism, and renal colic; used in Britain chiefly as a cure for ringworm in conjunction with glycerine. Used in Mauritius Islands for syphilis, leprosy, and various skin diseases.

¶ *Dose*: 10 minims of the fluid extract.

SILVERWEED

Potentilla anserina (LINN.)
N.O. Rosaceæ

Synonyms. Prince's Feathers. Trailing Tansy. Wild Tansy. Goosewort. Silvery Cinquefoil. Goose Tansy. Goose Grey. Moor Grass. Wild Agrimony

Part Used. Herb

The Silverweed, one of the commonest of the *Potentillas*, is very abundant in Great Britain and throughout the temperate regions, extending from Lapland to the Azores, and is equally at home in regions as remote as Armenia, China, New Zealand and Chile.

All soils are congenial to its growth. It spreads rapidly by means of long, creeping runners and thrives in moist situations, especially in clay, where the water is apt to stagnate, and is common by waysides, though on dusty ground it becomes much dwarfed.

It has a slender, branched root-stock, dark brown outside, which has been eaten in the Hebrides in times of scarcity.

The leaves are covered on both sides with a silky, white down of soft hairs, mostly marked on the underside, hence its English name of Silverweed. They are 2 to 5 inches long, much cut or divided, interruptedly pinnate, i.e. divided into twelve to fifteen pairs of oval, toothed leaflets along the mid-rib, each pair being separated by a shorter pair all the way up.

The buttercup-like flowers, in bloom from early summer till later autumn, are borne singly on long footstalks from the axils of the leaves on the slender runners. They are large, with five petals of a brilliant yellow colour and the calyx is cleft into ten divisions.

The Silverweed is a favourite food of cattle, horses, goats, pigs and geese. Only sheep decline it.

Older writers call it *Argentina* (Latin, *argent*, silver) from its appearance of frosted silver. The name Anserina (Latin, *anser*, a goose) was probably given it because geese were fond of it.

The generic name, *Potentilla*, is derived from the Latin adjective, *potens*, powerful, in allusion to the medicinal properties of some of the species.

¶ *Parts Used.* All parts of the plant contain tannin.

In modern herbal medicine the whole herb is used, dried, for its mildly astringent and tonic action. It has an astringent taste, but no odour.

The roots, which are even more astringent, have been used, also the seeds.

The herb is gathered in June, all shrivelled, discoloured or insect-eaten leaves being rejected. Collect only in dry weather, in the morning, after the dew has been dried by the sun. Failing the convenience of a specially-fitted drying-shed, where drying is carried on by artificial heat, drying may be done in warm, sunny weather out of doors, but in half-shade, as leaves dried in the shade retain their colour better than those dried in the sun. They may be placed on wire sieves, or wooden frames covered with wire or garden netting, at a height of about 3 or 4 feet from the ground, to ensure a current of air. The herbs must be brought indoors to a dry room or shed at night, before there is any chance of them becoming damp by dew.

For drying indoors, a warm, sunny attic may be employed, the window being left open by day, so that there is a current of air for the moist, hot air to escape; the door may also be left open. The leaves and herbs can be placed on coarse butter-cloth, stented, i.e. if hooks are placed beneath the window and on the opposite wall, the butter cloth can be attached by rings sewn on each side of it and hooked on so that it is stretched quite taut. The temperature should be from 70° to 100° F. Failing sun, any ordinary shed, fitted with racks and shelves can be used, provided that it is ventilated near the roof, and has a warm current of air, caused by an ordinary coke stove or anthracite stove. The important point is rapidity and the avoidance of steaming; the quicker the process of drying, the more even the colour obtained, making the product more saleable.

All dried leaves should be packed away at once in wooden or tin boxes, in a dry place, as otherwise they re-absorb about 12 per cent. of moisture from the air, and are liable to become mouldy and to deteriorate in quality.

¶ *Medicinal Action and Uses.* A strong infusion of Silverweed, if used as a lotion, will check the bleeding of piles, the ordinary infusion (1 oz. to a pint of boiling water) being meanwhile taken as a medicine.

The same infusion, sweetened with honey, constitutes an excellent gargle for sore throat. A tablespoonful of the powdered herb may also be taken every three hours.

It is also an excellent remedy for cramps in the stomach, heart and abdomen. In addition to the infusion taken internally, it is advisable to apply it to the affected parts on compresses.

On the Continent, a tablespoonful of the herb, boiled in a cup of milk, has been recommended as an effective remedy in tetanus, or lockjaw. The tea should be drunk as hot as possible. If the patient dislikes milk, boiling water may be used.

The dried and powdered leaves have been successfully administered in ague: the more astringent roots have been given in powder in doses of a scruple and upwards.

As a diuretic, Silverweed has been considered useful in gravel. Ettmueller extolled it as a specific in jaundice. Of the fresh plant, 3 oz. or more may be taken three or four times daily.

The decoction has been used for ulcers in the mouth, relaxation of the uvula, spongy gums and for fixing loose teeth, also for toothache and preserving the gums from scurvy.

A distilled water of the herb was in earlier days much in vogue as a cosmetic for removing freckles, spots and pimples, and for restoring the complexion when sunburnt.

In Leicestershire, Silverweed fomentations were formerly used to prevent pitting by smallpox.

Salmon (1710) says:

'It is very cold and dry in the second degree, astringent, anodyne, vulnerary and arthritic. It stops all fluxes of the bowels, even the bloody flux, also spitting, vomiting of blood, or any inward bleeding. It helps the whites in women and is profitable against ruptures in children and is good to dissipate contusions, fastens loose teeth and heals wounds or ulcers in the mouth, throat or in any part of the body, drying up old, moist, corrupt and running sores. It resists the fits of agues, is said to break the stone, and is good to cool inflammation in the eyes, as eke to take away all discolourings of the skin and to cleanse it from any kind of depredation.'

See FIVE-LEAF GRASS, TORMENTIL.

SIMARUBA

Simaruba Amara (D. C.)
Simaruba officinalis
N.O. Simarubaceæ

Synonyms. Dysentery Bark. Mountain Damson. Bitter Damson. Slave Wood. Stave Wood. Sumaruppa. Maruba. Quassia Simaruba
Part Used. Dried root-bark
Habitat. French Guiana, the Islands of Dominica, Martinique, St. Lucia, St. Vincent and Barbados

¶ *Description.* The name given by the founder of the genus was Carib *Simarouba*, but later writers adopted the present spelling.

The tree is 60 feet or more in height, with many long, crooked branches covered with smooth, greyish bark, leaves 9 to 12 inches long, and flowers growing in small clusters, with rather thick, dull-white petals. The bark is usually found in pieces several feet long, the roots being long, horizontal, and creeping. Very often the outer bark has been removed, when it shows a pale yellowish or pinkish-brown surface. It is odourless, difficult to powder, and intensely bitter. It is usually imported from Jamaica, in bales.

¶ *Constituents.* Simaruba root-bark contains a bitter principle identical with quassin, a resinous matter, a volatile oil having the odour of benzoin, malic acid, gallic acid in very small proportion, an ammoniacal salt, calcium malate and oxalate, some mineral salts, ferric oxide, silica, ulmin, and lignin.

It readily imparts its virtues at ordinary temperatures to water and alcohol. The infusion is as bitter as the decoction, which becomes turbid as it cools.

¶ *Medicinal Action and Uses.* A bitter tonic. It was first sent from Guiana to France in 1713 as a remedy for dysentery. In the years 1718 and 1725 an epidemic flux prevailed in France, which resisted all the usual medicines. Simaruba was tried with great success, and established its medical character in Europe. It restores the lost tone of the intestines, promotes the secretions, and disposes the patient to sleep. It is only successful in the latter stage of dysentery, when the stomach is not affected. In large doses it produces sickness and vomiting. On account of its difficult pulverization, it is seldom given in substance, the infusion being preferred, but like many bitter tonics, it is now seldom used. From its use, it has been called 'dysentery bark.'

¶ *Dosage.* From 20 grains to a drachm. A ¼ oz. of simaruba may be infused for 12 hours in 12 oz. of cold or boiling water, and a wineglassful of the infusion taken every three or four hours.

Fluid extract, ½ to 1 drachm.

¶ *Other Species.*

Simaruba glauca of Jamaica, San Domingo, Bahama Islands, Panama and Guatemala has identical properties, and by some writers is regarded as the same tree, others distinguishing it by a slight difference in the flowers. It is also known as Winged-leaved Quassia, and *S. medicinalis.*

S. versicolor of Brazil, has similar properties, the fruit and bark being also used as anthelmintics, and an infusion of the latter being employed in cases of snake-bite. The plant is so bitter that insects will not attack it, on which account the powdered bark has been employed to kill vermin.

S. glauca of Cuba furnishes a glutinous juice, which is employed in certain skin diseases.

S. excelsa or Quassia Excelsa yields quassin from boiled slices of the wood, furnishing the Quassia of commerce, substituted for the true *Surinam Quassia.*

Samadera Indica contains a similar bitter principle in its bark.

See QUASSIA.

SKIRRET

Sium Sisarum
N.O. Umbelliferæ

Part Used. Root

Sium Sisarum, or Skirret, is a plant of Chinese origin, cultivated in Europe. It has a sweetish, somewhat aromatic root, which is used as a vegetable in much the same manner as the Oyster plant or Salsify (*Tragopogon porrifolius*) and the Parsnip. It is supposed to be a useful diet in chest complaints.

The name (*Sium*) is from the Celtic *siu* (water), in allusion to their habitat.

S. Sisarum has been cultivated in this country since A.D. 1548. When boiled and served with butter, the roots form a dish, declared by Worlidge, in 1682, to be 'the sweetest, whitest, and most pleasant of roots.'

Culpepper says:

'*Sisari, secacul.* Of Scirrets. – They are hot and moist, of good nourishment, something windy, as all roots; by reason of which they . . . stir up appetite . . .'

SKUNK-CABBAGE

Symplocarpus fœtidus
N.O. Araceæ

Synonyms. Dracontium. Dracontium fœtidum (Linn.). Skunkweed. Polecatweed. Meadow Cabbage. Spathyema fœtida. Ictodes fœtidus

Parts Used. Seeds, root

Habitat. United States

¶ *Description.* The plant grows in abundance in moist places of the northern and middle United States. All parts of it have a strong, fœtid odour, dependent upon a volatile principle, which is quickly dissipated by heat. The rhizome should be collected in the autumn or early spring, and should not be kept more than one season, as it deteriorates with age and drying. In commerce it is found in cylindrical pieces, 2 inches or more in length and about 1 in. in diameter, or, more commonly, in transverse slices, much compressed and corrugated. It is dark brown outside, white or yellowish within. The seeds are regarded as more energetic than the root, and preserve their virtues longer. They have an acrid taste, and emit the fœtid odour only when bruised. The acridity of the root is absent in the decoction.

¶ *Constituents.* A fixed oil, wax, starch, volatile oil, fat, salts of lime, silica, iron and maganese.

¶ *Medicinal Action and Uses.* Antispasmodic, diaphoretic, expectorant, narcotic. Large doses cause nausea, vomiting, headache, vertigo and dimness of vision. It has been used with alleged success in asthma, chronic catarrh, chronic rheumatism, chorea, hysteria and dropsy. It is said to be helpful in epilepsy, and convulsions during pregnancy and labour. It is an ingredient in well-known herbal ointments and powders. Externally, as an ointment, it stimulates granulations, eases pain, etc.

The powdered root may be used, alone, or mixed with honey ($\frac{1}{2}$ oz. to 4 oz. of honey), but the best method of use is probably a saturated tincture of the fresh root.

¶ *Dosage.* Of powder, 10 to 20 grains. Of tincture, 1 to 2 fluid drachms. Of fluid extract, $\frac{1}{2}$ to 1 drachm.

SLIPPERY ELM. *See* ELM

SMARTWEED

Polygonum Hydropiper (LINN.)
N.O. Polygonaceæ

Synonyms. Water Pepper. Biting Persicaria. Bity Tongue. Arcmart. Pepper Plant. Smartass. Ciderage. Red Knees. Culrage. Bloodwort. Arsesmart
Parts Used. Whole herb and leaves
Habitat. Great Britain and Ireland, rarer in Scotland; is a native of most parts of Europe, in Russian Asia to the Arctic regions. Found abundantly in places that are under water during the winter

¶ *Description.* Annual. The branched stem, 2 to 3 feet in length, creeps at first, then becomes semi-erect. The leaves are lance-shaped, shortly stalked, wavy, more or less acute, glandular below, fringed with hairs. The stipules form a short inflated ochrea. The greenish-pink flowers are in long, slender, loose racemes, that mostly droop at their tips. There are six to eight stamens, two of which are functionless; two to three styles to the pistil. The fruit is black and dotted, as long as the perianth, three-sided and nut-like. The leaves have a pungent, acrid, bitter taste (something like pepper-mint), which resides in the glandulat dots on its surface, no odour.

¶ *Constituents.* The' plant's irritant medi-cinal properties are due to an active princi-ple not fully understood, called Polygonic Acid (when discovered by Dr. C. J. Rade-maker in 1871), which forms in green de-liquescent crystals, having a bitter and acrid taste and strong acid reaction. It is destroyed by heating or drying. Other authorities later considered this body to be simply a mixture of impure tannic and gallic acids, together with chlorophyll, and failed to isolate a stable active principle. The plant contains 3 or 4 per cent. of tannin. It imparts its properties to alcohol or water. The tincture must be made from the fresh plant; heat and age destroy its qualities.

It is said that this herb, together with Arbor Vitæ, constituted the anti-venereo remedy of Count Mattei.

Linnæus observes that the Water Pepper-wort will dye woollen cloths of a yellow colour, if the material be first dipped in a solution of alum, and that all domestic quad-rupeds reject it.

¶ *Medicinal Action and Uses.* Stimulant, diuretic, diaphoretic, emmenagogue, effi-cacious in amenorrhœa. A cold water in-fusion is useful in gravel, colds and coughs.

In combination with tonics and gum myrrh, it is said to have cured epilepsy – probably dependent on some uterine de-rangement. The infusion in cold water, which may be readily prepared from the fluid extract, has been found serviceable in gravel, dysentery, gout, sore mouths, colds and coughs, and mixed with wheat bran, in bowel complaints. Antiseptic and desiccant virtues are also claimed for it. The fresh leaves, bruised with those of the Mayweed (*Anthemis Cotula*), and moistened with a few drops of oil of turpentine, make a speedy vesicant.

Simmered in water and vinegar, it has proved useful in gangrenous, or mortified conditions. The extract, in the form of in-fusion or fomentation, has been beneficially applied in chronic ulcers and hæmorrhoidal tumours, also as a wash in chronic ery-sipetalous inflammations, and as a fomenta-tion in flatulent colic.

A hot decoction made from the whole plant has been used in America as a remedy for cholera, a sheet being soaked in it and wrapped round the patient immediately the symptoms start.

In Mexico, the infusion is used not only as a diuretic, but also put into the bath of sufferers from rheumatism.

A fomentation of the leaves is beneficial for chronic ulcers and hæmorrhoids – in tym-panitis and flatulent colic, and as a wash in chronic inflammatory erysipelas.

It was once held that a few drops of the juice put into the ear would destroy the worms that it was believed caused earache.

There is a tradition, quoted in old Herbals, that if a handful of the plant be placed under the saddle, a horse is enabled to travel for some time without becoming hungry or thirsty, the Scythians having used this herb (under the name of Hippice) for that purpose.

It was an old country remedy for curing proud flesh in the sores of animals. Culpepper tells us also that 'if the Arsemart be strewed in a chamber, it will soon kill all the fleas.'

The root was chewed for toothache – probably as a counter-irritant – and the bruised leaves used as a poultice to whitlows.

A water distilled from the plant, taken in the quantity of a pint or more in a day, has been found serviceable in gravel and stone.

The expressed juice of the freshly gathered plant has been found very useful in jaundice and the beginning of dropsies, the dose being from 1 to 3 tablespoonfuls.

In Salmon's *Herbal*, it is stated:
'It is known by manifold and large experi-ence to be a peculiar plant against gravel and

stone. The Essence causes a good digestion, it is admirable against all cold and moist diseases of the brain and nerves, etc., such as falling sickness, vertigo, lethargy, apoplexy, palsy, megrim, etc., and made into a syrup with honey it is a good pectoral. The oil dissolves and discusses all cold swellings, scrofulous and scirrhous tumours, quinsies, congealed blood, pleurisies, etc.'

Waller recommends it also for 'hypochondriacal diseases.'

SMILAX, CHINA

Synonym. China
Part Used. Root
Habitat. Eastern Asia

It has a hard, large, knotty, uneven rhizome, blackish externally, pale coloured or whitish internally. Stem without support, about 3 feet high, but growing much taller if it has a bush to cling to. Leaves thin, membraneous, round, five-nerved acute or obtuse at each end, mucronate at points. Stipules distinct obtuse; umbels greenish yellow, small ten-flowered; fruit red, size of bird cherry. This is the commercial China root, used as a substitute for Sarsaparilla. It is in large ligneous pieces 2 to 6 inches long and about 2 inches in diameter. Odourless, taste at first slightly bitter and acrid like Sarsaparilla. The root-stocks yield a yellow dye with alum and a brown one with sulphate of iron.

Brazilian or Rio Negro or Lisbon Sarsaparilla is furnished by *Smilax Papyracea*.

S. Aspera (habitat, South of France, Italy, etc.) yields the Italian Sarsaparilla which has the same properties as the American ones.

S. ovalifolia is used medicinally in India.

S. lanceæfolia is used in India and has very large tuberous root-stocks.

S. glyciphylla is the Australian medicinal Sarsaparilla.

S. macabucha is used in the Philippines for dysentery and other complaints.

S. anceps is the medicinal Sarsaparilla of Mauritius.

¶ *Preparations and Dosage.* Infusion, 1 oz. to 1 pint – 1 tablespoonful three times daily. Fluid extract, 1 to 2 drachms. Tincture, 2 to 4 drachms.

¶ *Other Species.* From the AMERICAN SMARTWEED (*Polygonum*, Linn.), which possesses properties similar to those of the English species; a homœopathic tincture is prepared from the fresh plant, which has been used with great advantage in diarrhœa and dysentery, in doses of 20 to 60 minims.

Smilax, China (LINN.)
N.O. Liliaceæ

In Persia the young shoots of some of the species are eaten as asparagus.

S. pseudo-China and other species are used in basket-making.

S. rotundifolia – Mexican – is said to be a diaphoretic and depurative.

All the Sarsaparillas have medicinal properties and can be used in the same way. Sarsaparilla is efficacious in proportion to its acrid taste. The properties reside chiefly in the cortex, though the bark is generally used.

The name Smilax was used by the Greeks to denote a poisonous tree – others derive the name from *Smile*, i.e. a cutting or scratching implement, in allusion to the rough prickles on the stem.

In commerce the varieties of Sarsaparillas are grouped as mealy and non-mealy, according to the starch they contain. The farinaceous matter is found under the rind.

The mealy group include Smilax officinalis, Honduras, Caracas, Brazilian, Syphilitica and Papyraceæ.

The non-mealy species are Jamaica Sarsaparilla, Mexican, Media and Lima.

The most esteemed varieties are Jamaica and Lima on account of their acrid taste.

See (AMERICAN) SPIKENARD.

See SARSAPARILLA

SNAKEROOT

Aristolochia serpentaria (LINN.)
N.O. Aristolochiaceæ

Synonyms. Aristolochia reticulata. Serpentatiæ Rhizoma. Serpentary Rhizome. Serpentary Radix. Virginian Snakeroot. Aristolochia officinalis. Aristolochia sagittata. Endodeca Bartonii. Endodeca Serpentaria. Snakeweed. Red River or Texas Snakeroot. Pelican Flower. Virginia serpentaria. Snagrel. Sangrel. Sangree. Radix Colubrina. Radix Viperina
Parts Used. Dried rhizome and roots
Habitat. The Central and Southern United States

¶ *Description.* Many species of *Aristolochia* have been employed in medicine, the classical name being first applied to *A. Clem-* atitis and *A. rotunda*, from their supposed emmenagogue properties. *A. serpentaria* and *A. reticulata*, or Texas Snakeroot, differ slightly in leaves and flowers, the latter having a slightly coarser root. Both are recognized as official in the United States of America.

The plant is a perennial herb, growing in rich, shady woods, the roots being collected in Western Pennsylvania, West Virginia, Ohio, Indiana and Kentucky, where it is packed in bales containing about 100 lb., often mixed with leaves, stems and dirt.

It has a short, horizontal rhizome, giving off numerous long, slender roots below. The flowers are peculiar, growing from the joints near the root and drooping until they are nearly buried in the earth or in their dried leaves. They are small, and brownish-purple in colour. Attempts at cultivation are being made, as the rather large use of *serpentaria* has caused the drug to become scarcer. A specimen was grown in an English garden as far back as 1632. There is one in cultivation at Kew, but it has not flowered there. The genus *Endodeca* was defined from this species, but it has no characters to distinguish it. Serpentaria has a yellowish or brownish colour, and both smell and taste are aromatic and resemble a mixture of valerian and camphor. Several kinds are cultivated in hot-houses for the singularity and, in some cases, the handsome appearance of their flowers, though their colours are usually dingy. The bent shape causes some blossoms to act as a fly-trap. *A. sipho*, a native of the Alleghany Mountains, is cultivated as an outdoor climbing plant, for the sake of its large leaves, the shape of its flowers inspiring the name of Pipe-Vine or Dutchman's Pipe.

¶ *Constituents.* A volatile oil in the proportion of about ½ per cent., and a bitter principle – Aristolochin – an amorphous substance of yellow colour and bitter and slightly acrid taste, soluble in both water and alcohol. The medicinal properties are due to these two substances, but the root also contains tannic acid, resin, gum, sugar, etc.

A more recent analysis gives volatile oil, resin, a yellow, bitter principle considered analagous to the bitter principle of quassia, gum, starch, albumen, lignin, malate and phosphate of lime, oxide of iron and silica.

About ½ oz. of the oil is furnished by 100 lb. of the root, the coarser, *A. reticulata*, yielding rather more. The resinous aristinic acid has been obtained from a number of species, including *A. serpentaria*. The alkaloid Aristolochine, found in several varieties, requires fuller investigation.

¶ *Medicinal Action and Uses.* Stimulant, tonic and diaphoretic, properties resembling those of valerian and cascarilla. Too large doses occasion nausea, griping pains in the bowels, sometimes vomiting and dysen-

teric tenesmus. In small doses, it promotes the appetite, toning up the digestive organs. It has been recommended in intermittent fevers, when it may be useful as an adjunct to quinine. In full doses it produces increased arterial action, diaphoresis, and frequently diuresis. In eruptive fevers where the eruption is tardy, or in the typhoid stage where strong stimulants cannot be borne, it may be very valuable. An infusion is an effective gargle in putrid sore-throat. It benefits sufferers from dyspepsia and amenorrhœa.

Long boiling impairs its virtues. A cold infusion is useful in convalescence from acute diseases.

It is probable that as it does not disturb the bowels, it may often be used where *Guaiacum* is not easily tolerated, for stimulating capillary circulation and promoting recovery in chronic forms of gouty inflammation.

Many powers are claimed for the drug as an antidote to the bites of snakes and mad dogs, but though there is much direct testimony, the claim is not considered to be authoritatively proved.

¶ *Dosage.* Powdered root, 10 to 30 grains. Fluid extract, ½ to 1 drachm. Tincture, B.P. and U.S.P., ½ to 1 drachm. Infusion, B.P., ½ to 1 oz. Conc. solution, B.P., ½ to 2 drachms.

¶ *Poisonous, if any, with Antidotes.* According to Pohl, aristolochine in sufficient dose produces in the higher animals violent irritation of the gastro-intestinal tract and of the kidneys, with death in coma from respiratory paralysis.

The celebrated Portland powder for the cure of gout contained aristolochia, with gentian, centaury and other bitters in the dose of a drachm every morning for three months, afterwards diminishing for a year or more, but its prolonged use injured the stomach and nervous system, bringing on premature decay and death.

¶ *Other Species.*
Analyses have been made of *A. Clematitis*, *A. rotunda*, *A. longa*, *A. argentea*, *A. indica* and *A. bracteata*, yielding aristolochine, aristolin, or aristinic acid. A closely allied if not identical resinous acid has been obtained from the plant *Bragantia Wallichii*, besides an alkaloid, which, under the name of *Alpam*, has long been used in Western India as an antidote to snake-venom. The allied species, *Bragantia tomentosa*, is said to be employed in Java as an emmenagogue.

Several species are found in the herbalists' stores of India which do not enter commerce.

A. bracteata is employed as an emmenagogue. *Aristolochia* of the Br. Add. was the dried stem and root of *A. indica*, the stems with attached roots being used for the cure of snake-bite.

Of *A. rotunda*, the Br. Add. recognized the concentrated liquor, i.e. 1 in 2 of 20 per cent. alcohol (dose, ½ to 2 fluid drachms), and the tincture, i.e. 1 in 5 of 70 per cent. alcohol (dose, ½ to 1 fluid drachm).

A. Clematitis, *A. longa* and *A. rotunda* are still retained in official catalogues in Europe, where they are indigenous. *A. Pistolochia*, of Southern Europe, appears to have been the aristolochia of Pliny, and is still used under the name of Pistolochia.

A. Clematitis, or Birthwort, is found in England, usually near old ruins, as if it had been cultivated for its medical use, as an aid to parturition.

It is stated that Egyptian jugglers use some of these plants to stupefy snakes before they handle them, while it is related that the juice of the root of *A. anguicida*, if introduced into the mouth of a serpent, will stupefy it, and if it be compelled to swallow a few drops it will die in convulsions.

It is conjectured that the Guaco of South America, a root of which is carried by all Indians and Negroes who traverse the country, is some species of Aristolochia, probably *A. cymbifera*, known in Brazil as milhommen, jarra, and jarrinha.

In the Argentine Republic the root of *A. argentina* is used as a diuretic and diaphoretic, especially in rheumatism.

In Arabia, Forskhal states that the leaves of *A. sempervirens* are used as a counter-poison.

A. fœtida, of Mexico, or Yerba del Indio, is used as a local stimulant to foul ulcers.

For snake-bite, in addition to *A. serpentaria* in North America, *A. maxima* or *Contra Capitano* is employed in South America, *A. anguicida* in the Antilles, *A. brasiliensis*, *A. cymbifera*, *A. macroura*, *A. trilobata*, etc.

See BIRTHWORT

SNAKEROOT, BUTTON

Liatris spicata (WILLD.)
N.O. Compositæ

Synonyms. Gay Feather. Devil's Bite. Colic Root
Part Used. Root
Habitat. Southern Ontario southwards

¶ *Description.* An indigenous perennial composite plant, growing in moist fields and grounds, found from Southern Ontario and Minnesota southwards. Root tuberous; has a herbaceous erect stem, which in August gives a beautiful spike of crimson-purple compound flowers. The odour of the root is terebinic, taste bitterish; the plant grows well in the author's garden at Chalfont St. Peter.
¶ *Constituent.* Coumarin.

¶ *Medicinal Action and Uses.* Useful for its diuretic properties and as a local application for sore throat and gonorrhœa, for which it is exceedingly efficacious. Being an active diuretic it is valuable in the treatment of Bright's disease. Its agreeable odour is due to Coumarin, which may be detected on the surface of its spatulate leaves.
¶ *Dosage.* A decoction is taken three or four times daily in 2-oz. doses.
¶ *Other Species.* Several varieties of *Liatris* are largely used in Southern United States to flavour tobacco, and are said to keep moths away from clothing. All varieties are active diuretics, and *L. squarrosa* (syn. 'Rattlesnake Master') has been utilized to cure rattlesnake-bite.

SNAPDRAGON

Antirrhinum magus (LINN.)
N.O. Scrophularaceæ

Part Used. Leaves

Snapdragon is closely allied to the Toad-flaxes. It is really not truly a native herb, but has become naturalized in many places, on old walls and chalk cliffs, being an escape from gardens, where it has been long cultivated.

The botanical name, *Antirrhinum*, refers to the snout-like form of the flower.
¶ *Medicinal Action and Uses.* The plant has bitter and stimulant properties, and the leaves of this and several allied species have been employed on the Continent in cataplasms to tumours and ulcers.

It was valued in olden times like the Toad-flax as a preservative against witchcraft.

The numerous seeds yield a fixed oil by expression, said to be little inferior to olive oil, for the sake of which it has been cultivated in Russia.
¶ *Other Species.*
Antirrhinum Orontium (Linn.), the Calf's Snout or Small Snapdragon, an annual found occasionally in cornfields, in lime or chalk soil, with narrow, hairy leaves and small, reddish flowers, resembling those of the Snapdragon in form, is said to be poisonous, but the fact is not well established.

Its properties seem similar to those of the other species.

The name, *Orontium*, given it by Dodonæus, is an old mediæval generic name for the Snapdragon.

See TOADFLEX.

SNOWDROP

Galanthus nivalis (LINN.)
N.O. Amaryllidaceæ

Synonyms. Fair Maid of February. Bulbous Violet

Snowdrop, usually spoken of as the first flower of our year, though the Winter Aconite has perhaps a better title to be so considered, has never been of much account in physic, and has never been recognized. Gerard says 'nothing is set down hereof by the ancient Writers, nor anything observed by the moderne.' He calls it the Bulbous Violet, but adds that some call it the Snowdrop, the earliest mention of it by this name, and it was known to all the old botanists as a bulbous violet.

The generic name, *Galanthus*, is Greek in its origin and signifies Milkflower. *Nivalis* is a Latin adjective, meaning relating to or resembling snow.

Gerard speaks of it as not a native of England, though somewhat common in gardens, having been introduced from Italy. It is a native of Switzerland, Austria and of Southern Europe generally, but where naturalized here spreads into considerable masses, and is plentiful wherever it occurs, generally growing in shady pastures, woods and orchards. There is probably no bulbous plant, however, which for all its extreme hardiness in resisting cold, shows such a marked preference or distaste for certain localities, even though there may be little variation in soil or altitude. In some districts snowdrops will grow and spread in woods as readily as the wild hyacinth; in others, with apparently identical conditions, it is difficult to get them to grow and they will refuse to spread.

The bulbs grow in compact masses. Each sends up a one-flowered stem. The points of the leaves protecting the flower-head are thickened and toughened at the tips, enabling them to push through the soil. This simple device shows on the mature leaf like a delicate nail on a green finger.

The flowers remain open a long time; the bud is erect, but the open flowers pendulous and adapted to bees. The perianth is in two whorls, on the inner surface of the inner perianth leaves are green grooves secreting honey – the stamens dehisce, or open, by apical slots and lie close against the style, forming a cone. The stigma projects beyond the anther cone and is first touched by an insect, which in probing for nectar, shakes the stamens and receives a shower of pollen.

Gerard appears to be wrong in saying that the plant has no medicinal use.

An old glossary of 1465, referring to it as *Leucis i viola alba*, classes it as an emmenagogue, and elsewhere, placed under the narcissi, its healing properties are stated to be 'digestive, resolutive and consolidante.'

SOAP TREE

Quillaja saponaria (MOLINA.)
N.O. Rosaceæ

Synonyms. Soap Bark. Panama Bark. Cullay
Part Used. Dried inner bark
Habitat. Peru and Chile, and cultivated in Northern Hindustan

¶ *Description.* A tree 50 to 60 feet high. Leaves smooth, shiny, short-stalked, oval, and usually terminal white flowers, solitary, or three to five on a stalk. Bark thick, dark coloured, and very tough. In commerce it is found in large flat pieces $\frac{1}{3}$ inch thick, outer surface brownish-white, with small patches of brownish cork attached, otherwise smooth; inner surface whitish and smooth, fracture splintery, chequered with pale-brown vast fibres, embedded with white tissue; it is inodorous, very acrid and astringent.

¶ *Constituents.* Its chief constituent is saponin, which is a mixture of two glucosides, guillaic acid and guillaia-sapotoxin. The latter is very poisonous and possesses marked foam-producing properties. Calcium oxalate is also present in the bark. The drug also contains cane-sugar and a non-toxic modi-fication of guillaic acid. As the active principles of Soap Bark are the same as those of Senega, Quillaia has been suggested as a cheap substitute for Sarsaparilla.

¶ *Medicinal Action and Uses.* It can be used as a stimulating expectorant. As a decoction (5 parts to 200), adult-dose 1 tablespoonful. Syrup of guillaia can be utilized as a substitute for syrup of Senega, by adding 4 parts of the fluid extract to 21 parts of syrup, using diluted alcohol as the menstruum.

¶ *Doses of Quillaia Bark.* Fluid extract, 2 to 8 drops. Solid extract, $\frac{1}{2}$ to 2 grains. Tincture, B.P. and U.S.P., $\frac{1}{4}$ to 1 drachm.

Might be useful in cases of aortic disease with hypertrophy, its efficacy depending on the diminished action of the cardiac ganglia and muscle which its active principle, Saponine, produces. Saponin appears to be identical with Cyclamin, from Cyclamen European, and with primulin from *Primula officinalis*. Digitonin from Digitalis appears to be a kind of Saponin differing somewhat from the others. Saponin, when applied locally, is a powerful irritant, local anæsthetic and muscular poison. On account of its local irritation, when injected hypodermically it causes intense pain; sneezing when applied to the nose; vomiting, diarrhœa and gastro-enteritis if taken in large doses internally. Locally applied, it paralyses motor and sensory nerves, and voluntary and involuntary muscular fibre; in the voluntary muscles it produces a condition of *rigor mortis*, and the muscular substance becomes brittle and structureless. Saponin acts as an emeto-cathartic and a diuretic if it is absorbed; in its excretion it irritates the bronchial mucous membrane, and is a protoplasmic poison. In poisoning produced from it, digitalis is indi-cated, as it is antagonistic to Saponin. Saponin is contained in agrostemma seeds, and has caused death; the symptoms were headache, vertigo, vomiting, hot skin, rapid feeble pulse, progressive muscular weakness, and finally coma.

Quillaia bark is used in its native country for washing clothes, and in this country is used by manufacturers and cleaners for washing or cleaning delicate materials. For washing hair: Powdered Soap Tree bark, 100 parts; alcohol, 400 parts; essence of Bergamot, 20 drops; mix. It is said to promote the growth of the hair. Was once used in the production of foam on non-alcoholic beverages, but its use in this way is now generally prohibited by law.

¶ *Other Species.*
The Brazilian species, *Quillaia Selloniana*, or *Fontenellea braziliensis*, has similar properties to *Quillaia Saponaria*.

SOAPWORT

Saponaria officinalis (LINN.)
N.O. Caryophyllaceæ

Synonyms. Soaproot. Bouncing Bet. Latherwort. Fuller's Herb. Bruisewort. Crow Soap. Sweet Betty. Wild Sweet William
Parts Used. Dried root and leaves
Habitat. Central and Southern Europe. Grows well in English gardens

¶ *Description.* A stout herbaceous perennial with a stem growing in the writer's garden to 4 or 5 feet high. Leaves lanceolate, slightly elliptical, acute, smooth, 2 or 3 inches long and ⅛ inch wide. Large pink flowers, often double in paniculate fascicles; calyx cylindrical, slightly downy; five petals, unguiculate; top of petals linear, ten stamens, two styles; capsule oblong, one-celled, flowering from July till September. No odour, with a bitter and slightly sweet taste, followed by a persistent pungency and a numbing sensation in the mouth.

¶ *Constituents.* Constituents of the root, Saponin, also extractive, resin, gum, woody fibre, mucilage, etc.

Soapwort root dried in commerce is found in pieces 10 and 12 inches long, $\frac{1}{12}$ inch thick, cylindrical, longitudinally wrinkled, outside light brown, inside whitish with a thick bark. Contains number of small white crystals and a pale yellow wood.

¶ *Medicinal Action and Uses.* A decoction cures the itch. Has proved very useful in jaundice and other visceral obstructions. For old venereal complaints it is a good cure, specially where mercury has failed. It is a tonic, diaphoretic and alterative, a valuable remedy for rheumatism or cutaneous troubles resulting from any form of syphilis. It is also sternutatory. Should be very cautiously used owing to its saponin content.

Dose. – Decoction, 2 to 4 fluid ounces three or four times daily. Extract or the inspissated juice will be found equally efficacious: dose, 10 to 20 grains. As a sternutatory 2 to 6 grains. Fluid extract, ¼ to 1 drachm.

SOAPWORT ROOT, EGYPTIAN

Gypsophila struthium (LINN.)
N.O. Caryophyllaceæ

Habitat. Europe and United States of America

¶ *Description.* The root is generally in lengths of 4 to 6 inches, ½ to 1½ inches in diameter; colour a yellowish white, furrowed down its length externally with lighter places where the cortex has been rubbed. The section is of a radiate and concentric structure. Taste bitter, then acrid; odour slight; powder irritating to the nostrils. This variety is rarely used medicinally, the Soapwort (*Saponaria officinalis*) being used as a sub-stitute. This is a perennial herbaceous plant with a stem 1 to 2 feet in height, growing in Europe and United States of America.

¶ *Medicinal Action and Uses.* Tonic, diaphoretic, alterative. A valuable remedy in the treatment of syphilitic, scrofulous and cutaneous diseases, also in jaundice, liver affections, rheumatism and gonorrhœa, the decoction is generally used. Saponin is produced from this plant.

SOLOMON'S SEAL

Polygonatum multiflorum (ALLEM.)
N.O. Liliaceæ

Synonyms. Lady's Seals. St. Mary's Seal. Sigillum Sanctæ Mariæ
(*French*) Scean de Solomon
(*German*) Weusswurz
Part Used. Root

A close relative to the Lily-of-the-Valley, and was formerly assigned to the same genus, *Convallaria*. It is a popular plant in gardens and plantations; a native of Northern Europe and Siberia, extending to Switzerland and Carniola. In England it is found, though rarely, growing wild in woods in York, Kent and Devon, but where found in Scotland and Ireland is regarded as naturalized. The Dwarf Solomon's Seal is found in the woods of Wiltshire.

¶ *Description.* The creeping root-stock, or underground stem, is thick and white, twisted and full of knots, with circular scars at intervals, left by the leaf stems of previous years. It throws up stems that attain a height of from 18 inches to 2 feet, or even more, which are for some considerable portion of their length erect, but finally bend gracefully over. They are round, pale-green in colour, and bare half-way up; from thence to the top, large and broadly-oval leaves grow alternately on the stem, practically clasping it by the bases. All the leaves have the character of turning one way, being bent slightly upward, as well as to one side, and have very marked longitudinal ribbing on their surfaces.

The flowers are in little drooping clusters of from two to seven, springing from the axils of the leaves, but hanging in an opposite direction to the foliage. They are tubular in shape, of a creamy or waxy white, topped with a yellowish-green, and sweet-scented, and are succeeded by small berries about the size of a pea, of a blackish-blue colour, varying to purple and red, and containing about three or four seeds.

The generic name *Polygonatum* signifies many-angled, and is supposed to be derived either from the numerous knots or swellings of the root or from the numerous nodes or joints of the stem, but the characteristics are not very marked ones. The specific name, *multiflorum*, serves to distinguish this many-flowered species from another in which the blossoms are solitary, or only in pairs from each axil.

The origin of the common English name of the plant is variously given. Dr. Prior tells us it comes from 'the flat, round scars on the rootstocks, resembling the impressions of a seal and called Solomon's, because his seal occurs in Oriental tales.'

Another explanation is that these round depressions, or the characters which appear when the root is cut transversely, and which somewhat resemble Hebrew characters, gave rise to the notion that Solomon 'who knew the diversities of plants and the virtues of roots,' has set his seal upon them in testimony of its value to man as a medicinal root.

Gerard maintained that the name Sigillum Solomons was given to the root 'partly because it bears marks something like the stamp of a seal, but still more because of the virtue the root hath in sealing and healing up green wounds, broken bones and such like, being stamp't and laid thereon.'

The name Lady's Seal was also conferred on the plant by old writers, as also St. Mary's Seal (*Sigillum Sanctæ Mariæ*).

¶ *Cultivation.* Solomon's Seal is a very hardy plant. It prefers a light soil and a shady situation, being a native of woods. If in a suitable soil and situation and not crowded by shrubs, it will thrive and multiply very rapidly by the creeping rootstocks. It will be better for occasional liberal dressings of leafmould, or an annual top dressing of decayed manure in March.

Seeds, sown as soon as gathered in the autumn, germinate in early spring, or the roots may be divided to any extent. The best time to transplant or part the roots is in autumn, after the stalks decay, but it may safely be done at any time, if taken up with plenty of soil, until they begin to shoot in the spring, when the ground should be dug about them and kept clean from weeds. They should also have room to spread and must not be removed oftener than every third or fourth year.

To give Solomon's Seal a good start when planting, the soil should be well broken up with a fork and have a little mild manure worked in.

¶ *Part Used.* The root dug in autumn and dried.

¶ *Constituents.* The rhizome and herb contain Convallarin, one of the active constituents of Lily-of-the-Valley, also Asparagin, gum, sugar, starch and pectin.

¶ *Medicinal Action and Uses.* Astringent, demulcent and tonic. Combined with other remedies, Solomon's Seal is given in pulmonary consumption and bleeding of the lungs. It is useful also in female complaints. The infusion of 1 oz. to a pint of boiling water is taken in wineglassful doses and is also used as an injection. It is a mucilaginous tonic, very

healing and restorative, and is good in inflammations of the stomach and bowels, piles, and chronic dysentery.

A strong decoction given every two or three hours has been found to cure erysipelas, if at the same time applied externally to the affected parts.

The powdered roots make an excellent poultice for bruises, piles, inflammations and tumours. The bruised roots were much used as a popular cure for black eyes, mixed with cream. The bruised leaves made into a stiff ointment with lard served the same purpose. Gerard says:

'The roots of Solomon's Seal, stamped while it is fresh and greene and applied, taketh away in one night or two at the most, any bruise, blacke or blew spots gotten by fals or women's wilfulness in stumbling upin their hastie husband's fists, or such like.'

A decoction of the root in wine was considered a suitable beverage for persons with broken bones, 'as it disposes the bones to knit.' On this point, Gerard adds:

'As touching the knitting of bones and that truly which might be written, there is not another herb to be found comparable to it for the purposes aforesaid; and therefore in briefe, if it be for bruises inward, the roots must be stamped, some ale or wine put thereto and strained and given to drinke . . . as well unto themselves as to their cattle,'
it being applied 'outwardly in the manner of a pultis' for external bruises.

Parkinson says, 'The Italian dames, however, doe much use the distilled water of the whole plant of Solomon's Seal' – for their complexions, etc.

In Galen's time, the distilled water was used as a cosmetic, and Culpepper says:
'the diluted water of the whole plant used to the face or other parts of the skin, cleanses it from freckles, spots or any marks whatever, leaving the place fresh, fair and lovely, for

which purpose it is much used by the Italian ladies and is the principal ingredient of most of the cosmetics and beauty washes advertised by perfumers at high price.'

The roots macerated for some time in water yield a substance capable of being used as food and consisting principally of starch. The young shoots form an excellent vegetable when boiled and eaten like Asparagus, and are largely consumed in Turkey. The roots of another species have been made into bread in times of scarcity, but they require boiling or baking before use.

The flowers and roots used as snuff are celebrated for their power of inducing sneezing and thereby relieving head affections. They also had a wide vogue as aphrodisiacs, for love philtres and potions.

The berries are stated to excite vomiting, and even the leaves, nausea, if chewed.

The properties of these roots have not been very fully investigated. It is stated that a decoction will afford not only relief but ultimate cure in skin troubles caused by the poison vine, or poisonous exalations of other plants. Dosage of the decoction: 1 to 4 oz. three times daily.

As a remedy for piles the following has been found useful: 4 oz. Solomon's Seal, 2 pints water, 1 pint molasses. Simmer down to 1 pint, strain, evaporate to the consistence of a thick fluid extract, and mix with it from ½ to 1 oz. of powdered resin. Dosage: 1 teaspoonful several times daily.

¶ *Other Species.*
Polygonatum biflorum, an American Solomon's Seal, has characters and constitution similar to the European.

P. uniflorum, now *P. officinale*, is said to be no longer used. The plant bears a single fragrant flower.

P. verticillatum, bearing its leaves in whorls, is only found in Scotland, and then rarely.

Smilacina Racemosa is known as False Solomon's Seal.

SORREL, COMMON   Rumex acetosa
SORREL, FRENCH   Rumex scutatus
SORREL, MOUNTAIN   Oxyria reniformis
                                  N.O. Germaniaceæ

SORREL, SHEEP'S   Rumex acetosella
SORREL, WOOD   Oxalis acetosella

Synonyms. Wood Sour. Sour Trefoil. Stickwort. Fairy Bells. Hallelujah. Cuckowes Meat. Three-leaved Grass. Surelle. Stubwort
(*Scotch*) Gowke-Meat   (*French*) Pain de Coucou
(*Irish*) Seamsog   (*Italian*) Iuliole
Parts Used. Leaves and herb

The Sour Docks or Sorrels, cultivated for pot-herbs, *Rumex acetosa* (Common Sorrel) and *R. scutatus* (French Sorrel), as well as the smaller *R. acetosella* (Sheep's Sorrel) and

Oxyria reniformis (Mountain Sorrel), owe the grateful acidity of their herbage to the presence of a special salt, binoxalate of potash, which is also present in Rhubarb. This, however, is absent in the common Docks. We find it to a marked degree in the WOOD SORREL (*Oxalis acetosella*), which indeed receives its name on this account, and not for any similarity in the structure of the plant, which is in no way related to the Sorrels and Docks.

¶ *Description.* It is a little plant of a far more delicate, even dainty character, growing abundantly in woods and shady places. From its slender, irregular creeping rootstock covered with red scales, it sends up thin delicate leaves, each composed of three heart-shaped leaflets, a beautiful bright green above, but of a purplish hue on their under surface. The long slender leaf-stalks are often reddish towards the base. The leaflets are usually folded somewhat along their middle, and are of a peculiarly sensitive nature. Only in shade are they fully extended: if the direct rays of the sun fall on them they sink at once upon the stem, forming a kind of three-sided pyramid, their under surfaces thus shielding one another and preventing too much evaporation from their pores. At night and in bad weather, the leaflets fold in half along the midrib, and the three are placed nearly side by side to 'sleep,' a security against storm and excessive dews.

The flowers, each set on long stalks, are fragile, in form somewhat like the Crane's-bills, to which they are closely allied, being bell-shaped, the corolla composed of five delicate white petals, veined with purple, enclosed in a five-scalloped cup of sepals and containing ten stamens, and in the centre, five green, thread-like columns, arising from a single five-celled ovary. At the base of the petals, a little honey is stored, but the flower seems to find favour with few insects.

As the flower fades, its stalk bends towards the ground and conceals the seed capsule under the leaves, till ripe, when it straightens again. The case of the capsule is elastic and curls back when the fruit is quite ripe, jerking the seeds out several yards, right over the leaves.

A second kind of flower is also produced. These are hidden among the leaves and are inconspicuous, their undeveloped petals never opening out. The ripening and seed scattering processes of these self-fertilized cleistogamous (or hidden) flowers are the same as with the familiar white-petalled ones. Wood Sorrel droops its blossoms in stormy weather, and also folds its leaves.

Neither the flowers nor any part of the plant has any odour, but the leaves have a pleasantly acid taste, due to the presence of considerable quantities of binoxalate of potash. This, combined with their delicacy, has caused them to be eaten as a spring salad from time immemorial, their sharpness taking the place of vinegar. They were also the basis of a green sauce, that was formerly taken largely with fish. 'Greene Sauce,' says Gerard, 'is good for them that have sicke and feeble stomaches . . . and of all Sauces, Sorrel is the best, not only in virtue, but also in pleasantness of his taste.'

Both botanical names *Oxalis* and *acetosella* refer to this acidity, *Oxalis* being derived from the Greek *oxys*, meaning sour or acid, and *acetosella*, meaning vinegar salts. Salts of Lemon, as well as Oxalic acid, can be obtained from the plant: 20 lb. of fresh herb yield about 6 lb. of juice, from which, by crystallization, between 2 and 3 oz. of Salts of Lemon can be obtained.

An old writer tells us:

'The apothecaries and herbalists call it Alleluya and Paniscuculi, or Cuckowes meat, because either the Cuckoo feedeth thereon, or by reason when it springeth forth and flowereth the Cuckoo singeth most, at which time also Alleluya was wont to be sung in Churches.'

It flowers between Easter and Whitsuntide.

By many, the ternate leaf has been considered to be that with which St. Patrick demonstrated the Trinity to the ancient Irish, though a tiny kind of clover is now generally accepted as the 'true Shamrock.'

The early Italian painters often depicted the blossom. Ruskin writes: 'Fra Angelico's use of the Oxalis acetosella is as faithful in representation as touching in feeling.'

¶ *Cultivation.* If roots are planted in a moist, shady border, they will multiply freely, and if kept clean from weeds will thrive and need no other care.

¶ *Part Used Medicinally.* The leaves, fresh or dried.

¶ *Medicinal Action and Uses.* It has diuretic, antiscorbutic and refrigerant action, and a decoction made from its pleasant acid leaves is given in high fever, both to quench thirst and to allay the fever. The Russians make a cooling drink from an infusion of the leaves, which may be infused with water or boiled in milk. Though it may be administered freely, not only in fevers and catarrhs, but also in hæmorrhages and urinary disorders, excess should be guarded against, as the oxalic salts are not suitable to all constitutions, especially those of a gouty and rheumatic tendency.

The old herbalists tell us that Wood Sorrel is more effectual than the true Sorrels as a blood cleanser, and will strengthen a weak stomach, produce an appetite, check vomiting, and remove obstructions of the viscera.

The juice of the leaves turns red when clarified and makes a fine, clear syrup, which was considered as effectual as the infusion. The juice used as a gargle is a remedy for ulcers in the mouth, and is good to heal wounds and to stanch bleeding. Sponges and linen cloths saturated with the juice and applied, were held to be effective in the reduction of swellings and inflammation.

An excellent conserve, *Conserva Ligulæ*, used to be made by beating the fresh leaves up with three times their weight of sugar and orange peel, and this was the basis of the cooling and acid drink that was long a favourite remedy in malignant fevers and scurvy.

In Henry VIII's time this plant was held in great repute as a pot-herb, but after the introduction of French Sorrel, with its large succulent leaves, it gradually lost its position as a salad and pot-herb.

From *Le Dictionnaire des Ménages* (Paris, 1820):

'*Limonade sans Citrous, Limonade Sèche*

'Take three drachms of *Salt of Sorrel* and one pound of white sugar; reduce them to powder separately, and then mix them. Keep the powder, which is known as dry lemonade, in a well-corked bottle. Substitute tartaric acid for Salt of Sorrel, divide the powder into suitable portions, and you have "lemonade powders without lemons."' '

From *A Plain Plantain*:

'*A Sirrup for a Feaver*

'Take Sirrup of Violets two ounces; Sirrup of Woodsorrell two ounces; Sirrup of Lemmon two ounces, mixed altogether, and drink it.'

¶ *Other Species.*
R. Conglomeratus (Clustered Dock). *R. obtusifolin. R. pulcher*, the Fiddle Dock, so called from the resemblance in the form of its leaves to a violin.

SORRELS

SORREL, FRENCH

Rumex scutatus (LINN.)

Synonym. Buckler-shaped Sorrel
Part Used. Herb
Habitat. It is a common plant in mountainous districts, being a native of the South of France, Italy, Switzerland, Germany and Barbary

This has a more grateful acid than Common Sorrel, and is therefore preferred for kitchen use in soups, especially by the French. Their Sorrel soup is made from this species.

It is distinguished from the Common Sorrel by the form of the leaves, which are cordate-hastate, very succulent, fleshy and brittle. The whole plant is intensely glaucous. The flowers are hermaphrodite, the stamens and pistils not on separate plants as in the Common Sorrel.

It is sometimes met with in Scotland, or in the North of England, but is a doubtful native.

It is said to have been introduced into this country in 1596.

SORREL, GARDEN

Rumex acetosa (LINN.)
N.O. Polygoneceæ

Synonyms. Green Sauce. Sour Sabs. Sour Grabs. Sour Suds. Sour Sauce. Cuckoo Sorrow. Cuckoo's Meate. Gowke-Meat
Part Used. Leaves

Of the two kinds of Sorrel cultivated for use as vegetables or salads, *Rumex acetosa*, the Garden Sorrel, is an indigenous English plant, common, too, in the greater part of Europe, in almost all soils and situations. It grows abundantly in meadows, a slender plant about 2 feet high, with juicy stems and leaves, and whorled spikes of reddish-green flowers, which give colour, during the months of June and July, to the grassy spots in which it grows.

It is generally found in pastures where the soil contains iron.

The leaves are oblong, the lower ones 3 to 6 inches in length, slightly arrow-shaped at the base, with very long petioles. The upper ones are sessile. They frequently become a beautiful crimson.

As the flowers increase in size, they become a purplish colour. The stamens and pistils are on different plants. The seeds, when ripe, are brown and shining. The perennial roots run deeply into the ground.

Sorrel is well known for the grateful acidity of its herbage, which is most marked when the plant is in full season, though in early spring it is almost tasteless.

The plant is also called 'Cuckoo's-meate'

752

from an old belief that the bird cleared its voice by its agency. In Scotland it is 'gowke-meat.'

Domestic animals are fond of this and other species of Sorrel. The leaves contain a considerable quantity of binoxalate of potash, which gives them their acid flavour and medicinal and dietetic properties. They have been employed from the most distant time as a salad. In France, Sorrel is put into ragouts, fricassées and soups, forming the chief constituent of the favourite *Soupe aux herbes*.

In the time of Henry VIII, this plant was held in great repute in England, for table use, but after the introduction of French Sorrel, with large succulent leaves, it gradually lost its position as a salad and a potherb, and for many years it has ceased to be cultivated.

John Evelyn thought that Sorrel imparted 'so grateful a quickness to the salad that it should never be left out.' He wrote in 1720:

'Sorrel sharpens the appetite, assuages heat, cools the liver and strengthens the heart; is an antiscorbutic, resisting putrefaction and in the making of sallets imparts a grateful quickness to the rest as supplying the want of oranges and lemons. Together with salt, it gives both the name and the relish to sallets from the sapidity, which renders not plants and herbs only, but men themselves pleasant and agreeable.'

Culpepper tells us

'Sorrel is prevalent in all hot diseases, to cool any inflammation and heat of blood in agues pestilential or choleric, or sickness or fainting, arising from heat, and to refresh the overspent spirits with the violence of furious or fiery fits of agues: to quench thirst, and procure an appetite in fainting or decaying stomachs: For it resists the putrefaction of the blood, kills worms, and is a cordial to the heart, which the seed doth more effectually, being more drying and binding. . . . Both roots and seeds, as well as the herb, are held powerful to resist the poison of the scorpion. . . . The leaves, wrapt in a colewort leaf and roasted in the embers, and applied to a large imposthume, botch, boil, or plague-sore, doth both ripen and break it. The distilled water of the herb is of much good use for all the purposes aforesaid.'

In this country, the leaves are now rarely eaten, unless by children and rustics, to allay thirst, though in Ireland they are still largely consumed by the peasantry with fish and milk. Our country people used to beat the herb to a mash and take it mixed with vinegar and sugar, as a green sauce with cold meat, hence one of its popular names: Green-sauce.

Because of their acidity, the leaves, treated as spinach, make a capital dressing with stewed lamb, veal or sweetbread. A few of the leaves may also with advantage be added to turnips and spinach. When boiled by itself, without water, it serves as an excellent accompaniment to roast goose or pork, instead of apple sauce.

'To Stew Sorrel for Fricandean and Roast Meat.

'Wash the Sorrel, and put it into a silver vessel, or stone jar, with no more water than hangs to the leaves. Simmer it as slow as you can, and when done enough, put a bit of butter and beat it well.'

Unless cooked carefully, Sorrel is likely to disagree with gouty persons, from the acid oxalate of potash it contains, but this may be got rid of if it is plunged for two or three minutes in boiling water, before cooking, this first water being then thrown away.

In Scandinavia, Sorrel has sometimes been used in time of scarcity to put into bread. The leaves contain a little starch and mucilage, and the root is rather farinaceous.

The juice of the leaves will curdle milk as well as rennet, and the Laplanders use it as a substitute for the latter.

The dried root affords a beautiful red colour when boiled and used for making barley water look like red wine, when in France they wish to avoid giving anything of a vinous nature to the sick.

The salt of Sorrel, binoxalate of potash, is much used for bleaching straw and removing ink stains from linen, and is often sold in the shops under the name of 'essential salt of lemons.'

¶ *Cultivation.* Sorrel of two kinds is cultivated, *R. acetosa*, or Garden Sorrel, and *R. scrutatus*, or French Sorrel. Garden Sorrel likes a damp situation, French Sorrel a dry soil and an open situation.

The finest plants are propagated from seed, sown in March, though it may be sown in any of the spring months. Sow moderately thin, in drills 6 inches apart, and thin out when the plants are 1 or 2 inches high. When the stalks run up in July, they should be cut back. The roots will then put out new leaves, which will be tender and better for kitchen use than the older leaves, so that by cutting down the shoots of some plants at different times, there will always be a supply of young leaves.

Both varieties are generally increased by dividing the roots, which may be done either in spring or autumn, the roots being planted about a foot apart each way, and watered.

¶ *Parts Used Medicinally.* The leaves both dried and fresh.

¶ *Constituents.* The sour taste of Sorrel is due to the acid oxalate of potash it contains; tartaric and tannic acids are also present.

¶ *Medicinal Action and Uses.* The medicinal action of Sorrel is refrigerant and diuretic, and it is employed as a cooling drink in all febrile disorders.

It is corrective of scrofulous deposits: for cutaneous tumours, a preparation compounded of burnt alum, citric acid, and juice of Sorrel, applied as a paint, has been employed with success.

Sorrel is especially beneficial in scurvy.

Both the root and the seed were formerly esteemed for their astringent properties, and were employed to stem hæmorrhage.

A syrup made with the juice of Fumitory and Sorrel had the reputation of curing the itch, and the juice, with a little vinegar, was considered a cure for ringworm, and recommended as a gargle for sore throat.

A decoction of the flowers, made with wine, was said to cure jaundice and ulcerated bowels, the root in decoction or powder being also employed for jaundice, and gravel and stone in the kidneys.

Gerard enumerated eight different kinds of Sorrel – the Garden, bunched or knobbed, Sheep, Romane, Curled, Barren and Great Broad-leaved Sorrel, and said of them:

'The Sorrells are moderately cold and dry. Sorrell doth undoubtedly cool and mightily dry, but because it is sour, it likewise cutteth tough humours. The juice thereof in summer time is a profitable sauce in many meats and pleasant to the taste. It cooleth a hot stomach. The leaves are with good success added to decoctions, and are used in agues. The leaves are taken in good quantity, stamped and stained into some ale and cooleth the body. The leaves are eaten in a tart spinach. The seed of Sorrell drunk in wine stoppeth the bloody flow.'

SORREL, MOUNTAIN

Oxyria reniformis (HOOK)

Part Used. Herb

The Mountain Sorrel is found distributed in the Arctic regions and the Alps of the north temperate zone, and grows by streams in Wales, Yorks and northwards.

It has the characters of the allied genus *Rumex*, approaching the Common Sorrel in habit, but is shorter and stouter. The leaves are all from the root, fleshy and kidney-shaped. The flowers are green, growing in clustered spikes. The generic name, *Oxyria*, is derived from the Greek *oxys* (sharp), from the acid flavouring of the stem and leaves, which make it, like the other Sorrels, an excellent pot-herb and antiscorbutic.

SORREL, SHEEP'S

Rumex acetosella

Synonym. Field Sorrel
Part Used. Herb

Sheep's Sorrel is much smaller than either French or Garden Sorrel, and is often tinged, especially towards the end of the summer, a deep red hue. It is a slender plant, the stems from 3 to 4 inches to nearly a foot high, often many and tufted, decumbent at the base. The leaves, $\frac{1}{2}$ to 2 inches in length, have long petioles and are variable in breadth, mostly narrow-lanceolate, the lower ones hastate and the lobes of the base usually spreading and often divided.

It grows in pastures and dry gravelly places in most parts of the globe, except the tropics, penetrating into Arctic and Alpine regions, and is abundant in Britain, where it is sometimes called Field Sorrel.

Like the other Sorrels, it is highly acid, though is less active in its properties than the French or Garden species.

¶ *Medicinal Action and Uses.* The whole herb is employed medicinally, in the fresh state. The action is diuretic, refrigerant and diaphoretic, and the juice extracted from the fresh plant is of use in urinary and kidney diseases.

SOUTHERNWOOD

Artemisia abrotanum (LINN.)
N.O. Compositæ

Synonyms. Old Man. Lad's Love. Boy's Love. Appleringie
(*French*) Garde Robe
Part Used. Herb

The Southernwood is the southern Wormwood, i.e. the foreign, as distinguished from the native plant, being a native of the South of Europe, found indigenous in Spain and Italy. It is a familiar and favourite plant in our gardens, although it rarely if ever flowers in this country. It has finely-divided, greyish-green leaves. It was introduced into this country in 1548. An ointment made with its ashes is used by country lads to promote the growth of a beard. St. Francis de Sales says: "To love in the midst of sweets, little children could do that, but to love in the bitterness of Wormwood is a sure sign of our affectionate fidelity.' This refers to the habit of including a spray of the plant in country bouquets presented by lovers to their lasses.

The volatile essential oil contained in the plant consists chiefly of Absinthol and is common in other Wormwoods. The scent is said to be disagreeable to bees and other insects, for which reason the French call the plant *Garderobe*, as moths will not attack clothes among which it is laid.

It used to be the custom for women to carry to church large bunches of this plant and Balm, that the keen, aromatic scent might prevent all feeling of drowsiness. Southernwood in common with Wormwood was thought to ward off infection. Even in the early part of last century, a bunch of Southernwood and Rue was placed at the side of the prisoner in the dock as a preventive from the contagion of jail fever.

It Italy, Southernwood, like Mugwort, is employed as a culinary herb.

¶ *Part Used.* The whole herb, collected in August and dried in the same manner as Wormwood.

¶ *Medicinal Action and Uses.* Tonic, emmenagogue, anthelmintic, antiseptic and deobstruent.

The chief use of Southernwood is as an emmenagogue. It is a good stimulant tonic and possesses some nervine principle. It is given in infusion of 1 oz. of the herb to 1 pint of boiling water, prepared in a covered vessel, the escape of steam impairing its value. This infusion or tea is agreeable, but a decoction is distasteful, having lost much of the aroma.

Fluid extract, ½ to 1 drachm.

Considerable success has also attended its use as an anthelmintic, being chiefly used against the worms of children, teaspoonful doses of the powdered herb being given in treacle morning and evening.

The branches are said to dye wool a deep yellow.

Culpepper says:

'Dioscorides saith that the seed bruised, heated in warm water and drunk helpeth those that are troubled in the cramps or convulsions of the sinews or the sciatica. The same taken in wine is an antidote and driveth away serpents and other venomous creatures, as also the smell of the herb being burnt doth the same. The oil thereof annointed on the backbone before the fits of agues come, preventeth them: it taketh away inflammation of the eyes, if it be put with some part of a wasted quince or boiled in a few crumbs of bread, and applied. Boiled in barley meal it taketh away pimples . . . that rise in the face or other parts of the body. The seed as well as the dried herb is often given to kill worms in children. The herb bruised helpeth to draw forth splinters and thorns out of the flesh. The ashes thereof dry up and heal old ulcers that are without inflammation, although by the sharpness thereof, it makes them smart. The ashes mingled with old salad oil helps those that have their hair fallen and are bald, causing the hair to grow again, either on the head or beard. A strong decoction of the leaves is a good worm medicine, but is disagreeable and nauseous. The leaves are a good ingredient in fomentation for easing pain, dispersing swellings or stopping the progress of gangrenes. The distilled water of the herb is said to helpe . . . diseases of the spleen. The Germans commend it for a singular wound herb. . . . Wormwood has thrown it into disrepute.'

SOUTHERNWOOD, FIELD

Artemisia campestris

Part Used. Herb

The Field Southernwood is common in most parts of Europe, but rare in Britain, occurring only on sandy heaths in Norfolk and Suffolk. It is perennial, like the other species of Artemisia, with a rather thick, tapering root, but unlike them, its foliage is not aromatic. The slender, grooved stems, until flowering, are prostrate; the leaves are silky when young, but nearly smooth when mature, the segments few in number, but very slender, ¼ to ½ inch long, terminating in a point with their margins recurved. The flower-heads are small and numerous, in long, slender, drooping racemes, the florets yellow and are in bloom in August and September.

¶ *Medicinal Action and Uses.* Dr. John Hill says of Field Southernwood that it is of a

'warm, fine, pleasant, aromatic taste, with a little bitterness, not enough to be disagreeable. It wants but to be more common and more known to be very highly valued . . . and one thing it is in particular, it is a composer; and always disposes the person to sleep. Opiates weaken the stomach and must not be given often where we wish for their assistance; this possesses the soothing quality without the mischief.'

This species of Artemisia has the same qualities, in a lesser degree, as the garden Southernwood, and Linnæus recommended an infusion of it as of use in pleurisy.

¶ *Cultivation of Species of Artemisia.* The Common Wormwood, Mugwort and Southernwood are regularly cultivated on some of the old established drug farms. They are grown in rows about 2 feet apart each way, and need no further care than to be kept free from weeds, growing in almost any soil. Mugwort and Common Wormwood may also be collected in the wild state.

Artemisia Dracunculus is the well-known culinary herb 'Tarragon,' a native of Siberia. It differs from the majority of its fellows in that its leaves are narrow and lance-shaped, of a bright green colour, and possess a peculiar aromatic taste, without the characteristic bitterness of the genus.

The Wormwood so frequently mentioned in Scripture is most probably *A. judaica*, growing in the Southern Desert.

See MUGWORT, TARRAGON, WORMWOOD.

SOW-THISTLES

N.O. Compositæ

SOW-THISTLE, COMMON

Sonchus oleraceus (LINN.)

Synonyms. Hare's Thistle. Hare's Lettuce
Parts Used. Leaves, stems, milky juice

The Sow-Thistle is a well-known weed in every field and garden. It is a perennial, growing from 1 to 3 feet high, with hollow, thick, branched stems full of milky juice, and thin, oblong leaves, more or less cut into (pinnatifid) with irregular, prickly teeth on the margins. The upper leaves are much simpler in form than the lower ones, clasping the stem at their bases.

The flowers are a pale yellow, and when withered, the involucres close over them in a conical form. The seed vessels are crowned with a tuft of hairs, or pappus, like most of this large family of Compositæ.

This plant is subject to great variations which are merely owing to soil and situation, some being more prickly than others.

The name of the genus, *Sonchus*, is derived from the Greek word for *hollow*, and bears allusion to the hollow nature of the succulent stems.

The Sow Thistles are sometimes erroneously called Milk Thistles from the milky juice they contain; the true Milk Thistle is, however, a very different plant (*see* THISTLES).

The Latin name of the species, *oleraceus*, refers to the use to which this weed has been put as an esculent vegetable. Its use as an article of food is of very early date, for it is recorded by Pliny that before the encounter of Theseus with the bull of Marathon, he was regaled by Hecale upon a dish of Sow-Thistles. The ancients considered them very wholesome and strengthening, and administered the juice medicinally for many disorders, considering them to have nearly the same properties as Dandelion and Succory.

The young leaves are still in some parts of the Continent employed as an ingredient in salads. It used in former times to be mingled with other pot herbs, and was occasionally employed in soups; the smoothest variety is said to be excellent boiled like spinach.

Its chief use nowadays is as food for rabbits. There is no green food they devour more eagerly, and all keepers of rabbits in hutches should provide them with a plentiful supply. Pigs are also particularly fond of the succulent leaves and stems of the Sow-Thistle.

One of the popular names of the Sow-Thistle: 'Hare's Thistle' or 'Hare's Lettuce,' refers to the fondness of hares and rabbits for this plant. An old writer tells us: 'when fainting with the heat she (the hare) recruits her strength with this herb: or if a hare eat of this herb in the summer when he is mad, he shall become whole.' Sheep and goats also eat it greedily, but horses will not touch it.

There are three or four other kinds of Sow Thistle, and as an old herbal tells us: 'They have all the same virtue, but this has them in perfection.'

SOW-THISTLE, CORN

Sonchus arvensis (LINN.),

Parts Used. Leaves, milky juice

The Corn Sow-Thistle is a perennial, with a large fleshy, creeping root. It is found in similar situations as the common species, though mainly in cornfields, where its large, bright golden flowers, externally tinged with red, showing above the corn, make it a conspicuous plant. It is readily distinguished from the Common Sow-Thistle by its stem, which is 3 to 4 feet high – being unbranched and by the much larger size of its flowers, the involucres and stalks of which are covered by numerous glandular hairs. The leaves, like those of the Common Sow-Thistle, applied outwardly by way of cataplasm, have been found serviceable in inflammatory swellings.

SOW-THISTLE, MARSH
Sonchus palustris (LINN.)

Part Used. Milky juice

The Marsh Sow-Thistle is a much taller species than either of the preceding, attaining a height of 6 to 8 feet, being one of the tallest of our English herbaceous plants. The root is perennial, fleshy and branched, but not creeping; the leaves, arrow-shaped at the base, large, shiny on the under surfaces; the flowers, large and pale yellow, with hairy involucres, are in bloom in September and October, much later than the last species, which it somewhat resembles, though the edges of the leaves are minutely toothed, not waved. It grows in marshy places but is rare in this country, being now extinct in most of the places in Norfolk, Suffolk, Kent and Essex where it was formerly found, and only occurring on the Thames below Woolwich. This thistle was placed by mediæval botanists under the planetary influences of Mars: 'Mars rules it, it is such a prickly business.'

SOW-THISTLE, MOUNTAIN
Sonchus alpinus (LINN.)

Synonym. Blue Sow-Thistle
Parts Used. Milky juice, leaves

The Blue or Mountain Sow-Thistle, a tall, handsome plant with very large blue flowers, but also very rare in these islands (it grows on the Clova Mountains), has been used as a salad in Lapland, the young shoots being stripped of their skin and eaten raw, but Linnæus informs us that it is somewhat bitter and unpalatable.

Of the Siberian Sow-Thistle (*Sonchus Tartaricus*), Anne Pratt, in *Flowers and Their Associations* (1840) says:

'This plant during that clear weather which is generally favourable to flowers, never uncloses; but let a thick mist overspread the atmosphere or a cloud arise large enough to drive home the Honey Bee, and it will soon unfold its light blue blossoms.'

¶ *Medicinal Action and Uses.* Culpepper considers that the Sow-Thistles possess great medicinal virtues, which lie chiefly in the milky juice. He tells us:

'They are cooling and somewhat binding, and are very fit to cool a hot stomach and ease the pain thereof. . . . The milk that is taken from the stalks when they are broken, given in drink, is very beneficial to those that are short-winded and have a wheezing.'

He goes on to inform us, on the authority of Pliny, that they are efficacious against gravel, and that a decoction of the leaves and stalks is good for nursing mothers; that the juice or distilled water is good 'for all inflammation, wheals and eruptions, also for hæmorrhoids.' Also that

'the juice is useful in deafness, either from accidental stoppage, gout or old age. Four spoonsful of the juice of the leaves, two of salad oil, and one teaspoonful of salt, shake the whole well together and put some on cotton dipped in this composition into the ears and you may reasonably expect a good degree of recovery.'

Again, that

'the juice boiled or thoroughly heated in a little oil of bitter almonds in the peel of a pomegranite and dropped into the ears is a sure remedy for deafness.'

Finally, he informs us that the juice 'is wonderfully efficacious for women to wash their faces with to clear the skin and give it lustre.'

Another old herbalist also says:

'The leaves are to be used fresh gathered; a strong infusion of them works by urine and opens obstructions. Some eat them in salads, but the infusion has more power.'

The whole plant has stiff spines on the leaf margin, and the seeds and roots are used in homœopathic medicine.

The milky juice of all the Sow-Thistles is an excellent cosmetic. The leaves are said to cure hares of madness.

See HAWKWEED, OX-TONGUE.

SPAGHNUM. *See* MOSS

SPEARMINT. *See* MINTS

SPEARWORT, LESSER
Ranunculus flammula (LINN.)
N.O. Ranunculaceæ

Part Used. Whole plant

The Lesser Spearwort has been used in the Isle of Skye and in many parts of the Highlands of Scotland to raise blisters, the leaves being well bruised in a mortar and applied in one or more limpet shells to the part where the blister is to be raised.

It was used in the fourteenth century under the name of 'flame' for 'cankers,' a term probably used for ulcers. Its distilled water has been employed as a harmless emetic.

This plant is very common throughout Britain, growing in wet and boggy parts of heaths and commons, where it flowers from June to September.

The stems often root at the lower joints, being more or less horizontal to start with, but afterwards rising to a foot or more in height, being terminated by a few loose flower-bearing branches. It has undivided, lanceolate (lance-shaped) leaves, the uppermost being the narrowest and smallest. The flowers are numerous, on long stalks, a light golden-yellow, $\frac{1}{2}$ to $\frac{3}{4}$ inch across.

¶ *Medicinal Action and Uses.* A tincture is used to cure ulcers.

See BUTTERCUP, CELANDINE.

SPEEDWELL, COMMON
Part Used. Herb

Veronica officinalis (LINN.)

N.O. Scrophulariaceæ

The Common Speedwell is a native of the Old World, but is abundantly naturalized in the eastern United States, where it grows in open, grassy places.

In this country, it is generally found on heaths, moors, dry hedgebanks and in coppices, where it is very common and generally distributed.

¶ *Description.* The plant is a perennial, of a prostrate habit, with ascending branches, bearing erect, spike-like clusters of blue flowers, the stems 3 to 18 inches long, varying very much in length according to soil. The leaves are opposite, shortly stalked, generally about an inch long, oval and attenuated into their foot-stalks, their margins finely toothed. The flowers are in dense, axillary, many-flowered racemes, $1\frac{1}{2}$ to 6 inches long, the individual flowers nearly stalkless on the main flower-stalk, their corollas only $\frac{1}{6}$ inch across, pale blue with dark blue stripes and bearing two stamens with a very long style. The capsule is inversely heart-shaped and notched, longer than the oblong, narrow sepals. The plant is of a dull green and is generally slightly hairy, having short hairs, sometimes smooth.

The fresh herb is faintly aromatic. After drying, it is inodorous. It has a bitterish, warm, and somewhat astringent taste.

¶ *Constituents.* Enz found a bitter principle, soluble in water and alcohol, but scarcely so in ether, and precipitated by the salts of lead, but not by tannic acid; an acrid principle; red colouring matter; a variety of tannic acid, producing a green colour with ferric salts; a crystallizable, fatty acid, with malic, tartaric, citric, acetic and lactic acids; mannite; a soft, dark green bitter resin.

Mayer, of New York (in 1863), found evidences of an alkaloid and of a saponaceous principle. Vintilesco (1910) found a glucoside both in this species and in *Veronica chamædrys.*

¶ *Medicinal Action and Uses.* This species of Veronica retained a place among our recognized remedies until a comparatively late period, and is still employed in herbal medicine.

Its leaves possess astringency and bitterness.

Among the Welsh peasantry, great virtues are attributed to the Speedwell. The plant has diaphoretic, alterative, diuretic, expectorant and tonic properties, and was formerly employed in pectoral and nephritic complaints, hæmorrhages, diseases of the skin and in the treatment of wounds. Modern herbalists still consider that an infusion of the dried plant is useful in coughs, catarrh, etc., and is a simple and effective remedy in skin diseases.

¶ *Other Species.*

In *Familiar Wild Flowers* (and also in Lindley's *Treasury of Botany*) mention is made of another Speedwell called 'Buxbaum's Speedwell' (*V. Buxbaumii*) which the author states is sometimes mistaken for *V. Agrestis,* but is a distinct species. It branches freely and attains to a height of a foot or so; its stem and leaves are thickly clothed with soft and silky hairs. The leaves are placed singly at irregular intervals along the stem, but are more numerous towards the summit; they are broadly heart-shaped, with margins deeply-cut into teeth, each leaf has a short leaf-stalk; all leaves are of the same character. The flower-bearing stems that spring from the axils of the leaves are very long, and give a decided character to the plant, while the flowers themselves have the curious Veronica character – three large and fairly equal segments and then a lower and narrower one. The blossoms are a clear blue in colour, and for a Veronica are decidedly large. The fruit or capsule that succeeds the flower is twice as broad as it is long, and this flattened-out character is a specific feature. It derived its name from a distinguished botanist of the eighteenth century.

Buxbaum's Speedwell is a plant of cultivation, springing up in gardens and fields, and never far from human society and influence. It is a southerner, and though found throughout England and even Southern Scot-

758

land, it is more at home in less northern latitudes, and was probably introduced with some kind of foreign seed.

V. Serpyllifolia (Thyme-leaved Speedwell); the Marsh Speedwell (*V. scutellata*); the Ivy-leaved Speedwell (*V. hederifolia*); the Procumbent Speedwell (*V. agrestis*); and the Wall Speedwell (*V. arvensis*).

The Spiked Speedwell (*V. spicata*) is decidedly rare, but a handsome species; the Rock Veronica (*V. saxatilis*), a fine species with few flowers, is chiefly found in the highlands of Scotland.

Three other extremely rare species are *V. verna* (Vernal Speedwell), *V. alpina* (Alpine Speedwell) and *V. triphyllos* (The Finger Speedwell).

See VERONICAS.

SPEEDWELL, GERMANDER

Veronica chamædrys (LINN.)
N.O. Scrophulariaceæ

Synonyms. Fluellin the Male. Veronique petit Chêne. Paul's Betony. Eye of Christ. Angels' Eyes. Cat's Eye. Bird's Eye. Farewell
Part Used. Herb

Speedwell, Germander, is the commonest British species of Speedwell, found everywhere, on banks, pastures, in copses, etc., flowering in spring and early summer.

The name Germander is a corruption of the Latin *chamædrys*. Gerard commenting on the name says: 'The Germander from the form of the leaves like unto small oak leaves, has the name chamædrys given it, which signifieth a dwarf oak' – though the likeness is not very pronounced.

¶ *Description.* This little plant has a creeping, branched root-stock, passing insensibly into the stem, which is weak and decumbent to the point where the leaves commence, and then raises itself about a foot, to carry up the flowers. The leaves are in pairs, nearly stalkless, ½ to 1½ inches long, egg-shaped to heart-shaped, deeply furrowed by the veins, the margins coarsely toothed. On the whole length of the stem are two lines of long hairs running down between each pair of leaves, shifting from side to side wherever they arrive at a fresh pair of leaves. These hairy lines act as barriers to check the advance of unwelcome crawling insects. The leaves themselves bear jointed hairs, and the flower-stalks, calyx and capsule also have long, gland-tipped hairs. The leaves are sometimes attacked by a gall mite, *Cecidomyia Veronica*, and white galls like white buttons are the result on the ends of the shoots.

The numerous flowers are in loose racemes, 2 to 6 inches long in the axils of the leaves, the flowers are rather close together on first expanding, but become distant after the fall of the corolla, which is ½ inch across, bright blue with darker lines, and a white eye in the centre, where the four petals join into the short tube. The corolla is so lightly attached that the least jarring causes it to drop, so that the plant at the slightest handling loses its bright blossom – hence, perhaps, its name Speedwell and similar local names, 'Farewell' and 'Good-bye.' The under lip of the corolla covers the upper in bud. The flower closes at night and also in rainy weather, when the brightness of the blossoms quite disappears, only the pale and pearly underside of its petals being visible.

The cross fertilization of the flower is performed chiefly by drone flies. On either side of the big, double, top petal, a little stamen stretches outward like a horn. When an insect approaches, it grasps the stamens with its front legs and they are thus drawn forwards and onwards, so that they dust the under-side of the insect with their pollen. He steadies himself for a moment, probing the flower for the nectar round the ovary and then flies away. As the stamens in any flower do not discharge their pollen until after the stigma, which projects over the lower petal, has been ready for some time to receive it, and since the stigmas also rub on the insect's abdomen, it is evident that it will probably be fertilized from some neighbouring flower before its own pollen is ready for use. When before and during rain the flower is closed, in the absence of insect visitors, it then, however, successfully carries on self-fertilization. Kerner, in *Flowers and their Unbidden Guests*, notes this fact in referring to the Speedwells, saying: 'In the mountainous districts of the temperate zones, it often happens that rainy weather sets in just at the time when the flowers are about to open, and that it lasts for weeks. Humble and hive-bees, butterflies and flies retire to their hiding-places, and for a considerable time cease to pay any visits to flowers. The growth of the plants is not, however, arrested during this period, and even in the flowers themselves, development quietly progresses if the temperature be not too low. The stigmatic tissue becomes receptive, the anthers attain to maturity, dehisce, and liberate their pollen, notwithstanding that no ray of sunshine penetrates the clouds, and that rain falls continuously. In such circumstances the mouth of the flower is not opened, self-fertilization takes place in the closed flower, and all the adjustments evolved with the object of securing cross-fertilization are ineffectual.'

The two-celled ovary matures into a flattened capsule, deeply notched at the top, which opens round the edges by two valves. The *Seeds* are said to be specially good as food for birds.

¶ *Medicinal Action and Uses.* Old writers of all countries speak highly of the virtues of the Speedwell as a vulnerary, a purifier of the blood, and a remedy in various skin diseases, its outward application being considered efficacious for the itch. It was also believed to cure smallpox and measles, and to be a panacea for many ills. Gerard recommends it for cancer, 'given in good broth of a hen,' and advocates the use of the root as a specific against pestilential fevers.

It is not to be confused with Germander (*Teucrium chamædrys*), the celebrated specific for gout, used by the Emperor Charles V.

The Germander Speedwell has a certain amount of astringency, and an infusion of its leaves was at one time famous for coughs, the juice of the fresh plant also, boiled into a syrup with honey, was used for asthma and catarrh, and a decoction of the whole plant was employed to stimulate the kidneys.

SPIKENARD, AMERICAN

Aralia racemosa (LINN.)
N.O. Araliaceæ

Synonyms. Spignet. Life of Man. Pettymorell. Old Man's Root. Indian Spikenard. Indian Root
Part Used. Root
Habitat. North America, New Zealand, Japan

¶ *Description.* The much-branched stem grows from 3 to 6 feet high. Very large leaves, consisting of thin oval heart-shaped, double saw-toothed leaflets. Small greenish flowers in many clusters – blooming later than *Aralia medicaulis* (for which it is often substituted), July to August. Has roundish red-brown berries going dark purple. Root-stock thick and large, spicy and aromatic. Fracture of cortex short, of the wood also short and fibrous. Odour aromatic, taste mucilaginous, pungent and slightly acrid. Transverse section of root shows thick bark, several zones containing oil. The plant grows freely in the author's garden.

¶ *Constituents.* Volatile oil, resin, tannin, etc.

¶ *Medicinal Action and Uses.* Stimulant, diaphoretic, alterative for syphilitic, cutaneous and rheumatic cases, and used in same manner and dosage as genuine Sarsaparilla. Much used also for pulmonary affections, and enters into the compound syrup of Spikenard. Fluid extract, ½ to 1 drachm. Infusion of ½ oz. to a pint of water in wineglassful doses.

See ARALIAS, SARSAPARILLAS.

SPIKENARD, CALIFORNIAN

Aralia Californica or Californian Spikenard may be used for same purposes as the other species. It is very like *A. racemosa*, but bigger in herbage and root.

See ANGELICA TREE, DWARF ELDER (AMERICAN), SARSAPARILLAS.

SPIKENARD, PLOUGHMAN'S

Inula Conyza
N.O. Compositæ

Synonyms. Conyza Squarrosa (Linn.). Cloron's Hard. Horse Heal. Cinnamon Root. Great Fleabane
Part Used. Herb
Habitat. It is found on dry banks and in copses, principally on limestone or chalky soil.

Ploughman's Spikenard is another member of this genus that – as its name implies – has had a popular reputation for its curative powers.

¶ *Description.* Its upright stems, rising from a biennial root, generally only a foot or two in height, often purplish in colour and downy, are branched and terminated by numerous small flower-heads of a dingy yellow or dusky purple, only about two-thirds of an inch across, the ray florets inconspicuous and the leaf-like scales of the involucre rolled back. The leaves of the plant are narrow, of a dull green, egg-shaped and downy. Their margins are either entire, or toothed, the teeth ending in horny points.

The plant has a slight, but not unpleasant, aromatic odour, hence, perhaps, one of its local names: Cinnamon Root.

¶ *Medicinal Action and Uses.* The older herbalists considered Ploughman's Spikenard a good wound herb, and it was frequently taken in decoction for bruises, ruptures, inward wounds, pains in the side and difficulty of breathing. It also had a reputation as an emmenagogue, and the juice of the while plant was applied externally to cure the itch.

The very smell of the plant was said to destroy fleas, and the leaves have been used, burnt, as an insecticide. Great Fleabane is one of its popular names.

Its specific name, *Conyza*, is derived from the Greek word for dust or powder, and refers to its power of killing noxious insects.

The leaves are sometimes substituted for

Digitalis, but may be readily distinguished by their entire margins to the leaves or, when toothed, by the horny points terminating the teeth.

Inula of several species (especially *Inule Britannica*, Linn.) has been used to adulterate Arnica flowers. *En masse*, this spurious drug is pale and dull-looking, and its rays are small and narrow and of a pale yellow, whereas Arnica flower rays are broad and bright yellow. Also Inula has the involucral scales in several series, the receptacle is not hairy, and the anther-bases are long-tailed.

See ELECAMPANE, FLEABANE.

SPINACH

Spinacia oleracea (LINN.)
N.O. Chenopodiaceæ

Part Used. Leaves

Habitat. The Spinach is an annual plant, long cultivated for the sake of its succulent leaves, a native of Asia, probably of Persian origin, being introduced into Europe about the fifteenth century

¶ *Constituents.* Spinach is relatively rich in nitrogenous substances, in hydrocarbons, and in iron sesqui-oxide, which last amounts to 3·3 per cent. of the total ash. It is thus more nourishing than other green vegetables. It is a valuable part of the diet in anæmia, not only on account of its iron, but also for its chlorophyll. Chlorophyll is known to have a chemical formula remarkably similar to that of hæmoglobin, and it is stated that the ingestion of chlorophyll will raise the hæmoglobin of the blood without increasing the formed elements. The plant contains from 10 to 20 parts per 1,000 by weight of chlorophyll. During the war, wine fortified with Spinach juice (1 in 50) was given to French soldiers weakened by hæmorrhage.

According to Chick and Roscoe (*Biochem. Journal*, 1926, XX, 137), fresh leaves of Spinach are a rich source of vitamin A, a small daily ration (0·1 gram and upward) encouraging growth and lessening or preventing xerophthalmia in young rats on diets devoid of fat-soluble vitamins. Spinach grown in the open in winter, spring or autumn possesses no antirachitic properties that can be demonstrated by the methods employed. Spinach leaves when irradiated with ultra-violet rays from a Hg vapour quartz lamp become powerfully antirachitic.

Boas (*Biochem. Journal*, 1926, XX, 153) found that the fresh leaves of winter-grown Spinach added to an experimental diet caused an even greater improvement in the well-being of rats and in the rate of growth than was caused by the addition of cod-liver oil. The weight of the skeleton was not, however, proportionally increased. The conclusion was drawn by Boas that winter Spinach con-

tains an amount of vitamin D which is negligible compared with its content of vitamin A.

The leaves contain a large proportion of saltpetre. The water drained from Spinach, after cooking, is capable of making as good match-paper as that made by a solution of nitre.

¶ *Cultivation.* Spinach should be grown on good ground, well worked and well manured, and for the summer crops abundant water will be necessary.

To afford a succession of Summer Spinach, the seeds should be sown about the middle of February and again in March. After this period, small quantities should be sown once a fortnight, as Summer Spinach lasts a very short time. The seeds are generally sown in shallow drills, between the lines of peas. If occupying the whole of a plot, the rows should be 1 foot apart.

The Round-seeded is the best kind for summer use.

The Prickly-seeded and the Flanders kinds are the best for winter and should be thinned out early in the autumn to about 2 inches apart, and later on to 6 inches. The Lettuce-leaved is a good succulent winter variety but not quite so hardy.

The first sowing of Winter Spinach should be made early in August and again towards the end of that month, in some sheltered but not shaded situation, in rows 18 inches apart, the plants as they advance being thinned and the ground hoed. By the beginning of winter, the outer leaves will have become fit for use, and if the weather is mild successive gatherings may be obtained up to the baginning of May.

SPINACH, NEW ZEALAND

Tetragonia expansar
N.O. Picoideæ

New Zealand Spinach is a half-hardy annual, a native of New Zealand, sometimes used as a substitute for Spinach during the summer months, but decidedly inferior to it. It is unrelated to the Spinach, belonging to the *Picoideæ*.

When cultivated in this country, seeds are sown in March on a gentle hot-bed. They must be previously steeped in water for several hours. The seedlings should be potted and placed in a frame till the end of May and then planted out in light, rich soil.

Only the young leaves are gathered for use, a succession being produced during summer and autumn.

See ARRACHS, CHENOPODIUMS, GOOSEFOOTS.

SPINDLE TREE

Euonymus atropurpureus
Euonymus Europœus (JACQ.)
N.O. Celastraceæ

Synonyms. Fusanum. Fusoria. Skewerwood. Prickwood. Gatter. Gatten. Gadrose. Pigwood. Dogwood. Indian Arrowroot. Burning Bush. Wahoo
(*French*) Fusain. Bonnet-de-prêtre
(*German*) Spindelbaume
Parts Used. Root, bark, berries

¶ *Description.* The Spindle Tree found in our hedges and copses is a smooth-leaved shrub. The leaves have very short stalks, are opposite in pairs and have minute teeth on the margin. It bears small greenish-white flowers, in loose clusters, during May and June, followed by an abundance of fruits. The fruit is three or more lobed, and becomes a beautiful rose-red colour; it bursts when ripe, disclosing ruddy-orange-coloured seeds, which are wrapped in a scarlet arillus. This yields a good yellow dye when boiled in water, and a green one with the addition of alum, but these dyes are fugitive. The berries attract children, but are harmful, for they are strongly emetic and purgative: they have proved fatal to sheep. The bark, leaves and fruit are all injurious, and no animal but the goat will browse upon them.

The Latin name for Spindle is *Fusus*, and by some of the old writers this plant is called Fusanum and the Fusoria. By the Italians it is still called Fusano. The fruit is given three or four as a dose, as a purgative in rural districts; and the decoction, adding some vinegar, is used as a lotion for mange in horses and cattle. In allusion to the actively irritating properties of the shrub, its name *Euonymus* is associated with that of Euonyme, the mother of the Furies. In old herbals it is called Skewerwood or prickwood (the latter from its employment as toothpicks), and *gatter, gatten*, or *gadrose*. Chaucer, in one of his poems, calls it *gaitre*.

Prior says:

Gatter is from the Anglo-Saxon words, *gad* (a goad) and *treow* (a tree); *gatten* is made up of *gad* again and *tan* (a twig); and *gadrise* is from *gad* and *hris* (a rod).'

The same hardness that fitted it for skewers, spindles, etc., made it useful for the ox-goad.

Turner apparently christened the tree Spindle Tree. He says:

'I coulde never learne an Englishe name for it. The Duche men call it in Netherlande, *spilboome*, that is, spindel-tree, because they use to make spindels of it in that country, and me thynke it may be as well named in English seying we have no other name. . . . I know no goode propertie that this tree hath, saving only it is good to make spindels and brid of cages (bird-cages).'

The wood, which is of a light yellow hue, strong, compact and easily worked, fulfils many uses. On the Continent it is used for making pipe-stems, and an excellent charcoal is made from the young shoots, which artists approve for its smoothness, and the ease with which it can be erased. It is also employed in the making of gunpowder.

¶ *Cultivation.* It is found in woods and hedgerows. The green and variegated Spindle Trees are familiar in British gardens. They all grow freely in any kind of soil, and are easily increased by inserting the ripened tips of the branches, about 3 inches long, into a fine, sandy loam in autumn, keeping them damp and fresh with a frequent spraying overhead. A species from South Europe and another from Japan are cultivated.

¶ *Parts Used.* The variety of Spindle Tree (*Euonymus atropurpureus*), common in the eastern United States, is known there as Wahoo, Burning Bush, or Indian Arrowwood. This is the kind generally used in medicine.

It is a shrub about 6 feet high, with a smooth ash-coloured bark, and has small dark purple flowers and leaves purple-tinged at the serrated edges.

Wahoo bark, as it is called commercially, is the dried root-bark of this species.

The root-bark is alone official, but the stem-bark is also collected and used as a substitute.

The root-bark, when dried, is in quilled or curved pieces, $\frac{1}{12}$ to $\frac{1}{6}$ inch thick, ash-grey, with blackish ridges or patches, outer surface whitish, or slightly tawny and quite smooth. Fracture friable, smooth, whitish, the inner layer appearing tangentially striated. The taste is sweetish, bitter and acrid. It has a very faint, characteristic odour, resembling liquorice.

The stem-bark is in longer quills, with a smooth outer surface, with lichens usually present on it, and a greenish layer under the epidermis.

¶ *Constituents.* Little is definitely known of the chemical constituents of Euonymus Bark. Its chief constituent is a nearly colourless intensely bitter principle, a resin called Euonymin. There are also present euonic acid, a crystalline glucoside, asparagin, resins, fat, dulcitol, and 14 per cent. of ash.

Commercial Euonymin is a powdered extract.

¶ *Medicinal Action and Uses.* Tonic, alterative, cholagogue, laxative and hepatic stimulant.

SPERGULARIA. *See* SANDSPURRY

SPURGES

Genera more than 200, species more than 3,000, representing almost all habits of growth and exhibiting a high degree of adaptability to varying environments. The valuable rubbers produced by the family are of great importance, notably that from the prepared milk juice of several species of *Hevea*, known in commerce as Para rubber.

The medicinal properties of the family depend chiefly upon two classes of constituents; first, fixed oils, or the fatty acids freed by their decomposition, typical properties of which are castor oil, from *Recinus communis*, and Croton oil, from *Croton tigilum*; also valuable drying oils, the artists' oil or lambang from the seeds of *Aleurites moluccana*, tung oil, said to be the most perfect drying oil known, from seeds of *A. cordata*. From *A. laccifera* gum-lac, of a very superior quality, is obtained; another excellent drying oil is obtained from *Sapium sebiferum*, known as Chinese tallow. Besides the cathartic properties resident in the fixed oils of these seeds,

In small doses, Euonymin stimulates the appetite and the flow of the gastric juice. In larger doses, it is irritant to the intestine and is cathartic. It has slight diuretic and expectorant effects, but its only use is as a purgative in cases of constipation in which the liver is disordered, and for which it is particularly efficacious. It is specially valuable in liver disorders which follow or accompany fever. It is mildly aperient and causes no nausea, at the same time stimulating the liver somewhat freely, and promoting a free flow of bile.

To make the decoction, add an ounce to a pint of water and boil together slowly. A small wineglassful to be given, when cold, for a dose, two or three times a day.

Of the tincture made with spirit from the bark, 5 to 10 drops may be taken in water or on sugar.

Euonymin is generally given in pill form and in combination with other tonics, laxatives, etc.

¶ *Preparations.* Fluid extract, $\frac{1}{2}$ to 1 drachm. Powdered extract, B.P. and U.S.P., 2 grains. Euonymin, 1 to 4 grains.

¶ *Other Species.* The green leaves of one species of *Euonymus* are said to be eaten by the Arabs to produce watchfulness, and a sprig of it is believed to be – to the person who carries it – a protection from plague. Another species is said to inflict painful wounds.

Euphorbias
N.O. Euphorbiaceæ

somewhat similar properties, almost always accompanied by more or less emesis, exists in the plant-parts generally, the active constituents being usually carried in the milk juices, so that the family has yielded a large number of drugs used somewhat like Ipecacuanha.

The genus *Euphorbia* comprises nearly a thousand species, and a large number of these species yield a milky juice. Some are herbaceous or shrubby, with or without leaves, the leafless varieties flourishing on African deserts like the cactus, having spiny stems. The milky juice of the stem coagulates on exposure to the air, forming a resinous mass which is generally marketed in the form of tears.

For external use it is of service in chronic rheumatism and paralysis as a counter-irritant, alone, or combined with cantharides, merezeon bark, etc., or as a plaster when mixed with Burgundy pitch or resin.

It is a violent irritant and caustic poison. At the Cape, the capsules are used for destroying animals. It may produce delirium.

(POISON)
SPURGE, OFFICIAL

Euphorbia resinifera
N.O. Euphorbiaceæ

Synonyms. Euphorbia officinarum. Poisonous Gum-Thistle. Dergmuse. Darkmous. Euphorbium Bush. Gum Euphorbium
Part Used. Concrete resinous juice
Habitat. The slopes of the Great Atlas range in Morocco

¶ *Description.* Resembling a cactus in appearance, this leafless perennial plant has a stem about 4 feet in height, and many branches. The flowers are small, simple, and bright yellow, and the fruit a small capsule with one seed in each cell. Specimens sent to Kew in 1870 have never flowered, but others have done so in Paris. Both Pliny and Dioscorides knew the drug, and its name is classical.

The milky juice is collected from incisions made in the fleshy branches, and is so acrid that it burns the fingers. It flows down the stems and encrusts them as it hardens in the sun. Poor Arabs bring in the resinous masses for sale in Morocco, whence it is chiefly exported from Mogador. The dust is so intensely irritant to the mucous membrane, that the mouth and nose of those handling it must be covered by a cloth.

In commerce the drug is found in yellowish-brown 'tears' that have a waxy appearance. They are almost transparent, slightly aromatic only when heated, and often pierced with holes made by the prickles of the plant while drying. The taste is slight, but becomes very acrid.

SPURGES, VARIOUS

Euphorbia cerifera is one of the sources of Candelilla wax which occurs as a coating on all parts of the plant.

'PILLBEARING SPURGE' (*E. pilulifera*) is commonly known as Queensland asthma weed, cat's hair, in allusion to its globular, axillary inflorescences. Is very common in all tropical countries. Its principal constituents are resins described as glucosidal, wax, and volatile matter; it is collected whilst flowering and fruiting, and has been utilized by some practitioners with a certain success in the treatment of subacute and chronic inflammation of the respiratory duct. Toxic doses have killed small animals through failure of respiration. The decoction is taken in asthmatic conditions, chronic bronchitis, and emphysema, the tincture being used in coryza and hay fever.

¶ *Dosage.* Compound Elixir of Euphorbia, C.F., from *E. pilulifera*. Tincture of Euphorbia, B.P.C., from *E. pilulifera*, 10 to 30 minims. Fluid extract of *E. pilulifera*, ½ to 1 drachm. Decoction of *E. pilulifera*, 1 in 40, 1 tablespoonful.

It is said to be employed as an ingredient of paint used for preserving ships' bottoms.

At Mogador, the branches are used for tanning leather.

¶ *Constituents.* The chief constituent is resin, and it also contains wax, calcium malate, potassium malate, lignin, bassorin, volatile oil, and water, with no soluble gum. Another analysis gives euphorbone, euphorbo-resene, euphorbic acid, calcium malate, a very acrid substance not yet isolated, and vegetable debris.

The acrid resin is soluble in alcohol, and will burn brilliantly, becoming very aromatic.

The powder is yellowish, and violently sternatatory.

¶ *Medicinal Action and Uses.* The internal use of the drug has been abandoned, owing to the severity of its action. It is an irritant emetic and cathartic. Its chief use is as a vesicant, and principally in veterinary practice. It has been used in dropsy; mixed with cantharides as a 'gout plaister'; and as an errhine in chronic brain, ear, or eye complaints, sometimes mitigated with the powder of *Convallaria maialis*, but accidents have led to its use being discontinued.

E. corollata: dose of dried root as an emetic, 10 to 20 grains; as a cathartic, 3 to 10 grains.

E. hypericifolia: an infusion of the dried leaves, ½ oz. infused in a pint of boiling water for ½ hour and a tablespoonful taken for a dose.

¶ *Other Species.*
E. tetragona, E. antiquorum of the African coast, and *E. canariensis* of the Canary Islands also supply the drug.

WHITE IPECACUANHA (*E. ipecacuanha*), the root of which is used, contains a fixed oil, starch, glucose, and various salts, also resin. Its medicinal properties are similar to *E. corollata*.

WHITE PURSLANE (*E. corollata*). Syn. White Parsley, Purging or Emetic Root, Apple Root, Wild Hippo. The whole plant is used, including the root. Its habitat is east and central North America. It abounds in lactiferous ducts, which contain starch; the resin is or carries the actual principle, the presence of glucoside is conjecture. Formerly it was used as an emetic in 10 to 20 grains, and as a cathartic in 3 to 10 grains, but because of its irritating and uncertain properties its use has been practically abandoned; the recent root bruised and applied to the skin produces vesication.

CAPER SPURGE (*E. lathyris*). (Syn. Mole Plant.) Has a milky juice of an acrid nature. Its seeds yield an abundance of fine clear oil called oil of Euphorbia; this is obtained by expression or by the action of alcohol or ether, and is colourless, inodorous, and almost insipid; it rapidly becomes rancid, and acquires a dangerous acrimony. The oil is a very violent poison, producing violent purgation and having an irritating effect upon the mucous membrane of the intestinal canal, and especially on the larger intestines; the oil resembles croton oil. In doses of 5 drops it is said to be less acrid and irritating than croton oil; it must be recently extracted. The seeds to the number of twelve or fifteen are used by country people in France as a purgative. The root of the plant is equally purgative and emetic; the leaves are vesicant and are used by beggars to produce ulcers by which to excite pity; the juice is depilatory; the seeds contain æsculetin in the free state.

E. hypericifolia is regarded in tropical America as a powerful astringent and has a reputation in the cure of diarrhœa and dysentery; it has also narcotic properties. The juice is said to cause temporary blindness when applied to the eyes; it contains caoutchouc, gallic acid, resin and tannin.

SPOTTED SPURGE (*E. maculata*) represents a group used by eclectics and homœopaths with claims for properties more or less special. It has been used in cholera, diarrhœa and dysentery in the form of an infusion of the leaves, and has been found to contain caoutchouc resin, tannin, and apparently euphorbon. Is said to be a valuable astringent; an infusion may be employed as an injection in the treatment of leucorrhœa. To this medicinal group belongs:

E. esula (Linn.) (Leafy Spurge) of Europe.
E. peplus (Linn.) of Europe.
E. helioscopia (Linn.) of Europe (Sun or Wart Spurge, Churnstaff, Seven Sisters).
E. humistrata (Engl.) of central North America.
E. hypericifolia (Linn.) of North America.
E. portulacoides of Chile.
E. iata (Eng.) of U.S.A.
E. marginata (Pursh.) (Mountain Snow) of western U.S.A.
E. Drummondii, the juice, has caused many fatalities to sheep and cattle in Australia.
E. cremocarpus is used in Australia for the poisoning of fish in calm pools and streams.

E. heterodoxa, a Brazilian species, said to have been used with extraordinary success against cancerous and syphilitic ulcers. It is a powerful irritant, mildly caustic; the milky juice preserved with salicylic acid is used.

E. prostata grows in the south-western portions of the U.S.A., and has the reputation of being a specific against the bite of the rattlesnake, spiders, etc.; the juice is used.

E. parviflora and *E. hirta*. Both used in India as antisyphilitics, and *E. canescens* similarly in Spain.

The juice of *E. linearis* is employed in Brazil for syphilitic ulcers of the cornua. *E. hiberna* was formerly much used in syphilis before the introduction of mercury. The plant is extensively employed by the peasantry of Kerry for stupefying fish, and so powerful are its qualities that a small basket filled with the bruised leaves will poison the fish for several miles down the river. The same properties are possessed by *E. platyphylla*, and in Brazil *E. cotinifolia* is used for the same purpose, and the acrid juice which drops from it is used by the natives to poison their arrows.

The seeds and leaves of *E. thymifolia* of India are given by the Tamuls as an anthelmintic and in bowel affections of children.

E. balsamifera, when cooked, is eaten in the Canaries.

The juice of *E. Mauritanica*, when dried, is employed as a condiment, and forms one of the adulterations of Scammony.

In countries bordering on the Mediterranean, *E. Peplis*, *E. spinosa*, *E. Dendroides*, *E. Aleppica*, *E. Apois*, are used as purgatives in domestic practice.

E. peplus, *E. peploides*, *E. pilosa*, *E. palustris* have the reputation of being remedies in hydrophobia.

E. Helisscopia juice is commonly applied to warts, and sometimes, though improperly, used to cure sore eyelids, causing in many instances intolerable pain and inflammation.

The bark of the roots of *E. Gerardiane*, *E. amydaloides* and *E. Cyparissias* have febrifuge reputations; but the latter is known to possess dangerous properties. It is destructive to sheep, and La Motte has seen a woman perish from having taken a lavement prepared with the plant. In France it is used as a popular purgative, under the name of *Rhubarbe des pauvres*. Orfila regards it as a poison.

The milky juice of *E. amydaloides* is very acrid, and though not highly poisonous, corrodes and ulcerates the flesh wherever it is applied.

Warts and corns anointed with it are said soon to disappear, but great caution is needed in using it, or injury is likely to result to the surrounding skin. Though said to be a remedy for toothache, it is not to be recommended on account of its very acrid nature.

The juice of *E. tribuloides,* a small cactus-shaped species growing in the Canaries, is there used as a diaphoretic.

It is reported by Scopoli, in his *Flora Carnoilica,* that he has seen death occasioned by the administration of 30 grains of the seed of *E. esula,* and gangrene caused on the belly by the application of the plant on that part; he also adds that people have lost their eyesight by rubbing their eyes with its juice.

E. buxifolia in the West Indies, *E. papillosa*

in Brazil, *E. laurifolia* in Peru, and *E. portulacoides* in Chile are used as purgatives.

E. tirucalli is employed in India as a vesicant, and in Java as a powerful emetic and purgative. It is said that exhalations from the tree cause the loss of eyesight; the juice is considered sudorific and, according to Sonnerat, is administered in India, in doses of a drachm, mixed with flour, daily as an antisyphilitic.

E. ligularia, another native of India, is held sacred to Munsa, the goddess of serpents; the root of the tree, mixed with black pepper, is employed for the cure of snake-bites, both internally and externally.

SQUAW VINE

Mitchella repens (LINN.)
N.O. Rubiaceæ

Synonyms. Partridgeberry. Checkerberry. Winter Clover. Deerberry. One-berry
Part Used. Herb
Habitat. United States

¶ *Description.* The plant grows in dry woods, among hemlock timber, and in swampy places; in flower in June and July. The leaves resemble those of clover and remain green throughout the winter. The fruit or berry also remains bright scarlet, is edible, and nearly tasteless, dry, and full of stony seeds. The use of the drug is peculiarly American.

¶ *Constituents.* It has been found to contain resin, wax, mucilage, dextrin, and what appears to be saponin.

¶ *Medicinal Action and Uses.* Parturient, diuretic, tonic, astringent. Beneficial in all uterine complaints. It resembles in its action pipsissewa (Chimaphila), for which it is often substituted. It is taken by Indian women for

weeks before confinement, in order to render parturition safe and easy. A herbal physician should be consulted for a safe and effectual preparation.

It is used in dropsy, suppression of urine, and diarrhœa. The following preparation is a cure for sore nipples: 2 oz. of the herb (fresh, if possible), 1 pint of water. Make a strong decoction, strain, and add an equal quantity of good cream. Boil the whole down to the consistency of a soft salve, and when cool, anoint the nipple every time the child is removed from the breast.

¶ *Dosages.* Of a strong decoction, 2 to 4 fluid ounces, two or three times a day. Fluid extract, ½ to 1 drachm.

SQUILL

Urginea scilla (STEINHEIL)
N.O. Liliaceæ

Synonyms. Maritime Squill. Scilla maritima (Linn.). Urginea maritima. Urginea Indica. White Squill. Red Squill
Part Used. Bulb, cut into slices, dried and powdered
Habitat. The Squill is found in dry, sandy places, especially the seacoast in most of the Mediterranean districts, being abundant in southern Spain, where it is by no means confined to the coast, and is found in Portugal, Morocco, Algeria, Corsica, southern France, Italy, Malta, Dalmatia, Greece, Syria and Asia Minor. In Sicily, where it grows most abundantly, it ascends to an elevation of 3,000 feet. Its range also includes the Canary Islands and the Cape of Good Hope. It is often grown under fig-trees in the Italian Riviera, and is grown in many botanical gardens, having first been recorded as cultivated in England in 1648, in the Oxford Botanic Gardens

¶ *Description.* It is a perennial plant with fibrous roots proceeding from the base of a large, tunicated, nearly globular bulb, 4 to 6 inches long, the outer scales of which are thin and papery, red or orange-brown in colour. The bulb, which is usually only half immersed in the sand, sends forth several long, lanceolate, pointed, somewhat undulated, shining, dark-green leaves, when fully grown

2 feet long. From the middle of the leaves, a round, smooth, succulent flower-stem rises, from 1 to 3 feet high, terminating in a long, close spike of whitish flowers, which stand on purplish peduncles, at the base of each of which is a narrow, twisted, deciduous floral leaf or bract. The flowers are in bloom in April and May and are followed by oblong capsules.

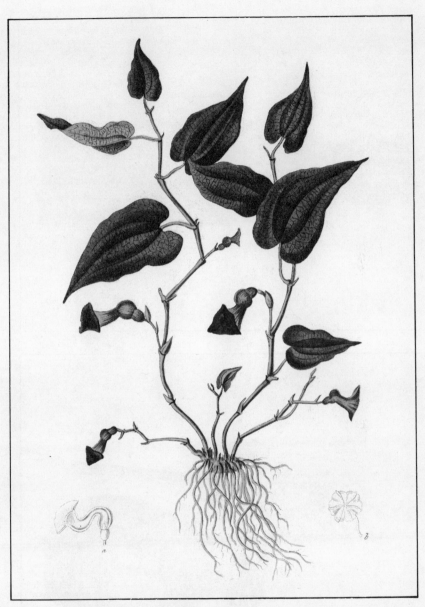

SNAKEROOT
Aristolochia Serpentaria

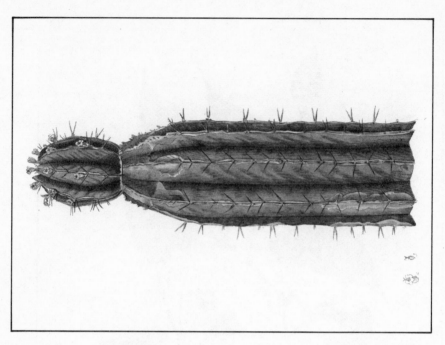

SPURGE (EUPHORBIUM)
Euphorbia Resinifera

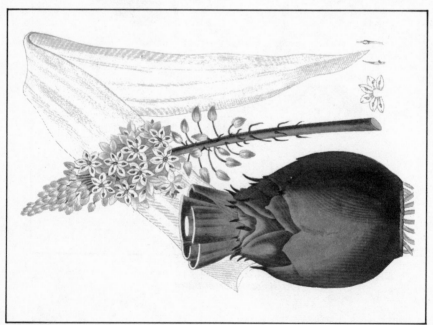

SQUILL
Urginea Scilla

It is a very variable plant, the bulb differing greatly in size and colour, and the leaves of the flower presenting similar varieties, which has led to the formation of several species, about twenty-five species having been described. Two varieties of Squill, termed respectively *white* and *red*, are distinguished by druggists. In the first named, the bulb scales are whitish or yellowish in colour, whereas the red species has deep, reddish-brown outer scales and yellowish white inner scales, covered with a pinkish epidermis, intermediate forms also occurring. No essential difference exists in the medicinal properties of the two kinds.

The White Squill, collected in Malta and Sicily, is preferred in England, while the Red Squill, collected in Algeria, is used in France. Both varieties are mentioned by Pliny and other ancient writers: the white is more mentioned in mediæval literature, though the medical school of Salerno preferred the red variety of the drug.

The United States Pharmacopœia defines the drug Scilla as the inner scales of the bulb of the white variety of *Urginea maritima* (Linn.).

Scilla, the classical name of the plant, is derived from a Greek word meaning to excite or disturb, as an emetic does the stomach. *Scilla maritima* was the name given by Linnæus, but this was changed to *Urginea*, in allusion to the Algerian tribe Ben Urgin, near Boma, where Steinheil in 1834 examined this plant, removing it from the genus *Scilla*. The main difference between the genera is that the genus *Urginea* has flat, discoid seeds, while in *Scilla* proper they are triquetrous (three-angled, with three concave faces). Baker named it *Urginea maritima*, but it now retains *Scilla* as its specific name.

As seen in commerce, the undried bulb is somewhat pear-shaped, and generally about the size of a man's fist, but often larger, weighing from $\frac{1}{2}$ lb. to more than 4 lb.

It has the usual structure of a bulb, being formed of smooth juicy scales, closely wrapped over one another. It has little odour, but its inner scales have a mucilaginous, bitter, acrid taste, owing to the presence of bitter glucosides.

In its home, it is frequently used fresh, but in other countries it is directed by the pharmacopœias to be deprived of its dry membraneous outer scales (which are destitute of activity), cut into thin, transverse slices and carefully dried, either in the sun, or by artificial heat, the inmost part being rejected, as this central portion, being the youngest growth, is deficient in activity.

Owing to the mucilaginous nature of the tissue, drying is tedious and difficult. When fresh, the bulb abounds in a viscid, very acrid juice, which is capable of causing inflammation of the skin. On drying, the bulb loses four-fifths of its weight, and its acridity is largely diminished, with slight loss of medicinal activity.

Squill is generally imported in ready-dried slices, packed in casks, from Malta, where the largest collections are made.

The dried slices are narrow, flattish, curved, yellowish-white, or with a roseate hue, according to the variety of Squill from which they are obtained, from 1 to 2 inches long, more or less translucent.

When quite dry, the strips are brittle and can easily be powdered, but they are tough and flexible when moist and dried. Squill should be kept in well-stoppered bottles, on account of its readiness to absorb moisture, when the slices become tough and cannot be reduced to powder. When kept in a dry place, Squill retains its virtues for a long time. When powdered, unless carefully preserved in a dried state by absorption of moisture, it forms a hard mass, and it is therefore officially recommended that powdered Squill should be kept quite dry over quicklime.

Occasionally, entire bulbs are imported, but are difficult to keep in the fresh state as they preserve their vitality for a long time, and if allowed to remain in a warm place, rapidly develop an aerial shoot. Professor Henslow reports (*Poisonous Plants in Field and Garden*) that a bulb was found attempting to grow after being stowed away for more than twenty years in the museum of St. Bartholomew's Hospital Medical School.

¶ *Constituents.* The chemical constituents of Squill are imperfectly known. Merck, in 1879, separated the three bitter glucosidal substances Scillitoxin, Scillipicrin and Scillin. The first two are amorphous and act upon the heart, the former being the more active; Scillin is crystalline and causes numbness and vomiting. Other constituents are mucilaginous and saccharine matter, including a peculiar mucilaginous carbohydrate named Sinistrin, an Inulin-like substance, which yields Lævulose on being boiled with dilute acid. The name Sinistrin (in 1834, first proposed by Macquart for Inulin) has also been applied to a mucilaginous matter extracted from barley, but it remains to be proved that the latter is identical with the Sinistrin of Squill. Calcium oxalate is also present, in bundles of long, acicular crystals, which easily penetrate the skin when the bulbs are handled, and causes intense irritation, sometimes eruption, if a piece of fresh Squill is rubbed on the skin.

The toxicity of Squills has more recently been ascribed to a single, bitter, non-nitrogenous glucoside, to which the name Scillitin is given, and which is the active diuretic and expectorant principle.

The bulbs also yield when distilled in a current of steam, a slightly coloured liquid oil of unpleasant odour.

The chemistry of Squills cannot yet be regarded as fully worked out, since most of the glucosides described have only been prepared in an amorphous condition of uncertain chemical identity.

¶ *Medicinal Action and Uses.* The Medicinal Squill was valued as a medicine in early classic times and has ever since been employed by physicians, being official in all pharmacopœias. Oxymel of Squill, used for coughs, was invented by Pythagoras, who lived in the sixth century before Christ.

It is mentioned by Theophrastus in the third century before Christ, and was known to all the ancient Greek physicians. Epimenides, a Greek, is said to have made much use of it, from which circumstance we find it called *Epimenidea.*

It is considered to be the Sea Onion referred to by Homer. Pliny was acquainted with it, and Dioscorides, who lived about the same time, describes the different varieties of the bulb and the method of making vinegar of Squills. A similar preparation, as well as compounds of Squill with honey, was administered by the Arabian physicians of the Middle Ages, who introduced the drug into European medicine, these preparations still remaining in use.

The mediæval reputation of Squill was originally as a diuretic, the older authorities attributing its diuretic action to a direct stimulant effect upon the kidney.

As a diuretic, it is frequently employed in dropsy, whether due to chronic disease of the kidneys or to the renal congestion consequent to chronic cardiac disease. Squill is not employed, however, when the kidneys are acutely inflamed. In the treatment of cardiac dropsy, Squill is frequently combined with digitalis.

Squill stimulates the bronchial mucous membrane and is given in bronchitis after subsidence of the acute inflammation. It is generally used in combination with other stimulating expectorants, its effects being thereby increased, and is considered most useful in chronic bronchitis, catarrhal affections and asthma. The tincture is administered combined with other expectorants, especially ipecacuanha and ammonium carbonate. Vinegar, Oxymel and Syrup of Squill are also common constituents of expectorant cough mixtures.

It is largely sued for its stimulating, expectorant and diuretic properties, and is also a cardiac tonic, acting in a similar manner to digitalis, slowing and strengthening the pulse, though more irritating to the gastro-intestinal mucous membrane. On account of its irritant qualities it is not administered in diseases of an acute inflammatory nature. It has also been given as an emetic in whooping-cough and croup, usually combined with ipecacuanha, but as an emetic is considered very uncertain in its action.

To prevent its too great action on the stomach, it is frequently combined with a portion of opium. With calomel, it forms a powerful stimulant of the urinary organs. (A pill containing 1 grain each of Squill, digitalis and calomel is popularly known as Niemeyer's pill.)

In poisonous doses, Squill produces violent inflammation of the gastro-intestinal and genito-urinary tracts, manifested by nausea, vomiting, abdominal pains and purging, and, in addition, dullness, stupour, convulsions, a marked fall in temperature, enfeebled circulation and sometimes death.

The powdered drug and extracts made from it have been largely used as rat poisons and are said to be very efficacious, the red variety being preferred for this purpose, although there would not seem to be sufficient evidence of its superiority

¶ *Dosage.* When given in substance, Squill is most conveniently administered in the form of pill. Dose: 1 to 3 grains.

Vinegar of Squill, B.P. Dose: 5 to 15 minims.

Vinegar of Squill, U.S.P. Average dose: 15 minims.

Liquid Extract of Squill, B.P. Codex. Dose: 1 to 3 minims.

Fluid Extract of Squill, U.S.P. Average dose: 1½ minim.

Opiate Linctus, B.P.C. Dose: ½ to 1 fluid drachm.

Linctus of Squill, B.P.B. Dose: ½ to 1 fluid drachm. (Used as cough linctus for children.)

Syrup of Squill, B.P. Used as an expectorant in acid cough mixtures. Dose: ½ to 1 fluid drachm.

Syrup of Squill, U.S.P. (The preparation commonly administered in bronchitis.) Average dose: 30 minims.

Compound Syrup of Squill, U.S.P. Average dose: 30 minims.

Compound Squill Tablets, B.P.C. Dose: 1 to 2 tablets.

Tincture of Squill, B.P. (Used with other expectorants to relieve cough and in chronic bronchitis.) Dose: 5 to 15 minims.

Tincture of Squill, U.S.P. Average dose: 15 minims.

Compound Linctus of Squill, B.P.C. (Gee's Linctus.) Dose: ½ to 1 fluid drachm.

Squill Mixture, B.P.C. (Fothergill's Cough Mixture.) Given for coughs. Dose: 2 to 4 fluid drachms.

Compound Squill Mixture, B.P.C. (Used as diaphoretic and expectorant.) Dose: ½ to 1 fluid ounce.

Squill and Ipecacuanha Mixture, B.P.C. Dose: ½ to 1 fluid ounce.

Squill and Opium Mixture (Abercrombie's Cough Mixture), B.P.C. Dose: 2 to 4 fluid drachms.

Oxymel of Squill, B.P. (Vinegar of Squill 20, purified honey 50.) Employed in coughs and colds to assist expectoration. Dose: ½ to 1 fluid drachm.

Compound Squill Pill, B.P. Dose: 4 to 8 grains.

Compound Syrup of Squill, B.P.C. (For coughs.) Dose: ½ to 1 fluid drachm.

¶ *Substitutes.* There are several bulbs used in place of the official Squill which, owing to the abundance and low price of the latter, do not appear in the European market.

Indian Squill consists of the younger bulbs of *Urginea indica* (Knuth), or of *Scilla indica* (Baker), which is also known as *Ledebouria hyacinthina* (Roth.).

U. indica, Knuth (*S. indica,* Roxb.) is a widely diffused plant occurring in northern India, Abyssinia, Nubia and Senegambia. It is known by the same Arabic and Persian names as *U. scilla* and its bulbs are used for similar purposes, but are considered to have no action when old and large. The bulbs consist of whitish, fleshy coats or scales, which enclose each other completely. They resemble common onions in shape.

S. indica, Baker (*L. hyacinthina,* Roth.), a native of India and Abyssinia, has a bulb often confused in the Indian bazaars with the preceding, but easily distinguished when entire by being *scaly,* not *tunicated,* its cream-coloured scales overlapping one another. The bulbs are about the size and shape of a small pear, somewhat smaller than those of *U. indica.* It is considered a better representative of the European Squill.

The bulbs of both species have a nauseous odour and a bitter acrid taste. They are collected soon after the plants have flowered, divested of their dry, outer, membraneous coats, cut into slices and dried.

The chief constituents in each case are bitter principles, similar to the glucosidal substances found in ordinary Squill, and needle-shaped crystals of calcium oxalate are also present.

The drug possesses stimulant, expectorant and diuretic principles, and is official in the India and Colonial Addendum for use in India and the Eastern Colonies as an equivalent of ordinary Squill.

U. altissima, Baker (*Ornithogalum altissimum,* Linn.), a South African species very closely related to the common Squill, has apparently the same properties.

The bulb of *S. Peruviana* (Linn.) has also been used and exported as a substitute for Squill.

Drimia ciliaris (Jacq.), native of the Cape of Good Hope, much resembles the official Squill, but has a juice so irritating if it comes into contact with the skin, that it was called by the Dutch colonists *Jeukbol,* i.e. Itch-bulb. It is used medicinally as an emetic, expectorant and diuretic.

Crinum asiaticum, var. *toxicarium* (Hubert), is a large plant with handsome white flowers and showy leaves, cultivated in Indian gardens and growing wild in low, humid spots in various parts of India and on the coast of Ceylon. The bulb was admitted in 1868 to the Pharmacopœia of India as a valuable emetic, but is not widely used.

The European Squills belonging to the genus *Scilla* possess in a milder form the same active principle, and some of the species are deleterious, if not absolutely dangerous. The bulbs of *S. lilio-hyacinthus* are used as a purgative by the inhabitants of the Pyrenees.

SQUIRTING CUCUMBER. *See* CUCUMBER

STAR ANISE. *See* ANISEED

STAR OF BETHLEHEM [1]

Ornithogalum umbellatum (LINN.)
N.O. Liliaceæ

Synonyms. Bath Asparagus. Dove's Dung. Star of Hungary. White Filde Onyon
Part Used. Bulb

The Star of Bethlehem is a bulbous plant nearly allied to the Onion and Garlic.

The leaves are long and narrow and dark-green; the flowers, in bloom during April and May, are a brilliant white internally, but with the petals striped with green outside. They expand only in the sunshine.

The bulbs, in common with those of many Liliaceous plants, are edible and nutritious. They were in ancient times eaten, both raw

The homœopaths make a tincture from the bulbs which is useful in some cases of cancer. – EDITOR.

and cooked, as Dioscorides related, and form a palatable and wholesome food when boiled. They are still often eaten in the East, being roasted like chestnuts, and Linnæus and others considered that they were probably the 'Dove's Dung' mentioned in the Second Book of Kings, vi. 25, as being sold at a high price during the siege of Samaria by the King of Syria, when 'the fourth part of a cab of dove's dung was sold for five pieces of silver.' The Greek name, *Ornithogalum*, signifies the 'birds' milk flower.' The plains of Syria and Palestine are sheeted in spring with the white flowers of a species of Star of Bethlehem, the bulbs of which are used as food, and are still called by the Arabs, 'Dove's Dung,' a name in common use among them for vegetable substances. Bochart tells us that the Arabs give this name to a moss that grows on trees and stony ground, and also to a pulse or pea, which appears to have been common in India. Large quantities of the bulb, it is stated, were parched and dried and stored at Cairo and Damascus, being much used during journeys, and especially by the great pilgrim caravans to Mecca.

In Lyte's *Dodoens* (1578) it is described as 'the white filde onyon,' growing in plenty near Malines. In Turner's *Herbal* (1548) it is not mentioned, but in Gerard's six species are enumerated. He says: 'There be sundry sorts of wild field Onions, called "Starres of Bethlehem," differing in stature, taste and smell, as shall be declared,' and calls them 'the Star of Hungary,' 'the Lesser Spanish Star,' 'the Star of Bethlehem,' 'the great Arabische star floure,' etc.

Though there are numerous species in this genus, only one is truly native to Great Britain, the spiked Ornithogalum, *O. pyrenaicum* (Linn.), and is not common, being a local plant, found only in a few counties. It is abundant, however, in woods near Bath, and the unexpanded inflorescence used to be collected and sold in that town under the name of 'Bath Asparagus,' and was cooked and served as a vegetable.

A leafless stalk, about 2 feet high, rises from the bulb, bearing greenish-white flowers in a long, erect spike.

¶ *Other Species.*
O. divaricatum (Lindl.) is the CALIFORNIAN SOAPROOT, Soap Bulb, Soap Apple or Amole. Its large bulb, resembling that of Squill, is universally used by the Indians of the regions where it grows as a detergent and as a fish poison. It has other uses dependent upon the action of its Saponin, and it is an emetico-cathartic poison.

O. thyroides (Jacq.), of South Africa, is a fatal stock poison.

O. Capense (Linn.), also of South Africa, yields a tuber used as an emmenagogue: the action is due to saponin.

Over the deserts of the south-western United States and Mexico, the tuberous rhizomes of large species of *Yucca* (also belonging to the order Liliaceæ) are called Soap Root, and have the same uses as those of the Californian variety of *Ornithogalum*. There is said to be no better tonic or stimulant for the hair than a free application of a solution of this juice in alcohol, water, or glycerine. Besides the Saponin, it contains a large number of raphides, which probably add mechanically to the stimulation.

Yucca filamentosa (Linn.), of the south-eastern United States, commonly known as 'Adam's Needle,' has a large rhizome which contains nearly 2 per cent. of Saponin, and which is used as a stimulant owing to the action of this constituent.

Gagea lutea (Ker Gawl.), the YELLOW STAR OF BETHLEHEM, has a small, egg-shaped or nearly round bulb, about the size of a large pea.

It flowers from March to May, and is a plant 6 to 10 inches high, with narrow leaves and yellow flowers (arranged in an umbel), which only open in the middle of the day. It occurs in woods and pastures in this country, but is not common.

It is recorded that the Swedes have eaten this bulb in times of scarcity. Round the main small bulb there are usually a number of bulbules about the size of sago grains, but only the parent bulb is enclosed in a yellowish outer skin.

Some species of Gagea have been used as diuretics, much like Squill, and probably contain related, if not identical, substances.

The tuberous root-stock of *Melanthium Virginicum* (Linn.), the Bunch Flower of the eastern and central United States, is poisonous and is used as a parasiticide.

(*POISON*)
STAVESACRE

Synonym. Lousewort
Part Used. Seeds
Habitat. Asia Minor and Europe

Stavesacre is a species of Larkspur, a stout, erect herb attaining 4 feet in height, indigenous to Asia Minor and southern Europe. It

Delphinium Staphisagria (LINN.)
N.O. Ranunculaceæ

is cultivated in France and Italy, our supplies having before the War been drawn chiefly from Trieste and from the south of Italy.

Stavesacre was well known to both the Greeks and Romans. Dioscorides mentions it, and Pliny describes its use as a parasiticide. It continued to be extensively employed throughout the Middle Ages.

This Delphinium is an annual, with a hairy stem and hairy palmate leaves, composed of five to seven oblong lobes, which have frequently one or two acute indentures on their sides. The flowers form a loose spike at the upper part of the stalk, each on a short peduncle, and are of a pale-blue or purple colour.

¶ *Cultivation.* The seeds of this species should be sown in April, where the plants are intended to remain and require no special treatment, growing in almost any soil or situation, but the plants are most luxuriant when given a deep, yellow loam, well enriched with rotted manure and fairly moist. They should be thinned to a distance of 2 feet apart.

¶ *Part Used.* The dried, ripe seeds. Shake the seeds out of the pods on trays and spread them out to dry in the sun. Then pack away in airtight boxes or tins. The dried, ripe seeds are brown when fresh, changing to a dull, earthy colour on keeping. In shape they are irregularly quadrangular, one side being curved and larger than the others, and the surface of the seed is wrinkled and pitted. They average about 6 mm. (nearly $\frac{1}{4}$ inch) long and rather less in width, ten weighing about 6 grains. The seed coat is nearly tasteless, but the endosperm is oily and has a bitter and acrid taste. The seeds have no marked collour.

¶ *Constituents.* The chief constituents of Stavesacre seeds are from 20 to 25 per cent. of alkaloidal matter, which consists chiefly of the bitter, acrid, crystalline, alkaloid Delphinine, an irritant poison, and a second crystalline alkaloid named Delphisine, and the amorphous alkaloid Delphinoidine. Less important are staphisagroine, of which traces only are present, and staphisagrine, which appears to be a mixture of the first three elements.

¶ *Medicinal Action and Uses.* Vermifuge and vermin-destroying. Stavesacre seeds are extremely poisonous and are only used as a parasiticide to kill pediculi, chiefly in the form of the official ointment, the expressed oil, the powdered seeds, or an acid aqueous extract containing the alkaloids.

These seeds are so violently emetic and cathartic that they are rarely given internally, though the powdered seeds have been given as a purge for dropsy, in very small quantities at first and increased till the effect is produced. The dose at first should not exceed 2 or 3 grains, given in powder or decoction, but the administration of the drug must always be accompanied by great caution, as staphisagrine paralyses the motor nerves like curare.

The seeds are used as an external application to some cutaneous eruptions, the decoction, applied with a linen rag, being effectual in curing the itch. It is made by boiling the seeds in water.

Delphinine has also been employed similarly to aconite, both internally and externally, for neuralgia. It resembles aconite in causing slowness of pulse and respiration, paralysis of the spinal cord and death from asphyxia. By depressing the action of the spinal cord it arrests the convulsions caused by strychnine.

See ACONITE, LARKSPUR (FIELD).

STONECROPS

Sedums
N.O. Crassulaceæ

STONECROP, WHITE

Sedum album
N.O. Crassulaceæ

Synonym. Small Houseleek (Culpepper)
Parts Used. Leaves, stalks

Culpepper's Small Houseleek is now generally called the White Stonecrop. It is not very common, and is found wild on rocks and walls. As a rule, however, when growing on garden walls and the roofs of cottages and outhouses, it owes its presence indirectly to human agency, and is to be considered a garden escape. The root is perennial and fibrous, the flowerless stems prostrate, of a bluish-green colour, round and leafy. The leaves are bright green and very succulent, oblong, cylindrical, blunt and spreading, $\frac{1}{3}$ to $\frac{1}{2}$ inch long. The flowering stems are 6 to 10 inches high, with a few leaves growing alternately on them and terminated by much-branched, flat tufts (cymes) of numerous, small, star-like flowers, about $\frac{1}{6}$ inch in diameter, the white petals twice as large as the green sepals.

This Stonecrop, which flowers in July and August, is not to be confounded with another white-flowered Stonecrop (*Sedum Anglicum*), which flowers earlier – June and July – and is an annual. It is a plant of smaller and compacter growth, the leaves shorter and less cylindrical, with less numerous flowers, the white petals of which are spotted with red.

The White Stonecrop is said to be indigenous in the Malvern Hills and Somerset, but a garden escape elsewhere, being grown as rock-plants.

S. Anglicum is abundant on the bank of a hedge close to Poole Harbour.

The older herbalists considered the White Stonecrop to possess all the virtues of the Houseleek. The leaves and stalks were recommended and used for all kinds of inflammation, being especially applied as a cooling plaster to painful hæmorrhoids. Culpepper tells us: 'it is so harmless an herb you can scarce use it amiss.' It was the custom, too, to prepare and eat it as a pickle, in the same way as the juicy Samphire.

STONECROP, COMMON
Sedum acre
N.O. Crassulaceæ

Synonyms. Biting Stonecrop. Wallpepper. Golden Moss. Wall Ginger. Bird Bread. Prick Madam. Gold Chain. Creeping Tom. Mousetail. Jack-of-the-Buttery
(*French*) Pain d'oiseau
Part Used. Herb

The Common or Biting Stonecrop is the commonest of the Stonecrops, growing freely upon walls and cottage roofs, on rocks and in sandy places, especially near the sea, forming tufts or cushions, 3 to 10 inches across, which in June and July are a mass of golden blossom, but its flowering season is very soon over.

The root is perennial and very fibrous, its minute threads penetrating into the smallest crevices. The stalks are numerous, many of them trailing and flowerless, others erect – generally 3 to 5 inches high – bearing the clusters of flowers. When growing among other foliage, or on rockwork, the flowerstalks are often drawn up to some height, at other times much dwarfed. They branch and are clothed with numerous leaves. The little upright and very succulent leaves that closely overlap on the flowerless stems are a distinguishing characteristic from the other yellow-flowering species of *Sedum*; they are so fleshy as to be almost round. The starlike flowers are of a brilliant yellow colour, the five sepals small and inconspicuous, but the five petals, spreading and acutely pointed, are a striking feature. There are ten stamens, with anthers the same tint as the petals.

The pungency of the leaves has obtained for the plant its specific name of *acre*, and the popular English name of Wallpepper and Wall Ginger. Gerard tells us it was known in his day as Mousetail, or Jack of the Butterie. As regards the latter name, Dr. Fernie says: 'this and the Sedums *album* and *reflexum* were ingredients in a famous worm-expelling medicine or "theriac" (treacle), and "Jack of the Buttery" is a corruption of *Bot. theriaque.*'

De Lobel called it *vermicularis*, partly – we are told – from the grub-like shape of the leaves, and partly from its medical efficacy as a vermifuge.

Some old writers considered this species to possess considerable virtues, but others, from the durability of its acrimony and the violence of its operation, have thought it unsafe to be administered. Culpepper tells us:

'Its qualities are directly opposite to the other Sedums, and more apt to raise inflammations than to cure them; it ought not to be put into any ointment, nor any other medicine.'

He considered it, however, good for scurvy, both inwardly in decoction and outwardly, bathed as a fomentation, and he also commended it for King's Evil. Other writers have likewise considered it to be a beneficial remedy in some scorbutic diseases, when properly and carefully used, recommending it in the form of a gargle for scurvy of the gums, and as a lotion for scrofulous ulcers. It has been considered useful in intermittent fever and in dropsy. In large doses it is emetic and cathartic, and applied externally will sometimes produce blisters.

Pliny recommends it as a means of procuring sleep, for which purpose he says it must be wrapped in a black cloth and placed under the pillow of the patient, without his knowing it, otherwise it will not be effectual.

STONECROP, CROOKED YELLOW
Sedum reflexum
N.O. Crassulaceæ

Synonym. Stonecrop Houseleek
Parts Used. Leaves, young shoots

The Stonecrop Houseleek of the old herbalists goes now by the name of Crooked Yellow Stonecrop.

¶ *Description.* It is not considered truly indigenous, though often found on rocks, old walls, house-tops, and sometimes on dry

772

banks, in many parts of the British Isles. The slender but tough stems, tinged with pink, are elongated, lying on the ground, sending up numerous ascending, short, leafy, barren shoots and erect, and somewhat flexuous flowering stems, 9 inches to 1 foot high, clothed with spreading and reflexed leaves, which are cylindrical and pointed, $\frac{1}{2}$ to $\frac{3}{4}$ inch long, spurred at their bases. The leaves are distant towards the lower ends of the barren shoots, but crowded towards the apex, forming a kind of tuft: they are only curved back, or reflexed, on the flowering stems. This Stonecrop also blossoms in July and August:

STONECROP, ORPINE

Synonyms. Live Long. Life Everlasting (*French*) Herbe aux charpentiers
Parts Used. Whole plant, leaves

The Orpine, the largest British species of this genus, is readily distinguished from most of the other plants allied to it by its large, broad, flattened leaves and terminal heads of pinkish flowers, being the only British species with flat leaves.

It has a wide distribution: in warmer countries it is a mountain plant. Lindley gives its true habitat as mountainous woods, and Cesalpinus, an early Italian botanist, calls it *Crassula montana*, but in this country it grows freely in lower situations. It is probable that it was originally an introduced plant, though it is now not uncommonly found in hedgebanks on shady sides of fields and in woods, though probably escaped from cultivation in many of its localities. In its wild state, the plant is from 1 to 2 feet high, though in gardens it may attain as much as 3 feet.

The root-stock is perennial, large and fleshy, producing small parsnip-shaped tubers, with a whitish-grey rind, containing a considerable store of nourishment. The stalks are numerous, erect, unbranched, round and solid, generally of a reddish tint, spotted and streaked with a deeper red above. The flat, fleshy leaves, bluish-green in colour, are numerous, placed alternately on the stem at very short intervals, and coarsely toothed. The upper leaves are rounded at their bases and without foot-stalks, the lower ones taper at the base to a short stalk, being almost wedge-shaped; they are largest and closest together about the middle of the stem, where they are $1\frac{1}{2}$ to 3 inches long.

The flowers are in compact heads at the top of the stems, forming a brilliant mass of crimson, in most cases, though sometimes whitish, suffused with dull purplish rose. They are spreading and acutely pointed, three times as long as the calyx. In their

the flowers are in terminal cymes as in the previous species, but are bright yellow.

In Holland, the leaves and young shoots of this species are used for salad.

Culpepper considered that as 'it is more frequent than the white stonecrop, flowering at the same time, it may very well supply its place.' He goes on to tell us that the House-leek, 'though not given inwardly, yet is recommended by some to quench thirst in fever.' Mixed with posset drink, 3 oz. of the juice of this and *Persicaria maculata*, boiled to the consistence of a julep, are recommended to allay the heat of inflammation.

Sedum Telephium
N.O. Crassulaceæ

centre are ten conspicuous stamens, with reddish anthers, and the ovaries they surround are also reddish.

The whole plant is smooth and somewhat shiny. It flowers in July and seeds in August.

The specific name is derived from Telephus, the son of Hercules, who is said to have discovered its virtues. Its most familiar English name, Orpine, is derived from *Auripigmentum*, the gold-coloured pigment, called Orpiment, or Orpin, a yellow sulphuret of the metal arsenic. This name, which might have been appropriate enough for the brilliant yellow flowers of the last two species described, is quite out of place applied to the crimson blossoms of this *Sedum*.

Its tenacity of life has earned it the name of 'Live Long' and 'Life Everlasting,' the length of time it will continue fresh after being gathered being remarkable. It will live a long time if uprooted and hung up in a room without earth or water, subsisting on the store of nourishment in its fleshy leaves and swollen roots.

¶ *Constituents.* The whole plant is mucilaginous and slightly astringent. It contains lime, sulphur, ammonia and probably mercury.

The leaves have sometimes been used as a salad, like the other *Sedums*, but though sheep and goats eat it, horses will refuse it.

¶ *Medicinal Action and Uses.* It has been used as a popular remedy for diarrhœa. The leaves are boiled in milk, and a large teacupful of the decoction taken three or four times a day is said also to stimulate the action of the kidneys, and to be serviceable for piles and hæmorrhages. Orpine has also an anti-cancerous reputation.

Culpepper stated that it was seldom used internally in his days, but that the celebrated

German herbalist, Tragus, considered its distilled water –

'profitable for gnawings or excoriation in the stomach or bowels, for ulcers in the lungs, liver or other inward parts and cures those diseases, being drunk for days together,'

and that the root has the same action, even stronger. He says that it is

'used outwardly to cool inflammations upon

any hurt or wound, and easeth the pain of them; as also to heal scaldings and burnings, the juice thereof being beaten with some green salad oil and anointed. The leaf bruised and laid to any green wound in the head or legs doth heal them quickly, and being bound to the throat cureth the quinsy; and it reduceth ruptures. If you make the juice into a syrup with honey or sugar, you may safely take a spoonful or two at a time for sore throat and quinsy.'

STONECROP, VIRGINIAN

Penthorum sedoides (LINN.)
N.O. Crassulaceæ

Synonyms. Ditch Stonecrop. Penthorum
Part Used. Herb

The Virginian Stonecrop is a native of America.

¶ *Description*. It is a biennial, with stems about a foot high, on which the leaves are placed on alternate sides, on short stalks. They are oblong, 2 to 3 inches long and about a third as broad, smooth and thin, the apex pointed and the margins finely toothed. The flowers are small and greenish, on short flower-stalks, in rows along the upper sides of the branches of the terminal cyme: there are five very small petals and five sepals, and the ovary is five-cleft and five-celled, surrounded by ten stamens with filaments twice as long as the calyx. The genus *Penthorum* differs from the genus *Sedum*, in having no nectaries in its flowers.

This plant has of late attracted much notice, especially in America, as a remedy for catarrh, catarrhal inflammation of the larynx, chronic bronchitis, with increased secretion of mucus and catarrhal affections of the stomach and bowels. It has also been employed with success in the treatment of diarrhœa, hæmorrhoids and infantile cholera.

It is demulcent, laxative and somewhat astringent in its action. A fluid extract is prepared from the whole herb and administered

in doses of from 10 to 20 drops. It has a slightly astringent taste.

¶ *Other Species*.

Among other species of *Sedum* are the HAIRY STONECROP (*Sedum villosum*), frequent in Scotland and the North of England, a small species with viscid stems and leaves and pinkish-white flowers. The THICK-LEAVED STONECROP (*S. dasyphyllum*), also a small species, but very rare, distinguished from the preceding by its fleshy, almost globular leaves, viscid flower-stalks and blunt petals. Other British species belonging to this group are: TASTELESS YELLOW STONECROP (*S. sexangulare*), distinguished from *S. acre* by its leaves, which are six in a whorl, growing in Greenwich Park, the Isle of Sheppey and a few other places. ST. VINCENT'S ROCK STONECROP (*S. rupestre*), a species allied to *S. reflexum*, with slightly flattened leaves, which grow five in a whorl, found on St. Vincent's Rocks and other limestone cliffs, rare; and WELSH STONECROP (*S. Fosterianum*), another species allied to *S. reflexum*, with leaves flattened at the base and compact cymes of flowers – which grows on the rocks in Wales and Shropshire.

See HOUSELEEK, KIDNEYWORT.

STONE ROOT

Collinsonia Canadensis (LINN.)
N.O. Labiatæ

Synonyms. Horseweed. Richweed. Richleaf. Knob-Root. Knobweed. Horsebalm. Hardback. Heal-all. Oxbalm. Knot-Root. Baume de Cheval. Guérit-tout
Parts Used. Whole plant, fresh root
Habitat. North America, from Canada to the Carolinas

¶ *Description*. The plant has a four-sided stem, from 1 to 4 feet in height, and bears large, greenish-yellow flowers. It grows in moist woods and flowers from July to September. The rhizome is brown-grey, about 4 inches long, knobby, and very hard. The whole plant has a strong, disagreeable odour and a pungent and spicy taste. The chief virtue of the plant is in the root, which should always be used fresh. The

name is derived from its discoverer, Peter Collinson.

¶ *Constituents*. In the root there is resin, starch, mucilage and wax. In the leaves, resin, tannin, wax and volatile oil. The alkaloid discovered in the root appears to be a magnesium salt.

¶ *Medicinal Action and Uses*. Sedative, antispasmodic, astringent, tonic, diaphoretic, diuretic.

A decoction of the fresh root has been given in catarrh of the bladder, leucorrhœa, gravel and dropsy. It is largely used by American veterinary surgeons as a diuretic. It is valuable in all complaints of urinary organs and rectum, and is best combined with other drugs.

It can be used externally, especially the leaves, for poultices and fomentations, bruises, wounds, sores, cuts, etc., and also as a gargle, in the strength of 1 part of fluid extract to 3 of water.

¶ *Preparations and Dosages.* Of fluid extract, 15 to 60 drops. Of Collinsonin, 2 to 4 grains.

STORAX

Liquidambar orientalis (MILL.)
N.O. Hamamelaceæ

Synonyms. Liquidambar imberbe. Styrax Præparatus. Prepared Storax. Styrax liquidus. Flussiger Amber. Liquid Storax. Balsam Styracis
Part Used. Balsam obtained from the wood and inner bark
Habitat. Asia Minor

¶ *Description.* A tree of 40 feet or more in height, with many branches, and a thick, purplish-grey bark; leaves palmately cut into five, three-lobed sections, and white flowers arranged in little, round solitary heads. The name *Liquidambar* was given by Monardes in the sixteenth century as the name of the resin obtained in Mexico from the American species, now *L. styraciflua*. *L. orientalis* was not known botanically until the middle of the last century, when it was grown in Chelsea, Kew, and other botanical gardens from seed brought from the Levant via Paris. It forms forests near Budrum, Melasso, Moughla, Marmorizza and a few places near, but does not appear to be found wild in any other district. The genus *Liquidambar* is very similar to that of *Platanus*, and this species to *L. styraciflua*.

Styrax officinale has been proved to be the source of the solid Storax of the Ancients, which was always scarce and valuable, and is now never found in commerce, though it is probable that the cultivated *S. officinale* of Europe is capable of yielding Storax. Storax appears to be a pathological rather than a physiological product; when the young wood is injured, oil-ducts are formed in which the Storax is produced. Its extraction is chiefly carried on by a tribe of wandering Turcomans called Yuruks. The outer bark of the tree is removed, the inner bark is stripped off and thrown into pits until a sufficient quantity has been collected. It is then packed in strong, horse-hair bags and pressed in a wooden press. After removal, hot water is thrown on the bags, which are pressed a second time, when the greater part of the balsam will be extracted. Another account says that the bark is first boiled in water in a large copper over a brick fire, by which process the balsam is separated, and can then be skimmed off. The boiled bark is then put into bags over which hot water is thrown, and submitted to pressure as described above, by which an additional quantity of balsam

(Yagh, or oil) is obtained. In either mode of procedure the product is the semi-liquid, opaque substance called Liquid Storax. This is chiefly forwarded in barrels to Constantinople, Smyrna, Syria and Alexandria; some to Smyrna, in goat-skins, with a certain proportion of water; thence it is forwarded to Trieste in barrels. Much goes to Bombay for India and China, but little comes to the United States or Britain. Liquid Storax is known in the East as Rosemalloes or Rosemalles. The residual bark left after the extraction of the balsam constitutes the fragrant, leaf-like cakes known as *Cortex Thymiamatis, Cortex Thuris* and *Storax Bark*.

The quality of Storax now on the market appears to be much inferior to that of a few years ago, and is usually much adulterated. As imported, Liquid Storax is a soft, viscid, opaque substance, about the consistence of honey, of a greyish-brown colour, and containing a variable quantity of water, which, after it has been allowed to stand for a time, floats on the surface. It has an agreeable, balsamic odour, though, when fresh, this is a little contaminated by naphthalin or bitumen. Its taste is burning, pungent, and aromatic.

The Prepared Storax is obtained from Liquid Storax by means of rectified spirit and straining. It is then described officially as 'a semi-transparent, brownish-yellow, semi-fluid balsam, of the consistence of thick honey, agreeable fragrance, and aromatic, bland taste.' The odour is slightly less agreeable than that of the balsam of Peru. It is imported in jars holding 14 lb. each.

¶ *Constituents.* The most abundant constituent of Storax is Storesin, in two forms, called alpha and beta, both free and in the form of a cinnamic ester. It is an amorphous substance, melting at 168° C. (334·4° F.), and readily soluble in petroleum benzin. Cinnamic esters of phenylprophyl, of ethyl, of benzyl, and especially cinnamate of cinnamyl, the so-called Styrasin, have also been observed. The yield of cinnamic acid varies from 6 to 12 per cent., or even as much as 23 per cent. of crystallized cinnamic acid can be obtained.

Another analysis gives free cinnamic acid, vanillin, styrol, styracin, cinnamic acid-ethyl ester, cinnamic acid-phenylprophyl ester, and storesinol partly free and partly as cinnamic acid ester.

Crude Storax contains from 1 to 9 per cent. of matter insoluble in alcohol, and up to 30 per cent. of water. When purified, it is brownish-yellow, viscous, and transparent in thin layers; entirely soluble in alcohol (90 per cent.) and in ether. Boiled with solution of potassium chromate and sulphuric acid, it evolves an odour of benzaldehyde. It loses not more than 5 per cent. of its weight when heated in a thin layer on a water-bath for one hour.

Owing to the demand for the cinnamic esters of Storax for perfumery purposes, much of the commercial drug has been deprived of these before it is put on the market.

¶ *Medicinal Action and Uses.* A stimulating expectorant and feeble antiseptic, at present very seldom used except as a constituent of the compound tincture of benzoin. Externally, mixed with 2 or 3 parts of olive oil, it has been found a useful local remedy in scabies. It has the same action as balsams of Tolu and Peru and benzoin. It has been recommended as a remedy in diphtheria, in pulmonic catarrhs, and as a substitute for South American copaiba in gonorrhœa and leucorrhœa. Combined with tallow or lard, it is valuable for many forms of skin disease, such as ringworm, especially in children. The taste and smell of opium is well concealed by the addition of Storax in pills, its fragrance being used frequently also in ointments.

¶ *Dosage.* 10 to 20 grains.

¶ *Adulterations, Substitutes, Allied Balsams.* L. *styraciflua*, or Sweet Gum, the American variety, is sometimes confused because its product, obtained by spontaneous exudation, is often called Liquidambar, as well as Liquid Storax or copalm balsam. It contains cinnamyl cinnamate, with ethyl, benzyl, and other esters of cinnamic acid. Another of its products, obtained by boiling the young branches, has also been confounded with Liquid Storax, which it resembles. It is used in Texas for coughs. A syrup of the bark is used for diarrhœa and dysentery in the Western States.

L. *storesin* is said to be known also in Eastern markets.

Aromatic resins are also obtained in China from L. *Formosana*, and in Java and Burma from L. *Altingea* (*Altingia excelsa*), where the Storax-like substance varies in colour from white to red.

Styrea reticulata and other species in Brazil have a fragrant secretion similar to benzoin, which is used in churches as frankincense.

The commonest adulterations are sawdust and turpentine.

STRAMONIUM. *See* THORNAPPLE

STRAWBERRY

Fragaria vesca (LINN.)
N.O. Rosaceæ

Part Used. Leaves

Habitat. The whole of the Northern Hemisphere, exclusive of the tropics

¶ *Description.* The Wild Strawberry, a delicate, thin-leaved plant, with small, scarlet berries, cone-shaped and studded with tiny, brown 'seeds,' has a fragrance and flavour more delicate even than the cultivated Strawberry. It chooses a slightly sheltered position, and, being very small, considerable labour goes to the collection of its fruit, which is much more used and appreciated in France than in Great Britain.

1629 is the date assigned to the introduction of the Scarlet Strawberry from Virginia, and the earliest mention of the Strawberry in English writings is in a Saxon plant list of the tenth century, and in 1265 the 'Straberie' is mentioned in the household roll of the Countess of Leicester. 'Strabery ripe,' together with 'Gode Peascode' and 'Cherrys in the ryse,' were some of the London cries mentioned by Lydgate in the fifteenth century. Ben Jonson, in a play written in 1603, speaks of

'A pot of Strawberries gathered in the wood
To mingle with your cream.'

The common idea that the word Strawberry is derived from the habit of placing straw under the cultivated plants when the berries are ripening is quite erroneous. The name is older than this custom, and preserves the obsolete preterit 'straw' of the verb 'to strew,' referring to the tangle of vines with which the Strawberry covers the ground.

¶ *Constituents.* Cissotanic, malic, and citric acids, sugar, mucilage and a peculiar volatile aromatic body uninvestigated.

Bacon found in the odour of the dying

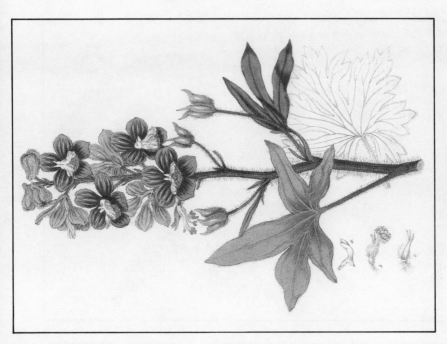

STAVESACRE.
Delphinium Staphisagria

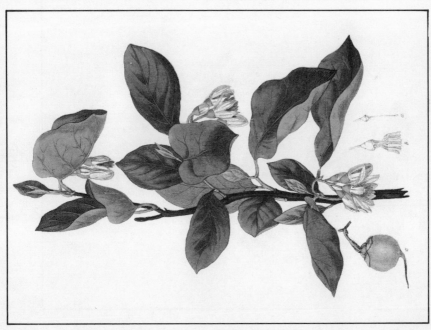

STORAX.
Liquidambar Orientalis

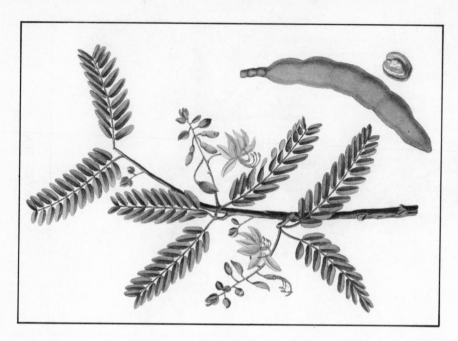

TAMARIND
Tamarindus Indica

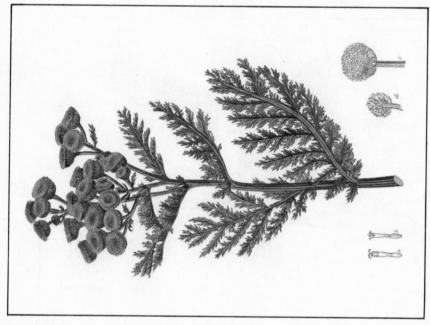

TANSY
Tanacetum Vulgare

leaves 'a most excellent cordial smell,' next in sweetness to the muskrose and violet.

¶ *Medicinal Action and Uses*. Laxative, diuretic, astringent. Both the leaves and the fruit were in early pharmacopœias, though the leaves were mostly used. The fruit contains malic and citric acids, a volatile matter, sugar, mucilage, pectin, woody fibre and water. It is easily digested and is not subject to acetous fermentation in the stomach. In feverish conditions the fruit is invaluable, and is also recommended for stone. Strawberry vitamins are of value in sprue. Culpepper declares the plant to be 'singularly good for the healing of many ills,' but Linnæus was the first to discover and prove the efficacy of the berries as a cure for rheumatic gout.

The root is astringent and used in diarrhœa. The leaves have the same property, and a tea made from them checks dysentery. The stalks only entered into the composition of the once-famous Antioch drink and vulnerary. Some recipes order that the drink should be prepared between the feasts of St. Philip and St. James and the Nativity of St. John the Baptist.

The Strawberry is a useful dentifrice and cosmetic. The fresh fruit removes discoloration of the teeth if the juice is allowed to remain on for about five minutes and the teeth are then cleansed with warm water, to which a pinch of bicarbonate of soda has been added. A cut Strawberry rubbed over the face immediately after washing will whiten the skin and remove slight sunburn. For a badly sunburnt face it is recommended to rub the juice well into the skin, to leave it on for half an hour, and then wash off with warm water to which a few drops of simple tincture of benzoin have been added; no soap should be used.

¶ *Dosage*. Infusion, 1 to 2 tablespoonsful.

AN OLD RECIPE

'Gather strawberry leaves on Lamas Eve, press them in the distillery until the aromatick perfume thereof becomes sensible. Take a fat turkey and pluck him, and baste him, then enfold him carefully in the strawberry leaves. Then boil him in water from the well, and add rosemary, velvet flower, lavender, thistles, stinging nettles, and other sweet-smelling herbs. Add also a pinte of canary wine, and half a pound of butter and one of ginger passed through the sieve. Sieve with plums and stewed raisins and a little salt. Cover him with a silver dish cover.'

(*POISON*)
STROPHANTHUS

Strophanthus Kombé (OLIV.)
N.O. Apocynaceæ

Synonyms. Strophanthus hispidus. Kombé Seeds. Strophanti Semina
Part Used. Dried, ripe seeds, deprived of their awns
Habitat. Tropical East Africa

¶ *Description*. The name *Strophanthus* is derived from the Greek *strophos* (a twisted cord or rope) and *anthos* (a flower), thus expressing the chief peculiarity of its appearance, the limb of the corolla being divided into five, long, tail-like segments. The official description of the seeds is 'lance-ovoid, flattened and obtusely-edged; from 7 to 20 mm. in length, about 4 mm. in breadth, and about 2 mm. in thickness; externally of a light fawn colour with a distinct greenish tinge, silky lustrous form, a dense coating of flat-lying hairs (*S. Kombé*) or light to dark brown, nearly smooth, and sparingly hairy (*S. hispidus*), bearing on one side a ridge running from about the centre to the summit; fracture short and somewhat soft, the fractured surface whitish and oily; odour heavy when the seeds are crushed and moistened; taste very bitter.'

In Germany the seeds of *S. hispidus* are preferred because of their guaranteed purity. This plant when growing alone is in the form of a bush, but is usually found as a woody climber inhabiting the forests between the coasts and the centre of the African continent. It then reaches to the tops of the highest trees, coiling on the ground and hanging in festoons from tree to tree. The stem is several inches in diameter. The flowers are cream-coloured, yellow at the base, purple-spotted above.

The British, French and Swiss officially favour *S. Kombé*, while the United States Pharmacopœia recognizes both. There is a voluminous literature on the subject.

The seeds of all species of the genus possess hairs that have a characteristic, thickened base, somewhat like those of nux vomica seeds; those of several species are used for the preparation of arrow poison in Africa, at Kombé in the Manganja country, in the Gaboon district, and in Guinea and Senegambia. In Gaboon the poison is called inée, onayé, or onage. Some of the poisons closely resemble those of the genus *Acocanthera*, which are used for a similar purpose. The plant yielding the arrow poison of Kombé was first brought to Europe by Sir John Kirke, and described as a new species by

Oliver, of Kew, under the name of *S. Kombé*. In preparing the arrow poison, the seeds, deprived of their hairs, are pounded to a pulp, the adhesive sap of another plant is added, and the mixture smeared for 6 inches along the point of the arrow. Game wounded by such an arrow is said to be rarely able to move 100 yards, while the flesh can be eaten without bad effect.

Strophanthus is found in commerce either in pods or as clean seeds. It must be preserved in tightly-closed containers, adding a few drops of chloroform or carbon tetrachloride from time to time, to prevent attacks by insects.

The usual course for the qualitative examination has been found insufficient, and a supplementary microscopical test is recommended. The question of its relative variability of strength as compared with digitalis is not definitely settled.

The seeds are reduced to powder with great difficulty. They are sometimes bruised in an iron mortar with broken glass, after drying.

As the active principle of Strophanthus is most abundant in the seeds, but is also found in the husks and hairs, pharmaceutical preparations of the drug should be made from the separated seeds, while other parts may be employed for the manufacture of Strophanthin.

¶ *Constituents.* A glucoside, Strophanthin, an alkaloid, Incëine, and fixed oil.

Sulphuric acid, diluted with one-fifth of its volume of water, colours the endosperm, and sometimes the cotyledons, dark green (presence of Strophanthin).

Herr Lampart and Müller received the Hagen Bucholz prize of the German Apothecaries Society for the proposed assay method following, based upon the preliminary extraction of the drug with absolute alcohol, the removal of oil from the precolate with petroleum ether, the conversion of the glucosides into strophanthidin by boiling with hydrochloric acid, and the subsequent extraction with chloroform, weighing, and calculating to strophanthin by multiplying by the factor 2·187.

The strophanthins from different species were found to vary somewhat in chemical composition, and Thoms proposes to name them as follows: *k*-strophanthin when obtained from *S. Kombé*, *g*-strophanthin when obtained from *S. gratus*, *e*-strophanthin when obtained from *S. Emini*, *h*-strophanthin when obtained from *S. hispidus*.

g-strophanthin is the one appearing to be identical with the glucoside Ouabain of Acocanthera.

Strophanthinum, a mixture of glucosides prepared from *S. Kombé*, is a whitish, crystalline powder freely soluble in water and giving a green coloration with sulphuric acid. Warmed with dilute acids it is readily hydrolized into Strophanthidin and a sugar.

Great care must be used in tasting it, and then only in very dilute solutions.

¶ *Medicinal Action and Uses.* The sole official use of Strophanthus in medicine is for its influence on the circulation, especially in cases of chronic heart weakness. As its action is the same as that of digitalis, although more likely to cause digestive disturbances,[1] it is often useful as an alternative or adjuvant to the drug. Believed to have greater diuretic power, it is esteemed of greater value in cases complicated with dropsies.

In urgent cases, the effects upon the circulation can be obtained almost immediately by means of the intravenous injection of its active principle. The hypodermic injection of Strophanthin is not recommended, owing to the intense local irritation it causes, and because of its strength it should be used with great care and under medical direction.

¶ *Dosages.* Of Extractum Strophanthi of the B.P., from $\frac{1}{4}$ to 1 grain. This extract takes the place of a solid preparation and can be administered in pills and capsules, 1 grain being equal to 5 minims of the United States tincture.

Of tincture of Strophanthus, B.P. and U.S.P., 5 to 15 drops.

Of Strophanthin, $\frac{1}{300}$ of a grain.

The maximum *daily* dose should not exceed: For *g*-strophanthin, intravenously, $\frac{1}{64}$ grain; by mouth, $\frac{1}{2}$ grain. For *k*-strophanthin, intravenously, $\frac{1}{40}$ grain; by mouth, $\frac{1}{20}$ grain.

¶ *Poisonous, if any, with Antidotes.* The greatest caution should always attend the use of strophanthin, though, unlike digitalis, its effects are not cumulative.

¶ *Varieties and Substitutions.* There are twenty-eight recognized species of the genus in Africa and Asia, extending to China, the East Indies and the Philippines. The commercial drug is often largely compounded of other than the recognized species, and may contain the seeds of related varieties, especially those of *Kickxia* (*Funtumia*) *africana*, which are beardless and spindle-shaped. They turn brown, then red, instead of green, when treated with concentrated sulphuric acid.

S. Kombé grows solely in East Africa, but the seeds from different regions are often mixed before they are shipped.

S. hispidus, S. glabra, S. Emini, S. courmontii (both var. *Kerkii* and var. *Fallax*), *S.*

Many practitioners are of opinion that Strophanthus does not cause digestive disturbances. – EDITOR.

gratus of Sierra Leone, and *S. Nicholsoni*, all contribute seeds.

The two most mixed with the official drug before exportation are those of *S. gratus* from the Senegal and Congo, where *S. hispidus* is found, and which are recommended by some authorities because easily recognized and yielding strophanthin readily in crystalline form, and *S. Thallone*.

At present Strophanthus seeds are less mixed than formerly. In 1892 the commercial seeds were classified as follows:

1. The official products of *S. Kombé* and *S. hispidus*, which contain strophanthin and no crystals of calcium oxalate.

2. Those resembling the official seeds, but coming from Mozambique and Sierra Leone.

3. Those containing calcium oxalate crystals but no strophanthin (from Senegal, Lagos, Niger, German East Africa, Togoland, and Baol of Senegal).

4. A very hairy seed from the Upper Niger, varying from a silky white to brown; the embryo contains calcium oxalate crystals, but the seeds do not contain strophanthin.

5. Seeds said to be glabrous, but having hairs in the region of the raphe, come from Lagos and Zambesi and contain neither calcium oxalate crystals nor strophanthin.

SUMACHS

N.O. Anacardiaceæ

The American Poison Ivy (*Rhus Toxicodendron*, Linn.) is one of the species of Sumachs, an attractive group of plants widely distributed in Europe, Asia and North America, varying much in habit from low bushes to moderately-sized trees, many of them familiar denizens of our gardens, for the sake of their ornamental foliage, which assumes beautiful tints in autumn, some of the varieties also bearing showy fruits.

Several species are of considerable importance, their value being chiefly in their leaves and sap, and in the large galls that are found on their leaves after they have been punctured by a tiny insect. The so-called Chinese Galls, of an irregular shape and astringent taste, which are imported into this country from China for tanning purposes, are formed by the puncture of the leaves of *Rhus semialata*, a species of aphis, and are of considerable economic value, containing 70 to 80 per cent. of gallotannic acid.

SUMACH, SMOOTH

Rhus glabra (LINN.)
N.O. Anacardiaceæ

Synonyms. Upland Sumach. Pennsylvania Sumach. Rhus copallinum (Mountain Sumach). Rhus typhinum (Staghorn or Velvet Sumach)

Parts Used. Bark of branches and root, dried, ripe berries, and exudation

Habitat. Almost all parts of the United States and Canada

¶ *Description.* There are several varieties of the plant, such as *Rhus typhinum* (Staghorn or Velvet Sumach), the berries of which now often replace those of *R. glabra* and *R. copallinum* (Mountain or Dwarf Sumach), and they should be carefully distinguished from the poisonous species. The non-poisonous have their fruit clothed with acid, crimson hairs, and their panicles are compound, dense, and terminal; the poisonous varieties have axillary panicles, and smooth fruit.

The flowers of *R. glabra* are greenish-red, and the fruit grows in clusters of small berries. It is a shrub from 6 to 15 feet high, with straggling branches and a pale-grey bark, sometimes slightly red. It grows in thickets and waste places. The berries should be gathered before the rain has removed their downy covering, for they are no longer acid when this has been washed off. They have a sour, astringent, not unpleasant taste, and are eaten freely by the country people. Their powder is a brownish-red.

When broken on the plant, a milky fluid is exuded from both bark and leaves, which forms later a solid gum-like body.

Excrescences are produced under the leaves containing quantities of tannic and gallic acid. They have been used as a substitute for imported Chinese galls, and found preferable.

The leaves, and, to a less extent, the bark, are largely used in tanning leather and dyeing. This Sumach, for the manufacture of extract for tanner's use, is largely cultivated in Virginia, where the annual crop amounts to from 7,000 to 8,000 tons. The percentage of tannin in Virginian Sumach varies from 16 to 25 per cent. That in the European or Sicilian Sumach (*R. coriaria*) falls from 6 to 8 per cent. below the percentage of the Virginian Sumach, yet the European is preferred by tanners and dyers, since by its use it is possible to make the finer, white leathers for gloves and fancy shoes.

The American product gives the leather a yellow colour, apparently due to the presence of quercitrin and quercitin.

Large quantities of a dark-red, semi-fluid, bitter, astringent extract are prepared in Virginia from Sumach, and is said to contain 25 to 30 per cent. of tannin. It is used both in

Europe and America. An infusion of the berries affords an excellent black dye for wool. A medicinal wine can also be prepared from them.

Oil of Rhus may be extracted from the seeds of this and other species of the genus. It will attain a tallow-like consistency on standing, and can be made into candles, which burn brilliantly, though they emit a pungent smoke.

¶ *Constituents.* The berries contain free malic acid and acid calcium malate coexist, with tannic and gallic acids, fixed oil, extractive, red colouring matter, and a little volatile oil. The active properties of both bark and berries yield to water.

¶ *Medicinal Action and Uses.* The bark is tonic, astringent, and antiseptic; the berries refrigerant and diuretic.

A strong decoction, or diluted fluid extract, affords an agreeable gargle in angina, especially when combined with potassium chlorate. Where tannin drugs are useful, as in diarrhœa, the fluid extract is an excellent astringent.

The bark, in decoction or syrup, has been found useful in gonorrhœa, leucorrhœa, diarrhœa, dysentery, hectic fever, scrofula and profuse perspiration from debility. Combined with the barks of slippery elm and white pine and taken freely, the decoction is said to have been greatly beneficial in syphilis. As an injection for prolapsus uteri and ani, and for leucorrhœa, and as a wash in many skin complaints, the decoction is valuable. For scald-head it can be simmered in lard, or the powdered root-bark can be applied as a poultice to old ulcers, forming a good antiseptic.

A decoction of the inner bark of the root is helpful for the sore-mouth resulting from mercurial salivation, and also for internal use in mercurial diseases. A free use of the bark will produce catharsis.

The berries may be used in infusion in diabetes, strangury bowel complaints, and febrile diseases; also as a gargle in quinsy and ulcerations of the mouth and throat, and as a wash for ringworm, tetters, offensive ulcers, etc.

The astringent excrescences, when powdered and mixed with lard or linseed oil, are useful in hæmorrhoids.

The mucilagic exudation, if the bark be punctured in hot weather, has been used advantageously in gleet and several urinary difficulties.

¶ *Dosages.* Of the fluid extract of bark, 1 to 2 drachms. Of the fluid extract of berries, 1 to 2 drachms. Of the decoction of bark, or infusion of berries, 1 to 4 fluid ounces. Rhusin, 1 to 2 grains.

The following has been recommended for gonorrhœa: Take 1 scruple each of the exudation and Canada balsam. Form into a pill mass with a sufficient quantity of powdered pokeroot, and divide into 10 pills, of which 1 or 2 may be taken three or four times daily.

SUMACH, SWEET

Rhus aromatica (AIT.)
N.O. Anacardiaceæ

Synonyms. Fragrant Sumach
Part Used. Bark

This species of Sumach, usually growing about 4 feet high, was introduced into England as an ornamental shrub in 1759.

The bark is used in tanning.

¶ *Medicinal Action and Uses.* The root-bark is astringent and diuretic. Used in diabetes and excessive discharge from kidneys and bladder. The wood exudes a peculiar odour and is used by the Indians in Arizona, California and New Mexico for making baskets.

¶ *Other Species.*

Rhus Diversilobe (CALIFORNIAN POISON OAK).

¶ *Medicinal Action and Uses.* A tincture of the fresh leaves is used for eczema and skin diseases.

The American species, *R. venenata* and *R. toxicodendron*, produce effects imputed to the Upas-tree of Java. The hands and arms, and sometimes even the whole body, becomes greatly swollen from simply touching or carrying a branch of one of these plants, and the swelling is accompanied with intolerable pain and inflammation, ending in ulceration. Some people, however, are able to handle the plants with impunity. *R. venenata*, called the POISON SUMACH or POISON ELDER, is a tall shrub with pinnate leaves composed of eleven or thirteen smoothish leaflets.

From the sap of *R. vernicifera*, the VARNISH SUMACH or Lacquer-tree of China and Japan, the varnish used in the manufacture of the famous Japanese lacquer-ware is prepared. The leaves and galls are also rich in tannin, and are used extensively for tanning various kinds of leather, and the expressed oil of the seed serves for candles. Japan Wax is obtained in Japan by expression and heat, or by the action of solvents from the fruit of another Sumach, *R. succedanea*. It consists almost entirely of palmitin and free palmitic acid, and is not a true wax; it is used in candle-making, for adulterating white beeswax and in making pomades.

R. copallina, a North American tree, provides copal resin, a transparent substance with a slight tinge of brown, which when dissolved in any volatile liquid, generally in oil of turpentine, forms one of the most perfect and beautiful of all the varnishes (known by the name of Copal Varnish).

The VENETIAN SUMACH, *R. cotinus*, though a native of Southern Europe, is so hardy a shrub as not to be injured by the frost of our winters, and is a familiar plant in our gardens, being cultivated for the very singular and ornamental appearance of its elongated, feathery fruit-stalks, which, combined with its blue-green leaves, have led to its common name of SMOKE PLANT. Both root and stem have been used for dyeing a yellow, approaching to orange, the colour obtained being, however, somewhat fugitive. The leaves are largely used for tanning.

Sumac Yellow is obtained from the dried and powdered branches of *R. coriana*, the ELM-LEAVED SUMACH, a shrub indigenous to the Mediterranean region, where it is culti-vated for dyeing yellow and for tanning leather, the SICILIAN SUMACH being considered the best quality. The shoots are cut down every year close to the root, and after being dried are reduced to powder by means of a mill. An infusion of this yields a fawn colour, bordering on green, which may be improved by the judicious application of mordants. The principal use, however, of Sumach in dyeing is the production of black, by means of the large quantity of gallic acid which it affords. The bark is used instead of the oak for tanning leather, and it is said that all Turkey leather is tanned with this plant. The leaves and seeds are used in medicine and are considered astringent and styptic: the Tripoli merchants sell the seeds at Aleppo, where they are used to provoke an appetite before meals. The shrub is frequent in our gardens, retaining its dense clusters of deep red, rough berries till winter, after the leaves have fallen. It is quite hardy, and like most of the Sumachs is easily propagated by seed. *See* (POISON) IVY.

SUMBUL

Ferula Sumbul (HOOK, F.)
N.O. Umbelliferæ

Synonyms. Euryangium Musk Root. Jatamansi. Ouchi. Ofnokgi. Sumbul Radix. Racine de Sumbul. Sumbulwurzel. Moschuswurzel
Parts Used. Root and rhizome
Habitat. Turkestan, Russia, Northern India

¶ *Description.* The plant reaches a height of 8 feet, and has a solid, cylindrical, slender stem which gives rise to about twelve branches. The root-leaves are 2½ feet long, triangular in outline, while the stem-leaves rapidly decrease in size until they are mere sheathing bracts. The pieces of root, as met with in commerce, are from 1 to 3 inches in diameter and ¾ to 1 inch in thickness. They are covered on the outside with a dusky-brown, papery, transversely-wrinkled cork, sometimes fibrous; within they are spongy, coarsely fibrous, dry, and dirty yellowish-brown, with white patches and spots of resin. The odour is strong and musk-like, the taste bitter and aromatic.

Sumbul – a Persian and Arabic word applied to various roots – was discovered in 1869 by the Russian Fedschenko, in the mountains south-east of Samarkand near the small town of Pentschakend on the River Zarafshan, at an elevation of 3,000 to 4,000 feet. A root was sent to the Moscow Botanical Gardens, and in 1872 two were sent from there to Kew, one arriving alive. In 1875 the plant died after flowering. The genus *Euryangium* (i.e. 'broad reservoir') was based by Kauffmann on the large, solitary dorsal vittæ, or oil tubes, which are filled with a quantity of latex – the moisture surounding the stigma – which pours out freely when a section is made, smelling strongly of musk, especially if treated with water, but they almost disappear in ripening, making the plant difficult to classify.

The root has long been used in Persia and India medicinally and as incense in religious ceremonies.

The physicians of Moscow and Petrograd were the first to employ it on the Continent of Europe, and Granville first introduced it to Great Britain and the United States.

The root of *Ferula suaveolens*, having only a faint, musky odour, is one of the species exported from Persia to Bombay by the Persian Gulf. It is the Sambul Root of commerce which differs from the original drug, being apparently derived from a different species of Ferula than that officially given.

The recognized source in the United States Pharmacopœia is *F. Sumbul* (Hooker Fil.). False Sumbul is the root of *Dorema Ammoniacum*; it is of closer texture, denser, and more firm, of a red or yellow tinge and feeble odour.

¶ *Constituents.* Volatile oil, two balsamic resins, one soluble in alcohol and one in ether; wax, gum, starch, a bitter substance soluble in water and alcohol, a little angelic and valeric acid. The odour seems to be con_ nected with the balsamic resins. The volatile oil has a bitter taste like peppermint, and on dry distillation yields a bluish oil containing umbelliferone. A 1916 analysis shows moisture, starch, pentrosans, crude fibre, protein, dextrin, ash, sucrose, reducing sugar, volatile oil and resins. Alkaloids were not detected. The volatile oil did not show the presence of sulphur. Both betaine and umbelliferon were detected. In the resin, vanillic acid was identified and a phytosterol was present. Among the volatile acids were acetic, butyric, angelic and tiglic acid, and among the non-volatile oleic, linoleic, tiglic, cerotic, palmitic and stearic.

¶ *Medicinal Action and Uses.* Stimulant and antispasmodic, resembling valerian in its action, and used in various hysterical conditions. It is believed to have a specific action on the pelvic organs, and is widely employed in dysmenorrhœa and allied female disorders.

It is also a stimulant to mucous membranes, not only in chronic dysenteries and diarrhœas, but in chronic bronchitis, especially with asthmatic tendency, and even in pneumonia.

Half an ounce of a tincture produced narcotic symptoms, confusing the head, causing a tendency to snore even when awake, and giving feelings of tingling, etc., with a strong odour of the drug from breath and skin which only passed off after a day or two.

The tincture of 10 per cent. Sumbul, with 2 volumes of alcohol and 1 of water, is used as an antispasmodic and nervine. The fluid extract, being superior, superseded the tincture. (Sumbul, in No. 30 powder, 1,000 grams, with a mixture of 4 volumes of alcohol and 1 of water as the menstruum.)

¶ *Dosages.* B.P., ½ to 1 drachm. Of fluid extract, ½ to 1 fluid drachm. Of extract of Sumbul or Muskroot, 2 to 5 grains. Solid extract, U.S.P., 4 grains.

SUNDEW

Drosera rotundifolia (LINN.)
N.O. Droraceæ

Synonyms. Dew Plant. Round-leaved Sundew. Red Rot. Herba rosellæ. Sonnenthau rosollis. Rosée du Soleil

Part Used. The flowering plant dried in the air, *not* artificially

Habitat. Britain, and in many parts of Europe, India, China, Cape of Good Hope, New Holland, North and South America, Russian Asia

¶ *Description.* This little insectivorous plant is found growing in muddy edges of ponds, bogs and rivers, where the soil is peaty. It is a small herbaceous, perennial, aquatic plant, with short and slender fibrous root, from which grow the leaves. These are remarkable for their covering of red glandular hairs, by which they are readily recognized, apart from their flowers which only open in the sunshine. Their leaves are orbicular on long stalks, depressed, lying flat on ground and have on upper surface long red viscid hairs, each having a small gland at top, containing a fluid, which looks like a dewdrop, hence its name. This secretion is most abundant when the sun is at its height. Flower-stems erect, slender, 2 to 6 inches high, at first coiled inward bearing a simple raceme, which straightens out as flowers expand; these are very small and white, appearing in summer and early autumn. Seeds numerous, spindle-shaped in a loose chaffy covering contained in a capsule. These hairs are very sensitive, they curve inward slowly and catch any insects which alight on them; the fluid on the

points also retains them. After an insect has been caught, the glandular heads secrete a digestive fluid which dissolves all that can be absorbed from the insect. It has been noted that secretion does not take place when inorganic substances are imprisoned.

¶ *Constituents.* The juice is bitter, acrid, caustic, odourless, yielding not more than 30 per cent. ash, and contains citric and malic acids.

¶ *Medicinal Action and Uses.* Used with advantage in whooping-cough, exerting a peculiar action on the respiratory organs; useful in incipient phthisis, chronic bronchitis, asthma, etc., the juice is said to take away corns and warts, and may be used to curdle milk. In America it has been advocated as a cure for old age; a vegetable extract is used together with colloidal silicates in cases of arterio sclerosis.

¶ *Dosages.* 2 fluid drachms of the saturated tincture added to 4 fluid drachms of water or wine and a teaspoonful taken for a dose. Fluid extract, 10 to 20 drops. Solid extract, 2 to 5 grams.

SUNFLOWER

Helianthus annuus
N.O. Compositæ

Synonyms. Marigold of Peru. Corona Solis. Sola Indianus. Chrysanthemum Peruvianum

The common Sunflower is a native of Mexico and Peru, introduced into this country in the sixteenth century and now one of our most familiar garden plants.

It is an annual herb, with a rough, hairy

stem, 3 to 12 feet high, broad, coarsely-toothed, rough leaves, 3 to 12 inches long, and circular heads of flowers, 3 to 6 inches wide in wild specimens and often a foot or more in cultivation. The flower-heads are composed of many small tubular flowers arranged compactly on a flattish disk: those in the outer row have long strap-shaped corollas, forming the rays of the composite flower.

The genus *Helianthus*, to which the Sunflower belongs, contains about fifty species, chiefly natives of North America; many are indigenous to the Rocky Mountains, others to tropical America, and a few species are found in Peru and Chile.

They are tall, hardy, annual or perennial herbs, several of which are grown in gardens, being of easy cultivation in moderately good soil, and that useful plant of the kitchen garden, the Jerusalem Artichoke (*Helianthus tuberosus*), is also a member of the genus.

The name *Helianthus*, being derived from *helios* (the sun) and *anthos* (a flower), has the same meaning as the English name Sunflower, which it is popularly supposed has been given these flowers from a supposition that they follow the sun by day, always turning towards its direct rays. But since the word 'Sunflower' existed in English literature before the introduction of *H. annuus*, or at any rate before its general diffusion in English gardens, it is obvious that some other flower must have been intended. The Marigold (*Calendula officinalis*) is considered by Dr. Prior to have been the plant described by Ovid as turning to the sun, likewise the *solsæce* the Anglo-Saxon, a word equivalent to *solsequium* (sun-following). The better explanation for the application of the name to a flower is its resemblance to 'the radiant beams of the sun.'

In Peru, this flower was much reverenced by the Aztecs, and in their temples of the Sun, the priestesses were crowned with Sunflowers and carried them in their hands. The early Spanish conquerors found in these temples numerous representations of the Sunflower wrought in pure gold.

In some of the old Herbals we find the Rock-rose (*Helianthemum vulgare*) also termed Sunflower, its flowers opening only in the sunshine. The so-called 'Pigmy sunflower' is *Actinella grandiflora*, a pretty perennial 6 to 9 inches high, from the Colorado mountains.

The Sunflower is valuable from an *economic*, as well as from an ornamental point of view. Every part of the plant may be utilized for some economic purpose. The *leaves* form a cattle-food and the *stems* contain a fibre which may be used successfully in making paper. The *seed* is rich in oil, which is said to approach more nearly to olive oil than any other vegetable oil known and to be largely used as a substitute. In pre-war days, Sunflower seed was sometimes grown in this country, especially on sewage farms, as an economical crop for pheasants, as well as poultry. The *flowers* contain a yellow dye.

One of the many effects of the War in its relation to agriculture was the increase in the use of the Sunflower.

It forms one of the well-known crops in Russia, Spain, France, Germany, Italy, Egypt, India, Manchuria and Japan. The average acre will produce about 50 bushels of merchantable seeds, and each bushel yields approximately 1 gallon of oil, for which there is a whole series of important uses.

The oil is produced mainly in Russia, but to an increasing extent also in Roumania, Hungary, Bulgaria and Poland. In 1913 some 180,000 tons of oil were produced, practically all of which was consumed locally.

The oil pressed from the seeds is of a citron yellow colour and a sweet taste and is considered equal to olive oil or almond oil for table use. The resulting oil-cake when warm pressed, yields a less valuable oil which is used largely for technical purposes, such as soap-making, candle-making and in the art of wool-dressing. As a drying oil for mixing paint, it is equal to linseed oil and is unrivalled as a lubricant.

The residue after the oil is expressed forms an important cattle-food. This oil-cake is relished by sheep, pigs, pigeons, rabbits and poultry.

The seed makes excellent chicken-food and feeding fowls on bruised Sunflower seeds is well known to increase their laying power.

The seeds of the large-seeded varieties are also much liked by Russians and are sold in the street as are chestnuts in this country. Big bowls of Sunflower seeds are to be seen in the restaurants of railway stations, for people to eat. Indian natives are also fond of the seeds.

Roasted in the same manner as coffee, they make an agreeable drink, and the seeds have been used in Portugal and Russia to make a wholesome and nutritious bread.

The pith of the sunflower stalk is the lightest substance known; its specific gravity is 0·028, while that of the Elder is 0·09 and of Cork 0·24. The discovery of the extreme lightness of the pith of the stalk has essentially increased the commercial value of the plant. This light cellular substance is now carefully removed from the stalks and applied to a good many important uses, chiefly in the making of life-saving appliances. The pith has been recommended for moxa, owing to the nitre its contains.

¶ *Chemical Constituents.* The black-seeded variety yield between 50 and 60 per cent. of the best grade of oil.

The oil has a specific gravity of from 0·924 to 0·926, solidifies at 5° F., is slightly yellowish, limpid, of a sweetish taste and odourless. It dries slowly and forms one of the best burning oils known, burning longer than any other vegetable oil.

Ludwig and Kromayer obtained a tannin which they called Helianthitanic acid, and gave it the formula $C_{14}H_9O_8$. On boiling with moderately diluted hydrochloric acid, they obtained a fermentable sugar and a violet colouring matter. E. Diek found only small quantities of Inulin, large quantities of Levulin and a dextro-rotatory sugar.

All parts of the plant contain much carbonate of potash.

¶ *Extraction.* For the extraction of the oil, the seeds are bruised, crushed and ground to meal in a five-roller mill, under chilled iron or steel cylinders. The meal, after being packed in bags, is placed in hydraulic presses, under a pressure of 300 atmospheres or more, and allowed to remain under pressure for about seven minutes. All edible oils are thus obtained and are known in commerce as 'cold-drawn oils' or 'cold pressed oils.' As a preliminary operation, the seeds are freed from dust, sand and other impurities by sifting in an inclined revolving cylinder or sieving machine, covered with woven wire, having meshes varying according to the size and nature of the seeds operated upon. This preliminary purification is of the greatest importance. The seeds are then passed through a hopper over the rollers, which are finely grooved, so that the seed is cut up whilst passing in succession between the first and second rollers in the series, then between the second and the third, and so on to the last, when the grains are sufficiently bruised, crushed and ground. The distance between the rollers can be easily regulated, so that the seed leaving the bottom roller has the desired fineness. The resulting more or less coarse meal is either expressed in this state, or subjected to a preliminary heating, according to the quality of the product to be manufactured. The oil exuding in the cold dissolves the smallest amount of colouring matter, etc., and hence has suffered least in its quality.

By pressing in the cold, only part of the oil or fat is recovered. A further quantity is obtained by pressing the seed meal at a somewhat elevated temperature, reached by warming the crushed seeds either immediately after they leave the five-roller mill, or after the 'cold-drawn oil' has been taken off. The cold pressed cakes are first disintegrated, generally under an edge-runner. This oil is of a second-grade quality.

Vertical hydraulic presses are at present almost exclusively in use, the Anglo-American type of press being most employed. It represents an open press, fitted with a number (usually sixteen) of iron press plates, between which the cakes are inserted by hand. A hydraulic ram then forces the table carrying the cakes against a press-head and the exuding oil flows down the sides into a tank below.

According to the care exercised by the manufacturer in the range of temperature to which the seed is heated, various grades of oils are obtained.

¶ *Cultivation.* In growing crops of the Sunflower, various methods of planting and spacing are recommended in different countries. It is best, says a scientific American authority, to plant in rows running north and south, the seeds to be placed 9 inches apart, in rows 30 inches apart.

But in this country, instead of sowing in the open, the most successful growers sow in boxes, or singly in pots under glass, afterwards planting the seedlings out in ground that has been well prepared and enriched with manure. Not that rich soil is essential, practically any kind of soil is suitable so long as it is open to sun and light and splendid returns of seed have been obtained from waste land without any preparation beyond digging the soil.

A well-tilled soil is, however, desirable for successful Sunflower cultivation, preferably with not too much clay in its composition. It should be well ploughed in the autumn and harrowed in the spring. A certain depth is necessary, as the roots will spread from 12 inches to 15 inches in each direction.

In the latter years of the War, the Ministry of Food and the Food Production Department supplied full information as to cultivation and harvesting and undertook to purchase the ripened seed in quantities of $\frac{1}{2}$ cwt. and upwards: they were used in the manufacture of margarine and other essential fats used in the making of munitions.

The seed should be sown thinly in boxes in March and when the plants have made three or four leaves, they should be potted off into small pots and grown on if possible in gentle heat. Where no heat is available, a cold frame is the next best thing. Provided that frost can be excluded, a cool, unheated glasshouse may be used.

When established, they should be gradually hardened off for planting out in May, after all danger of late spring frosts is past.

Suitable compost for seeds and potting off is: 1 part leaf mould, 1 part sand, 2 parts loam. If this is not available, any good garden soil will do and it need not be very finely sifted. The seeds germinate readily and grow very rapidly.

Ordinary farmyard manure should be dug into the soil at the rate of 3 cwt. per rod, as they are gross feeders. The Sunflower plants should be planted 3 feet apart between the rows and 2 feet from plant to plant in good soils, and slightly closer on poor soils.

An application of superphosphate before or at the time of planting, at the rate of 1½ oz. per square yard will encourage early maturing of the seed.

It is of interest to note that the plant assimilates a large quantity of potash and therefore it must not be planted in the same soil the second year.

Seeds should not be sown *in the open* until late in April, only a sunny border being chosen.

The Food Production Department advised cultivators who intended growing largely for munitions to sow seed early in May, in drills 1 to 1½ inch deep and stated the amount of seed required to be at the rate of 1 oz. to 8 rods, or 1½ lb. per acre.

In exposed positions, the plants will require support and this is best done by placing a good strong stake each end and one in centre of row, and running a length of wire or thick string from stake to stake and tying the plants to this loosely.

¶ *Harvesting.* No more attention will be needed until the heads commence to ripen, when they should be looked to daily, as the seed soon falls if left too long and also, as the seed ripens, garden pests of the larger sort, birds and squirrels in particular, are always troublesome.

Some growers prevent the loss caused by the attacks of birds to whom the seeds are particularly attractive and by the shaking out of the ripe seeds, by surrounding the heads with bags of rough muslin, but this can only be done when growing on a small scale. With a large plantation, scare away birds by any of the usual methods.

It is, of course, impossible to say exactly when the harvesting should commence. Everything depends upon climatic conditions. If the weather is warm and dry, so that the best plan is to leave the plants alone, so that the ripening process can be carried out naturally, the heads being cut when about to shed their seeds. In a fine autumn, Sunflower seed will ripen well in the open and the best re-

sults are got when the seed can thus be allowed to mature.

When the head shrivels and the seeds are ripe, cut the plants at the ground level, standing them with their heads uppermost, like shocks or sheaves of corn. When the heads are thoroughly dry, cut them off and thresh out the remaining seeds by standing each head on its side and hammering it with a mallet. Store the seeds in bags, in a dry place.

If the weather is dull or wet, unfavourable for ripening of the seed out-of-doors, hasten the ripening by cutting the plants at ground level as soon as the seeds are plump.

Stand them shock-wise, if possible under cover, in a damp-proof outside house, barn or room, and wind being as good a drying agent as the sun, see that the store is well ventilated and leave windows and doors wide open when the weather is propitious. When the heads shrivel, cut them off and complete drying in a very slow oven. Place the heads in single layers on the shelves of the oven in the evening, leaving the door slightly open. Remove them when the fire is made up in the morning and replace them in the evening.

If a kiln or hop oast is available, it may be used for finishing off the drying, but if the seeds are exposed to a high temperature, they will be useless for next year's sowing.

The important things to remember are that the seeds are not ready if they cannot be removed from the heads without difficulty, and they will not keep very long if not dry when stored.

In Russia, where Sunflowers are extensively grown for human food the method adopted by the peasants for removing the seed from the heads is interesting. A wooden disk is made, through which nails are hammered in rows radiating from the centre. The disk is attached to a handle and the seed-head is held in contact with the nails when the disk is turned, with the result that the seed, which is collected in sacks, is raked out very quickly. The disk is so arranged that one man can hold the seed-head in position and at the same time turn the handle to extract the seeds.

The Mammoth or Giant Sunflower, which comes from Russia and is called the Russian Sunflower, is the best kind to grow, these being nearly double the size of the ordinary variety. During the War, the only seed available was the American Giant, which was said, however, to be equal to the Russian.

The tall Mammoth Sunflower, bearing heads of an average width of 15 inches, containing 2,000 seeds, yields about 50 bushels an acre, producing 50 gallons of oil and about 150 lb. of oil-cake, the stems giving 10 per cent. of potash.

It has been estimated in Denmark, that the crops of one season in that country would produce 2,000 tons of seed, yielding 350 tons of oil, and about 1,550 tons of oil-cake and oil waste to be used as fodder.

With the exception of Cambridgeshire, the Sunflower grows best in England in the Southern and South-Western counties.

They have been proved to do best on deep, stony soil, and it is an advantage to grow them where bees are kept, as they are much visited by the honey-bee, fertilization of the flowers ensuing.

¶ *Sunflower-seeds as Poultry and Cattle Food.* Sunflower seeds have a high feeding value – the analysis in round figures is 16 per cent. albumen and 21 per cent. fat.

Being so rich in oil, they are too stimulating to use alone and should only be used in combination with other feeding stuffs. Fed with oats in equal quantities, they make a perfectly balanced ration. Since both of these articles contain a big proportion of indigestible matter, particularly in the husks, grit must on no account be withheld, if the birds are to derive full benefit.

As food for laying poultry, it ought in the opinion of some authorities, not to be used in excess of one-third of the total mixture of corn, owing to its fat-producing properties.

The seeds are palatable to poultry and greedily devoured by them. A very common way to supply the birds with the seeds is to hang up the ripe heads just high enough to compel the chicks to pick them out, for when the heads are thrown into the yard, they are trodden on and wasted.

Sunflower-seed oil-cake is a valuable article for bringing up the feeding value of some of the poultry foods and was specially in demand for this purpose in war-time, when the supply of good cereals ran short. It is more fattening to cattle than Linseed cake, being richer in nitrogenous substances, containing 34 per cent. albumen. As well as being an excellent food for poultry, and also for rabbits, it keeps both horses and cattle in good condition. It is said that cows, fed on Sunflower-seed oil-cake, mixed with bran, will have an increased flow of good, rich milk.

It is largely exported by Russia to Denmark, Sweden and elsewhere for stock feeding.

¶ *Sunflower Plants as Green Food.* With Sunflowers there need be little waste. The green leaves, when gathered young, make a good succulent green food for poultry stock of all ages. They can be finely minced up and added – raw – to the mash for young or adult stock, or they can be boiled and put in the soft food. The leaves are much appreciated by rabbits, horses, cows and other stock.

The dried leaves can be rubbed up or reduced to a meal form and be well scalded prior to inclusion in the mash, and the ripe seeds can also be ground into a meal if desired.

¶ *Litter.* Even the stems and seedless heads need not be wasted where fowls are kept. Many may prefer to use them as fire-kindlers, but they will, when thoroughly dry, come in useful as litter for the laying-houses. When dry, they can be passed through a chaff-cutting machine and be added to the other litter – peat-moss or dried leaves. They need to be made into a scratchable material for hens, but for ducks, the material can be placed deeply in the house as a bedding. Ducks need litter to 'squat' on rather than to scratch in.

¶ *Silage.* The value of the Giant Sunflower as a silage crop is discussed in the March, 1918, number of *The Journal of Heredity*, by F. B. Linfield, the Director of the Montana Agricultural Station. Trials were made of this plant in the higher valleys, where Beans and Maize were not well adapted, owing to the uncertainty of their yield. In three successive years, the yield of the Sunflower varied from 22 to 30 tons of green fodder per acre, being about two and a half times that of Maize, and more than twice as great as that of Lucerne, for the season. It had, moreover, the advantage of so shading the ground as to keep all weeds under. Feeding experiments were made with it, both as a green crop and as silage. Cows were found to eat it as readily as Maize fodder, and control experiments showed that the milk flow was maintained as readily as with the latter crop; nor was there evidence of any taint in the milk. A portion of the Sunflower fodder was put into the silo and fed in the winter, both to cows and fattening steers, with satisfactory results. It matures in the English climate better than Maize, and, consequently, would not be so liable to become sour in the silo and its relatively high oil content would probably render it valuable.

¶ *As Fuel. As Source of Potash for Manure.* Sunflowers, when the stalks are dry, are as hard as wood and make an excellent fire.

Those who undertake to grow Sunflowers should, however, bear in mind that the ash obtained from the plants after the seed has been harvested is, owing to its richness in potash, a manure of considerable value, so that it is really wasteful to use up the dry stems merely on the domestic fire; it is of more advantage to make them up in heaps on the ground, burn them there and save the ash.

At the time of cutting, strip off the leaves and feed them to rabbits or poultry. When the stems are dry and after the seed crop has been gathered, choose a fine day to burn both stems and empty seed-heads.

Of the ash obtained from burning the Sunflower stems and heads (apart from seeds) 62 per cent. consists of potash, and as an acre of Sunflowers produces from 2,500 to 4,000 lb. of top, the total yield of potash is considerable. Allowing 3,000 lb. of top, there would be produced 160 lb. of ashes per acre of crop, which should contain upwards of 50 lb. of potash.

The ash should either be spread at once or stored under cover; if left exposed to rain, the potash will be washed away and the ash rendered of little manurial value. It can be used with advantage for the potato or other root crop in the following year, being spread a little while before the crop is planted, at the rate of from $\frac{1}{2}$ to 1 oz. to the square yard.

¶ *As Soil Improver.* The growing herb is extremely useful for drying damp soils, because of its remarkable ability to absorb quantities of water. Swampy districts in Holland have been made habitable by an extensive culture of the Sunflower, the malarial miasma being absorbed and nullified, whilst abundant oxygen is emitted.

¶ *Textile Use.* The Chinese grow this plant extensively, and it is believed that a large portion of its fibre is mixed with their silks.

¶ *A Bee Plant.* The Sunflower is a good bee plant, as it furnishes hive bees with large quantities of wax and nectar.

¶ *As Vegetable.* The unexpanded buds boiled and served like Artichokes form a pleasant dish.

¶ *Medicinal Action and Uses.* The seeds have diuretic and expectorant properties and have been employed with success in the treatment of bronchial, laryngeal and pulmonary affections, coughs and colds, also in whooping cough.

The following preparation is recommended: Boil 2 oz. of the seeds in 1 quart of water, down to 12 oz. and then strain. Add 6 oz. of good Holland gin and 6 oz. of sugar. Give in doses of 1 to 2 teaspoonsful, three or four times a day.

The oil possesses similar properties and may be given in doses of 10 to 15 drops or more, two or three times a day.

A tincture of the flowers and leaves has been recommended in combination with balsamics in the treatment of bronchiectasis.

The seeds, if browned in the oven and then made into an infusion are admirable for the relief of whooping cough.

Tincture of Helianthus has been used in Russia. Kazatchkoft says that in the Caucasus the inhabitants employ the Sunflower in malarial fever. The leaves are spread upon a bed covered with a cloth, moistened with warm milk and then the patient is wrapped up in it. Perspiration is produced and this process is repeated every day until the fever has ceased.

A tincture prepared from the seed with rectified spirit of wine is useful for intermittent fevers and ague, instead of quinine. It has been employed thus in Turkey and Persia, where quinine and arsenic have failed, being free from any of the inconveniences which often arise from giving large quantities of the other drugs.

The leaves are utilized in herb tobaccos.

SWAMP MILKWEED

Asclepias incarnata (LINN.)
N.O. Asclepiadaceæ

Synonyms. Flesh-coloured Asclepias. Swamp Silkweed. Rose-coloured Silkweed
Part Used. Root

¶ *Description.* A herb growing in wet places, flowering in the United States in July and August. Stem erect, smooth, with two downy lines above, about $2\frac{1}{2}$ feet high, branched above, very leafy; leaves opposite, petiolate, oblong, lanceolate, hairy, acute, cordate at base, 4 to 7 inches long, 1 to 2 inches wide; flowers rose-purple, fragrant, disposed in terminal-crowded umbels two to six on a peduncle 2 inches long, consisting of ten to twenty small flowers; pods smooth; rhizome oblong, 1 inch in diameter, knotty, surrounded with rootlets, 4 to 6 inches long, yellow-brown externally, white internally; bark thin, wood with fine medullary rays.

The roots exudes a milky juice with a heavy odour, which is lost in drying.

Solvents: Alcohol, water.

¶ *Constituents.* Asclepiadin (the emetic principle), an alkaloid, two acrid resins, volatile oil, fixed oil, albumen, starch, pectin and glucose.

¶ *Medicinal Action and Uses.* Emetic, diuretic, anthelmintic, stomachic. Swamp Milkweed strengthens the heart in the same way as digitalis and is a quick and certain diuretic. It is given in dropsy as a diuretic in place of digitalis, also in coughs, colds, rheumatism from cold, threatened inflammation of the lungs. Also in diarrhœa, gastric catarrh, certain skin eruptions of an erysipelatous nature and in asthma and dyspnœa. It may also be used with advantage in the early stages of dysentery.

It acts as a vermifuge in doses of 10 to 20 grains.

Preparations and Dosages. Specific Swamp Milkweed, 1 to 20 minims. The infusion is made of ½ oz. of the powdered root to a pint of boiling water. Dose of the powder, 15 to 60 grains.

TAG ALDER. *See* ALDER

TALLOW TREE

Sapium Salicifolium
N.O. Euphorbiaceæ

Synonym. Sapium
Parts Used. Leaves, fruit
Habitat. Tropics of both Hemispheres and cultivated in China and Paraguay

Description. It yields a milky juice, which is acrid and even poisonous, the leaves are willow-like, and at their point of union with the stalk have two round glands; the flowers are small and greenish, and grow in terminal spikes, the lower portion bearing the fertile, and the upper ones the sterile flowers. The bark of *Sapium Salicifolium* yields a substance for tanning which is used instead of oak; most modern writers unite this genus with *Stillingia*, from which there are no reliable characters to distinguish it. In America, *S. Biglandulosum* is a source for rubber. Sapium or *S. Indicum* is known in Borneo under the name of Booroo; the leaves are used for dye-ing and staining rotang a dark colour; the acrid milky juice burns the mouth as Capsicum does; the young fruit is acid and eaten as a condiment; the fruit is also used to poison alligators; the ripe fruit are woolly, trilobed capsules, about 1 inch across, three-celled and containing only one seed in each.

S. sebiyerum, the Chinese Tallow Tree, gives a fixed oil which envelops the seeds. The tallow occurs in hard brittle opaque white masses, which consists of palmatin and stearin. The oil is used for lighting and manure. The waste from the nuts for fuel and manure.

See QUEEN'S DELIGHT.

TAMARAC

Larix Americana (MICHX.)
N.O. Coniferæ

Synonyms. American Larch. Black Larch. Hackmatack. Pinus Pendula (Salisb.)
Part Used. Bark
Habitat. Eastern North America

Description. The tree has a straight slender trunk with thin horizontal branches growing to 80 to 100 feet high; leaves short, 1 or 2 inches long, very fine, almost thread-form, soft deciduous, without sheaths in fascicles of from twenty to forty, being developed early in the spring from lateral scaly and globular buds which produce growing shoots on which the leaves are scattered. Cones oblong of a few rounded scales widening upward from ½ to 1 inch in length, deep purple colour, scales thin, inflexed on the margin. Bracts elliptical, often hollowed at the sides, abruptly acuminate, with a slender point and, together with the scales, persistent.

Medicinal Action and Uses. The bark used as a decoction is laxative, tonic, diuretic and alterative, useful in obstructions of the liver, rheumatism, jaundice and some cutaneous diseases. A decoction of the leaves has been used for piles, hæmoptysis, menorrhagia, diarrhœa and dysentery.

Dosage. 2 tablespoonsful of the bark decoction.

See PINES.

TAMARINDS

Tamarindus Indica (LINN.)
N.O. Leguminosæ

Synonyms. Imlee. Tamarindus officinalis (Hook)
Part Used. The fruits freed from brittle outer part of pericarp
Habitat. India; tropical Africa; cultivated in West Indies

Description. A large handsome tree with spreading branches and a thick straight trunk, ash-grey bark, height up to 40 feet. Leaves alternate, abruptly pinnated; leaflets light green and a little hairy, in twelve to fifteen pairs. In cold damp weather and after sunset the leaflets close. Flowers fragrant, yellow-veined, red and purple filaments, in terminal and lateral racemes. Legume oblong, pendulous, nearly linear, curved, somewhat compressed, filled with a firm acid pulp. Bark hard and scabrous, never separates into valves; inside the bark are three fibres, one down, on the upper concave margin, the other two at equal distances from the convex edge. Seeds six to twelve, covered with a shiny smooth brown shell, and inserted into the convex side of the pericarp. There are three varieties of Tamarinds. The East Indian, with long pods containing six to twelve seeds, the West Indian, with shorter pods containing about four seeds, and a third, with the pulp of the pod a lovely rose colour. West Indian Tamarinds are usually imported in syrup, the outer shell having been removed; East Indian Tamarinds are exported in a firm black mass of shelled legumes; the third kind are usually preserved in syrup.

¶ *Constituents.* Citric, tartaric and malic acids, potassium, bitartrate, gum, pectin, some grape sugar, and parenchymatous fibre.

¶ *Medicinal Action and Uses.* Cathartic, astringent, febrifuge, antiseptic, refrigerant. There are no known constituents in Tamarinds to account for their laxative properties; they are refrigerant from the acids they contain, an infusion of the Tamarind pulp making a useful drink in febrile conditions, and the pulp a good diet in convalescence to maintain a slightly laxative action of the bowels; also used in India as an astringent in bowel complaints. The pulp is said to weaken the action of resinous cathartics in general, but is frequently prescribed with them as a vehicle for jalap, etc. Tamarind is useful in correcting bilious disorders; 3 drachms up to 2 oz. of the pulp to render it moderately cathartic are required according to the case. The leaves are some-

times used in subacid infusions, and a decoction is said to destroy worms in children, and is also useful for jaundice, and externally as a wash for sore eyes and ulcers. A punch is made from the fruit in the West Indies, mixed with a decoction of borage to allay the scalding of urine. Tamarind Whey, made by boiling 1 oz. of the pulp in 1 pint of milk and then strained, makes a cooling laxative drink. In some forms of sore throat the fruit has been found of service. In Mauritius the Creoles mix salt with the pulp and use it as a liniment for rheumatism and make a decoction of the bark for asthma. The Bengalese employ Tamarind pulp in dysentery, and in times of scarcity use it as a food, boiling the pods or macerating them and removing the dark outer skin. The natives of India consider that the neighbourhood in which Tamarind trees grow becomes unwholesome, and that it is unsafe to sleep under the tree owing to the acid they exhale during the moisture of the night. It is said that no plant will live under the shade of it, but in the Author's experience some plants and bulbs bloomed luxuriantly under the Tamarind trees in her garden in Bengal. The wood is very hard and durable, valuable for building purposes and furnishes excellent charcoal for gunpowder; the leaves in infusion give a yellow dye. Tamarinds in Indian cookery is an important ingredient in curries and chutneys, and makes a delicious sauce for duck, geese and water fowl, and in Western India is used for pickling fish, Tamarind fish being considered a great delicacy.

TANSY

Tanacetum vulgare (LINN.)
N.O. Compositæ

Synonym. Buttons
Part Used. Herb
Habitat. Tansy, a composite plant very familiar in our hedgerows and waste places, is a hardy perennial, widely spread over Europe

¶ *Description.* The stem is erect and leafy, about 2 to 3 feet high, grooved and angular. The leaves are alternate, much cut into, 2 to 6 inches long and about 4 inches wide. The plant is conspicuous in August and September by its heads of round, flat, dull yellow flowers, growing in clusters, which earn it the name of 'Buttons.' It has a very curious, and not altogether disagreeable odour, somewhat like camphor.

It is often naturalized in our gardens for ornamental cultivation. The feathery leaves of the Wild Tansy are beautiful, especially when growing in abundance on marshy ground, and it has a more refreshing scent than the Garden Tansy.

¶ *Cultivation.* Tansy will thrive in almost any soil and may be increased, either in

spring or autumn, by slips or by dividing the creeping roots, which if permitted to remain undisturbed, will, in a short time, overspread the ground. When transplanting the slips or portions of root, place therefore at least a foot apart.

The name Tansy is probably derived from the Greek *Athanaton* (immortal), either, says Dodoens, because it lasts so long in flower, or, as Ambrosius thought, because it is capital for preserving dead bodies from corruption. It was said to have been given to Ganymede to make him immortal.

Tansy was one of the Strewing Herbs, mentioned by Tusser in 1577, and was one of the native plants dedicated to the Virgin Mary.

Perhaps it found additional favour as a 'Strewing Herb' because it was said to be effectual in keeping flies away, particularly if mixed with elder leaves.

Parkinson grew Tansy amongst other aromatic and culinary herbs in his garden.

It is connected with some interesting old customs observed at Easter time, when even archbishops and bishops played handball with men of their congregation, and a Tansy cake was the reward of the victors. These Tansy cakes were made from the young leaves of the plant, mixed with eggs, and were thought to purify the humours of the body after the limited fare of Lent. In time, this custom obtained a kind of symbolism, and Tansies, as these cakes were called, came to be eaten on Easter Day as a remembrance of the bitter herbs eaten by the Jews at the Passover. Coles (1656) says the origin of eating it in the spring is because Tansy is very wholesome after the salt fish consumed during Lent, and counteracts the ill-effects which the 'moist and cold constitution of winter has made on people . . . though many understand it not, and some simple people take it for a matter of superstition to do so.'

'This balsamic plant,' says Boerhaave (the Danish physician), 'will supply the place of nutmegs and cinnamon,' and the young leaves, shredded, serve as a flavouring for puddings and omelets. Gerard tells us that Tansy Teas were highly esteemed in Lent as well as Tansy puddings.

From an old cookery book:

'A Tansy.

'Beat seven eggs, yolks and whites separately; add a pint of cream, near the same of spinach-juice, and a little tansy-juice gained by pounding in a stone mortar; a quarter of a pound of Naples biscuit, sugar to taste, a glass of white wine, and some nutmeg. Set all in a sauce-pan, just to thicken, over the fire; then put it into a dish, lined with paste, to turn out, and bake it.'

Culpepper says: 'Of Tansie. The root eaten, is a singular remedy for the gout: the rich may bestow the cost to preserve it.'

Cows and sheep eat Tansy, but horses, goats and hogs refuse to touch it, and if meat be rubbed with this plant, flies will not attack it. In Sussex, at one time, Tansy leaves had the reputation of curing ague, if placed in the shoes.

The Finlanders employ it in dyeing green.

¶ *Parts Used.* The leaves and tops. The plant is cut off close above the root, when first coming into flower in August.

¶ *Constituents.* Tanacetin, tannic acid, a volatile oil, mainly thujone, waxy, resinous and protein bodies, some sugar and a colouring matter.

¶ *Medicinal Action and Uses.* Anthelmintic, tonic, stimulant, emmenagogue.

Tansy is largely used for expelling worms in children, the infusion of 1 oz. to a pint of boiling water being taken in teacupful doses, night and morning, fasting.

It is also valuable in hysteria and in kidney weaknesses, the same infusion being taken in wineglassful doses, repeated frequently. It forms an excellent and safe emmenagogue, and is of good service in low forms of fever, in ague and hysterical and nervous affections. As a diaphoretic nervine it is also useful.

In moderate doses, the plant and its essential oil are stomachic and cordial, being anti-flatulent and serving to allay spasms.

In large doses, it becomes a violent irritant, and induces venous congestion of the abdominal organs.

In Scotland, an infusion of the dried flowers and seeds ($\frac{1}{2}$ to 1 teaspoonful, two or three times a day) is given for gout. The roots when preserved with honey or sugar, have also been reputed to be of special service against gout, if eaten fasting every day for a certain time.

From 1 to 4 drops of the essential oil may be safely given in cases of epilepsy, but excessive doses have produced seizures.

Tansy has been used externally with benefit for some eruptive diseases of the skin, and the green leaves, pounded and applied, will relieve sprains and allay the swelling.

A hot infusion, as a fomentation to sprained and rheumatic parts, will in like manner give relief.

¶ *Preparations and Dosages.* Fluid extract, $\frac{1}{2}$ to 2 drachms. Solid extract, 5 to 10 grains.

In the fourteenth century we hear of Tansy being used as a remedy for wounds, and as a bitter tonic, and Tansy Tea has an old reputation in country districts for fever and other illnesses.

Gerard also tells us that cakes were made of the young leaves in the spring, mixed with eggs,

'which be pleasant in taste and good for the stomache; for if bad humours cleave thereunder, it doth perfectly concoct them and carry them off. The roote, preserved in honie, or sugar, is an especiall thing against the gout, if everie day for a certaine space, a reasonable quantitie thereof be eaten fasting.'

See COSTMARY.

TAPIOCA

Manihot utilissima (POHL.)
Jatropha Manihot (LINN.)
N.O. Euphorbiaceæ

Synonyms. Cassara. Manioc. Manihot. Brazilian Arrowroot. Cassara Starch. Janipha Manihot (Kunth.)

Part Used. The starch grains obtained from the Bitter and Sweet Cassara Root

Habitat. Brazil and tropical America

¶ *Description.* Irregular hard white rough grains possessing little taste, partially soluble in cold water and affording a fine blue colour when iodine solution is added to its filtered solution. Many of the starch grains are swollen by the heat of drying. The root of the Sweet Cassara may be eaten with impunity; that of the Bitter, which is the more extensively cultivated, contains an acrid milky juice, which renders it highly poisonous if eaten in the recent state; this poison is entirely eliminated in the process of washing and drying for the production of Tapioca.

The name 'Tapioca' is that used by the Brazilian Indians.

¶ *Medicinal Action and Uses.* A nutritious diet for invalids; is baked into bread by the natives of Central America; it is used to adulterate arrowroot.

¶ *Other Species.*

Arum arrowroot derived from *Arum Dracunculus (see* ARUM).

East India arrowroot, or Aircuma arrowroot, is derived from the tubers of *Aircuma angustifolia* and *C. Leucophiza*, belonging, like the true arrowroot, to the order Marantaceæ, according to some botanists, and by others assigned to the same order as the ginger, viz. Zingiberaceæ.

See MANDIOCA.

TARRAGON

Artemisia Dracunculus (LINN.)
N.O. Compositæ

Synonyms. Little Dragon, Mugwort
(*French*) Herbe au Dragon

Parts Used. Leaves, herb

Tarragon, a member of the Composite tribe, closely allied to Wormwood, is a perennial herb cultivated for the use of its aromatic leaves in seasoning, salads, etc., and in the preparation of Tarragon vinegar.

It grows to a height of about 2 feet and has long, narrow leaves, which, unlike other members of its genus, are undivided. It blossoms in August, the small flowers, in round heads, being yellow mingled with black, and rarely fully open. The roots are long and fibrous, spreading by runners.

Tarragon is more common in Continental than in English cookery, and has long been cultivated in France for culinary purposes.

The name Tarragon is a corruption of the French *Esdragon*, derived from the Latin *Dracunculus* (a little dragon), which also serves as its specific name. It was sometimes called little Dragon Mugwort and in French has also the name *Herbe au Dragon*. To this, as to other Dragon herbs, was ascribed the faculty of curing the bites and stings of venomous beasts and of mad dogs. The name is practically the same in most countries.

One of the legends told about the origin of Tarragon, which Gerard relates, though without supporting it, is that the seed of flax put into a radish root, or a sea onion, and set in the ground, will bring forth this herb.

¶ *Cultivation.* Two kinds of Tarragon are cultivated in kitchen gardens. The French Tarragon, with very smooth, dark green leaves and the true Tarragon flavour, which is a native of the South of Europe, and Russian Tarragon, a native of Siberia, with less smooth leaves of a fresher green shade and somewhat lacking the peculiar tartness of the French variety.

As Tarragon rarely produces fertile flowers, either in England or France, it is not often raised by seed, but it may be readily propagated by division of roots in March or April, or by cuttings struck when growth is commencing in spring or later in the summer, under a hand-glass, placed outside. A few young plants should be raised annually to keep up a supply.

It loves warmth and sunshine and succeeds best in warm, rather dry situations, and a little protection should also be afforded the roots through the winter, as during severe frost they are liable to be injured. Both varieties need a dry, rather poor soil, for if set in a wet soil, they are likely to be killed by our winter.

The green leaves should be picked between Midsummer and Michaelmas. The foliage may also be cut and dried in early autumn for use in a dry state afterwards. The beds should then be entirely cut down and top-dressed, to protect from frost. If green leaves are required during winter, a few roots should be lifted in the autumn and placed in heat: it will only need a small quantity to maintain a succession.

If the herb is required dried, for winter use, gather in August, choosing a fine day, in the morning after the sun has dried off the dew. Cut off close above the root and reject any stained or insect-eaten leaves. Tie in bunches – about six stalks in a bunch – spread out fanwise, so that the air may penetrate freely to all parts and hang over strings, either on a hot, sunny day, in the open, but in half-shade, or indoors, in a sunny room, or failing sun, in a well-ventilated room by artificial heat, care being taken that the window be left open by day, so that there is a free current of air and the moisture-laden air may escape. If dried in the open, bring in before there is any risk of damp from dew or showers. A disused green-house may be used as drying-shed, provided that the glass is shaded and that there is no tank in the house to cause steaming. Heating may be either by pipes or by any ordinary coke or anthracite stove, should sun fail, but ventilation is in all cases essential. The drying temperature for aromatic herbs should never exceed 80°.

The bunches of herbs should be of uniform size and length, to facilitate packing, and when quite dry and crisp, must be packed away at once, in airtight boxes or tins, otherwise moisture will be re-absorbed from the air.

¶ *Medicinal Action and Uses.* John Evelyn says of Tarragon: ' 'Tis highly cordial and friend to the head, heart and liver.'

In Continental cookery its use is advised to temper the coolness of other herbs in salads. The leaves, which have a fragrant smell in addition to their aromatic taste, make an excellent pickle.

Fresh Tarragon possesses an essential volatile oil, chemically identical with that of Anise, which becomes lost in the dried herb.

To make Tarragon vinegar, fill a wide-mouthed bottle with the freshly-gathered leaves, picked just before the herb flowers, on a dry day. Pick the leaves off the stalks and dry a little before the fire. Then place in a jar, cover with vinegar, allow to stand some hours, then strain through a flannel jelly bag and cork down in the bottles. The best white vinegar should be used.

Tarragon vinegar is the only correct flavouring for Sauce Tantare, but must never be put into soups, as the taste is too strong and pungent. French cooks usually mix their mustard with Tarragon vinegar.

Russian Tarragon is eaten in Persia to induce appetite.

The root of Tarragon was formerly used to cure toothache.

See MUGWORT, WORMSEED.

TEA
Camellia Thea (LINK.)
N.O. Camelliaceæ

Synonyms. Thea sinensis (Sims). Thea Veridis. Thea bohea. Thea stricta Jassamica. Camellia theifera (Griff.)

Part Used. Dried leaf

Habitat. Assam; cultivated in Ceylon, Japan, Java, and elsewhere where climate allows

¶ *Description.* A small evergreen shrub cultivated to a height of 7 to 8 feet, but growing wild up to 30 feet high, much branched. Bark rough, grey. Leaves dark green, lanceolate or elliptical, on short stalks, blunt at apex, base tapering, margins shortly serrate, young leaves hairy, older leaves glabrous. Flowers solitary or two or three together on short branchlets in the leaf axils, somewhat drooping, on short stalks with a few small bracts, 1 to 1½ inches wide; sepals five, imbricate, slightly united below, ovate or rounded, blunt smooth, persistent; petals usually five or up to nine, unequal, strongly rounded, concave, spreading, white, caducous; stamens indefinite, adherent to petals at base in two rows, filaments flexuose, half the length of petals; anthers large, versatile; ovary small, free, conical, downy, three-celled with three or four pendulous ovules in each cell; styles three distinct or combined at base, slender simple stigmas. Fruit a smooth, flattened, rounded, trigonous three-celled capsule; seed solitary in each cell; size of a small nut.

It was formerly supposed that black and green tea were the produce of distinct plants, but they are both prepared from the same plant. Green tea is prepared by exposing the gathered leaves to the air until superfluous moisture is eliminated, when they are roasted over a brisk wood fire and continually stirred until they become moist and flaccid; after this they pass to the rolling table, and are rolled into balls and subjected to pressure, which twists them and gets rid of the moisture; they are then shaken out on flat trays, again roasted over a slow and steady charcoal fire, and kept in rapid motion for an hour to an hour and a half, till they assume a dullish green colour. After this they are winnowed, screened, and graded into different varieties. With black tea, the gathered leaves are exposed to the air for a longer period, then gathered up and tossed until soft and flaccid, and after further exposure, roasted in an iron pan for about five minutes. After rolling and pressing, they are shaken out, exposed to the outer air for some hours, re-roasted for three or four minutes, re-rolled, spread out in baskets and exposed to the heat of a charcoal fire for five or six minutes and then rolled for the third time and again heated, and finally dried in baskets over charcoal fires, from which process they become black in colour. China is the great tea-producing country, over four million acres of ground being devoted to its cultivation. In India also it is a very important product.

¶ *Constituents.* Caffeine (theine), tannin (10 to 20 per cent. gallotannic acid), boheic acid, volatile oil, aqueous extract, protein wax, resin, ash and theophylline.

¶ *Medicinal Action and Uses.* Stimulant, astringent. It exerts a decided influence over the nervous system, generally evinced by a feeling of comfort and exhilaration; it also causes unnatural wakefulness when taken in quantity. Taken moderately by healthy individuals it is harmless, but in excessive quantities it will produce unpleasant nervous and dyspeptic symptoms, the green variety being decidedly the more injurious. Tea is rarely used as a medicine, but, the infusion is useful to relieve neuralgic headaches.

TEAZLES
N.O. Dipsaceæ

The Fuller's Thistle was an old name for the Teazle, of which there are three varieties in this country, *Dipsacus Fullonum*, the FULLER'S TEAZLE, the COMMON TEAZLE (*D. sylvestris*), and the SMALL TEAZLE (*D. pilosus*), a distinct species sometimes found in moist hedgerows, but not generally distributed, being in height, shape of its flower-heads and form of the foliage, quite distinct from the two first named species and having more the habit of a Scabious than of a Teazle.

Many botanists consider the Fuller's Teazle only a variety of the Common Wild Teazle, in which the spines of the flower-heads are strongly developed into a hooked form, a feature preserved by cultivation and apt to disappear by neglect, or on poor soil, causing it to relapse into the ordinary wild variety.

TEAZLE, COMMON
Dipsacus sylvestris
N.O. Dipsaceæ

Synonyms. Venus' Basin. Card Thistle. Barber's Brush. Brushes and Combs. Church Broom

Parts Used. Root, heads

Habitat. The Common Teazle is to be found on waste land, in hedgerows and dykesides, mainly in the south of England, being rarer in the north

¶ *Description.* It is a biennial, with a tall, rigid, prickly, furrowed stem, generally attaining the height of 4 or 5 feet, bearing cylindrical flower-heads, globular when young, but lengthening out to a cone-like shape when in full flower. The whole plant is very harsh and prickly to the touch.

For some distance below the head, the stems are bare except for prickles, then small pairs of leaves appear, joined directly by their bases to the main stem, with a shining, white midrib, on the back of which are many prickles. In the lower and larger pairs of leaves the bases are joined round the stem and form deep cups, which are capable of holding dew and rain. This conspicuous feature has earned the plant its older name of Venus' Basin, and it was held that the water which collects there acquired curative properties. It was regarded as a remedy for warts, and was also used as a cosmetic and an eye-wash. The generic name of the plant, *Dipsacus*, also refers to this peculiarity in structure, being derived from the Greek verb, *to be thirsty*.

The English name, Teazle, is from the Anglo-Saxon *tæsan*, signifying to tease cloth, and refers to the use of the flower-heads by cloth-workers. These heads are a mass of semi-stiff spines, the spines longest at the top of the head, each head being enclosed by curving, narrow, green bracts, set with small prickles, arising in a ring at the base of the head and following the line of the head, though a little outside it, curved inward at the tip. When the head commences to flower, the purple petals of the floret show in a ring about one-third of the way down and then spread upward and downwards simultaneously.

¶ *Medicinal Action and Uses.* Culpepper tells us that the medicinal uses of both the Wild and Fuller's Teazle are the same, and that 'the roots, which are the only parts used, are said to have a cleansing faculty.' He refers to the use of the water in the leaf-basins as a cosmetic and eye-wash, and tells us, on the authority of Dioscorides, that an ointment made from the bruised roots is good, not only for warts and wens, but also against cankers and fistulas.

Other old writers have recommended an infusion of the root for strengthening the stomach and creating an appetite. Also for removing obstructions of the liver, and as a remedy for jaundice.

Lyte, in his translation of Dodoens, 1586, says that the small worms found often within the heads 'do cure and heale the quartaine ague, to be worne or carried about the necke or arme,' a theory which Gerard contemptuously discards, from his own personal experience.

But the principal use of the Teazle, dating from long before Gerard's time, still remains unchallenged, and that is for wool 'fleecing,' or raising the nap on woollen cloth. The cultivated variety, *D. Fullonum*, Gerard's 'tame Teasell' is used, because, as already mentioned, its spines are crooked, not straight. These heads are fixed on the rim of a wheel, or on a cylinder, which is made to revolve against the surface of the cloth to be 'fleeced,' thus raising the nap. No machine has yet been invented which can compete with the Teazle in its combined rigidity and elasticity. Its great utility is that while raising the nap, it will yet break at any serious obstruction, whereas all metallic substances in such a case would cause the cloth to yield first and tear the material.

This particular Teazle is grown largely in the west of England, and also imported from France, Germany, Italy, Africa and America, to meet the needs of our manufacturers. One large firm uses 20,000 Teazle heads in a year.

The heads are cut as soon as the flowers wither, about 8 inches of stem remaining attached to them, and they are then dried and sorted into qualities.

The arms of the Clothworkers' Company are three Teazle-heads.

Closely allied to the Teazle, though very different in appearance, is the Scabious, also belonging to the natural order Dipsaceæ, a family of plants having affinities with the large order Compositæ, to which the Thistles belong.

See KNAPWEED, CENTAURY, STAR THISTLE, SCABIOUS.

THAPSIA

Thapsia Garganica
N.O. Umbelliferæ

Synonym. Drias
Habitat. Southern Europe, from Spain to Greece, also Algeria

¶ *Description.* The plant was well known to the Ancients who gave it its peculiar name, believing it to be obtained originally from the Isle of Thapsus. It is considered by the Algerians to be a specific against pain, every part of the plant being efficacious, though deadly poisonous to Camels. The root is a strong purgative. Thapsia Silphion is thought to be identical with *Thapsia Garganica*, is found on the mountains near the site of Ancient Cyrene, and is said to have yielded the gum resin to the Ancients as *Laser Cyrenaicum* or *Asa Dulces*, the Greek name being *Silphion*. Representations of it occur on Cyrene coins.

¶ *Medicinal Action and Uses.* Theophrastus speaks of the purgative and emetic properties of the root, and modern French doctors recognize its value and include it in their Codex as *Resin Thapsiæ*. An extract is made from the bark of the root with alcohol, the moisture is evaporated and made into a plaster with 7 per cent. of the resin combined with yellow wax, turps and colophony. Great caution has to be exercised in unpacking the commercial bales of the roots because the dust or powder arising in the process causes itching and swelling of the face and hands. The French Thapsia plaster is a very drastic counter-irritant, creating much inflammation with an eczematous eruption (and intolerable itching) which leaves scars. Another variety, *T. Villosa*, also contains in its root a vesicant resin which acts more gently than *T. Garganica*.

THISTLES

N.O. Compositæ

Thistle is the old English name – essentially the same in all kindred languages – for a large family of plants occurring chiefly in Europe and Asia, of which we have fourteen species in Great Britain, arranged under the botanical groups Carduus, Carlina, Onopordon and Carbenia, or Cnicus.

In agriculture the Thistle is the recognized sign of untidiness and neglect, being found not so much in barren ground, as in good ground not properly cared for. It has always been a plant of ill repute among us; Shakespeare classes 'rough Thistles' with 'hateful Docks,' and further back in the history of our race we read of the Thistle representing part of the primeval curse on the earth in general, and on man in particular, for – 'Thorns also and Thistles shall it bring forth to thee.'

Thistles will soon monopolize a large extent of country to the extinction of other plants, as they have done in parts of the American prairies, in Canada and British Columbia, and as they did in Australia, till a stringent Act of Parliament was passed, about twenty years ago, imposing heavy penalties upon all who neglected to destroy Thistles on their land, every man being now compelled to root out, within fourteen days, any Thistle that may lift up its head, Government inspectors being specially appointed to carry out the enforcement of the law.

The growth of weeds in Great Britain, having, in the opinion of many, also reached disturbing proportions, it is now proposed to enact a similar law in this country, and the Smallholders' Union is bringing forward a 'Bill to prevent the spread of noxious weeds in England and Wales,' the provisions being similar to the Australian law – weed-infested roadsides, as well as badly-cleared cultivated land, to come within the scope of the enactment.

Among the thirteen noxious weeds enumerated in the proposed Bill, the name of Thistle is naturally to be found. And yet in medicine Thistles are far from useless.

When beaten up or crushed in a mill to destroy the prickles, the leaves of all Thistles have proved excellent food for cattle and horses. This kind of fodder was formerly used to a great extent in Scotland before the introduction of special green crops for the purpose. The young stems of many of the Thistles are also edible, and the seeds of all the species yield a good oil by expression.

Two or three of our native species are handsome enough to be worthy of a place in gardens. Some species which flourish in hotter and drier climates than our own, such as the handsome Yellow Thistles of the south of Europe, *Scolymus*, are cultivated for that purpose, and have a classical interest, being mentioned by Hesiod as *the* flower of summer. This striking plant, crowned with its golden flowers, is abundant throughout Sicily. The Fish-bone Thistle (*Chamæpeuce diacantha*), from Syria, is also a very handsome plant. A grand Scarlet Thistle from Mexico (*Erythrolena conspicua*) was grown in England some fifty years ago, but is now never seen.

THISTLE, HOLY

Carbenia benedicta (BERUL.)

Synonyms. Blessed Thistle. Cnicus benedictus (Gætn.). Carduus benedictus (Steud.)
Part Used. Herb

A Thistle, however, that has been cultivated for several centuries in this country for its medicinal use is known as the Blessed or Holy Thistle. It is a handsome annual, a native of Southern Europe, occurring there in waste, stony, uncultivated places, but it grows more readily in England in cultivation.

It is said to have obtained its name from its high reputation as a heal-all, being supposed even to cure the plague. It is mentioned in all the treatises on the Plague, and especially by Thomas Brasbridge, who in 1578 published his *Poore Man's Jewell, that is to say, a Treatise of the Pestilence, unto which is annexed a declaration of the vertues of the Hearbes Carduus Benedictus and Angelica.* Shakespeare in *Much Ado about Nothing,* says: 'Get you some of this distilled Carduus Benedictus and lay it to your heart; it is the only thing for a qualm. . . . I mean plain Holy Thistle.' The 'distilled' leaves, it says 'helpeth the hart,' 'expelleth all poyson taken in at the mouth and other corruption that doth hurt and annoye the hart,' and 'the juice of it is outwardly applied to the bodie' ('lay it to your heart,' *Sh.*), 'therefore I counsell all that have Gardens to nourish it, that they may have it always to their own use, and the use of their neighbours that lacke it.'

It has sometimes been stated that the herb was first cultivated by Gerard in 1597, but as this book was published twenty years previously it would appear to have been in cultivation much earlier, and in fact it is described and its virtues enumerated in the *Herbal* of Turner in 1568.

¶ *Description.* The stem of the Blessed Thistle grows about 2 feet high, is reddish, slender, very much branched and scarcely able to keep upright under the weight of its leaves and flowerheads. The leaves are long, narrow, clasping the dull green stem, with prominent pale veins, the irregular teeth of the wavy margin ending in spines. The flowers are pale yellow, in green prickly heads, each scale of the involucre, or covering of the head, ending also in a long, brown bristle. The whole plant, leaves, stalks and also the flowerheads, are covered with a thin down. It grows more compactly in some soils than in others.

¶ *Cultivation.* Being an annual, Blessed Thistle is propagated by seed. It thrives in any ordinary soil. Allow 2 feet each way when thinning out the seedlings. Though

795

occurring sometimes in waste places in England as an escape from cultivation, it cannot be considered indigenous to this country. The seeds are usually sown in spring, but if the newly-ripened seeds are sown in September or October in sheltered situations, it is possible to have supplies of the herb green, both summer and winter.

¶ *Part Used*. The whole herb. The leaves and flowering tops are collected in July, just as the plant breaks into flower, and cut on a dry day, the best time being about noon, when there is no longer any trace of dew on them.

About 3½ tons of fresh herb produce 1 ton when dried, and about 35 cwt. of dry herb can be raised per acre.

¶ *Chemical Constituents*. Blessed Thistle contains a volatile oil, and a bitter, crystalline neutral body called Cnicin (soluble in alcohol and slightly also in water) which is said to be analogous to salicin in its properties.

¶ *Medicinal Action and Uses*. Tonic, stimulant, diaphoretic, emetic and emmenagogue. In large doses, Blessed Thistle acts as a strong emetic, producing vomiting with little pain and inconvenience. Cold infusions in smaller draughts are valuable in weak and debilitated conditions of the stomach, and as a tonic, creating appetite and preventing sickness. The warm infusion – 1 oz. of the dried herb to a pint of boiling water – in doses of a wineglassful, forms in intermittent fevers one of the most useful diaphoretics to which employment can be given. The plant was at one time supposed to possess very great virtues against fevers of all kinds.

Fluid extract, ½ to 1 drachm.

It is said to have great power in the purification and circulation of the blood, and on this account strengthens the brain and the memory.

The leaves, dried and powdered, are good for worms.

It is chiefly used now for nursing mothers, the warm infusion scarcely ever failing to procure a proper supply of milk. It is considered one of the best medicines which can be used for the purpose.

Turner (1568) says:

'It is very good for the headache and the megram, for the use of the juice or powder of the leaves, preserveth and keepeth a man from the headache, and healeth it being present. It is good for any ache in the body and strengtheneth the members of the whole body, and fasteneth loose sinews and weak. It is also good for the dropsy. It helpeth the memory and amendeth thick hearing. The leaves provoke sweat. There is nothing better for the canker and old rotten and festering sores than the leaves, juice, broth, powder and water of Carduus benedictus.'

Culpepper (1652) writes of it:

'It is a herb of Mars, and under the Sign Aries. It helps swimmings and giddiness in the head, or the disease called vertigo, because Aries is the House of Mars. It is an excellent remedy against yellow jaundice and other infirmities of the gall, because Mars governs choller. It strengthens the attractive faculty in man, and clarifies the blood, because the one is ruled by Mars. The continual drinking the decoction of it helps red faces, tetters and ringworm, because Mars causeth them. It helps plague-sores, boils and itch, the bitings of mad dogs and venomous beasts, all which infirmities are under Mars. Thus you see what it doth by sympathy.

'By Antypathy to other Planets: it cures the French Pox by Antypathy to Venus who governs it. It strengthens the memory and cures deafness by Antypathy to Saturn, who hath his fall in Aries which Rules the Head. It cures Quarten Agues and other diseases of Melancholy, and a dust Choller by Sympathy to Saturn, Mars being exalted in Capricorn. Also it provokes Urine, the stopping of which is usually caused by Mars or the Moon.'

Mattheolus and Fuschius wrote also of *Carduus benedictus:*

'It is a plant of great virtue; it helpeth inwardly and outwardly; it strengthens all the principal members of the body, as the brain, the heart, the stomach, the liver, the lungs and the kidney; it is also a preservative against all disease, for it causes perspiration, by which the body is purged of much corruption, such as breedeth diseases; it expelleth the venom of infection; it consumes and wastes away all bad humours; therefore, give God thanks for his goodness, Who hath given this herb and all others for the benefit of our health.'

Four different ways of using Blessed Thistle have been recommended: It may be eaten in the green leaf, with bread and butter for breakfast, like Watercress; the dried leaves may be made into a powder and a drachm taken in wine or otherwise every day; a wineglassful of the juice may be taken every day, or, which is the usual and the best method, an infusion may be made of the dried herb, taken any time as a preventive, or when intended to remove disease, at bed time, as it causes copious perspiration.

Many of the other Thistles may be used as

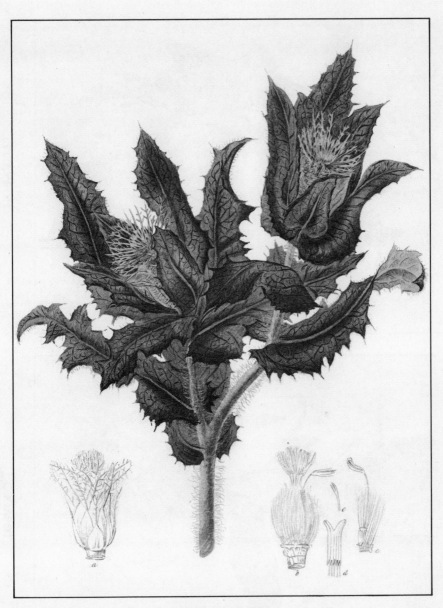

HOLY THISTLE
Carbenia Benedicta

XC

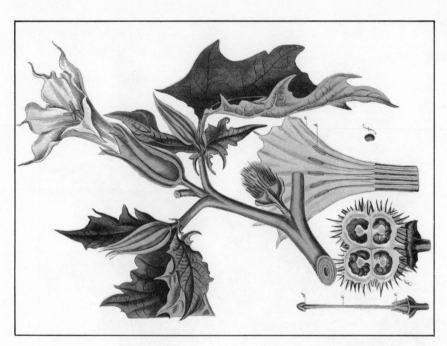

THORNAPPLE
Datura Stramonium

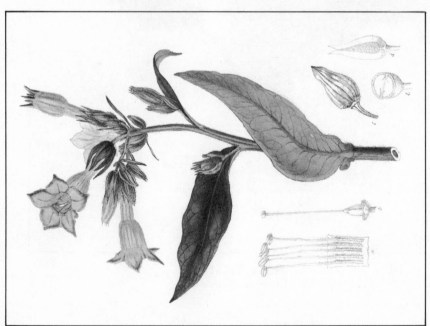

TOBACCO
Nicotiana Tabacum

substitutes for the Blessed Thistle. The seeds of the Milk Thistle (*Carduus Marianus*), known also as *Silybum Marianum*, have similar properties and uses, and the Cotton Thistle, Melancholy Thistle, etc., have also been employed for like purposes.

THISTLE, MILK

Silybum Marianum

Synonym. Marian Thistle

Parts Used. Whole herb, root, leaves, seeds and hull

The Marian, or Milk Thistle, is perhaps the most important medicinally among the members of this genus, to which all botanists do not, however, assign it, naming it *Silybum Marianum.*

¶ *Description.* It is a fine, tall plant, about the size of the Cotton Thistle, with cut-into root-leaves, waved and spiny at the margin, of a deep, glossy green, with milk-white veins, and is found not uncommonly in hedgebanks and on waste ground, especially by buildings, which causes some authorities to consider that it may not be a true native. In Scotland it is rare.

This handsome plant is not unworthy of a place in our gardens and shrubberies and was formerly frequently cultivated. The stalks, like those of most of our larger Thistles, may be eaten, and are palatable and nutritious. The leaves also may be eaten as a salad when young. Bryant, in his *Flora Dietetica*, writes of it: 'The young shoots in the spring, cut close to the root with part of the stalk on, is one of the best boiling salads that is eaten, and surpasses the finest cabbage. They were sometimes baked in pies. The roots may be eaten like those of Salsify.' In some districts the leaves are called 'Pig Leaves,' probably because pigs like them, and the seeds are a favourite food of goldfinches.

The common statement that this bird lines its nest with thistledown is scarcely accurate, the substance being in most cases the down of Colt's-foot (*Tussilago*), or the cotton down from the willow, both of which are procurable at the building season, whereas thistledown is at that time immature.

Westmacott, writing in 1694, says of this Thistle: 'It is a Friend to the Liver and Blood: the prickles cut off, they were formerly used to be boiled in the Spring and eaten with other herbs; but as the World decays, so doth the Use of good old things and others more delicate and less virtuous brought in.'

The heads of this Thistle formerly were eaten, boiled, treated like those of the Artichoke.

There is a tradition that the milk-white veins of the leaves originated in the milk of the Virgin which once fell upon a plant of Thistle, hence it was called Our Lady's Thistle, and the Latin name of the species has the same derivation.

¶ *Medicinal Action and Uses.* The seeds of this plant are used nowadays for the same purpose as Blessed Thistle, and on this point John Evelyn wrote: 'Disarmed of its prickles and boiled, it is worthy of esteem, and thought to be a great breeder of milk and proper diet for women who are nurses.'

It is in popular use in Germany for curing jaundice and kindred biliary derangements. It also acts as a demulcent in catarrh and pleurisy. The decoction when applied externally is said to have proved beneficial in cases of cancer.

Gerard wrote of the Milk Thistle that

'the root if borne about one doth expel melancholy and remove all diseases connected therewith. . . . My opinion is that this is the best remedy that grows against all melancholy diseases,'

which was another way of saying that it had good action on the liver. He also tells us:

'Dioscorides affirmed that the seeds being drunke are a remedy for infants that have their sinews drawn together, and for those that be bitten of serpents:'

and we find in a record of old Saxon remedies that 'this wort if hung upon a man's neck it setteth snakes to flight.' The seeds were also formerly thought to cure hydrophobia.

Culpepper considered the Milk Thistle to be as efficient as *Carduus benedictus* for agues, and preventing and curing the infection of the plague, and also for removal of obstructions of the liver and spleen. He recommends the infusion of the fresh root and seeds, not only as good against jaundice, also for breaking and expelling stone and being good for dropsy when taken internally, but in addition, to be applied externally, with cloths, to the liver. With other writers, he recommends the young, tender plant (after removing the prickles) to be boiled and eaten in the spring as a blood cleanser.

A tincture is prepared by homœopathists for medicinal use from equal parts of the root and the seeds with the hull attached.

It is said that the empirical nostrum, *antiglaireux*, of Count Mattaei, is prepared from this species of Thistle.

Thistles in general, according to Culpepper, are under the dominion of Jupiter.

Synonyms. Cotton Thistle. Woolly Thistle

Parts Used. Leaves, root

The Scotch Thistle, or Cotton Thistle (*Onopordon Acanthium*) is one of the most beautiful of British plants, not uncommon in England, by roadsides and in waste places, particularly in chalky and sandy soils in the southern counties.

¶ *Description.* It is a biennial, flowering in late summer and autumn. The erect stem, 18 inches to 5 feet high, is very stout and much branched, furnished with wing-like appendages (the decurrent bases of the leaves) which are broader than its own diameter. The leaves are very large, waved and with sharp prickles on the margin. The flowers are light purple and surrounded with a nearly globular involucre, with scales terminating in strong, yellow spines.

The whole plant is hoary with a white, cottony down, that comes off readily when rubbed, and causes the young leaves to be quite white. From the presence of this covering, the Thistle has obtained its popular name of Cotton or Woolly Thistle.

This species is one of the stiffest and most thorny of its race, and its sharp spines well agree with Gerard's description of the plant as 'set full of most horrible sharp prickles, so that it is impossible for man or beast to touch the same without great hurt and danger.'

Which is the true Scotch Thistle even the Scottish antiquarians cannot decide, but it is generally considered to be this species of Thistle that was originally the badge of the House of Stuart, and came to be regarded as the national emblem of Scotland. The first heraldic use of the plant would appear to be in the inventory of the property of James III of Scotland, made at his death in 1458, where a hanging embroidered with 'thrissils' is mentioned. It was, undoubtedly, a national badge in 1503, in which year Dunbar wrote his poetic allegory, 'The Thrissill and the Rose,' on the union of James IV and Princess Margaret of England. The Order of the Thistle, which claims, with the exception of the Garter, to be the most ancient of our Orders, was instituted in 1540 by James V, and revived by James VII of Scotland and Second of England, who created eight Knights of the Order, *Nemo me impune lacessit* (which

would seem to apply most aptly to the species just described), appears surrounding the Thistle that occupies the centre of the coinage of James VI. From that date until now, the Thistle has had a place on our coins.

Pliny states, and mediæval writers repeat, that a decoction of Thistles applied to a bald head would restore a healthy growth of hair.

¶ *Medicinal Action and Uses.* The Ancients supposed this Thistle to be a specific in cancerous complaints, and in more modern times the juice is said to have been applied with good effect to cancers and ulcers.

A decoction of the root is astringent and diminishes discharges from mucous membranes.

Gerard tells us, on the authority of Dioscorides and Pliny, that 'the leaves and root hereof are a remedy for those that have their bodies drawn backwards,' and Culpepper explains that not only is the juice therefore good for a crick in the neck, but also as a remedy for rickets in children. It was considered also to be good in nervous complaints.

The name of the genus is derived from the Greek words *onos* (an ass) and *perdon* (I disperse wind), the species being said to produce this effect in asses.

The juicy receptacle or disk on which the florets are placed was used in earlier times as the Artichoke – which is also a member of the Thistle tribe. The young stalks, when stripped of their rind, may be eaten like those of the Burdock.

The cotton is occasionally collected from the stem and used to stuff pillows, and the oil obtained from the seeds has been used on the Continent for burning, both in lamps and for ordinary culinary purposes. Twelve pounds of the seeds are said to produce, when heat is used in expression, about 3 lb. of oil.

The greater number of the Thistles are assigned to the genus *Carduus*. The derivation of the name of this genus is difficult to determine; by some orders it is said to come from the Greek *cheuro*, a technical word denoting the operation of carding wool, to which process the heads of some of the species are applicable.

THISTLE, DWARF   Carduus acaulis

Synonyms. Ground Thistle. Dwarf May Thistle (Culpepper)

Part Used. Root

Carduus acaulis, the Dwarf Thistle, is found in pastures, especially chalk downs, and is rather common in the southern half of

England, particularly on the east side. It is a perennial, with a long, woody root-stock. The stem in the ordinary form is so short that the flowers appear to be sessile, or sitting, in the centre of the rosette of prickly leaves, but very occasionally it attains the length of a foot or 18 inches, and then is usually slightly branched. The leaves are spiny and rigid, with only a few hairs on the upper side, and on the veins beneath, and are of a dark, shining green. The flowers are large and dark crimson in colour, and are in bloom from July to September.

THISTLE, CREEPING PLUME

Synonym. Way Thistle
Parts Used. Root, leaves

Carduus arvensis, the Creeping Plume Thistle, or Way Thistle, has many varieties. It is found in cultivated fields and waste places, and is very common and widely distributed. The root-stock is perennial, creeping extensively and sending up leafy barren shoots and flowering stems about 3 feet high.

THISTLE, WELTED

Synonym. Field Thistle
Parts Used. Root, leaves

Carduus crispus, the Welted Thistle, or Field Thistle, is one of the taller species. The stem, 3 to 4 feet high, is erect, branched, continuously spinous-winged throughout. The leaves are green on both sides, downy on the veins beneath, narrow, cut into numerous lobes and very prickly. The flowers are purplish-crimson, not very large, sometimes clustered three or four together on short stalks. The plant varies much in the degree

THISTLE, WOOLLY-HEADED

Parts Used. Root, leaves

Carduus eriophorus, the Woolly-headed Thistle, is a biennial. The stem is elongated, branched, not winged, short and furrowed, woolly, 3 to 5 feet high. The lowest leaves are very large, often 2 feet long, the stem leaves much smaller, all deeply cut into, with strap-shaped lobes joined together in pairs in the lower ones. The flowers are light reddish-purple, the large woolly heads covered with reddish curled hairs. The

THISTLE, MELANCHOLY

Parts Used. Root, leaves

Carduus heterophyllus, the Melancholy Thistle, is said by some to have been the original badge of the House of Stuart, instead of the Cotton Thistle; it is the *Cluas an fleidh* of the Highlanders, and is more common in Scotland than in England, where it only occurs in the midland and northern counties, growing no farther south than the

The Thistle is very injurious in pastures; it kills all plants that grow beneath it, and ought not to be tolerated, even on the borders of fields and waste places. At one time the root used to be chewed as a remedy for toothache.

Johns (*Flowers of the Field*) calls this the Ground Thistle, and Culpepper calls it the Dwarf May Thistle, and says that 'in some places it is called the Dwarf Carline Thistle.'

Carduus arvensis

The leaves are attenuated, embracing the stems at their base, with strong spines at their margins. The flowers are in numerous small heads, and are pale purple in colour. The plant is bright green, the leaves often white beneath, but varying much in this respect.

Carduus crispus

of soft hairiness, and consequently in the green or whitish colour of the leaves. It is common and generally distributed in England, growing in hedgebanks, borders of fields and by roadsides, occurring less frequently in Scotland. This is one of the least troublesome of the Thistles, being an annual and less abundant than some others. Like the last species, it has many variations of form.

Carduus eriophorus

whole plant is a deep dull green. It flowers in August.

This Thistle is eaten when young as a salad. The young stalks, peeled and soaked in water to take off the bitterness, are excellent, and may be eaten either boiled or baked in pies after the manner of Rhubarb, though Gerard says: 'concerning the temperature and virtues of these Thistles we can allege nothing at all.'

Carduus heterophyllus

northern counties of Wales. It is a perennial, with a long and creeping root. The stems are tall and stout, often deeply furrowed, and more or less covered with a white or cotton-like down. The leaves clasp the stem at their bases and white dark green above, have their under-surfaces thickly covered with white and down-like hairs.

Unlike most of the Thistles, the leaves are not continued down the stem at all, and are much simpler in form than the ordinary type of Thistle foliage. Their edges have small bristle-like teeth. The flowerheads are borne singly on long stalks, the bracts that form the involucre being quite destitute of prickles.

Culpepper considered that a decoction of this Thistle in wine 'being drank expels superfluous melancholy out of the body and makes a man as merry as a cricket.'

And he further adds:

'Dioscorides saith, the root borne about one doth the like, and removes all diseases of melancholy: Modern writers laugh at him: *Let them laugh that win*: my opinion is, that it is the best remedy against all melancholy diseases that grows; they that please may use it.'

THISTLE, SPEAR

Carduus lanceolatus

Parts Used. Root, leaves

Carduus lanceolatus, the Spear Thistle, is one of our most striking and common Thistles. It grows in waste places, by roadsides, in pastures and cultivated ground, and is generally distributed over the whole kingdom. The plant is a biennial, the stem 1 to 5 feet high, stout and strong, more or less woolly with narrow, spinous wings. The leaves have the segments elongated or lance-shaped, palmately cleft sometimes in large plants, but short and scarcely cleft at all in weaker specimens, each lobe terminating in a long and acute prickle. They are dark, dull green above, paler beneath, where they are sometimes nearly white from the abundance of hair present. The flowerheads stand singly and are large and conspicuous. The flowers are a beautiful purple and, like those of the Artichoke, have the property of curdling milk.

THISTLE, MUSK

Carduus nutans

Synonym. Nodding Thistle
Parts Used. Root, seeds

Carduus nutans, the Musk Thistle, or Nodding Thistle, occurs in waste places, and is particularly partial to chalky and limestone soils. It is not uncommon in England, but is rare in Scotland, where it is confined to sandy seashores in the southern counties. The stem is erect, 2 to 3 feet high, branched only in larger plants, furrowed, interruptedly winged. The leaves are long, undulated, with scattered hairs on both surfaces, somewhat shiny, green and very deeply cut. This is a common Thistle on a dry soil, and may be known by its large drooping, crimson-purple flowers, the largest of all our Thistle blooms, handsome both in form and colour, and by its faint, musky scent.

The down of this, as of some other species, may be advantageously used as a material in making paper.

THISTLE, MARSH PLUME

Carduus palustris

Synonym. Cirsium palustre
Parts Used. Root, leaves

Carduus palustris, or *Cirsium Palustre*, the Marsh Plume Thistle, is very common in meadows, marshes and bogs, by the sides of ditches, etc., and is generally distributed over the country. It is a biennial, the stem stout, erect, furrowed, 1 to 5 feet high, scarcely branched at all, the branches, when occurring, being much shorter than the main stem, which is narrowly winged, the wings having numerous, long slender spines. The spines on the edges of the narrow, long leaves are similar to those on the wings of the stem.

The flowers are dark, dull, crimson purple, small in themselves, but grouped together in large clusters, which distinguish it from most of our thistles, though one or two others exhibit their characteristic in a lesser degree. The plant is a deep dull green, the leaves sometimes slightly hoary beneath.

The stalks of this species are said to be as good as those of the Milk Thistle, and in Evelyn's time were similarly employed.

Culpepper tells us that, in his day, it was 'frequent in the Isle of Ely.'

THISTLE, CARLINE

Carlina vulgaris

Parts Used. Root, leaves

Carlina vulgaris, the Carline Thistle, closely related to the last-named Thistles, but assigned to a special genus, of which it is the sole representative in this country, is found on dry banks and pastures, being rather scarce except on chalk, where it is plentiful. It is rare in Scotland. It is a biennial, the root, a taproot, producing in the first year a tuft of strap-shaped, nearly flat leaves, hoary, especially beneath, very spinuous, but with the spines short and weak. The flower stem, appearing in the second year, is from 3 inches to 2 feet high, purple, not winged, the leaves on it decreasing in length and increasing in width from bottom to top, strongly veined, spinous and waved at the edges. The whole plant is pale green, the leaves rigid and scarcely altering after the plant is dead, except in colour. The flowers are straw yellow, the inner florets purplish, the heads distinguished by the straw-coloured, glossy, radiating long inner scales of the involucre, or outer floral cup. The outer bracts are very prickly. The flowers expand in dry and close in moist weather. They retain this property for a long time and form rustic hygrometers, being often seen on the Continent nailed over cottage doors for this purpose. The presence of the Carline Thistle indicates a very poor soil; it particularly infests dry, sandy pastures.

Culpepper describes the 'Wild Carline Thistle (*C. vulgaris*)' as having flowers 'of a fine purple,' so he must have confused it with another species, or given it a wrong name.

The original name of this plant was Carolina, so called after Charlemagne, of whom the legend relates that

'a horrible pestilence broke out in his army and carried off many thousand men, which greatly troubled the pious emperor. Wherefore he prayed earnestly to God, and in his sleep there appeared to him an angel who shot an arrow from a crossbow, telling him to mark the plant upon which it fell, for with that plant he might cure his army of the pestilence.'

The herb so miraculously indicated was this Thistle. Its medicinal qualities appear to be very like those of Elecampane, it has diaphoretic action, and in large doses is purgative. The herb contains some resin and a volatile essential oil of a camphoraceous nature, like that of Elecampane, which has made it of use for similar purposes as a cordial and antiseptic.

In Anglo-Saxon, the plant was called from the bristly appearance of its flowerheads, *ever throat*, i.e. boar's throat. It was formerly used in magical incantations.

The texture of Carline Thistles is like that of Everlasting Flowers; they scarcely alter their appearance when dead; and the whole plant is remarkably durable.

Other Thistles are the SLENDER-FLOWERED THISTLE (*C. pycnocephalous*) which has stems 2 to 4 feet high, slightly branched, hoary, with broad continuous, deeply-lobed, spinous wings; leaves cottony underneath; heads many, clustered, cylindrical, small; florets pink. It grows in sandy, waste places, especially near the sea: frequent. Biennial.

The TUBEROUS PLUME THISTLE (*C. tuberosus*). The root is spindle-shaped with tuberous fibres; stem 2 feet high, single, erect, round, hairy, leafless above; leaves not decurrent, deeply pinnatifid, fringed with minute prickles; heads generally solitary, large, egg-shaped; florets crimson. Grows only in Wiltshire. Perennial.

The MEADOW PLUME THISTLE (*C. pratensis*). A small plant, 12 to 18 inches high, with fibrous roots; a cottony stem, giving off runners; few leaves, mostly radical, soft, wavy, fringed with minute spines, not decurrent; and generally solitary heads, with adpressed, slightly cottony bracts and crimson florets. Found in wet meadows; not general. Flowers in August. Perennial.

The SOW THISTLE is in no sense a Thistle, but is more nearly allied to the Dandelion.

The Star Thistles belong to the genus *Centaurea*.

See KNAPWEEDS, TEAZLE, SCABIOUS, CORNFLOWER, SOW THISTLE

THISTLE, COMMON STAR

Centaurea Colcitrapa
N.O. Compositæ

Parts Used. Herb, seeds, root
Habitat. South-east England

Centaurea Calcitrapa, the Common Star Thistle, occurs in waste places and by roadsides, but is somewhat rare and chiefly found in south-east England.

¶ *Description*. The stem is branched, not winged, like most of the true Thistles; the lower leaves are much cut into, almost to the midrib, but the uppermost are merely toothed or with entire margins. On the flowerheads are long sharp spines, $\frac{1}{2}$ inch to 1 inch long. The flowers themselves are pale, purplish rose, the ray florets no longer than the central ones. The plant is a dull green, somewhat hairy, and flowers in July.

The specific name of this species is due to the resemblance of the flower-head to the *Caltrops*, or iron ball covered with spikes, formerly used for throwing under horses' feet to lame them on a field of battle.

It is a troublesome weed to agriculturists in certain districts, and is only eradicated by breaking up the ground.

THISTLE, YELLOW STAR

> Synonym. St. Barnaby's Thistle
> Parts Used. Herb, seeds, root

Centaurea solstitialis, the Yellow Star Thistle, St. Barnaby's Thistle, is rare and hardly to be considered a native, though found in dry pastures in south-east Kent.

¶ *Description.* The plant forms a scrubby bush, 18 inches to 2 feet high, with the lower part of the stems very stiff, almost woody, the branches when young very soft, with broad wings, decurrent from the short, strap-shaped leaves. The lower leaves are deeply cut into, the upper ones narrow and with entire margins. The spines of the flower-heads are very long, $\frac{1}{2}$ inch to 1 inch in length, pale yellow. The whole plant is hoary.

This plant obtains its name from being

(POISON) [1]
THORNAPPLE

> Synonyms. Stramonium. Datura. Devil's Apple. Jamestown-weed. Jimson-weed. Stinkweed. Devil's Trumpet. Apple of Peru
> Parts Used. Leaves, seeds
> Habitat. Throughout the world, except the colder or Arctic regions

The Thornapple is, like the Henbane, a member of the order Solanceæ. It belongs to the genus *Datura*, which consists of fifteen species, distributed throughout the warmer portion of the whole world, the greatest number being found in Central America. Nearly all of them are used locally in medicine, and are characterized by similar properties to those of the official species, *Datura Stramonium*. The plants vary from herbs to shrubs, and even trees.

The question of the native country and early distribution of *D. Stramonium* has been much discussed by botanical writers. It is doubtful to what country this plant originally belonged. Many European botanists refer it to North America, while there it is looked on as a denizen of the Old World. Nuttall considers it originated in South America or Asia, and it is probable that its native country is to be found in the East. Alphonse de Candolle, *Géographie Botanique* (1855), gives it as his opinion that *D. Stramonium* is indigenous to the Old World, probably to the borders of the Caspian Sea or adjacent regions, but certainly not India; it grows wild abundantly in southern Russia from the

¶ *Medicinal Action and Uses.* The seeds used to be made into powder and drunk in wine as a remedy for stone, and the powdered root was considered a cure for fistula and gravel.

Centaurea solstitalis
N.O. Compositæ

supposed to flower about St. Barnabas' Day, June 11 (old style). It is an annual.

¶ *Medicinal Action and Uses.* It has been used for the same purposes as the Common Star Thistle.

Many species of *Centaurea* grow wild in Palestine, some of formidable size. Canon Tristram mentions some in Galilee through which it was impossible to make way till the plants had been beaten down. 'Thistle' mentioned several times in the Bible refers to some member of this family (*Centaurea*), probably *C. Calcitrapa*, which is a Palestinian weed.

See CENTAURY, KNAPWEEDS.

Datura Stramonium (LINN.)
N.O. Solanaceæ

borders of the Black Sea eastward to Siberia. Its seeds are very retentive of life, and being often in the earth put on shipboard for ballast, from one country to another, the plant is thus propagated in all regions, and it is now spread throughout the world, except in the colder or Arctic regions. Gypsies are also said to have had a share in spreading the plant by means of its seeds from western Asia into Europe. In the United States, it is now a familiar weed, found everywhere in the vicinity of cultivation, especially about barnyards, timber-yards, docks and waste places, frequenting dung-heaps, the roadsides and commons, and other places where a rank soil is created by the deposited refuse of towns and villages. Where the plant grows abundantly, its vicinity may be detected by the rank odour which it diffuses. Notwithstanding the abundance of the plant in North America, it is cultivated there in order to obtain a drug of uniform quality. The Bureau of Plant Industry, United States Department of Agriculture, has conducted experiments on a large scale: several hundred pounds of leaf were grown and cured by artificial heat in a tobacco barn, proving of excellent quality,

The dried leaves are not regarded as poisonous. – EDITOR.

being marketed at a price in advance of the highest quoted figures.

In Great Britain, it is only occasionally found and can scarcely be considered naturalized here, though it is sometimes met with in the south of England, generally in rich, waste ground, chiefly near gardens or dwellings. It is sometimes grown in private gardens in England as an ornamental plant. It was cultivated in London towards the close of the sixteenth century.

The name Stramonium is of uncertain origin: some authorities claim that it is derived from the Greek name of the madapple. *Stramonia* was the name of *D. metel* at Venice, in the middle of the sixteenth century, and the plant is figured under that title in the great Herbals of Tragus and Fuchsius. *D. Stramonium* seems to have been a later introduction into Europe than *D. metel*, not becoming general till after the middle of the sixteenth century, but as it rapidly spread and became a common plant, the name of the latter was transferred to it.

The generic name, *Datura*, is from the Hindoo *Dhatura*, derived from the Sanskrit, *D'hustúra*, applied to the Indian species *fastuosa*, well known to the mediæval Arabian physicians under the name of *Tatorea*.

¶ *Description.* The Thornapple is a large and coarse herb, though an annual, branching somewhat freely, giving a bushy look to the plant. It attains a height of about 3 feet, its spreading branches covering an area almost as broad. On rich soil it may attain a height of even 6 feet.

The root is very long – thick and whitish, giving off many fibres. The stem is stout, erect and leafy, smooth, a pale yellowish-green in colour, branching repeatedly in a forked manner, and producing in the forks of the branches a leaf and a single, erect flower. The leaves are large and angular, 4 to 6 inches long, uneven at the base, with a wavy and coarsely-toothed margin, and have the strong, branching veins very plainly developed. The upper surface is dark and greyish-green, generally smooth, the under surface paler, and when dry, minutely wrinkled.

The plant flowers nearly all the summer. The flowers are large and handsome, about 3 inches in length, growing singly on short stems springing from the axils of the leaves or at the forking of the branches. The calyx is long, tubular and somewhat swollen below, and very sharply five-angled, surmounted by five sharp teeth. The corolla, folded and only half-opened, is funnel-shaped, of a pure white, with six prominent ribs, which are extended into the same number of sharp-pointed segments. The flowers open in the evening for the attraction of night-flying moths, and emit a powerful fragrance.

The flowers are succeeded by large, egg-shaped seed capsules of a green colour, about the size of a large walnut and covered with numerous sharp spines, hence the name of the plant. When ripe, this seed-vessel opens at the top, throwing back four valve-like forms, leaving a long, central structure upon which are numerous rough, dark-brown seeds. The appearance of the plant when in flower and fruit is so peculiar that it cannot be mistaken for any other native herb.

The plant is smooth, except for a slight downiness on the younger parts, which are covered with short, curved hairs, which fall off as growth proceeds. It exhales a rank, very heavy and somewhat nauseating narcotic odour. This fœtid odour arises from the leaves, especially when they are bruised, but the flowers are sweet-scented, though producing stupor if their exhalations are breathed for any length of time.

The plant is strongly narcotic, but has a peculiar action on the human frame which renders it very valuable as a medicine. The whole plant is poisonous, but the seeds are the most active; neither drying nor boiling destroys the poisonous properties. The usual consequences of the poison when taken in sufficient quantity are dimness of sight, dilation of the pupil, giddiness and delirium, sometimes amounting to mania, but its action varies greatly on different persons. Many fatal instances of its dangerous effects are recorded: it is thought to act more powerfully on the brain than Belladonna and to produce greater delirium. The remedies to be administered in case of poisoning by Stramonium are the same as those described for Henbane poisoning, and also Belladonna poisoning. It is classed in Table II of the poison schedule. The pupils have become widely dilated even by accidentally rubbing the eyes with the fingers after pulling the fresh leaves of Stramonium from the plant.

The seeds have in several instances caused death, and accidents have sometimes occurred from swallowing an infusion of the herb in mistake for other preparations, such as senna tea.

Browsing animals as a rule refuse to eat Thornapple, being repelled by its disagreeable odour and nauseous taste, so that its presence is not really dangerous to any of our domestic cattle. Among human beings the greater number of accidents have occurred among children, who have eaten the half-ripe seeds which have a sweetish taste.

The poisonous properties of the seeds are well known in India, where the Datura is abundant, the thieves and assassins not unfrequently administering them to their victims to produce insensibility.

In America it is called the 'Devil's Apple,' from its dangerous qualities and the remarkable effects that follow its administration. When the first settlers arrived in Virginia, some ate the leaves of this plant and experienced such strange and unpleasant effects that the colonists (so we are told) gave it this name by which it is still known in the United States. It is also known very commonly there by the name of 'Jamestown (or Jimson) Weed,' derived probably from its having been first observed in the neighbourhood of that old settlement in Virginia.

There are two varieties of this species of Datura, one with a green stem and white flowers, the other with a dark-reddish stem, minutely dotted with green and purplish flowers, striped with deep purple on the inside. The latter is now considered as a distinct species, being the *D. Tatula* of Linnæus. The leaves are mostly of a deeper green, and have purplish foot-stalks and mid-ribs.

De Candolle considered *D. Tatula* to be a native of Central America, whence it was imported into Europe in the sixteenth century, and naturalized first in Italy and then in South-west Europe, where it is very common. It occurs in England more rarely than *D. Stramonium*, under similar conditions and seems a more tender plant. It is sometimes cultivated here. The properties of both species are the same.

In early times, the Thornapple was considered an aid to the incantation of witches, and during the time of the witch and wizard mania in England, it was unlucky for anyone to grow it in his garden.

¶ *Cultivation.* Thornapple is easily cultivated, growing well in an open, sunny situation. It will flourish in most moderately good soils, but will do best in a rich calcareous soil, or in a good sandy loam, with leaf mould added.

Seeds are sown in the open in May, in drills 3 feet apart, barely covered. Sow thinly, as the plants attain a good size and grow freely from seed. Thin out the young plants to a distance of 12 to 15 inches between each plant in the drill. From 10 to 15 lb. of seed to the acre should be allowed.

The soil should be kept free from weeds in the early stages, but the plants are so umbrageous and strong that they need little care later. If the summer is hot and dry, give a mulching of rotted cow-manure.

The plants may also be raised from seeds,

sown in a hot-bed in February or March, or in April in boxes in a cool greenhouse, the seedlings, when large enough, being transferred to small pots, in which they are grown with as much light and air as possible till June, when they are planted in the open. Thornapple transplants readily.

If grown for leaf crop, the capsules should be picked off as soon as formed, as in a wind the spines tear the leaves. Some seed, for propagation purposes, should always be collected from plants kept specially for the purpose.

Though cultivated in this country, on some of the herb farms, such as Long Melford and Brentford, Thornapple was not much grown on a commercial scale before the War, considerable quantities of the dried leaves having always been imported from Germany and Hungary.

¶ *Parts Used, Harvesting and Preparation for Market.* All parts of the Thornapple have medicinal value, but only the leaves and seeds are official. The United States Pharmacopœia formerly recognized leaves, root and seeds, but since 1900 the leaves alone are recognized as official. They are used in the dried state and are referred to as *Stramonium*.

Stramonium leaves are official in all Pharmacopœias. Many require that they be renewed annually. The Belgian excludes discoloured leaves. The Portuguese directs the use of the entire plant except the root, and allows the substitution of *D. Tatula*. To how great an extent it is true that the quality deteriorates on being kept is conjectural.

The commercial drug as imported into Great Britain consists of the leaves and young shoots, collected while the plant is in flower, and subsequently dried, and containing the shrivelled, bristly young fruits, tubular calyx, and yellowish corolla, but the official description, for medicinal purposes, permits of the use of the leaves only.

The leaves should be gathered when the plant is in full bloom and carefully dried. The United States Pharmacopœia considers that they may be gathered at any time from the appearance of the flowers till the autumnal frosts. In this country they are generally harvested in late summer, about August, the crop being cut by the sickle on a fine day in the morning, after the sun has dried off the dew, and the leaves stripped from the stem and dried carefully as quickly as possible, as for Henbane.

The dried leaves are usually much shrivelled and wrinkled, and appear in commerce either loose, or more or less matted together, of a dark-greyish green colour, especially on the upper surface, stalked and often unequal at the base, and are characterized by the very coarse pointed teeth. About 34 parts of dried leaves are produced from 100 parts of fresh leaves.

The fresh leaves, when bruised, emit a fœtid, narcotic odour, which they lose on drying. Their taste is bitter and nauseous. These properties, together with their medicinal virtues, are imparted to water and alcohol and the fixed oils. The leaves if carefully dried retain their bitter taste.

The inspissated juice of the *fresh* leaves was formerly commonly prescribed, but the alcoholic extract is now almost exclusively used.

Stramonium *seeds* are official in a number of Pharmacopœias. The thorny capsules are gathered from the plants when they are quite ripe, but still green. They should then be dried in the sun for a few days, when they will split open and the seeds can be readily shaken out. The seeds can then be dried, either in the sun or by artificial heat.

The dried, ripe seeds are dark brown or dull black in colour, flattened, kidney-shaped in outline, wrinkled and marked with small depressions, and average about $\frac{1}{6}$ inch in length. Though ill-smelling when fresh, when dry they have a scarcely perceptible odour till crushed, but a bitter, oily taste. They should not be stored in a damp place, or will mildew. *Kiln-dried* seeds, it should be noted, are no use for cultivation.

The demand for the seed is very limited, but the dry leaves find a ready market. The south of Europe furnishes a quantity, but owing to careless collection and neglect of botanical characters, the South European product is often mixed with other leaves of no value, which are sometimes entirely substituted for it, especially species of *Xanthium*, which has spiny though smaller fruits. Spanish Stramonium which contains no Stramonium at all has been offered in London and Liverpool. The imported commercial Stramonium leaves are also frequently found freely adulterated with those of *Carthamus helenoides*.

¶ *Constituents.* Stramonium *leaves* contain the same alkaloids as Belladonna, but in somewhat smaller proportion, the average of commercial samples being about 0·22 per cent.: the percentage may, however, rise to as much as 0·4 per cent. The mid-rib and footstalk of the leaf contain a far larger proportion than the blade. It is generally considered that the main stems and the root contain little alkaloid, and should, therefore, not be present in the drug. The *American Journal of Pharmacy* (January, 1919) directs attention to the fact that if the stems could be

utilized, the cost of labour in harvesting a crop of Stramonium would be only one-fourth or one-fifth of what it is where the leaves alone are gathered, since machinery for the purpose could be employed. Dr. G. B. Koch, of the Biological Laboratories of the H.K. Mulford Co., Philadelphia, has been making careful experiments on the relative value of the stem and root of this plant, and has arrived at the following conclusions:

1. The whole plant, either with or without the root, can be harvested and used for the commercial preparations without fear of the total alkaloid content falling below 0·25 per cent., which is the desired standard of the United States Pharmacopœia.

2. The total mydriatic (pupil-dilating) alkaloids of the leaf and secondary stems when analysed individually, or the leaves with 10 per cent. of the secondary stems, run much higher than the United States Pharmacopœia requirement.

3. Of the whole plant, including stem, root and leaf, the leaf represents about 41 per cent.

4. Excluding the root, the ratio of the leaf to the stem is about 47·5 to 52·3 per cent.

In general it has been found that fresh parts yielded more alkaloid than the dried parts. The alkaloid consists chiefly of hyoscyamine, associated with atropine and hyoscine (scopolamine), malic acid also being present. The Daturin formerly described as a constituent is now known to be a mixture of hyoscyamine and atropine. The leaves also yield 17 to 20 per cent. of ash, and are rich in potassium nitrate, to which, doubtless, part of the antispasmodic effects are due, and they contain also a trace of volatile oil, gum, resin, starch, and other unimportant substances.

Seeds. Except that they contain about 25 per cent. of fixed oil, the constituents of the seeds are practically the same as those of the leaves, though considered to contain a much greater proportion of alkaloid, which renders them more powerful than the leaves. But the presence of the large amount of fixed oil makes it difficult to extract the alkaloids or to make stable preparations and the leaves have, therefore, greatly taken the place of the seeds.

¶ *Medicinal Action and Uses.* Antispasmodic, anodyne and narcotic. Its properties are virtually those of hyoscyamine. It acts similarly to belladonna, though without constipating, and is used for purposes similar to those for which belladonna is employed, dilating the pupil of the eyes in like manner. It is considered slightly more sedative to the central nervous system than is belladonna.

Stramonium is, in fact, so similar to belladonna in the symptoms produced by it in small or large doses, in its toxicity and its general physiological and therapeutic action, that the two drugs are practically identical, and since they are about the same strength in activity, the preparations may be used in similar doses.

Stramonium has been employed in all the conditions for which belladonna is more commonly used, but acts much more strongly on the respiratory organs, and has acquired special repute as one of the chief remedies for spasmodic asthma, being used far more as the principal ingredient in asthma powders and cigarettes than internally. The practice of smoking *D. ferox* for asthma was introduced into Great Britain from the East Indies by a certain General, and afterwards the English species was substituted for that employed in Hindustan. Formerly the roots were much used: in Ceylon, the leaves, stem and fruit are all cut up together to make burning powders for asthma, but in this country the dried *leaves* are almost exclusively employed for this purpose. The beneficial effect is considered due to the presence of atropine, which paralyses the endings of the pulmonary branches, thus relieving the bronchial spasm. It has been proved that the smoke from a Stramonium cigarette, containing 0·25 grams of Stramonium, leaves contains as much as 0·5 milligrams of atropine. The leaves may be made up into cigarettes or smoked in a pipe, either alone, or with a mixture of tobacco, or with cubebs, sage, belladonna and other drugs. More commonly, however, the coarsely-ground leaves are mixed into cones with some aromatic and with equal parts of potassium nitrate, in order to increase combustion and are burned in a saucer, the smoke being inhaled into the lungs. Great relief is afforded, the effect being more immediate when the powdered leaves are burnt and the smoke inhaled than when smoked by the patient in the form of cigars or cigarettes, but like most drugs, after constant use, the relief is not so great and the treatment is only palliative, the causation of the attack not being affected. Accidents have also occasionally happened from the injudicious use of the plant in this manner. Dryness of the throat and mouth are to be regarded as indications that too large a quantity is being taken.

The *seeds*, besides being employed to relieve asthma in the same manner as the leaves, being smoked with tobacco, are employed as a narcotic and anodyne, generally used in the form of an extract, prepared by boiling the seeds in water, or macerating them in alcohol. A tincture is sometimes preferred. The extract is given in pills to allay cough in spasmodic bronchial asthma, in whooping-cough and spasm of the bladder, and is considered a better cough-remedy than opium, but should only be used with extreme care, as in over-doses it is a strong narcotic poison.

Applied locally, in ointment, plasters or fomentation, Stramonium will palliate the pain of muscular rheumatism, neuralgia, and also pain due to hæmorrhoids, fistula, abscesses and similar inflammation.

¶ *Preparations and Dosages.* Powdered leaves, $\frac{1}{10}$ to 5 grains. Fluid extract leaves, 1 to 3 drops. Fluid extract seeds, 1 to 2 drops. Tincture leaves, B.P. and U.S.P., 5 to 15 drops. Powdered extract, U.S.P., $\frac{1}{8}$ grain. Solid extract, B.P., $\frac{1}{4}$ to 1 grain. Ointment, U.S.P.

Gerard declared that

'the juice of Thornapple, boiled with hog's grease, cureth all inflammations whatsoever, all manner of burnings and scaldings, as well of fire, water, boiling lead, gunpowder, as that which comes by lightning and that in very short time, as myself have found in daily practice, to my great credit and profit.'

It has been conjectured that the leaves of *D. Stramonium* were used by the priests of Apollo at Delphi to assist them in their prophecies, and in the Temple of the Sun, in the city of Sagomozo the seeds of the Floripondio (*D. Sanguinea*) are used for a similar purpose. The Peruvians also prepare an intoxicating beverage from the seeds, which induces stupefaction and delirium if partaken of in large quantities. The Arabs of Central Africa are said to dry the leaves, the flowers, and the rind of the rootlet, which is considered the strongest preparation, and to smoke them in a common bowl, or in a water-pipe. It is esteemed by them a sovereign remedy for asthma and influenza, and although they do not use it like the Indian Datura poisoners, accidents nevertheless occur from its narcotic properties.

Stramonium was at one time esteemed as a sedative in epilepsy, and in acute mania and other forms of active insanity, but its action is very uncertain.

The introduction of Stramonium into medicine is due chiefly to the exertions of Baron Storch, in the latter half of the eighteenth century, who was also instrumental in re-introducing Henbane into modern medicine.

In a recent issue of an American medical journal, the opinion was expressed that Stramonium was a remedy for hydrophobia, the writer saying 'there is no drug so far proven that deserves as thorough and careful a trial in this dread disease as Stramonium.'

The poorer Turks are said to use Stramonium instead of opium, for smoking.

¶ *Other Species.*
In India and the Eastern and West Indian Colonies, the leaves and seeds of *D. fastuosa* var. *alba* are also official, under the name of Datura. They possess similar properties, and are regarded as of equal strength.

D. fastuosa is a small shrub indigenous to tropical India. There are said to be several varieties of this species, and it is generally conceded to be the most toxic of the Indian Daturas. The leaves are ovate and more or less angular, the flowers being mostly purplish, sometimes white.

Of the varieties of *D. fastuosa*, the British Pharmacopœia recognizes that known as *alba*. From it the Thugs prepared the poison *Dhât*, with which they used to stupefy their victims. It is used in India as a criminal poison, the professional poisoners being called *Dhatureeas*.

The drug has a slight, unpleasant odour and a bitter taste. It contains the alkaloid Hyoscine, a resin and a fixed oil, hyoscyamine being also present and a small proportion of atropine.

It is used by the native doctors (India) for the relief of rheumatic and other painful affections.

While this drug produces effects more or less similar to those of belladonna, its precise action has not been clearly determined.

This species of Datura grows in abundance in almost all the islands of the Philippine group, in some localities reaching a height of 6 feet, and might afford a favourable source of atropine and hyoscyamine, though it has not so far been made use of commercially, there being no attempt at cultivation or even systematic collection of the

drug, though attention was drawn to its latent possibilities during the War.

Under the names of *Man t'o lo fa, Wan t'o hua* and *Nau Yeung fa* the Chinese use as a medicine the flowers of the *D. alba*.

D. metel is also an Indian plant and resembles *D. fastuosa*; it differs in that the leaves are heart-shaped, almost entire and downy, and the flowers always white. The leaves contain 0·55 per cent. alkaloid, the seeds 0·5 per cent., all hyoscine.

D. alba or *D. metel* also produce similar effects. The Rajpoot mothers are said to smear their breasts with the juice of the leaves, to poison their newly-born female infants.

D. arborea, a South American species (the Tree Datura), growing freely in Chile, contains about 0·44 per cent. alkaloid, nearly all hyoscine. A tincture of the flowers is used to induce clairvoyance.

D. quercifolia, of Mexico, contains 0·4 per cent. in the leaves and 0·28 per cent. of alkaloids in the seeds, about half hyoscyamine and half hyoscine.

El Bethene, a Datura of the Sahara Desert, is capable of causing delirium, coma and death.

D. Tatula, Purple Stramonium has already been mentioned. It owes its activity to the same alkaloids as *D. Stramonium*, and its leaves are also much used in the form of cigarettes as a remedy for spasmodic asthma.

D. ferox, Chinese Datura, is used in homœopathy.

A tincture is made from the unripe fruit and a trituration of the seeds.

An Old Recipe 'for A Burne'

'Take of the plant called *Thorneaple*, and Elder leaves, 2 good handfuls; pound both leaves and apples very small in A stone mortar; then take a pound of Barow hogs lard watered and putt them altogether in an earthen pan, working them well together; lett itt stand till it begins to hoare [grow musty], and then sett itt over A soft fire, not letting it boyle; then strain it, and putt in fresh herbs; order itt as before; this doe three times; and then keep itt for your use; it will keep seven years.'—(*A Plain Plantain*.)

THUJA. *See* CEDAR

THYME, BASIL   Calamintha acinos
N.O. Labiatæ

Synonyms. Common Calamint. Calamintha officinalis. Calamintha menthifolia. Thymos acinos. Acinos vulgaris. Mountain Mint
Part Used. Herb
Habitat. Rather scarce in England, though fairly generally distributed over the country; it is rare in Scotland and very rare in Ireland
¶ *Description.* This species is found on dry banks and in fields, in chalky, gravelly and sandy soils: a small, bushy herb, its stems 6 to 8 inches high, branching at the base, slender and leafy.

The shortly stalked leaves, ¼ to ½ inch long,

with the veins prominent beneath, are egg-shaped and hairy. The flowers, in bloom in July and August, are ½ inch long and grow in whorls from the axils of the leaves, like in the preceding species, as well as at the summit of the stem. The corollas are bluish-purple, variegated with white on the lower lip, in the middle of which there is a purple spot. The calyx is distinctly two-lipped, the lower lip bulged at the base and has prominent ribs, fringed with bristly hairs.

The plant varies much in degree of hairiness. It has a pleasant, aromatic smell, somewhat similar, though weaker, than that of Thyme, to which, however, in general appearance, it bears little resemblance.

Basil Thyme was a great favourite with the old herbalists. Gerard enumerates twelve uses to which it can be applied without fear of failure. Among them he states that

'it cureth them that are bitten of serpents; being burned or strewed, it drives serpents away; it taketh away black and blew spots that come by blows or by beatings, making

the skinne faire and white; but for such things, saith Galen, it is better to be laid to greene than dry.'

Externally, its use has been recommended as an addition to warm baths, especially for children, as a strengthener and nerve soother.

The oil, which is very heating, is of service as a rubefacient, applied to the skin in sciatica and neuralgia.

One drop of the oil, on cotton wool, put into a decayed tooth, will alleviate the pain.

The flowering tops are used to flavour jugged hare, etc., they have a milder and rather more grateful flavour than the common Thyme.

Although it has been stated that animals will seldom eat this plant and that rabbits do not touch it, it has been alleged that sheep love to crop its fragrant leaves and that, as a consequence, a fine flavour is imparted to their flesh.

It is said that Wild Thyme and Marjoram laid by milk in the dairy will prevent it being turned by thunder.

THYME, CAT

Teucrium Marum (LINN.)
N.O. Labiatæ

Synonym. Marum
Parts Used. Leaves, root-bark, whole herb

The Cat Thyme, or Marum, is not a British plant, but a native of Spain, though with care it can be grown here and will live through the winter in the open, on a dry soil and in a good situation, when the frosts are not severe, though it is frequently killed in hard winters, if unprotected by mats or other covering.

In the southern countries of Europe, this species of *Teucrium* forms a shrub 3 or 4 feet high, but in England it rarely attains even half that height. It has oval leaves, broader at the base, downy beneath, with uncut margins. The flowers are in one-sided spikes, the corollas crimson in colour.

The leaves and younger branches when fresh, on being rubbed emit a volatile, aromatic smell, which excites sneezing, but in taste they are somewhat bitter, accompanied with a sensation of heat.

¶ *Medicinal Action and Uses.* The plant is supposed to possess very active powers,

having been recommended in many diseases requiring medicine of a stimulant, aromatic and deobstruent quality. It has been considered good in most nervous complaints, the leaves being powdered and given in wine. The powdered leaves, either alone, or mixed with other ingredients of a like nature, when taken as snuff, have been recommended as excellent for 'disorders of the head,' under the name of compound powder of Assarabacca, but lavender flowers are now generally substituted for Cat Thyme.

Cat Thyme is more nearly related to the Germanders and to Wood Sage than to the Thymes.

The bark of the root is considerably astringent and has been used for checking hæmorrhages.

A homœpathic tincture is made from the whole herb, said to be effectual against small thread-worms in children.

THYME, GARDEN

Thymus vulgaris (LINN.)
N.O. Labiatæ

Synonym. Common Thyme
Part Used. Herb

The Garden Thyme is an 'improved' cultivated form of the Wild Thyme of the mountains of Spain and other European countries bordering on the Mediterranean, flourishing also in Asia Minor, Algeria and Tunis, and

is a near relation to our own Wild Thyme (*Thymus serpyllum*), which has broader leaves (the margins not reflexed as in the Garden Thyme) and a weaker odour.

It is cultivated now in most countries with

temperate climates, though we do not know at what period it was first introduced into northern countries. It was certainly commonly cultivated in England before the middle of the sixteenth century, and is figured and described by Gerard.

¶ *Description.* *T. vulgaris* is a perennial with a woody, fibrous root. The stems are numerous, round, hard, branched, and usually from 4 to 8 inches high, when of the largest growth scarcely attaining a foot in height. The leaves are small, only about ⅛ inch long and ₁⁄₁₆ inch broad, narrow and elliptical, greenish-grey in colour, reflexed at the margins, and set in pairs upon very small foot-stalks. The flowers terminate the branches in whorls. The calyx is tubular, striated, closed at the mouth with small hairs and divided into two lips, the uppermost cut into three teeth and the lower into two. The corolla consists of a tube about the length of the calyx, spreading at the top into two lips of a pale purple colour, the upper lip erect or turned back and notched at the end, the under lip longer and divided into three segments. The seeds are roundish and very small, about 170,000 to the ounce, and 24 oz. to the quart: they retain their germinating power for three years. The plant has an agreeable aromatic smell and a warm pungent taste. The fragrance of its leaves is due to an essential oil, which gives it its flavouring value for culinary purposes, and is also the source of its medicinal properties. It is in flower from May to August.

There are three varieties usually grown for use, the broad-leaved, narrow-leaved and variegated: the narrow-leaved, with small, greyish-green leaves, is more aromatic than the broad-leaved, and is also known as Winter or German Thyme. The fragrant Lemon Thyme, likewise grown in gardens, has a lemon flavour, and rather broader leaves than the ordinary Garden Thyme, is not recurved at the margins, and ranks as a variety of *T. serpyllum*, the Wild Thyme. It is of a more trailing habit and of still smaller growth than the common Garden Thyme, and keeps its foliage better in the winter, though is generally considered to be not as hardy as the common Thyme. Another variety, the Silver Thyme, is the hardiest of all and has perhaps the best flavour. There is a variety, also, called the Orange Thyme, which Dr. Kitchener, in *The Cook's Oracle*, describes as a delicious herb that deserves to be better known. This and other varieties of Thyme, including the Caraway Thyme, which was used to rub the baron of beef, before it was roasted, and so came to be called 'Herbe Baronne,' are all worth cultivating.

The name Thyme, in its Greek form, was first given to the plant by the Greeks as a derivative of a word which meant 'to fumigate,' either because they used it as incense, for its balsamic odour, or because it was taken as a type of all sweet-smelling herbs. Others derive the name from the Greek word *thumus*, signifying courage, the plant being held in ancient and mediæval days to be a great source of invigoration, its cordial qualities inspiring courage. The antiseptic properties of Thyme were fully recognized in classic times, there being a reference in Virgil's *Georgics* to its use as a fumigator, and Pliny tells us that, when burnt, it puts to flight all venomous creatures. Lady Northcote (in *The Herb Garden*) says that among the Greeks, Thyme denoted graceful elegance; 'to smell of Thyme' was an expression of praise, applied to those whose style was admirable. It was an emblem of activity, bravery and energy, and in the days of chivalry it was the custom for ladies to embroider a bee hovering over a sprig of Thyme on the scarves they presented to their knights. In the south of France, Wild Thyme is a symbol of extreme Republicanism, tufts of it being sent with the summons to a Republican meeting.

This little plant, so familiar also in its wild form, has never been known in England by any familiar name, though occasionally 'Thyme' is qualified in some way, such as 'Running Thyme,' or 'Mother-of-Thyme.' 'Mother Thyme' was probably derived from the use of the plant in uterine disorders, in the same way that 'Motherwort' (*Leonurus Cardiaca*) has received its popular name for use in domestic medicine.

The affection of bees for Thyme is well known and the fine flavour of the honey of Mount Hymettus near Athens was said to be due to the Wild Thyme with which it was covered (probably *T. vulgaris*), the honey from this spot being of such especial flavour and sweetness that in the minds and writings of the Ancients, sweetness and Thyme were indissolubly united. 'Thyme, for the time it lasteth, yieldeth most and best honie and therefor in old time was accounted chief,' says an old English writer. Large clumps of either Garden or Wild Thyme may with advantage be grown in the garden about 10 feet away from the hives.

Though apparently not in general use as a culinary herb among the ancients, it was employed by the Romans to give an aromatic flavour to cheese (and also to liqueurs).

¶ *Cultivation.* Sow about the middle of March or early April, in dry, mild weather, moderately thin, in shallow drills about ½ inch deep, and 8 or 9 inches apart, in good, light soil, in a warm position. Cover in evenly with the soil. Some of the plants may remain where planted, after a thinning for early use, others plant out in the summer. Thyme thrives best with lots of room to spread in. It is well to make new beds annually. Self-sown plants will answer for this where found.

Stocks may also be increased by dividing old roots, or making cuttings, by slipping pieces off the plants with roots to them and planting out with trowel or dibber, taking care to water well. This may be done as soon as the weather is warm enough, from May to September. The old clumps may be divided to the utmost extent and provided each portion has a reasonable bit of root attached, success is assured. The perfume of Lemon Thyme is sweeter if raised from cuttings or division of roots, rather than from seed.

Although Thyme grows easily, especially in calcareous light, dry, stony soils, it can be cultivated in heavy soils, but it becomes less aromatic. It dislikes excess of moisture. To form Thyme beds, choose uncultivated ground, with soil too poor to nourish cereals. If Thyme grows upon walls or on dry, stony land, it will survive the severest cold of this country. If the soil does not suit it very well and is close and heavy, some material for lightening it, such as a little road-sand or sweepings, ensuring reasonable porosity, will be welcomed, and should be thoroughly incorporated – in a gritty soil it will root quickly, but it does not like a close, cold soil about its roots.

According to Gattefosse, the Thyme is 'a faithful companion of the Lavender. It lives with it in perfect sympathy and partakes alike of its good and its bad fortune.' Generally speaking, the conditions most suitable to the growth of Thyme are identical with those favoured by Lavender.

The plant is often overrun by Dodder (*Cuscuta epithymum*). If this happens, cut off the affected plants and burn them, or use a solution of sulphate of iron.

At the close of the summer, as soon as the herbs have been cut sufficiently, the beds should be attended to, all weeds cleared away and the soil well forked on the surface.

In winter, protect the plants from frost by banking up with earth.

Thyme roots soon extract the goodness from the soil, hence whatever is sown or planted afterwards will seldom thrive unless the ground is first trenched deeper than the Thyme was rooted, and is well manured.

The whole herb is used, fresh and dried. Though cultivated in gardens for culinary use, Common Thyme is not grown in England on a large scale, most of the dried Thyme on the market having been imported from the Continent, mainly from Germany.

Its essential oil is distilled in the south of France, the flowering herb being used for the production of oil of Thyme. In the neighbourhood of Nîmes, the entire plant is used and the distillation is carried on at two periods of the year, in May and June, and again in the autumn. In England, only a comparatively small amount of the essential oil is distilled, but it is considered to be of a high quality. For distilling, the fresh herb should be collected on a dry day, when just coming into flower; the lower portions of the stem, together with any yellow or brown leaves, should be rejected and the herbs conveyed to the distillery as soon as possible.

¶ *Constituents*. Oil of Thyme is the important commercial product obtained by distillation of the fresh leaves and flowering tops of *T. vulgaris*. Its chief constituents are from 20 to 25 per cent. of the phenols Thymol and Carvacrol, rising in rare cases to 42 per cent. The phenols are the principal constituents of Thyme oil, Thymol being the most valuable for medicinal purposes, but Carvacrol, an isomeric phenol, preponderate in some oils. Cymene and Pinene are present in the oil, as well as a little Menthone. Borneol and Linalol have been detected in the high boiling fractions of the oil and a crystalline body, probably identical with a similar body found in Juniper-berry oil.

Two commercial varieties of Thyme oil are recognized, the 'red,' the crude distillate, and the 'white' or colourless, which is the 'red' rectified by re-distilling. The yield of oil is very variable, from 2 per cent. to 1 per cent. in the fresh herb (100 lb. of the fresh flowering tops yielding from ½ to 1 lb. of essential oil) and 2·5 per cent. in the dried herb, the yield of oil from the dried German herb being on the average 1·7 per cent. and from the dried French herb 2·5 to 2·6 per cent. The phenols present in French and German oils consist mainly of Thymol, but under certain conditions the latter may be replaced by Carvacrol. The value of Thyme oil depends so much upon the phenols it contains, that it is important that these should be estimated, as the abstraction of Thymol is by no means uncommon.

Red oil of Thyme is frequently imported and sold under the name of oil of Origanum: it is often adulterated with oils of turpentine, spike lavender and rosemary, and coloured with alkanet root, and is not infrequently more or less destitute of Thymol. *True* oil of Origanum is extracted from Wild Marjoram, *Origanum vulgare*, and other species of *Origanum*.

French oil of Thyme is the most esteemed variety of the oil known. A considerable quantity of Thyme oil is also distilled in Spain, but probably from mixed species of Thyme oil, the origin of Spanish Thyme oil not having been definitely proved; a certain amount is also distilled in Algeria from *T. Algeriensis*. French oil (specific gravity 0·905 to 0·935) contains 20 to 36 per cent. of phenols, chiefly Thymol, on which the value of the oil chiefly depends. Spanish oil contains a much higher percentage of phenols, 50 to 70 per cent., mostly Carvacrol, but sometimes a fairly large proportion of Thymol is present. The production of Thymol or Carvacrol seems to depend on some variation in the soil or climatic conditions which favours the formation of one or the other. The specific gravity of Spanish oil is 0·928 to 0·958.

T. capitans also yields an oil of a specific gravity about 0·900, closely resembling that obtained from *T. vulgaris*. A similar oil is obtained from *T. camphoratus*. A somewhat different oil is obtained from the Lemon Thyme, *T. serpyllum*, var *citriodorus*. This oil has an odour resembling Thyme, Lemon and Geranium. It contains only a very small amount of phenols. Admixture with the oil of *T. serpyllum* does not alter the specific gravity of Thyme oil. *T. mastichina*, the so-called Spanish Wood Marjoram, also yields an oil of Thyme, of a bright yellow colour, turning darker with age and with a camphoraceous odour like Thyme.

¶ *Medicinal Action and Uses.* Antiseptic, antispasmodic, tonic and carminative.

The pounded herb, if given fresh, from 1 to 6 oz. daily, mixed with syrup, has been employed with success as a safe cure for whooping cough. An infusion made from 1 oz. of the dried herb to 1 pint of boiling water, sweetened with sugar or honey, is also used for the same purpose, as well as in cases of catarrh and sore throat, given in doses of 1 or more tablespoonsful, several times daily. The wild plant may be equally well used for this.

Thyme tea will arrest gastric fermentation. It is useful in cases of wind spasms and colic, and will assist in promoting perspiration at the commencement of a cold, and in fever and febrile complaints generally.

In herbal medicine, Thyme is generally used in combination with other remedies.

Fluid extract, ½ to 1 drachm. Oil, 1 to 10 drops.

According to Culpepper, Thyme is

'a noble strengthener of the lungs, as notable a one as grows, nor is there a better remedy growing for hooping cough. It purgeth the

body of phlegm and is an excellent remedy for shortness of breath. It is so harmless you need not fear the use of it. An ointment made of it takes away hot swellings and warts, helps the sciatica and dullness of sight and takes away any pains and hardness of the spleen: it is excellent for those that are troubled with the gout and the herb taken anyway inwardly is of great comfort to the stomach.'

Gerard says it will 'cure sciatica and pains in the head,' and is healing in leprosy and the falling sickness.

Oil of Thyme is employed as a rubefacient and counter-irritant in rheumatism, etc.

Thyme enters into the formula for Herb Tobacco, and employed in this form is good for digestion, headache and drowsiness.

In Perfumery, Essence of Thyme is used for cosmetics and rice powder. It is also used for embalming corpses.

The dried flowers have been often used in the same way as lavender, to preserve linen from insects.

In this country, Thyme is principally in request for culinary requirements, for its use in flavouring stuffings, sauces, pickles, stews, soups, jugged hare, etc. The Spaniards infuse it in the pickle with which they preserve their olives.

All the different species of Thyme and Marjoram yield fragrant oils extensively used by manufacturing perfumers for scenting soaps. When dried and ground, they enter into the composition of sachet powders.

THYMOL, a most valuable crystalline phenol, is the basis of the fragrant volatile Essence of Sweet Thyme, and is obtainable from *Carum copticum, Monarda punctata* and various other plants, as well as from *T. vulgaris*, being present to the extent of from 20 to 60 per cent. in the oils which yield it. Ajowan oil, its principal commercial source (from the seeds of *C. copticum*), contains from 40 to 55 per cent. of Thymol; the oil of *T. vulgaris* contains from 20 to 30 per cent. as a rule of Thymol and Carvacrol in varying proportions, while the oil of *M. punctata* contains 61 per cent. of Thymol.

The extraction of Thymol is effected by treating the oil with a warm solution of sodium hydroxide: this alkali dissolves the Thymol, and on dilution with hot water the undissolved oil (terpenes, etc.) rises to the surface. The alkaline thymol compound is decomposed by treatment with hydrochloric acid and subsequent crystallization of the oily layer into large, oblique, prismatic crystals. Thymol (*methyl-propyl-phenol*) has been prepared synthetically.

When treated with caustic potash and

iodine, it yields iodo-thymol, commonly known as 'Aristol.'

Camphor of Thyme was noticed first by Neumann, apothecary to the Court at Berlin in 1725. It was called Thymol and carefully examined in 1853 by Lallemand and recommended instead of Phenol (carbolic acid) in 1868 by Bouilhon, apothecary, and Paquet, M.D., of Lille.

Thymol is a powerful antiseptic for both internal and external use; it is also employed as a deodorant and local anæsthetic. It is extensively used to medicate gauze and wool for surgical dressings. It resembles carbolic acid in its action, but is less irritant to wounds, while its germicidal action is greater. It is therefore preferable as a dressing and during recent years has been one of the most extensively used antiseptics.

Thymol is also a preservative of meat.

In respect of its physiological action, Thymol appears to stand between carbolic acid and oil of turpentine. Its action as a disinfectant is more permanent and at the same time more powerful than that of carbolic acid. It is less irritating to the skin, does not act as a caustic like carbolic acid, and is a less powerful poison to mammals. In the higher animals it acts as a local irritant and anæsthetic to the skin and mucous membrane. It is used as an antiseptic lotion and mouth wash; as a paint in ringworm, in eczema, psoriasis, broken chilblains, parasitic skin affections and burns; as an ointment, half-strength, perfumed with lavender, to keep off gnats and mosquitoes. Thymol in oily solution is applied to the respiratory passages by means of a spray in nasal catarrh, and a spirituous solution may be inhaled for laryngitis, bronchial affections and whooping cough. It is most useful against septic sore throat, especially during scarlet-fever. Internally, it is given in large doses, to robust adults, in capsules, as a vermifuge, to expel parasites, especially the miner's worm, and it has also been used in diabetes and vesical catarrh.

Thymol finds no place in perfumery, but the residual oil after extracting the crystalline Thymol from Ajowan oil, which amounts to about 50 per cent. of the original oil, is generally sold as a cheap perfume for soap-making and similar purposes, under the name of 'Thymene.'

Till the outbreak of war, Thymol was manufactured almost exclusively in Germany. One of the chief commercial sources of Thymol, Ajowan seed (*C. copticum*), is an annual umbelliferous plant, a kind of caraway, which is abundant in India, where it is widely cultivated for the medicinal properties of its seeds. Almost the whole of the exports of Ajowan seed from India, Egypt, Persia and Afghanistan went to Germany for the distillation of the oil and extraction of Thymol, the annual export of the seed from India being about 1,200 tons, from which the amount of Thymol obtainable was estimated at 20 tons. On the outbreak of war the export of Ajowan seed dropped to 2 tons per month, and there was a universal shortage of Thymol, just when it was urgently needed for the wounded.

As a result of investigations by the Imperial Institute, Thymol is now being made by several firms in this country, and the product is equal in quality and appearance to that previously imported from Germany. In India, also, good samples were obtained as a result of experiments conducted in Government laboratories in the early months of the War, and by the close of 1915 companies were already established at Dehra and Calcutta for its manufacture on a large scale. In the two years ending June, 1919, as much as 10,500 lb. of Thymol were exported from Calcutta.

Several other plants can be utilized as sources of Thymol, although none yield such high percentages as Ajowan seed. The following new sources of Thymol were suggested when the scarcity of the valuable antiseptic made itself so severely felt on curtailment of Continental supplies: Garden Thyme and Wild Thyme (*T. vulgaris* and *serpyllum*), American Horse Mint (*M. punctata*), *Cunila mariana*, *Mosla japonica*, *Origanum hirtum*, *Ocimim viride* and *Satureja thymbra*.

The oil of Thyme obtained by distilling the fresh-flowering herb of *T. vulgaris* is already an article of commerce, and contains varying amounts of Thymol, but the actual amount present is not very high, varying, as already stated, from 20 to 25 per cent., only in very rare cases amounting to more; and the methods of separation in order to obtain a pure compound are necessarily more complicated than in the manufacture from Ajowan oil.

The American Horsemint (*M. punctata*), native to the United States and Canada, seems likely to prove a more valuable source of Thymol than *T. vulgaris*. It yields from 1 to 3 per cent. of a volatile oil, which contains a large proportion of Thymol, up to 61 per cent. having been obtained; Carvacrol also appears to be a constituent. The oil has a specific gravity of 0·930 to 0·940, and on prolonged standing deposits crystals of Thymol.

Another species also found in America (*M. didyma*) (called also 'Oswego tea' from the use sometimes made of its *leaves* in America) is said to yield an oil of similar composition, though not to the same degree, and so far *M. punctata* is considered the only plant indigenous to North America which can be looked upon as a fruitful source of Thymol, though from *C. mariana*, also found in North America, an oil is derived – Oil of Dittany – which is stated to contain about 40 per cent. of phenols, probably Thymol.

Thymol is also contained in the oil distilled from the dry herb of *Mosla japonica*, indigenous to Japan. It is stated to yield about 2·13 per cent. of oil, containing about 44 per cent. of Thymol.

Satureja thymbra, which is used in Spain as a spice and is closely allied to the Savouries grown in the English kitchen garden, yields an oil containing about 19 per cent. of Thymol. Other species of *Satureja* contain Carvacrol.

A new source of Thymol is also *Ocimum viride*, the 'Mosquito Plant' of West Africa and the West Indies, which yield 0·35 to 1·2 of oil from which 32 to 65 per cent. of Thymol can be extracted. This plant occurs wild on all soils in every part of Sierra Leone, and is also grown in the Seychelles. In Sierra Leone it bears the name of 'Fever-plant' on account of its febrifugal qualities; a decoction is made from the leaves.

The Origanum oils shipped from Trieste and Smyrna generally contain only Carvacrol, the only species yielding Thymol exclusively and to a considerable degree being *Origanum hirtum*, which may be regarded as a promising source of Thymol.

Recently a Spanish species of Thyme has been used as a source of Thymol (*T. zygis*, Linn.), known to Theophrastus as *Serpyllum zygis*. It is common throughout Spain and Portugal, occurring in oak and other woods, in desert and dry gravelly places among the sierras of the central, eastern and southern provinces. In consequence of its wide distribution, the common names for the plant vary greatly; in Portugal it is known as Wood Marjoram, *ouregao do mato*; but the most frequently recurring name in Spain is *Tomillo salsero* or Sauce Thyme, from its use as a condiment. The species is very similar to *T. vulgaris*, but is easily distinguished by the comparatively large white hairs at the base of the leaves. The flowers are either purple or white, the white form being the only one occurring in the Balearic Islands, where it is called *Senorida de flor blanca*. There are two well-known varieties, var. *floribunda* and var. *gracillis*, a simpler, less-branched form, and it is the latter (not such a decided alpine as *floribunda*) which is now being used by a British manufacturer as a source of Thymol. See *Chemist and Druggist*, June 12th and July 17th, 1920. Var. *gracilis* is more easily collected on account of its lower station, and further unguarded exploitation of the wild plant might result in the substitution of var. *floribunda*, which it seems probable yields an oil with quite different characters and content from those of the oil obtained from var. *gracilis*.

Carvacrol has not hitherto been employed in medicine, but the antiseptic properties of Origanum oil, consisting principally of Carvacrol, as well as of the phenol itself, have been investigated and Iodocrol – iodide of Carvacrol – a reddish-brown powder, has been used lately as an antiseptic in place of iodoform in treatment of eczema and other skin diseases.

If required, a British Possession can provide Carvacrol as a substitute for Thymol. It can be obtained from oils derived from a variety of plants, but most profitably from the Origanum of Cyprus (*Origanum dubium*), which contains 82·5 per cent. of Carvacrol. At the instance of the Imperial Institute, this Cyprus Origanum oil has been produced in commercial quantities from wild plants in Cyprus, and already in 1913 was exported thence to the United Kingdom to the value of £980. It is believed that the plant can be cultivated profitably and on a large scale in Cyprus, and experiments in this direction were begun shortly after the outbreak of war. The oil from *O. onites*, var. *Symrnæum* – Smyrna Origanum oil – contains 68 per cent. phenols, almost wholly Carvacrol. Other sources of Carvacrol are *Monarda fistulosa* (Wild Bergamot), which yields 52 to 58 per cent. of Carvacrol; *Satureja montana* (Winter Savoury or White Thyme), oil from wild plants of this species containing 35 to 40 per cent. of Carvacrol; while that from cultivated plants has been found to contain as much as 65 per cent. A sample of Dalmatian *Satureja*, a form of *S. montana*, yielded at the Imperial Institute 68·75 of phenolic constituents, consisting mostly of Carvacrol.

THYME, WILD

Thymus serpyllum (LINN.)
N.O. Labiatæ

Synonyms. Mother of Thyme. Serpyllum
Part Used. Herb

The Wild Thyme is indigenous to the greater part of the dry land of Europe, though is a great deal less abundant than the Common Thyme so widely cultivated. It is found up to a certain height on the Alps, on high plateaux, and in valleys, along ditches and roads, on rocks, in barren and dry soil, and also in damp clay soil destitute of chalk. It is seen in old stony, abandoned fields, dried-up lawns and on clearings. In England it is found chiefly on heaths and in mountainous situations, and is also often cultivated as a border in gardens or on rockeries and sunny banks. It was a great favourite of Francis Bacon, who in giving us his plan for the perfect garden, directs that alleys should be planted with fragrant flowers: 'burnet, wild thyme and watermints, which perfume the air most delightfully being trodden upon and crushed,' so that you may 'have pleasure when you walk or tread.'

The herb wherever it grows wild denotes a pure atmosphere, and was thought to enliven the spirits by the fragrance which it diffuses into the air around. The Romans gave Thyme as a sovereign remedy to melancholy persons.

Wild Thyme is a perennial, more thickset than the Garden Thyme, though subject to many varieties, according to the surroundings in which it grows. In its most natural state, when found on dry exposed downs, it is small and procumbent, often forming dense cushions; when growing among furze or other plants which afford it shelter, it runs up a slender stalk to a foot or more in height, which gives it a totally different appearance. The specific name, *serpyllum*, is derived from a Greek word meaning to creep, and has been given it from its usually procumbent and trailing habit.

¶ *Description.* The root is woody and fibrous, the stems numerous, hard, branched, procumbent, rising from 4 inches to 1 foot high, ordinarily reddish-brown in colour. The bright green oval leaves ⅛ inch broad, tapering below into very short foot-stalks, are smooth and beset with numerous small glands. They are fringed with hairs towards the base and have the veins prominent on the under surfaces. Their margins are entire and not recurved as in Garden Thyme. As with all other members of the important order Labiatæ, to which the Thymes belong, the leaves are set in pairs on the stem. The plant flowers from the end of May or early June to the beginning of autumn, the flowers, which are very similar to those of the Garden Thyme, being purplish and in whorls at the top of the stems.

Bees are especially fond of the Thyme blossoms, from which they extract much honey. Spenser speaks of the 'bees-alluring time,' and everyone is familiar with Shakespeare's the 'bank whereon the wild thyme blows,' the abode of the queen of the Fairies. It was looked upon as one of the fairies'

flowers, tufts of Thyme forming one of their favourite playgrounds.

In some parts it was a custom for girls to wear sprigs of Thyme, with mint and lavender, to bring them sweethearts!

Thyme has also been associated with death. It is one of the fragrant flowers planted on graves (in Wales, particularly), and the Order of Oddfellows still carry sprigs of Thyme at funerals and throw them into the grave of a dead brother. An old tradition says that Thyme was one of the herbs that formed the fragrant bed of the Virgin Mary.

Wild Thyme is the badge of the Drummond clan.

¶ *Cultivation.* Wild Thyme will grow on any soil, but prefers light, sandy or gravel ground exposed to the sun.

Propagate by seeds, cuttings, or division of roots. Care must be taken to weed. Manure with farmyard manure in autumn or winter and nitrates in spring.

Cut when in full flower, in July and August, and dry in the same manner as Common Thyme.

It is much picked in France, chiefly in the fields of the Aisne, for the extraction of its essential oil.

¶ *Constituents.* When distilled, 100 kilos (about 225 lb.) of dried material yield 150 grams of essence (about 5 or 6 oz.). It is a yellow liquid, with a weaker scent than that of oil of Thyme extracted from *T. vulgaris*, and is called oil of Serpolet. It contains 30 to 70 per cent. of phenols: Thymol, Carvacrol, etc. It is made into an artificial oil, together with the oil of Common Thyme. In perfumery, oil of Serpolet is chiefly used for soap.

The flowering tops, macerated for 24 hours or so in salt and water, are made into a perfumed water.

¶ *Medicinal Action and Uses.* In medicine, Wild Thyme or Serpolet has the same properties as Common Thyme, but to an inferior degree. It is aromatic, antiseptic, stimulant, antispasmodic, diuretic and emmenagogue.

The infusion is used for chest maladies and for weak digestion, being a good remedy for flatulence, and favourable results have been obtained in convulsive coughs, especially in whooping cough, catarrh and sore throat. The infusion, prepared with 1 oz. of the dried herb to a pint of boiling water, is usually sweetened with sugar or honey and made demulcent by linseed or acacia. It is given in doses of 1 or more tablespoonfuls several times daily.

The infusion is also useful in cases of drunkenness, and Culpepper recommends it as a certain remedy taken on going to bed for 'that troublesome complaint the nightmare,' and says: 'if you make a vinegar of the herb as vinegar of roses is made and annoint the head with it, it presently stops the pains thereof. It is very good to be given either in phrenzy or lethargy.'

Wild Thyme Tea, either drunk by itself or mixed with other plants such as rosemary, etc., is an excellent remedy for headache and other nervous affections.

Formerly several preparations of this plant were kept in shops, and a distilled spirit and water, which were both very fragrant.

TIGER LILY. *See* LILY

TOADFLAX

Linaria vulgaris (MILL.)
N.O. Scrophulariaceæ

Synonyms. Fluellin. Pattens and Clogs. Flaxweed. Ramsted. Snapdragon. Churnstaff. Dragon-bushes. Brideweed. Toad. Yellow Rod. Larkspur Lion's Mouth. Devils' Ribbon. Eggs and Collops. Devil's Head. Pedlar's Basket. Gallwort. Rabbits. Doggies. Calves' Snout. Eggs and Bacon. Buttered Haycocks. Monkey Flower

Part Used. Herb

Habitat. The genus *Linaria*, to which it belongs, contains 125 species, native to the Northern Hemisphere and South America, seven of which are found in England

The Toadflax grows wild in most parts of Europe, on dry banks, by the wayside, in meadows by hedge sides, and upon the borders of fields. It is common throughout England and Wales, though less frequent in Ireland. In Scotland, it is found, as a rule, only in the southern counties. Having been introduced into North America, probably originally with grain, it has become there a troublesome weed. It is especially abundant in sandy and gravelly soil and in chalk and limestone districts.

¶ *Description.* From a perennial and creeping root, the Toadflax sends up several slender stems, erect and not much branched, generally between 1 and 2 feet long, bearing numerous leaves, which are very long and narrow in form. Both stems and leaves are glaucous, i.e. of a pale bluish tint of green, and are quite destitute of hairs.

The stems terminate in rather dense spikes of showy yellow flowers, the corolla in general shape like that of the Snapdragon, but with a long spur, and with the lower lip orange. The Toadflax flowers throughout the summer, from late June to October.

The mouth of the flower is completely closed and never opens until a bee forces its entrance. The only visitors are the large bees – the humble-bee, honey-bee, and several wild bees – which are able to open the flower, and whose tongues are long enough to reach the nectar, which is so placed in the spur that only long-lipped insects can reach it. The closing of the swollen lower lip excludes beetles from the spur. When the bee alights on the orange palate, the colour of which is specially designed to attract the desired visitor, acting as a honey-guide, it falls a little, disclosing the interior of the flower, which forms a little cave, on the floor of which are two ridges of orange hairs, a track between them leading straight to the mouth of the long, hollow spur. Above this is the egg-shaped seed-vessel with the stamens. Between the bases of the two longer stamen filaments, nectar trickles down along a groove to the spur, from the base of the ovary where it is secreted. The bee pushes into the flower, its head fitting well into the cavity below the seed-vessel and thrusting its proboscis down the spur, sucks the nectar, its back being meanwhile well coated by the pollen from the stamens, which run along the roof, the stigma being between the short and long stamens. It is reckoned that a humble-bee can easily take the nectar from ten flowers in a minute, each time transferring pollen from a previous flower to the stigma of the one visited, and thus effecting cross-fertilization.

The Toadflax is very prolific. Its fruit is a little rounded, dry capsule, which when ripe, opens at its top by several valves, the many minute seeds being thrown out by the swaying of the stems. The seeds are flattened and lie in the centre of a circular wing, which, tiny as it is, helps to convey the seed some distance from the parent plant.

Sometimes a curiously-shaped Toadflax blossom will be found: instead of only one spur being produced, each of the five petals whose union builds up the toad-like corolla forms one, and the flower becomes of regular, though almost unrecognizable shape. This phenomenon is termed by botanists, 'peloria,' i.e. a monster. As a rule it is the terminal flower that is thus symmetrical in structure, but sometimes flowers of this type occur all down the spike.

The name Toadflax originated in the resemblance of the flower to little toads, there being also a resemblance between the mouth of the flower and the wide mouth of a toad. Coles says that the plant was called Toadflax, 'because Toads will sometimes shelter themselves amongst the branches of it.'

The general resemblance of the plant in early summer to a Flax plant, accounts for the latter part of its name, and also for another of its country names, 'Flaxweed.' The Latin name, *Linaria*, from *linum* (flax), was given it by Linnæus, from this likeness to a flax plant before flowering. The mixture of light yellow and orange in the flowers has gained for it the provincial names of 'Butter and Eggs,' 'Eggs and Bacon,' etc.

Gerard says:

'Linaria being a kind of Antyrrhinum, hath small, slender, blackish stalks, from which do grow many long, narrow leaves like flax. The floures be yellow with a spurre hanging at the same like unto a Larkesspurre, having a mouth like unto a frog's mouth, even such as is to be seene in the common Snapdragon; the whole plant so much resembleth Esula minor, that the one is hardly knowne from the other but by this olde verse: "Esula lactescit, sine lacte Linaria crescit."

' "Esula with milke doth flow,
Toadflax without milke doth grow." '

This *Esula* is one of the smaller spurge, *Euphorbia esula*, which before flowering so closely resembles Toadflax that care must be taken not to collect it in error; the milky juice contained in its stems (as in all the Spurges) will, however, at once reveal its identity.

The leaves of the Toadflax also contain an acrid, rather disagreeable, but not *milky* juice, which renders them distasteful to cattle, who leave them untouched. Among the many old local names given to this plant we find it called 'Gallwort,' on account of its bitterness, one old writer affirming that it received the name because an infusion of the leaves was used 'against the flowing of the gall in cattell.' The larvæ of several moths feed on the plant, and several beetles are also found on it.

¶ *Part Used Medicinally. Cultivation.* For medicinal purposes, Toadflax is generally gathered in the wild condition, but it can be cultivated with ease, though it prefers a dry soil. No manure is needed. Seeds may be sown in spring. All the culture needed is to thin out the seedlings and keep them free of weeds. Propagation may also be carried out by division of roots in the autumn.

The whole herb is gathered just when coming into flower and employed either fresh or dried.

When fresh, Toadflax has a peculiar, heavy, disagreeable odour, which is in great measure dissipated by drying. It has a weakly saline, bitter and slightly acrid taste.

¶ *Constituents.* Toadflax abounds in an acrid oil, reputed to be poisonous, but no harm from it has ever been recorded. Little or nothing is known of its toxic principle, but its use in medicine was well known to the ancients.

Its constituents are stated to be two glucosides, Linarin and Pectolinarian, with linarosin, linaracin, antirrhinic, tannic and citric acids, a yellow colouring matter, mucilage and sugar.

¶ *Medicinal Action and Uses.* Astringent, hepatic and detergent. It has some powerful qualities as a purgative and diuretic, causing it to be recommended in jaundice, liver, skin diseases and scrofula; an infusion of 1 oz. to the pint has been found serviceable as an alterative in these cases and in incipient dropsy. The infusion has a bitter and unpleasant taste, occasioned by the presence of the acrid essential oil. It was at one time in great reputation among herb doctors for dropsy. The herb distilled answers the same purpose, as a decoction of both leaves and flowers in removing obstructions of the liver. It is very effectual if a little Peruvian bark or solution of quinine and a little cinnamon be combined with it. Gerard informs us that 'the decoction openeth the stopping of the liver and spleen, and is singular good against the jaundice which is of long continuance,' and further states that 'a decoction of Toadflax taketh away the yellownesse and deformitie of the skinne, being washed and bathed therewith.'

The fresh plant is sometimes applied as a poultice or fomentation to hæmorrhoids, and an ointment of the flowers has been employed for the same purpose, and also locally in diseases of the skin. A cooling ointment is made from the fresh plant – the whole herb is chopped and boiled in lard till crisp, then strained. The result is a fine green ointment, a good application for piles, sores, ulcers and skin eruptions.

The juice of the herb, or the distilled water, has been considered a good remedy for inflammation of the eyes, and for cleansing ulcerous sores.

Boiled in milk, the plant is said to yield an excellent fly poison, and it is an old country custom in parts of Sweden to infuse Toadflax flowers in milk, and stand the infusion about where flies are troublesome.

The flowers have been employed in Germany as a yellow dye.

TOADFLAX, IVY-LEAVED

Linaria Cymbalaria
N.O. Scrophulariaceæ

Synonyms. Ivywort. Aaron's Beard. Climbing Sailor. Creeping Jenny. Mother of Millions. Mother of Thousands. Thousand Flower. Oxford-weed. Pedlar's Basket. Pennywort. Rabbits. Roving Jenny. Wandering Jew
Part Used. Herb

Ivy-leaved Toadflax (Mill.) (*Linaria Cymbalaria*). This little trailing plant, with ivy-like leaves and small lilac flowers, was not originally a British plant, but a native of the Mediterranean region, but it has become naturalized over almost the whole of Europe, from Holland southwards, except in Turkey, and is now thoroughly at home in England, having first been introduced into the Chelsea Botanic Gardens from Italy.

It is mostly found near houses, on old garden walls, where it hangs down from the interstices between the stones, the roots being thin and fibrous, and finding their way into crevices. The stems are purple in colour and very numerous, slender and stringy, rooting at intervals and very long, growing to a length of 2 or 3 feet.

¶ *Description.* The ivy-like leaves, somewhat thick in texture, and smooth, are cut up into five prominent, rounded lobes or divisions, and are on long stalks. The backs of the leaves are of a reddish-purple. The flower-stalks, about equal in length to the leaf-stalks, arise singly from the axils of the leaves and bear small flowers similar in form to those of the common Toadflax, of a delicate lilac colour, the palate being bright yellow and each blossom ending in a spur, which in this case is only as long as the calyx. Before fertilization each flower pushes itself out into the light and sun, standing erect, but when the seeds are mature, it bends downward, buries the capsule in the dark crannies between the stones on which it grows, the seeds being thus dispersed by direct action of the plant itself.

This little Toadflax is in flower from May right up to November, and is visited only by bees. It has become a favourite garden flower for planting on rockeries.

Gerard illustrates the plant in his *Herbal*, springing from brickwork, but the block of his illustration was incorrectly placed upside down, so that the plant instead of being represented as growing downwards, stands erect. Parkinson, in 1640, also figures this plant in the same way, and names it *Cymbalaria hederacea*.

In Italy it is the 'plant of the Madonna.'

¶ *Medicinal Action and Uses.* The Ivy-leaved Toadflax has anti-scorbutic properties, and has been eaten as a salad in southern Europe, being acrid and pungent like Cress.

It is reported to have been successfully administered in India for diabetes.

The flowers yield a clear but not permanent yellow dye.

TOBACCO

Nicotiana Tabacum (LINN.)
N.O. Solanaceæ

Synonyms. Tabacca. Tabaci Folia (B.P.C.)
Part Used. Leaves, cured and dried
Habitat. Virginia, America; and cultivated with other species in China, Turkey, Greece, Holland, France, Germany and most sub-tropical countries

¶ *Description.* The genus derives its name from Joan Nicot, a Portuguese who introduced the Tobacco plant into France. The specific name being derived from the Haitian word for the pipe in which the herb is smoked. Tobacco is an annual, with a long fibrous root, stem erect, round, hairy, and viscid; it branches near the top and is from 3 to 6 feet high. Leaves large, numerous, alternate, sessile, somewhat decurrent, ovate, lanceolate, pointed, entire, slightly viscid and hairy, pale-green colour, brittle, narcotic odour, with a nauseous, bitter acrid taste. Nicotine is a volatile oil, inflammable, powerfully alkaline, with an acrid smell and a burning taste. By distillation with water it yields a concrete volatile oil termed nicotianin or Tobacco camphor, which is tasteless, crystalline, and smells of Tobacco; other constituents are albumen, resin, gum, and inorganic matters.

¶ *Constituents.* The most important constituent is the alkaloid Nicotine, nicotianin, nicotinine, nicoteline. After leaves are smoked the nicotine decomposes into pyridine, furfurol, collidine, hydrocyanic acid, carbon-monoxide, etc. The poisonous effects of Tobacco smoke are due to these substances of decomposed nicotine.

¶ *Medicinal Action and Uses.* A local irritant; if used as snuff it causes violent sneezing, also a copious secretion of mucous; chewed, it increases the flow of saliva by

817

irritating the mucous membrane of the mouth; injected into the rectum it acts as a cathartic. In large doses it produces nausea, vomiting, sweats and great muscular weakness.

The alkaloid nicotine is a virulent poison, producing great disturbance in the digestive and circulatory organs. It innervates the heart, causing palpitation and cardiac irregularities and vascular contraction, and is considered one of the causes of arterial degeneration.

Nicotine is very like coniine and lobeline in its pharmacological action, and the pyridines in the smoke modify very slightly its action.

Tobacco was once used as a relaxant, but is no longer employed except occasionally in chronic asthma. Its active principle is readily absorbed by the skin, and serious, even fatal, poisoning, from a too free application of it to the surface of the skin has resulted.

The smoke acts on the brain, causing nausea, vomiting and drowsiness.

Medicinally it is used as a sedative, diuretic, expectorant, discutient, and sialagogue, and internally only as an emetic, when all other emetics fail. The smoke injected into the rectum or the leaf rolled into a suppository has been beneficial in strangulated hernia, also for obstinate constipation, due to spasm of the bowels, also for retention of urine, spasmodic urethral stricture, hysterical convulsions, worms, and in spasms caused by lead, for croup, and inflammation of the peritoneum, to produce evacuation of the bowels, moderating reaction and dispelling tympanitis, and also in tetanus. To inject the smoke it should be blown into milk and injected; for croup and spasms of the rima glottides it is made into a plaster with Scotch snuff and lard and applied to throat and breast, and has proved very effectual. A cataplasm of the leaves may be used as an ointment for cutaneous diseases. The leaves in combination with the leaves of belladonna or stramonium make an excellent application for obstinate ulcers, painful tremors and spasmodic affections. A wet Tobacco leaf applied to piles is a certain cure. The inspissated juice cures facial neuralgia if rubbed along the tracks of the affected nerve. The quantity of the injection must never exceed a scruple to begin with; half a drachm has been known to produce amaurosis and other eye affections, deafness, etc.

The Tobacco plant was introduced into England by Sir Walter Raleigh and his friends in 1586, and at first met with violent opposition.

Kings prohibited it, Popes pronounced against it in Bulls, and in the East Sultans condemned Tobacco smokers to cruel deaths. Three hundred years later, in 1885, the leaves were official in the British Pharmacopœia.

Externally nicotine is an antiseptic. It is eliminated partly by the lungs, but chiefly in the urine, the secretion of which it increases. Formerly Tobacco in the form of an enema of the leaves was used to relax muscular spasms, to facilitate the reduction of dislocations.

A pipe smoked after breakfast assists the action of the bowels.

The pituri plant contains an alkaloid, Pitarine, similar to nicotine, and the leaves are used in Australia instead of Tobacco. An infusion of Tobacco is generally used in horticulture as an insecticide.

In cases of nicotine poisoning, the stomach should be quickly emptied, and repeated doses of tannic acid given, the person kept very warm in bed, and stimulants such as caffeine, strychnine, or atropine given, or if there are signs of respiratory failure, oxygen must be given at once.

¶ *Other Species.*

Tobacco (*Nicotiana rustica*). Turkish Tobacco is grown in all parts of the globe.

N. quadrivalis, affording Tobacco to the Indians of the Missouri and Columbia Rivers, has, as the name implies, four-valved capsules.

N. fruticosa – habitat, China – is a very handsome plant and differs from the other varieties in its sharp-pointed capsules.

N. persica. Cultivated in Persia; is the source of Persian Tobacco.

N. repandu. Cultivated in Central and southern North America. Havannah is used in the manufacture of the best cigars.

Latakria Tobacco (syn. *N. Tabacum*) is the only species cultivated in Cuba.

N. latissima yields the Tobacco known as Orinoco.

N. multivulvis has several valved capsules.

TOLU BALSAM. *See* BALSAM

TONKA BEANS. *See* TONQUIN

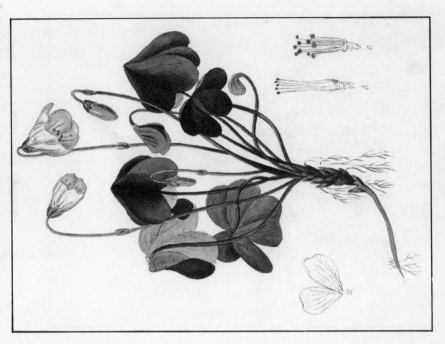
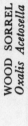

WOOD SORREL
Oxalis Acetosella

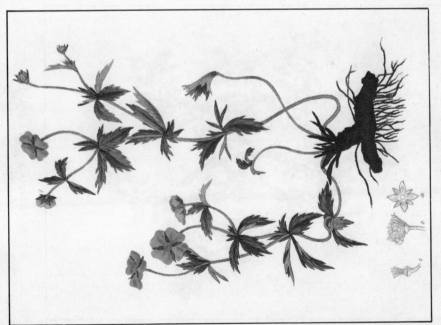

TORMENTIL
Potentilla Tormentilla

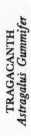

TRAGACANTH
Astragalus Gummifer

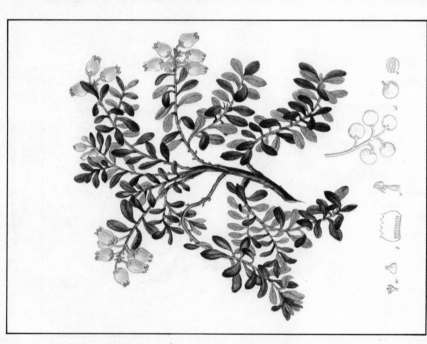

BEARBERRY (UVA-URSI)
Arbutus Uva-Ursi

TONQUIN BEAN

Dipteryx odorata (WILLD.)
N.O. Leguminosæ

Synonyms. Tonka Bean. Coumarouna odorata
Part Used. Seeds
Habitat. A forest tree native to Brazil and British Guiana and called there 'Rumara'

¶ *Description.* The odour of coumarin, which distinguishes the Tonka Bean, is found in many plants, especially in Melilotus, sweet vernal grass, and related grasses.

One pound of the beans has yielded 108 grains of coumarin, which is the anhydride of coumaric acid. In addition to its use in perfumery as a fixative, coumarin is used to flavour castor-oil and to disguise the odour of iodoform.

The fatty substance of the beans is sold in Holland as *Tonquin butter.*

¶ *Medicinal Action and Uses.* Aromatic, cardiac, tonic, narcotic. The fluid extract has been used with advantage in whooping cough, but it paralyses the heart if used in large doses.

¶ *Dosage.* For children of five years' old, 5 to 8 grains.

TORMENTIL

Potentilla Tormentilla (NECK.)
N.O. Rosaceæ

Synonyms. Septfoil. Thormantle. Biscuits. Bloodroot. Earthbank. Ewe Daisy. Five Fingers. Flesh and Blood. Shepherd's Knapperty. Shepherd's Knot. English Sarsaparilla
Parts Used. Root, herb

In *Potentilla Tormentilla* the flowers are yellow as in *P. reptans,* but smaller, and have four petals instead of five, and eight sepals, not ten, so separated as to form a Maltese cross when regarded from above.

From the root-stock come leaves on long stalks, divided into three or five oval leaflets (occasionally, but rarely, seven, hence the names Septfoil and Seven Leaves), toothed towards their tips. The stem-leaves, in this species, are stalkless with three leaflets.

A small-flowered form is very frequent on heaths and in dry pastures, a larger-flowered, in which the slender stems do not rise, but trail on the ground, is more general in woods, and on hedge-banks. From the ascending form, 6 to 12 inches high, this species has been called *P. erecta,* but even in this case the long stems are more often creeping and ascending rather than actually erect.

The name Tormentil is said to be derived from the Latin *tormentum,* which signifies such gripings of the intestines as the herb will serve to relieve, likewise the twinges of toothache.

The plant is very astringent, and has been used in some places for tanning.

It has been official in various Pharmacopœias and was formerly in the Secondary List of the United States Pharmacopœia.

It is considered one of the safest and most powerful of our native aromatic astringents, and for its tonic properties has been termed 'English Sarsaparilla.'

All parts of the plant are astringent, especially the red, woody rhizome.

The rhizome is 1 to 2 inches long, as thick as the finger, or smaller, tapering to one end,

usually with one to three short branches near the larger end, ridged, with several strong, longitudinal wrinkles between them, bearing numerous blunt indentations. It is brown or blackish externally; internally, light brownish red; the fracture short and somewhat resinous, showing a thin bark, one or two circles of small, yellowish wood-wedges, broad medullary rays and a large pith. It has a peculiar faint, slightly aromatic odour and a strongly astringent taste.

¶ *Chemical Constituents.* It contains 18 to 30 per cent. of tannin, 18 per cent. of a red colouring principle – Tormentil Red, a product of the tannin and yielding with potassium hydroxide, protocatechuic acid and phloroglucin. It is soluble in alcohol, but insoluble in water. Also some resin and ellagic and kinovic acids have been reported.

¶ *Medicinal Action and Uses.* There is a great demand for the rhizome, which in modern herbal medicine is used extensively as an astringent in diarrhœa and other discharges, operating without producing any stimulant effects. It also imparts nourishment and support to the bowels.

It is employed as a gargle in sore, relaxed and ulcerated throat and also as an injection in leucorrhœa.

It may be given in substance, decoction or extract. The dose of the powdered root or fluid extract is ½ to 1 drachm.

The fluid extract acts as a styptic to cuts, wounds, etc.

A strongly-made decoction is recommended as a good wash for piles and inflamed eyes. The decoction is made by boiling 2 oz. of the bruised root in 50 oz. of water till it is reduced one-third. It is then strained and taken in doses of $1\frac{1}{2}$ oz. It may be used as an astringent gargle.

If a piece of lint be soaked in the decoction and kept applied to warts, they will disappear.

The decoction for internal use should be made with 4 drachms to $\frac{1}{2}$ pint of water, boiled for 10 minutes, adding $\frac{1}{2}$ drachm of cinnamon stick at the end of boiling. Dose, 1 or 2 tablespoonsful.

Compound Powder of Tormentil. (A very reliable medicine in diarrhœa and dysentery.) Powdered Tormentil, 1 oz; Powdered Galangal, 1 oz.; Powdered Marshmallow root, 1 oz.; Powdered Ginger, 4 drachms.

An infusion is made of the powdered ingredients by pouring 1 pint of boiling water upon them, allowing to cool and then straining the liquid. Dose, 1 or 2 fluid drachms, every 15 minutes, till the pain is relieved – then take three or four times a day.

A *simple infusion* is made by scalding 1 oz. of the powdered Tormentil with 1 pint of water and taking as required in wineglassful doses for chronic diarrhœa, fluxes, etc.

A continental recipe for an astringent decoction is equal parts of Tormentilla, Bistort and Pomegranate.

Dr. Thornton declared that in fluxes of blood, 1 drachm of Tormentil given four times a day in an infusion of Hops did wonders.

Thornton tells of a poor old man who made wonderful cures of ague, smallpox, whooping cough, etc., from an infusion of this herb and became so celebrated locally that Lord William Russell gave him a piece of ground in which to cultivate it, which he did, keeping it a secret for long.

It was much given for cholera, and also sometimes in intermittent fevers, and used in a lotion for ulcers and long-standing sores. The juice of the fresh root, or the powder of the dried, was used in compounding ointments and plasters for application to wounds and sores.

The fresh root, bruised, and applied to the throat and jaws was held to heal the King's Evil.

Culpepper says:

'Tormentil is most excellent to stay all fluxes of blood or humours, whether at nose, mouth or belly. The juice of the herb and root, or the decoction thereof, taken with some Venice treacle and the person laid to sweat, expels any venom or poison, or the plague, fever or other contagious disease, as the pox, measles, etc., for it is an ingredient in all antidotes or counterpoisons.' . . . 'It resisteth putrefaction.' . . . 'The root taken inwardly is most effectual to help any flux of the belly, stomach, spleen or blood and the juice wonderfully opens obstructions of the spleen and lungs and cureth yellow jaundice. Tormentil is no less effectual and powerful a remedy against outward wounds, sores and hurts than for inward and is therefore a special ingredient to be used in wound drinks, lotions and injections. . . . It is also effectual for the piles. . . . The juice or powder of the root, put into ointments, plasters and such things that are applied to wounds or sores is very effectual.'

In the Western Isles of Scotland and in the Orkneys the roots were used for tanning leather and considered superior even to oak bark, being first boiled in water and the leather steeped in the cold liquor. The Laplanders employed the thickened red juice of the root for staining leather red.

The Americans use the name Tormentil for *Geranium maculatum*, the Spotted Cranesbill, which has similar properties.

Many other of the 150 species of Potentilla have been similarly used in medicine.

See FIVE-LEAF GRASS, SILVERWEED, CINQUEFOILS.

TRAGACANTH

Astragalus gummifer (LABILL.)
N.O. Leguminosæ

Synonyms. Gum Tragacanth. Syrian Tragacanth. Gum Dragon (known in commerce as Syrian Tragacanth)
Part Used. Gummy exudation
Habitat. Asia Minor, Persia and Kurdistan

¶ *Description.* The plant is a small branching thorny shrub, the stem of which exudes a gum, vertical slits giving flat ribbon-shaped pieces and punctures giving tears; these have a horny appearance, are nearly colourless or faintly yellow, marked with numerous concentric ridges; the flakes break with a short fracture, are odourless and nearly tasteless; soaked in cold water, they swell and form a gelatinous mass 8 or 10 per cent. only dissolving.

¶ *Constituents.* The portion soluble in water contains chiefly polyarabinan-trigalætangeddic acid; the insoluble part is called bassorin. Tragacanth also contains water, traces of starch, cellulose, and nitrogenous substances, yielding about 3 per cent. ash.

¶ *Medicinal Action and Uses.* Demulcent, but owing to its incomplete solubility is not often used internally. It is much used for the suspension of heavy, insoluble powders to impart consistence to lozenges, being superior to gum arabic, also in making emulsions, mucilago, etc. Mucil-age of Tragacanth has been used as an application to burns; it is also employed by manufacturers for stiffening calico, crape, etc.

Mucilage, B.P. and U.S.P. Comp. Powder, B.P., 20 to 60 grains.

¶ *Adulterants.* The Indian gum, the product of *Coplospermum gossypium*, also acacia, dextrin wheat and corn starch.

TRAVELLERS' JOY. *See* CLEMATIS

TREE OF HEAVEN
Ailanthus glandulosa (DESF.)
N.O. Simarubeæ

Synonyms. Chinese Sumach. Vernis de Japon. Ailanto. (Trans. as Tree of the Gods. – Götterbaum.)

Parts Used. Inner bark of tree, root

Habitat. China and India. Cultivated throughout Europe and the United States

¶ *Description.* A large, handsome tree of rapid growth, bearing leaves from 1 to 2 feet long, and greenish flowers of a disagreeable odour. Was introduced into England in 1751 and is frequently found in gardens as a shade tree.

The *Ailanthus imberiflora* occurs in Australia, and in India the *A. excelsa* has a bark used as a bitter tonic.

In France it is cultivated for its leaves, on which the caterpillar of the silk-spinning Ailanthus Moth (*Bombyx Cynthia*) is fed, yielding a silk more durable and cheaper than Mulberry silk, though inferior to it in fineness and gloss. Its name of Japan Varnish shows that it was mistaken for the true Japanese Varnish Tree, a species of Sumach. At one time it was classed as a Rhus.

The wood is satiny, yellowish-white, and well suited for cabinet-making when climates permit of adequate growth.

The bark has a nauseating, bitter taste, and, when fresh, a sickening odour.

The leaves have been found in commerce adulterated with those of senna.

¶ *Constituents.* Lignin, chlorophyll, a yellow colouring matter, a gelatinous substance (pectin), quassin, an odorous resin, traces of a volatile oil, a nitrogenous, fatty matter, and several salts. A later analysis found starch, tannin, albumen, gum, sugar, oleoresin, and a trace of volatile oil, potash, phosphoric acid, sulphuric acid, iron, lime, and magnesia.

All the characteristic properties of either the fresh or carefully dried bark can be exhausted by alcohol, to which a deep, green colour will be imparted, changing to yellowish-brown with age and more quickly if exposed to air.

¶ *Medicinal Action and Uses.* Antispasmodic, cardiac depressant, astringent. The effect produced by Hetet when experimenting on dogs, was copious stools and the discharge of worms. The resin purges, but rarely acts as an anthelmintic. In China the bark is popular for dysentery and other bowel complaints. A smaller dose of the oleoresin produces similar results, and keeps better than the bark.

The vapours of the evaporating extract have a prostrating effect, as have the emanations from the blossoms, while the action upon patients of powder or extract is disagreeable and nauseating, though they have been successfully used in dysentery and diarrhœa, gonorrhœa, leucorrhœa, prolapsus ani, etc., and also as a tænifuge.

The infusion may be given in sweetened orange-flower or other aromatic water, to lessen the bitterness and resultant sickness. Though it produces vomiting and great relaxation, it is stated not to be poisonous.

A tincture of the root-bark has been used successfully in cardiac palpitation, asthma and epilepsy.

The action of the trees in malarial districts is considered to resemble that of the Eucalyptus.

The statement that the resin is purgative has been disputed, some asserting that it is inert.

¶ *Dosages.* From 7 to 20 grains. Of the tincture, 5 to 60 drops from two to four times a day. Of the infusion, a teaspoonful, night and morning, cold. (50 grams of the root-bark infused for a short time in 75 grams of hot water, then strained.)

TURKEY CORN

Dicentra Canadensis (D.C.)
N.O. Fumariaceæ

Synonyms. Turkey Pea. Squirrel Corn. Staggerweed. Bleeding Heart. Shone Corydalis. Corydalis. Corydalis Canadensis (Goldie). Bicuculla Canadensis (Millsp.)
Part Used. Dried tubers
Habitat. Westward and south of New York to North Carolina

¶ *Description.* This plant is essentially indigenous to America, a perennial 6 to 10 inches high, with a tuberous root, flowering in early spring (often in March) having from six to nineteen nodding, greenish-white, purple-tinged flowers, the root or tuber small and round. It should be collected only when the plant is in flower. It grows in rich soil on hills and mountains. The tubers are tawny yellow-coloured, the colour being a distinctive character. The plant must not be confounded with *Corydalis (Dicentra) Cuccularia* (Dutchman's Breeches), which flowers at the same time and very much resembles it (though smaller), except in the root, the rind of which is black with a white inside, and when dried, turns brownish-yellow, and under the microscope is full of pores. It has also a peculiar faint odour, the taste at first slightly bitter, then followed by a penetrating taste, which influences the bowels and increases the saliva; the differences in the colour after drying may be caused by the age of the root. Under the miscroscope, it is porous, spongy, resinous, with a glistening fracture. Another *Corydalis* also somewhat like Turkey Corn is *C. Formosa*, the fresh root of which is darkish yellow throughout and has a fracture much resembling honeycomb. The true Turkey Corn is much used by American eclectic practitioners. It is slightly bitter in taste and almost odourless. Tannic acid and all vegetable astringents are incompatible with preparations containing Turkey Corn, or with its alkaloid, Corydalin.
¶ *Constituents.* The amount of alkaloids in the dried tubers is about 5 per cent.; they have been found to contain corydalin, fumaric acid, yellow bitter extractive, an acrid resin and starch. The constituents of the drug have not been exactly determined, but several species of the closely allied genus *Corydalis* have been carefully studied and *C.*

tuberosa, cava and *bulbosa* have been found to yield the following alkaloids: Corycavine, Bulbocapnine and Corydine; Corydaline is a tertiary base, Corycavine is a difficult soluble base; Bulbocapnine is present in largest amount and was originally called Corydaline. Corydine is a strong base found in the mother liquor of Bulbocapnine and several amorphous unnamed bases have been found in it. All these alkaloids have narcotic action. Protopine, first isolated from opium, has been found in several species of *Dicentra* and in *C. vernyi, ambigua* and *tuberosa.*
¶ *Medicinal Action and Uses.* Tonic, diuretic and alterative; useful in chronic cutaneous affections, syphilis and scrofula and in some menstrual complaints. The corydalin sold by druggists is often impure.

Turkey Corn is often combined with other remedies, such as Stillingia, Burdock or Prickly Ash.
¶ *Dosages.* An infusion is prepared of 5 grams of the powdered Corydalin in 100 c.c. of hot distilled water stirred for 10 minutes and then filtered. This gives a light amber fluid and a precipitate with mercuric-potassium iodide T.S. and a dark blue colour with Iodine T.S.

Infusion, $\frac{1}{2}$ oz. in 1 pint of boiling water, in wineglassful doses three or four times daily. Fluid extract, $\frac{1}{2}$ to 1 drachm. Corydalin, in $\frac{1}{2}$ grains, three or four times daily. Saturated tincture, $\frac{1}{2}$ drachm to 2 fluid drachms.
¶ *Other Species.*
Dicentra pusilla (Sieb et Zuce), of Japan, is there popularly used for dysentery.

C. ambigua, used by the Chinese in medicine. A number of the same alkaloids are found in it and others closely allied.

As commonly understood in medicine, the name Corydalis applies to the tubers of Turkey Corn, but several others of the genus *Dicentra* and *Corydalis* are used.

TURMERIC

Curcuma longa (LINN.)
N.O. Zingiberaceæ

Synonyms. Curcuma. Curcuma rotunda (LINN.). Amomum curcuma (Jacq.)
Part Used. Dried rhizome
Habitat. Southern Asia. Cultivated in China, Bengal and Java

¶ *Description.* A perennial plant with roots or tubers oblong, palmate, and deep orange inside; root-leaves about 2 feet long, lanceolate, long, petioled, tapering at each end, smooth, of a uniform green; petioles

sheathing spike, erect, central, oblong, green; flowers dull yellow, three or five together surrounded by bracteolæ. It is propagated by cuttings from the root, which when dry is in curved cylindrical or oblong

822

tubers 2 or 3 inches in length, and an inch in diameter, pointed or tapering at one end, yellowish externally, with transverse, parallel rings internally deep orange or reddish brown, marked with shining points, dense, solid, short, granular fracture, forming a lemon yellow powder. It has a peculiar fragrant odour and a bitterish, slightly acrid taste, like ginger, exciting warmth in the mouth and colouring the saliva yellow. It yields its properties to water or alcohol.

¶ *Constituents.* An acrid, volatile oil, brown colouring matter, gum, starch, chloride of calcium, woody fibre and a yellowish colouring matter named curcumin; this is obtained by digesting tumeric in boiling alcohol,

filtering and evaporating the solution to dryness, the residue being digested in ether, filtered and evaporated.

¶ *Medicinal Action and Uses.* Tumeric is a mild aromatic stimulant seldom used in medicine except as a colouring. It was once a cure for jaundice. Its chief use is in the manufacture of curry powders. It is also used as an adulterant of mustard and a substitute for it and forms one of the ingredients of many cattle condiments. Tincture of Turmeric is used as a colouring agent, but the odour is fugitive. It dyes a rich yellow. Turmeric paper is prepared by soaking unglazed white paper in the tincture and then drying. Used as a test for alkaloids and boric acid.

TURPETH

Ipomœa Turpethum
N.O. Convolvulaceæ

Synonyms. Turpeth Root. Indian Jalap. Trivrit. Nisoth. Operculina Turpethum
Parts Used. Dried root, stem
Habitat. India. Ceylon, Pacific Islands, China, Australia

¶ *Description.* There are two varieties of this convolvulaceous plant, the Sveta, or White Turpeth, preferred as a mild cathartic, and the black or Kirshna, a powerful drastic. The pieces of root are cylindrical, somewhat twisted, and dull grey outside. The drug has a faint odour, and the taste becomes nauseous after it has been in the mouth for some time, though less so than the true jalap. The genus *Ipomœa* are closely related to the *Batatas.*

¶ *Constituents.* Resin, a fatty substance, volatile oil, albumen, starch, a yellow colouring matter, lignin, salts, and ferric oxide. The root contains 10 per cent. of resin, which is a glucoside, Turpethin, insoluble in ether, but soluble in alcohol, to which it gives a brown colour not removable by animal charcoal. To obtain pure, the alcoholic solution is concentrated; the resin is precipitated by, and afterwards boiled with,

water, then dried, reduced to powder, digested with ether, and finally redissolved by absolute alcohol and deposited by ether. After being treated several times in this way, it is obtained in the state of a brownish resin, yielding on pulverization a grey powder, which irritates the mucous membrane of the nostrils and mouth. It is inflammable, burning with a smoky flame and emitting irritant vapours. With strong bases it acts like jalapin, takes up water, and is transferred into a soluble acid, while with dilute acids it is decomposed into turpetholic acid, and glucose.

¶ *Medicinal Action and Uses.* Cathartic and purgative. It is rather slow in its action, less powerful and less unpleasant than jalap.

¶ *Dosage.* 5 to 20 grains.

See BINDWEED, CONVOLVULUS.

UNICORN ROOT, FALSE

Chamælirium luteum (A. GRAY)
N.O. Liliaceæ

Synonyms. Starwort. Helonias. Helonias dioica (Pursh.). Helonias lutea (Ker-Gawl). Chamælirium Carolinianum (Willd.). Veratrum luteum (Linn.)
Part Used. Root

¶ *Description.* A herbaceous perennial found in low moist ground east of the Mississipi and flowering in May and June. Stem 1 to 3 feet high, simple, smooth, angular; leaves alternate, spatulate below, lanceolate above, radical leaves, 8 inches long, ½ inch wide, narrow at base and formed into a whorl; flowers numerous, small, greenish white, bractless, diœcious, in a dense, terminal raceme, nodding like a plume, 6 inches long,

petals of such flowers narrow, stamens longer than the petals, filaments tapering; anthers terminal, two lobed; petals of female flowers linear; stamens short; ovary ovate, triangular, furrowed; stigmas three-capsule, oblong, three-furrowed, opening at summit; fruit many, compressed, acute; rhizome bulbous, terminating abruptly, 1 inch long; odour faint; taste bitter. Solvents: alcohol, water.

¶ *Constituents.* Chamælirin, fatty acid.

¶ *Medicinal Action and Uses.* Emetic, tonic, diuretic, vermifuge. In large doses a cardiac poison. Of the greatest value in female disorders of the reproductive organs. The indication for its use is a dragging sensation in the extreme lower abdomen. It is useful in impotence, as a tonic in genito-urinary weakness or irritability, for liver and kidney diseases. Especially in diseases due to poor action of the liver and not to weakness of the heart or circulation. It is a good remedy in albuminaria.

¶ *Preparations.* Fluid extract, 5 to 30 drops. Helonin, 2 to 4 grains. Specific helonias, 1 to 20 drops.

UNICORN ROOT, TRUE

Aletris farinosa (LINN.)
N.O. Hæmodoraceæ

Synonyms. Colic-root. Stargrass. Starwort. Star-root. Blazing Star. Ague-root. Aloe-root. Ague Grass. Black-root. Bitter Grass. Crow Corn. Bettie Grass. Devil's Bit
(*French*) Aletris Farinseu
(*German*) Mehlige Aletria
Parts Used. Root, dried rhizome
Habitat. North America. Found at edges of swampy or wet sandy woods, from Florida northward, specially on seashore

¶ *Description.* A low-growing, spreading perennial herb, with tuberous cylindrical, somewhat horizontal root, having many fibres from its lower surface. No stem, leaves lanceolate, acute, ribbed, sessile, or slightly sheathing at base, smooth and flat, pale coloured, thin and coriaceous. Flower-stem simple with remote scales, 1 to 3 feet high, topped with a spiked raceme of short-stalked, white, bell-shaped oblong flowers blooming May to August; the outer surface of these has a mealy frosted appearance. Fruit is an ovate, tapering, coriaceous capsule, enclosed in a persistent envelope. Seeds numerous, ovate, ribbed, albuminous, fleshy, and oily.

In commerce the rhizome is found dried in pieces about 2 inches long and ⅖ inch thick, light brown colour, flattish on upper surface and densely tufted with the remains of the leaves, fracture yellow and slightly fibrous; the roots from the rhizome are wiry about 3 inches long and of a glossy black colour, but when first dried brownish. Taste intensely bitter, peculiar; it loses a great part of its nauseous bitterness with age. Odour very faint.

¶ *Constituents.* The bitter principle in the root has not yet been determined. Its best solvent is alcohol. It contains a large percentage of bitter extractive, colouring matter and resin, and a quantity of starch.

¶ *Medicinal Action and Uses.* The fresh root in large doses is somewhat narcotic, emetic and cathartic; when dried, these properties are lost. In smaller doses it gives colic in hypogastrium, and a sense of stupefaction and vertigo. When dried it becomes a valuable bitter tonic and its tincture or decoction has been used in flatulence, colic, hysteria, and to tone up the stomach; of value in dyspepsia and where there is an absence of urinary phosphates. Its most valuable property is its tonic influence on the female generative organs, proving of great use in cases of habitual miscarriage and as a general tonic. *Extractio Aletridis alcoholicum* is the official preparation.

¶ *Dosages.* The dried powdered root, 5 to 10 grains. Saturated tincture, 5 to 15 drops in water. Fluid extract, ½ to 1 drachm.

UVA URSI. *See* BEARBERRY

VALERIAN

Valeriana officinalis (LINN.)
N.O. Valerianaceæ

Synonyms. Phu (Galen). All-Heal. Great Wild Valerian. Amantilla. Setwall. Setewale Capon's Tail
Part Used. Root
Habitat. Europe and Northern Asia

Two species of Valerian, *Valeriana officinalis* and *V. dioica*, are indigenous in Britain, while a third, *V. pyrenaica*, is naturalized in some parts. The genus comprises about 150 species, which are widely distributed in the temperate parts of the world.

In medicine, the root of *V. officinalis* is intended when Valerian is mentioned. It is supposed to be the *Phu* (an expression of aversion from its offensive odour) of Dioscorides and Galen, by whom it is extolled as an aromatic and diuretic.

It was afterwards found to be useful in

certain kinds of epilepsy. The plant was in such esteem in mediæval times as a remedy, that it received the name of All Heal, which is still given it in some parts of the country.

The plant is found throughout Europe and Northern Asia, and is common in England in marshy thickets and on the borders of ditches and rivers, where its tall stems may generally be seen in the summer towering above the usual herbage, the erect, sturdy growth of the plant, the rich, dark green of the leaves, their beautiful form, and the crowning masses of light-coloured flowers, making the plant conspicuous.

¶ *Description.* The roots tend to merge into a short, conical root-stock or erect rhizome, the development of which often proceeds for several years before a flowering stem is sent up, but slender horizontal branches which terminate in buds are given off earlier, and from these buds proceed aerial shoots or stolons, which produce fresh plants where they take root. Only one stem arises from the root, which attains a height of 3 or 4 feet. It is round, but grooved and hollow, more or less hairy, especially near the base. It terminates in two or more pairs of flowering stems, each pair being placed at right angles to those above and below it. The lower flowering stems lengthen so as to place their flowers nearly or often quite on a level with the flowers borne by the upper branches, forming a broad and flattened cluster at the summit, called a *cyme.* The leaves are arranged in pairs and are united at their bases. Each leaf is made up of a series of lance-shaped segments, more or less opposite to one another on each side of the leaf (pinnate). The leaflets vary very much in number, from six to ten pairs as a rule, and vary also in breadth, being broad when few in number and narrower when more numerous; they are usually 2 to 3 inches long. The margins are indented by a few coarsely-cut teeth. The upper surface is strongly veined, the under surface is paler and frequently more or less covered with short, soft hairs. The leaves on the stem are attached by short, broad sheaths, the radical leaves are larger and long-stemmed and the margins more toothed.

The flowers are in bloom from June to September. They are small, tinged with pink and flesh colour, with a somewhat peculiar, but not exactly unpleasant smell. The corolla is tubular, and from the midst of its lobes rise the stamens, only three in number, though there are five lobes to the corolla. The limb of the calyx is remarkable for being at first inrolled and afterwards expanding in the form of a feathery pappus, which aids the dissemination of the fruit. The fruit is a capsule containing one oblong compressed seed. Apart from the flowers, the whole plant has a fœtid smell, much accentuated when bruised.

Although more often growing in damp situations, Valerian is also met with on dry, elevated ground. It is found throughout Britain, but in the northern counties is more often found on higher and dryer ground – dry heaths and hilly pastures – than in the south, and then is usually smaller, not more than 2 feet high, with narrow leaves and hairy, and is often named *sylvestris.* The medicinal qualities of this form are considered to be especially strong.

Though none of the varieties differ greatly from the typical form, Valerian is more subject than many plants to deviations, which has caused several more or less permanent varieties to be named by various botanists. One of the chief is *V. sambucifolia* (Mikan), the name signifying 'Elder-leaved,' from the form of its foliage, the segments being fewer (only four to six pairs) and broader than in the type form, and having somewhat of the character of the elder.

V. celtica is supposed to be the *Saliunca* of ancient writers. It is used by Eastern nations to aromatize their baths. The roots are collected by the Styrian peasants, and are exported by way of Trieste to Turkey and Egypt, whence they are conveyed to India and Ethiopia. *V. sitchensis*, a native of north-western America, is considered by the Russians the most powerful of all species.

Valerian is cultivated for the sake of the drug in England (in Derbyshire), but to a much greater extent in Prussia, Saxony (in the neighbourhood of Colleda, north of Weimar), in Holland and in the United States (Vermont, New Hampshire and New York). English roots have always commanded about four times the price of the imported. In Derbyshire, the cultivation of Valerian takes place in many villages near Chesterfield, the wild plants occurring in the neighbourhood not being sufficient to supply the demand. Derbyshire Valerian plants are of two varieties: *V. Milkanii* (Syme), on limestone, and *V. sambucifolia* (Mikan) on the coal measures. The former yields most of the cultivated Derbyshire rhizome.

The derivation of the name of this genus of plants is differently given. It is said by some authors to have been named after Valerius, who first used it in medicine; while others derive the name from the Latin word *valere* (to be in health), on account of its medicinal qualities. The word *Valeriana* is not found in the classical authors; we first meet with it in the ninth or tenth century, at which period and for long afterwards it was used as synonymous with *Phu* or *Fu*; *Fu, id est valeriana*, we find it described in ancient medical works of that period. The word *Valerian* occurs in the recipes of the Anglo-Saxon leeches (eleventh century). Valeriana, Amantilla and Fu are used as synonymous in the *Alphita*, a mediæval vocabulary of the important medical school of Salernum. Saladinus of Ascoli (about 1450) directs the collection in the month of August of *radices fu, id est Valerianæ*. Referring to the name *Amantilla*, by which it was known in the fourteenth century, Professor Henslow quotes a curious recipe of that period, a translation of which runs as follows: 'Men who begin to fight and when you wish to stop them, give to them the juice of Amantilla *id est Valeriana* and peace will be made immediately.' *Theriacaria, Marinella, Genicularis* and *Terdina* are other old names by which Valerian has been known in former days. Another old name met with in Chaucer and other old writers is 'Setwall' or 'Setewale,' the derivation of which is uncertain. Mediæval herbalists also called the plant 'Capon's Tail,' which has rather fantastically been explained as a reference to its spreading head of whitish flowers.

Drayton (*Polyolbion*) mentions the use of Valerian for cramp; and a tea was made from its roots.

¶ *Cultivation.* Valerian does well in all ordinary soils, but prefers rich, heavy loam, well supplied with moisture.

In Derbyshire, cultivation is from wild plants collected in local woods and transplanted to the prepared land. Preference is given in collecting to root offsets – daughter plants and young flowering plants, which develop towards the close of summer, at the end of slender runners given off by the perennial rhizomes of old plants. These should be set 1 foot apart in rows, 2 or 3 feet apart. The soil should first be treated with farmyard manure, and after planting it is well to give liquid manure from time to time, as well as plenty of water. The soil must be well manured to secure a good crop. Weeding requires considerable attention.

Propagation may also be by seed, either sown when ripe in cold frames, or in March in gentle heat, or in the open in April. In the first two cases, transplant in May to permanent quarters. But to ensure the best alkaloidal percentage, it is best to transplant and cultivate the daughter plants of the wild Valerian.

¶ *Harvesting and Preparation for Market.* The flowering tops must be cut off as they appear, thus enabling the better development of the rhizome. Many of the young plants do not flower in the first year, but produce a luxuriant crop of leaves, and yield rhizome of good quality in the autumn.

In September or early October, all the tops are cut off with a scythe and the rhizomes are harvested, the clinging character of the Derbyshire soil not allowing them to be left in the ground longer.

The drug as found in commerce consists usually of the entire or sliced erect rhizome, which is dark yellowish-brown externally, about 1 inch long and $\frac{1}{2}$ inch thick, and gives off numerous slender brittle roots from $2\frac{1}{2}$ to 4 inches long, whilst short, slender, lateral branches (stolons) are also occasionally present. The root-stock, which is sometimes crowned with the remains of flowering stems and leaf-scales is usually firm, horny and whitish or yellowish internally, but old specimens may be hollow. A transverse section is irregular in outline and exhibits a comparatively narrow bark, separated by a dark line from an irregular circle of wood bundles of varying size.

The drug may also consist of small, undeveloped rhizomes about $\frac{1}{4}$ inch long, crowned with the remains of leaves and bearing short slender roots, the young rhizome having been formed where the stolons given off from mature root-stocks have taken root and produced independent plants.

The roots of Valerian are of similar colour to the erect rhizome, about $\frac{1}{10}$ inch thick, striated longitudinally and usually not shrivelled to any great extent; a transverse section shows a thick bark and small wood.

The drug has a camphoraceous, slightly bitter taste and a characteristic, powerful, disagreeable odour, which gradually develops during the process of drying, owing to a change which occurs in the composition of the volatile oil contained in the sub-epidermal layer of cells: the odour of the fresh root, though not very agreeable, is devoid of the unpleasant valerianaceous odour.

The colour and odour of Valerian rhizome distinguish it readily from other drugs. The rhizome somewhat resembles Serpentary rhizome (*Aristolochia Serpentaria*, Virginian Snakeroot), but may be distinguished therefrom by its odour, erect method of growth, and by the roots being thicker, shorter and less brittle.

¶ *Substitutes.* Valerian root is often fraudulently adulterated with those of other species, notably with those of *V. dioica* (Linn.) (Marsh Valerian), which are smaller and of much feebler odour, and not possessed of such active properties. This Valerian is also a native of Great Britain, found in wet meadows and bogs, but rather scarce. It is a smaller plant than the official Valerian, its stem only growing 6 to 18 inches high. The leaves are very variable, the lower ones generally entire, oval but broader at the base, the upper ones cut into pairs of leaflets, and the flowers *diœcious*, i.e. stamens and pistil, or seed-producing organs in different flowers, the male flowers being arranged rather loosely, and the female flowers, which are smaller and darker, being in more compact heads.

The roots of *V. Phu* (Linn.) are also frequently found mingled with those of the official plant in the imported drug. This species is a native of Southern Europe and Western Asia, often grown in gardens for its decorative golden foliage, being easy of culture. Its rhizome is sometimes known as *V. Radix Majoris*. It is from 4 to 6 inches long, ½ inch in thickness, brown and with a feeble, valerian-like odour and taste. Its thicker rhizome lies obliquely in the earth instead of being erect like that of *V. officinalis*, and is rooted at the bottom only, the roots being numerous and yellowish.

It is stated also that in Germany various Ranunculaceous (or Buttercup) roots are a dangerous adulterant of Valerian; they may be readily detected by their want of the peculiar odour of the official root. The Valerian in the markets of Paris is often largely adulterated with the roots of Scabious (*Scabiosus succisa*, Linn.) and *S. arvensis* (Linn.). They are shorter than the genuine root, less rough, very brittle, not striated, or channelled, and with a white fracture. Though inodorous in themselves, they are very apt to acquire odour from contact with the Valerian. The roots of *Geum urbanum*, or Avens, which in themselves are pleasingly aromatic, but may also on contact acquire some of the odour, have also occasionally been found in parcels of imported Valerian root.

¶ *Chemical Constituents*. The chief constituent of Valerian is a yellowish-green to brownish-yellow oil, which is present in the dried root to the extent of 0·5 to 2 per cent. though an average yield rarely exceeds 0·8 per cent. This variation in quantity is partly explained by the influence of locality, a dry, stony soil, yielding a root richer in oil than one that is moist and fertile.

Lindley's *Treasury of Botany* states: 'What is known to chemists as volatile oil of Valerian seems not to exist naturally in the plant, but to be developed by the agency of water.'

The oil is contained in the sub-epidermal ayer of cells in the root, not in isolated cells or glands. It is of complex composition, containing valerianic, formic and acetic acids, the alcohol known as borneol, and pinene. The valerianic acid present in the oil is not the normal acid, but isovalerianic acid, an oily liquid to which the characteristically unpleasant odour of Valerian is due. It is gradually liberated during the process of drying, being yielded by the decomposition of the chief constituent, bornyl-isovalerianate, by the ferment present. It is strongly acid, burning to the palate and with the odour of the plant. The oil is soluble in 30 parts of water and readily in alcohol and ether. It is found in nature in the oil of several plants, also in small proportion in train oil and the oil of *Cetacea* (whales, porpoises, etc.), which owe their smell to it. It is also one of the products of oxidation of animal matters and of fat oils, and is secreted in certain portions of animal bodies. Its salts are soluble and have a sweetish taste and fatty aspect.

The root also contains two alkaloids – Chatarine and Valerianine – which are still under investigation and concerning which little is known, except that they form crystalline salts. There are also a glucoside, alkaloid and resin all physiologically active, discovered in the fresh rhizome by Chevalier as recently as 1907. He claims that the fresh root is of greater medicinal value than the dry on this account.

On incineration, the drug, if free from adherent earthy matter, yields about 8 or 9 per cent. of ash.

The chief preparation of the British Pharmacopœia is the *Tinctura Valerianæ Ammoniata*, containing Valerian, oil of Nutmeg, oil of Lemon and Ammonia: it is an extremely nauseous and offensive preparation. An etherial tincture and the volatile oil are official in some of the Continental Pharmacopœias, and a distilled water and syrup in the French Codex.

Valerianate of oxide of ethyl, or valerianic ether is a fragrant compound occurring in some vegetable products. The valerianic acid in use is not prepared from the root, but synthetically from amyl alcohol. Valerianic acid combines with various bases (the oxides of metals) to form salts called Valerianates. Valerianate of zinc, prepared by double decomposition, is used as an antispasmodic and is official in the British Pharmacopœia.

¶ *Medicinal Action and Uses*. Valerian is a powerful nervine, stimulant, carminative and antispasmodic.

It has a remarkable influence on the cerebro-spinal system, and is used as a sedative to the higher nerve centres in conditions of nervous unrest, St. Vitus's dance, hypochrondriasis, neuralgic pains and the like.

The drug allays pain and promotes sleep. It is of especial use and benefit to those suffering from nervous overstrain, as it possesses none of the after-effects produced by narcotics.

During the recent War, when air-raids were a serious strain on the overwrought nerves of civilian men and women, Valerian, prescribed with other simple ingredients, taken in a single dose, or repeated according to the need, proved wonderfully efficacious, preventing or minimizing serious results.

Though in ordinary doses, it exerts an influence quieting and soothing in its nature upon the brain and nervous system, large doses, too often repeated, have a tendency to produce pain in the head, heaviness and stupor.

It is commonly administered as *Tinctura Valerianæ Ammoniata*, and often in association with the alkali bromides, and is sometimes given in combination with quinine, the tonic powers of which it appreciably increases.

Oil of Valerian is employed to a considerable extent on the Continent as a popular remedy for cholera, in the form of cholera drops, and also to a certain extent in soap perfumery.

Ettmuller writes of its virtues in strengthening the eyesight, especially when this is weakened by want of energy in the optic nerve.

The juice of the fresh root, under the name of Energetene of Valerian, has of late been recommended as more certain in its effects, and of value as a narcotic in insomnia, and as an anti-convulsant in epilepsy. Having also some slight influence upon the circulation, slowing the heart and increasing its force, it has been used in the treatment of cardiac palpitations.

Valerian was first brought to notice as a specific for epilepsy by Fabius Calumna in 1592, he having cured himself of the disease with it.

¶ *Preparations and Dosages.* Fluid extract, ½ to 1 drachm. Solid extract, 5 to 10 grains. Tincture, B.P. and U.S.P., 1885, 1 to 2 drachms. Ammoniated tincture, B.P. and U.S.P. 1898, ½ to 1 drachm.

Culpepper (1649) joins with many old writers to recommend the use both of herb and root, and praises the herb for its longevity and many comforting virtues, reminding us that it is 'under the influence of Mercury, and therefore hath a warming faculty.' Among other uses, he adds:

'The root boiled with liquorice, raisons and aniseed is good for those troubled with cough. Also, it is of special value against the plague, the decoction thereof being drunk and the root smelled. The green herb being bruised and applied to the head taketh away pain and pricking thereof.'

Gerard tells us that herbalists of his time thought it 'excellent for those burdened and for such as be troubled with croup and other like convulsions, and also for those that are bruised with falls.' He relates that the dried root was held in such esteem as a medicine among the poorer classes in the northern counties and the south of Scotland, that 'no broth or pottage or physicall meats be worth anything if Setewale (the old name for Valerian) be not there.'

Sutherland describes many varieties of Valerian, and himself grew the Indian Valerian which is still sent to Mincing Lane, and offered on the British market. Hanbury states that, according to its habitat, it has many variations which some botanists take as separate species. In the south of England, when once it obtains a hold of the ground, nothing will eradicate it. It was well known to the Anglo-Saxons, who used it as a salad.

Valerian has an effect on the nervous system of many animals, especially cats, which seem to be thrown into a kind of intoxication by its scent. It is scarcely possible to keep a plant of Valerian in a garden after the leaves or root have been bruised or disturbed in any way, for cats are at once attracted and roll on the unfortunate plant. It is equally attractive to rats and is often used by rat-catchers to bait their traps. It has been suggested that the famous Pied Piper of Hamelin owed his irresistible power over rats to the fact that he secreted Valerian roots about his person.

In the Middle Ages, the root was used not only as a medicine but also as a spice, and even as a perfume. It was the custom to lay the roots among clothes as a perfume (*vide* Turner, *Herbal*, 1568, Pt. III, p. 56), just as some of the Himalayan Valerians are still used in the East, especially *V. Jatamansi*, the Nard of the Ancients, believed to be the Spikenard referred to in the Scriptures. It is still much used in ointments. Its odour is not so unpleasant as that of our native Valerians, and this and other species of Valerian are used by Asiatic nations in the manufacture of precious scents. Several aromatic roots were known to the Ancients under the name of *Nardus*, distinguished according to their origin or place of growth by the names of

Nardus indica, N. celtica, N. montana, etc., and supposed to have been derived from different valerianaceous plants. Thus the *N. indica* is referred to *V. Jatamansi* (Roxb.), of Bengal, the *N. celtica* to *'V. celtica* (Linn.), inhabiting the Alps and the *N. montana* to *V. tuberosa,* which grows in the mountains of the south of Europe.

¶ *Other Species.*

JAPANESE VALERIAN, or Kesso Root, was formerly believed to be the product of *Patrinia scabiosæfolia* (Link.), but is now known to be obtained from a Japanese variety of *V. officinalis.* It yields a volatile oil. By the absence of a well-marked, upright rhizome, it widely differs from true Valerian, though at first sight agrees to some extent with it. In colour and taste it is almost identical.

The roots of *V. Mexicana* (D.C.), MEXICAN VALERIAN, which occurs in Mexican commerce in slices, or fleshy disks, contain a large percentage of valerianic acid, which they yield readily and economically. As much as 3·3 per cent. of oil has been extracted from the roots of this species.

V. pyrenaica (Linn.), the HEART-LEAVED VALERIAN, a native of the Pyrenees, is occasionally found in Great Britain naturalized in plantations. It is a large, coarse herb, the stem 2 to 4 feet high, the radical leaves sometimes very large, often a foot in diameter, heart-shaped, the upper ones smaller, with a few basal leaflets, the flowers much as in *V. officinalis.* It is not employed medicinally.

V. montana and *V. angustifolia* are Alpine varieties, but can be grown in this country with a little care. They are almost entirely grown for decorative purposes, flowering from May to August, and possessing none of the unpleasant smell of Valerian.

Culpepper describes a plant which he calls 'Water Valerian' (*V. Aquatica*), with 'much larger' flowers than the garden Valerian, which, however, they resemble, and of a 'pale purple colour.' He states it grows 'promiscuously in marshy grounds and moist meadows' and flowers in May.

VALERIAN, AMERICAN

Cypripedium pubescens (WILLD.)
Cyprepedium parviflorum
N.O. Orchidaceæ

Synonyms. Lady's Slipper. Cypripedium hirsutum. American Valerian. Noah's Ark. Yellow Lady's Slipper. Nerve-root
Part Used. Root

American Valerian is one of the names given to the Yellow Lady's Slipper (*Cypripedium*). The roots of several varieties, the principal being *Cypripedium pubescens* and *Cyprepedium parviflorum*, are employed in hysteria, being a gentle, nervous stimulant and antispasmodic, less powerful than Valerian.

American Valerian is official in the United States Pharmacopœia for the production of a fluid extract. *Cypridenin* is a complex, resinoid substance, obtained by precipitating with water a concentrated tincture of the rhizome.

¶ *Preparations and Dosages.* Powdered root, 1 drachm. Fluid extract, ½ to 1 drachm. Cypripedin, 1 to 3 grains. Solid extract alc., 5 to 10 grains.

VALERIAN, INDIAN

Valeriana Wallichii (DE CANDOLLE)
N.O. Valerianaceæ

Synonym. Tagar.

Indian Valerian is a perennial, herbaceous plant, indigenous to India, being found in the temperate Himalayan region. The dried rhizome and rootlets are used for medicinal purposes, and the drug is known in India as 'tagar.' It possesses stimulant and antispasmodic properties, and is official in the Indian and Colonial Addendum for use in the Eastern Colonies. The chief preparation of the drug is *Tinctura Valerianæ Indicæ Ammoniata.* Indian Valerian is practically identical in its composition with the European drug, but contains a slightly larger amount of volatile oil. It may be employed in the same way as Valerian, but is more used as a perfume than in medicine. It is largely employed in preparations for the hair, and the dried rhizome is used as incense.

It occurs in commerce in crooked pieces of a dull brown colour, about 2 inches long, and from ¼ to ½ inch in diameter, with a number of bracts at the crown and blunt at the lower extremity. The rhizome is marked with transverse ridges and studded thickly with prominent circular tubercles to a few of which thick rootlets may be attached. The crown usually bears the remains of the leafstalks. In transverse section it is dark, with a large pith and diffuse ring of small woodbundles. The drug is very hard and tough, and shows a greenish-brown surface when fractured. This and its crooked form distinguish it from Common Valerian. Its colour, due to the presence of volatile oil resembles that of ordinary Valerian rhizome, but is much stronger. The chief constituent of the drug is this oil, but it also contains valerianic and other organic acids, together with resin, tannin, etc. As in the case of ordinary Valerian, the valerianic acid is probably formed by the gradual decomposition of other constituents present in the volatile oil.

¶ *Preparations*. Tincture Valerianæ Indicæ Ammoniata.

The INDIAN NARD, or Spikenard, sometimes called Syrian Nard, is still occasionally to be found in commerce. It is a small, delicate root, from 1 to 3 inches long, beset with a tuft of soft, light brown, slender fibres, of an agreeable odour and a bitter aromatic taste. It was formerly very much esteemed as a medicine, but is now almost out of use. Its properties are analogous to those of Valerian, but it must not be confused with Indian Valerian.

VALERIAN, RED-SPUR

Centranthus rubra (D. C.)
N.O. Valerianaceæ

Synonyms. Pretty Betsy. Bouncing Bess. Delicate Bess. Drunken Sailor. Bovisand Soldier

Habitat. England, Scotland and the Mediterranean countries

The Red-Spur Valerian, a plant with lance-shaped, untoothed leaves and red flowers with a spur at the base, grouped in dense clusters, must not be confounded with the true medicinal Valerian, though the mistake is often made. It is destitute of the properties of the official Valerian, and is not usefully applied in England, though in some parts of Continental Europe the leaves are eaten. They are exceedingly good in salad, or cooked as a vegetable, and in France there is a sale for the roots for soups.

This plant is not truly British, but is perfectly naturalized in the south of England, being found quite often growing on rocks or walls, in old chalk-pits, railway cuttings and waste places in Kent and Devonshire, though less frequently in the northern counties and only in a few places in Scotland. It is naturally a native of the Mediterranean countries, and was probably originally introduced as a decorative plant. It is mentioned by many of the older writers as a garden flower. Gerard, writing in 1597, saying: 'It groweth plentifully in my garden, being a great ornament to the same.' Parkinson (1640) says that it grows 'in our gardens chiefly, for we know not the natural place.'

¶ *Description.* The root-stock is perennial and very freely branching, enabling it to take a firm hold in the crevices in which it

has once gained possession. The stems are stout, somewhat shrubby at the base, between 1 and 2 feet long, hollow and very smooth in texture. The leaves 2 to 4 inches long and pointed, opposite one another in pairs, are somewhat fleshy, their outlines generally quite entire. The very numerous flowers are in masses, either of a rich crimson colour, a delicate pink, or much more rarely, white, and are in bloom from June to September. The spur to the long, tubular corolla is a marked feature. Each flower only contains one stamen. The fruit is small and dry, the border of the surrounding calyx forming a feathery rosette or pappus.

Linnæus included this species with the Valerians, as *Valeriana rubra*, but De Candolle assigned it to a separate genus, *Centranthus*, in which all later botanists have followed him. The name of the genus comes from the Greek *kentron* (a spur) and *anthos* (a flower), in reference to the corolla being furnished with a spur at the base, which absolutely distinguishes it from the true Valerian, apart from other differences.

'Pretty Betsy' and 'Bouncing Bess' are popular names for the Red Valerian. Near Plymouth, we find the names 'Drunken Sailor' and 'Bovisand Soldier,' and in West Devon, the smaller, paler kind is known as 'Delicate Bess.'

VERBENA, LEMON

Lippia citriodora
N.O. Verbenaceæ

Synonyms. Aloysia citriodora. Verveine citronelle or odorante. Herb Louisa. Lemon-scented Verbena. Verbena triphylla. Lippia triphylla

Parts Used. Leaves, flowering tops

Habitat. Chile and Peru. Cultivated in European gardens

¶ *Description.* This deciduous shrub was introduced into England in 1784, reaching a height of 15 feet in the Isle of Wight and in sheltered localities. The leaves are very fragrant, lanceolate, arranged in threes, 3 to

4 inches long, with smooth margins, pale green in colour, having parallel veins at right-angles to the mid-rib and flat bristles along the edges. The many small flowers are pale purple, blooming during August in slim,

terminal panicles. The leaves, which have been suggested to replace tea, will retain their odour for years and are used in perfumery. They should be gathered at flowering time.

All the species of Lippia abound in volatile oil.

¶ *Constituents*. The odour is due to an essential oil obtainable by distillation. It has not been analysed in detail.

¶ *Medicinal Action and Uses*. Febrifuge, sedative. The uses of Lemon Verbena are similar to those of mint, orange flowers, or melissa, as a stomachic and antispasmodic in dyspepsia, indigestion and flatulence, stimulating skin and stomach.

¶ *Dosage*. The decoction may be taken in several daily doses of three tablespoonsful.

¶ *Other Species*.

Lippia Scaberrima, or Beukessboss of South Africa, yields an essential oil with an odour like lavender, named Lippianol. It has a peculiar crystalline appearance, with the qualities of a monohydric alcohol.

From *L. mexicana* or possibly *Cedronella mexicana*, an essential oil resembling that of fennel was separated, and also a substance like camphor, called Lippioil.

The essence of Lemon-Grass, or *Andropogon Schœnanthus*, should not be confused with that of Lemon-Scented Verbena.

SWEET VERNAL GRASS. *See* GRASSES

VERONICAS

The genus *Veronica* includes some of our most beautiful native flowers, the Speedwells, which differ from the other British *Scrophulariceæ* in having only two stamens, which project horizontally from the rotate, or wheel-shaped corolla, which has only four unequal spreading lobes, the lower segment being the smallest, the two posterior petals, according to the theory of botanists, being united into one large one. The numerous species found in England have generally blue petals with dark diverging lines at the base, though in a few cases, pinkish flowers are found.

All the species of Veronica possess a slight degree of astringency, and many of them were formerly used in medicine, some

N.O. Scrophulariaceæ

20 of them have been employed as drugs, those with the chief reputaticn being *Veronica Chamædrys*, *V. officinalis*, and *V. Beccabunga*, all natives of Great Britain; the American species *V. leptandra*, now known as *Leptandra veronica* and another species, native to Asia Minor, called *V. peduncularis* (Bieb.) or *V. nigricans* (Koch.), the root of which is used there under the name Batitjoe.

The name of this genus of plants is said to have been derived from the Saint; others say it is from the Greek words *phero* (I bring) and *nike* (victory), alluding to its supposed efficacy in subduing diseases.

See BROOKLIME, SPEEDWELL, GERMANDER SPEEDWELL.

VERVAIN

Verbena officinalis (LINN.)
Verbena hastata
N.O. Verbenaceæ

Synonyms. Herb of Grace. Herbe Sacrée. Herba veneris
Parts Used. Leaves, flowering heads
Habitat. Europe, Barbary, China, Cochin-China, Japan

¶ *Description*. In England the Common Vervain is found growing by roadsides and in sunny pastures. It is a perennial bearing many small, pale-lilac flowers. The leaves are opposite, and cut into toothed lobes. The plant has no perfume, and is slightly bitter and astringent in taste. The name *Vervain* is derived from the Celtic *ferfaen*, from *fer* (to drive away) and *faen* (a stone), as the plant was much used for affections of the bladder, especially calculus. Another derivation is given by some authors from *Herba veneris*, because of the aphrodisiac qualities attributed to it by the Ancients. Priests used it for sacrifices, and hence the name *Herba Sacra*. The name *Verbena* was the classical Roman name for 'altar-plants' in general, and

for this species in particular. The druids included it in their lustral water, and magicians and sorcerers employed it largely. It was used in various rites and incantations, and by ambassadors in making leagues. Bruised, it was worn round the neck as a charm against headaches, and also against snake and other venomous bites as well as for general good luck. It was thought to be good for the sight. Its virtues in all these directions may be due to the legend of its discovery on the Mount of Calvary, where it staunched the wounds of the crucified Saviour. Hence, it is crossed and blessed with a commemorative verse when it is gathered. It must be picked before flowering, and dried promptly.

831

¶ *Constituents.* The plant appears to contain a peculiar tannin, but it has not yet been properly analysed.

¶ *Medicinal Action and Uses.* It is recommended in upwards of thirty complaints, being astringent, diaphoretic, antispasmodic, etc. It is said to be useful in intermittent fevers, ulcers, ophthalmia, pleurisy, etc., and to be a good galactogogue. It is still used as a febrifuge in autumn fevers.

As a poultice it is good in headache, earneuralgia, rheumatism, etc. In this form it colours the skin a fine red, giving rise to the idea that it had the power of drawing the blood outside. A decoction of 2 oz. to a quart, taken in the course of one day, is said to be a good medicine in purgings, easing pain in the bowels. It is often applied externally for piles. It is used in homœopathy.

Fluid extract, ½ to 1 drachm.

¶ *Other Species.*

Verbena Jamaicensis (JAMAICA VERVAIN) grows in Jamaica, Barbados, and other West Indian islands, bearing violet flowers.

The juice is used in dropsy and for children as an anthelmintic and cooling cathartic. The negroes use it as an emmenagogue, and for sore and inflamed eyes. As a poultice, with wheat-flour, the bruised leaves are used for swelling of the spleen, and for hard tumours at their commencement.

V. Lappulaceæ (BURRY VERVAIN), another West Indian herb, with pale blue flowers, is a vulnerary sub-astringent, being used even for very severe bleeding wounds in men and cattle, especially in Jamaica.

V. hastata (BLUE VERVAIN, Wild Hyssop, Simpler's Joy) is indigenous to the United States, and is used unofficially as a tonic, emetic, expectorant, etc., for scrofula, gravel, and worms. A fluid extract is prepared from the dried, over-ground portion.

V. Urticifolia. The root, boiled in milk and water with the inner bark of *Quercus Alba*, is said to be an antidote to poisoning by *Rhus Toxicodendron*.

V. Sinuata. An infusion of the root, taken as freely as possible, is said to be a valuable antisyphilitic.

VINE

Vitis vinifera (LINN.)
N.O. Vitaceæ

Synonym. Grape Vine
Parts Used. Fruit, leaves, juice
Habitat. Asia, Central and Southern Europe, Greece, California, Australia, and Africa

¶ *Description.* The name vine is derived from *viere* (to twist), and has reference to the twining habits of the plant which is a very ancient one; in the Scriptures the vine is frequently mentioned from the time of Noah onward. Wine is recorded as an almost universal drink throughout the world from very early times. The vine is a very long-lived plant. Pliny speaks of one 600 years old, and some existent in Burgundy are said to be 400 and over.

The stem of old vines attains a considerable size in warm climates, planks 15 inches across may be cut therefrom, forming a very durable timber.

Artificial heat for forcing the grapes was not used till the early part of last century and the first accounts of vineries enclosed by glass date from the middle of that period.

The vine is propagated by seeds, layers, cuttings and grafting and succeeds in almost any gravelly soil; that of a volcanic nature produces the finest wines. It is a climbing shrub with simple, lobed, cut or toothed leaves (seldom compound) with thyrsoid racemes of greenish flowers, the fruit consisting of watery or fleshy pulp, stones and skin, two-celled, four-seeded.

¶ *Constituents.* The leaves gathered in June contain a mixture of cane sugar and glucose, tartaric acid, potassium bi-tartrate, quercetine, quercitrin, tannin, amidon, malic acid, gum, inosite, an uncrystallizable fermentable sugar and oxalate of calcium; gathered in the autumn they contain much more quercetine and less trace of quercitrin.

The ripe fruit juice termed 'must' contains sugar, gum, malic acid, potassium bi-tartrate and inorganic salts; when fermented this forms the wine of commerce.

The dried ripe fruit commonly called raisins, contain dextrose and potassium acid tartrate.

The seeds contain tannin and a fixed oil.

The juice of the unripe fruit, 'Verjuice,' contains malic, citric, tartaric, racemic and tannic acids, potassium bi-tartrate, sulphate of potash and lime.

¶ *Medicinal Action and Uses.* Grape sugar differs from other sugars chemically. It enters the circulation without any action of the saliva. The warming and fattening action of grape sugar is thus more rapid in increasing strength and repairing waste in fevers but is unsuitable for inflammatory or gouty conditions.

The seeds and leaves are astringent, the leaves being formerly used to stop hæmorrhages and bleeding. They are used dried and powdered as a cure for dysentery in cattle.

832

The sap, termed a tear or lachryma, forms an excellent lotion for weak eyes and specks on the cornea.

Ripe grapes in quantity influence the kidneys producing a free flow of urine and are apt to cause palpitation in excitable and full-blooded people. Dyspeptic subjects should avoid them.

In cases of anæmia and a state of exhaustion the restorative power of grapes is striking, especially when taken in conjunction with a light nourishing diet.

In cases of small-pox grapes have proved useful owing to their bi-tartrate of potash content; they are also said to be of benefit in cases of neuralgia, sleeplessness, etc.

Three to 6 lb. of grapes a day are taken by people undergoing the 'grape cure,' sufferers from torpid liver and sluggish biliary functions should take them not quite fully ripe, whilst those who require animal heat to support waste of tissue should eat fully ripe and sweet grapes.

Dried grapes; the raisins of commerce, are largely used in the manufacture of galencials, the seeds being separated and rejected as they give a very bitter taste. Raisins are demulcent, nutritive and slightly laxative.

¶ *Other Species.*

Vitis labrusca, indigenous to North America, is the Wild Vine or Foxgrape.

V. cordifolia, the Heart-leaved Vine or Chickengrape.

V. riparia, the Riverside or Sweet-scented Vine.

VIOLET, DOG

Viola canina (LINN.)
N.O. Violaceæ

Parts Used. Leaves and flowers

¶ *Description.* The Dog Violet differs principally from the Sweet Violet in its long straggling stems and paler blue flowers. It possesses the same properties, being powerfully cathartic and emetic. At one time a medicine made from it had some reputation in curing skin diseases. It may be found on dry hedge-banks and in the woods, flowering from April to August, a longer flowering period than the Sweet Violet. It is a very variable plant in size of leaf and blossom, form of leaf and other parts, but there seem to be no permanent and reliable differences to justify the division into distinct sub-species. The root-stock of the Dog Violet is short and from it rises a tuft of leaves. The flowering stems are at first short, but as time goes on they elongate considerably until sometimes they may be found nearly a foot long. The leaves are heart-shaped and with serrated edges, but vary much in their proportions. They are ordinarily, like the stems, quite smooth, while in the Sweet Violet we often get them more or less covered with soft hairs. The flowers are scentless, generally larger than those of the Sweet Violet, not only paler in colour, but like most purple flowers, occasionally varying to white.

The popular name of this plant is a reproach for its want of perfume.

VIOLET, HAIRY

Viola hirta
N.O. Violaceæ

Part Used. Whole plant

The Hairy Violet (*Viola hirta*), the Dog Violet (*V. canina*), the Marsh Violet (*V. palustris*) (which has pale lilac flowers) and the Heartsease or Pansy (*V. tricolor*) are other well-defined species of indigenous Violets, most of them, however, being subject to variations, which have been described by botanists as sub-species.

Henslow says *V. palustris* is not uncommon in the north, but rarer in southern counties. It has very smooth leaves, as is usually the case with semi-aquatic plants; the flowers are scentless. The same authority mentions another variety, *V. calcarea,* a dwarfed, starved form of *V. hirta.*

¶ *Description.* The Hairy Violet bears a very considerable resemblance to *V. odorata,* the Sweet Violet. The main points of difference are as follows: in the Hairy Violet the flowers are almost or quite scentless; it but rarely throws out the trailing shoots that are so characteristic a feature in the Sweet Violet; the hairs on the stem are in the Sweet Violet deflexed, while in the Hairy Violet they are spreading and are thus more conspicuous, sufficiently so to give the popular name to the plant. The little scales on the flower-stems, called bracts, are in Sweet Violet ordinarily above the middle of the stalk, while in the Hairy Violet they are ordinarily (in neither case invariably) below this point. This species is more frequently found in the east of England than the west, and is common in chalk and limestone districts or near the sea.

VIOLET, SWEET

Viola odorata (LINN.)
N.O. Violaceæ

Synonyms. Sweet-Scented Violet
Parts Used. Flowers and leaves dried, and whole plant fresh
Habitat. The Violet family comprises over 200 species, widely distributed in the temperate and tropical regions of the world, those natives of Europe, Northern Asia and North America being wholly herbaceous, whilst others, native of tropical America and South America, where they are abundant, are trees and shrubs. The genus *Viola* contains about 100 species, of which five are natives of Great Britain

¶ *Description.* The sweet-scented Violet appears at the end of February and has finished blooming by the end of April.

The familiar leaves are heart-shaped, slightly downy, especially beneath, on stalks rising alternately from a creeping rhizome or underground stem, the blades of the young leaves rolled up from each side into the middle on the face of the leaf into two tight coils. The flower-stalks arise from the axils of the leaves and bear single flowers, with a pair of scaly bracts placed a little above the middle of the stalk.

The flowers are generally deep purple, giving their name to the colour that is called after them, but lilac, pale rose-coloured or white variations are also frequent, and all these tints may sometimes be discovered in different plants growing on the same bank.

They bear five sepals extended at their bases, and five unequal petals, the lower one lengthened into a hollow spur beneath and the lateral petals with a hairy centre line. The anthers are united into a tube round the three-celled capsule, the two lower ones furnished with spurs which are enclosed within the spur of the corolla.

The flowers are full of honey and are constructed for bee visitors, but bloom before it is really bee time, so that it is rare that a Violet flower is found setting seed. There is indeed a remarkable botanical curiosity in the structure of the Violet: it produces flowers both in the spring and in autumn, but the flowers are different. In spring they are fully formed, as described, and sweet-scented, but they are mostly barren and produce no seed, while in autumn, they are very small and insignificant, hidden away amongst the leaves, with no petals and no scent, and produce abundance of seed. This peculiarity is not confined to the Violet. It is found in some species of *Oxalis*, *Impatiens*, *Campanula*, *Eranthemum*, etc. Such plants are called *cleistogamous* and are all self-fertilizing. The cleistogamous flowers of the Violet are like flowers which have aborted instead of developing, but within each one are a couple of stamens and some unripe seeds. In warmer climates, like Italy, these 'cleistogamous' buds develop into perfect flowers. Only

occasionally do they do so in England. In the woodland species (*Viola sylvatica*) all the flowers on the plant may be cleistogamous.

The Violet propagates itself, also, in another way by throwing out scions, or runners, from the main plant each summer after flowering, and these in turn send out roots and become new plants, a process that renders it independent of seed.

The Violet is very abundant in the neighbourhood of Stratford-on-Avon, where it is nowadays much cultivated for commercial purposes.

Violet is the diminutive form of the Latin *Viola*, the Latin form of the Greek name *Ione*. There is a legend that when Jupiter changed his beloved Io into a white heifer for fear of Juno's jealousy, he caused these modest flowers to spring forth from the earth to be fitting food for her, and he gave them her name. Another derivation of the word Violet is said to be from *Vias* (wayside).

Other flowers besides the Violet formerly bore that name, e.g. the Snowdrop was called the 'bulbous or narcissus Violet'; the plant now called 'Honesty' (or Moonwort) had the apellation of 'Strange Violet'; and two species of Gentian were called 'Autumn Bell-flower' or 'Calathian Violet,' and another 'Marion's Violet.' The periwinkle, now generally known in France by the name of *Pervenche*, in other times was known as '*du lisseron*' or '*Violette des sorciers*'; and our own Violet was called, in distinction from the others, 'March Violet,' and in French *Violette de Mars*.

At Pæstum, which has been and still is famous for its Violets as well as for its roses, several kinds of Violets are found, and one species that grows in the woods has exceedingly large leaves and seed-vessels; but the flower is so small that it can hardly be seen; this has given rise to the idea that it blooms underground. The flowers are of a pale yellow.

The Violet of India bears its blossom in an erect position, while our own native plant hangs down its head. It has been suggested by Professor Rennie that the drooping position of the purple petals shaded still more by the large green flower-cup, serves as an umbrella to protect the seed while unripe, from the rains and dews, which would injure it. As soon as the seed is matured and the little canopy no longer wanted, the flower rises and stands upright on its stem.

Some butterflies feed entirely on Violet, and the stem of the plant is often swelled and spongy in appearance, due to insects, whose eggs were deposited on the stalk during the preceding summer. The little animal, on hatching out, finds its food ready for it, and penetrating the plant, disturbs its juices and causes this excrescence.

Violets were mentioned frequently by Homer and Virgil. They were used by the Athenians 'to moderate anger,' to procure sleep and 'to comfort and strengthen the heart.' Pliny prescribes a liniment of Violet root and vinegar for gout and disorder of the spleen, and states that a garland or chaplet of Violets worn about the head will dispel the fumes of wine and prevent headache and dizziness. The ancient Britons used the flowers as a cosmetic, and in a Celtic poem they are recommended to be employed steeped in goats' milk to increase female beauty, and in the Anglo-Saxon translation of the Herbarium of Apuleius (tenth century), the herb *V. purpureum* is recommended 'for new wounds and eke for old' and for 'hardness of the maw.'

In Macer's *Herbal* (tenth century) the Violet is among the many herbs which were considered powerful against 'wykked sperytis.'

Askham's *Herbal* has this recipe for insomnia under Violet:

'For thē that may not slepe for sickness seeth this herb in water and at even let him soke well hys feete in the water to the ancles, whā he goeth to bed, bind of this herbe to his temples.'

Violets, like Primroses, have been associated with death, especially with the death of the young. This feeling has been constantly expressed from early times. It is referred to by Shakespeare in *Hamlet* and *Pericles* and by Milton in *Lycidas*.

In parts of Gloucestershire the country people have an aversion to bringing Violets into their cottages because they carry fleas. This idea may have arisen from these insects in the stem.

When Napoleon went to Elba his last message to his adherents was that he should return with Violets. Hence he was alluded to and toasted by them in secret as Caporal Violette, and the Violet was adopted as the emblem of the Imperial Napoleonic party.

Violets were also and still are used in cookery, especially by the French. '*Vyolette:*

Take flowrys of Vyolet, boyle hem, presse hem, bray (pound) hem smal,' and the recipe continues that they are to be mixed with milk and floure of rys and sugar or honey, and finally to be coloured with Violets. A recipe called *Mon Amy* directs the cook to 'plant it with flowers of Violets and serve forth.'

A wine made from the flowers of the Sweet Violet was much used by the Romans.

Violets impart their odour to liquids, and vinegar derives not only a brilliant tint, but a sweet odour from having Violet flowers steeped in it.

The chief use of the Violet in these days is as a colouring agent and perfume, and as the source of the medicinally employed Syrup of Violets, for which purposes the plant is largely cultivated, especially in Warwickshire. The Syrup can be made as follows: To 1 lb. of Sweet Violet flowers freshly picked, add $2\frac{1}{2}$ pints of boiling water, infuse these for twenty-four hours in a glazed china vessel, then pour off the liquid and strain it gently through muslin; afterwards add double its weight of the finest loaf sugar and make it into a syrup, but without letting it boil. This is an old-fashioned recipe.

Another recipe, from a seventeenth century recipe book:

'*Sirrup of Violets*

'Take a quantity of Blew Violets, clip off the whites and pound them well in a stone morter; then take as much fair running water as will sufficiently moysten them and mix with the Violets; strain them all; and to every halfe pint of the liquor put one pound of the best loafe sugar; set it on the fire, putting the sugar in as it melts, still stirring it; let it boyle but once or twice att the most; then take it from the fire, and keep it to your use. This is a daynty sirrup of Violets.'

Syrup of Violet with Lemon Syrup and acetic acid makes an excellent dish in summer. The Syrup forms a principal ingredient in Oriental sherbet.

¶ *Cultivation.* The Wild Violet has been developed by cultivation till its blossoms in some varieties are many times the original size.

One of the essential points for the successful cultivation of Violets, either for the sake of marketing the cut blooms, or for medicinal purposes, is clear atmosphere. They seldom do well near a town, because the undersides of the leaves are covered with hairs, which catch the grit, thus blocking the breathing pores.

Neglect of a few simple rules is invariably the cause of failure. One frequently finds a bed of Violets which produces nothing but leaves. The plants may have been healthy enough to begin with and they were probably well and truly planted, but after the first season of bloom they were allowed to spread and become overcrowded. The Violet must be renewed and replanted every year. Failure to perform this operation spells failure.

If the amateur contemplates growing Violets in order to obtain bloom during autumn and winter, April is a favourable time to set about the task of making a Violet bed. The Violet in summer time delights in partial shade, therefore the bed should be made if possible under the north-east side of a fence or hedge. The bed should be, however, placed fairly well in the open, and if grown in private gardens not in the dense shadow cast by house walls, nor under trees, though shade to a certain amount is absolutely essential in summer, as when exposed to sun the plants become overrun with red spider, an insect pest to which the Violet is specially liable. At the same time, it is as essential that the plants be exposed to the full sun in the autumn. If grown on a large scale, a suitable situation for summer quarters is between rows of sweet peas.

Ordinary garden soil will suffice for successful Violet culture, but the soil must be carefully prepared and deep digging is essential. This should be done some time before planting-out time; if possible in autumn, so that the ground may be left open to the effects of winter. Avoid, if possible, stiff clay, as in very wet soil Violets are apt to become diseased. Violets flourish best on a good medium soil, neither too heavy, nor too light. The ideal soil is a deep, sandy soil. Where the soil is heavy, it can be improved by an admixture of well-decayed manure, road grit, leaf-mould and burnt vegetable refuse. Rank stable manure must be avoided or the roots will produce any quantity of foliage and very few flowers. A dressing of leaf-mould is advantageous, as it will prevent the surface from becoming cracked in hot weather and will at the same time supply the roots with the medium in which they are most at home naturally.

The young plants should be rooted runners; plant not less than a foot apart each way. Choose a moist, dull day for planting, or if dry, puddle in the roots. If an inverted flower-pot be placed over each young Violet during the day in hot sunshine and lifted off during rain and at night, the plants will become established at much greater ease than if the ground were allowed to become baked by the sun. Water must be given copiously in

dry weather, and the plants will also benefit at such times from a mulching or top dressing of leaf-mould or decayed manure, old mushroom-bed manure being useful for this purpose.

If the foliage assumes a yellow tint, it is almost an indication of the presence of red spider. The plants should then be sprinkled at frequent intervals with a mixture of sulphur and well-seasoned soot and a thorough syringing such as will reach the under-part of the foliage should also be given, using a solution of Gishurst compound, repeating the operation at intervals of a day or two, until the pest is eradicated.

The soil between the rows should be hoed frequently and the runners of most varieties must be removed in the summer. The single varieties, on account of their stronger growth, require more room than the double forms. Single varieties of the more modern kinds, such as the Princess of Wales, flower freely on the runners which issue from the parent plant, and for this reason such runners may be left. The double varieties, on the contrary, must have the runners removed so as to strengthen the crowns which give the finest blooms. Good single varieties besides the Princess of Wales are Wellsiana, La France, Admiral Avellan and California, and among the doubles Mrs. J. J. The double garden variety, especially the pale blue Neapolitan Violet which forms a stem 6 inches in height, is often called the Tree Violet.

From plants thus established in the open, a plentiful supply of blooms will be forthcoming in the following spring. It is, however, only in sheltered places that Violets will thrive in the open during winter. It is generally found necessary to transfer the plants to cold frames for flowering, and to grow the flowers for the sake of marketing the cut blooms for profit; this is absolutely essential, as without glass, Violets can only be obtained in March and April, when they are plentiful, cheap and unprofitable. Frames in which melon or cucumbers have been grown during the summer will be found eminently suitable for the purpose. A foundation of stable litter and leaves, a foot deep or more, turned frequently to allow the volatile gases to escape from the litter, and then well trodden, and covered with a layer of about 6 inches of rich loamy soil, makes a very suitable bed. A great point to bear in mind is the desirability of keeping the crowns of plants as near to the glass as possible. If therefore it is necessary to raise the bed this should be done before the plants are put in the winter quarters.

Water the Violets from the outdoor bed a day before lifting; by taking this precaution, it will be possible to lift the roots so that they bring away with them a good-sized ball of earth. All straggling runners should be cut away, leaving only two or three, already rooted probably, and showing flowers close up to the old plants. These reserved runners, if not already rooted, should be pegged down, and, in addition to flowering freely, will be just what are wanted for planting out next spring. There must be no crowding of the plants as, unless they are kept perfectly clear of each other, damping off is likely to take place, especially if the ventilation is faulty. They should be planted a foot apart, firmly and deeply, or sufficiently to bury the stems, keeping the crowns well out of the soil. Level all and give a good watering immediately to settle the roots, and keep the frame closed for a few days until the plants begin to make roots, but no longer. Plenty of air must be supplied day and night, as long as the weather remains mild. In frost keep the lights down, and when severe cover with mats, but do not keep the frames too close or dark from excessive covering. For Violets in frames, light and air cannot be overstudied, and whilst not allowing the frost to exercise a too severe influence upon them, it is advisable to expose them to all the fresh air and light obtainable, to keep the plants in healthy condition. The leaves when the plants are kept close and in darkness will turn yellow and lose their vitality, and under such conditions the plants soon become weakened and rendered incapable of producing flowers. It is a good plan to sprinkle the soil around the plants with a little finely-powdered charcoal, as the latter will absorb the moisture that unavoidably arises through the frames being kept closed and darkened during severe weather. Application of water to the roots of Violets in midwinter is not necessary, but later, when the sun exercises a greater evaporative influence and air in abundance can be admitted to the plants, it will be necessary to occasionally apply water as well as manure in liquid form. Care must be taken to keep the glass clean and free from any smoky deposit which obscures the light; in cleaning the glasses both sides regularly, avoid any drip on to the plants. Remove all decaying foliage and constantly watch for slugs. Fog is bad for Violets in frames: it causes the leaves to damp off and sometimes kills the plants outright.

Plants removed to frames in the latter half of September, if properly attended to, will begin to bloom early in October and continue to flower till April. In this month, after suitable cuttings and runners have been taken from them for next season's use, they may be thrown or given away, for each season young plants alone should be cultivated. If a little fresh soil is given early in March as a top-dressing to the plants in the frames, the runners become stronger and better rooted for planting out-of-doors. Besides being kept moist at the roots by occasional watering, their growth is much benefited by an overhead sprinkling in the evening during the summer, when the surrounding soil is hot and dry. While this promotes a healthy growth, it tends also to keep down red spider.

Some growers raise their young plants from cuttings taken early in October, when lifting the plants to put them into frames or cool greenhouses. At this time, it is easy to secure a few hundreds of the healthiest cuttings, heeling them in till time permits of their being dealt with. Inserted in boxes of soil or preferably under spare lights, model plants for putting out in March or early April will result, which in turn give the finest flowering clumps.

¶ *Parts Used Medicinally.* The flowers *dried* and the leaves and whole plant *fresh.*

The odour of the flowers is in a great measure destroyed by desiccation and the degree to which they retain their colour depends on the method of collecting and drying them.

The Violet flowers used for Syrup of Violets are not always the ordinary wild *V. odorata,* the colour of which soon fades, except under special treatment. Other species with deeper-coloured and larger blue flowers, and also deep-coloured garden Violas and Pansies are often substituted for the Sweet Violet, for upon the colour their value depends.

¶ *Constituents.* The chief chemical constituents of the flowers are the odorous principle and the blue colouring matter, which may be extracted from the petals by infusion with water and turns green and afterwards yellow with alkalis and red with acids. The flowers yield their odour and slightly bitter taste to boiling water and their properties may be preserved for some time by means of sugar in the form of Syrup of Violets.

A glucoside, Viola-quercitin, is also a constituent, found throughout the plant and especially in the rhizome. It may be isolated by exhausting the fresh plant with warm alcohol, removing the alcohol by distillation and treating the residue with warm distilled water, from which it crystallizes in fine yellow needles, which are soluble in water, less so in alcohol and insoluble in ether. On boiling with mineral acids, the glucoside is split up into quercitin and a fermentable sugar. The activity of the plant, according to the British

Pharmacopœia, is probably due to this glucoside and its products of decomposition, or a ferment associated with it.

Salicylic acid has also been obtained from the plant.

The scientist Boullay discovered in the root, leaves, flowers and seeds of this plant an alkaloid resembling the Emetin of Ipecacuanha (which also belongs to the same group of plants), which he termed Violine. The same alkaloid was found by the French physician Orfila (1787–1853) to be an energetic poison, which may be identical with Emetin.

It has been found that the Toulouse Violet, which is *without scent* when cultivated in the land from which it takes its name, develops a very agreeable and pronounced perfume when raised at Grasse.

The growth of Violet flowers for the extraction of their perfume is not carried out to such an extent as formerly, as the natural perfume is suffering severely from the competition of the artificial product which forms the greater part of the Violet perfume of commerce. The natural perfume is very expensive to extract, an enormous quantity of flowers being required to scent a pomade. The largest Violet plantations are at Nice. The species used are the double Parma Violet and the Victoria Violet. A certain amount of perfume of a distinctive character is also now made from the green leaves of Violet plants, taken just before flowering.

¶ *Medicinal Action and Uses*. The Violet is still found in the Pharmacopœias.

Violet flowers possess slightly laxative properties. The best form of administration is the Syrup of Violets. *Syrop Violæ* of the British Pharmacopœia directs that it may be given as a laxative to infants in doses of ½ to 1 teaspoonful, or more, with an equal volume of oil of Almonds.

Syrup of Violets is also employed as a laxative, and as a colouring agent and flavouring in other neutral or acid medicines.

The older writers had great faith in Syrup of Violets: ague, epilepsy, inflammation of the eyes, sleeplessness, pleurisy, jaundice and quinsy are only a few of the ailments for which it was held potent. Gerard says: 'It has power to ease inflammation, roughness of the throat and comforteth the heart, assuageth the pains of the head and causeth sleep.'

The flowers are crystallized as an attractive sweetmeat, and in the days of Charles II, a favourite conserve, Violet Sugar, named then 'Violet Plate,' prepared from the flowers, was considered of excellent use in consumption, and was sold by all apothecaries. The flowers have undoubted expectorant qualities.

The fresh flowers have also been used as an addition to salads; they have a laxative effect.

An infusion of the flowers is employed, especially on the Continent, as a substitute for litmus, as a test of acids and alkalis.

Of the *leaves*, Gerard tells us that they

'are used in cooling plasters, oyles and comfortable cataplasms or poultices, and are of greater efficacies amongst other herbs as Mercury, Mallowes and such like in clisters for the purposes aforesaid.'

They are an old popular remedy for bruises.

Culpepper says:

'It is a fine pleasing plant of Venus, of a mild nature and no way hurtful. All the Violets are cold and moist, while they are fresh and green, and are used to cool any heat or distemperature of the body, either inwardly or outwardly, as the inflammation in the eyes, to drink the decoction of the leaves and flowers made with water or wine, or to apply them poulticewise to the grieved places; it likewise easeth pains in the head caused through want of sleep, or any pains arising of heat if applied in the same manner or with oil of Roses. A drachm weight of the dried leaves or flowers of Violets, but the leaves more strongly, doth purge the body of choleric humours and assuageth the heat if taken in a draught of wine or other drink; the powder of the purple leaves of the flowers only picked and dried and drank in water helps the quinsy and the falling sickness in children, especially at the beginning of the disease. It is also good for jaundice. The flowers of the Violets ripen and dissolve swellings. The herbs or flowers while they are fresh or the flowers that are dry are effectual in the pleurisy and all diseases of the lungs. The green leaves are used with other herbs to make plasters and poultices for inflammation and swellings and to ease all pains whatsoever arising of heat and for piles, being fried with yoke of egg and applied thereto.'

The underground stems or rhizomes (the so-called roots) are strongly emetic and purgative. They have occasionally been used as adulterants to more costly drugs, notably to ipecacuanha. A dose of from 40 to 50 grains of the powdered root is said to act violently, inciting nausea and great vomiting and nervous affection, due to the pronounced emetic qualities of the alkaloid contained.

The seeds are purgative and diuretic and have been given in urinary complaints, and are considered a good corrective of gravel,

A modern homœopathic medicinal tincture is made from the whole fresh plant, with proof spirit, and is considered useful for a spasmodic cough with hard breathing, and also for rheumatism of the wrists.

The glucosidal principles contained in the leaves have not yet been fully investigated, but would appear to have distinct antiseptic properties.

Of late years, preparations of fresh Violet leaves have been used both internally and externally in the treatment of cancer, and though the British Pharmacopœia does not uphold the treatment, it specifies how they are employed. From other sources it is stated that Violet leaves have been used with benefit to allay the pain in cancerous growths, especially in the throat, which no other treatment relieved, and several reputed cures have been recorded.

An infusion of the leaves in boiling water (1 in 5) has been administered in doses of 1 to 2 fluid ounces. A syrup of the petals and a liquid extract of the fresh leaves are also used, the latter taken in teaspoonful doses, or rubbed in locally. The fresh leaves are also prepared as a compress for local application.

The *infusion* is generally drunk cold and is made as follows: Take 2½ oz. of Violet leaves, freshly picked. Wash them clean in cold water and place them in a stone jar and pour over them 1 pint of boiling water. Tie the jar down and let it stand for twelve hours, till the water is green. Then strain off the liquid into a well-stoppered bottle and the tea is ready for drinking cold at intervals of every two hours during the day, taking a wineglassful at a time till the whole has been consumed each day. It is essential that the tea should be made fresh every day and kept in a cool place to prevent it turning sour. If any should be left over it should be thrown away.

As a cure for cancer of the tongue, it is recommended to drink half this quantity daily at intervals and apply the rest in hot fomentations.

Injection. – About a couple of wineglassfuls made tepid can be used, if required, as an injection, night and morning, but this infusion should be made separate from the tea and should not be of greater strength than 1 oz. of leaves to ½ pint of water.

As a hot *Compress*, for external use, dip a piece of lint into the infusion, made the same strength as the tea, of which a sufficient quantity must be made warm for the purpose. Lay the lint round or over the affected part and cover with oilskin or thin mackintosh. Change the lint when dry or cold. Use flannel, not oilskin, for open wounds, and in cold weather it should be made fresh about every alternate day. Should this wet compress cause undue irritation of the skin, remove at once and substitute the following compress or *poultice*: Chop some fresh-gathered young Violet leaves, without stems, and cover with boiling water. Stand in a warm place for a quarter of an hour and add a little crushed linseed.

A *concentrated preparation* is also recommended, made as follows: Put as many Violet leaves in a saucepan as can boil in the water. Boil for ½ hour, then strain, squeezing tightly. Evaporate this decoction to one-fourth its bulk and add alcohol (spirits of wine 1 in 15); 1½ oz. or 3 tablespoonsful of spirits of wine will keep 24 oz. for a month. This syrupy product is stated to be extremely efficacious, applied two or three times a day, or more, on cotton-wool about the throat. This will not cause irritation unless applied to the skin with waterproof over for a considerable time, as under such circumstances moisture will cause irritation.

For *lubricating* the throat, dry and powder Violet leaves and let them stand in olive oil for six hours in a water bath. Make strong. It will keep any time.

A continuous daily supply of fresh leaves is necessary and a considerable quantity is required. It is recorded that during the nine weeks that a nurseryman supplied a patient suffering from cancer in the colon – which was cured at the end of this period – a Violet bed covering six rods of ground was almost entirely stripped of its foliage.

Violet Ointment. – Place 2 oz. of the best lard in a jar in the oven till it becomes quite clear. Then add about thirty-six fresh Violet leaves. Stew them in the lard for an hour till the leaves are the consistency of cooked cabbage. Strain and when cold put into a covered pot for use. This is a good old-fashioned Herbal remedy which has been allowed to fall into disuse. It is good as an application for superficial tubercles in the glands of the neck, Violet Leaves Tea being drunk at the same time.

VIOLET, WATER

Hottonia palustris
N.O. Violaceæ

Synonyms. Water Milfoil. Water Yarrow. Feather Foil

The Water Violet, an aquatic plant, is in no wise related to the familiar Violets and Pansies, but is a member of the Primrose tribe – named after Hotton, an early Leyden professor of Botany.

Description. It is common in ponds and

ditches. From the abundance of its finely-divided leaves, which are all submersed, it was also called Millefolium by older writers and Water Milfoil, Water Yarrow and Feather Foil popularly. It flowers in May and June, the flowers being large and handsome, pink or pale purple, with a yellow eye, arranged in whorls one above the other around a leafless stalk, which rises several inches out of the water and forms a handsome spike.

VIRGINIA CREEPER

Vitis Hederacea (WILLD.)
N.O. Vitaceæ

Synonyms. American Ivy. Five-leaved Ivy. Ampolopsis quinquefolia (Mich.). Cissus Hederacea (Ross.). Cissus quinquefolia (Desf.). Vitis quinquefolia (LINN.). Wood Vine

Parts Used. Bark, twigs, fresh leaves, berries, resin

This common creeper is familiar to all on account of its rapid growth and the magnificence of its autumn colouring. It is specially useful in town gardens, where it is not affected by the smoky atmosphere.

The stem is extensively climbing, reaching out in all directions and fastening itself by the disk-like appendages of the tendrils, and also by rootlets. It will shoot about 20 feet in one year, and in time it becomes very woody.

The flowering branches become converted into tendrils, as in the case of the Vine. An inspection of any vine in summer will generally show some tendrils with buds upon them, revealing their origin. Occasionally, what *ought* to have been a tendril becomes a flowering branch and bears a full bunch of grapes. The two together are called a 'double cluster.'

¶ *Description.* The leaves have long petioles, or foot-stalks, and are divided into five leaflets. The flowers are in small clusters – yellowish-green in colour and open in July, a few at a time. They are much liked by bees, and are succeeded by dark purplish-blue berries, which are ripe in October, being then about the size of a pea.

Under the name of *Hedera quinquefolia*, this creeper was first brought to Europe from Canada, and was cultivated here as early as 1629. Parkinson, in whose days it was introduced, described it –

'The leaves are crumpled or rather folded together at the first coming forth and very red, which after growing forth are very fair, large and green, divided into four, five, six or seven leaves standing together upon a small foot-stalk – set without order on the branches, at the ends whereof, as also at other places sometimes, come forth short tufts of buds for flowers, but we could never see them open themselves to show what manner of flower it would be or what fruit would follow in our country.'

¶ *Part Used.* Bark and twigs. A tincture is made of the fresh young shoots and bark, which are chopped and pounded to a pulp, mixed with 2 parts by weight of alcohol, and left for 8 days in the dark before being strained and filtered off. The tincture is not official in either the United States or the British Pharmacopœia.

The generic name *Hedera* is supposed to be derived either from the Celtic *hædra* (a cord), or from the Greek *hedra* (a seat). The specific name *Helix* was given by Linnæus, on account of its being a great harbourer of snails, Helix being the scientific name of the Snail family. The English name of Ivy is said to be from *iw* (green), from its evergreen character. Yew is derived from the same word.

¶ *Constituents.* The properties depend on the special balsamic resin contained in its leaves and stems, as well as in its particular aromatic gum. The berries contain a very bitter principle somewhat like quinine. The alkaloid contained in it is termed Hederin.

¶ *Medicinal Action and Uses.* Stimulating, diaphoretic and cathartic. Many virtues were attributed by our forefathers to this plant. Its berries have been found of use in febrile disorders, and were regarded as a specific against the plague and similar disorders, for which they were infused in vinegar. During the Great Plague of London, Ivy berries were given with some success for their antiseptic virtues and to induce perspiration.

In India the leaves are used as an aperient, and a resinous matter that in warm climates exudes from the bark of the main stems (and may be procured by wounding them) is considered a useful stimulant, antispasmodic and emmenagogue. This gum possesses mildly aperient properties, and was at one time included as a medicine in the Edinburgh Pharmacopœia, but has now fallen out of use. Dissolved in vinegar it had the reputation of being a good filling for a hollow tooth causing neuralgic toothache.

The leaves have a very unpleasant taste. Taken inwardly in infusion, they act as an aperient and emetic, but are sudorific. They have been given on the Continent to children suffering from atrophy. The juice is said to cure headache, when applied to the nostrils. An infusion of the leaves and berries will also mitigate a severe headache.

The fresh leaves of Ivy, boiled in vinegar and applied warm to the sides of those who are troubled with the spleen, or stitch in the sides, will give much ease. The same applied with Rose-water, and oil of Roses to the temples and forehead eases headaches. Cups made from Ivywood have been employed, from which to sip hot or cold water for diseases of the spleen.

A decoction of the leaves applied externally will destroy head lice in children, and fresh Ivy leaves bruised and applied will afford great relief to bunions and shooting corns, a remedy to the excellence of which John Wesley has testified.

The leaves have also been employed as poultices and fomentations in glandular enlargements, indolent ulcers, etc.

A decoction of the leaves has been used as a black dye.

The berries possess much the same properties as the leaves, being strongly purgative and emetic. An infusion of the berries has been frequently found serviceable in rheumatic complaints and is reported to have cured the dropsy.

The dried bark is also used in a decoction. When stripped from the branches (after the berries have ripened) and dried in the sun, it occurs in quilled pieces 2 to 3 inches long and from ¼ to ½ inch in diameter, externally brown with enlarged transverse scars, the fracture showing a white bark with coarse flattened fibres in the inner portion. One ounce of the bark to a pint of boiling water is taken in wineglassful doses.

A fluid extract is also prepared from the bark and twigs, of which the dose is ½ to 1 drachm; another preparation, Ampelopsin, is taken in doses of 2 to 4 grains.

¶ *Constituents.* Pyrocatachin (Oxyphenic acid) in the green leaves. Cisso-tannic acid has been determined as the pigment of the red coloration in the autumnal coloured leaves, and has an astringent, bitter taste. The leaves when green contain also free tartaric acid and its salts, with sodium and potassium. Glycollic acid and calcium glycollate exist in the ripe berries.

In scrofulous affections the drug is principally employed in the form of a syrup.

WAFER ASH. *See* ASH

WAHOO. *See* SPINDLE

(POISON)
WAKE ROBIN, AMERICAN
Arum triphyllum (LINN.)
N.O. Araceæ

Synonyms. Dragon Root. Wild Turnip. Devil's Ear. Pepper Turnip. Indian Turnip. Jack-in-the-Pulpit. Memory Root. Arisamæ triphyllum (Schott.)
(*French*) Gouet à trois feuilles
(*German*) Dreiblattiger Aron
Part Used. The root (fresh corm)
Habitat. Eastern North America in damp places. Indigenous almost all over United States and Canada

¶ *Description.* The plant has a round flattened perennial rhizome, the upper part tunicated as in the onion, the lower and larger portion tuberous and fleshy, with numerous long white radicles in a circle from its upper edge, the under-side covered with a dark, loose, wrinkled epidermis. Spathe ovate, acuminate, convoluted into a tube at the bottom, flattened and bent at top like a hood, varying in colour internally, supported by an erect scape inverted at base by petioles and their acute sheaths. Spadix club-shaped, shorter than spathe, rounded at end, contracted at base, surrounded by stamens or ovaries; the upper portions of the spadix withers together with the spathe, whilst the ovaries grow into a large compact bunch of shining scarlet berries. Leaves, one or two standing on long sheathing foot-stalks, ternate. Leaflets oval, mostly entire, acuminate, smooth, paler on under-side, becoming glaucous with growth, the two lateral ones rhomboidal.

¶ *Constituents.* In the recent state it has a peculiar odour and is violently acrid. It has been found to contain besides the acrid principle, 10 to 17 per cent. of starch, albumen, gum, sugar, extractive, lignin and salts of potassium and calcium.

¶ *Medicinal Action and Uses.* Acrid, expectorant, and diaphoretic. Used in flatulence, croup, whooping-cough, stomatitis, asthma, chronic laryngitis, bronchitis and pains in chest.

In the fresh state it is a violent irritant to the mucous membrane, when chewed burning the mouth and throat; if taken internally this plant causes violent gastro-enteritis which may end in death.

¶ *Dosage.* Powdered root, 10 grains two or three times daily.

The perfectly fresh root should not be used and the fully dried root is inactive.

¶ *Antidote.* Strong tea and stimulants.
See CUCKOO PINT.

WALLFLOWER [1]

Cherranthus cheiri (LINN.)
N.O. Cruciferæ

Synonyms. Gillyflower. Wallstock-gillofer. Giroflier. Gillyflower. Handflower. Keiri. Beeflower. Baton d'or

Parts Used. Flowers, stems

Habitat. All Southern Europe, on old walls, quarries and seacliffs

¶ *Description.* This homely perennial plant of the cabbage family was introduced into this country over 300 years ago, and its delightful fragrance soon made it a general favourite. It has single flowers, yellowy orange in its wild state, and quickly spreads abundantly from seed, commencing to bloom in early spring, and continuing most of the summer. In olden times this flower was carried in the hand at classic festivals, hence it was called Cherisaunce by virtue of its cordial qualities.

¶ *Constituents.* Oil, a powerful glucoside, of the digitalis group, and cherinine, a crystalline alkaloid.

¶ *Medicinal Action and Uses.* The oil has a pleasing perfume if diluted, but in full strength a disagreeable odour. The alkaloid is useful acting on nerve centres and on the muscles.

WALL RUE. *See* FERNS

WALNUT

Juglans nigra (LINN.)
N.O. Juglandaceæ

Synonyms. Carya. Jupiter's Nuts
(*Dutch*) Walnoot
(*Greek*) Carya persica. Carya basilike
(*Roman*) Nux persica. Nux regia

Parts Used. Leaves, bark

Habitat. According to Dr. Royle *Juglans regia* extends from Greece and Asia Minor, over Lebanon and Persia, probably all along the Hindu-Kush to the Himalayas. It is abundant in Kashmir, and is found in Sirmore, Kumdon and Nepal. The walnuts imported into the plains of India are chiefly from Kashmir. Dr. Hooker states that in the Sikkim Himalaya, the Walnut inhabits the mountain slopes at an elevation of 4,000 to 7,000 feet.

According to Pliny, it was introduced into Italy from Persia, and it is mentioned by Varro, who was born B.C. 116, as growing in Italy during his lifetime.

There is no certain account of the time it was brought into this country. Some say 1562; but Gerard, writing about thirty years later, mentions the Walnut as being very common in the fields near common highways, and in orchards.

The Common Walnut, a large and handsome tree, with strong, spreading boughs, is not a native of Britain. Its native place is probably Persia. Other varieties of Walnut, the Black Walnut, the various kinds of Hickory, etc., are mostly natives of North America.

The Romans called the tree *nux*, on account of its fruit. The English name Walnut is partly of Teutonic origin, the Germans naming the nut *Wallnuss*, or *Welsche Nuss* – *Welsche* signifying foreign.

It was said that in the 'golden age,' when men lived upon acorns the gods lived upon Walnuts, and hence the name of *Juglans*, *Jovis glans*, or Jupiter's nuts.

¶ *Description.* The tree grows to a height of 40 or 60 feet, with a large spreading top, and thick, massive stem. One accurately measured by Professor du Breuil, in Normandy, was upwards of 23 feet in circumference; and in some parts of France there are Walnut trees 300 years old, with stems of much greater thickness. In the southern parts of England the trees grow vigorously and bear abundantly, when not injured by late frosts in spring.

The flowers of separate sexes are borne upon the same tree and appear in early spring before the leaves. The male flowers have a calyx of five or six scales, surrounding from eighteen to thirty-six stamens; whilst the

[1] In homœopathic medicine a tincture of the whole plant has been found useful in the effects of cutting the wisdom tooth. – EDITOR.

calyx of the female flowers closely envelops the ovary, which bears two or three fleshy stigmas. The deciduous leaves are pinnate.

For drying indoors, a warm, sunny attic, or loft may be employed, the window being left open by day, so that there is a current of air and the moist, hot air may escape: the door may also be left open. The leaves can be placed on coarse butter-cloth, stented – if hooks are placed beneath the window and on the opposite wall the butter-cloth can be attached by rings sewn on each side of it and hooked on so that it is stretched taut. The temperature should be from 70° to 100°.

Failing sun, any ordinary shed, fitted with racks and shelves, can be used, provided it is ventilated near the roof and has a warm current of air, caused by an ordinary coke or anthracite stove. Empty glasshouses can readily be adapted into drying-sheds (especially if heated by pipes) if the glass is shaded. Ventilation is essential, and there must be no open tank in the house to cause steaming.

The leaves should be spread in a single layer, preferably not touching, and may be turned during drying.

All dried leaves should be packed away at once, in airtight, wooden or tin boxes in a dry place, otherwise they re-absorb moisture from the air.

Walnut leaves are parchment-like when dry, and the leaf-stalks brown, but the leaves themselves keep their good colour when dried. They have a bitter and astringent taste. By long keeping, the leaves become brown and lose their characteristic, aromatic odour.

The bark is dried in the same manner as the leaves. When dry, it occurs in quilled or curbed pieces, 3 to 6 inches long or more, and ¾ inch broad, dull blackish-brown, with traces of a thin, whitish epidermal layer, tough and fibrous and somewhat mealy. The inner fibres are tough and flattened, the outer ones, white and silky. The taste is bitter and astringent, but it has no odour.

¶ Constituents. The active principle of the whole Walnut tree, as well as of the nuts, is Nucin or Juglon. The kernels contain oil, mucilage, albumin, mineral matter, cellulose and water.

¶ Medicinal Action and Uses. The bark and leaves have alterative, laxative, astringent and detergent properties, and are used in the treatment of skin troubles. They are of the highest value for curing scrofulous diseases, herpes, eczema, etc., and for healing indolent ulcers; an infusion of 1 oz. of dried bark or leaves (slightly more of the fresh leaves) to the pint of boiling water, allowed to stand for six hours, and strained off is taken in wineglassful doses, three times a day, the same infusion being also employed at the same time for outward application. Obstinate ulcers may also be cured with sugar, well saturated with a strong decoction of Walnut leaves.

The bark, dried and powdered, and made into a strong infusion, is a useful purgative.

The husk, shell and peel are sudorific, especially if used when the Walnuts are green. Whilst unripe, the nut has worm-destroying virtues.

The fruit, when young and unripe, makes a wholesome, anti-scorbutic pickle, the vinegar in which the green fruit has been pickled proving a capital gargle for sore and slightly ulcerated throats. Walnut catsup embodies the medicinal virtues of the unripe nuts.

It is much cultivated in some parts of Italy, France, Germany and Switzerland, and formerly also in England, particularly on the chalk-hills of Surrey, for the sake of its timber, as well as for its fruit.

On the Continent, the wood is still in great request for furniture, but when mahogany became a favourite wood in this country, in the early part of last century, the old walnut trees that were cut down were not always replaced by young ones, so that plantations of this tree diminished.

At one time as much as £600 was given for a single Walnut tree.

The leaves have a very strong, characteristic smell, aromatic and not unpleasant, but said to be injurious to sensitive people. They have three, sometimes four pairs of leaflets and a terminal one, the leaflets varying in size on the same leaf, being 2¼ to 4 inches in length and 1 to 1½ inch wide, entire, smooth, shining, and paler below.

The flowers begin to open about the middle of April and are in full bloom by the middle of May, before which time the tree is in full leaf.

Even in the south of France, this tree is frequently injured by spring frosts.

The wood has been much used, not only for furniture and wainscoting, but for the wheels and bodies of coaches, for making gun-stocks, and by the cabinet-maker for inlaying. It is unfit for use as beams because of its brittleness.

The oil yielded by the kernel of the fruit (the part eaten) is used to polish the wood. Not congealing by cold, it is found on this account most useful for painters for mixing gold-size and varnish with white and delicate colours. The oil has been used in some parts of France for frying, eaten as butter and employed as lamp oil. One bushel of nuts, producing about 15 lb. of peeled kernels, will yield about 7 lb. of the oil.

The green husks of the fruit, boiled, make a good yellow dye.

No insects will touch the leaves of the Walnut, which yield a brown dye, which gypsies use to stain their skin. It is said to contain iodine.

The husks and leaves, macerated in warm water impart to it an intense bitterness, which will destroy all worms (if the liquid be poured on to lawns and grass walks) without injuring the grass itself.

¶ *Parts Used Medicinally*. The leaves and bark. The leaves are stripped off the tree singly, in June and July and dried.

Gather the leaves only in fine weather, in the morning, after the dew has been dried by the sun. The prevalence of an east wind is favourable, as the dry air facilitates the process of drying. Reject all stained leaves.

Drying may be done in warm, sunny weather, out-of-doors, but in half-shade as leaves dried in the shade retain their colour better than those dried in the sun and do not become so tindery. They may be placed on wire sieves, or frames covered with wire or garden netting – at a height of about 3 or 4 feet from the ground, to ensure a current of air – and must be taken indoors to a dry room or shed, before there is any chance of them becoming damp from dew or showers.

The juice of the green husks, boiled with honey, is also a good gargle for a sore mouth and inflamed throat, and the distilled water of the green husks is good for quinsy and as an application for wounds and internally is a cooling drink in agues.

The thin, yellow skin which clothes the inner nut is a notable remedy for colic, being first dried, and then rubbed into powder. It is administered in doses of 30 grains, with a tablespoonful of peppermint water.

The oil extracted from the ripe kernels, taken inwardly in ½ oz. doses, has also proved good for colic and is efficacious, applied externally, for skin diseases of the leprous type and wounds and gangrenes.

¶ *Preparations*. Fluid extract leaves, 1 to 2 drachms. Walnut oil.

The Walnut has been termed 'vegetable arsenic,' on account of its curative effect in eczema and other skin diseases.

William Cole, an exponent of the doctrine of signatures, says in *Adam in Eden*, 1657:

'Wall-nuts have the perfect Signature of the Head: The outer husk or green Covering, represent the *Pericranium*, or outward skin of the skull, whereon the hair groweth or barks, and therefore salt made of those husks or barks,

are exceeding good for wounds in the head. The inner wooddy shell hath the Signature of the Skull, and the little yellow skin, or Peel, that covereth the Kernell, of the hard *Meninga* and *Pia-mater*, which are the thin scarfes that envelope the brain. The Kernel hath the very figure of the Brain, and therefore it is very profitable for the Brain, and resists poysons; For if the Kernel be bruised, and moystned with the quintessence of Wine, and laid upon the Crown of the Head, it comforts the brain and head mightily.'

Culpepper says of Walnuts :

'if they' [the leaves] 'be taken with onions, salt, and honey, they help the biting of a mad dog, or the venom or infectious poison of any beast, etc. Caius Pompeius found in the treasury of Mithridates, King of Pontus, when he was overthrown, a scroll of his own handwriting, containing a medicine against any poison or infection; which is this: Take two dry walnuts, and as many good figs, and twenty leaves of rue, bruised and beaten together with two or three corns of salt and twenty juniper berries, which take every morning fasting, preserves from danger of poison, and infection that day it is taken. . . . The kernels, when they grow old, are more oily, and therefore not fit to be eaten, but are then used to heal the wounds of the sinews, gangrenes, and carbuncles. . . . The said kernels being burned, are very astringent . . . being taken in red wine, and stay the falling of the hair, and make it fair, being anointed with oil and wine. The green husks will do the like, being used in the same manner. . . . A piece of the green husks put into a hollow tooth, eases the pain.'

RECIPES

'To preserve green Walnuts in Syrup

'Take as many green Walnuts as you please, about the middle of July, try them all with a pin, if it goes easily through them they are fit for your purpose; lay them in Water for nine days, washing and shifting them Morning and Night; then boil them in water until they be a little Soft, lay them to drain; then pierce them through with a Wooden Sciver, and in the hole put a Clove, and in some a bit of Cinnamon, and in some the rind of a Citron Candi'd: then take the weight of your Nuts in Sugar, or a little more; make it into a syrup, in which boil your Nuts (scimming them) till they be tender; then put them up in Gally potts, and cover them close. When you lay them to drain, wipe them with a Course cloth to take off a thin green Skin. They are Cordial and Stomachal.' – (From *The Family*

Physician, 'by Geo. Hartman, Phylo Chymist, who liv'd and Travell'd with the Honourable Sir Kenelm Digby, in several parts of Europe, the space of Seven Years till he died.')

The next is from a seventeenth-century household MS. Receipt Book inscribed *Madam Susanna Avery, Her Book, May ye 12th, Anno Domini* 1688.

'To Pickel Wallnutts Green

'Let your nutts be green as not to have any shell; then run a kniting pin two ways through them; then put them into as much ordinary vinegar as will cover them, and let them stand thirty days, shifting them every too days in ffrech vinegar; then ginger and black peper of each ounce, rochambole two ounces slised, a handfull of bay leaves; put all togeather cold; then wrap up every wall nutt singly in a vine leaf, and put them in putt them into [*sic*] the ffolloing pickel: for 200 of walnutts take two gallans of the best whit vineager, a pint of the best mustard seed, fore ounces of horse radish, with six lemons sliced with the rin(d)s on, cloves and mace half an ounce, a stone jar, and put the pickel on them, and cork them close up; and they will be ffitt for use in three months, and keep too years.'

WALNUT, WHITE

Synonyms. Oil Nut
See BUTTERNUT

Juglans cinerea (LINN.)
N.O. Juglandaceæ

WATER BETONY. *See* BETONY

WATERCRESS

Nasturtium officinale
N.O. Cruciferæ

Parts Used. Leaves, flowers, seeds
Habitat. Europe and Russian Asia

¶ *Description.* A hardy perennial found in abundance near springs and open running watercourses, of a creeping habit with smooth, shining, brownish-green, pinnatifid leaves and ovate, heart-shaped leaflets, the terminal one being larger than the rest. Flowers small and white, produced towards the extremity of the branches in a sort of terminal panicle.

The true nasturtium or Indian Cress cultivated in gardens as a creeper has brilliant orange-red flowers and produces the seeds which serve as a substitute for capers in pickles.

The poisonous Marshwort or 'Fool's Cress' is often mistaken for Watercress, with which it is sometimes found growing. It may readily be distinguished by its hemlock-like white flowers, and when out of flower, by its finely toothed and somewhat pointed leaves, much longer than those of the watercress

and of a paler green. The Latin name 'Nasturtium' is derived from the words *nasus tortus* (a convulsed nose) on account of its pungency.

¶ *Constituents.* A sulpho-nitrogenous oil, iodine iron, phosphates, potash, with other mineral salts, bitter extract and water. Its volatile oil rich in nitrogen combined with some sulphur in the sulpho-cyanide of allyl.

¶ *Medicinal Action and Uses.* Watercress is particularly valuable for its antiscorbutic qualities and has been used as such from the earliest times. As a salad it promotes appetite. Culpepper says that the leaves bruised or the juice will free the face from blotches, spots and blemishes, when applied as a lotion.

¶ *Dosage.* Expressed juice, 1 to 2 fluid ounces.

Watercress has also been used as a specific in tuberculosis. Its active principles are said to be at their best when the plant is in flower.

WATER DOCK. *See* DOCK

WATER DROPWORT. *See* DROPWORT, HEMLOCK WATER

WATER FENNEL. *See* FENNEL

WATER SOLDIER

Stratiotes aloides
N.O. Hydrocharidaceæ

Synonyms. Water Houseleek. Water Aloe. Water Sengren. Sea Green. Crab's Claws. Knight's Pondweed. Freshwater Soldier. Water Parsnip
(*French*) Aloides
(*German*) Wasserfeder
Part Used. Herb

Culpepper describes under the name of Water Houseleek, Water Sengren or Sea-

green, a plant that has nothing to do with any of these other succulent plants, and that nowadays generally goes by one of its other popular names, Water Soldier, and is botanically known as *Stratiotes aloides*.

It is an aquatic plant, the only British representative of its genus, and is found growing in ditches in the Eastern counties of England, mostly in the Fen district. The roots extend some distance into the mud and throw up numerous deep-green, spreading, narrow, rigid and brittle leaves, from 6 to 18 inches long, very sharply pointed, with sharp prickles on each margin. They are strikingly similar to the foliage of an aloe, hence its specific name, *aloides*, and another of its popular English names, Water Aloe. The name of the genus is derived from the Greek word for a soldier, in reference to its crowded, sword-like leaves.

¶ *Description.* The flower-stalk is stout and short, about 6 inches high, bearing at its summit a two-leaved sheath, which is likened by old writers to the claws of a crab, from which another of its names, Crab's Claws, is derived. Stamens and pistils are on different plants. In the case of the staminate flowers, the sheath contains several delicate white flowers, with three petals and numerous stamens, twelve of which are perfect, as well as many other imperfect ones. The flowers containing the ovary – which is six-celled and six-angled, and develops into a pulpy, flask-shaped berry – are solitary on the stem.

After flowering in the month of July, the plant sinks to the bottom and ripens its fruit while submerged. It is a perennial and propagates itself freely by stolons as well as by seed. Although each root only flowers once, the parent plant rooted in the mud at the bottom of the ditch, after flowering, sends out buds of leaves at the end of long runners, which rise to the surface in the spring, and become separate plants, forming roots, flower, and then sink to the bottom, where they fix themselves in the mud, ripen their seeds and become, in their turn, parents of another race of young offsets, which in turn rise in the spring and float on the surface, sometimes eight or ten in a circle, so thick as to entirely fill up the surface of the ditches, and prevent all other plants from growing.

¶ *Medicinal Action and Uses.* Culpepper tells us that the herb 'is good against St. Anthony's Fire, and assuages swelling and inflammations in wounds; an ointment made of it is good to heal them.' He also informs us it is good for 'bruised kidneys.' It had in olden times the reputation of being an unfailing cure for all wounds made by iron weapons.

WHITE POND LILY. *See* LILY

WILD CARROT. *See* CARROT

WILD CHERRY. *See* CHERRY

WILD GINGER. *See* GINGER

WILD INDIGO. *See* INDIGO

WILD YAM. *See* YAMS

WILD MINT. *See* MINTS

WILLOW, BLACK AMERICAN

Salyx nigra (MARCH)
N.O. Salicaceæ

Synonym. Pussy Willow
Parts Used. Bark, berries
Habitat. America (New York and Pennsylvania)

¶ *Description.* A tree growing on banks of rivers up to 15 to 25 feet high, with a rough blackish bark. Leaves narrowly lanceolate, pointed, tapering at each end, serrulate, smooth, and green on both sides, petioles and midveins tomentose. Stipules small, deciduous, dentate; aments erect, cylindric, villous. Scales oblong, very villous. Sterile aments 3 inches long, glands of sterile flowers two large and deeply two or three cleft. Stamens four to six, often but three in the upper scales, filaments bearded at base. Ovary pedicillate, smooth, ovoid. Style very short, stigmas bifid.

¶ *Constituents.* The bark contains tannin and about 1 per cent. of Salinigrin, a white crystalline glucoside soluble in water and alcohol.

¶ *Medicinal Action and Uses.* An aphrodisiac, sedative, tonic. The bark has been prescribed in gonorrhœa and to relieve ovarian pain; a liquid extract is prepared and used in mixture with other sedatives. Largely used in the treatment of nocturnal emissions.

Fluid extract, $\frac{1}{2}$ to 1 drachm.

WILLOW, WHITE

Salix alba (LINN.)
N.O. Salicaceæ

Synonym. European Willow
Part Used. Bark
Habitat. Central and Southern Europe

¶ *Description.* A large tree with a rough greyish bark, the twigs being brittle at the base; the leaves are pubescent on both surfaces and finely serrulate; it hybridizes with other species of *Salix,* it flowers in April and May and the bark is easily separable throughout the summer; flowers and leaves appear coincidently from March to June.

¶ *Constituents.* The bark contains up to 13 per cent. of tannin as its chief constituent, also a small quantity of salicin.

¶ *Medicinal Action and Uses.* Tonic, antiperiodic and astringent. It has been used in dyspepsia connected with debility of the digestive organs. In convalescence from acute diseases, in worms, in chronic diarrhœa and dysentery, its tonic and astringent combination renders it very useful.

¶ *Dosages.* 1 drachm of the powdered root. 1 or 2 fluid ounces of the decoction.

WILLOW-HERBS

N.O. Onagrariaceæ

The Willow-herbs (*Epilobium*), nine species of which are natives of Great Britain, belong to the order Onagraceæ, to which belong also the familiar garden flowers the Fuchsia, Clarkia and Godetia, and the Evening Primrose (*Œnothera biennis*) (a native of North America, which, as a garden escape, is sometimes found apparently wild). The insignificant wild plant *Circæa lutetiana,* the Enchanter's Nightshade, also belongs to the same family. Many of the members of the order, being rich in tannin, find considerable domestic use as astringents.

The name of the genus *Epilobium* is from two Greek words *epi* (upon) and *lobos* (a pod), from the fact that the flowers stand upon the top of long, thin, pod-like seed-vessels, having somewhat the appearance of rather thick flower-stems. The name Willow-herb refers to the willow-like form of the leaves.

WILLOW-HERB, ROSE BAY

Epilobium angustifolium (LINN.)
N.O. Onagrariaceæ

Synonyms. Flowering Willow. French Willow. Persian Willow. Rose Bay Willow. Blood Vine. Blooming Sally. Purple Rocket. Wickup. Wicopy. Tame Withy
Part Used. Herb

Epilobium angustifolium (Linn.), the Rose Bay Willow-herb, is one of our handsomest wild flowers, and like the Foxglove, is for its beauty often cultivated as a garden plant.

Its tall, erect stems, 4 to 8 feet high, densely clothed with long, narrow, minutely-toothed leaves, terminate in long, showy spikes of flowers of a light rose-purple, hence the name Rose Bay, the leaves having likewise been compared to those of the Bay Laurel. The plant has also been named Blood Vine, because it has a red appearance. In Ireland, we find it called 'Blooming Sally,' Sally being a corruption of the Latin *Salix,* the Willow, really a reference to the willow-like leaves.

Gerard calls it:

'A goodly and stately plant having leaves like the greatest willow or osier, garnished with brave flowers of great beautie, consisting of four leaves apiece of an orient purple colour.'

It is a native of most countries of Europe. In this country, it has apparently become more common than it was in Gerard's day.

He tells us he had received some plants of this species from a place in Yorkshire, apparently as a rarity, 'which doe grow in my garden very goodly to behold, for the decking up of houses and gardens.'

It is to be found by moist riversides and in copses, but will sometimes spring up in a town, self-sown, on waste ground recently cleared of buildings: the site of Kingsway and Aldwych in London, adjoining the Strand, where many buildings, centuries old, had been pulled down, was the following summer covered by the Rose Bay Willow-herb, as by a crimson mantle, though no one could explain where the seeds had come from. The same phenomenon was repeated, in Westminster, when other old buildings were demolished for improvements and the ground remained waste for a considerable time. In America, it springs up on ground recently cleared by firing, being one of the plants called 'Fireweed' in the United States where it is known as the Great or Spiked Willowherb, Bay Willow, Flowering Willow, Purple Rocket, Wickup and Wicopy.

The plant is in bloom for about a month. The individual flowers are about an inch in diameter, calyx and corolla each four-parted; the stamens, eight in number, standing up, form an arch or dome over the ovary, on the green, fleshy, upper surface of which nectar is secreted. Sprengel, in 1790, showed that the flowers, which open soon after sunrise, are protenandrous, i.e. the anthers ripen first, and self-pollination would occur if insects did not visit them. Bees, who much visit the flowers in search of nectar, get smeared by the pollen, which is sticky. It is not left by them on the stigma of the same flower, however, which at this stage is a mere knob, immature and unable to receive the pollen grains. On reaching another flower, further advanced, the stigma, ripe for reception of pollen, has opened out to become a white, four-rayed cross of great distinctness and perforce receives any pollen the insect visitor may have collected as he pushes by to get to the nectar below, and the ovules thus become fertilized.

The dead flowers, when fertilization has been effected, fall off cleanly from the long, projecting, quadrangular pods, which later split into four long strands, which stretch wide apart, disclosing a mass of silky white hairs, in which are embedded the very tiny seeds, a few hairs being attached to the top of each seed. The slightest wind scatters them broadcast over the neighbourhood. All the Willow-herbs distribute their seeds in the same manner, and as the plant spreads extensively by creeping stems it is very difficult to keep it within bounds.

¶ *Uses.* The leaves of the Rose Bay Willow-herb have been used as a substitute and adulterant of Tea. Though no longer so employed in England, the leaves of both this species and of the Great Hairy Willow-herb (*E. hirsutum*, Linn.) are largely used in Russia, under the name of Kaporie Tea.

Green (*Universal Herbal*, 1832) reports:

'The young shoots are said to be eatable, although an infusion of the plant produces a stupifying effect.

'The pith when dried is boiled, and becoming sweet, is by a proper process made into ale, and this into vinegar, by the Kamtschatdales; it is also added to the Cow Parsnip, to enrich the spirit that is prepared from that plant.

'As fodder, goats are said to be extremely fond of it and cows and sheep to eat it.

'The down of the seeds, mixed with cotton or fur, has been manufactured into stockings, etc.'

The young shoots are boiled and eaten like asparagus.

The ale made from the plant in Kamchatka is rendered still more intoxicating with a toadstool, the Fly Agaric, *Agaricus muscarius.*

¶ *Medicinal Action and Uses.* The roots and leaves have demulcent, tonic and astringent properties and are used in domestic medicine in decoction, infusion and cataplasm, as astringents.

Used much in America as an intestinal astringent.

The plant contains mucilage and tannin.

The dose of the herb is 30 to 60 grains. It has been recommended for its antispasmodic properties in the treatment of whooping-cough, hiccough and asthma.

In ointment, it has been used locally as a remedy for infantile cutaneous affections.

By some modern botanists, this species is now assigned to a separate genus and designated: *Chamænerion angustifolium* (Scop.).

WILLOW-HERB, GREAT HAIRY

Epilobium hirsutum (LINN.)
N.O. Onagrariaceæ

Synonyms. Son-before-the-Father. Codlings and Cream. Apple Pie. Cherry Pie. Gooseberry Pie. Sod Apple and Plum Pudding
Part Used. Herb

The Great Hairy Willowherb, though it has not so conspicuous a flower as the Rose Bay, is yet a striking plant, growing in great masses by pond sides, along the margins of lakes and rivers and in marshes and pools.

It is tall and erect, branched, with underground creeping shoots, like the Rose Bay. The leaves are placed opposite one another on the stem, are 3 to 5 inches long, their bases clasping the stem and like it, very woolly, hence the specific Latin name *hirsutum,* and the common English name.

The flowers are numerous and large, rose-purple, though not so brilliant as those of the Rose Bay, bell-shaped and partly drooping, the petals broad and notched.

In this species, stigmas and anthers ripen together and the plant is capable of self-pollination, but cross-pollination is ensured by insect visitors by the more prominent position of the stigmas. Insect visitors are, however, not very numerous, and in their absence the stigmas curl back and touch the anthers. (In another smaller species, *Epilobium parviflorum* (Schreb.) rarely visited by insects, four stamens are shorter, four longer than the style; the former are only useful for cross-pollination, the latter self-pollinate the flower. Stamens and stigma ripen simultaneously.)

The seeds, contained in similar long pods, are provided as in the Rose Bay, with a tuft of hairs which aid in wind dispersal.

The leaves, and particularly the top-shoots, when slightly bruised, have a delicate, cool fragrance, resembling scalded codlings, whence its popular name of Codlings and Cream, but this fragrance is very soon lost after the plant is gathered. It is also called, in allusion to this delicate scent, Apple Pie, Cherry Pie, Gooseberry Pie, Sod Apple and Plum Pudding. It is said to be the 'St. Anthony's Herb' of antiquity.

The old English country name of 'Son-before-the-Father' arises because, as Lyte says: 'the long huskes in which the seede is contained doe come forth and waxe great before that the floure openeth.'

The name 'Hooded Willow-herb' does not refer to one of these species, but is another name for the Scullcap (*Scutellaria*), and the 'Purple Willow-herb' is also not this species, but another name for *Lythrum Salicaria*, the Purple Loosestrife, a plant that is often present in the same riverside situations.

Although the leaves of *E. hirsutum* have also been used as astringents there are reports of violent poisoning with epileptic-like convulsions having been caused by its employment.

WINTERGREEN

Gaultheria procumbens (LINN.)
N.O. Ericaceæ

Synonyms. Teaberry. Boxberry. Mountain Tea. Checkerberry. Thé du Canada. Aromatic Wintergreen. Partridge Berry. Deerberry

Part Used. Leaves

Habitat. Northern United States from Georgia to Newfoundland; Canada

¶ *Description.* A small indigenous shrubby, creeping, evergreen plant, growing about 5 to 6 inches high under trees and shrubs, particularly under evergreens such as Kalmias and Rhododendrons. It is found in large patches on sandy and barren plains, also on mountainous tracts. The stiff branches bear at their summit tufts of leaves which are petiolate, oval, shiny, coriaceous, the upper side bright green, paler underneath. The drooping white flowers are produced singly from the base of the leaves in June and July, followed by fleshy, bright red berries (with a sweetish taste and peculiar flavour), formed by the enlargement of the calyx. The *leaves* were formerly official in the United States Pharmacopœia, but now only the oil obtained from them is official, though in some parts the whole plant is used. The odour is peculiar and aromatic, and the taste of the whole plant astringent, the leaves being particularly so.

¶ *Constituents.* The volatile oil obtained by distillation and to which all the medicinal qualities are due, contains 99 per cent. Methyl Salicylate: other properties are 0·3 of a hydrocarbon, Gaultherilene, and an aldehyde or ketone, a secondary alcohol and an ester. To the alcohol and ester are due the characteristic odour of the oil. The oil does not occur visibly in the plant, but as a non-odorous glucoside, and before distillation, the leaves have to be steeped for twelve to twenty-four hours for the oil to develop by fermentation – a reaction between water and a neutral principle: Gaultherin.

¶ *Medicinal Action and Uses.* Tonic, stimulant, astringent, aromatic. Useful as a diuretic and emmenagogue and for chronic mucous discharges. Is said to be a good galactogogue. The oil of Gaultheria is its most important product. It has all the properties of the salicylates and therefore is most beneficial in acute rheumatism, but must be given internally in capsules, owing to its pungency, death from inflammation of the stomach having been known to result from frequent and large doses of it. It is readily absorbed by the skin, but is liable to give rise to an eruption, so it is advisable to use for external application the synthetic oil of Wintergreen, Methyl Salicylate, or oil from the bark of *Betula lenta*, which is almost identical with oil of Gaultheria. In this form, it is a very valuable external application for rheumatic affections in all chronic forms of joint and muscular troubles, lumbago, sciatica, etc. The leaves have found use as a substitute for tea and as a flavouring for genuine tea. The berries form a winter food for animals, partridges, deer, etc. They have been used, steeped in brandy, to produce a bitter tonic taken in small quantities. The oil is a flavouring agent for tooth powders, liquid dentifrices, pastes, etc., especially if combined with menthol and eucalyptus.

¶ *Dosage.* Capsules of oil of Gaultheris, 10 minims in each, 1, three times daily.

¶ *Other Species.*
Gaultheria hispidula, or Cancer Wintergreen, supposed to remove the cancerous

taint from the system. Is also used for scrofula and prolapsus of the womb.

G. Shallon is the Sallol of North-west America, whose edible fruit deserves to be more widely known and cultivated.

Pyrola rotundifolia, known as False Wintergreen or British Wintergreen, was formerly considered a vulnerary.

With *Chimophila umbellata*, the Bitter Wintergreen, Rheumatism Weed or Pipsissewa, *C. maculata*, the Spotted Wintergreen was used internally by North American Indians for rheumatism and scrofula. For its diuretic action it is occasionally prescribed, in fluid extract, for cystitis and considered useful in disordered digestion.

Trientalis Europæa, the Chickweed Wintergreen, a British plant, was formerly esteemed in ointment as a wound salve, and an infusion taken internally for blood poisoning or eczema. The root is emetic.

See PYROLA.

WINTER'S BARK

Drimys winteri (FORST.)
N.O. Magnoliaceæ

Synonyms. True Winter's Bark. Winter's Cinnamon. Wintera aromatica. Wintera
Part Used. Bark
Habitat. Antarctic America, southern parts of South America, along the Straits of Magellan and north to Chile, Brazil

¶ *Description.* This very large evergreen tree took its name from Captain Winter, who discovered its medicinal properties while attending Drake in his voyage round the world. It will grow to 50 feet high. The bark is green and wrinkled, that of the branches smooth and green, erect and scarred, leaves alternate, oblong, obtuse, with a midrib veinless, glabrous and finely dotted underside. Flowers small on terminal peduncles, approximately one-flowered, simple. Fruits up to six obovate, baccate, and many seeded. The bark is the official part and is found in small carved pieces ¼ inch thick, dull yellow grey externally. Both Canella and Cinnamodendron are found in its transverse section, exhibiting radiating white lines at the end of the last rays, diverging towards the circumference; odour aromatic with a warm pungent taste.

¶ *Constituents.* An inodorous acrid resin, pale yellow volatile oil, tannic acid, oxide of iron, colouring matter and various salts.

¶ *Medicinal Action and Uses.* Stimulant, aromatic tonic, antiscorbutic, may be substituted in all cases for canella and cinnamon barks. Dose, 30 grains powdered bark; this bark is becoming very scarce and is seldom imported into Britain.

¶ *Other Species.*
Under the name of *Winter's Bark* Malambo Bark was imported into the United States (or Croton Malambo) or Matias bark, is the product of a small shrubby tree, found on the coast of Venezuela and Columbia. It has an aromatic smell and a pungent bitter taste with a calamus flavour. Active contents, a volatile oil, and bitter extractive, found most useful for dyspepsia, hemicrania, intermittent fever, and as a general aromatic tonic, also a useful adjuvant to diuretics and a good substitute for Peruvian bark.

Drimys Chilensis, growing in Chile, has analogous properties to Winter's Bark.

Cinnamodendron axillaris. The bark is used in fevers and called Casca Paratuds.

D. aromatica. An Australian species.
See (WHITE) CINNAMON.

WINTER'S BARK, FALSE

Cinnamodendron corticosum
N.O. Canallaceæ

Synonyms. Red Canella. Mountain Cinnamon
Part Used. Dried bark
Habitat. Jamaica

¶ *Description.* This is pungent like Winter's Bark, but a much paler brown colour, resembling canella bark, but without its chalky white inner surface. It has a ferruginous grey-brown colour, darker externally, with scars of the nearly circular subereous warts smooth and finely striated on the inner surface. Like canella bark in odour and pungent taste but is not bitter.

¶ *Constituents.* Volatile oil and tannic acid, it may be distinguished from canella bark by its decoction becoming blackened by a persalt of iron, can be used for the same diseases as Winter's Bark. In South America it is much used for diarrhœa, etc.

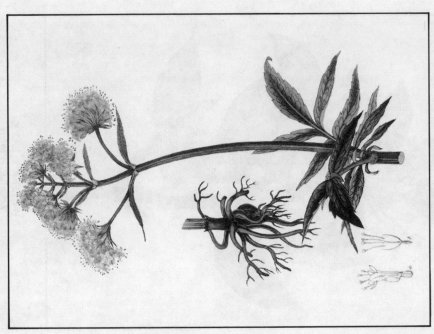
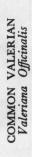

COMMON VALERIAN
Valeriana Officinalis

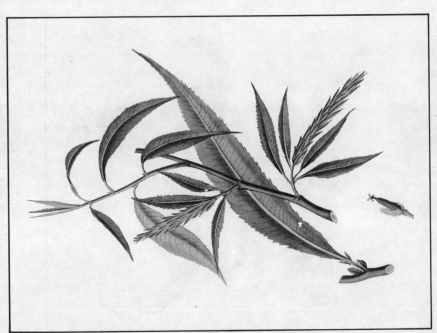

WILLOW
Salix Russeliana

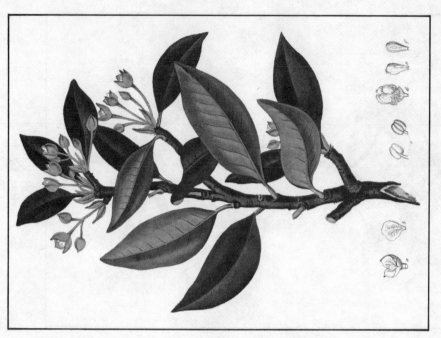

WINTER'S BARK
Drimys Winteri

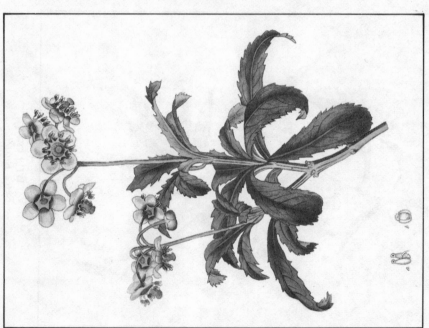

WINTERGREEN
Chimophila Umbellata

WITCH HAZEL   Hamamelis virginiana (LINN.)
                               N.O. Hamamelideæ

Synonyms. Spotted Alder. Winterbloom. Snapping Hazelnut
Parts Used. Bark, dried; leaves, fresh and dried
Habitat. The Eastern United States and Canada

¶ *Description.* The name *Hamamelis* was adopted from a Greek word to indicate its resemblance to an apple-tree.

This shrub, long known in cultivation, consists of several crooked branching trunks from one root, 4 to 6 inches in diameter, 10 to 12 feet in height, with a smooth grey bark, leaves 3 to 5 inches long and about 3 inches wide, on short petioles, alternate, oval or obovate, acuminate, obliquely sub-cordate at the base, the margin crenate, dentate, scabrous, with raised spots underneath, pinnately veined and having stellate hairs. The leaves drop off in autumn, then the yellow flowers appear, very late in September and in October, in clusters from the joints, followed by black nuts, containing white seeds which are oily and edible. In Britain, the nut does not bear seeds, but in America, they are produced abundantly, but often do not ripen till the following summer. The seeds are ejected violently when ripe, hence the name Snapping Hazelnut. The leaves are inodorous, with an astringent and bitterish aromatic taste. The twigs are flexible and rough, colour externally, yellowish-brown to purple, wood greeny white, pith small. The bark as found in commerce is usually in quilled pieces $\frac{1}{16}$ inch thick, 2 to 8 inches long, with silvery grey, scaly cork; longitudinally striated; fracture fibrous and laminated; taste and odour slight.

¶ *Constituents.* Of the *leaves* (official in the United States Pharmacopœia), tannic and gallic acids, an unknown bitter principle and some volatile oil.

The *bark* contains tannin, partly amorphous and partly crystal, gallic acid, a physterol, resin, fat and other bitter and odorous bodies.

¶ *Medicinal Action and Uses.* The properties of the leaves and bark are similar, astringent, tonic, sedative, valuable in checking internal and external hæmorrhage, most efficacious in the treatment of piles, a good pain-killer for the same, useful for bruises and inflammatory swellings, also for diarrhœa, dysentery and mucous discharges.

It has long been used by the North American Indians as poultices for painful swellings and tumours.

The decoction has been utilized for incipient phthisis, gleet, ophthalmia, menorrhagia and the debilitated state resulting from abortion.

A tea made of the leaves or bark may be taken freely with advantage, being good for bleeding of the stomach and in complaints of the bowels, and an injection of this tea is excellent for inwardly bleeding piles, the relief being marvellous and the cure speedy. An ointment made of 1 part fluid extract of bark to 9 parts simple ointment is also used as a local application, the concentration Hamamelin being also employed, mainly in the form of suppositories.

Witch Hazel has been supposed to owe its utility to an action on the muscular fibre of veins. The distilled extract from the fresh leaves and young twigs forms an excellent remedy for internal or external uses, being beneficial for bleeding from the lungs and nose, as well as from other internal organs. In the treatment of varicose veins, it should be applied on a lint bandage, which must be constantly kept moist: a pad of Witch Hazel applied to a burst varicose vein will stop the bleeding and often save life by its instant application.

Pond's Extract of Witch Hazel was much used in our grandmother's days as a general household remedy for burns, scalds, and inflammatory conditions of the skin generally and it is still in general use.

In cases of bites of insects and mosquitoes a pad of cotton-wool, moistened with the extract and applied to the spot will soon cause the pain and swelling to subside.

Diluted with warm water, the extract is used for inflammation of the eyelids.

¶ *Dosage.* Liquor Hamamelidis, $\frac{1}{2}$ to 3 drachms (a distillate of the fresh leaves). Used also with equal parts of glycerine as injection for piles.

Liquid extract, 5 to 15 minims (preparation of the dried leaves made with alcohol) externally for varicose veins. Injection for piles, 2 to 5 minims.

Hamamelin, $\frac{1}{2}$ to 2 grains, in pill (powdered extractive from the bark). 1 to 3 grains with cacao butter is useful for piles.

Tincture (from the bark), 30 to 60 minims. 1 drachm in 3 oz. cold water given as enema for piles. Lotion of 1 or 2 drachms with water to an ounce useful for bruises.

Ointment: employed externally for piles.

WOAD

Ivatis tinctoria (LINN.)
N.O. Cruciferæ

Synonyms. (*Anglo-Saxon*) Wad.
  (*French*) Guède
  (*Italian*) Guado
  (*Spanish and French*) Pastel
  (*Dutch*) Weat
Part Used. Leaves

Dyer's Woad, French *Guède* (supposed to be derived from Gaudum, now Gualdo, the name of a town in the Roman States, where it was extensively cultivated), was formerly much cultivated in Britain for the dye extracted from the leaves. It is now nearly superseded by indigo, but is still cultivated in the south of France and in Flanders, as its dye is said to improve the quality and colour of indigo, when mixed in certain proportions. Woad is cultivated to a small extent in Lincolnshire and Woad mills are still worked at Wisbech, but not for the dye itself, the produce *fixes* true indigo, and is also used to form a base, or mordant, for a black dye.

Woad belongs to a genus spread over Southern Europe and Western Asia, and from having been much cultivated in many parts of Asia and Europe, has become established in stony and waste places as far north as Sweden. It is found in many parts of Great Britain, but not fully naturalized, except near Tewkesbury, where, according to Hooker, it appears to be indigenous. At the earliest time in the history of Britain it must have been plentiful in the country, since Cæsar found the natives stained with it, but afterwards, probably from its extensive use, it became less common, and we find our Saxon forefathers importing Woad to dye their home-spun cloth. Their name for it was *Wad* or *Waad*, whence the English name woad.

¶ *Description.* Gerard tells us:

'Glaston or Guadon, Woad is about three feet high, with long, bluish-green leaves growing round and out of the stalk, growing smaller as they reach the top, when they branch out with small yellow flowers, which in turn produce seed like little black tongues. The root is white and single. The Wild Woad is similar except that the stalk is softer, smaller and browner, and the leaves and tongues narrower. Where Woad is cultivated in fields, the wild Woad grows. It flowers from June to September. Cæsar in his fifth book of the French wars mentions that the British stained themselves blue with woad. Pliny in his 22nd book, Chapter I, says the French call it *Glastum* and British women and girls colouring themselves with it went naked to some of their sacrifices.

'Garden Woad is dry but not sharp, Wild Woad is drier and sharper and biting. The decoction made of Woad is good for hardness of the spleen, also good for wounds and ulcers to those of strong constitution and those accustomed to much physical labour and coarse fare. It is used as a dye, profitable to some, hurtful to many.'

Culpepper says:

'Some people affirm the plant to be destructive to bees, and fluxes them, which if it be, I cannot help it. I should rather think, unless bees be contrary to other creatures, it possesses them with the contrary disease, the herb being exceeding dry and binding. . . . A plaister made thereof, and applied to the region of the spleen which lies on the left side, takes away the hardness and pains thereof. The ointment is excellently good for such ulcers as abound with moisture, and takes away the corroding and fretting humours: It cools inflammations, quenches St. Anthony's fire, and stays defluxion of the blood to any part of the body.'

He also says that the seeds, if chewed, turn the saliva blue.

¶ *Cultivation.* The cultivation of Woad was formerly carried on by people who devoted themselves entirely to it, and as crops of the plant are not successful for more than two years on the same piece of land, they never stayed long in one place, but hiring land in various districts, led a wandering life with their families and gained their living by their crops. Later, many farmers devoted a portion of their land to the growth of Woad, alternating the spots year after year.

Good loam soil is needed, land in good heart, repeatedly ploughed and harrowed from autumn till the following August, when the seeds are sown in drills, being thinned out by hoeing when about a fortnight old, to a distance of about 6 inches apart. In the spring, careful hoeing to remove weeds is necessary. The first crop can be gathered as soon as the leaves are fully grown, while perfectly green. The leaves are picked off when the plant is coming into flower. If the land be good and the crop well husbanded, it will produce three or more gatherings, repeated at intervals of a few weeks, but the first two gatherings are the best. An acre of land will produce a ton of Woad, and in good seasons, a ton and a half. If the land in which the seed is sown should have been in culture before for other crops, it will require dressing before it is sown – about twenty loads of stable manure to the acre being laid on and ploughed in with the last ploughing before the seeds are sown, this being enough to keep the ground in heart till the final crop of Woad is gathered.

¶ *Treatment of the Crop.* The leaves are dried a little in the sun, then ground in a mill to a pasty mass, which is formed into heaps exposed to the air but protected from rain, until it ferments. A crust which forms over it is carefully prevented from breaking, and when fermentation is complete, usually in about a fortnight, the mass is again mixed up and formed into cakes. Before being used by the dyer, these cakes have to be again broken up, moistened and subjected to further fermentation. Much of the quality of the dye is said to depend on the way in which this operation is performed.

The colour is brought out by mixing an infusion of the Woad thus prepared with limewater.

The best Woad used to be worth £20 or more a ton, till its price declined on the introduction of indigo, to which it is inferior in richness of colour, but is more permanent.

It is stated, also, that Woad leaves, covered with boiling water, weighted down for half an hour and the water poured off, treated with caustic potash and subsequently with hydrochloric acid, yield a good indigo dye. If the time of infusion be increased, greens and browns are obtained.

How the Ancients prepared the blue dye is not known.

¶ *Medicinal Action and Uses.* The herb is so astringent, that it is not fit to be given internally as a medicine, and has only been used medicinally as a plaster, applied to the region of the spleen, and as an ointment for ulcers, inflammation and to stanch bleeding.

Ivatis indigotica is cultivated as a tinctorial plant in the north of China, where it is called Tein-ching. It is a small, half-shrubby plant, with a decumbent stem, bearing at its extremity several long drooping racemes of small yellow flowers, and smooth black fiddle-shaped pods about ½ inch long. The lower leaves are rather fleshy, on long stalks, oval, lance-shaped, and pointed, with the edges slightly toothed, the upper ones very much narrower and smaller. In the north of China, this plant takes the place of the indigo of the south, and its colouring matter is obtained by a process closely analogous to that employed in the preparation of indigo, but instead of being thoroughly inspissated so as to form solid cakes, it is used by the Chinese dyers in a semi-liquid or pasty state. It is commonly employed for dyeing cotton cloth, to which it imparts a dark-blue colour.

WOOD ANEMONE. *See* ANEMONE

WOOD BETONY. *See* BETONY

WOODRUFF, SWEET

Asperula odorata (LINN.)
N.O. Rubiaceæ

Synonyms. (*Old English*) Wuderove. Wood-rova
(*Old French*) Muge-de-boys
Part Used. Herb

The Sweet Woodruff, a favourite little plant growing in woods and on shaded hedgebanks, may be readily recognized by its small white flowers (in bloom in May and June) set on a tender stalk, with narrow, bright-green leaves growing beneath them in successive, star-like whorls, just as in Clivers or Goosegrass, about eight leaves to every whorl. Unlike the latter, however, its stems are erect and smooth: they rarely exceed a foot in height, their average being 8 or 9 inches. The plant is perennial, with creeping, slender root-stock.

Being a lover of woods and shady places, its deep-green foliage develops best in the half-shade, where the sunlight penetrates with difficulty. Should the branches over-shadowing it be cut away, and the full light fall upon it, it loses its colour and rapidly becomes much paler.

When the seed is quite ripe and dry, it is a rough little ball covered thickly with flexible, hooked bristles, white below, but black-tipped, and these catch on to the fur and feathers of any animal or bird that pushes through the undergrowth, and thus the seed is dispersed.

The name of the plant appears in the thirteenth century as 'Wuderove,' and later as 'Wood-rove' – the *rove* being derived, it is said, from the French *rovelle*, a wheel, in allusion to the spoke-like arrangement of the leaves in whorls. In old French works it appears as *Muge-de-boys*, musk of the woods.

Some of the old herbalists spelt the name Woodruff with an array of double consonants: Woodderowffe. Later this spelling was written in a rhyme, which children were fond of repeating:

WOODDE,
ROWFFE.

Cultivation. As a rule, the plant is not cultivated, but collected from the woods, but it might be grown under orchard trees and can be propagated, (1) by seeds, sown as soon as ripe, in prepared beds of good soil, in the end of July or beginning of August, (2) by division of roots during the spring and early summer, just after flowering. Plant in moist, partially shaded ground, 1 foot apart.

Chemical Constituents. The agreeable odour of Sweet Woodruff is due to a crystalline chemical principle called Coumarin, which is used in perfumery, not only on account of its own fragrance, but for its property of fixing other odours. It is the odorous principle also present in melilot, tonka beans, and various other plants belonging to the orders Leguminosæ, Graminæ and Orchidaceæ. It is employed in pharmacy to disguise disagreeable odours, especially that of iodoform, for which purpose 1 part of coumarin is used to 50 parts of iodoform. The plant further contains citric, malic and rubichloric acids, together with some tannic acid.

The powdered leaves are mixed with fancy snuffs, because of their enduring fragrance, and also put into *potpourri*.

WOOD SAGE. *See* SAGE

WOOD SANICLE. *See* SANICLE

WOOD SORREL. *See* SORREL

WORMSEED, AMERICAN

Medicinal Action and Uses. Woodruff was much used as a medicine in the Middle Ages.

The fresh leaves, bruised and applied to cuts and wounds, were said to have a healing effect, and formerly a strong decoction of the fresh herb was used as a cordial and stomachic. It is also said to be useful for removing biliary obstructions of the liver.

The plant when newly gathered has but little odour, but when dried, has a most refreshing scent of new-mown hay, which is retained for years. Gerard tells us:

'The flowers are of a very sweet smell as is the rest of the herb, which, being made up into garlands or bundles, and hanged up in houses in the heat of summer, doth very well attemper the air, cool and make fresh the place, to the delight and comfort of such as are therein. It is reported to be put into wine, to make a man merry, and to be good for the heart and liver, it prevaileth in wounds, as *Cruciata* and other vulnerary herbs do.'

In Germany, one of the favourite hock-cups is still made by steeping the fresh sprigs in Rhine wine. This forms a specially delightful drink, known as *Maibowle*, and drunk on the first of May.

The dried herb may be kept among linen, like lavender, to preserve it from insects. In the Middle Ages it used to be hung and strewed in churches, and on St. Barnabas Day and on St. Peter's, bunches of box, Woodruff, lavender and roses found a place there. It was also used for stuffing beds.

Chenopodium anthelminticum (BERT.)
N.O. Chenopodiaceæ

Synonyms. Chenopodium Ambrosioides (Linn.). Mexican Tea. Jesuit's Tea. Herba Sancti Mariæ
Part Used. Seeds
Habitat. Indigenous to Mexico and South America, Missouri, New England, and eastern United States

The American Wormseed plant (*Chenopodium ambrosioides*, Linn.), and still more a variety of it, *C. ambrosioides*, var. *anthelminticum* (Bert), furnishes the important drug Chenopodium.

It is indigenous to Mexico and South America, but has become thoroughly naturalized as far north as Missouri and New England, where it grows about dwellings and in manured soils. It is now found in almost all parts of the eastern United States, a coarse,

perennial weed of the roadside and waste places, smoothish, more or less viscid-glandular, the stout, erect, angular and grooved stem growing to a height of about 2 feet.

Description. The leaves are slightly petioled, oblong-lanceolate, toothed, the upper ones entire and tapering at both ends. The small, very numerous flowers are yellowish-green in colour and occur in numerous small clusters, or globular spikes,

854

arranged in the axils of slender, lateral, leafy branches. The calyx is five-cleft, the lobes ovate, pointed. Stamens five, ovary covered on the top with small, oblong, stalked glands; styles, two to three. The fruit is perfectly enclosed in the calyx, obtusely angled, the seed smooth and shining, the embryo forming about three-quarters of a ring around the mealy albumen.

The drug consists of these small, irregular, globular fruits, not larger than the head of a pin. They are very light and of a greenish-yellow or brown colour. On rubbing the fruit, the membraneous pericarp is removed and the single, small, brownish-black seed is exposed.

The odour of the fruit is strong, resembling somewhat that of eucalyptus; the taste, pungent and bitter.

The fruit of *C. ambrosioides*, var. *anthelminticum* is even more aromatic.

Both varieties of the plant flower from July to September and the fruits ripen successively through the autumn and are collected in October.

The whole herb has a strong, peculiar, somewhat aromatic odour, which is due to the presence of a volatile oil and is retained on drying. The leaves have been used in place of tea in Mexico.

The American aborigines used the whole herb in decoction in painful menstruation, but its principal use has been — both leaves and seeds – as a vermifuge, and it is to-day considered one of the best expellents of lumbricoids.

Though all parts of the plant possess anthelmintic properties, the fruits and the oil extracted from them are alone employed, being official in the United States Pharmacopœia. It was long customary for the seeds to be administered in the form of a powder, or an electuary, but although the activity of the seed is unquestioned, it has now been entirely displaced in America by the volatile oil obtained by distillation from the crushed fruits, to which the medicinal importance of the fruit is due.

The oil was first isolated in 1895 by a German pharmacist who lived in Brazil, where the seeds had long been used as a vermifuge.

Most of this oil is distilled in Maryland, and since Baltimore is the commercial centre of that state, this oil is commonly known as Baltimore oil, in distinction from Western Missouri oil, which has at times played a rôle in the market. The plant is now cultivated in large quantities near Baltimore.

¶ *Constituents of the Oil.* American Wormseed oil, known as Chenopodium oil, is colourless or yellowish, when freshly distilled, becoming deeper yellow and even brownish by use. It has a peculiar, penetrating, somewhat camphoraceous odour (the peculiar odour of the plant), and a pungent, bitter taste.

The yield of oil from the crushed fruits is 0·6 to 1·0 per cent.

Its chief constituent is Ascaridole, to the high percentage of 60 to 70 per cent., an unstable substance, allied to cineal, readily decomposed on heating, with the production of a hydrocarbon. It also contains *p*-cymene, *a*-perpinene, probably dihydro-*p*-cymene and possibly sylvestrene. Betzine and choline have also been reported.

According to the researches of De Langen, Flue and Welhuizen, of the Dutch-Indian Medical Service, in 1919, the oil contains Glycol and Safrol, and these authors ascribe the powerful effect of the oil to the combination of Ascaridole and Safrol.

The characters of the oil are:

Specific gravity, 0·950 to 0·990.
Optical rotation, $- 5°$ to 10°.
Refraction index, 1·4723 to 1·4726.
Saponification number, 246 to 280.
Soluble in three volumes of 70 per cent. alcohol.

Adulteration with American turpentine oil causes lowering of the specific gravity and insolubility in alcohol.

The fresh plant yields the alkaloid Chenopodine, a white tasteless and odourless crystalline powder, soluble in 11 parts of cold water, 3 of boiling water and 20 per cent. of alcohol.

¶ *Medicinal Action and Uses.* Chenopodium, being a very active anthelmintic, is frequently used for the expulsion of lumbricoid (round) worms, especially in children. Because of its efficacy, ease of administration and low toxicity, it is perhaps the most valuable of all the vermifuge remedies.

The bruised fruit may be given in doses of 20 grains, in the form of an electuary.

A fluid extract is prepared, of which the dose is $\frac{1}{2}$ to 1 drachm.

The expressed juice of the fresh plant is also employed, in tablespoonful doses. A decoction made by boiling 1 oz. of the fresh plant with 1 pint of milk or water has sometimes been given in doses of a wineglassful.

The volatile oil is now much used, the dose of which, for a child, is from 5 to 10 minims.

The drug should be given in one full dose, fasting, and then be followed, in about two hours, by an active purgative, such as castor oil. When the purge has acted, the patient can take food. The treatment should be repeated ten days later. In view of the uncertain ascaridole contents of some samples, small doses should be given at first.

Toxic symptoms are transient dizziness and vomiting.

The oil has been recommended in the treatment of malaria, chorea, hysteria and other nervous diseases.

The plant has been employed, under the name of *Herba Sancti Mariæ*, in pectoral complaints, as an expectorant, in catarrh and asthma.

Although oil of Chenopodium has been official in the United States Pharmacopœia for many years, it does not appear to have received official recognition elsewhere. It owes its modern popularity to the investigations of Brüning, who repeatedly drew attention to it (see *Zeitschrift für exot. Path.,* 1906).

In 1912 two Dutch physicians, both working in Delhi (Dutch East Indies), stated that this essential oil is the most effective remedy against *ankylostomiasis,* the Hookworm disease. Originally, this disease was exclusively a tropical and subtropical one, but about thirty years ago, it appeared in mine-workers in Europe north of the Alps.

The Hookworm, which causes the disease, is called *Ankylostos duodenale,* the male of which attains a length of 10 mm., the female 14 mm. The living hookworm is flesh-coloured, the dead one has a grey or white colour. At the foot of the hook-formed teeth, glands, each consisting of a single cell, pour their contents into the wounds which the worm makes in the mucous membrane of the intestinal canal and into the blood-vessels by means of the teeth. It is supposed that the phenomena of the disease must be attributed to the mechanical changes brought about by the hookworm, as well as to a poisonous substance secreted by the worm. The worm deposits its eggs in the intestinal canal of its host. Together with the fæces, these eggs leave the body of the host. At a temperature of 25° to 30° C., the larva develops, and after two changes of skin, enters into the body of the new host by means of vegetables, drinking-water, or through the skin.

Several medicaments have been tried against the hookworm; thymol had appeared to be the only remedy that had been used with some success, but it is much surpassed by Chenopodium oil, which gives better results than eucalyptus, betanaphthol, or thymol.

The use of this oil commenced when thymol was not available during the early days of the Great War. It proved to be satisfactory in every way and is the drug commonly used in Ceylon since 1917. Statistics indicate that in three treatments, about 95 per cent. of the worms are removed from the body. It has also been used in Fiji and has proved an anthelmintic of great potency. It is said there that over 80 per cent. of the worms are expelled after a single dose.

The maximum individual dose would appear to be 1 c.c., but it is best given in three cacheta of 0·5 c.c. each, at two-hourly intervals, followed three hours later by a saline purge of 1 oz. of magnesium sulphate.

The observances of the two Dutch physicians Schüffner and Vervoort have been confirmed by other medical men, and at present, Chenopodium oil has become the specific remedy against the Hookworm disease.

It is, however, a dangerous remedy in the hands of the layman on account of its activity, for unfortunately, the oil as it appears in commerce contains markedly varying quantities of the active principle Ascaridole, and the amount lessens with keeping, making it desirable that dealers should always mention the Ascaridole percentage of the oil they are selling and the date of distillation. The freshly-distilled oil in cases of overdoses has been known to cause symptoms of poisoning. Ascaridole, extracted and administered in place of the whole oil, is effective, and the use of it eliminates uncertainty of the strength of a dose of the oil, but it is relatively costly.

Carbon tetrachloride, recently introduced as a remedy for Hookworm, has proved most efficient. It is the cheapest of all advocated treatments, but the dose of 3 mils., at present given, sometimes proves dangerous and would appear to require reduction. A combination of this drug with Ascaridole is being now tested.

Chenopodium oil has also been shown to be of great service against the tapeworm and is employed in veterinary practice in a worm mixture for dogs, combined with oil of turpentine, oil of aniseed, castor oil and olive oil.

Since this oil has proved so important, steps have been taken to cultivate the plant in the Dutch East Indies, and these endeavours have met with great success, and manufacture of the oil in Netherlands India is now being extensively carried on.

¶ *Other Species.*

From *C. glaucum* (Linn.), the Oak-leaved Goosefoot of the United States, a medicinal tincture is made, which is used for expelling round-worms. There exists some doubt as to whether the properties of the tincture are not also due in part to the aphis that infests the plant.

This species is also a native of Great Britain. The European and Asiatic *C. Botrys*, Jerusalem Oak, or Feather Geranium, is considered an expectorant in France.

See ARRACHS, BEETS, CHENOPODIUMS, GOOSEFOOT, GLASSWORTS, QUINOA SPINACH.

WORMSEED, LEVANT

Artemisia cina (BERG.)
N.O. Compositæ

Synonyms. Sea Wormwood. Santonica. Semen Sanctum. Semen Cinæ. Semen Contra. Semen Santonici. Artemesia Lercheana. Artemisia maritima, var. Stechmanniana. Artemisia maritima, var. pauciflora. Artemesia Chamæmelifolia

(Italian) Semenzina

Part Used. Seeds

The Levant Wormseed, largely imported into Britain, is derived from a variety of the Sea Wormwood. Several species of Wormwood are mentioned by Dioscorides as being effective as a vermifuge, one of which was reported as growing in the country of the Santones in Gaul. Its ancient reputation has been maintained in modern times, for the universally employed vermifuge Santonin (the very name derived from classic days) is produced from Santonica – popularly called Wormseed – which consists of the minute, dried, unexpanded flower-heads of a Russian variety of the Sea Wormwood (*Artemisia maritima*, var. *Stechmanniana*, Bess.). This variety, which some botanists consider to be a distinct species, under the name of *A. Cina* (Berg.), or *A. chamæmelifolia* (Vill.), grows in profusion in Siberia, Turkestan and Chinese Mongolia. The greater part of the Wormseed is used in Turkestan, where it grows in enormous quantities in the desert of the Kirghiz, especially near the town of Chimkent, where a factory has been erected in which large quantities of Santonin are produced from the Wormseed collected in the vicinity, not more than 10 per cent. of the drug being now exported in the crude state, in which condition it is known in this country as Levant Wormseed. The plant is low and shrubby, throwing up a number of erect stems on which the little greenish-yellow, oblong flower-heads are borne. Each head is about ⅛ inch long and 1/16 inch in diameter, and contains three to five minute, tubular flowers. In July and August, before the flowers expand, they are stripped from the stems and dried, being brought into Chimkent by the Kirghiz and other tribes.

Wormseed has long been used as an anthelmintic. Tragus, in 1531, in Brunfels' *Herbal*, mentions Wormseed as being imported by way of Genoa; it was employed in Italy under the name of Semenzina (diminutive of *Semenza*, seed), in the belief that it consisted of small seeds. From this word is derived the name of *Semen cinæ*, by which the drug is often known: *Semen contra* (another of its names) is an abbreviation of *Semen contra vermes*. The drug at first sight appears to consist of a number of small brownish, ridged seeds, and it is not till they are closely examined that their true nature becomes apparent.

The drug exhales when crushed an agreeable aromatic odour, and possesses a bitter, aromatic camphoraceous taste. As imported, it frequently contains considerable fragments of the leaves and slender flower-stalks.

¶ *Constituents.* The chief constituent of Wormseed is a crystalline principle, Santonin, to which the anthelmintic property of the drug is due. Santonin attains its maximum 2·3 to 3·6 per cent. in July and August; after the flowerheads have expanded, it rapidly diminishes in quantity. It is extracted from the flower-heads by treating them with Milk of Lime, the Santonin being converted into soluble calcium santonate. It occurs in colourless, shining, flat prisms, without odour and almost tasteless at first, but afterwards developing a bitter taste. It is sparingly soluble in water, but soluble in alcohol and ether.

Wormseed also contains a crystalline substance, Artemisin, and a yellow volatile oil consisting of Cineol, to which its odour is due.

¶ *Medicinal Action and Uses.* Wormseed is one of the oldest and most common anthelmintics, especially for children. In domestic practice the seeds are used powdered, combined with honey or treacle, the dose of the seeds taken thus in substance being 10 to 30 grains. The seeds have also been employed in infusion or decoction, but in these forms their bitterness is a strong objection. As a general rule, however, the crude drug Wormseed is seldom administered, its active constituent Santonin being employed. It acts as a direct poison to parasites, and is used as a remedy for round-worms, which it rapidly expels; it has also an effect on thread-worms

857

to a lesser degree, but has no action on tape-worms. It is usually administered as a powder or in lozenges, not in solution, and is often given with calomel, or compound powder of scammony.

¶ *Preparations.* Santonin, 2 to 5 grains. Santonin lozenges, B.P.

Several cases are on record of fatal poisoning by Santonin, and Santonin rendered yellow by exposure to direct sunlight is sometimes preferred, it being stated to be less poisonous. It is known as yellow Santonin, or Photosantonin.

Even small doses of Santonin will produce remarkable effects on the vision, appreciation of colour being so disturbed that objects appear to have a yellowish tinge, which is sometimes preceded by a faint colour. Santonin may also cause headache, nausea and vomiting, and in large doses, epileptiform convulsions.

See MUGWORT, WORMWOOD.

WORMWOODS

N.O. Compositæ

The Wormwoods are members of the great family of Compositæ and belong to the genus *Artemisia*, a group consisting of 180 species, of which we have four growing wild in England, the Common Wormwood, Mugwort, Sea Wormwood and Field Wormwood. In addition, as garden plants, though not native, Tarragon (*A. dracunculus*) claims a place in every herb-garden, and Southernwood (*A. abrotanum*), an old-fashioned favourite, is found in many borders, whilst others, such as *A. sericea, A. cana* and *A. alpina*, form pretty rockwork shrubs.

The whole family is remarkable for the extreme bitterness of all parts of the plant: 'as bitter as Wormwood' is a very Ancient proverb.

In some of the Western states of North America there are large tracts almost entirely destitute of other vegetation than certain kinds of *Artemisia*, which cover vast plains. The plants are of no use as forage: and the few wild animals that feed on them are said to have, when eaten, a bitter taste. The Artemisias also abound in the arid soil of the Tartarean steppes and in other similar situations.

The genus is named *Artemisia* from Artemis, the Greek name for Diana. In an early translation of the *Herbarium* of Apuleius we find:

'Of these worts that we name Artemisia, it is said that Diana did find them and delivered their powers and leechdom to Chiron the Centaur, who first from these Worts set forth a leechdom, and he named these worts from the name of Diana, Artemis, that is Artemisias.'

WORMWOOD, COMMON

Artemisia Absinthium (LINN.)
N.O. Compositæ

Synonym. Green Ginger
Part Used. Whole Herb
Habitat. Europe, Siberia, and United States of America

The Common Wormwood held a high reputation in medicine among the Ancients. Tusser (1577), in *July's Husbandry*, says:

'While Wormwood hath seed get a handful or twaine
To save against March, to make flea to refraine:
Where chamber is sweeped and Wormwood is strowne,
What saver is better (if physick be true)
For places infected than Wormwood and Rue?
It is a comfort for hart and the braine,
And therefore to have it it is not in vaine.'

Besides being strewn in chambers as Tusser recommended, it used to be laid among stuffs and furs to keep away moths and insects.

According to the Ancients, Wormwood counteracted the effects of poisoning by hemlock, toadstools and the biting of the sea-dragon. The plant was of some importance among the Mexicans, who celebrated their great festival of the Goddess of Salt by a ceremonial dance of women, who wore on their heads garlands of Wormwood.

With the exception of Rue, Wormwood is the bitterest herb known, but it is very wholesome and used to be in much request by brewers for use instead of hops. The leaves resist putrefaction, and have been on that account a principal ingredient in antiseptic fomentations.

An Old Love Charm

'On St. Luke's Day, take marigold flowers, a sprig of marjoram, thyme, and a little *Wormwood*; dry them before a fire, rub them

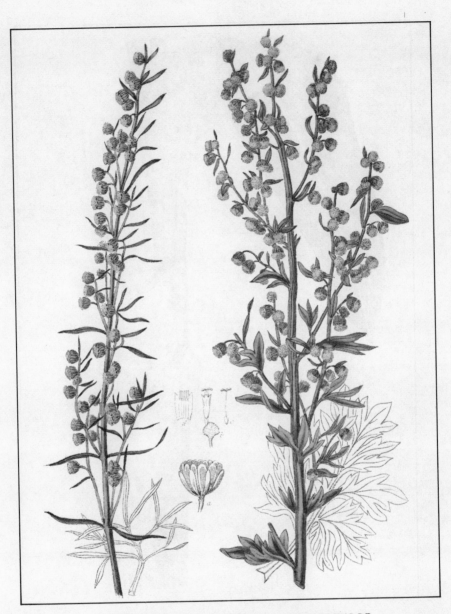

LEVANT WORMSEED AND LEVANT WORMWOOD
Artemisia Cina and *Artemisia Absinthium*

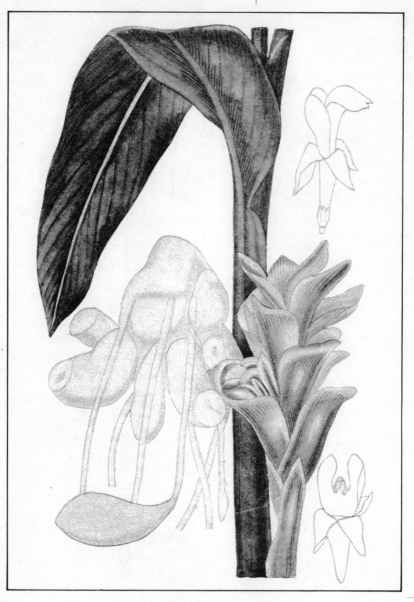

ZEDOARY
Curcuma Zedoaria

to powder; then sift it through a fine piece of lawn, and simmer it over a slow fire, adding a small quantity of virgin honey, and vinegar. Anoint yourself with this when you go to bed, saying the following lines three times, and you will dream of your partner "that is to be":

"St. Luke, St. Luke, be kind to me,
In dreams let me my true-love see." '

Culpepper, writing of the three Wormwoods most in use, the Common Wormwood, Sea Wormwood and Roman Wormwood, tells us: 'Each kind has its particular virtues' ... the Common Wormwood is 'the strongest,' the Sea Wormwood, 'the second in bitterness,' whereas the Roman Wormwood, 'to be found in botanic gardens' – the first two being wild – 'joins a great deal of aromatic flavour with but little bitterness.'

The Common Wormwood grows on roadsides and waste places, and is found over the greater part of Europe and Siberia, having been formerly much cultivated for its qualities. In Britain, it appears to be truly indigenous near the sea and locally in many other parts of England and Scotland, from Forfar southwards. In Ireland it is a doubtful native. It has become naturalized in the United States.

¶ *Description.* The root is perennial, and from it arise branched, firm, leafy stems, sometimes almost woody at the base. The flowering stem is 2 to 2½ feet high and whitish, being closely covered with fine silky hairs. The leaves, which are also whitish on both sides from the same reason, are about 3 inches long by 1½ broad, cut into deeply and repeatedly (about three times pinnatifid), the segments being narrow (linear) and blunt. The leaf-stalks are slightly winged at the margin. The small, nearly globular flower-heads are arranged in an erect, leafy panicle, the leaves on the flower-stalks being reduced to three, or even one linear segment, and the little flowers themselves being pendulous and of a greenish-yellow tint. They bloom from July to October. The ripe fruits are not crowned by a tuft of hairs, or pappus, as in the majority of the Compositæ family.

The leaves and flowers are very bitter, with a characteristic odour, resembling that of thujone. The root has a warm and aromatic taste.

¶ *Cultivation.* Wormwood likes a shady situation, and is easily propagated by division of roots in the autumn, by cuttings, or by seeds sown in the autumn soon after they are ripe. No further care is needed than to keep free from weeds. Plant about 2 feet apart each way.

¶ *Parts Used.* The whole herb – leaves and tops – gathered in July and August, when the plant is in flower and dried.

Collect only on a dry day, after the sun has dried off the dew. Cut off the upper green portion and reject the lower parts of the stems, together with any discoloured or insect-eaten leaves. Tie loosely in bunches of uniform size and length, about six stalks to a bunch, and spread out in shape of a fan, so that the air can get to all parts. Hang over strings, in the open, on a fine, sunny, warm day, but in half-shade, otherwise the leaves will become tindery; the drying must not be done in full sunlight, or the aromatic properties will be partly lost. Aromatic herbs should be dried at a temperature of about 70°. If no sun is available, the bunches may be hung over strings in a covered shed, or disused greenhouse, or in a sunny warm attic, provided there is ample ventilation, so that the moist heated air may escape. The room may also be heated with a coke or anthracite stove, care being taken that the window is kept open during the day. If after some days the leaves are crisp and the stalks still damp, hang the bunches over a stove, when the stalks will quickly finish drying. Uniformity in size in the bunches is important, as it facilitates packing. When the drying process is completed, pack away at once in airtight boxes, as otherwise the herbs will absorb about 12 per cent. moisture from the air. If sold to the wholesale druggists in powdered form, rub through a sieve as soon as thoroughly dry, before the bunches have had time to absorb any moisture, and pack in tins or bottles at once.

¶ *Constituents.* The chief constituent is a volatile oil, of which the herb yields in distillation from 0·5 to 1·0 per cent. It is usually dark green, or sometimes blue in colour, and has a strong odour and bitter, acrid taste. The oil contains thujone (absinthol or tenacetone), thujyl alcohol (both free and combined with acetic, isovalerianic, succine and malic acids), cadinene, phellandrene and pinene. The herb also contains the bitter glucoside *absinthin*, absinthic acid, together with tannin, resin, starch, nitrate of potash and other salts.

¶ *Medicinal Action and Uses.* Tonic, stomachic, febrifuge, anthelmintic.

A nervine tonic, particularly helpful against the falling sickness and for flatulence. It is a good remedy for enfeebled digestion and debility.

¶ *Preparations*. Fluid extract, $\frac{1}{2}$ to 1 drachm. Wormwood Tea, made from 1 oz. of the herb, infused for 10 to 12 minutes in 1 pint of boiling water, and taken in wineglassful doses, will relieve melancholia and help to dispel the yellow hue of jaundice from the skin, as well as being a good stomachic, and with the addition of fixed alkaline salt, produced from the burnt plant, is a powerful diuretic in some dropsical cases. The ashes yield a purer alkaline salt than most other vegetables, except Beanstalks and Broom.

The juice of the larger leaves which grow from the root before the stalk appears has been used as a remedy for jaundice and dropsy, but it is intensely nauseous. A light infusion of the tops of the plant, used fresh, is excellent for all disorders of the stomach, creating an appetite, promoting digestion and preventing sickness after meals, but it is said to produce the contrary effect if made too strong.

The flowers, dried and powdered, are most effectual as a vermifuge, and used to be considered excellent in agues. The essential oil of the herb is used as a worm-expeller, the spirituous extract being preferable to that distilled in water. The leaves give out nearly the whole of their smell and taste both to spirit and water, but the cold water infusions are the least offensive.

The intensely bitter, tonic and stimulant qualities have caused Wormwood not only to be an ingredient in medicinal preparations, but also to be used in various liqueurs, of which absinthe is the chief, the basis of absinthe being absinthol, extracted from Wormwood. Wormwood, as employed in making this liqueur, bears also the name 'Wermuth' – preserver of the mind – from its medicinal virtues as a nervine and mental restorative. If not taken habitually, it soothes spinal irritability and gives tone to persons of a highly nervous temperament. Suitable allowances of the diluted liqueur will promote salutary perspiration and may be given as a vermifuge. Inferior absinthe is generally adulterated with copper, which produces the characteristic green colour.

The drug, *absinthium*, is rarely employed, but it might be of value in nervous diseases such as neurasthenia, as it stimulates the cerebral hemispheres, and is a direct stimulant of the cortex cerebri. When taken to excess it produces giddiness and attacks of epileptiform convulsions. Absinthium occurs in the British Pharmacopœia in the form of extract, infusion and tincture, and is directed to be extracted also from *A. maritima*, the Sea Wormwood, which possesses the same virtues in a less degree, and is often more used as a stomachic than the Common Wormwood. Commercially this often goes under the name of Roman Wormwood, though that name really belongs to *A. Pontica*. All three species were used, as in Culpepper's time.

Dr. John Hill (1772) recommends Common Wormwood in many forms. He says:

'The Leaves have been commonly used, but the flowery tops are the right part. These, made into a light infusion, strengthen digestion, correct acidities, and supply the place of gall, where, as in many constitutions, that is deficient. One ounce of the Flowers and Buds should be put into an earthen vessel, and a pint and a half of boiling water poured on them, and thus to stand all night. In the morning the clear liquor with two spoonfuls of wine should be taken at three draughts, an hour and a half distance from one another. Whoever will do this regularly for a week, will have no sickness after meals, will feel none of that fulness so frequent from indigestion, and wind will be no more troublesome; if afterwards, he will take but a fourth part of this each day, the benefit will be lasting.'

He further tells us that if an ounce of these flowers be put into a pint of brandy and let to stand six weeks, the resultant tincture will in a great measure prevent the increase of gravel – and give great relief in gout. 'The celebrated Baron Haller has found vast benefit by this; and myself have very happily followed his example.'

WORMWOOD, ROMAN

Artemesia Pontica
N.O. Compositæ

Part Used. Herb

Roman Wormwood (*Artemesia Pontica*) is not indigenous to this country, being a native of Southern Europe. It grows about the same height as the Common Wormwood, but has smaller and more finely cut leaves, the segments being narrower, the upper leaves more resembling those of Southernwood; the leaves are white with fine hairs on both upper and under surfaces. The flowers, which blossom in July, are numerous, at the tops of the branches, and are darker and much smaller than those of Common Wormwood.

This is the most delicate though the least strong of the Wormwoods; the aromatic flavour with which its bitterness is mixed causes it to be employed in making the liqueur *Vermuth*.

Medicinally, the fresh tops are used, and also the whole herb, dried. Much of the *A. Pontica* in commerce is *A. maritima*.

Culpepper considered the Roman Wormwood 'excellent to strengthen the stomach.' Also that 'the juice of the fresh tops is good against obstructions of the liver and spleen. . . . An infusion of the flowering tops strengthens digestion. A tincture is good

against gravel and gives great relief in the gout.'

Dr. John Hill says of this plant that it is the 'most delicate, but of least strength. The Wormwood wine, so famous with the Germans, is made with Roman Wormwood, put into the juice and work'd with it; it is a strong and an excellent wine, not unpleasant, yet of such efficacy to give an appetite that the Germans drink a glass with every other mouthful, and that way eat for hours together, without sickness or indigestion.'

WORMWOOD, SEA

Artemesia maritima
N.O. Compositæ

Synonym. Old Woman
Parts Used. Young flowering tops and shoots
Habitat. In Britain it is found as far as Wigton on the West and Aberdeen on the East; also in north-east Ireland and in the Channel Islands

The Sea Wormwood, in its many variations of form, has an extremely wide distribution in the northern hemisphere of the Old World, occurring mostly in saltish soils. It is found in the salt marshes of the British Isles, on the coasts of the Baltic, of France and the Mediterranean, and on saline soils in Hungary; thence it extends eastwards, covering immense tracts in Southern Russia, the region of the Caspian and Central Siberia to Chinese Mongolia.

¶ *Description.* It somewhat resembles *Artemesia Absinthium*, but is smaller. The stems rise about a foot or 18 inches in height. The leaves are twice pinnatifid, with narrow, linear segments, and, like the whole plant, are covered on both sides with a white cottony down. The small, oblong flower-heads – each containing three to six tubular florets – are of a yellowish or brownish tint; they are produced in August and September, and are arranged in racemes, sometimes drooping, sometimes erect.

Popularly this species is called 'Old Woman,' in distinction to 'Old Man' or Southernwood, which it somewhat resembles, though it is more delicate-looking and lacks the peculiar refreshing scent of 'Old Man.'

Dr. Hill says of this species:

'This is a very noble bitter: its peculiar province is to give an appetite, as that of the Common Wormwood is to assist digestion; the flowery tops and the young shoots possess the virtue: the older Leaves and the Stalk should be thrown away as useless. . . . The apothecaries put three times as much sugar as of the ingredient in their Conserves; but the virtue is lost in the sweetness, those will not keep so well that have less sugar, but 'tis easy to make them fresh as they are wanted.'

The plant abounds in salt marshes in which cattle have been observed to fatten

quickly, and thus the herb has acquired the reputation of being beneficial to them, but they do not eat it generally, and the richness of maritime pasturage must be regarded as the true reason of their improvement under such circumstances.

¶ *Part Used.* The flowering tops and young shoots are used, collected and dried in the same manner as Wormwood.

¶ *Medicinal Action and Uses.* The plant possesses the same properties as the other Wormwoods, but is less powerful. It is a bitter tonic and aromatic.

Although it is not now employed in regular medical practice, it is often made use of by country people for intermittent fever, and for various other medicinal purposes instead of the true Wormwood.

Thornton, in his *Family Herbal*, tells us that

'beat up with thrice its weight of fine sugar, it is made up into a conserve ordered by the London College, and may be taken where the other preparations disgust too much.'

It acts as a tonic and is good in worm cases, and Culpepper gives the following uses for it:

'Boiling water poured upon it produces an excellent stomachic infusion, but the best way is taking it in a tincture made with brandy. Hysteric complaints have been completely cured by the constant use of this tincture. In the scurvy and in the hypochondriacal disorders of studious, sedentary men, few things have a greater effect: for these it is best in strong infusion. The whole blood and all the juices of the body are effected by taking this herb. It is often used in medicine instead of the Roman Wormwood, though it falls far short of it in virtue.'

See MUGWORT, SOUTHERNWOOD, WORMSEED (LEVANT).

WOUNDWORT, HEDGE

Stachys sylvatica (LINN.)
N.O. Labiatæ

Part Used. Herb

The Hedge Stachys, or Hedge Woundwort, the most frequent of the *Stachys*, is a coarse, hairy, malodorous plant, common in woods and hedges. It has thick, creeping roots that throw up tall stems, 2 or 3 feet high. Like the rest of the genus and labiate plants in general, these are quadrangular, but instead of being hollow (like the Deadnettles) they are filled with pith and solid; they are very hairy and often more or less red in colour.

The stem branches a good deal, though the upright character of the plant is preserved, the branches being very similar in character to the main stem and issuing from it in pairs, opposite to each other, at the same spot from which the leaf-stalks arise, the leaves being thrown off from the stem in pairs, each at right angles to the pair above and below it. The blades of the leaves are heart-shaped, similar in form to those of the nettle, with bold, saw-like teeth to the margins, and are on rather long footstalks.

The flowers grow in rings or whorls upon the stem, as in the other species of *Stachys*, each ring having narrow, leafy bracts beneath it, and being separated from the other by an intervening space of stem, the whole forming a long, terminal spike. There are rarely more than six flowers in each whorl. The lower lip of each flower is entire, beautifully variegated with white upon the dull crimson-purple ground and with its sides folded back. The upper lip is also entire and very convex, slightly viscid to the touch. The four stamens are beneath the protecting hood formed by the upper part of the flower, two of them longer than the others, their anthers first dull violet, then becoming black and containing pure white pollen. When in seed, the calyx teeth become rigid, and as the calyx tube dries and contracts, the four little nutlets enclosed are shot out. The corolla tube is often half filled with honey, and the mouth of the tube is provided with stiff white hairs to keep insect visitors to the centre of the channel, this flower laying itself out to be fertilized by hive bees, humble bees and long-tongued flies, who settle on the lower lip, and as they creep up the channel of the petal tube, get dusted with the pollen from the stamens in the hooded petal.

An old authority tells us that this herb 'stamped with vinegar and applied in manner of a pultis, taketh away wens and hard swellings, and inflammation of the kernels under the eares and jawes,' and also that the distilled water of the flowers 'is used to make the heart merry, to make a good colour in the face, and to make the vitall spirits more fresh and lively.'

It is said that a yellow dye can be obtained from the plant, and it has been suggested that the very tough fibres of its stem might be utilized commercially; it has also been classed among the Woundworts good for stanching blood. Referring to its pungent fœtid smell when rubbed, Green, in his *Universal Herbal* (1832), considers that 'being one of those that powerfully affect the nerves, it might prove no contemptible stimulant if judiciously used.' He informs us also that toads are thought to be fond of living under its shade, and that though sheep and goats eat it, cows and hogs refuse it.

WOUNDWORT, MARSH

Stachys palustris (LINN.)
N.O. Labiatæ

Synonyms. All-Heal. Panay. Opopanewort. Clown's Woundwort. Rusticum Vulna Herba. Downy Woundwort
Part Used. Herb

The Marsh Woundwort is common in marshy meadows and by the sides of rivers and ditches in most parts of Great Britain.
¶ *Description.* From its root-stock, which is perennial, with numerous, white, fleshy, subterranean stolons, which creep in all directions, it throws up stout stems, 2 or 3 feet high, quadrangular, having many pairs of rather elongated, oblong leaves, tapering to a point and usually clasping the stem at the base. The light purple labiate flowers are arranged in a long spike terminating the stem, usually with only six flowers in each whorl. The long-stalked leaves that spring directly from the root, as in the Wood Betony, have mostly faded off by the time the flowers appear in late summer. The whole plant is very hairy.

This plant had formerly a great reputation as a vulnerary, being strongly recommended by Gerard in his *Herbal*. He tells us that once being in Kent, visiting a patient, he accidentally heard of a countryman who had cut himself severely with a scythe, and had bound a quantity of this herb, bruised with grease and 'laid upon in manner of a poultice' over the wound, which healed in a week, though it would 'have required forty daies with balsam itself.' Gerard continues:

'I saw the wound and offered to heal the same for charietie, which he refused, saying I could not heal it so well as himself – a clownish answer, I confess, without any thanks for my good-will: whereupon I have named it "Clown's Woundwort." '

Parkinson gives the same origin of the name.

Gerard himself, according to his own account, afterwards 'cured many grievous wounds, and some mortale with the same herbe.' The plant was regarded as a valuable remedy in such cases long before Gerard's time, having long borne the names, among country people, All-heal and Woundwort. The Welsh have an ancient name for it bearing the same signification.

It has edible roots. These are tuberous and attain a considerable size; when boiled they form a wholesome and nutritious food, rather agreeable in flavour. The young shoots may likewise be eaten cooked like Asparagus, but though pleasant in taste they have a disagreeable smell.

In modern herbal medicine this plant (which is collected in July, when just coming into flower and dried in the same manner as Wood Betony) is employed for its antiseptic and antispasmodic properties. It relieves gout, cramp and pains in the joints and vertigo. The bruised leaves, which have an unpleasant odour and an astringent taste, when applied to a wound will stop bleeding and heal the wound, as is claimed for them by old tradition, and the fresh juice is made into a syrup and taken internally to stop hæmorrhages, dysentery, etc.

See BETONY, WOOD.

YAM, WILD

Dioscorea Villosa (LINN.)
N.O. Dioscoreaceæ

Synonyms. Dioscorea. Colic Root. Rheumatism Root. Wilde Yamwurzel
Part Used. Dried rhizome
Habitat. Southern United States and Canada

¶ *Description*. There are upwards of 150 varieties of Dioscorea, many, like the potato, being edible. An Indo-Chinese species is used as a dye in Southern China. *Dioscorea Villosa* is a perennial, twining plant, with long, knotty, matted, contorted, ligneous root-stocks. The root is long, branched, crooked, and woody, the taste being insipid, afterwards acrid, and having no odour. It is usually sold in pieces of various lengths, which are difficult to pulverize, as the root flattens out when this is attempted. The therapeutical value is lost after the first year, so that it should be freshly gathered and carefully dried each year.

¶ *Constituents*. Much saponin has been found in the roots, and a substance improperly called *dioscorein*, obtained by precipitating the tincture with water.

¶ *Medicinal Action and Uses*. Antispasmodic. Perhaps the best relief and promptest cure for bilious colic, especially helpful in the nausea of pregnant women. Valuable also in painful cholera morbus with cramps, neuralgic affections, spasmodic hiccough and spasmodic asthma.

¶ *Dosage*. ½ to 1 drachm of fluid extract. Dioscorein, ¼ to 4 grains.

¶ *Poisonous, if any, with Antidotes*. An alkaloid separated from the Javanese *D. hirsuta* has been found to be a convulsive poison, resembling picrotoxin, but much feebler.

YARROW

Achillea millefolium (LINN.)
N.O. Compositæ

Synonyms. Milfoil. Old Man's Pepper. Soldier's Woundwort. Knight's Milfoil. Herbe Militaris. Thousand Weed. Nose Bleed. Carpenter's Weed. Bloodwort. Staunchweed. Sanguinary. Devil's Nettle. Devil's Plaything. Bad Man's Plaything. Yarroway.
(*Saxon*) Gearwe
(*Dutch*) Yerw
(*Swedish*) Field Hop
Part Used. Whole Herb
Habitat. Yarrow grows everywhere, in the grass, in meadows, pastures, and by the roadside. As it creeps greatly by its roots and multiplies by seeds it becomes a troublesome weed in gardens, into which it is seldom admitted in this country, though it is cultivated in the gardens of Madeira

The name *Yarrow* is a corruption of the Anglo-Saxon name for the plant – *gearwe*; the Dutch, *yerw*.

¶ *Description*. The stem is angular and rough, the leaves alternate, 3 to 4 inches long and 1 inch broad, clasping the stem at the base, bipinnatifid, the segments very finely cut, giving the leaves a feathery appearance.

It flowers from June to September, the flowers, white or pale lilac, being like minute daisies, in flattened, terminal, loose heads, or cymes. The whole plant is more or less hairy, with white, silky appressed hairs.

Yarrow was formerly much esteemed as a vulnerary, and its old names of Soldier's Wound Wort and Knight's Milfoil testify to this. The Highlanders still make an ointment from it, which they apply to wounds, and Milfoil tea is held in much repute in the Orkneys for dispelling melancholy. Gerard tells us it is the same plant with which Achilles stanched the bleeding wounds of his soldiers, hence the name of the genus, *Achillea.* Others say that it was discovered by a certain Achilles, Chiron's disciple. It was called by the Ancients, the *Herba Militaris,* the military herb.

Its specific name, *millefolium,* is derived from the many segments of its foliage, hence also its popular name, Milfoil and Thousand Weed. Another popular name for it is Nosebleed, from its property of stanching bleeding of the nose, though another reason given for this name is that the leaf, being rolled up and applied to the nostrils, causes a bleeding from the nose, more or less copious, which will thus afford relief to headache. Parkinson tells us that 'if it be put into the nose, assuredly it will stay the bleeding of it' – so it seems to act either way.

It was one of the herbs dedicated to the Evil One, in earlier days, being sometimes known as Devil's Nettle, Devil's Plaything, Bad Man's Plaything, and was used for divination in spells.

Yarrow, in the eastern counties, is termed *Yarroway,* and there is a curious mode of divination with its serrated leaf, with which the inside of the nose is tickled while the following lines are spoken. If the operation causes the nose to bleed, it is a certain omen of success:

'Yarroway, Yarroway, bear a white blow,
If my love love me, my nose will bleed now.'

An ounce of Yarrow sewed up in flannel and placed under the pillow before going to bed, having repeated the following words, brought a vision of the future husband or wife:

'Thou pretty herb of Venus' tree,
  Thy true name it is Yarrow;
Now who my bosom friend must be,
  Pray tell thou me to-morrow.'
      (Halliwell's *Popular Rhymes,* etc.)

It has been employed as snuff, and is also called Old Man's Pepper, on account of the pungency of its foliage. Both flowers and leaves have a bitterish, astringent, pungent taste.

In the seventeenth century it was an ingredient of salads.

¶ *Parts Used.* The whole plant, stems, leaves and flowers, collected in the wild state, in August, when in flower.

¶ *Constituents.* A dark green, volatile oil, a peculiar principle, *achillein,* and achilleic acid, which is said to be identical with aconitic acid, also resin, tannin, gum and earthy ash, consisting of nitrates, phosphates and chlorides of potash and lime.

¶ *Medicinal Action and Uses.* Diaphoretic, astringent, tonic, stimulant and mild aromatic.

Yarrow Tea is a good remedy for severe colds, being most useful in the commencement of fevers, and in cases of obstructed perspiration. The infusion is made with 1 oz. of dried herb to 1 pint of boiling water, drunk warm, in wineglassful doses. It may be sweetened with sugar, honey or treacle, adding a little Cayenne Pepper, and to each dose, a teaspoonful of Composition Essence. It opens the pores freely and purifies the blood, and is recommended in the early stages of children's colds, and in measles and other eruptive diseases.

A decoction of the whole plant is employed for bleeding piles, and is good for kidney disorders. It has the reputation also of being a preventative of baldness, if the head be washed with it.

¶ *Preparations.* Fluid extract, ½ to 1 drachm.

An ointment made by the Highlanders of Scotland of the fresh herb is good for piles, and is also considered good against the scab in sheep.

An essential oil has been extracted from the flowers, but is not now used.

Linnæus recommended the bruised herb, fresh, as an excellent vulnerary and styptic. It is employed in Norway for the cure of rheumatism, and the fresh leaves chewed are said to cure toothache.

In Sweden it is called 'Field Hop' and has been used in the manufacture of beer. Linnæus considered beer thus brewed more intoxicating than when hops were used.

It is said to have a similar use in Africa.

Culpepper spoke of Yarrow as a profitable herb in cramps, and Parkinson recommends a decoction to be drunk warm for ague.

The medicinal values of the Yarrow and the Sneezewort (*A. millefolium* and *A. ptar-*

mica), once famous in physic, were discarded officially in 1781.

Woolly Yellow Yarrow (*A. tomentosa*) is very rare, and a doubtful native; its leaves are divided and woolly, the flowers bright yellow.

YELLOW DOCK. *See* DOCKS

YELLOW FLAG. *See* IRISES

YELLOW PARILLA. *See* PARILLA

YERBA REUMA

Frankenia grandifloria (CHAM. and SCHLECHT)
N.O. Frankeniaceæ

Synonyms. Frankenia. Flux Herb
Part Used. Herb
Habitat. California, Nevada, Arizona and Northern Mexico

¶ *Description.* A small, shrubby plant, with a prostrate, much-branched stem, about 6 inches long, growing in sandy places. It is salty to the taste, leaving an astringent after-taste. It has no odour.

¶ *Constituents.* It contains about 6 per cent. of tannin.

¶ *Medicinal Action and Uses.* Astringent. The herb is used as a remedy in catarrhal affections, especially of the nose and genito-urinary tract.

When diluted with from two to five times its volume of water, it may be used as an injection or spray.

It may also be taken internally.

¶ *Dosage.* Of fluid extract, 10 to 20 minims.

YERBA SANTA

Eriodictyon glutinosum (BENTH.)
N.O. Hydrophyllaceæ

Synonyms. Mountain Balm. Consumptive's Weed. Gum Bush. Bear's Weed. Holy or Sacred Herb. Eriodictyon Californicum (Hook and Arn.)
Part Used. Dried leaves
Habitat. California, Northern Mexico

¶ *Description.* A low, shrubby evergreen plant, 2 to 4 feet high, found growing abundantly in clumps on dry hills in California and Northern Mexico. The stem is smooth, usually branched near the ground, and covered with a peculiar glutinous resin, which covers all the upper side of the plant. Leaves, thick and leathery, smooth, of a yellowish colour, their upper side coated with a brownish varnish-like resin, the under surface being yellowish-white reticulated and tomentose, with a prominent midrib, alternate, attached by short petioles, at acute angle with the base; shape, elliptical, narrow, 2 to 5 inches long, ¾ inch wide, acute and tapering to a short leaf-stalk at the base. The margin of the leaf, dentate, unequal, bluntly undulate. The flowers, bluish, in terminal clusters of six to ten, in a one-sided raceme, the corolla funnel-like, calyx sparsely hirsute.

¶ *Constituents.* The chief constituents are five phenolic bodies, eriodictyol, homœriodictyol, chrysocriol, zanthœridol and eridonel. Free formic and other acids, glycerides of fatty acids; a yellow volatile oil; a phytosterol, a quantity of resin, some glucose. Taste, balsamic and sweetish, afterwards acrid, but not bitter, recalls Dulcamara and creates a flow of saliva. Odour, aromatic. The leaves are brittle when dry, but flexible in a warm, moist atmosphere. *Eriodictyon Californicum* is official in the United States Dispensary. Alcohol is the best agent for the fluid extract of the dried plant.

¶ *Medicinal Action and Uses.* Recommended for bronchial and laryngeal troubles and in chronic pulmonary affections, in the treatment of asthma and hay-fever in combination with *Grindelia robusta*. Likewise advised for hæmorrhoids and chronic catarrh of the bladder. Much used in California as a bitter tonic and a stimulating balsamic expectorant and is a most useful vehicle to disguise the unpleasant taste of quinine. Male fern and Hydrastis. In asthma, the leaves are often smoked. Aromatic syrup is the best vehicle for quinine.

¶ *Dosage.* 15 to 60 grains.

¶ *Other Species.* E. tomentosum, often found growing next to *E. Californicum*, especially in South California, but is easily distinguished from *E. Californicum*, being a larger shrub, and having a dense coat of short, villous hairs, colouring with age, whity-rusty; corolla, salver-shaped; leaves oval or oblong, and obtuse.

(*POISON*)
YEW [1]

Taxus Baccata
N.O. Taxaceæ and Coniferæ

Poisonous Parts. Leaves, seed and fruit
Habitat. Europe, North Africa, Western Asia

¶ *Description.* A tree 40 to 50 feet high, forming with age a very stout trunk covered with red-brown, peeling bark and topped with a rounded or wide-spreading head of branches; leaves spirally attached to twigs, but by twisting of the stalks brought more or less into two opposed ranks, dark, glossy, almost black-green above, grey, pale-green or yellowish beneath, $\frac{1}{2}$ to $1\frac{1}{2}$ inches long, $\frac{1}{15}$ to $\frac{1}{12}$ inch wide. Flowers unisexual, with the sexes invariably on different trees, produced in spring from the leaf axils of the preceding summer's twigs. Male, a globose cluster of stamens; female, an ovule surrounded by small bracts, the so-called fruit bright red, sometimes yellow, juicy and encloses the seed.

No tree is more associated with the history and legends of Great Britain than the Yew. Before Christianity was introduced it was a sacred tree favoured by the Druids, who built their temples near these trees – a custom followed by the early Christians. The association of the tree with places of worship still prevails.

Many cases of poisoning amongst cattle have resulted from eating parts of the Yew.

¶ *Constituents.* The fruit and seeds seem to be the most poisonous parts of the tree. An alkaloid taxine has been obtained from the seeds; this is a poisonous, white, crystalline powder, only slightly soluble in water; another principle, Milossin, has also been found.

¶ *Uses.* The wood was formerly much valued in archery for the making of long bows. The wood is said to resist the action of water and is very hard, and, before the use of iron became general, was greatly valued.

ZEDOARY

Curcuma Zedoaria (ROSCOE)
N.O. Zingiberaceæ

Synonyms. Turmeric. Zitterwurzel
Part Used. Dried rhizome
Habitat. East Indies and Cochin-China

¶ *Description.* There are two kinds of Zedoary, the long and the round, distinguished by the names of *radix zedoaria longæ* (Curcuma Zerumbet, the Long Zedoary of the shops) and *radix zedoaria rotundæ*. The long is in slices, or oval fingers; the round in transverse, rounded sections, twisted and wrinkled, greyish-brown in colour, hairy, rough, and with few root scars. The odour is camphoraceous, and the taste warm, aromatic, and slightly bitter, resembling ginger. The five commercial varieties come from China, Bengal, Madras, Java and Cochin-China, and vary in size and colour. When chewed they turn the saliva yellow. The powder is coloured brown-red by alkalis and boric acid. The Zerumbet has been erroneously confused with the round Zedoary.

Curcuma Starch, or East Indian Arrowroot, is prepared from the rhizomes of *Curcuma angustifolia.*

Some varieties of Zedoary are used as an ingredient in condiments and curries.

¶ *Constituents.* A volatile oil, when distilled with water, fixed oil, pungent resin, curcumin (an orange-yellow, tasteless, resinous principle), starch, mucilage, and an alkaloid.

¶ *Medicinal Action and Uses.* Aromatic, stimulant. Useful in flatulent colic and debility of the digestive organs, though it is rarely employed, as ginger gives the same, or better results. It is used as an ingredient in bitter tincture of Zedoary, antiperiodic pills (with and without aloes) bitter tincture, antiperiodic tincture (with and without aloes).

¶ *Dosages.* From 10 grains to $\frac{1}{2}$ drachm. Fluid extract, 10 to 30 drops. Infusion of $\frac{1}{2}$ oz. to a pint of boiling water, 1 tablespoonful.

---

[1] In homœopathy a tincture of the young shoots and also of the berries is used in a variety of diseases: cystitis, eruptions, headache and neuralgia, affections of the heart and kidneys, dimness of vision, and gout and rheumatism. – EDITOR.

Aaron's Beard, 817
Aaron's Rod, 361, 562
Ab-el-mosch, 566
Abelmoschus Moschatus, 566
Abies Canadensis, 638
Abies Larix, 636
Achweed, 368
Acinos Vulgaris, 807
Aconitum pardalianches, 610
Adam's Flannel, 562
Adder's Eyes, 632
Adder's Root, 236
Adderwort, 105
Adonis, 389
Adulsa Bakas, 506
African Pepper, 175
Agraphis nutans, 116, 424
Agrimony, Common, 12
Ague-grass, 824
Ague-root, 824
Ailanto, 821
Ailum, 159
Aivelle, 99
Alder – Red, Smooth, 18
Alecost, 226
Al-henna, 404
Alkekengi officinale, 191
Al-Khanna, 404
Alehoof, 442
Aletris Farinsen, 824
Alexanders, 500
Algaroba, 450
Alisanders, 500
Allgood, 365
All-Heal, 731, 824, 862
Allseed, 457
Alnus Rubra, 18
Aloe-root, 824
Aloysia citriodora, 830
Alsidium Helminthocorton, 551
Alsine media, 195
Alum Bloom, 233
Alum Root, 233
Amantilla, 824
Ambrakorner, 566
Ambretta, 566
Ambroise, 351
American Calumba, 214
American Dogwood, 122
American Everlasting, 477
American Greek Valerian, 3
American Ground Pine, 550
American Hellebore, 390
American Ipecacuanha, 431
American Nightshade, 648
American Spinach, 648
American Valerian, 829
Amomum Cardamomum, A. Repans, 159
Amomum Curcuma, 822

Amplopsis quinquefolia, 840
Amyris Gileadensis, A. Opobalsamum, 78
Amygdalis Persica, 619
Anchusa, 18
Anise, 201
Anemone grœnlandica, 361
Anethum graveolus, 255
Angels' Eyes, 759
Anhalonium Williamsii, 531
Aniseed Stars, 43
Annotta Orellana Orleana, 43
Apalachine à feuilles de Prunier, 16
Aplopappus, 249
Apple of Peru, 802.
Apple of Sodom, 417
Apple Pie, 848
Appleringre, 754
Apricock, 51
Aralia quinquefolia, 354
Araroba Powder, 51
Araruta, 57
Arbor Vitæ, 176
Arbor Vitæ, American, 176
Arbor Vitæ, Western, 176
Arbre à Suif, 87
Arbutus uva-ursi, 89
Archangel, 579
Archangelica officinalis, 35
Arcmart, 743
Arillus Myristicae, 504
Arisamae triphyllum, 841
Aristolochia reticulata, A. officinalis, A.
    sagittata, 744
Armstrong, 457
Aromatic Quinquina, 166
Aromatic Wintergreen, 849
Arrowroot – East, West Indian, Indian, 57
Arruda brava, 444
Arruda do Mato, 444
Arryan, 189
Arsesmart, 743
Artanthe elongata, 522
Artanthe hixagona, 96
Artemesia Lercheana, A. Maritima, A.
    Chamæmelifolia, 857
Artetyke, 229
Arthritica, 229
Arum, 236
Arusa, 506
Asa's Foot, 212
Asagræa officinalis, 697
Ash – Weeping, Common, 65
Ash-coloured Ground Liverwort, 494
Ashweed, 368
Aspen – American, Quaking, 650
Asphodel – White, Branched, 72
Asphodele Rameux, 72
Ass Ear, 215
Asteracantha Longifolia, 425

Asthma Weed, 494
Asthyrium Felix-fœmina, 302
Auld Man's Bell, 116
Auld Wife's Huid, 6
Australian Fever Bush, 257
Australian Quinine, 30
Ava, Ava Pepper, 454
Avegreen, 422
Avens – Nodding, Drooping, 75
Ayron, 422

Bachelor's Buttons, 309
Baconweed, 366
Badiana, 43
Bad Man's Plaything, 863
Bahama Cascarilla, 166
Bahia Powder, 51
Bairnwort, 247
Baldmoney, 349
Balessan, 78
Balm – Sweet, Lemon, 76
Balsam Copaiba, 221
Balsam Herb, 226
Balsam Styracis, 775
Balsam-weed, 449
Balsamina, 49
Balsamita, 226
Balsamodendron Myrrha, 571
Balsamodendrum Opobalsamum, 78
Balsamum Meccæ, B. Gileadense, 78
Balsamum Tolutanum, B. Americanum, 80
Balsumodendron Gileadensis, 78
Bamboo Brier, 714
Bamia Moschata, 566
Bananas, 646
Banksia Abyssinica, 459
Banwort, Banewort, 386
Baptisia, 432
Barbe de Capucin, 197
Barberry – Ophthalmic, 84
Barber's Brush, 793
Barweed, 206
Basam, 124
Base-broom, 375
Basil Thyme, 152
Bastard, 147
Bastard Cabbage Tree, 150
Bath Asparagus, 769
Baton d'Or, 842
Baume de Cheval, 774
Baume de la Mecque, 78
Bay, 464
Bayberry, 341
Bead Tree, 75
Bearbind, 101
Bear's Bed, 552
Bear's Foot, 462
Bear's Grape, 648
Bear's Weed, 865
Bearwind, 219
Beaver Poison, 391

Bechan, 78
Becky Leaves, 123
Bee Balm, 95
Beechwheat, 137
Beeflower, 842
Bees' Nest, 165
Beet – Garden, Sea, White, 93
Beggar's Blanket, 562
Beggar's Buttons, 143
Beggar's Stalk, 562
Beggarweed, 260
Beggary, 329
Bel, 76
Belæ Fructus, 76
Belladonna, 583
Belladonna, Japanese, 722
Belladonna, Scopola, 722
Benthamidian Florida, 122
Berberis Dumetorum, 82
Berbery, 82
Bereza, 103
Berke, 103
Bermuda Arrowroot, 57
Berry-bearing Orache, 115
Betel Nut, 54
Bettie Grass, 824
Betula Alnus, 17
Bharout, 450
Bicuculla Canadensis, 822
Bigaradier, 601
Bigelovia Veneta, 249
Bignonia Caroba, 160
Birang-i-Kabuli, 286
Birda rubra, 711
Bird Bread, 772
Birdlime Mistletoe, 547
Bird Pepper, 175
Bird's Eye, 386, 759
Bird's Foot, 299
Bird's Neat, 161
Bird's Nest, 165
Bird's Tongue, 457
Birthroot, 96
Biscuits, 819
Bishop's Elder, 368
Bishop's Leaves, 314
Bishopsweed, 368
Bishopswort, 97, 368
Bisom, 124
Bisornkorner, 566
Bissy Nuts, 458
Biting Persicaria, 743
Biting Stonecrop, 772
Bitter Ash, 662
Bitter Bark, 29, 257
Bitter Cucumber, 49
Bitter Damson, 741
Bitter Grass, 824
Bitter Herb, 77
Bitter Redberry, 122
Bitterroot, 350

Bittersweet, 589
Bitter Wood, 662
Bitterwort, 349
Bity Tongue, 743
Bizzom, 124
Black-berried White Bryony, 131
Black Cherry, 191, 583
Black Dogwood, 135
Blackeye Root, 130
Black Haw, 381
Black Indian Hemp, 395
Black Jack, 644
Black Maidenhair, 303
Black Pot-herb, 500
Black Root, 824
Black Sampson, 265
Black Snake Root, 211
Black Stinking Horehound, 416
Black-Tang, 111
Black Whortles, 99
Blackwort, 215
Bladder Fucus, 111
Bladderpod, 494
Blanket Herb, 562
Blasentang, 111
Blatterdock, 148
Blazing Star, 824
Bleaberry, 99
Bleeding Heart, 822
Blindweed, 738
Blitum Americanum, 648
Blood Hilder, 276
Bloodroot, 819
Blood Vine, 847
Bloodwood, 496
Bloodwort, 743, 863
Bloody Fingers, 322
Blooming Sally, 496, 847
Blue Bell, 3
Bluebells, 424
Blueberries, 99, 605
Blueberry Root, 212
Bluebottle, Bluebow, 223
Blue Cap, 223
Blue Curls, 731
Blue Flag, 439
Blue Gum Tree, 287
Blue Magnolia, 505
Blue Rocket, 6
Blue Sow-Thistle, 757
Blueweed, 142
Blume, 262
Blunt-leaved Everlasting, 80
Bly, 108
Bobbins, 236
Boden Chloigin, 673
Bog, 92
Bog, Moss, 552
Bog, Onion, 308
Bog, Rhubarb, 148
Bogshorns, 148

Bois de Campechy, 496
Bok, Boke, 92
Bolas, 142
Boldoa Fragrans, 118
Boldu, Boldus, 118
Boltsede, 456
Boneset, 215
Bore Tree, 265
Bottle-brush, 419
Bottleweed, 456
Bouleau, 103
Boule d'Or, 358
Bouncing Bess, 830
Bouncing Bet, 386, 748
Bourse de Pasteur, 738
Bour Tree, 265
Bovisand Soldier, 830
Bowl, 571
Bowman's Root, 431
Boxberry, 849
Box Tree, 122
Boy's Love, 754
Braamboss, 671
Brake Fern, 305
Brake Root, 307
Bramble, Brambleberry, Bramble-Kite, 108
Bramble of Mount Ida, 671
Brameberry, 108
Brank, 137
Bras Paddy, 680
Brassica sinapioides, 568
Brassica sinapistrum, 570
Braune Weiderich, 496
Brazil Powder, 51
Brazil Tea, 609
Brazilian Arrowroot, 791
Brazilian Cocoa, 381
Bread and Cheese Tree, 385
Breeam, 124
Bridewort, 524
Brideweed, 815
Brimstonewort, 298
British Myrrh, 201
Broad-leaved Elm, 282
Brooklembe, 123
Brombeere, 110
Broom, 366
Broom Tops, 124
Browme, 124
Brown Radiant Knapweed, 457
Brownwort, 314
Bruisewort, 215, 247, 748
Brum, 124
Brummel, 108
Brunella, 731
Brushes and Combs, 793
Brustbeeren, 451
Buche, 92
Buchweizen, 137
Buckbean, 117
Buckles, 229

Buckshorne, 642
Bugbane, 81, 211
Buk, Buke, 92
Bulbous Violet, 747
Bullies, Bullions, 142
Bull Nettle, 417
Bullock's Eye, 422
Bullock's Lungwort, 562
Bull's Eyes, 519
Bullsfoot, 212
Bullweed, 386, 456
Bully-bloom, 142
Bumble-Kite, 108
Bur-Marigold, 15
Burnet – Garden, Common, 145
Burnet – Lesser, 720
Burning Bush, 762
Burrage, 119
Burra Gokhru, 147
Butter Dock, 148, 258
Buttered Haycocks, 815
Butterfly-weed, 647
Butter Winter, 639
Buttonhole, 304
Buttons, 789

Caaroba, 160
Cactus – Vanilla, Sweet-scented, Large-
    flowered, 184
Caffea, 210
Calamus, 726
Calamus Draco, 262
Calamintha officinalis, C. menthifolia, 807
Calico Bush, 466
Californian Feverbush, 309
Californian Gum Plant, 376
Call-me-to-you, 386
Calsfoot, 80
Caltha officinalis, 517
Calverkeys, 116
Calves' Snout, 815
Camellia theifera, 792
Cammock, 674
Camolea, 531
Camomille puante, 523
Canada Pitch, 638
Canada Snakeroot, 354
Canadian Moonseed, 610
Canadisches Sonnenroschen, 328
Cancer-root, 648
Canchalagua, 184
Candle Berry, 87
Candlewick Plant, 562
Canella, Canellæ Cortex, 202
Cankerwort, 668
Cannabis Indica, C. Chinense, 396
Canton Cassia, 168
Capalaga, 159
Capdockin, 148
Cape Gooseberry, 191
Capon's Tail, 824

Capu Kanassa, 566
Carberry, 364
Cardamomi Semina, 159
Cardamomum – Alpinia, Matonia, 159
Cardamomum minus, 159
Cardoon Artichoke, 61
Card Thistle, 793
Carduus benedictus, 795
Carob, 450
Carob Tree, 160
Carobinha, 160
Carpenter's Herb, 139
Carpenter's Square, 313
Carpenter's Weed, 863
Carragreen, 552
Carrahan, 552
Carya, 842
Carya basilike, C. persica, 842
Casca Bark, 716
Cascara Sagrada, 136
Cascarillæ cortex, 166
Case-weed, 738
Cassara, Cassara Starch, 791
Casse-lunette, 290
Cassia aromaticum, C. bark, C. lignea, 168
Cassia æthiopica, C. Angustifolia C. Lan-
    ceolata, C. Lenitiva, C. officinalis, C.
    senna, 734
Cassavium pomiferum, 167
Cassilago, Cassilata, 397
Catchword, 206
Catnep, 173
Cat's Eye, 759
Catsfoot, 442
Cedrus Lycea, 176
Celandine – Common, Garden, 178
Celandine, Small, 179
Centaury gentian, 182
Centinode, 457
Centory, Century, 182
Cephaelis Ipecacuanha, 432
Ceterach, 302
Cetraria, 552
Cevadilla, 697
Chamælirium Carolinianum, 823
Chamomile – Dog, Stinking, Wild, 523
Chamomile, Spanish, 621
Chanvre, 396
Charity, 446
Charlock, 570
Chasse fièvre, 352
Chavica Betel, 96
Cheat, 372
Checkerberry, 766, 849
Cheese Rennet, C. Renning, 91
Cheeses, 507
Chelone, C. Obliqua, 77
Chelone, White, 77
Chenopodium Ambrosioides, 854
Cherry Bay, 465
Cherry Pie, 387, 848

Chervil – Great Sweet, Sweet, Cow, 201
Chèvre-feuille, 409
Chicken Toe, 233
Chien-dent, 371
Chillies, 175
China, 744
China Root, 339
Chinese Anise, 43
Chionathus, 328
Chirata, 199
Chocolate Flower, 233
Chocolate Tree, 151
Chondrus, 552
Chongras, 648
Chop Nut, 152
Christe Herbe, 388
Christmas Rose, 388
Christ's Eye, 707
Christ's Ladder, 182
Christ's Spear, 308
Christ's Thorn, 405
Chrusa borealis, 361
Chrysanthemum Peruvianum, 782
Chrysatobine, 51
Chucklusa, 298
Church Broom, 793
Church Steeples, 12
Churls Head, 456
Churnstaff, 815
Ciderage, 743
Cinchona Bark, 631
Cingulum Sancti Johannis, 556
Cinnamon – Bastard, Chinese, 168
Cinnamon Root, 760
Cinnamon Sedge, 726
Cinquefoil, 316
Cirsium palustre, 800
Cissampelos Pareira, 609
Cissus Hederacea, 840
Cissus quinquefolia, 840
Cistus, C. Canadensis, 328
Cistus Chamærhodendros, 466
Citronnier, 474
Citrus acris, 485
Citrus aurantium amara, C. bigaradia, C. dulcis, C. vulgaris, 601
Citrus limonum, C. medica, 474
City Avens, 73
Cives, 200
Clappe de pouch, 738
Clarry, 203
Clary, 705
Clear Eye, 203, 705
Cleavers, 206
Climbing Sailor, 817
Cloron's Hard, 760
Clot, 562
Clot-Bur, 143
Clover – King's, Sweet, Plaster, 525
Clove Root, 73
Clown's Lungwort, 562

Clown's Woundwort, 862
Clutia Eleuteria, 166
Cnicus benedictus, 795
Coakum, 648
Cocaine, 208
Cocculus Palmatus, 154
Cockle Buttons, 143
Cockeburr, 12
Cocks, 644
Cock's Comb, 673
Cocoa, 151
Codlings and Cream, 848
Cokan, 648
Cokil, 372
Cola acuminata, 458
Cola Nuts, 458
Cole Seed, 570
Colewort, 73
Colic Root, 339, 647, 746, 863
Colic Tree, 824
Colocynth Pulp, 49
Colombo, 154
Colombo, American, Faux, Radix, 214
Coltsfoot, 354
Coltstail, 320
Common Calamint, 807
Common Lilac, 477
Common Lime, 485
Common Mallow, 508
Common Shrubby Everlasting, 359
Common Wayside Dock, 258
Compass Weed, C. Plant, 681, 694
Coneflower, 265
Consolida, 215
Consound, 215
Consumptive's Weed, 865
Convallaria, 480
Convall-lily, 480
Conyza Squarrosa, 760
Coon Root, 115
Copaiva, 221
Coptide, 361
Coptis, 361
Coqueret, 191
Coral Root, 233
Cornbind, 219
Cornel, 122
Corn Feverfew, 524
Corn Poppy, Corn Rose, 651
Cornouiller à grandes fleurs, 122
Cornu Cervinum, 642
Corona Solis, 782
Cortezade Granada, 649
Cortex erythrophelei, 716
Cortex granati, 649
Cortex Thuris, 166
Corydalis, C. Canadensis, 822
Corydalis, Shone, 822
Cossoo, 459
Costa Canina, 644
Cotton Weed, 242

Cotula Maruta fœtida, 523
Coughwort, 212
Couhage, 228
Coumarouna odorata, 819
Couage, 228
Cowbane, 394
Cow Cress, 123
Cowcumber, 239
Cowede, 456
Cowgrass, 457
Cowitch, 228
Crab's Claw, 845
Cramp Bark, 381
Creeping Jenny, 549, 817
Creeping Joan, 549
Creeping Tom, 772
Crest Marine, 709
Crete-de-coq, 673
Crewel, 229
Crivell Melyn, 673
Crocus, 698
Crowberry, 648
Crow Corn, 824
Crowdy Kit, 314
Crowfoot, 34, 149, 233
Crow Soap, 748
Crude Chrysarobin, 51
Cuca, 208
Cuckoo's Bread, 640
Cuckoo's Meat, 751
Cuckoo Sorrow, 752
Cuckowes Meat, 752
Cucumber Tree, 505
Cuddle Me, 386
Cuddy's Lungs, 562
Cudweed, 175, 477
Cullay, 747
Cull Me, 386
Culrage, 743
Culverkeys, 116
Culver's Physic, 111
Culver's Root, 111
Culverwort, 214
Cumino aigro, 242
Curcuma, C. rotunda, 822
Cure All, 75
Curled Dock, 259
Cusparia Bark, 41
Cusso, 459
Custard Apple, 608
Cutch, 173
Cutweed, 111
Cydonia Vulgaris, 664
Cypripedium hirsutum, 829

Daffy-down-dilly, 245
Dagger Flower, 439
Daggers, 437
Daisy – Butter, Dun, Field, Horse, Maudlin,
    Moon, 248
Danewort, 276

Dame's Violet, 681
Daphne, 464
Darkness, 764
Darlahad, 84
Darnel Grass, 372
Datura, 802
Dead Men's Bells, 322
Dead Tongue, 263
Deberries, 364
Deerberry, 766, 849
Deilen Ddu, 313
Delicate Bess, 830
Dentallaria, 648
Dergmuse, 764
Deus Caballinus, 397
Devil's Apple, 802
Devil's Bit, 257, 824
Devil's Bite, 746
Devil's Cherries, 583
Devil's Dung, 62
Devil's Ear, 841
Devil's Garters, 219
Devil's Guts, 260
Devil's Head, 815
Devil's Herb, 583
Devil's Nettle, 863
Devil's Plaything, 863
Devil's Ribbon, 815
Devil's Trumpet, 802
Devil Tree, 29, 257
Dew Plant, 782
Dhan, 680
Dioscorea, 863
Didin, 571
Didthin, 571
Diosma betulina, 133
Dirtweed, 366
Dirty Dick, 366
Dita Bark, 29
Ditch Stonecrop, 774
Divale, 583
Dog Chamomile, 188
Dog-Fennel, 188
Doggies, 815
Dog-grass, 370
Dog Parsley, 614
Dog Poison, 614
Dog Rowan Tree, 381
Dogsbane, 108, 395
Dog Standard, 668
Dog's Fennel, 523
Dog's Tongue, 421
Dog's Tooth Violet, 11
Dog-Tree, 122
Dogwood, 762
Dogwood, Female, Swamp's, 605
Dolichos pruriens, 228
Dolloff, 524
Donnesbart, 422
Donnhove, 212
Doom Bark, 716

Dorstenia Houstoni, 219
Dossemo, 78
Doucette, 225
Dove's Dung, 769
Dove's-foot, 233
Draconis Resina, 262
Dracontium, D. fœtidum, 742
Dragon-bushes, 815
Dragon Flower, 437, 439
Dragon Root, 841
Dragon's Blood Palm, 262
Dragon's Claw, 233
Drake, 372
Dreiblättiger Aron, 841
Drelip, 229
Drias, 794
Drunken Sailor, 830
Duboisia, 223
Duck's Foot, 512
Dudgeon, 121
Duffle, 562
Dulcamara, 589
Dusty Miller, 202
Dutch Honeysuckle, 409
Dutch Myrtle, 341
Dutch Rushes, 419
Dwarf Bay, 531
Dwayberry, 583
Dyers' Broom, 375
Dyer's Bugloss, 18
Dyer's Greenwood, 129
Dyer's Madder, 504
Dyer's Weed, 129, 492
Dysentery Bark, 741

Earthbank, 819
Earth Smoke, 329
East Indian Catarrh Root, 339
Easter Flower, 32
Easter Mangiant, 105
Ebil, 159
Echino cactus Lewinii, E. Williamsii, 531
Echites Scholaris, 29
Ecorce de Granade, 649
Edellebere, 493
Eggs and Bacon, 815
Eggs and Collops, 815
Egyptian Alcée, 566
Egyptian Onion, 598
Egyptian Privet, 404
Egyptian's Herb, 357
Elder – Black, Common, 265
Elder, Red, Rose, Water, 381
Elf Dock, 278
Elm – Indian, Moose, Red, 283
Eltroot, 368
Elutheria, 166
Enebro, 452
English Bog Myrtle, 341
English Mandrake, 132
English Masterwort, 368

English Mercury, 365
Englishman's Foot, 640
Ephedrine, 286
Epitomin, 286
Erba Santa Maria, 533
Erect Knotgrass, 458
Eriffe, 206
Eriodictyon Californicum, 865
Eruca Sativa, 681
Eryngo, 407
Erysimum officinale, 570
Eternal Flower, 359
Eudodeca Bartonii, E. Serpentaria, 744
Eugenia Aromatica, 208
Eupatorium maculatum, E. purpureum, E. ternifolium, E. trifoliatum, E. verticillatum, 374
Euphorbia officinarum, 764
Euphorbium Bush, 764
Euphrasia, 290
European Globe Flower, 358
European Ground Pine, 141
European Larch, 636
European White Bryony, 131
Euryangium, 781
Eustachya Alba, E. Purpurea, 111
Everlasting Friendship, 206
Eve's Cups, 640
Ewe Daisy, 819
Eye Balm, 362
Eyebright, 203, 494
Eye of Christ, 759
Eye of the Day, 247
Eye Root, 362

Faba Ignatic, 431
Fabiana, 632
Faggio, 92
Fagos, 92
Fagus Castanea, 193
Fair Maid of February, 747
Fairy Bells, 752
Fairy Caps, 322
Fairy Cups, 229
Fairy's Glove, 322
Fairy Thimble, 322
False Dittany, 147
False Jacob's Ladder, 3
False Quinquina, 166
False White Cedar, 176
Färberginster, 375
Farewell, 759
Farinhade Mandioca, 510
Fat Hen, 365, 366
Faya, 92
Fea, Feabes, Feaberry, 364
Featherfew, 309
Featherfoil, 309, 834
Felon Herb, 556
Felonwood, Felonwort, 589
Feltwort, 562

Felwort, 349, 350
Female Fern, 305
Female Fern Herb, 552
Female Horsetail, 516
Fenkel, 293
Fennel – Sea, 709
Fennel – Sweet, Wild, 293
Fever Bark, 30
Feverberry, 364
Feverbush, 16
Feverwort, 182
Fiddler, 314
Fiddlewood, 314
Field Hop, 863
Fieldhove, 212
Field Lady's Mantle, 615
Figwort, 179
Filwort, 182
Fingerberry, 110
Finger Fern, 302
Finnochio, 297
Fiore d'ogni mese, 517
Fish Berry, 209
Five-Finger Blossom, 316
Five-Finger Root, 263
Five Fingers, 316, 354, 819
Flaggon, 437
Flag Lily, 439
Flake Manna, 67
Flammula Jovis, 205
Flapperdock, 148
Flax – Dwarf, Fairy, Purging, 319
Flaxweed, 815
Fleaseed, 643
Fleawort, 320
Flesh and Blood, 819
Flesh-coloured Asclepias, 787
Fleur de Coucou, 245
Fleur de Luce, 437
Fliggers, 437
Flirtwort, 309
Flores Carthami, 698
Flores Rhœados, 651
Flores Tiliæ, 485
Flower o' Luce, 386
Flowering Dogwood, 122
Flowering Sally, 496
Flowering Spurge, 531
Fluellin, 815
Fluellin, the Male, 759
Fluffweed, 562
Flussiger Amber, 775
Flux Herb, 865
Fly-Catcher, 640
Fly-Trap, 108, 640
Foalswort, 212
Foam Flower, 220
Folk's Glove, 322
Food of the Gods, 62
Fox's Clote, 143
Fragrant Everlasting, 80

Francisea Uniflora, 509
Frangula Bark, 135
Frankenia, 865
Frasera Canadensis, F. Walteri, 214
Frauenmantle, 462
Frauen Munze, 533
Fraxinella, 147
French Wheat, 137
Freshwater Soldier, 845
Frey, 366
Friar's Cap, 6
Friar's Cowl, 236
Fringe Tree Bark, 328
Frogsfoot, 149
Frost Blite, 366
Frostplant, Frostweed, 328
Fructus Anethi, 255
Fucus, 111
Fuller's Herb, 748
Fumus, Fumus Terræ, 329
Furze, 366
Fusanum, 762
Fusoria, 762

Gadrose, 762
Gagroot, 494
Gaitre Berries, 381
Galipea officinalis, 41
Gallitricum, 705
Gallwort, 815
Galu gasturi, 566
Gambier, 173
Gambodia, 341
Ganeb, 396
Ganja, 396
Garcinia Morella, 341
Garden Angelica, 35
Garden Hollyhock, 409
Garden Nightshade, 582
Garden Patience, 680
Garden Rue, 694
Gargant, 339
Garget, 648
Garlic Sage, 351
Gatten, Gatter, 762
Gay Feather, 746
Gazels, 385
Gearwe, 863
Gelsemium Sempervirens, 345
Gemeiner Wachholder, 452
Genet des Teinturiers, 375
Genevrier, 452
Genista Scoparius, 124
Georgina, 246
Gillenia, 431
Gill-go-by-the-Hedge, 442
Gill-go-over-the-Ground, 442
Gillyflower, 842
Ginepro, 452
Gingilly, 94
Gipsyweed, 141

Gipsy-wort, 357
Giroflier, 842
Gladdon, 726
Gladwin, 357
Gladyne, 437
Glandulæ Rotteleræ, 453
Glassworts, 189
Glatte, 77
Gleditschine, 358
Globe Crowfoot, 358
Globe Ranunculus, G. Trollius, 358
Gloves of Our Lady, 322
Gnaphalium, 359
Gnaphalium dioicum, 175
Gnaphalium Connoideum, G. Obtusifolium, 80
Goa, Goa Powder, 51
Goat's Arrach, 55
Goat's Leaf, 409
Goatweed, 368
Godfathers and Godmothers, 386
God'shair, 304
Gold Chain, 772
Goldcup, 149, 235
Golden Maidenhair, 552
Golden Moss, 772
Golden Rod, 562
Goldens, 248
Goldilocks, 359
Goldruthe, 361
Golds, 517
Goldy Star, 73
Gon Gouha, 609
Goonteh, 492
Gooseberry Pie, 848
Goosebill, 206
Goosefools, 189
Goosegogs, 364
Goosegrass, 206
Goose Grey, Goose Tansy, 740
Goosewort, 740
Goss, 366
Gouet à trois feuilles, 841
Gowan, 248
Gowke-Meat, 752, 753
Grains of Paradise, 628
Granadilla, 618
Grana Moschata, 566
Granat Wurzelrinde, 649
Grape Vine, 832
Gravel Plant, 53
Gravelweed, 374
Great Fleabane, 760
Great Morel, 583
Great Ox-eye, 248
Great Raifort, 417
Great Wild Valerian, 824
Greek Hay-seed, 299
Greek Valerian, 446
Green Broom, 124
Green Endive, 476

Green Ginger, 858
Green Sauce, 752
Greenweed, Greenwood, 375
Grenadier, 649
Grenouillette, 235
Grindelia – Hardy, Scaly, 376
Grip Grass, 206
Groats, 597
Groseille, 364
Groser, Grozet, 364
Ground Ash, 368
Ground Elder, 368
Ground Furze, 674
Ground Glutton, 377
Ground Holby, 639
Ground Laurel, 53
Ground Lily, 96
Ground Moss, 552
Ground Raspberry, 362
Grozet, 364
Grundy Swallow, 377
Guado, 852
Guarana Bread, 381
Guarea trichiliodes, 210
Guede, 852
Guérit-tout, 774
Guinea Corn, 130
Gujatatti elachi, 159
Gum Ammoniac, 31
Gum Benjamin, 95
Gum Benzoin, 95
Gum Bush, 865
Gum Camphor, 155
Gum Dragon, 820
Gum Euphorbium, 764
Gum Plant, 215, 376
Gum Resin, 340
Gummigutta, 341
Gunga, 492
Gura Nut, 458
Gurru Nuts, 458
Gutta gamba, 341
Gyrotheca capitata, G. tinctoria, 461

Hackmatack, 176, 788
Hæmatoxylon Lignum, 496
Hag's Taper, 562
Hagthorn, 385
Hair of Venus, 303
Hallelujah, 752
Hallfoot, 212
Halves, 385
Handflower, 842
Hant, 396
Haplopappus Baylahuen, 427
Happy Major, 143
Hardback, 774
Hardhead, 456
Hard Irons, 456
Hare's Beard, 562
Hare's Lettuce, 756

Hare's Thistle, 756
Hartshorne, 642
Hartsthorn, 134
Hart's Tree, 525
Hat-ta-wa-no-min-schi, 122
Haw, 385
Hawkweed, 384
Haya, 92
Haymaids, 442
Hayriffe, 206
Hayruff, 206
Hazels, 385
Hazelwort, 63
Heal-all, 774
Headache, 651
Heart of Osmund, 308
Heart of the Earth, 731
Hedge Basil, 87
Hedge Bills, 219
Hedge Calamint, 87
Hedge Convolvulus, 101
Hedgeheriff, 206
Hedgemaids, 442
Heidekorm, 137
Helianthemum Ramultoflorum, 328
Helleborus triflius, H. trilobus, H. pumilus, 261
Hellweed, 260
Helmet Flower, 724
Helonias, H. dioica, H. lutea, 823
Helonias officinalis, 697
Hemidesmus, 714
Hemlock – Lesser, Smaller, 614
Hemlock, Water, 617
Hemlock Bark, 638
Hemlock Gum, 638
Hemlock Pitch, 638
Hemlock Spruce, 638
Hempweed, 374
Hen Plant, 644
Hendibeh, 197
Hepatica triloba, 493
Herb Bennet, 73, 391
Herb Christopher, 81
Herb Constancy, 386
Herb Gerard, 368
Herb Ivy, 642
Herb Louisa, 830
Herb of Grace, 831, 694
Herb Patience, 258
Herb Peter, 229
Herb Trinitatis, 386
Herb Trinity, 493
Herb Twopence, 549
Herb Willow, 497
Herba di San Pietra, 709
Herba Myrti Rabanitini, 341
Herba Paris, 610
Herba rosellæ, 782
Herba ruta caprariæ, 696
Herba Sancti Mariæ, 854

Herba Stella, 642
Herba Veneris, 831
Herbe de la Croix, 547
Herbe de la langue, 648
Herbe du Siège, 313
Herbe Militaris, 863
Herbe Sacrée, 831
Herbe Sainte-Marie, 226
Herby grass, 694
Hercules Club, 40
Heterameris Canadensis, 328
Hetre, 92
High Cranberry, 381
Highwaythorn, 134
Hindberry, 671
Hindebar, Hindbeer, Hindbur, 671
Hind Heal, 351
Hind's Tongue, 304
Hippocastanum Vulgare, 192
Hirtentasche, 738
Hoarhound, 415
Hoar Strange, Hoar Strong, 298
Hog Apple, 512
Hog's-bean, 397
Hogweed, 457
Holly-leaved Barberry, 369
Holm, 405
Holme Chase, 405
Holy Herb, 739, 865
Holy Rope, 15
Holy Tree, 75, 405
Honeyblobs, 364
Honey locust, 358
Hooded Bindweed, 101
Hoodwort, 724
Hook-Heal, 731
Hop Tree, 71
Horminum, 705
Horsebalm, 774
Horsebane, 263, 264
Horse Blobs, 519
Horse Cress, 123
Horse Floure, 232
Horse-fly Weed, 432
Horse Gowan, 248
Horse Heal, 278, 760
Horsehoof, 212
Horse Knops, 456
Horse Tongue, 304
Horseweed, 774
Houseleek – Small, Stonecrop, 771
Housewell Grass, 123
Huckleberry, 99
Hulm, 405
Hulver Bush, 405
Humming-bird Tree, 77
Huntsman's Cup, 640
Hurtleberry, 99
Hurts, 99
Hurtsickle, 223
Husked Nut, 193

Hylantree, 265
Hylder, 265
Hyoscyamus, 397

Iceland Lichen, 552
Ice Vine, 609
Ictodes fœtidus, 742
Ignatia amara, 431
Ilachi, 159
Ilex Verticillata, 16
Imlee, 788
Impatiens pallida, 449
Incensier, 681
Indian Arrowroot, 762
Indian Bael, 76
Indian Balm, 96
Indian Balmony, 199
Indian Chocolate, 75
Indian Cup Plant, 243
Indian Dye, 362
Indian Gentian, 199
Indian Ginger, 354
Indian Hippo, 431
Indian Lilac Tree, 75
Indian Paint, 115, 362
Indian Pennywort, 425
Indian Pink, 637
Indian Poke, 390
Indian Posy, 80
Indian Root, 339, 760
Indian Shamrock, 96
Indian Spikenard, 760
Indian Tobacco, 494
Indian Turnip, 841
Indigo-weed, 432
Ink Root, 474
Insect Flowers, Insect Plants, 622
Intoxicating Pepper, 454
Ipomœa, I. purga, 101
Iris Aquatica, I. Lutia, 437
Iris Minor, 439
Irish Tops, 124
Ironhead, 456
Ispaghula, 643
Is'-ze-kn, 57
Italian Fitch, 696
Itch-weed, 390
Iuliole, 752
Ivy – American, Five-leaved, 840
Ivywort, 817

Jacaranda Caroba, 160
Jacinth, 116
Jack-by-the-Hedge, 571
Jack-go-to-bed-at-noon, 360
Jack-in-the-Pulpit, 841
Jack-jump-about, 368
Jack-jump-up-and-kiss-me, 386
Jack-of-the-Buttery, 772
Jack-run-in-the-Country, 219
Jackstraw, 644
Jacob's Ladder, 480

Jacob's Staff, 562
Jacob's Sword, 437
Jalap, 648
Jalap, Indian, 823
Jalap, Wild, 656
Jamaica Cabbage Tree, 150
Jamaica Mignonette, 404
Jamaica Pepper, 19
Jamaica Quassia, 67, 662
Jambul, 446
Jamestown-weed, 802
Jamguarandi, 444
Jamum, 446
Janipha Manihot, 791
Japanese Isinglass, 12
Jasmine – Carolina, False, Yellow, 345
Jatamansi, 781
Jaundice Root, 362
Jaunet, 149
Java Plum, 446
Jequirity, 492
Jerusalem Cowslip, 502
Jesuit's Powder, 153, 631
Jesuit's Tea, 609, 854
Jew's Myrtle, 128
Jimson-weed, 802
Joe-pye Weed, 374
Joubarbe des toits, 422
Jopi Weed, 374
Juarandi, 444
Judendornbeeren, 451
Judenkirsche, 191
Jungle Weed, 215
Jupiter's Bean, 397
Jupiter's Beard, 422
Jupiter's Eye, 422
Jupiter's Nuts, 193, 842
Jupiter's Staff, 562
Justica adhatoda, 506

Kæmpferia Galanga, 339
Kakelah seghar, 159
Kamcela, 453
Karcom, 698
Kecksies, 391
Keiri, 842
Kellerhals, 531
Kelp-Ware, 111
Kemps, 644
Kernelwort, 313
Ketmie odorante, 566
Kex, 391
Key Flower, 229
Key of Heaven, 229
Kidneywort, 493
Kif, 396
Kingcups, 519
Kings and Queens, 236
King's Crown, 381
King's Cure, 639
King's Spear, 72

Kinnikinnik, 605
Kiss-her-in-the-Buttery, 386
Kit-run-about, 386
Kit-run-in-the-Fields, 386
Kiwach, 228
Klotzsch, 234
Kneeholm, Kneeholly, Kneeholy, 128
Knight's Pondweed, 845
Knight's Spur, 464
Knitback, Knitbone, 215
Knob-Root, Knob-Weed, 774
Knotgrass, 457
Knot-Root, 774
Knotted Marjoram, 519
Kola Seeds, 458
Kombé Seeds, 777
Kooso, 459
Kosso, 459
Krameria Root, 674
Krapp, 504
Krausdistel, 407
Krokos, 698
Krusbaar, 364
Kusso, 459

Lacca cærulea, L. musica, 492
Lacmus, 492
Lacris, Lacrisse, 487
Lactuca agnina, 225
Lactucarium, 476
Ladder-to-Heaven, 480
Ladies' Meat, 385
Ladies' Seal, 132
Lad's Love, 754
Lady of the Meadows, 524
Laitue vireuse, 476
Lady's Purse, 738
Lady's Seal, 749
Lady's Slipper, 829
Lamb's Lettuce, 225
Lamb's Quarter's, 96, 366
Lamb's Tongue, 644
Land Whin, 674
Langwort, 148
Lappa, 143
Laquebleu, 492
Larch – American, Black, 788
Large-leaved Germander, 351
Lark's Claw, Lark's Heel, Lark's Toe, 464
Laricis Cortex, 636
Larix Europœa, L. decidua, 636
Larkspur Lion's Mouth, 815
Latherwort, 748
Laurel, Broad-leafed, 466
Laurel, Common, 465
Laurel, Noble, Roman, True, 464
Laurel, Camphor, 155
Laureole gentille, 531
Laurier armande, L. aux Crêmes, L. Cerise, 465
Laurier d'Apollon, 464

Laurier Sauce, 464
Laurocerasifolia, 465
Laurus Cinnamomum, 202
Laurus Sassafras, 715
Leadwort, 648
Leaf Cup, 91
Lebensbaum, 176
Le Blé Noir, 137
Lechea Major, 328
Ledum Grœnlandicum, 460
Leemoo, 474
Lemon-scented Verbena, 830
Lent Lily, 245
Lentisk, 522
Leontopodium, 462
Leopard's Bane, 55
Leopard's Foot, 519
Leptandra-Wurzel, 111
Lesser Red Rattle, 672
Lettuce – Acrid, Strong-Scented, 476
Lettuce Opium, 476
Leucanthemum Vulgare, 248
Levant Nut, 209
Levers, 437
Lichen Caninus, L. Cinerens Terrestis, 494
Lichen Roccella, 492
Lichwort, 624
Life Everlasting, 175, 773
Life of Man, 760
Lignum Campechianum, L. cœruleum, 496
Lignum Crucis, 547
Lignum rubrum, 717
Lignum vitæ, 380
Ligna cervina, 304
Ligusticum Levisticum, 499
Lily Constancy, 480
Lily May, Male, 480
Lily – Large White Water, Sweet-scented, Sweet Water, 484
Lily, White, 482
Limettæ Fructus, 485
Limewort, 123
Limone, 474
Limoun, 474
Limpwort, 123
Lindefolia Spectabilis, 421
Linden Flowers, 485
Link, 116
Linn Flowers, 485
Linseed, 317
Lion's Foot, 462
Lippia triphylla, 830
Liquidambar imberbe, 775
Liquirita, officinalis, 487
Little Dragon Mugwort, 791
Live-in-Idleness, 386
Live Long, 773
Liverleak, 493
Liver Lily, 439
Livers, 437
Liverweed, 493

Lizzy-run-up-the-Hedge, 442
Loblollie, 225
Locust Tree, 4
Logger Head, 456
L'Oignon d'Egypte, 600
Long-rooted Birthroot, 104
Lopophora Lewinii, 531
Lorbeer, 464
Lords and Ladies, 236
Lousewort, 672, 770
Lovage – Cornish, Italian, Old English, 499
Lovage, Sea, 501
Love-in-Idleness, 386
Love Idol, Loving Idol, 386
Love-in-Winter, 639
Love Leaves, 143
Love-lies-Bleeding, 30, 386
Loveman, 206
Lucerne – Sweet, 525
Lucken-Gowans, 358
Lung Moss, 502
Lurk-in-the-Ditch, 624
Lycorys, 487
Lysimaque rouge, 496
Lythrum, 496

Mace, 226
Mâche, 225
Macis, 504
Macleaya, 650
Mad-Dog Weed, 645
Madweed, 724
Mahonia Aquifolia, 369
Ma Huang, 286
Maid's Hair, 91
Maithen, Maithes, 523
Maize, 224
Malabar Cardamums, 159
Malicorio, 649
Mallards, 507
Malus communis, 44
Mamæire, 607
Manchineel, 513
Mancona Bark, 716
Mandragon, 510
Mangel Wurzel, 93
Manihot, 791
Man-in-the-Earth, 656
Man-in-the-Ground, 656
Man's Health, 354
Manioc, 510, 791
Manroot, 656
Manseed, 651
Manzanilla, 185
Manzanilla loca, 523
Mapato, 674
Maple – Curled, Swamp, 516
Maracoc, 618
Maranta Arrowroot, M. Indica, M. ramosis-
    sima, M. Starch, 57
March Everlasting, 242

Margosa, 75
Marguerite, 248
Marigold of Peru, 782
Marjorana hortensis, 519
Maronte, 523
Marrubium nigrum, 416
Marsadenia Condurango, 219
Marsh Barren Horsetail, 516
Marsh Clover, 117
Marsh Crowfoot, 235
Marsh Parsley, 298
Marsh Penny, 425
Marsh Rosemary, 474
Marsh Samphire, 357
Marsh Smallage, 298
Marsh Trefoil, 117
Maruba, 741
Marum, 808
Maruta Cotula, 188, 523
Maruta Fœtida, 188
Marygold, 517
Mary Gowles, 517
Maryland Pink, 637
Maté, 609
Maté, Houx, Ilex, Yerba, 609
Mathor, 523
Matte Felon, 456
Maudlinwort, 248
Mauls, 507
May, 385
May Apple, 512
Mayblossom, 385
Mayflower, 53, 229
Maypops, 618
May Rose, 381
Maythen, 185
Mayweed, 188
Meadow Anemone, 32
Meadow Cabbage, 742
Meadow Runagates, 549
Meadow Routs, 519
Meadsweet, 524
Mechameck, 656
Méchoacan du Canada, 648
Meefenchel, 709
Meeriche, 111
Meet-me-in-the-Entry, 386
Mehlige Aletria, 824
Mehndi, 404
Meklin, 437
Melampode, 388
Melanthium Sabadilla, 697
Meleze, 636
Melilot – Corn, White, Yellow, 525
Melo Granato, 649
Melon Tree, 607
Memory Root, 841
Mendee, 404
Mentha Odorata, 545
Mentha Spicata, 533
Menthe de Notre Dame, 533

Mercury Goosefoot, 365
Mexican Lippia, 486
Mexican Tea, 854
Mezerei Cortex, M. officinarum, 531
Midden Myles, 366
Middle Comfrey, 139
Middle Fleabane, 321
Milfoil, 863
Milfoil, Knight's, 863
Milk Parsley, 298
Milkweed, 108
Milkwort, 733
Mill Mountain, 152, 319
Miltwaste, 302
Minnari Asclepias, 714
Mint – Brandy, 537
Mint, Egyptian, 545
Mint, Fish, Garden, Green, Lamb's, Mackerel, Our Lady's, Spire, 533
Mint, Hairy, Marsh, Whorled, 543
Mirra, 571
Mitrewort, 220
Mix Moschata, 591
Moho-moho, 522
Monarda lutea, 546
Mon-ha-can-ni-nun-schi, 122
Monkey Flower, 815
Monkshood, 6
Monk's Rhubarb, 258
Monœcia triandria, 103
Moorgrass, 740
Morelle à Grappes, 648
Mormodica Elaterium, 241
Morning Glory, 103
Morr, 571
Mortification Root, 507
Moschuswurzel, 781
Mother of Thyme, 813
Mother of Millions, 817
Mother's Heart, 738
Mountain Balm, 152, 865
Mountain Cinnamon, 850
Mountain Damson, 741
Mountain Balm Bark, 166
Mountain Everlasting, 175
Mountain Flax, 733
Mountain Mint, 152, 807
Mountain Pink, 53
Mountain Radish, 417
Mountain Spinach, 56
Mountain Tea, 849
Mountain Tobacco, 55
Mouse Ear, 384
Mousetail, 772
Moutarde des Allemands, 417
Mouthroot, 361
Mucuna prurita, 228
Mudar Yercum, 154
Muge-de-boys, 852
Mullein Dock, 562
Muscadier, 504

Muscal Buttons, 531
Muscus Terrestris Repens, 551
Musk Ranunculus, 550
Musk Root, 781
Musk Melon, 527
Musquash Root, 391
Mutton Chops, 206
Mutton Tops, 366
Myrica, 87
Myristica Moschata, 504
Myristica officinalis, 504, 591
Myrosperum Pereira, 79
Myrtle Flower, 437
Myrtle Grass, 726
Myrtle Sedge, 726
Myrtus Chekan, 189
Mystyldene, 547

Naked ladies, 700
Narcissus, 245
Naughty Man's Cherries, 583
Neem, 75
Neemoo, 474
Nepenthes distillatoria, 640
Nepeta Glechoma, 442
Nerve-root, 824
Netchweed, 55
Nettle – Dummy, 582
Nettle, Bee, Blind, Deaf, Dumb, White, Dead, 579
Nettle, Stinging, 574
New England Boxwood, 122
New Jersey Tea, 673
Nidor, 329
Niggerhead, 265
Nigrobaccus, 110
Nim, 75
Nine Hooks, 462
Nine-joints, 457
Ninety-knot, 457
Nisoth, 823
Nivarra, 680
Nkasa, 716
Noah's Ark, 829
Noble Liverwort, 493
Nodding Squill, 424
None-so-Pretty, 80
Noon Flower, 360
Nose Bleed, 863
Nutmeg Flower, 297
Nux persica, Nux regia, 842

Oak Fern, 307
Oak Lungs, 502
Oatmeal, 597
Oculus Christi, 205, 517, 707
Oderwort, 105
Ofbit, 722
Ofnokgi, 781
Oil Nut, 150, 845
Old Field Balsam, 80

Old Maid's Nightcap, 233
Old Man, 754
Old Man's Beard, 328
Old Man's Flannel, 562
Old Man's Nightcap, 101
Old Man's Pepper, 863
Old Man's Root, 760
Old Woman, 861
Olea Oleaster, O. Lancifola, O. Gallica, 598
Olibanum, 326
Olivier, 598
One Berry, 610, 766
Operculina Turpethum, 823
Opium Poppy, 651
Opopanewort, 862
Or, 110
Or Seille, 492
Orache – Spreading, 56
Orange – Bigarde, Bitter, China, Seville, Sweet Portugal, 601
Orange Milkweed, 647
Orange Root, 362
Orchanet, 18
Orchella Weed, 492
Ordeal Bark, 152, 716
Oregon Grape Root, 369
Orvale, 203
Oryza latifolia, O. montana, O. setegera, 680
Osmund the Waterman, 308
Osterick, 105
Oswego Tea, 95
Ouchi, 781
Our Lady's Bedstraw, 91
Our Lady's Flannel, 562
Our Lady's Keys, 229
Our Lady's Tears, 480
Oxford-weed, 817

Paddock-pipes, 419
Paederota Virginica, 111
Paigle, 229
Pain de Coucou, 752
Pain d'Oiseau, 772
Paint, 461
Pale Mara, 29
Pale-touch-me-not, 449
Pali-mara, 257
Palma Christi, 169
Palsywort, 229
Pancon, 115
Panais, Le, 615
Panama Bark, 747
Panicant, 407
Papaya Vulgaris, 607
Pappoose Root, 212
Paprika, 628
Paraguay, P. Herb, 609
Parisette, 610
Parsley Breakstone, 615
Parsley Piercestone, 615
Parson and Clerk, 236

Partridge Berry, 766, 849
Partyke, 496
Pasque Flower, 32
Passe Flower, 32
Passerina, 195
Passion Vine, 618
Passion's Dock, 258
Password, 229
Pastel, 852
Pastinaca Opoponax, 600
Pastinake, 615
Pattens and Clogs, 815
Paul's Betony, 759
Paullinia, P. Sorbilis, 381
Peachwood, 496
Pearl Barley, 84
Pedlar's Basket, 815, 817
Peggle, 229
Pelican Flower, 744
Pellitory of Spain, 621
Pellitory, Roman, 621
Pellote, 531
Pennycress, 571
Pennygrass, 673
Penny Pies, 455
Pennywort, 817
Pensée, 386
Penthorum, 774
Pepper – Black, 627
Pepper Sweet, 628
Pepper and Salt, 738
Pepper Plant, 743
Pepper Turnip, 841
Periploca Indica, 714
Perlatum, 84
Persele, Persely, 611
Persica Vulgaris Null, 619
Persio, 492
Personata, 143
Pestilenzkraut, 696
Peter's Staff, 562
Petersylinge, 611
Petit Chêne, 352
Pettigree, 128
Pettymorell, 582, 760
Pewterwort, 419
Pheasant's Eye, 389
Phellandrium aquaticum, 264
Philanthropium, 143
Philanthropos, 12
Philtron, 161
Phu, 284
Physic Root, 111
Phytolacca – Branching, 648
Phytolacca Americana, P. Berry, P. Root, P. Vulgaris, 648
Phytolaque, 648
Pick-Pocket, 738
Pick-Purse, 738
Pied-de-Lion, 462
Pied-de-Poule, 371

Pigeon Berry, 648
Pigmentum Indicum, 432
Pigrush, 437
Pigweed, 366, 368, 457, 660, 762
Pilewort, 179
Piliolerial, 624
Pilosella, 384
Pimento, 19
Pimpinella Sanguisorba, 146
Pin du Lord, 637
Pinang, 54
Pink-eyed John, 386
Pink-o'-the-Eye, 386
Pinus Alba, 637
Pinus Canadensis, 638
Pinus Pendula, 788
Pipe Tree, 265
Piper, 627
Piper elongatum, P. granulosum, 522
Pipperidge Bush, 82
Pix Canadensis, 638
Plantago decumbens, P. Ispaghula, 643
Plantain – Black, Long, Snake, 644
Plaintain, Broad-leaved, 640
Plantula Marilandica, 733
Plumrocks, 229
Plum Tree, 659
Pocan, 648
Podalyria tinctoria, 432
Poison Ash, 328
Poison Flag, 439
Poison Hemlock, 391
Poison Nut, 592
Poison Oak, 443
Poison Parsley, 391
Poison Vine, 443
Poisonous Gum-Thistle, 764
Poisonous Potato, 417
Polar Plant, 681, 694
Polecatweed, 742
Polygala Virginiana, 733
Polypody of the Oak, 307
Poolroot, 711
Poor Man's Parmacettie, 738
Poor Man's Treacle, 342
Poor Man's Weatherglass, 632
Porillon, 245
Pot Marigold, 517
Prairie Turnip, 655
Prayer Beads, 492
Premorse Scabious, 722
Pretty Betsy, 830
Pretty Mugget, 91
Pretty Mulleins, 229
Prickly Ash (Angelica Tree), 40
Prickly Broom, 366
Prickly Elder, 40
Prick Madam, 772
Prickwood, 762
Pride of China, 75
Prideweed, 320

Priest's Crown, 249
Prince's Feathers, 740
Prince's Pine, 639
Prinos Confertus, P. Gronovii, 16
Protium Gileadense, 78
Prunella, 731
Pseudosarsa, 714
Psyllion, Psyllias, 643
Pterocarpi Lignum, 717
Pucha-pat, 618
Pudding Grass, 624
Pukeweed, 494
Pulegium, 624
Pulicaria dysenterica, 321
Pulsatilla Nuttaliane, 34
Pumacuchu, 674
Purple Archangel, 580
Purple Boneset, 374
Purple Clover, 207
Purple Goat's Beard, 708
Purple Medicle, 501
Purple Rocket, 847
Purple Side-Saddle Flower, 640
Purple Willow Herb, 496
Pussy Willow, 846
Pyrethree, 621
Pyrethri Radix, 621
Pyrethrum, P. officinarum, 621
Pyrethrum, Anthemis, Matricaria, 621
Pyrethrum, Parthenium, 309
Pyrola umbellata, 639
Psyllium Seeds, 643

Quaker, 236
Quaker Buttons, 592
Quassia Simaruba, 741
Queen Anne's Pocket Melon, 528
Queen of the Meadow, 524
Queen-of-the-Meadow Root, 374
Queen's Root, 664
Quercus Marina, 111
Quick, 385
Quick-grass, 370
Quick-in-the-hand, 449
Quinquenervia, 644
Quinsy Berries, 243

Rabbit Root, 712
Rabbits, 815, 817
Racine de Sumbul, 781
Racoonberry, 512
Radix Colubrina, R. Viperina, 744
Ragged Cup, 243
Rag Paper, 562
Ragweed, 668
Raisin d'Amerique, 648
Raizpara los dientes, 674
Ramp, 236, 670
Ramsted, 815
Ramsthorn, 134
Rapuntium inflatum, 494

Raspbis, 671
Rasura Satalum ligni, 717
Rati, 492
Rattlebush, 432
Rattle Grass, Yellow, 673
Rattle Pouches, 738
Rattle Root, 211
Rattlesnake Root, 733
Ray-grass, 372
Red Bark, 631
Red Berry, 354
Red Canella, 850
Red Centaury, 182
Red Chamomile, 389
Red Cockscomb, 30
Red Cole, 417
Red Ink Plant, 648
Red Knees, 743
Red Mathes, 389
Red Morocco, 389
Red Pucoon, 115
Red Rattle Grass, 672
Red River Snakeroot, 744
Red Robin, 457
Red Root, 115, 461
Red Rot, 782
Red Sandalwood, 717
Red Texas Snakeroot, 744
Red Water Bark, 716
Reglisse, 487
Reps, 244
Rhamnus Zizyphus, 451
Rhatamy – Peruvian, Red, 674
Rhatanhiawurzel, 674
Rheumatism Root, 863
Rheumatism Weed, 639
Rhizoma Galangæ, 339
Rhubarb – Bastard, Garden, 677
Rhubarb, China, East Indian, 675
Rhus copallinum, R. typhinum, 779
Ribble Grass, 644
Ribs, 244
Ribwort, 644
Richleaf, 774
Richweed, 774
Rigolizia, 487
Ring-o'-Bells, 116
Ringworm Powder, 51
Ripplegrass, 640
Risp, 244
Roast Beef Plant, 357
Robbia, 504
Robin-run-in-the-Grass, 206
Robin-run-in-the-Hedge, 442
Robin's Eye, 552
Roccella phycopsis, R. Pygmæa, 492
Rock Brake, 307
Rock Brake Herb, 552
Rocket – Dame's, White Purple, 681
Rock Moss, 492
Rock of Polypody, 307

Rock Rose, 328
Roman Coriander, 297
Roman Plant, 201
Ropebind, 219
Roquette, 681
Rosage Alpenrose, 675
Rose Apple, 446
Rose-a-Rubie, 389
Rosebay, 675
Rose Noble, 313
Rosée du Soleil, 782
Rosin Weed, 376
Rother Weiderich, 496
Rottlera tinctoria, 453
Round-leaved Hepatica, 493
Round-leaved Sundew, 782
Roving Jenny, 817
Rowan Tree, 69
Royal Staff, 72
Rubus Cuneifolus, 110
Rubywood, 717
Rucchette, 681
Rudbeckia, 265
Ruddes, 517
Ruffet, 366
Run-by-the-Ground, 624
Running Jenny, 549
Rusticum Vulna Herba, 862
Ryntem Root, 349

Sabadillermer, 697
Sabal, S. Serrulata, 719
Sabline rouge, 711
Sacred Bark, 136
Sacred Herb, 865
Saffron – American, Bastard, Dyer's, Fake, 698
Sage – Broad-leaved, Garden, Marrow, Red, 700
Sage of Bethlehem, 533
Sahlep, 602
St. Anthony's Turnip, 149
St. Barbara's Hedge Mustard, 570
St. James's Tea, 460
St. James-wort, 668
St. John's Herb, 15
St. John's Plant, 556
St. Mary's Seal, 749
Salad Burnet, 146
Salade de Chanoine, 225
Salade de Prêtre, 225
Salep, 602
Salicaire, 496
Sallowthorn, 137
Saloop, 602
Salt-rheum Weed, 77
Salsipis des prés, 708
Salvia Salvatrix, 700
Sampier, 709
Sanctæ Mariæ, 749
Sand Brier, 417

Sanders-wood, 710
Sangree, Sangrel, 744
Sanguinary, 738, 863
Sanguis draconis, 262
Sanpetra, 709
Santalum rubrum, 717
Santolina, 473
Santonica, 857
Sapium, 788
Sapium Sylvaticum Yaw Root, 664
Sappan, 717
Saracen Corn, 137
Sarazina Gibbosa, 640
Sardian Nut, 193
Sarothamnus scoparius, 124
Sarracenie, 640
Sarrasin, 137
Sarsaparilla – English, 819
Sarsaparilla, False, Wild, 712
Sarsaparilla, Moonseed, Texas, 610
Sarsaparilla, Red-bearded, 713
Satan's Apple, 510
Satyrion, 602
Sauce Alone, 571
Saucy Bark, 716
Savine Tops, 717
Sawage, 700
Scabiosa arvensis, 721
Scabwort, 278
Scaldhead, 108
Scaldweed, 260
Scaly Fern, 302
Scammony, 102
Scarlet Berry, 589
Scarlet Monarda, 95
Scean de Solomon, 749
Schloss Tea, 507
Schlutte, 191
Schœnocaulon officinale, 697
Scilla maritima, 766
Scilla nutans, S. nonscriptus, 424
Scorzo de Melogranati, 649
Scotch Quelch, 370
Scratweed, 206
Scullcap – Greater, Mad-dog, 724
Sea Beets, 189
Sea Green, 845
Sea Holme, 407
Sea Hulver, 407
Sea Lavender, 474
Sea Wormwood, 857
Sea Wrack, 111
Seamsog, 752
See Bright, 203, 705
Seetang, 111
Segg, 437
Self-Heal, 711
Semen Abelmoschi, 566
Semen Cinæ, S. contra, S. sanctum, S. Santonici, 857
Semen Strychnos, 592

Seneca, Seneka, 733
Senecio hieracifolius, 315
Senegæ officinalis, S. radix, 733
Sengreen, 422
Senna – Alexandrian, East Indian, Egyptian, Nubian, Tinnevelly, 734
Sennacutifolia, 734
Sention, 377
Septfoil, 819
Serpentaria, 549
Serpentary Radix, S. Rhizome, 744
Serpent's Tongue, 11
Serpyllum, 813
Setæ Siliquæ Hirsutæ, 228
Setwale, Setwall, 824
Seven Barks, 424
Shalder, 437
Shameface, 233
Shave Grass, 419
Sheep's Herb, 645
Sheggs, 437
Shellflower, 77
Shepherd's Bag, 738
Shepherd's Barometer, 632
Shepherd's Clubs, 562
Shepherd's Knapperty, 819
Shepherd's Knot, 819
Shepherd's Needle, 201
Shepherd's Scrip, 738
Shepherd's Sprout, 738
Shepherd's Staff, 562
Shot Bush, 81, 712
Shrubby Sea Blite, 115
Shrubby Trefoil, 71
Shumach – Pennsylvania, Upland, 779
Siam Benzoin, 95
Sicklewort, 139
Side-saddle Plant, 640
Sigillum Sanctæ, 749
Silkweed – Rose-coloured, Swamp, 787
Silky Cornel, 605
Silver Bells, 381
Silver Leaf, 80, 382, 664
Silverweed, 449
Silvery Cinquefoil, 740
Simaruba Honduras Bark, 166
Simson, 377
Sinapis Alba, 566
Singer's Plant, 570
Skewerwood, 762
Skoke, 648
Skunk Bush, 309
Skunkweed, 742
Slan-lus, 640
Slave Wood, 741
Slipperweed, 449
Slippery Root, 215
Slough-Heal, 731
Smallage, 182
Small Spikenard, 712
Smallwort, 179

Smartgrass, 743
Smearwort, 365
Smell Fox, 34
Smilax Medica, 713
Smilax Sarsaparilla, 714
Smooth Cicely, 201
Smooth Lawsonia, 404
Snagul, 744
Snakebite, 115
Snake Cucumber, 528
Snake Head, 77
Snake Lily, 439
Snake Root, 733
Snakeweed, 105, 640, 744
Snapdragon, 815
Snapping Hazelnut, 851
Snowball Tree, 381
Snowdrop Tree, 328
Snow Rose, 675
Soap Bark, 747
Soap Root, 748
Sola Indianus, 782
Solanum quadrifolium, 610
Soldier's Herb, 522
Solidago, 361
Solis Sponsa, 517
Solsequia, 519
Son-before-the-Father, 848
Sonnenthau rosollis, 782
Sophora tinctoria, 432
Sorghum Seeds, S. Saccharatum, 130
Sorrel, Buckler-shaped, 752
Sorrel, Field, 754
Sour Grabs, Sour Sabs, Sour Sauce, Sour
    Suds, 752
Sour Trefoil, 752
Sowbane, 366
Sowbread, 245
Sow Fennel, 298
Spanish Bugloss, 18
Spanish Chestnut, 193
Sparrow Tongue, 457
Spartium Scoparium, 124
Spathyema fœtida, 742
Speckled Jewels, 449
Spergularia rubra, 711
Spignet, 760
Spiked Loosestrife, 496
Spinach, 189
Spinach Beet, 93
Spiny Cot Burr, 210
Spiræa stipulata, S. trifoliata, 431
Spirit Weed, 461
Spogel Seed, 643
Sponsa Solis, 519
Spoon Wood, 453, 466
Spoonwort, 725
Spotted Alder, 851
Spotted Corobane, 391
Spotted Cranesbill, 233
Spotted Hemlock, 391

Spotted Monarda, 546
Spotted-touch-me-not, 449
Spurge Laurel, 531
Spurge Olive, 531
Spurge Plant, 357
Squaw Root, 211, 212
Squill – Maritime, Red, White, 766
Squinancy Berries, 243
Squinancy-wort, 667
Squirrel Corn, 822
Staggerwood, 822
Staggerwort, Stammerwort, 668
Starbloom, 637
Star Chickweed, 195
Starch Hyacinth, 423
Starchwort, 236
Stargrass, Star-root, 824
Star of Hungary, 769
Starweed, 195
Starwort, 823, 824
Statice Limonium, 474
Staunchweed, 863
Stave Wood, 741
Steeple Bush, 382
Stellaria, 462
Stephensia elongata, 522
Stepmother, 386
Sterculia acuminata, 458
Sticklewort, 12
Stickwort, 752
Stinking Arrach, 55
Stinking Goosefoot, 55
Stinking Motherwort, 55
Stinking Nanny, 668
Stinking Tommy, 674
Stinkweed, 802
Stizolobium pruriens, 228
Stoechas, 359
Storax – Liquid, Prepared, 775
Storksbill, 233
Stramonium, 802
Strangle Tare, 260
Strawberry Blite, 30
Strawberry Spinach, 115
Strawberry Tomato, 191
String of Sovereigns, 549
Stringy Bark Tree, 287
Strophanti Semina, 777
Stubwort, 752
Styrax Liquidus, Præparatus, 775
Succory, 197
Sugar Pods, 450
Sulphurwort, 298
Sumach – Chinese, 821
Sumach Fragrant, 780
Sumaruppa, 741
Sumatra Benzoin, 95
Sumbul radix, S. wurzel, 781
Sunflower Artichoke, 58
Sunkfield, 316
Surelle, 752

Suterberry, 70
Swallow-wort, 647
Swamp Dogwood, 71
Swamp Hellebore, 390
Swamp Sassafras, 505
Swamp Tea Tree, 151
Sweatroot, 3
Sweet Bark, 166
Sweet Bay, 464
Sweet Betty, 748
Sweet Bracken, 201
Sweet Broom, 128
Sweet Bugle, 141
Sweet Cane, 726
Sweet Cus, 201
Sweet Fern, 201
Sweet Flag, 726
Sweet Humlock, 201
Sweet Myrtle, 726
Sweet Root, 726
Sweet Round-leaved Dock, 677
Sweet Rush, 726
Sweets, 201
Sweet-scented Life Everlasting, 80
Sweet Slumber, 115
Sweet Vernal, 389
Sweetwood Bark, 166
Swine's grass, 457
Swine's Snout, 249
Swynel Grass, 457
Sycocarpus Rusbyi, 210
Symphonica, 397
Synkefoyle, 316
Syzgium Jumbolana, 446

Tabacca, 817
Tabaci Folia, 817
Tagar, 824
Tailed Pepper, 236
Tallow-Shrub, 87
Tame Withy, 847
Tamus, 132
Tanner's Bark, 593
Target-leaved Hibiscus, 566
Tartar Root, 354
Teaberry, 849
Teel, 94
Tekrouri, 396
Tentwort, 303
Terra Japonica, 173
Tetterbury, 132
Tetterwort, 115
Thea bohea, T. sinensis, T. veridis, 792
Thé du Canada, 849
Thick-leaved Pennywort, 425
Thistle, Blessed, 795
Thistle – Dwarf May, Ground, 798
Thistle – Field, Way, 799
Thistle, Marian, 797
Thistle, Nodding, 800

Thistle, St. Barnaby's, 802
Thoho-Thoho, 522
Thormantle, 819
Thorn, 385
Thorny Burr, 143
Thoroughwort, 118
Thor's Beard, 422
Thousand Flower, 817
Thousand Weed, 863
Three-faces-under-a-Hood, 386
Three-leaved Grass, 752
Three-(t)horned Acacia, 358
Throatwort, 313
Thuia du Canada, 176
Thymosacinos, 807
Tiglium Seeds, 234
Tilia cordata, T. intermedia, platyphylla, T.
  vulgaris, 485
Tilleul, 485
Ti Namie, 621
Tipsinah, 655
Tissa rubra, 711
Toad, 815
Toadroot, 81
Tola Bona, 365
Toluifera Pereira, 79
Tolutanischer Balsam, 80
Tom Rong, 341
Tonka Bean, 819
Toothache Tree, 40, 70
Torches, 562
Touresol, 492
Toute-bonne, 203
Trackleberry, 99
Tragacanth – Gum, Syrian, 820
Trailing Tansy, 740
Treacle Wormseed, 571
Treadfoot, 417
Tree of Life, 176
Tree Primrose, 658
Trefoil, 207, 493
Trilissia odorata, 255
Triticum repens, 370
Triticum vaccinum, 232
Trivrit, 823
Truelove, 610
Trumpet-weed, 374
Tuahgu, 655
Tuber Root, 647
Tuberous Moschatel, 550
Tun-hoof, 442
Turmeric, 866
Turmeric Root, 362
Turnsole, 387, 492
Turtle-bloom, 77
Turtle-head, 77
Turkey Pea, 822
Twice Writhen, 105
Twitch-grass, 370
Two Penigrasse, 549
Twopenny Grass, 549

Uabano, 381
Uaranzeiro, 381
Ulmi Cortex, 282
Umbrella Plant, 148
Underground Onion, 599
Upright Virgin's Bower, 205
Urginea Indica, U. Maritima, 766
Uva-Ursi, 89
Uvaria triloba, 608
Uvedalia, 91

Vaccinium Frondosum, 99
Valerian Locusta, 225
Vanilla Leaf, 255
Vapor, 329
Vegetable Gold, 361
Vegetable Mercury, 509
Vegetable Oyster, 708
Vegetable Sulphur, 551
Velvet Dock, 278, 562
Velvet Flower, 30
Velvet Leaf, 609
Velvet Plant, 562
Venice Turpentine, 636
Venus' Basin, 793
Veratrum Californicum, V. Lobelianium, 391
Veratrum Luteum, 823
Veratrum Officinale, 697
Verbena triphylla, 830
Verge d'Or, 361
Vernis de Japon, 820
Veronica Purpurea, Virginia, 111
Veronique petit chêne, 759
Verrucaria, 519
Vervaim Sage, 205
Verveine citronelle, 830
Vesper Flower, 681
Vine Maple, 610
Violet Bloom, 589
Viranga, 286
Virginia Serpentaria, 744
Virginian Dogwood, 122
Virginian Poke, 648
Virginian Preene, 191
Virginian Snakeroot, 744
Virginian Water Horehound, 141
Virgin's Gloves, 322
Vitis quinquefolia, 840
Vomitroot, 494
Vona-nox, 103
Vouacapoua inermis, 150

Wachsgagle, 87
Wad, 852
Wahoo, 762
Wake-Robin, 96, 236
Walewort, 276
Wall Fern, 307
Wall Ginger, 772
Wall-Ink, 123

Wall Pennyroyal, 455
Wall Pennywork, 455
Wallpepper, 772
Wallstock-gillofer, 842
Walnoot, 842
Wandering Jenny, 549
Wandering Jew, 817
Wandering Tailor, 549
Wapatoo, 57
Warnera, 362
Water-Aloe, 845
Water Betony, 314
Water Blobs, 519
Water Bugle, 141
Water Cup, 640
Water Dock, 259
Water Fennel, 264
Water Fern, 308
Water Flag, 439
Water Horehound, 357
Water Houseleek, 845
Water Lovage, 263
Water Milfoil, 834
Water Nymph, 484
Water Parsnip, 845
Water Pepper, 743
Water Pimpernel, 123
Water-Pumpy, 123
Water Sengren, 845
Water Trefoil, 117
Water Yarrow, 834
Wattle Bark, 3
Wax Dolls, 329
Wax Myrtle, 87
Way Bennet, 73
Waybread, Waybroad, 640
Waythorn, 134
Weat, 852
Weazle Snout, 582
Weisze Nieszwurzel, 391
Weiszer Germer, 391
Well-Ink, 123
Wendles, 644
Weusswurz, 749
Weyl Ash, 368
Weymouth Pine, 637
Whin, 366
Whinberry, 99
White Ash, 368
White Birch, 103
White Cup, 382
White Dittany, 147
White Filde Onyon, 769
White Leaf, 382
White Gentian, 500
White Maidenhair, 303
White Man's Foot, 640
White Mullein, 562
White Poplar, 650
White Pot Herb, 225
White Rot, 425

White Tea Tree, 151
Whitethorn, 385
White Walnut, 150
White Weed, 248
White Wood, 151, 202
Whitsun Bosses, 381
Whitsun Rose, 381
Whortleberry, 99
Wickup, 847
Wicopy, 847
Wild Agrimony, 740
Wild Apple, 43
Wild Arrach, 55
Wild Balsam, 449
Wild Celandine, 449
Wild Celery, 182
Wild Cinnamon, 202
Wild Cranesbill, 233
Wild Cucumber, 241
Wild Curcuma, 362
Wild Damson, 142
Wild English Clary, 707
Wild Geranium, 233
Wild Hops, 132
Wild Ice Leaf, 562
Wild Laburnum, 525
Wild Lady's Slipper, 449
Wild Lemon, 512
Wild Liquorice, 81, 492, 674, 712
Wild Masterwort, 368
Wild Nard, 63
Wild Nep, 132
Wild Pansy, 386
Wild Rye, 73
Wild Sarsaparilla, 81
Wild Snowball, 673
Wild Sweet William, 748
Wild Sunflower, 278
Wild Tansy, 740
Wild Turnip, 841
Wild Vanilla, 255
Wild Vine, 132
Wild Woodbine, 345
Wilde Yamwurzel, 863
Willow – European, Flowering, French, Per-
    sian, Rose Bay, 847
Willow, Red, Rose, 605
Willow-wort, 497
Wind Flower, 32, 34
Windroot, 647
Wingseed, 71
Wintera, W. aromatica, 850
Winterberry – Black Alder, Deciduous, Vir-
    ginian, 16
Winterbloom, 851

Winter Clover, 766
Winter Green, 639
Winter, Round-leaved, 662
Winter Pink, 53
Winter's Cinnamon, 850
Witches' Gloves, 322
Witches' Pouches, 738
Withywind, 219
Woad, 375
Wood Bells, 116
Wood Pimpernel, 497
Wood-rova, 853
Wood Sage, 351
Wood Sour, 752
Wood Vine, 840
Wood Waxen, 129, 375
Wolfsbohne, 502
Wolf's Claw, 551
Wolt Schjeluke, 531
Wool Flower, 461
Woollen, 562
Worm Bark, 150
Wormgrass, Wormgrass (American), 637
Wormroot – American, Carolina, Maryland,
    637
Wormseed, 189, 571
Woundwort, 361
Woundwort, Downy, 862
Woundwort, Soldier's, 863
Wuderove, 853

Yalluc, 215
Yarroway, 863
Yellow Archangel, 582
Yellow Bedstraw, 91
Yellow Cabbage Tree, 150
Yellow Cinchona, 153
Yellow Flag, 437
Yellow Iris, 437
Yellow Laburnum, 460
Yellow Leaf Cup, 91
Yellow Puccoon, 362
Yellow Rod, 815
Yellow Root, 362
Yellow Snowdrop, 11
Yellow Water Dropwort, 263
Yellow Willow Herb, 497
Yellow Wood, 70
Yerba dulce, 486
Yerba Soldado, 522
Yerw, 863
Yuca, 510

Zitterwurzel, 866
Zizyphus sativa, 451

A SERVICE INDEX TO FACILITATE USE OF THIS HERBAL

Courtesy of the New York Botanical Garden

All entries without asterisks (*) are to be found in Index Kewensis and Index Filicum, excepting varietal names.

A

*Abaria kaffra 47
Abelmoschus esculentus 566
  moschatus 566
Abies alba 635
  balsamea 79, 635
  canadensis 635, 638
  larix 635, 636
  pectinata 635
  vulgaris 635
Abrus precatorius 492
Acacia abyssinica 5
  arabica 3, 4, 5, 173
  berteriana 496
  catechu 173
  concinna 3
  decurrens 3
  glaucophylla 5
  gummifera 5
  melanoxylon 3
  nilotica 4
  niopo 3
  senegal 3, 4, 5
  verek 3
Acer campestre 514
  platanoides 515
  pseudo-platanus 515
  rubrum 516
  saccharinum 514
Achillea ageratum 226, 227
  ligustica 500
  millefolium 271, 863, 864
  ptarmica 864
  tomentosa 865
Aconitum autumnale 7
  chasmanthum 10
  chinense 10
  cynoctonum 108

Aconitum ferox 9, 10
  fischeri 10
  hemsleyanum 10
  heterophyllum 10
  japonicum 7
  laciniatum 10
  lycoctonum 7
  napellus 6, 7, 8, 9, 10
  orientale 10
  palmatum 10
  paniculatum 7
  *pardalianches 610
  pyrenaicum 7
  spicatum 10
  uncinatum v. japonicum 10
  variegatum 7
  volubile 10
  *wilsoni 10
Acorus calamus 106, 438, 448, 726
Actaea alba 81
  spicata 81
Actinella grandiflora 783
Adhatoda vasica 506
Adiantum aethiopicum 304
  capillus veneris 303
  fragile 304
  lunulatum 304
  *nigrum 303
  pedatum 303, 304
  radiatum 304
  trapexiforme 304
Adonis amurensis 389
  autumnalis 389
  vernalis 389, 390
Adoxa moschatellina 331, 550
Aegle marmelos 76
Aegopodium podagraria 368
*Aeranthis hyemalis 11

Aesculus flava 193
  hippocastanum 192
  parviflora 193
  pavia 193
  rubicunda 193
Aethusa cynapium 394, 614
Agaricus melleus 447
Agathis dammara 635
Agathophyllum aromaticum 592
Agave Americana 26
Agraphis nutans 116, 424
Agrimonia agrimonoides 14
  eupatoria 12
  odorata 13
Agropyrum acutum 371
  junceum 371
  pungens 371
  repens 370, 371
Agrostemna githago 223
Ailanthus glandulosa 821
  imberbiflora 821
Ajuga chamaepytis 139, 141
  pyramidalis 139
  reptans 139
Alchemilla alpina 462, 463
  arvensis 462, 615
  conjuncta 463
  vulgaris 145, 462
Aletris farinosa 824
Aleurites cordata 763
  laccifera 763
  moluccana 763
Alhagi maurorum 68
Alisma plantago 645
*Alkanna officinalis 19
  *sempervirens 19
  tinctoria 18
Alkekengi officinarum 191
Allium cepa 599
  cepa v. aggregatum 599
  cepa v. proliferum 600
  fragrans 344
  macleanii 604
  odorum 344
  oleraceum 343
  sativum 342
  schoenoprasum 200
  ursinum 343
  vineale 343
Alnus glutinosa 17
  rubra 18
  serrulata 18
Aloe abyssinica 27
  africana 27
  chinensis 27
  ferox 27, 28

Aloe perryi 26, 27
  platylepis 27
  spicata 27
  vera 26, 27
  vulgaris 27
Aloysia citriodora 830
Alpinia calcarata 340
  cardamomum 159
  galanga 340
  officinarum 339, 340
*Alsidium helminthocorton 551
Alsine media 195
Alstonia constricta 30, 257, 258
  scholaris 29, 257
  spectabilis 29, 258
Althaea officinalis 507
  rosea 409
Altingea excelsa 776
Amanita caesarea 334
  muscaria 334
  pantherina 334
  phalloides 333, 334
  rubescens 333
Amaranthus blitum 30, 115
  campestris 30
  caudatus 30
  hypochondriacus 30
  oleraceus 30
  polygonoides 30
  spinosus 30
Ammi majus 369
Amomum angustifolium 160
  cardamomum 159, 160
  curcuma 822
  globosum 160
  *kararina 160
  maximum 160
  racemosum 160
  repens 159
  subulatum 160
  xanthioides 160
Amorphophallus campanulatus 238
*Ampelopsis grana habzeli 628
  *grana paradisi 628
  *hoggii 443
  *melegueta 629
  quinquefolia 840
Amygdalus communis v. amara 21, 22
  communis v. dulcis 21, 22
  nana 23
  persica 619
*Amyris bdellium 573
  gileadensis 78
  opobalsamum 78
Anacardium occidentale 47, 167, 168

Anacyclus officinarum 622
  pyrethrum 621, 622
Anagallis arvensis 632, 633
  caerulea 633
  tenella 634
Anagyris foetida 461
Anamirta paniculata 209, 465, 610
Anchusa officinalis 120
Andira araroba 51
  inermis 52, 150
  retusa 150
Andrographis paniculata 200
Andropogon arundinaceus v. saccharatus 516
  schoenanthus 374, 831
Anemone apennina 32
  blanda 32
  coronaria 32
  groenlandica 361
  hepatica 32, 493
  hortensis 32
  nemorosa 32, 33, 34, 35
  nemorosa v. apetala 35
  nemorosa v. robusta 35
  nuttalliana 33
  pratensis 32, 33
  pulsatilla 32
  ranunculoides 32
Anethum foeniculum 293
  graveolens 255
Angelica archangelica 35, 40
  atropurpurea 40
  heterocarpa 36, 499
  sylvestris 36, 40
Anhalonium jourdanianum 531
  lewinii 531
  williamsii 531
Anona glabra 47
  palustris 47
  squamosa 47
  tripetala 47
Antennaria dioica 175, 359
  margaritacea 81, 477
  plantaginifolia 359, 645
Anthemis arvensis 185, 188, 523
  cotula 185, 188, 523, 743
  nobilis 185, 187, 188, 524
  pyrethrum 621
  tinctoria 523
Anthoxanthum odoratum 373
  puelii 373
*Anthriscus cynapium 612
  sylvestris 394
Antiaris toxicaria 562
Antirrhinum majus 746
  orontium 746
Apium graveolens 182, 611

*Apium heleioselinon 611
  *hortense 611
  petroselinum 611
Aplopappus discoideus 249
  laricifolius 249
Aplotaxis auriculata 279
Apocynum androsaemifolium 108, 395
  cannabinum 108, 395
  hypericifolium 108
  venetum 108
Aquilaria agallocha 29
Aquilegia parviflora 214
  vulgaris 214
Aralia californica 760
  hispida 277, 278
  nudicaulis 81, 492, 712, 714, 760
  quinquefolia 354
  racemosa 760
  spinosa 40, 71, 277, 278
Arbuta rufescens 610
Arbutus unedo 52
  uva-ursi 89, 90
Archangelica officinalis 35
Arctium lappa 142
Arctostaphylos alpina 89
  glauca 90
  polifolia 90
  tomentosa 90
  uva-ursi 89, 122
Areca catechu 54
  dicksonii 54
  oleracea 54
Arenaria rubra 711
Arisaema triphyllum 841
Aristolochia anguicida 746
  argentina 104, 745, 746
  bracteata 745
  brasiliensis 746
  clematitis 744, 745, 746
  cymbifera 104, 746
  foetida 104, 746
  indica 104, 745
  longa 104, 745, 746
  macroura 746
  maxima 746
  officinalis 737
  pistolochia 746
  reticulata 744, 745
  rotunda 744, 745, 746
  sagittata 744
  sempervirens 104, 746
  serpentaria 63, 104, 211, 356, 744, 745, 746, 826
  sipho 745
  trilobata 746
Armeniaca vulgaris 51

Arnica montana 55
Arnoseris pusilla 199
Artanthe elongata 522
  hexagyna 96
Artemisia abrotanum 754, 858
  absinthium 858, 861
  alpina 858
  campestris 755
  cana 858
  chamaemelifolia 857
  chinensis 557
  cina 857
  dracunculus 756, 791, 858
  lercheana 857
  maritima 860, 861
  maritima v. pauciflora 857
  maritima v. stechmanniana 857
  moxa 557
  pontica 860, 861
  sericea 858
  vulgaris 556
Arum dioscoridis 238
  dracunculus 238, 239, 791
  esculentum 238
  indicum 238
  italicum 238
  lyratum 238
  maculatum 58, 236, 238
  montanum 238
  triphyllum 238, 841
Asagraea officinalis 697
Asarum arifolium 354
  canadense 354
  europaeum 63, 354
Asclepias acida 64
  cornuti 64
  curassavica 64, 65, 434
  incarnata 64, 787
  pulchra 64
  syriaca 64
  tuberosa 64, 647
  verticillata 65
  vincetoxicum 65, 734
Asimina triloba 608
Asparagus officinalis 71
Asperula cynanchica 667
  odorata 853
Asphodelus fistulosus 72
  luteus 72
  ramosus 72
Aspidium filix mas 300
  marginale 301
  oreopteris 301
  spinulosum 301, 302
Aspidosperma quebracho-blanco 663
Asplenium ceterach 302

Asplenium finix femina 301, 302
  nigrum 303
  ruta muraria 303
  scolopendrium 304
  trichomanes 303
Asteracantha longifolia 425
Astragalus gummifer 820
*Athalia annulata 123
Atherosperma moschatum 592, 716
Athyrium filix femina 302
Atriplex hastata 56
  hortensis 56, 661
  *olida 56
  patula 56
  pedunculata 661
  portulacoides 661
  rosea 661
Atropa belladonna 583, 584, 589, 723
  mandragora 510, 585
Aucuba japonica 640
*Auricula muris 384
Avena sativa 597
Avouacouapa retusa 150

B

Ballota nigra 416
*Balsamita foeminea 226
  *mas 226
Balsamodendron africanum 572
  gileadense 78
  myrrha 571
  opobalsamum 78
*Balsamus americanus 80
  *gileadense 78
  *meccae v. judaicum 78
  *tolutanum 80
Banksia abyssinica 459
Baphia nitida 717
Baptisia tinctoria 432
Barosma betulina 133, 134
  crenulata 133
  serratifolia 133
Bartsia latifolia 85
  odontites 85
  viscosa 85
*Batos idaia 671
*Bdellium kataf 572
  *mukul 573
  *playfairii 572
  *roxburghii 573
*Belladonna scopola 722
Bellis perennis 247
Berberis aquifolium 84, 369
  aristata 84
  asiatica 84

Berberis lycium 84
  nervosa 369
  repens 369
  vulgaris 82
Beta maritima 93
  vulgaris 93
  vulgaris v. cicla 93
Betonica officinalis 97
Betula alba 103
  alnus 17
  lenta 104, 849
  nana 104
  papyracea 104
  pubescens 103
  triphylla 104
  verrucosa 103
Bicuculla canadensis 822
Bidens bipinnata 16
  cernua 16
  tripartita 14, 15, 16
Bigelowia veneta 249
Bignonia caroba 160
*Bilocarpus microphyllus 737
Biota orientalis 177
*Birda rubra 711
Bixa orellana 43, 50
*Blitum americanum 648
*Blumea balcamferi 155
Bocconia arborea 650, 651
  cordata 650, 651
  frutescens 651
  integrifolia 651
Boehmeria nivea 576
Boerhaavia decumbens 434
*Bolax clebaria 601
  gilliesii 601
Boldoa fragrans 118
*Boletus cervinus 338
  *chirurgorum 335
  *edulis 334
  *laricis 335
  *purgans 335
  *sanatus 335
Bonnaya rotundifolia 427
Borago officinalis 119
Borreria ferruginea 433
  poaya 433
Bosea yervamora 362
Boswellia thurifera 326
Botrychium lunaria 309
*Botrytis cinerea 478, 479
Bragantia tomentosa 745
  wallichii 745
Brassica alba 566
  napus 570
  nigra 568

*Brassica sinapioides 568
  sinapistrum 570
Brauneria pallida 265
Brayera anthelmintica 459
Bromelia ananas 47
Brosimum alicastrum 562
  galactodendron 562
Broussonetia kaempferi 562
  kazinoki 562
  papyrifera 562
Brunfelsia hopeana 509
Bryonia alba 131
  dioica 131, 132, 513
*Buceras oliverii 173
Bulnesia sarmienti 686
Buphane disticha 246
Butea frondosa 455
Buxus sempervirens 90, 121
  suffruticosa 122

C

Cactus bonplandii 184
  divaricatus 184
  flagelliformis 184
  *giganteus 184
  grandiflorus 184
  *pilocereus 184
Cakile maritima 681
Caladium esculentum 238
Calamintha acinos 807
  clinopodium 87
  menthaefolia 807
  nepeta 153
  officinalis 152, 153, 807
  vulgaris 87
Calamus aromaticus 11, 726
  draco 262, 729
  rotang 263
Calendula officinalis 55, 517, 783
Callicarpa americana 560
Callitris robusta 177
Calotropis gigantea 154
  procera 47, 64, 154
Caltha palustris 519
*Calus jovis 203, 705
Calycanthus floridus 21
Calystegia sepium 101
  soldanella 102
Camellia thea 792
  theifera 792
Campanula persicifolia 670
  rapunculoides 670
  rapunculus 670
Canella alba 502

Canna achiras 58
  edulis 58
Cannabis chinensis 396
  indica 108, 395, 396
Capparis spinosa 426
Capsella bursa-pastoris 738
Capsicum frutescens 175
  minimum 175
Carbenia benedicta 795
Cardamomum minus 159
  *siberiense 160
Carduus acaulis 798
  arvensis 799
  benedictus 795, 796, 797
  crispus 799
  *eriophyllus 799
  heterophyllus 799
  lanceolatus 800
  marianus 797
  nutans 800
  palustris 800
Carex arenaria 371, 730
  vulpina 731
  vulpinoidea 731
Carica papaya 529, 607
*Carlina pratensis 801
  *pycnocephalous 801
  *tuberosus 801
  vulgaris 800, 801
Carthamus helenioides 805
  tinctorius 698
Carum carvi 157
  copticum 811, 812
  petroselinum 611
*Cassavium pomiferum 167
Cassia acutifolia 734, 735, 736
  aethiopica 734
  angustifolia 734, 736
  *aromaticum 168
  cathartica 737
  chamaecrista 737
  elongata 736
  fistula 737
  holosericea 737
  laevigata 737
  lanceolata 734, 737
  lenitiva 734
  *lignea 168
  marylandica 737
  montana 737
  multijuja 737
  nictitans 532
  obovata 736, 737
  *officinalis 734
  rugosa 737
  senna 734

Cassia splendida 737
  *vera 169
Cassine peragua 609
Castanea vesca 193
Catabrosa aquatica 374
*Catechu nigrum 173
Caulophyllum thalictroides 212, 357
Ceanothus americanus 673
  azureus 673
  chloroxylon 496
Cedrela odorata 177
  toona 177
Cedronella mexicana 486, 831
  triphylla 79
Cedrus atlantica 177
  deodara 177
  libani 177
  *lycea 176
*Centaurea colcitrapa 801, 802
  cyanus 223
  jacea 457
  nigra 456
  scabiosa 456
  solstitialis 802
Centranthus ruber 830
Centunculus minimus 229
Cephaelis ipecachuanha 432
Cephalanthus occidentalis 492
Ceradia furcata 573
Ceratonia siliqua 160, 450, 451
Cercis siliquastrum 266
Cereus caespitosus 184
  grandiflorus 184
*Cetraria islandica 552
Chamaelirium luteum 823
Chamaenerion angustifolium 848
Chamaepeuce diacantha 795
Cheiranthus cheiri 842
Chelidonium majus 178, 180
Chelone glabra 77
Chenopodium album 366
  ambrosioides 854
  ambrosioides v. anthelminticum 854, 855
  anthelminticum 854
  bonus-henricus 189, 365
  botrys 857
  glaucum 856
  hybridum 366
  olidum 55
  quinoa 189
  rubrum 366
  vulvaria 55
Chimaphila maculata 639, 850
  umbellata 639, 850
Chionanthus virginica 328
Chlorophora tinctoria 561

894

Chondrodendron tomentosum 609
*Chondrus crispus 114, 552
*Chrusa borealis 361
Chrysanthemum carneum 622
  cinerariaefolium 622
  leucanthemum 248
  maritium 310
  parthenium 156, 309
  *peruvianum 782
  roseum 622
  suaveolens 310
Chrysophyllum cainito 47
Cichorium intybus 197
Cicuta maculata 394
  virosa 392, 394
Cimicifuga racemosa 211
Cinchona calisaya
  officinalis 631
  succirubra 631
Cineraria canadensis 315
  maritima 379
Cinnamodendron axillare 203, 850
  corticosum 850
Cinnamomum burmanni 169
  camphora 155
  cassia 168, 202
  culilawan 169, 202
  iners 169, 202
  *inserta 169
  ligneum 169
  loureirii 169
  nitidum 169, 202
  obtusifolium 169
  pauciflorum 169
  rubrum 169
  sintok 169
  tamala 169
  zeylanicum 168, 169, 202
Circaea lutetiana 847
Cissampelos convolvulacea 609
  glaberrima 609
  pareira 609, 610
Cissus hederacea 840
  quinquefolia 840
Cistus canadensis 328
  *chamaerhodendros 466
  creticus 329
  ladaniferus 329
  laurifolius 329
  ledon 329
Citrullus colocynthis 49, 241, 527
  vulgaris 527, 528
*Citrus acris 485
  aurantium 601
  aurantium v. dulcis 601
  bigaradia 601

Citrus javanica 476
  limetta 47, 476, 485
  limonum 474
  lumia 476
  margarita 476
  medica 474, 476
  medica acida 476, 485
  medica cedra 476
  vulgaris 601
  vulgaris v. bigaradia 601
*Cladonia pyxidata 551
  *rangiferina 552
  *sanguinea 552
*Claviceps purpurea 338, 339
Claytonia tuberosa 660
Clematis crispa 206
  flammula 206
  recta 205, 206
  viorna 206
  virginiana 206
  vitalba 206
Clusia flava 47
Cluytia eluteria 166
Cnicus benedictus 795
Coccoloba uvifera 456
Cocculus indicus 465, 610
Cochlearia anglica 418
  armoracia 417, 418
  danica 418
  macrocarpa 417
  officinalis 418, 725
Cochlospermum gossypium 821
Codonopsis tangshen 356
Coffea arabica 206, 210
Cola acuminata 458, 459
  ballayi 459
  vera 459
Colchicum autumnale 700
Collinsonia canadensis 774
Colocasia antiquorum 238
  *caladium 238
  macrorrhiza 238
Colutea arborescens 737
Combretum sundaicum 215, 653
Commiphora erythraea v. glabrescens 572
  myrrha 571
  myrrha v. molmol. 571
  opobalsamum 78
  roxburghii 573
*Condurango blanco 219
  *cortex 219
Conium maculatum 391, 392
Convallaria majalis 480, 764
Convolvulus arvensis 103, 219
  batata 101
  dissectus 101

*Convolvulus duartinus 103
  jalapa 101
  minor 100
  panduratus 656
  purpureus 100
  *rhodorhiza 101
  scammonia 100, 102
  sepium 101
  soldanella 102
Conyza squarrosa 760
*Copaiba officinalis 221
Copaifera lansdorfii 221
Coptis anemonaefolia 361
  teeta 361
  trifolia 361
  trifolia v. chinensis 361
Corallorhiza innata 233
  multiflora 233
  odontorhiza 233
  verna 233
  wisteriana 233
Coriandrum sativum 221
Coriaria myrtifolia 737
Cornus amomum 123
  circinata 123, 605
  coerulea 123
  florida 122
  mascula 123
  sanguinea 123
  sericea 123, 605
  stolonifera 123
  suecica 123
Coronilla emerus 737
  scorpioides 130
Corrigiola littoralis 622
Cortusa matthioli 712
Corydalis ambigua 822
  bulbosa 822
  canadensis 822
  cava 822
  cucullaria 822
  formosa 822
  tuberosa 822
  vernyi 822
Coscinium fenestratum 215
*Cotula maruta foetida 523
Cotyledon umbilicus 455
Crassula montana 773
Crataegus aronia 386
  azarolus 386
  odoratissima 386
  oxyacantha 385, 386
Crinum asiaticum v. toxicarium 769
Crithmum maritimum 709, 710
Crocus sativus 698, 699
  sativus v. cartwrightianus 699

Crocus sativus v. elwesii 699
  sativus v. haus knechtii 699
  sativus v. orsinii 699
  sativus v. pallasii 699
Crotalaria juncea 395
  tenuifolia 395
*Croton annum 628
  cascarilla 167
  draco 263, 729
  eluteria 166, 167
  hibiscifolius 263
  micans 167
  niveus 167
  pseudo china 167
  sanguifluus 263
  suberosus 167
  tiglium 234, 763
*Cryptocarpus spiralis 433
Cucumis anguria 240
  cantalupensis 528
  chate 528
  colocynthis 133
  dudaim 528
  flexuosus 240, 528
  hardwickii 240
  melo 239, 527
  myriocarpus 240
  prophetarum 240
  sativus 239
  sativus v. sitkinensis 240
  trigonus 240
Cucurbita maxima 527, 529
  melopepo 529
  ovifera 529
  pepo 239, 529
Cuminum cyminum 242
Cunila mariana 812, 813
  origanoides 546
Cupressus thuioides 177
Curanga amara 427
Curcuma angustifolia 58, 791
  leucorhiza 791
  longa 822
  rotunda 822
  zedoaria 866
Cuscuta epilinum 261
  epithymum 261, 470, 810
  europaea 260, 261
  hassiaca 261
  trifolii 261
Cusparia febrifuga 41
Cyclamen europaeum 245
  hederaefolium 245
  *peraicum 245
Cydonia japonica 666
  maulei 667

896

Cymbalaria hederacea 817
Cymbopogan citratus 374
  martini 374
  nardus 374
Cynanchum argel 737
  oleaefolium 736
Cynara scolymus 60
Cynodon dactylon 371
Cynoglossum officinale 421
Cynosurus cristatus 374
Cyperus articulatus 11, 729
  bulbosus 730
  elegans 729
  esculentus 730
  hexastachyos 730
  longus 730
  odoratus 730
  papyrus 730
  pertenuis 729
  rotundus 730
  sanguineofuscus 729
  scariosus 730
  tegetum 729
Cypripedium hirsutum 829
  parviflorum 357, 829
  pubescens 734, 829
Cytisus laburnum 460, 461
  *purpurascens 461
  scoparius 124, 368

D

*Daemonorops cinnabari 263
  didymophylla 263
  draco 262, 729
  draconcellus 263
  micracanthus 263
  propinquus 263
Dahlia variabilis 246, 280
Daphne alpina 532
  gnidium 531, 532
  laureola 531, 532
  mezereum 531
  paniculata 532
  pontica 532
  tartonraira 532
  thymelaea 532
Datura alba 807
  arborea 807
  fastuosa 807
  fastuosa v. alba 807
  ferox 806, 807
  metel 803, 807
  quercifolia 807
  sanguinea 806
  stramonium 47, 589, 802, 803, 804, 806

Datura tatula 804, 807
Daucus carota 161, 165
  maritimus 162, 165
  *pastinaca 161
Delphinium consolida 464
  staphisagria 770
*Dendrographa leucophoea 493
Dicentra canadensis 822
  cucullaria 822
  pusilla 822
  spectabilis 331
Dictamnus albus 147
Diervilla diervilla 410
Digitalis purpurea 322, 324, 325
Dioon edule 58
Dioscorea hirsuta 863
  villosa 863
Diosma betulina 133
Dipsacus fullonum 793, 794
  pilosus 793
  sylvestris 793
Dipteryx odorata 819
Dirca palustris 532
Dolichos pruriens 228
  urens 229
Dorema ammoniacum 31, 781
Dorstenia brasiliensis 219
  contrajerva 219
  drakena 219
  houstoni 219
Dracaena draco 263, 729
  terminalis 263
Dracocephalum canariense 79
Dracontium foetidum 742
Drimia ciliaris 769
Drimys aromatica 850
  chilensis 850
  winteri 850
Drosera rotundifolia 782
Dryas octopetala 74
Dryobalanops aromatica 155
  camphora 155
Dryopteris abbreviata 300
  affinis 300
  borreri 300
  elongata 300
  filix mas 300, 301, 302
  *pumilum 300
Duboisia hopwoodii 223
  myoporoides 223

E

Ecballium elaterium 240, 241, 527
Echinacea angustifolia 265
  purpurea 265

Echinocactus lewisii 531
   williamsii 531
Echinocystis lobata 47
Echites scholaris 29
Echium vulgare 120, 142
Elettaria cardamomum 159, 160
   cardamomum v. major 160
*Elophomyces granulatus 337
Embelia basaal 286
   ribes 286
   robusta 286
*Emplastrum oxycroceum 698
Endodeca bartonii 744
   serpentaria 744
Ephedra vulgaris 286
Epifagus virginianus 93
Epigaea repens 53
Epilobium angustifolium 847
   hirsutum 848
   parviflorum 848
*Equisetum arvense 419, 420
   *debile 420
   elongatum 420
   fluviatile 420
   giganteum 420
   hyemale 419, 420
   maximum 419, 420, 421
   sylvaticum 419, 421
Erechtites hieracifolia 315, 540
Erica arborea 691
Erigeron acris 321
   canadensis 320, 540
Eriodictyon californicum 865
   glutinosum 865
   tomentosum 865
Eriophorum angustifolium 731
*Eruca marina 681
   sativa 681
Eryngium alpinum 409
   amethystinum 409
   aquaticum 409
   campestre 407, 408, 409
   maritimum 407
Erysimum cheiranthoides 571
   officinale 570
   orientale 571
*Erythraea acaulis 184
   centaurium 182
   chilensis 184
   latifolia 182
   littoralis 182
   pulchella 182
Erythrolaena conspicua 795
Erythronium americanum 11
Erythrophleum guineense 716
Erythroxylum coca 208, 209

Eucalyptus amygdalina 287, 288
   australiana 288
   bakeri 288
   citriodora 288
   dives 288
   globulus 287, 288, 289
   gunnii v. rubida 289
   macarthurii 288
   mannifera 289
   *nostrata 289
   odorata 288
   piperata 288
   *polybractea 288
   pulverulenta 289
   radiata 289
   resinifera 289
   smithii 288
   staigeriana 288
   stuartiana 288
   viminalis 289
*Euchema spinolum 12
Eugenia aromatica 208
   caryophyllata 208
   chekan 189
   jambolana 446
   jambos 47
   malaccensis 47
   pimenta 19
Euonymus atropurpureus 762
   europaeus 762
Eupatorium ageratoides 290
   *aquaticum mas 14
   aromaticum 212, 290
   ayapana 290
   cannabinum 14, 15
   collinum 290
   foeniculaceum 290
   glutinosum 290, 523
   hyssopifolium 290
   incarnatum 290
   leucolepis 290
   maculatum 374, 375
   nervosum 290
   perfoliatum 118, 290
   purpureum 119, 374
   rebaudianum 290
   rotundifolium 290
   ternifolium 374
   teucrifolium 290
   trifoliatum 374
   urticaefolium 290
   verbenaefolium 290
   verticillatum 374
   villosum 290
Euphorbia aleppica 765
   amygdaloides 765

Euphorbia antiquorum 764
   apios 765
   balsamifera 765
   buxifolia 766
   canariensis 764
   canescens 765
   cerifera 764
   corollata 764
   cotinifolia 765
   *cremocarpus 765
   cyparissias 765
   dendroides 765
   drummondii 765
   esula 765, 766, 816
   gerardiana 765
   helioscopia 765
   heterodoxa 765
   hiberna 765
   hirta 765
   humistrata 765
   hypericifolia 764, 765
   *iata 765
   ipecacuanha 434, 764
   lathyris 765
   laurifolia 766
   ligularia 766
   linearis 765
   maculata 765
   marginata 765
   mauritanica 765
   officinarum 764
   palustris 765
   papillosa 766
   parviflora 765
   peploides 765
   peplus 765
   pilosa 765
   pilulifera 764
   platyphyllos 765
   portulacoides 765, 766
   prostrata 765
   resinifera 764
   spinosa 765
   tetragona 764
   thymifolia 765
   tirucalli 766
   tribuloides 766
Euphrasia officinalis 290, 706
Eustachya alba 111
   purpurea 111

          F

Faba ignati 431
Fabiana imbricata 632
Fagara clava-herculis 70

Fagopyrum esculentum 138
Fagus castanea 193
   sylvatica 92
   sylvatica v. purpurea 93
*Fateorhiza palmata 610
Feronia elephantum 47, 76
Ferula communis 31
   foetida 62
   galbaniflua 340
   hermonis 341
   *sagapenum 63
   *serapinum 63
   suaveolens 781
   sumbul 781
Fibigia umbellata 373
Ficaria verna 180
Ficus carica 311
   sycomorus 313, 515
*Flammula jovis 205
Flemingia congesta 454
Foeniculum capillaceum 294
   dulce 294, 295, 297
   officinale 294
   piperitum 296
   vulgare 293, 294, 297
*Fomes fomentarius 336
Fontenellea braziliensis 748
Fragaria vesca 776
Franciscea uniflora 509, 510
Frankenia grandifolia 865
*Frasera canadensis 214
   carolinensis 214
   walteri 214
Fraxinus acuminata 67
   americana 67
   excelsior 65, 68
   lanceolata 67
   nigra 66
   ornus 67, 68
Fremontia californica 285
Fritillaria imperialis 480
   meleagris 328
*Fucus amylaceus 114
   *canaliculatus 114
   *crispus 114
   *helminthocorton 114, 551
   *natans 114
   *nodosus 112, 114
   *serratus 112, 114
   *siliquosus 114
   *vesiculeux 111
   *vesiculosis 111, 112, 114
Fumaria capnoides 331
   capreolata 331
   claviculata 331
   cucullaria 331

Fumaria densiflora 331
  enneaphylla 331
  fungosa 331
  indica 331
  lutea 331
  nobilis 331
  officinalis 329
  parviflora 331
  sempervirens 331
  sibirica 331
  spectabilis 331
  spicata 331
  vesicaria 331
Funtumia africana 778

G

Gagea lutea 231, 770
Galanthus nivalis 747
Gale palustris 341
Galega officinalis 696
  virginiana 697
Galeopsis tetrahit 581
Galipea officinalis 41
Galium aparine 91, 206
  cruciatum 234, 505
  elatum 91
  mollugo 92
  palustre 92
  saxatile 92
  tinctorium 92
  tricorne 92
  uliginosum 92
  verum 91, 92, 234
*Gallitricum alterum 203, 705
*Garania mangostana 76
Garcinia hanburyi 341
  kola 459
  morella 342
Gardenia campanulata 449
  florida 449
  grandiflora 449
Garrya fremontii 309
Gaultheria hispidula 849
  procumbens 849
  shallon 850
*Gelidium armansii 12
Gelsemium elegans 346
  nitidum 345, 449
  sempervirens 345
*Genista griot 376
  hispanica 376
  purgans 376
  scoparia 124, 376
  spinosa 366

Genista tinctoria 129, 375
Gentiana acaulis 348, 350
  amarella 349, 350
  andrewsii 348
  campestris 349, 350, 728
  centaurium 182
  cruciata 351
  lutea 108, 215, 347, 348
  nivalis 350
  pannonica 348
  pneumonanthe 350
  puberula 348
  punctata 348
  purpurea 348
  quinqueflora 351
  saponaria 348
  scabra 349
  verna 350
Geranium dissectum 233
  maculatum 233, 820
Geum coccineum 75
  elatum 75
  montanum 75
  reptans 75
  rivale 75
  sylvaticum 75
  urbanum 73, 75, 827
*Gigartina helminthocorton 114
  *mamillosa 114
  *spiciosa 12
Gillenia stipulacea 434
  stipulata 431
  trifoliata 431
Glaux maritima 229
Glechoma hederacea 174, 442, 630
Gleditschia ferox 358
  macracantha 358
  triacanthos 358
Globularia turbith 737
Glyceria aquatica 374
Glycyrrhiza echinata 487, 488, 491
  glabra 487, 488, 490, 491
  glandulifera 487, 488, 491
  lepidota 488
  uralensis 488
Gnaphalium arenarium 359
  citrinum 359
  cymosum 359
  dioicum 175
  margaritaceum 81
  plantaginifolia 359
  polycephalum 80, 359
  uliginosum 242
Gonolobus cundurango 219
Goodyera repens 645

Gossypium barbadense 228
  herbaceum 228
*Gracilaria lichenoides 12
*Graphium ulmus 282
Gratiola amara 427
  officinalis 427
  peruviane 427
Grindelia camporum 376, 377
  camporum v. paludosa 377
  cuneifolia 376, 377
  robusta 376, 865
  robusta v. latifolia 377
  squarrosa 376, 377
Guaiacum officinale 380
  sanctum 380
Guarea rusbyi 210
  trichilioides 210
Gynocardia odorata 189
Gypsophila struthium 748
Gyrotheca capitata 461
  tinctoria 461

H

Haematoxylon campechianum 496
  *lignum 496
Hagenia abyssinica 459
Hamamelis virginiana 851
Haplopappus baylahuen 427
Hedera chrysocarpa 441
  helix 440
  quinquefolia 840
Helianthemum canadense 328
  corymbosum 328, 329
  *michauxii 328
  ramuliflorum 328
  rosmarinifolium 328
  vulgare 783
Helianthus annuus 782, 783
  tuberosus 58, 783
Helichrysum stoechas 359
Heliconia bihai 646
Heliotropium peruvianum 387
Helleborus foetidus 388, 389, 390
  niger 388
  officinalis 388
  orientalis 391
  pumilus 361
  trifolius 361
  trilobus 361
  viridis 388
Helminthia echioides 360, 605
Helonias dioica 823
  lutea 823
  officinalis 697

Hemiesmus indicus 714
Hemprichia erythraea 572
Hepatica triloba 493
  triloba v. americana 493
  triloba v. obtusa 493
Herniaria glabra 697
  hirsuta 697
Herpestis amara 427
*Hertiera litorales 459
Hesperis matronalis 681
*Heterameris canadensis 328
Heudelotia africana 573
Hibiscus abelmoschus 566
  esculentus 566
Hieracium aurantiacum 383
  canadense 315
  murorum 383, 384
  pilosella 384
  sylvaticum 383
Hippocastanum vulgare 192
Hippomane mancinella 513
Hippophae rhamnoides 137
Hippuris vulgaris 516
*Hirneola auricula judae 269, 336
  *polytricha 336
Holcus lanatus 373
  mollis 373
Hordeum distichon 84
*Horminum commune 203, 705
  *hortense 203, 705
  *humile germanicum 203, 705
  pyrenaicum 705
  *sativum verum dioscorides 203, 705
  sylvestre 203, 705
Hottonia palustris 839
*Houckenya peploides 661
Humulus lupulus 411
Hyacinthus non-scriptus 116, 424
  orientalis 424
Hydrangea arborescens 424
  hortensis 424, 425
  quercifolia 424
  vulgaris 424
Hydrastis canadensis 362
Hydrocotyle asiatica 425
  vulgaris 425
Hygrophila spinosa 371, 425
Hyoscyamus albus 403
  muticus 404
  niger 397, 399, 401, 403, 404
Hypericum perforatum 707
Hyssopus officinalis 426
*Hysterionica baylahuen 427

I

Iberis amara 156
Ictodes foetidus 742
Ignatia amara 431
Ilex aquifolium 405
  dahoon 609
  gongonha 407
  macoucoua 407
  paraguayensis 407, 609
  theezans 407
  verticillata 16
  vomitoria 609
Illicium anisatum 42
  verum 43, 160
Impatiens aurea 449, 450
  balsamina 450
  biflora 449, 450
  cornuta 450
  noli-me-tangere 450
  pallida 449
  roylei 450
  sultani 450
Imperatoria ostruthium 522
Indigofera tinctoria 432
Inula britannica 55, 761
  campana 279
  conyza 324, 760
  crithmoides 710
  dysenterica 321
  helenium 278, 324
Iodina rhombifolia 663
Ionidium ipecacuanha 433
Ipomoea fastigiata 656
  jalapa 101
  purga 101
  purpurea 100
  turpethum 823
*Iris aquatica 437
  florentina 435, 436
  foetidissima 357, 435
  germanica 435, 436
  *lenax 439
  lutea 437
  *minor 439
  missouriensis 439
  pallida 435, 436
  pseudacorus 435, 437, 438, 729
  tuberosa 435
  versicolor 435, 436, 439
  xiphium 434
Isatis indigotica 853
  tinctoria 376, 852

J

Jacaranda caroba 160
  procera 160
Janipha manihot 791
Jasione montana 722
Jasminum angustifolium 448
  floribundum 449
  frutescens 449
  fruticans 345, 449
  grandiflorum 447, 448
  humile 449
  nervosum 449
  nudiflorum 449
  odoratissimum 345, 449
  officinale 447
  paniculatum 448
  pubescens 449
  sambac 448
Jateorhiza columba 154, 214
Jatropha manihot 791
Juglans cinerea 150, 845
  nigra 842
Juniperus communis 452, 453
  oxycedrus 177, 453
  phoenicea 178, 718
  sabina 717
  virginiana 47, 177, 453, 718
Justicia adhatoda 506

K

Kaempferia galanga 339
Kalmia angustifolia 467
  glauca 467
  latifolia 466, 467
Kickxia africana 778
Knautia arvensis 721
*Kola vera 458
Krameria argentea 674
  ixine 674
  lanceolata 675
  triandra 674
Kyllinga monocephala 730

L

*Lacca caerulea 492
  *musica 492
Lachnanthes tinctoria 461
*Lactuca agnina 225
  altissima 476
  canadensis 315, 476
  capitata 476
  sativa 476

Lactuca scariola 476
  virosa 476
*Laminaria digitata 112, 114
  *saccharina 114
  *stenophylla 114
Lamium album 579
  amplexicaule 581
  galeobdolon 582
  maculatum 581
  purpureum 580, 582
Larix americana 177, 635, 788
  decidua 635, 636
  europaea 68, 635, 636
  leptolepsis 335
  sibirica 335
Laserpitum latifolium 500
*Latakia tobacco 818
Laurus cinnamomum 202
  nobilis 464, 465
  sassafras 715
Lavandula delphinensis 467, 468, 470
  fragrans 467
  latifolia 468
  officinalis 467
  spica 468
  stoechas 473
  vera 467
Lavatera arborea 509
Lawsonia alba 404
  inermis 404
*Lecanora acharius 241
  *tartare 493
Lechea major 328
Ledebouria hyacinthina 769
*Ledum floribus bullates 466
  groenlandicum 460
  latifolium 460
Leontice chrysogonum 362
Leontodon autumnalis 383
  hispidus 253, 383
  taraxacum 249
Leonurus cardiaca 555, 809
Leptandra purpurea 111
  *veronica 831
  virginica 111
Levisticum officinale 499
Lewisia rediviva 108, 660
  *spathulum 108
Liatris odoratissima 255
  scariosa 255
  spicata 255, 746
  squarrosa 255, 746
Libocedrus bidwillii 177
  decurrens 177
*Lichen caninus 494
  *cinereus terrestris 494

Ligusticum filicinum 500
  levisticum 499, 500
  scoticum 500, 501
  sinense 500
Lilium auratum 484
  canadense 479
  candidum 478, 479, 482, 484
  candidum v. peregrinum 482
  chalcedonicum 479, 482
  hansoni 479
  japonicum 479
  kamtschatkaense 484
  martagon 478, 479, 484
  monadelphum 479
  pardalinum 479
  pomponium 484
  pomponium verum 479
  pyrenaicum 479
  superbum 479
  tigrinum 478, 479, 484
  *variegatum 328
Linaria cymbalaria 817
  vulgaris 815
Lindelofia spectabilis 421
Lindera benzoin 21
Linum catharticum 319
  perenne 318, 320
  usitatissimum 317
Lippia citriodora 476, 486, 830
  dulcis 486
  graveolens 486
  *mexicana 486
  nodiflora 486
  origanoides 486
  pseudo-thea 486
  scaberrima 486, 831
  triphylla 830
Liquidambar altingia 776
  formosana 776
  imberbis 775
  orientalis 775
  *storesin 776
  styraciflua 775, 776
Liquiritia officinalis 487
Lithospermum tinctorium 18
Lobelia cardinalis 495
  dortmanna 495
  erinus 495
  inflata 494, 495
  kalmii 495
  purpurascens 495
  syphillitica 495
  urens 495
Lochnera rosea 629, 631
Lolium perenne 372
  temulentum 372

Lonicera brachypoda repens 410
  caprifolium 409, 410
  japonica 410
  periclymenum 409, 410
  tartarica 410
  xylosteum 410
Lophophora lewinii 531
Lucuma glycyphloea 491
  mammosa 459
Luffa aegyptiaca 527
Lupinus albus 502, 503
  angustifolius 503
  *arabicus 503
  arboreus 503
  luteus 503
  *niger 503
  perennis 503
  polyphyllus 503
Lychnis githago 223
*Lycoperdon gigantea 337
Lycopersicum esculentum 47
Lycopodium clavatum 551
  complanatum 550
Lycopsis arvensis 120, 142
Lycopus europaeus 357
  virginicus 141
Lycoris radiata 246
Lysimachia nummularia 229, 549
  vulgaris 229, 497
Lythrum hyssopifolia 497
  salicaria 496, 849
  verticillatum 497

M

Maclura brasiliensis 562
  tinctoria 561
Magnolia acuminata 505, 506
  glauca 506, 716
  tripetala 505, 506
  virginiana 505, 506
  virginiana v. acuminata 241
Mahonia aquifolium 369
Mallotus philippinensis 453
Malus communis 43
  *henricus 365
  persica 619
  *punica 649
Malva moschata 509
  rotundifolia 509
  sylvestris 508
Mammea americana 47
Mammillaria retusa 531
Mandragora officinalis 47, 511
  officinalis v. autumnalis 511
  officinalis v. vernalis 511

Manihot palmata 58
  utilissima 58, 510, 791
Maranta allouia 58
  arundinacea 57, 58
  dichotoma 58
  galanga 340
  indica 57
  malaccensis 58
  *nobilis 58
  ramosissima 57, 58
Marchantia polymorpha 494
*Marjorana hortensis 519
Marrubium nigrum 416
  vulgare 415
*Marsdenia condurango 219
Maruta cotula 523
Massora aromatica 169, 716
Matonia cardamomum 159
Matricaria chamomilla 187, 341
  inodora 188, 524
  pyrethrum 621
Medeola virginica 240
Medicago sativa 501
Melaleuca decussata 151
  ericifolia 151
  hypericifolia 151
  latifolia 151
  leucadendron 151
  viridifolia 151
Melampyrum pratense 232
Melanthium sabadilla 697
  virginicum 770
Melia azadirachta 75
Melilotus alba 525, 526
  arvensis 525, 526
  officinalis 76, 525, 526
Melissa officinalis 76
Menispermum canadense 610
Mentha aquatica 544, 545
  aquatica v. crispa 536
  arvensis 541, 544
  arvensis v. glabrata 541
  arvensis v. javanesa 541
  arvensis v. piperascens 541
  cardiaca 534
  citrata 545
  *citriodora 546
  crispa 545
  *fistulosa 546
  incana 541
  longifolia 536
  odorata 545
  piperita 532, 537, 541
  piperita v. rubra 538
  pulegium 532, 624
  pulegium v. decumbens 625

Mentha pulegium v. erecta 625
  rotundifolia 545
  sativa 543, 544
  spicata 533
  *squarrosa 546
  sylvestris 534, 545, 546
  verticillata 536
  viridis 532, 533, 534, 536, 707
Menyanthes trifoliata 117
Mercurialis annua 530
  perennis 529
Meum athamanticum 500
Mezereum officinarum 531
*Mimosa fragifolia 532
  humilis 532
  *linguis 532
Mitchella repens 212, 477, 766
Molinia varia 374
Momordica balsamina 49, 450
  charantia 49
  elaterium 133, 241
  mixta 49
Monarda didyma 44, 95, 545, 546, 812
  fistulosa 813
  lutea 546
  punctata 95, 545, 546, 811, 812, 813
Monodora myristica 592
Monsonia ovata 550
Morinda tinctoria 561
Morus alba 558, 559, 560
  alba v. stylosa 562
  indica 561
  nigra 558, 560, 561
  rubra 560
  tinctoria 561
Mosla japonica 812, 813
Mucuna pruriens 228, 229
  prurita 228, 229
  urens 229
Musa acuminata 646
  cavendishii 646
  fehi 645
  paradisiaca 646
  sapientum 646
  textilis 395
Muscari comosum 424
  racemosum 423
*Muscus terrestris repens 551
*Myosotis symphytifolia 322
Myrica cerifera 87, 88, 341
  cordifolia 88
  gale 88, 341
  gale v. tomentosa 341
  nagi 88
  pennsylvanica 88
Myriophyllum alterniflorum 532

Myriophyllum spicatum 532
  verticillatum 532
Myristica argentea 504, 591
  aromatica 591
  fragrans 504, 591
  malabarica 504
  moschata 504
  officinalis 504, 591, 592
  otoba 504
  sebifera 592
  surinamensis 592
Myrospermum pereirae 79
  toluiferum 80
Myroxylon frutescens 80
  pereirae 79
Myrrhis odorata 201, 491
Myrtus cheken 189
  *tobasco 21

N

*Narcissus caparonius 328
  jonquilla 246, 573
  odorus 246, 573
  poeticus 246, 573
  princeps 573
  pseudo-narcissus 245, 246, 573
*Nardus celtica 829
  indica 829
  *montana 829
Narthecium ossifragu͏ 72
Narthex asafoetida
Nasturtium officin͏ 845
Nelumbium spe͏ ͏sum 58
Nepenthes disti͏ ͏toria 640
Nepeta catari͏ 73
  glechoma ͏ icosa 818
Nicotiana f͏ 18
  latissim͏ ͏is 818
  multi͏ 18
  persi͏ valvis 818
  qu͏ ͏da 818
  re͏ ͏ca 818
  ͏ acum 817, 818
  ͏ella sativa 297
  ͏phar advena 484
  ͏yctanthes arbor-tristis 449
Nymphaea odorata 484

O

Ocimum americanum 86
  basilicum 86
  canum 85, 86
  crispum 85

Ocimum gratissimum 85, 86
  guineense 85
  minimum 85
  tenuiflorum 85
  viride 85
Oculus Christi 205, 812, 813
Oenanthe crocata 263, 264
  fistulosa 264, 501
  fluviatilis 264
  phellandrium 264
  pimpinelloides 264
Oenothera biennis 658, 847
  biennis v. grandiflora 658
  biennis v. lamarkiana 658
  odorata 658
Olea europaea 598
  fragrans 599
  gallica 598
  lancifolia 598
  oleaster 598
Ononis arvensis 674
Onopordon acanthium 798
Operculina turpethum 823
Ophelia angustifolia 200
Ophioglossum vulgatum 308
Opopanax chironium 600
Opuntia cochinellifera 185
  decumana 185
  *grana-finegrah 185
  *sylvestre 185
  vulgaris 185
Orchis conopea 602, 603
  coriophora 602, 603
  latifolia 602, 603, 604
  longicruris 603
  maculata 602, 603
  mascula 602, 603
  militaris 602, 603
  morio 602, 603
  pyramidalis 602, 603
  saccifera 602, 603
  ustulata 603
Origanum dictamnus 147, 520
  dubium 813
  heracleoticum 521
  hirtum 812, 813
  majorana 519, 521
  maru 426
  onites 521
  onites v. smyrnaeum 813
  sipyleum 520
  vulgare 426, 520, 810
Ornithogalum altissimum 769
  capense 770
  divaricatum 770
  pyrenaicum 72, 770

Ornithogalum thyrsoides 770
  umbellatum 769
Orobanche virginiana 93
Oryza latifolia 680
  montana 680
  *setegera 680
Osmunda regalis 81, 308
Oxalis acetosella 750, 751, 754
*Oxylanathum britannicum 105
Oxyria reniformis 750, 751, 754

P

Paederota virginica 111
Paeonia albiflora 607
  corallina 606
  officinalis 606
Palicourea densiflora 227
Panax quinquefolium 354, 355, 734
Panicum glabrum 373
  sanguinale 373
Papaver argemone 654
  dubium 654
  hybridum 654
  rhoeas 651, 654
  somniferum 651, 653
  somniferum v. album 651, 653
Papaya vulgaris 607
Parietaria officinalis 624
Paris polyphylla 611
  quadrifolia 610
Passerina stelleri 449
Passiflora caerulea 618
  capsularis 618
  contrayerva 618
  edulis 618
  foetida 618
  incarnata 618
  laurifolia 476, 618
  macrocarpa 618
  maliformis 618
  normalis 618
  pallida 618
  quadrangularis 618
  rubra 618
Pastinaca opopanax 600
  sativa 615
Patrinia scabiosaefolia 829
Paullinia cupana 381
  sorbilis 381
Pavetta indica 449
Pedalium murex 147
Pedicularis sylvatica 672
Pelargonium antidysentericum 621
  capitatum 550, 621
  odoratissimum 621

Pelargonium roseum 550, 621
  triste 621
Penthorum sedoides 774
Peramium pubescens 645
  repens 645
Periploca indica 714
*Peronospora sordida 563
Persica vulgaris 619
Persicaria maculata 773
Petasites albus 148
  fragrans 148
  vulgaris 148
Petroselinum sativum 611
*Pettigora canina 494
Peucedanum graveolens 255, 257
  officinale 298
  palustre 298
  sowa 257
Peumus boldus 118
*Peziza oeriginosa 594
Phalaris canariensis 373
Phaseolus vulgaris 88
Phellandrium aquaticum 264
Phlomis fruticosa 707
Phlox carolina 638
  glaberrima 638
  ovata 638
*Phoma lavandulae 470
Phragmites communis 374
Physalis alkekengi 191
  peruviana 583
  somnifera 192
  viscosa 192
Physostigma venenosum 152
Phytolacca americana 648
  decandra 648
  drastica 649
  vulgaris 648
Picea abies 635
  mariana 635
  vulgaris 635
Picraena excelsa 67, 662
Picramnia antidesma 166
Picris hieracioides 606
Pilocarpus jaborandi 444
  microphyllus 445
  pennatifolius 445
  pinnatus 445
  racemosus 445
  selloanus 445
  simplex 445
  spicatus 445
  trachylophus 445
Pimenta acris 88, 465
  officinalis 19
Pimpinella anisum 41, 42

Pimpinella magna 720
  *sanguisorba 146
  saxifraga 146, 720
Pinguicula vulgaris 712
Pinus alba 635
  australis 635
  balsamea 635
  canadensis 635, 638
  cedrus 635
  cembra 635
  cubensis 635
  dammara 635
  densiflora 635
  echinata 635
  gerardiana 635
  halepensis 635
  heterophylla 635
  khasya 635
  larix 635, 636
  macrocarpa 635
  maritima 635
  merkusii 635
  montana 635
  mughus 635
  nigra 635
  palustris 635
  pendula 635, 788
  picea 635
  pinaster 635
  pinea 635
  ponderosa 635
  pumilio 635
  rigida 635
  *roxburghii 635
  sabiniana 635
  *scropica 635
  strobus 635, 637
  *succimifera 636
  sylvestris 176, 636
  taeda 636
  teocote 636
  thunbergii 636
Piper aduncum 523
  album 627
  angustifolium 290, 522
  betel 96, 628
  cubeba 236
  elongatum 522
  granulosum 522
  jaborandi 445
  longum 628
  methysticum 454
  nigrum 627, 628
  officinarum 628
  pellucidum 628

Piper rotundifolium 628
  trioicum 627
  umbellatum 628
Piscidia erythrina 123, 261
Pistacia lentiscus 522
*Planta genista 125
Plantago amplexicaulis 643
  arenaria 643
  coronopus 642
  cynops 643
  decumbens 643
  ispaghula 643
  lanceolata 644
  major 640, 642, 643, 644
  maritima 644
  media 643
  ovata 643
  psyllium 643, 644
Plumbago europaea 648
  zeylanica 648
Plumiera alba 449
  rubra 449
Podalyria tinctoria 432
Podophyllum emodi 513
  peltatum 476, 512
*Podosphoera castagnei 413
Pogonopus febrifugus 167
Pogostemon heyneanus 619
  patchouly 618
Poinciana pulcherrima 737
Polemonium caeruleum 446
  reptans 3, 446
Polygala alba 734
  boynkini 734
  latifolia 733
  senega 65, 356, 733, 734
  *virginiana 733
Polygonatum biflorum 750
  multiflorum 749
  officinale 750
  uniflorum 750
  verticillatum 750
Polygonum arifolium 458
  aviculare 457, 458
  bistorta 105, 260
  convolvulus 139
  cymosum 138
  erectum 458
  fagopyrum 137
  hydropiper 743
  sagittatum 139
  tartaricum 138
  viviparum 458
Polymnia uvedalia 91
Polypodium dryopteris 307
  vulgare 307, 491

*Polyporus annosus 335
  *anthelminticus 335
  *betulina 336
  *fomentarius 335, 336
  *giganteus 336
  *igniarius 336
  *marginiatus 336
  *officinalis 335
  *squamosus 335, 336
  *suaveolens 335
  *sulphureus 336
  *tinctorius 335
*Polystictus versicolor 336
*Polytrichium juniperum 552
Populus balsamifera 79
  candicans 79, 650
  grandidentata 650
  nigra 79
  tremula 650
  tremuloides 650
Portulaca oleracea 650
  sativa 660
Potentilla anserina 740
  erecta 819
  reptans 316, 819
  tormentilla 819
Poterium sanguisorba 145, 691
*Pragmidium subcorticium 685
Primula auricula 232, 659
  farinosa 231
  farinosa v. scotica 232
  grandiflora 658
  obconica 232, 659
  officinalis 748
  scotica 232
  veris 229, 657
  vulgaris 656
Prinos confertus 16
  gronovii 16
  verticillatus 16
Prosopis dulcis 161
  siliquastrum 161
Protium gileadense 78
Prunella vulgaris 731
Prunus armeniaca 51
  avium 190
  domestica 142, 659
  insititia 142
  laurocerasus 24, 190, 465
  persica 619
  serotina 191
  spinosa 142
Pseudotsuga taxifolia 639
Psoralea bituminosa 656
  corylifolia 656
  esculenta 47, 655

Psoralea glandulosa 609, 656
  melilotoides 655
  obliqua 656
  pedunculata 655
  physodes 656
Psychotria acuminata 433
  emetica 433
  ipecacuanha 432
Ptelea trifoliata 71
Pteris aquilina 305
  esculenta 306
Pterocarpus angolensis 717
  draco 263, 729
  erinaceus 455
  marsupium 289, 455
  santalinus 711, 717
Pterospora andromedea 93
*Puccinia mentha 535, 539
*Pulegium regium 624
Pulicaria dysenterica 321
Pulmonaria officinalis 707
Pulsatilla nuttaliana 34
Punica granatum 649
*Punicum malum 649
Pycnanthemum incanum 546
*Pyrethrum germanicum 622
  *officinarum 621
  parthenium 309
  roseum 622
• umbelliferum 622
Pyrola media 661
  minor 661, 662
  rotundifolia 662, 850
  secunda 661
  umbellata 639
  uniflora 661
Pyrus americana 70
  aucuparia 69
  cydonia 664
  japonica 666
  malus 43
  malus v. astracanica 47
  malus v. paradisiaca 47
  malus v. pendula 47

Q

Quamoclit coccinea 449
Quassia amara 67, 662
  simaruba 741
Quercus abelicea 595
  alba 595, 832
  cerris 595
  coccifera 594
  ilex 594, 595
  infectoria 596, 597

*Quercus marina 111
  pedunculata 594
  persica 68
  prinus 595
  robur 593, 594
  sessiliflora 594
  skinneri 594
  tinctoria 595
  vallonea 68
  virens 595
Quillaja saponaria 733, 747, 748
  sellowiana 748
*Quina morada 167

R

Radiola linoides 320
Ramona stachyoides 703
Ranunculus acris 149, 235
  bulbosus 33, 149
  ficaria 179
  flammula 33, 757
  sceleratus 33, 181, 235
*Raphanus agrios 417
  caudatus 668
  erucoides 668
  maritimus 668
  raphanistrum 667, 668
  rusticanus 417
  sativus 418, 667
  sibiricus 668
  tenellus 668
Rapuntium inflatum 494
Reseda luteola 376
Rhamnus frangula 135, 137
  infectoria 135
  purshiana 135, 136
Rheum emodi 667
  officinale 677, 678
  palmatum 675, 676, 677
  rhaponticum 675, 676, 677, 678
Rhinanthus crista-galli 672, 673
Rhododendron chrysanthum 675
Rhus aromatica 104, 444, 780
  copallina 779, 781
  coriaria 779, 781
  cotinus 562, 781
  diversiloba 780
  glabra 779
  semialata 597, 779
  succedanea 780
  toxicodendron 443, 444, 779, 780, 832
  typhina 779
  venenata 277, 444, 780
  vernicifera 277, 780
  vernix 277

Ribes grossularia 364
  nigrum 243
  rubrum 244
  uva-crispa 364
Richardsonia scabra 433
Ricinus africanus 171
  communis 169, 763
Robinia pseudo-acacia 4
*Roccella fuciformis 493
  *montagnei 493
  *phycopsis 492, 493
  *pygmaea 492, 493
  *tinctoria 241, 492
Rosa arvensis 690, 691
  canina 690
  centifolia 684, 685, 689, 692
  damascena 684, 686, 689
  gallica 684, 685, 687, 692
  indica 684
  *muscatta 686
  rubiginosa 690, 691
  rugosa 685
  spinosissima 690, 691
  villosa 690, 691
*Rosmarinus coronarium 681
  officinalis 681
Rottlera schimperi 454
  tinctoria 453
Rubia cordifolia 505
  peregrina 234, 505
  sylvestris 505
  tinctorum 91, 206, 234, 504, 505
Rubus caesius 109
  chamaemorus 109
  coryfolius 109
  cuneifolius 110
  fructicosus 108, 109
  idaeus 671
  laciniatus 109
  nigrobaccus 110
  occidentalis 109
  odoratus 109
  rhamnifolius 109
  saxatilis 109
  villosus 110
Rumex acetosa 258, 750, 752, 753
  acetosella 750
  acutus 259, 260
  alpinus 258, 680
  aquaticus 259, 260
  conglomeratus 752
  crispus 259
  ecklonianus 52
  hydrolapathum 258, 259, 260
  obtusifolius 258, 752
  pulcher 752

Rumex sanguineus 259
  scutatus 258, 750, 752, 753
Ruscus aculeatus 128
  alexandrinus 128
  androgynus 128
  hypoglossum 128
  hypophyllum 128
  racemosus 128
Ruta graveolens 694

S

Sabadilla officinarum 697
Sabal serrulatum 719
Sabatia angularis 184
  campestris 184
  elliottii 184
*Sabina cacumina 717
Sagittaria sagittifolia 57
Salicornia herbacea 357, 358
Salix alba 847
  nigra 846
Salsola kali 357, 358
  sativa 357
  soda 357
  tragus 357
Salvia candelabrum 701
  candicans 702
  cypria 703
  glutinosa 702
  grandiflora 702
  hians 701
  horminum 702
  lyrata 701
  *mellifer 703
  officinalis 700, 701
  pomifera 702
  pratensis 707
  *salvatrix 701
  sclarea 203, 204, 702, 703, 705
  triloba 703
  urticifolia 701
  verbenaca 205, 707
Samadera indica 742
Sambucus canadensis 270, 277
  ebulus 268, 276, 278
  glauca 277
  melanocarpa 277
  nigra 265, 270, 277
  racemosa 277
  *rubens 277
Sanguinaria canadensis 115, 364
Sanguisorba officinalis 145
Sanicula europaea 711
Sanseviera angolensis 395
  guineenesis 395

Sanseviera roxburghiana 395
Santalum album 710
  *rubrum 711, 717
Santolina chamaecyparissus 473
  fragrantissima 474
Sapium biglandulosum 788
  indicum 788
  salicifolium 788
  sebiferum 763, 788
  sylvaticum 664
Saponaria officinalis 733, 748
*Sarazina gibbosa 640
Sarcostemma glaucum 434
*Sargassum bacciferum 114
Sarothamnus scoparius 124
Sarracenia purpurea 640
*Sarsaparilla officinalis 713
  *papyracea 713
Sassafras goesianum 716
  officinale 715
  variifolium 715
Satureia hortensis 718
  montana 719, 813
  thymbra 719, 812, 813
Scabiosa arvensis 721, 827
  columbaria 721
  succisa 374, 722, 827
Scandix cerefolium 201
Schinopsis lorentzii 663
Schoenocaulon officinale 697
Scilla indica 769
  lilio-hyacinthus 769
  maritima 766
  nonscripta 424
  nutans 116, 424
  peruviana 769
Scirpus caespitosus 730
  capillaris 730
  cernuus 730
  fluitans 730
  holoschoenus 730
  lacustris 730
  nanus 730
  pauciflorus 730
  setaceus 730
*Sclerotium clavus 339
Scolopendrium vulgare 304
*Scolymus cardunculus 61
Scoparia dulcis 427
Scopolia atropoides 722
  carniolica 722, 723
  japonica 723
*Scorodosma foetida 63
Scorzonera humilis 55
Scrophularia aquatica 314
  nodosa 313, 314

Scrophularia scorodonia 314
  vernalis 314
Scutellaria coccinea 725
  galericulata 724, 725
  integrifolia 724
  lateriflora 724
  *micrantha 725
  minor 724
Secale cornutum 339
Sechium edule 527
Sedum acre 772, 774
  album 771, 772
  anglicum 771, 772
  dasyphyllum 774
  forsterianum 774
  reflexum 772, 774
  rupestre 774
  sexangulare 774
  telephium 773
  villosum 774
Semecarpus anacardium 168
Sempervivum tectorum 422, 423
Senecio aquaticus 669
  aureus 379, 482, 484
  campestris 379
  erucifolius 379
  hieracifolius 315
  jacobaea 668, 669
  latifolius 379, 669
  maritimus 202, 379
  populifolius 669
  *radiata 378
  sylvaticus 379, 380
  tussilaginis 669
  viscosus 380
  vulgaris 377, 378, 379, 380
Senna acutifolia 734
  *baladi 737
  *indica 736
  italica 737
  *jebeli 737
  obtusa 737
Serenoa serrulata 719
*Serpyllum zygis 813
Sesamum indicum 94
Siegesbeckia orientalis 739
Silphium gummiferum 243
  laciniatum 694
  laeve 243
  perfoliatum 243, 694
Silybum marianum 797
Simaba cedron 178
Simaruba amara 741
  excelsa 742
  glauca 166, 742
  medicinalis 742

Simaruba officinalis 741
  versicolor 166, 178, 742
Sinapis alba 566
  arvensis 570
  nigra 568
Sison amomum 612
Sisymbrium alliaria 571
  officinale 570
  sophia 576
Sium angustifolium 617
  latifolium 617
  sisarum 742
Smilacina racemosa 750
Smilax anceps 744
  aspera 744
  china 199, 744
  glyciphylla 744
  lanceaefolia 744
  macabucha 744
  medica 713, 715
  officinalis 713
  ornata 713
  ovalifolia 744
  papyracea 744
  pseudo-china 198, 744
  rotundifolia 744
  sarsaparilla 714
  spruceana 713
  syphilitica 713
Smyrnium olusatrum 225, 500
Solanum aethiopicum 583
  album 583
  anguivi 583
  arrebenta 591
  carolinense 417
  dulcamara 410, 589, 654
  esculentum 47, 583
  gnaphaloides 583
  indigoferum 583
  laciniatum 47, 583
  *lethale 585
  lycopersicum 47
  mammosum 591
  marginatum 583
  muricatum 583
  nigrum 582, 589
  oleraceum 583, 591
  pseudocapsicum 192, 591
  pseudoquina 583
  quadriflorum 610
  quitoense 583
  ramosum 583
  saponaceum 583
  sessiliflorum 583
  sodomeum 47
  toxicarium 583

Solanum tuberosum 654
  vescum 583
  vespertilio 583
Solenostemma argel 737
Solidago canadensis 362
  gigantea 362
  odora 362
  rigida 362
  sempervirens 362
  virgaurea 361
Sonchus alpinus 757
  arvensis 756
  oleraceus 756
  palustris 757
  tataricus 757
Sophia chirurgorum 570
Sophora tinctoria 432
Sorbus aucuparia 69
Sorghum saccharatum 130, 516
  vulgare 130
Spartina stricta 373
  townsendi 373
Spartium junceum 127, 130
  scoparium 124
Spathyema foetida 742
Spergularia marina 711
  rubra 711
*Sphaerococcus euchema 12
  *helminthocorton 551
*Sphagnum cymbifolium 552
Spigelia anthelmia 638
  marilandica 637
Spinacia oleracea 761
Spiraea bella 525
  filipendula 525
  fortunei 525
  prunifolia 525
  salicifolia 525
  stipulata 431
  tomentosa 382, 525
  ulmaria 524, 525
Spiranthes autumnalis 464
  diuretica 464
Spondias dulcis 47
Stachys arvensis 97
  betonica 97
  germanica 97
  palustris 97, 862
  sieboldi 61
  sylvatica 97, 862
Statice caroliniana 474
  limonium 474
  monopetala 361
Stellaria media 195
*Stephensia elongata 522

Sterculia acuminata 458
  chicha 459
  striata 459
*Sticta pulmonaria 502
Stillingia sylvatica 664
Stizolobium pruriens 228
Stratiotes aloides 845, 846
Strophanthus courmonti 778
  courmonti v. fallax 778
  courmonti v. kerkii 778
  emini 778
  glaber 778
  gratus 778, 779
  hispidus 777, 778, 779
  kombe 777, 778, 779
  nicholsoni 779
  tholloni 779
Strychnos ignatii 431, 593
  innocua 593
  ligustrina 593
  nux-vomica 592
  pseudo-quina 593
  tieute 593
  toxifera 593
Stylophorum diphyllum 357
Styrax benzoin 95
  officinale 775
  *praeparatus 775
  reticulatum 776
Suaeda fruticosa 115
  maritima 115
Sutherlandia frutescens 737
Swartzia decipiens 445
Swertia chirata 199
Sycocarpus rusbyi 210
Symphoricarpus racemosa 410
Symphytum asperrimum 216
  officinale 215, 216, 324
  officinale v. patens 216
  tuberosum 216
Symplocarpus foetidus 742
*Syringa baccifera 477
  vulgaris 477
Syzygium jambolanum 446

T

Tacca oceanica 58
  pinnatifida 58
Tamarindus indica 788
  officinalis 788
Tamarix gallica v. mannifera 68, 69
Tamus communis 130
  cretica 131
Tanacetum balsamita 226
  vulgare 500, 789

Taraktogenos kurzii 189
Taraxacum dens-leonis 249
  officinale 249, 253
Taxus baccata 866
Tephrosia apollinea 737
Tetragonia expansa 762
Teucrium chamaedrys 351, 352, 760
  marum 808
  scordium 351, 353
  scorodonia 351, 707
Thapsia garganica 794
Thea bohea 792
  sinensis 792
  stricta 792
Theobroma cacao 151
Thlaspi arvense 571
Thuya articulata 177, 453
  occidentalis 176
  orientalis 177
Thymus algeriensis 811
  camphoratus 811
  capitatus 811
  mastichina 811
  serpyllum 808, 809, 811, 812, 813
  serpyllum v. citriodorus 811
  vulgaris 808, 809, 810, 811, 812, 813
  vulgaris v. floribunda 813
  vulgaris v. gracilis 813
  zygis 813
Tiarella cordifolia 220
Tilia cordata 485
  europaea 485
  intermedia 485
  platyphylla 485
  vulgaris 485
Tissa rubra 711
Tofieldia palustris 72
Toluifera pereirae 79
Torreya californica 592
Toxylon pomiferum 562
Tragopogon porrifolius 708, 742
  pratensis 55, 360
Tribulus terrestris 147
Trientalis europaea 850
Trifolium pratense 207, 410
Trigonella foenum-graecum 299
  purpurascens 299
*Trilissia odorata 255
Trillium erectum 96
  erythrocarpum 97
  grandiflorum 97
  nivale 97
  pendulum 96
  sessile 97
Triosteum perfoliatum 357, 734
Triticum repens 370

*Triticum vaccinium 232
Trollius asiaticus 359
  europaeus 358
  laxus 359
Tsuga canadensis 638
*Tunatea decipiens 445
Turnera aphrodisiaca 249
  opifera 249
Tussilago farfara 212
  petasites 148

U

Ulex europaeus 366, 367, 461
  gallii 367
  nanus 367
  strictus 367
Ulmus alata 283
  campestris 282
  campestris v. suberosa 283
  chinensis 283
  fulva 283
  glabra 283
  montana 283
  suberosa 282
Umbellularia californica 716
Uncaria gambier 173
Urginea altissima 769
  indica 766, 769
  maritima 766, 767
  scilla 766, 769
*Uromyces alchemillae 463
Urtica canadensis 395
  cannabina 395
  crenulata 574
  dioica 574, 575, 576
  heterophylla 574
  pilulifera 575
  tuberosa 574
  urens 574, 575, 576
  urentissima 574
*Ustilago maydis 339
Uvaria cordata 608
  febrifuga 608
  longifolia 608
  narum 608
  *taminia 131
  triloba 608
  *tripetaloidea 608
  zeylanica 608

V

Vaccinium arboreum 100
  corymbosum 100
  dumosum 100

Vaccinium frondosum 98
  myrtillus 98, 100
  resinosum 100
  uliginosum 100
  vitis-idaea 90
Valeriana angustifolia 829
  aquatica 829
  celtica 825, 829
  dioica 824, 826
  jatamansi 828, 829
  locusta 225
  mexicana 829
  mikaniae 825
  officinalis 824, 827, 829
  phu 827
  pyrenaica 824, 829
  rubra 830
  sambucifolia 825
  sitchensis 825
  sylvestris 825
  tuberosa 829
  wallichii 829
Valerianella olitoria 225
Vandellia diffusa 427
Veratrum album 347, 390, 391
  californicum 391
  lobelianum 391
  luteum 823
  officinale 390, 697
  sabadilla 697
  viride 390
Verbascum blattaria 563
  nigrum 563
  phlomoides 566
  pulverulentum 566
  sinuatum 566
  thapsiforme 566
  thapsus 324, 562, 564
Verbena hastata 831, 832
  jamaicensis 832
  lappulacea 832
  officinalis 831
  *sinuata 832
  triphylla 486, 830
  urticifolia 832
Veronica agrestis 758, 759
  alpina 759
  arvensis 759
  beccabunga 123, 831
  buxbaumii 758
  chamaedrys 123, 758, 759, 831
  hederifolia 759
  nigricans 831
  officinalis 702, 703, 758, 831
  peduncularis 831
  purpurea 111

Veronica saxatilis 729
  scutellata 759
  serpyllifolia 759
  spicata 759
  triphyllos 759
  verna 759
  virginica 111
*Verrucaria albissima 166
Viburnum opulus 97, 381
  prunifolium 382
Vinca major 629, 631
  minor 629, 631
  rosea 629, 631
Vincetoxicum officinale 434
Viola arvensis 386
  *calcarea 833
  canina 833
  hirta 833
  lutea 386
  odorata 833, 834
  palustris 833
  purpurea 835
  sylvatica 834
  tricolor 386, 833
Viscum album 547
Vitex trifolia 188
Vitis cordifolia 833
  hederacea 840
  labrusca 833
  quinquefolia 840
  riparia 833
  vinifera 832
*Voucapoua araroba 51
  inermus 150

W

Waltheria glomerata 523

X

Xanthium spinosum 210
  strumarium 210

Y

Yucca filamentosa 770

Z

Zanthoxylum americanum 40, 70, 277
  carolinianum 70
  fraxineum 70
Zea mays 58, 224, 225
Zingiber officinale 353
Zizyphus agrestis 452
  baclei 451
  *barelei 452
  jujuba 451
  lotus 451
  napeca 452
  sativa 451
  spina-Christi 452
  vulgaris 451